TEXTBOOK OF
RADIOLOGY
AND IMAGING

TEXTBOOK OF
RADIOLOGY AND IMAGING

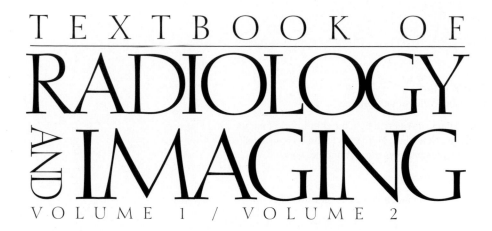

VOLUME 1 / VOLUME 2

SIXTH EDITION

EDITED BY

DAVID SUTTON MD FRCP FRCR DMRD MCAR(Hon)
Consulting Radiologist, St Mary's Hospital and The National Hospital
for Neurology and Neurosurgery, London, UK

ASSOCIATE EDITORS

CT
RICHARD W. WHITEHOUSE BSc MD MRCP FRCR

MRI
JEREMY P.R. JENKINS MB BCh MRCP DMRD FRCR

Nuclear Medicine
E. RHYS DAVIES CBE MB BChir (Cantab) FRCR FRCPE
FFRRCSI (Hon) FDSRCS

General Radiology
JANET MURFITT MB BS MRCP FRCR

Ultrasound
WILLIAM R. LEES MB BS FRCR

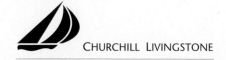

CHURCHILL LIVINGSTONE

New York, Edinburgh, London, Madrid, Melbourne, San Francisco, Tokyo 1998

CHURCHILL LIVINGSTONE
Medical Division of Pearson Professional Limited

Distributed in the United States of America by Churchill Livingstone Inc.,
650 Avenue of the Americas, New York, N.Y. 10011, and by associated
companies, branches, and representatives throughout the world

First Edition 1969
Second Edition 1975
Third Edition 1980
Fourth Edition 1987
Fifth Edition 1993
Sixth Edition 1998

ISBN 0 443 053685
International Student Edition ISBN 0 443 055629

British Library Cataloguing in Publication Data
A catalogue record for this book is available from the British Library

Library of Congress Cataloging in Publication Data
A catalog record for this book is available from the Library of Congress

Medical knowledge is constantly changing. As new information becomes
available, changes in treatment, procedures, equipment and the use of drugs
become necessary. The editors, contributors and the publishers have, as far as
it is possible, taken care to ensure that the information given in this text is
accurate and up to date. However, readers are strongly advised to confirm
that the information, especially with regard to drug usage, complies with the
latest legislation and standards of practice.

The Publishers have made every effort to trace the copyright holders for
borrowed material. If they have inadvertently overlooked any, they will be
pleased to make the necessary arrangements at the first opportunity.

Commissioning Editors: Gavin Smith, Sheila Khullar
Copy Editors: Ruth Swan, Rich Cutler
Project Manager: Nora Naughton
Design Direction: Jeanette Jacobs
Administration: Tracey Thompsett

Produced by Longman Asia Ltd, Hong Kong
SWT/01

CONTENTS

Cover Illustrations: Vol 1: Fig 25.5 and legend on p 675
Vol 2: Fig 34.120 and legend on p 1024

v

CONTRIBUTORS

Paul Allan BSc DMRD FRCR FRCPE
Senior Lecturer, Medical Radiology, University of Edinburgh; Honorary Consultant Radiologist, Royal Infirmary of Edinburgh NHS Trust, Edinburgh, UK

Otto Chan FRCR
Consultant Radiologist, The Royal London Hospital, London, UK

A H A Chapman MB MRCP FRCR
Consultant Radiologist, St James's University Hospital, Leeds, UK

Graham R Cherryman MBChB FRCR
Professor of Radiology, University of Leicester; Honorary Consultant Radiologist, Leicester Royal Infirmary and Glenfield Hospital, Leicester,UK

Roger Chisholm MA MB BChir MRCP FRCR
Consultant Radiologist, Hope Hospital, (University of Manchester), Salford, UK

Mark Cobby MB ChB MRCP FRCR
Consultant Radiologist, Frenchay Hospital, Bristol, UK

E Rhys Davies CBE MB BChir (Cantab) FRCR FRCPE FFRCSI (Hon) FDSRCS
Emeritus Professor of Clinical Radiology, University of Bristol, Bristol, UK

Robert Dick MB BS(Syd) FRCAR FRCR
Consultant Radiologist, Royal Free Hospital, London, UK

Claire Dicks-Mireaux MBBS MRCP FRCR DMRD
Consultant Paediatric Radiologist, Great Ormond Street Hospital for Children NHS Trust,London, UK

Robert M Donaldson MD FRCP FACC
Consultant Cardiologist, Royal Brompton National Heart and Lung Hospital, London, UK

Paul Dubbins BSc FRCR
Consultant Radiologist, Plymouth General Hospital Freedom Fields, Plymouth, UK

Stuart Field MA MB BChir DMRD FRCR
Consultant Radiologist and Clinical Director, Kent and Canterbury Hospital, Canterbury, UK

John A Fielding MD FRCR DMRD
Consultant Radiologist, Royal Shrewsbury Hospitals NHS Trust, Shrewsbury, UK

W Gedroyc MRCP FRCR
Consultant Radiologist, St Mary's Hospital, London, UK

Joseph A Gleeson FRCP FRCR
Consultant Radiologist, Chelsea and Westminster Hospital, London, UK

Roger H S Gregson BSc MB BS FRCR DMRD
Consultant Radiologist & Head of Training, University Hospital, Nottingham; Clinical Teacher in Radiology, Queen's Medical Centre, University of Nottingham, Nottingham, UK

H Highman MB FRCP FRCR DMRD
Consulting Radiologist, St Mary's Hospital; Honorary Clinical Senior Lecturer, Imperial College of Science, Technology and Medicine, (St Mary's Hospital Medical School), London, UK

Jeremy P R Jenkins MB BCh MRCP DMRD FRCR
Consultant Radiologist and Honorary Clinical Senior Lecturer, Manchester Royal Infirmary, Manchester, UK

Simon Jones MRCP FRCR
Consultant Radiologist, Poole and Royal Bournemouth NHS Trusts, Poole, UK

John Karani BSc MBBS FRCR
Consultant Radiologist, King's College Hospital, London, UK

Brian Kendall FRCR FRCP FRCS
Consulting Radiologist, The National Hospital for Neurology and Neurosurgery, and the Middlesex Hospital, London, UK.

William R Lees MB BS FRCR FRACR(Hon)
Professor of Medical Imaging, University College, London; Clinical Director of Medical Imaging, UCL Hospitals Trust, London, UK

Glyn A S Lloyd DM FRCR FRCOphth
Consulting Radiologist, Royal National Throat, Nose and Ear Hospital, London, UK

Richard Mason FRCS MRCP FRCR
Consulting Radiologist, Middlesex Hospital, University College of London Hospitals, London, UK

Michael J Michell FRCR
Consultant Radiologist, King's College Hospital, Denmark Hill, London, UK

Janet B Murfitt MB BS MRCP FRCR
Consultant Radiologist, The Royal London Hospital, Royal Hospitals Trust, London, UK

Julle Olliff MRCP FRCR
Consultant Radiologist, Queen Elizabeth Hospital, Edgbaston, Birmingham, UK

Simon P G Padley MRCP FRCR
Consultant Radiologist, Chelsea and Westminster Hospital, London, UK

Peter D Phelps MD FRCS FRCR
Consultant Radiologist, Royal National Throat Nose and Ear Hospital, London, UK

Maurice J Raphael MD FRCP FRCR
Consultant Radiologist, The Middlesex Hospital, London, UK

Peter Renton FRCR DMRD
Consultant Radiologist, Royal National Orthopaedic Hospital and University College Hospital; Honorary Senior Lecturer, Institute of Orthopaedics, University College London, London, UK

David Rickards FRCR FFRDSA
Consultant Uroradiologist, University College of London Hospitals, London, UK

Philip J A Robinson FRCP FRCR
Consultant Radiologist, St James University Hospital, Leeds, UK

Michael I Rothman MD
Assistant Professor of Radiology, Neurosurgery and Otolaryngology/Head and Neck Surgery, and Medical Director, Anna Gudelsky Magnetic Resonance Center, The University of Maryland Medical System, Baltimore, Maryland, USA

Michael B Rubens MB BS FRCR DMRD
Director of Imaging and Consultant Radiologist, Royal Brompton Hospital; Honorary Senior Lecturer, Imperial College School of Medicine at the National Heart and Lung Institute, London, UK

Donald Shaw MA MSc BH FRCP FRCR
Consultting Radiologist, Great Ormond Street Hospital for Children NHS Trust, London, UK

John A Spencer MA MD MRCP FRCR
Consultant Radiologist, St James's University Hospital, Leeds, UK

Fritz Starer FRCPEd FRCR
Consulting Radiologist (Ped), Westminster Hospital and Westminster Children's Hospital, London, UK

John M Stevens MBBS DRACR FRCR
Consultant Neuroradiologist, National Hospital for Neurology and Neurosurgery, Queen Square and St Mary's Hospital, London, UK

David Sutton MD FRCP FRCR DMRD MCAR(Hon)
Consulting Radiologist, St Mary's Hospital and The National Hospital for Neurology and Neurosurgery, London, UK

Brian M Thomas MB FRCP FRCR
Consulting Radiologist, University College of London Hospitals and St Mark˛s Hospital, London, UK

Iain Watt FRCP FRCR
Consultant Clinical Radiologist, Bristol Royal Infirmary, Bristol, UK

Richard W Whitehouse BSc MD MRCP FRCR
Consultant Radiologist, Manchester Royal Infirmary; Honorary Clinical Lecturer, University of Manchester, Manchester, UK

Peter Wilde BSc MRCP FRCR
Consultant Cardiac Radiologist, United Bristol Healthcare Trust, Bristol, UK

Jeremy W R Young MA BM BCh FRCR
Professor & Chairman of Radiology, Medical University of South Carolina, Charleston, South Carolina USA

Gregg Zoarski MD
Assistant Professor, Department of Radiology and Neurosurgery, University of Maryland Medical System, Baltimore, Maryland, USA

PREFACE

The first edition of this textbook was published in 1969 and achieved immediate success as a standard work. Further editions have followed at regular intervals since and served to consolidate its position as a popular and best selling major Textbook of Radiology and Imaging. Recent editions have been translated into Spanish and Arabic and sales of the 5th edition reached record figures, emphasizing the important place Medical Imaging now occupies in medical practice, and the student's need for guidance through the bewildering plethora of new information in the field.

The constant expansion of Imaging methods and potential is based on scientific and technical advances including improvements in computers and computer software. Although it is only five years since the last edition was published, further major technical advances have taken place since then. In CT helical (spiral) scanners have been introduced, improving the quality and scope of 3D CT and 3D CT angiography. The resolution of 3D MR and 3D MR angiography has also advanced to the stage where the replacement of conventional invasive angiography is now in sight. Interventional Radiology has expanded into new areas whilst interventional MR has now become increasingly practical and holds great promise for the future. Ultrasound has also advanced into wider areas with increasing use of Color Doppler and Power Doppler. Functional Neuroimaging with PET and SPECT is emerging from the research stages and when more freely available could have a major influence on clinical practice. MR spectroscopy however has failed to fulfil its early promise and still awaits routine clinical acceptance.

Also since the last edition the centenary of Roentgen's epoch making discovery was celebrated in 1995. The pioneer of X-rays thus initiated a branch of medical science which has lasted over 100 years and is still being exploited and improved.

This new edition contains some 2000 new or replacement figures. Apart from the general revision and the deletion of obsolete material, it also records the increasing use of MR in the skeletal system and the increasing use of high resolution CT in the respiratory section. Non invasive methods including Doppler Ultrasound and MR are being more widely applied to the investigation of the Cardiovascular System, the Abdomen and the CNS.

New chapters or sections added to this edition include Abdominal Trauma; Orbital Ultrasound; Color Doppler of Arteries, Veins, Liver and Gynecology; MR of Soft Tissues and Interventional MR. Some chapters have been completely rewritten by new authors, including those on Mammography, the Salivary Glands, Pharynx and Esophagus, the Stomach and Duodenum, the Biliary Tract, several Chest chapters and the Orbit. New Appendices contain Glossaries to help the student understand the technical advances in CT and MRI and the large number of new acronyms resulting from them. However, the emphasis throughout the text remains, as in previous editions, on clinical value rather than techniques and technical descriptions.

In previous editions we have emphasized that a large work with some 40 contributors takes several years to plan, edit and prepare for publication, so that it can never be entirely up to date with a rapidly advancing technically based specialty. The student is therefore again advised to monitor current specialist journals and to attend professional symposia and meetings, particularly when preparing for examinations.

London, 1998   *David Sutton*

1

CONGENITAL SKELETAL ANOMALIES; SKELETAL DYSPLASIAS; CHROMOSOMAL DISORDERS

Peter Renton
with contributions from W. R. Lees

CONGENITAL SKELETAL ANOMALIES

Very many congenital skeletal anomalies have been described. Some minor abnormalities are only discovered coincidentally or are never noticed. In many of these the skeleton is affected and often is the only system implicated. Many infective orthopedic conditions acquired in childhood have been wholly or partially eradicated. Congenital abnormalities are therefore assuming increasing importance and present tremendous challenges to orthopedic surgeons. However, only those of great importance to the radiologist will be dealt with in this section. Suggestions for further reading are given at the end of the Chapter.

UPPER LIMB

Many congenital anomalies exist. A short glossary of descriptive terms in common use is presented here.

Adactyly—absence of fingers

Amelia—absence of limbs

Brachydactyly—short phalanges

Brachymesophalangy—short middle phalanges

Clinodactyly—incurving of a finger, usually the fifth, in the coronal plane

Hemimelia—absence of part of a hand

Hyper- or *hypophalangism*—the presence of a greater or lesser number of phalanges

Longitudinal defect—absence of part of a limb along its longitudinal axis; this may be pre-axial (radial), post-axial (ulnar) or central

Macrodactyly—enlargement of a digit

Oligodactyly—absence of fingers

Phocomelia—absence of the proximal parts of a limb

Polydactyly—increased number of digits; may be pre- or post-axial

Symphalangism—fusion of phalanges in one digit

Syndactyly—fusion of adjacent digits. May involve soft tissues and/or bone.

(After Poznanski)

The lesions may be grouped into:

1. Failure of differentiation, e.g. syndactyly
2. Failure of development, which may be transverse, e.g. aphalangy, or longitudinal
3. Duplications
4. Overgrowth—as in neurofibromatosis
5. Generalized dysplasias
6. Congenital (Streeter's) bands.

Some lesions are solitary and of no significance, e.g. isolated clinodactyly, while others occur in combination so that clinodactyly is also seen as part of major syndromes, e.g. trisomy 21. Radial defects especially are associated with other anomalies, e.g. with atrial septal defects in the Holt–Oram syndrome. Some defects are attributable to drugs, such as thalidomide (Distaval) administered to the mother in the first three months of pregnancy. This may cause damage to the growing nerves and it may be that the sensory nerve is the tissue organizer (McCredie 1975). Epanutin, used in the treatment of maternal epilepsy, may cause

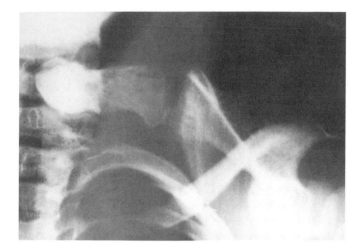

Fig. 1.1   The scapula is elevated and a large omovertebral bone is shown.

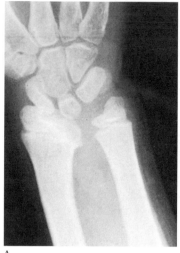

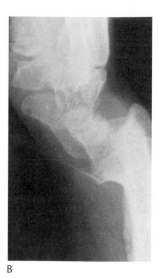

A   B

Fig. 1.2 A,B   Madelung's deformity—defective development of the inner third of the radial epiphysis, increase in interosseous space, backward projection of the ulna and anterior displacement of the hand.

hypoplasia of distal phalanges in utero. Many lesions are genetically inherited so that a harmless *congenital broad thumb* may be seen in different generations of the same family. Other defects may represent sporadic mutations of the gene.

Sprengel's Shoulder   This deformity consists of an abnormally high scapula. The deformity is due to failure of the shoulder girdle to descend from its embryonic position in the neck, a process which is normally completed by the end of the third fetal month. The lesion is usually unilateral, though it may be bilateral. Other congenital anomalies are frequently associated.

Radiographs show the characteristic elevated scapula. The scapula may be normal in shape, but usually there is some shortening of its vertebral border with the result that its shape approaches that of an equilateral triangle. Rotation of the scapula may often be observed; generally the inferior angle rotates toward the spine, though rotation in the opposite direction may occur.

From the upper part of the vertebral border or from the superior angle, an accessory bone—the omovertebral or suprascapular bone—may be found uniting this part of the scapula to the spine (Fig. 1.1). This structure may be represented only by fibrous tissue or cartilage and, if bony, may vary greatly in size and radiopacity.

Other anomalies which frequently coexist include *cervical spina bifida*, the *Klippel–Feil anomaly*, *cervical ribs* and *other rib lesions*, *scoliosis* and *hemivertebrae*.

No difficulties in diagnosis should arise. In old *paralytic lesions*, the scapula may be raised. If not evident from the history, the correct diagnosis should be suspected by noting the hypoplasia of bone typical of a paralytic lesion.

Radius and Ulna   Radial defects are much more common than ulnar and may occur in isolation or as part of major syndromes, in which case they are usually bilateral.

Radial defects may occur with:

- Ectodermal dysplasia
- Holt–Oram syndrome
- Fanconi syndrome
- Thrombocytopenia—absent radius syndrome

- Trisomy 18
- Thalidomide embryopathy
- Renal, ear and esophageal anomalies.

The defect may range from hypoplasia of the thumb to complete absence of radius, scaphoid, trapezium and thumb. The limb is shortened and a radial club hand results, with the hand deviated to the side of the absent bone.

Synostosis of the radius and ulna may be seen at the upper end and is usually associated with dislocation of the radial head. This lesion has marked hereditary tendencies.

Madelung's Deformity   This lesion is much commoner in girls and it is generally bilateral. It usually presents during adolescence. The cardinal abnormality is defective development of the inner third of the epiphysis of the lower end of the radius. As a consequence the radial shaft is bowed, so increasing the interosseous space. The lower end of the ulna is subluxed backward. The hand and carpus project forward at the wrist joint to produce a bayonet-like appearance in a lateral view (Fig. 1.2).

The lesion may be part of the *Léri–Weill syndrome* (dyschondrosteosis see below) and *Turner syndrome*. Similar appearances may follow trauma or infection to the growing epiphyseal plate (Fig. 1.3).

Hand and Wrist   Very many congenital abnormalities (and normal variants) may be found in the hands and feet. Specialist monographs should be consulted (see list at end of Chapter).

Carpal fusions may occur in isolation or as part of a syndrome. In isolation they are usually transverse, e.g. lunate–triquetrum and capitate–hamate, and are much commoner in blacks. In syndromes they are usually proximodistal and occur in *Apert syndrome, dyschondrosteosis, chondroectodermal dysplasia, Holt–Oram syndrome* and *Turner syndrome*. Similar appearances may follow trauma, infection and rheumatoid disease.

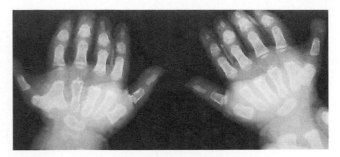

Fig. 1.4 Chondroectodermal dysplasia (Ellis–van Creveld syndrome). Polysyndactyly is demonstrated. In addition, the phalanges are abnormal in morphology.

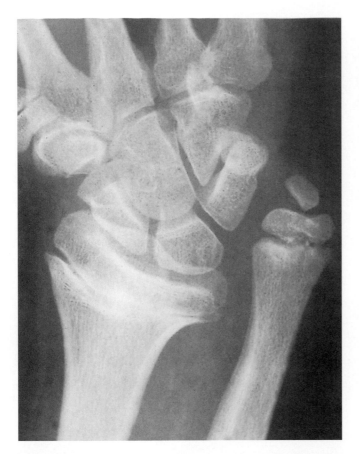

Fig. 1.3 Trauma to the distal radius has resulted in partial fusion of the epiphyseal plate and partial growth arrest. Avulsion of the ulnar styloid occurred at the same time.

Polydactyly Polydactyly is more common in blacks. It may be *postaxial* (ulnar) and may range from a minor ossicle to complete duplication of the little finger. *Preaxial* lesions (radial) range from minor partial duplication of the thumb distal phalanx to complete thumb duplication. On occasion the hand may be duplicated. Syndactyly may be associated with polydactyly.

Polydactyly may be associated with *Ellis–van Creveld syndrome* (chondroectodermal dysplasia) (Fig. 1.4), *Laurence–Moon–Biedl syndrome* (polysyndactyly, mental defect, obesity and retinitis pigmentosa), *trisomy 13* and asphyxiating thoracic dysplasia—all postaxial—and with *Holt–Oram syndrome* and *Fanconi's anemia* (preaxial).

Syndactyly occurs in *Apert syndrome, Fanconi's anemia, Laurence–Moon–Biedl syndrome, trisomy 13* and *trisomy 18*. (For fuller list consult specialist texts; see references at end of Chapter).

THE LOWER LIMB

Congenital Dislocation of the Hip

This is a very important condition because success in its treatment depends upon early recognition. The incidence of hip instability at birth is 5–10/1000, and of frank dislocation 1–1.5/1000. One-

third of cases of congenital dislocation of the hip are detected late, but these often have a family history of the disease.

Instability and dislocation is usually unilateral (L:R = 11:1) but both hips may be involved (unilateral:bilateral = 11:4). Females are more commonly affected (F:M = 5:1). Sixty per cent of affected children are first-born. These children are far more likely to have been breech presentations (breech:vertex = 6:1), possibly because the abnormal lie does not permit reduction in utero. Children born by cesarean section are thus also more likely to have associated instability and dislocation. A family or twin history is also common; a subsequent child has a 6% risk of involvement.

Congenital dislocation of the hip is more commonly found in the winter (winter:summer = 1.5:1), possibly because of tight swaddling of children in a position of dislocation in winter.

Imaging

Ultrasound (*Prof. W. R. Lees*) Using a high-frequency ultrasound transducer, it is possible to image the anatomy of the infant hip joint. The bone of the acetabulum impedes the passage of the ultrasound beam, producing a highly echogenic interface. Cartilage allows through transmission, with its internal structure returning low-level echoes. Muscles and tendons also show characteristic echo patterns (Figs. 1.5A,B).

The femoral head is seen as a spherical structure containing coarse low-level echoes. The triradiate cartilage presents similarly as an acoustic defect at the base of the acetabulum.

A stable hip joint does not permit posterior movement of the femoral head in the acetabulum. This defines the most commonly used scanning technique. The hip is scanned in the supine position with 90° flexion. Firm posterior pressure will result in subluxation of the unstable hip, which is best seen scanning in the transverse plane (Fig. 1.5C). Movement of 3–4 mm on the flexion stress maneuver is found with a loose joint. This corresponds to a slight click on clinical examination. Movement of more than 6 mm is significant subluxation.

The position of the limbic cartilage is important in complete dislocation, where it is interposed between the femoral head and the acetabulum (Fig. 1.5C).

The size, shape and symmetry of the femoral heads and acetabula can be monitored on treatment through windows cut in the hip spica. The ossification center develops between 1 and 6 months, and is seen as an echogenic focus within the poorly echogenic femoral head.

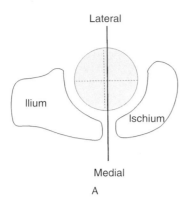

Lateral

Ilium

Ischium

Medial

A

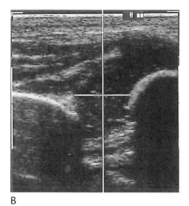

B

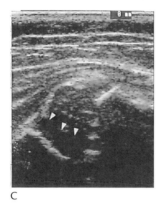

C

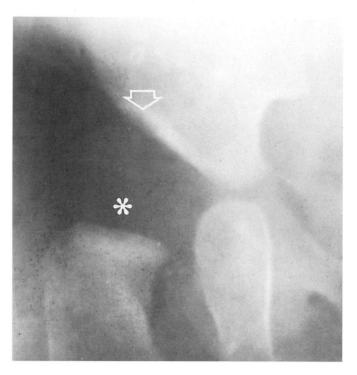

Fig. 1.6   A small defect with marginal sclerosis is seen above the acetabulum (arrow) in a neonate who later was shown to have a congenitally dislocated femoral head. The * marks the site of the projected femoral head.

Fig. 1.5   A. Diagram of a transverse section through the infant hip showing the normal relationship of the ball of the femoral head to the acetabulum. **B.** A normal transverse section indicating the important axes, as in 5A. **C.** Inferior subluxation with interposition of poorly echogenic limbic cartilage (small arrows) between the moderately echogenic femoral head and the floor of the acetabulum.

The acetabulum is best imaged in the coronal plane. If the acetabular cup accommodates less than one-third of the femoral head, then acetabular dysplasia is definitely present and it must be suspected if one-half to one-third only is accommodated.

Ultrasonography should be used whenever there is clinical suspicion of CDH. Conventional radiography has three shortcomings: cartilage is not directly visualized and its position has to be inferred from bony landmarks; the standard radiographic positions are those in which subluxation is least likely to occur; and the examination is static, with stress views rarely obtained. Ultrasonography is simple, rapid and free of hazard.

Plain Film Radiology   The advent of neonatal hip ultrasound, especially if it can be carried out as a screening test and again at three months, has limited the use of conventional radiology. The indications for conventional radiographs given below (taken from Catterall's work [personal communication, 1990]) of course apply also to ultrasound. Discussion of radiology is still necessary as access to ultrasound may be limited.

Absolute Indications   (If any one of these is present, the hips should be examined by imaging):

1. Family history of congenital dislocation of hip
2. Neonatal hip instability

3. Limb shortening
4. Limitation of hip abduction in flexion.

Relative Indications   (If any two of these are present, the hips should be examined by imaging):

1. Breech presentation
2. First-born child
3. Cesarean section
4. Other congenital abnormalities
5. Excessive fetal moulding.

At birth, neither femoral head is ossified but, occasionally, a notch above the acetabulum may be present (Fig. 1.6) and even in the absence of the femoral head, congenital dislocation of the hip can then be diagnosed.

Retarded ossification of the femoral ossific nucleus is a traditional sign of congenital dislocation of the hip. In some early cases, however, the femoral ossific nucleus may appear to be larger on the dislocated than on the normal side. Some incongruous findings are probably explicable by the lesion being bilateral.

Sometimes poor development of the acetabulum is obvious in cases of congenital dislocation of the hip. In our experience the acetabular angle is increased in congenital dislocations even in the neonatal period. The *acetabular angle* is the angle subtended by a line drawn through the centers of both Y-cartilages (Hilgenreiner's line) and a line parallel to the acetabular roof.

The eventual position of the femoral head and its relationship to the acetabulum can often be inferred from a film of the hips in the neutral position. The site of the non-ossified epiphysis may be inferred as lying superior to the epiphyseal plate. This in turn lies at right angles and proximal to the femoral neck (Fig. 1.6).

Seen later, from the age of 6 months onward, the radiological diagnosis is usually easy (Fig. 1.7). The femoral head will be displaced upward and outward and delayed ossification of its epiphysis will be observed. The acetabulum will be shallower than that of the normal hip and its roof will not be set horizontally but will slope upward and outward. Use of the many lines and coordinates described in this condition is not necessary, provided heed is paid to the possibility of a bilateral dislocation.

During management the radiologist will be asked to decide whether reduction has been attained or maintained. This decision

may be very difficult to make on radiographs taken through plaster, but ultrasound may give the answer.

Reduction may be impossible to obtain or the hip may be unstable. In such cases *arthrography* may be used to study the disposition of soft-tissue structures of the joint.

Possible abnormal findings are:

1. The fibrocartilaginous rim of the acetabulum, called the *limbus*, may become inverted into the joint and form a barrier to stable reduction. In an arthrogram of a normal hip a thorn-like projection marks a small gap between the outer part of the limbus and the capsular attachment. When the limbus is inverted, the 'thorn' is lost and the filling defect caused by the limbus is seen (Fig. 1.8).

2. The *ligamentum teres* may become so large that it may offer a barrier to reduction. A hypertrophic ligamentum teres may be visible on the arthrogram but estimation of its size by this means is unreliable.

3. The *psoas tendon* may become contracted and a notch for the tendon is seen inferiorly.

Arthrography is of particular service in deciding whether complete reduction of a dislocation has been achieved. There are times when it is not possible to obtain this information from examination of plain films—especially when the femoral ossific nucleus appears to be set eccentrically on the femoral neck.

The primary cause of unstable reduction of a dislocated femoral head has long been debated. Excessive anteversion of the femoral neck is often seen and the condition often necessitates a de-rotation osteotomy for reduction to be maintained. The femoral neck of a normal baby is usually anteverted to 35°; this diminishes to 15° in the adult. In congenital dislocation, the femoral neck may be anteverted to 70–80°. CT is useful for measuring the degree of anteversion.

In neglected dislocations, the misplaced femoral head may produce a depression on the side of the ilium above the acetabulum, constituting a *false acetabulum* (Fig. 1.7C). This may vary in size from a shallow depression to a deep socket. The original acetabular socket becomes progressively more shallow.

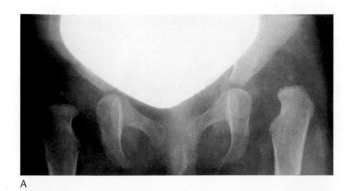

A

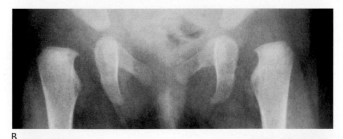

B

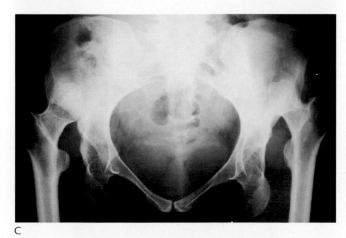

C

Fig. 1.7 A,B Bilateral congenital dislocation of the hip. The initial radiograph demonstrates lateral subluxation of both femoral heads with dysplastic acetabula. The ossifying nucleus can be seen developing at the mid point of the growth plate. Its eventual position could be predicted from the original plain film. **C.** End-stage undiagnosed bilateral CDH. The femoral heads have molded in their new situation and articulate with the iliac blades.

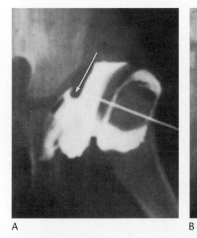

A

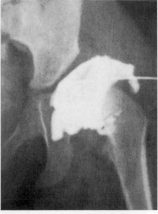

B

Fig. 1.8 A. Arthrogram of the left hip shows filling defect caused by inverted limbus (arrow). **B.** Appearances following limbectomy. (Courtesy of Mr A. C. Clark.)

Osteochondritis may complicate a congenital dislocation of the hip, particularly after vigorous methods of reduction or surgery. Not all cases of osteochondritis are attributable to the complications of treatment, for there does appear to be a true association between congenital dislocation and Perthes' disease of the hip.

Idiopathic Coxa Vara of Childhood: Proximal Femoral Focal Deficiency (PFFD)

Two types of idiopathic coxa vara are recognized:

1. A congenital form, generally present at birth, sometimes associated with other congenital lesions
2. An infantile form, not present at birth, recognized around the age of 4 years and often bilateral (33%).

PFFD (congenitally short femur) consists of failure of normal development of a lesser or greater part of the proximal femur. Some distal femur, by definition, is always present, thus distinguishing it from femoral agenesis.

Coxa vara is included as part of the PFFD spectrum if the varus is associated with congenital femoral shortening present at birth, i.e. Type 1 above. If PFFD is severe, coxa vara cannot arise at all, even in congenital cases.

The mean angle of the neck of the shaft at one year of age is 148°, decreasing to 135° at 5 years, and 120° in the elderly. Coxa vara is present when the angle is less than normal, but certainly if below 110°.

Radiographic Findings: Coxa Vara   The lesion is usually bilateral, though it may be unilateral. Coxa vara will usually be obvious. The femoral head will be situated low in the acetabulum and its outline may appear woolly. Secondary deformity of the acetabulum may result. A triangular fragment of bone may be seen at the lower part of the femoral neck. This wedge of bone, commoner in the infantile cases, is bounded by clear bands forming an inverted V (Fig. 1.9). The medial or inner band is the epiphyseal line. The outer one is, of course, abnormal. Some writers have regarded it as an area of osteochondritis, others as a stress fracture. In later cases the greater trochanter will be found to curve like a beak and it may articulate with the ilium. Not all these features are necessarily present in every case.

Acquired coxa vara may be found in conditions where bone is softened, e.g. in *rickets, fibrous dysplasia, osteogenesis imperfecta* and *cleidocranial dysplasia*, as well as in *Perthes' disease* and following *slipped epiphysis*.

In some cases which appear to have PFFD with no proximal femur in which to have coxa vara, arthrography of the hip may reveal a cartilaginous neck and head with varus deformity, as will ultrasound.

Radiographic Findings: PFFD (Fig. 1.10)   A short femur, which is laterally situated and proximally displaced, is demonstrated at birth. The distal femur is by definition present. Ossification of the proximal portion is delayed. A spectrum of proximal deficiencies exists.

Abnormalities of the Patella

The patella is frequently *bipartite* and sometimes *multipartite*. The upper, outer part is always involved. The anomaly is often bilateral and well corticated all round, which helps to distinguish it from a fracture. Not all cases, however, are bilateral.

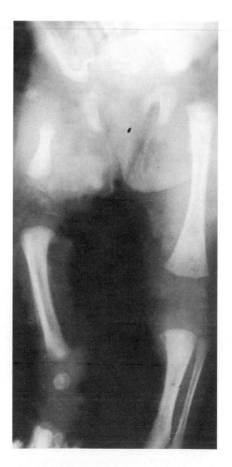

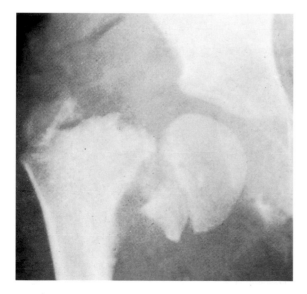

Fig. 1.9   Congenital coxa vara—extreme coxa vara with some slip of the epiphysis. A triangular fragment of bone is well shown.

Fig. 1.10   Proximal focal femoral deficiency. Only a hypoplastic portion of the distal right femur is apparent.

In the *nail–patella syndrome* the patella may be rudimentary or hypoplastic and set laterally (see Fig. 1.17B).

The patella may be *dislocated* due to a variety of congenital causes, e.g. *hypoplasia of the lateral femoral condyle, external rotation of the tibia* and *malattachment of the iliotibial tract*. The displacement is invariably outward.

Congenital Pseudarthrosis of the Tibia and Fibula

The pseudarthrosis of the tibia is seen at the junction of the middle and lower thirds. Often a similar lesion is found in the fibula.

Radiological examination of early cases may show a sclerotic or radiolucent zone in the affected area. This bows, resorbs and fractures and the severed ends of the bone become sclerotic. Still later, the proximal part becomes cupped and the distal part pointed, so forming a pseudarthrosis (Fig. 1.11). This uncommon lesion is notoriously resistant to treatment.

Neurofibromatosis is usually given as the most frequent cause of this condition. Other associations are with *fibrous dysplasia* and *idiopathic juvenile osteoporosis*. Occasionally, a similar lesion has been found affecting the *forearm bones*.

The Foot and Ankle

Accessory Bones of the Foot   Supernumerary centers of ossification are more common in the foot than in the hand. They should be identified to distinguish them from fractures. They may themselves fracture and be a cause of pain, or may be involved in rheumatoid arthritis, osteochondritis, osteoarthritis, infections and hyperparathyroidism. More than 50 have been described but most of them are rarities. As they become radiologically visible in adults, the incidence rises to 30%. The *os tibiale externum* is found in some 7% of feet, the *os trigonum* in 5% and the *os peroneum* in 8% but surveys differ as to their incidence.

Degenerative change, which may be painful, can occur between

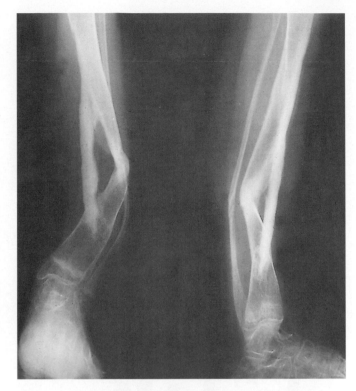

Fig. 1.11 Neurofibromatosis. Pseudarthroses are seen bilaterally. The fibulae are thin and bowed. Bony struts have been inserted at surgery.

the os tibiale externum and the adjacent navicular. An overlying bursitis arises over the bony prominence.

The os trigonum may be entrapped between the calcaneus and posterior tibia in ballet dancers and footballers, and this bone becomes the site of osteochondritis. Change can be seen on plain films, where the ossicle becomes sclerotic and fragmented. The bone scan is positive, and change is also seen at MR (Fig. 1.12).

The os peroneum may fracture.

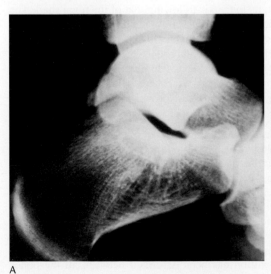

A

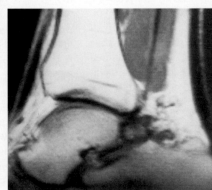

B

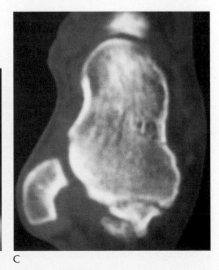

C

Fig. 1.12   Avascular necrosis of the os trigonum. **A.** This bone is sclerotic and would be grossly abnormal on a bone scan. **B.** MR scan. **C.** CT scan.

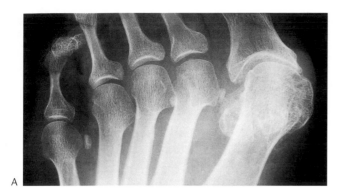

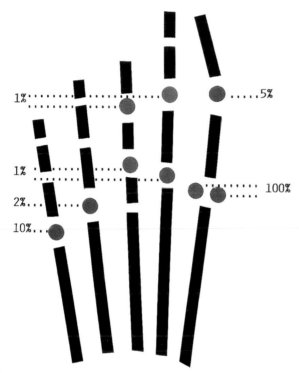

Fig. 1.13 **A.** Sesamoids at the metatarsal heads. Apart from the usual medial and lateral sesamoids at the great toe metatarsal head, sesamoids are also seen at the second, third, fourth and fifth metatarsal heads. **B.** To show the percentages of foot sesamoid incidence in Bizarro's (1921) series.

Two sesamoids are regularly seen at the head of the great toe metatarsal. Sesamoids may on occasion be seen at all the meta-tarsal heads (Fig. 1.13). The medial is bipartite in one-third of cases, the lateral in only 5%. A bipartite sesamoid is larger than its normal counterpart and corticated all round, while a fractured sesamoid shows non-corticated fracture parts. Pathology in meta-tarsal sesamoids can be demonstrated on axial views, and isotope bone scans will often be abnormal.

Congenital Talipes Equinovarus (*congenital club foot*) This condition is nearly always idiopathic but club foot is sometimes associated with other bony abnormalities.

The idiopathic type is of limited interest to the radiologist. The three cardinal abnormalities are: 1. adduction of the forefoot; 2. inversion of the foot; and 3. plantar flexion of the foot. Radio-logically, medial displacement of the navicular and cuboid in relation to the heads of the talus and calcaneus will be seen. The

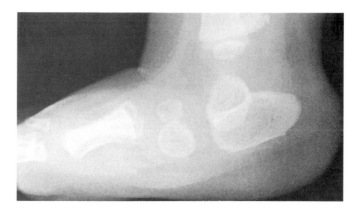

Fig. 1.14 Congenital vertical talus — note vertical position of the talus and elevation both of the calcaneus and of the forefoot.

calcaneus will rotate medially under the talus. Plantar flexion will be seen by posterior displacement of the calcaneus.

Ossification of the talus and navicular may be retarded. Usually secondary hypoplasia of the bones of the tarsus and of the soft tissue is seen.

Ball and Socket Ankle Joint In this condition the ankle joint is abnormally shaped and its range of movement increased. It is usually found when the midtarsal and subtaloid joints are rigid, generally caused by tarsal fusions; in such cases inversion and eversion of the ankle compensate for the loss of these movements at the midtarsal and subtaloid joints.

Some cases are seen in patients with a short leg—in a few no underlying cause is seen.

Radiographic features are characteristic. The trochlear surface of the talus, normally convex anteroposteriorly and concave from side to side, loses this concavity and approaches the shape of a sphere. The mortice of the talus becomes correspondingly molded into a cup-like cavity to form a ball and socket articulation.

Congenital Vertical Talus This is a rare cause of congenital flat foot in children. The radiographic appearances are diagnostic. The talus is vertical, its long axis following that of the tibial shaft. The vertical displacement of the talus remains constant whether the patient is standing or recumbent. The bones of the forefoot and the calcaneus are raised and produce the typical rocker-bottom foot (Fig. 1.14). When the navicular becomes ossified its shape will be seen to appear normal except for a little constriction of its waist. It will be seen obviously dislocated and lying in contact with the body of the talus.

Congenital Fusions Painful flat foot (the peroneal spastic flat foot) may be due to fusion of certain tarsal bones (Fig. 1.15). If the union is cartilaginous or fibrous, rather than bony, it is not seen radiologically. Flattening of the longitudinal arch of the foot is seen. Bony union is not directly demonstrable before adolescence but appears with ossification of the cartilaginous link between the bones. Fusion of the medial facet of the subtalar joint is the most common. It is well seen on an axial view of the foot. Calcaneonavicular fusion is shown on oblique views of the foot (Fig. 1.15). Coalition has been described between all the bones of the hind foot. Restriction of movement at the subtalar joint causes abnormal movement of the hind foot, with lipping at the

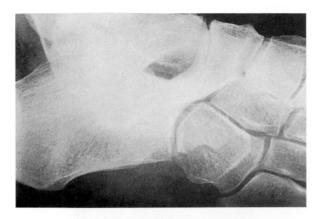

Fig. 1.15   Calcaneonavicular bar.

calcaneonavicular joint, seen together with longitudinal arch flattening and obliteration of subtalar joints on the lateral view of the foot. These changes result in a local increase in uptake on *radionuclide bone scanning*. *CT* and *isotope scanning* will also show foot fusions, as does *MRI* (Fig. 1.16).

THE PELVIS

Iliac Horns   These are bony processes projecting dorsally from the outer surface of the wings of the ilium. They may occur alone or be associated with the syndrome of rudimentary or absent patellae, deformity of the elbows (hypoplasia of capitellum and radial head) and dystrophy of the nails (*nail–patella syndrome—Fong's lesion* (Fig. 1.17).

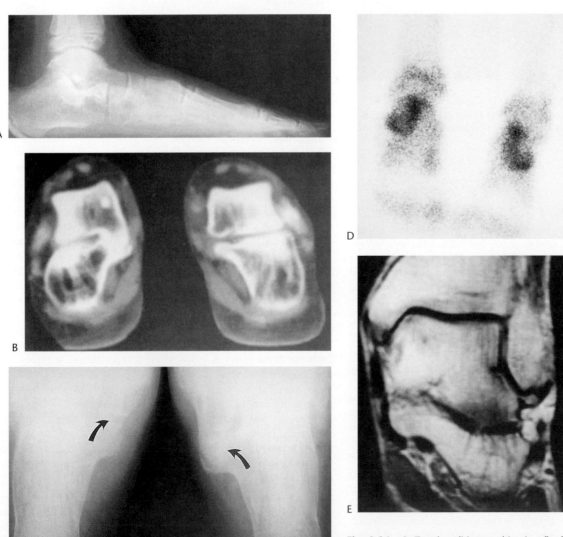

Fig. 1.16   **A.** Tarsal coalition resulting in a flat foot. The subtalar joints are no longer clearly visualized. **B.** CT scan of tarsal coalition showing right-sided fusion of the middle facet of the subtalar joint. **C.** Axial view showing unilateral coalition of the middle facet (arrows). **D.** The bone scan shows a site of symmetrically increased uptake away from the fusion—a stress phenomenon. **E.** The MR scan shows obliteration of the subtalar joint.

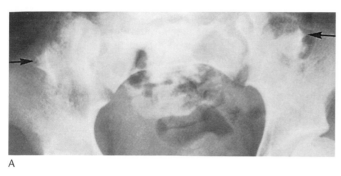

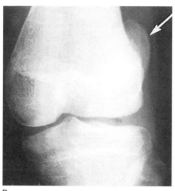

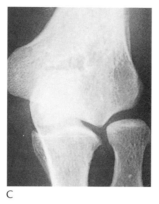

Fig. 1.17 Nail–patella syndrome. **A.** Iliac horns are seen (arrow). **B.** A small laterally placed patella is shown. **C.** Hypoplasia of the capitellum is shown.

THE SPINE

Spinal anomalies range from gross defects, incompatible with life, to minor anomalies which are no more than anatomic variants. Some of these may be mistaken for fractures, e.g. the unfused accessory ossification centers at the tips of inferior articular facets or those related to the anterosuperior part of the margins of vertebral bodies. Fractures are rarely seen at such sites and have ragged rather than smooth edges.

Coronal Cleft Vertebra   This anomaly is seen in vertebral bodies of newborn infants and is due to failure of fusion of two ossification centers. In about half the cases more than one vertebral body is affected. The abnormality has been seen on prenatal radiographs—it occurs more frequently in males.

The cleft is seen on a lateral radiograph as a linear or oval defect between a small posterior and larger anterior ossification centers. The anteroposterior diameter of the affected vertebral body is often increased. The cleft consolidates in a few months. These clefts are of no importance except that they are seen in some dysplasias (see *chondrodystrophia calcificans congenita*).

Butterfly Vertebra   In the affected vertebra, the upper and lower surfaces are deeply concave or V-shaped, so that the vertical dimension of the vertebral body in the midline is much reduced. In the frontal projection, it is seen that vertebrae above and below are molded into the deficient centers of the affected vertebra (Fig. 1.18).

Malfusions of Appendages   Epiphyses of the spinous processes, transverse processes and articular facets may remain unfused. The

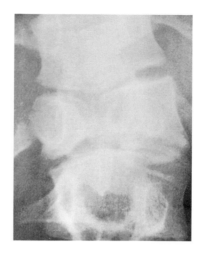

Fig. 1.18 Butterfly vertebra—upper and lower surfaces of affected vertebra are V-shaped, and contiguous vertebrae are moulded into the deficient center.

abnormality is without importance except that it may mimic a fracture.

Hemivertebrae   They may cause scoliosis unless an equal number appear on each side. In the thoracic region, a hemivertebra will bear a rib. Multiple hemivertebrae may cause dwarfism.

Congenital Vertebral Fusion   Many forms of congenital vertebral fusion may be found. Complete fusion of the bodies and neural arches may occur, or the fusion may be limited to parts of the bodies or neural arches. At times it may not be possible to decide whether a fusion is developmental or post-inflammatory. Fusion of neural arches, however, is almost always a developmental anomaly. The anteroposterior diameter of congenital block vertebrae may be reduced and an anterior concavity may be found. These features may also be found in old postinfective fusions or after juvenile chronic arthritis. A posterior concavity in addition may indicate a congenital lesion.

Complete vertebral fusions are often called 'block vertebrae'. They may be of no clinical significance but, frequently, disk degeneration develops above or below the fused vertebrae due to altered mechanics in the spine. Such lesions are relatively common in the cervical spine where a more severe anomaly, the *Klippel–Feil syndrome*, may be seen (Fig. 1.19). In this condition, many cervical vertebrae are fused, the neck is short and its movements limited, and hair grows low on the neck. Often there is torticollis and atrophy of facial musculature. Other congenital anomalies, such as spina bifida, rib lesions and Sprengel's shoulder, usually coexist.

Vertebral fusions are also found in *fibrodysplasia ossificans progressiva*.

Separate Odontoid   (*os odontoideum*) The odontoid peg may sometimes be completely detached from the body of the second cervical vertebra, and be situated in the region of the foramen magnum (Fig. 1.20). Posterior fossa symptoms may result.

It has been shown that in some cases at least the separate ossicle results from a fracture in childhood of the base of the odontoid peg, with subsequent failure to unite. The lesion is thus not always 'congenital'.

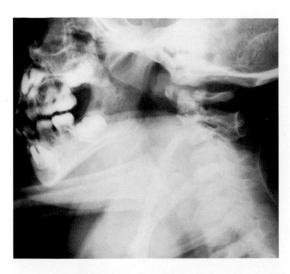

Fig. 1.19 Klippel–Feil deformity. Short neck with elevated shoulders and scapulae. Fusion is demonstrated at C2/3 level.

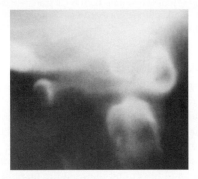

Fig. 1.20 Os odontoideum. The odontoid peg is clearly separate from the body of C2 but retains a normal relationship with the arch of the atlas. These lesions usually follow trauma in childhood.

Cervical Rib This is a common anomaly. The supplementary rib usually arises from the seventh cervical vertebra, rarely from the sixth and very rarely from the fifth.

The diagnosis is straightforward, though it may be necessary to count all the ribs in order to distinguish a rudimentary first thoracic rib from a cervical rib. Cervical ribs arise from cervical transverse processes. These slope downward from the neural arch in the cervical spine but upward in the thoracic spine. Cervical ribs vary greatly in size and shape, and clinical symptoms bear little relation to the radiographic abnormality. A very small cervical rib element may have a fibrous attachment to the first thoracic rib which causes much disability; this change may be seen at MRI. A large cervical rib may be asymptomatic.

Sacralization and Lumbarization It is often difficult to give a definite level to a particular vertebral body in the lumbar region, especially if the lumbosacral region is transitional. Again, it may be necessary to count all the vertebral bodies from C1 down. It has been said that the transverse processes of L3 are the lowest (most caudal) which lie transversely, while those for L4 are inclined upward. Various permutations occur. Small, or absent, ribs on T12 may occur with large transverse processes on L5

which fuse with the sacrum (sacralization of L5). This is known as cranial shift. Caudal shift implies the presence of ribs on L1 and lumbarization of S1, that is, it comes to bear free-floating transverse processes. A rudimentary disk is then seen between S1 and S2.

The sacralized transverse process may form a pseudarthrosis with the ilium and degenerative sclerosis may appear around the false joint. This may be a site of low back pain. In addition, the free disk above the pseudarthrosis shows early degeneration, especially if it lies high in relation to the iliac crest where it is said to be 'vulnerable' and susceptible to degeneration. Conversely, a low lumbosacral junction, buried deep between the crests, is less likely to degenerate. Similarly, a disk at the level beneath a transverse process–iliac blade fusion is 'protected' from early degeneration. The transverse process at L5 is usually the bulkiest and it may totally or partially articulate with the sacrum in 15–30%.

Anomalies of Lumbosacral Facets (*trophism*) The facet joints in the lumbar spine may be clearly seen in the anteroposterior projection. They should be symmetric but vary in their orientation. At L1 the facets have an almost vertical orientation but passing interiorly are re-orientated so that they face upward, inward and backward.

Facets are angled at around 52° in the sagittal midline at L5/S1 but 10° less at L4/5. The lower facets are asymmetric in around 20–30% of patients. It has been said that the direction of disk degeneration and protrusion is related to the orientation of the facet—usually on the side of the more oblique facet.

With degeneration, the lower lumbar facet joints cease to be symmetric, so that often one joint is seen and the other at that level is not (Fig. 1.21A). This rotational change is associated with much new bone around the narrowed facet joints and adjacent laminae, often with symptoms of nerve root impingement. The changes are well demonstrated with CT scanning (Fig. 1.21B), when the acquired asymmetry of the entire neural arch is seen as well as the local new bone formation.

Spina Bifida Incomplete fusion of neural arches is a common finding. In most cases only a minor midsagittal defect in the neural arch is seen. The rather misleading term 'spina bifida occulta' is applied to this condition. There is no true breach in such cases; the radiolucent area represents merely non-ossified cartilage. In children many of these areas become ossified as growth progresses.

True breaches in the neural arch do, of course, occur, and they may be accompanied by a meningocele protruding posteriorly and usually in the lumbar region. Occasionally, in the thorax and in the sacral region, the sac may protrude laterally and anteriorly through the intervertebral foramina and sacral foramina respectively. Other vertebral and rib anomalies are very frequent in the severe forms of spina bifida. The presence of hydrocephalus is a common feature in marked spina bifida.

Foot deformities, such as *pes cavus*, may be associated with spina bifida. Likewise, *perforating ulcers* causing absorption of metatarsal heads, *neuropathic joints* and *spontaneous fractures* accompanied by excessive callus may all occur. *Metaphyseal fractures* are sometimes seen in this condition.

In cases of alimentary reduplications, the possibility of associated malformations of the spine should be borne in mind. The reduplications or *neurenteric cysts* may be associated with severe

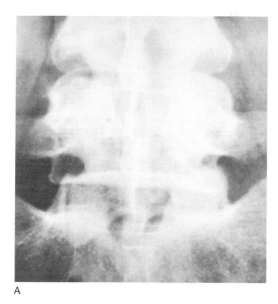
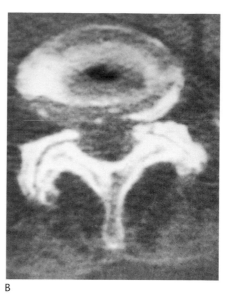

A   B

Fig. 1.21   A. The facet joints are no longer symmetric and show features of degeneration. **B.** The CT scan shows gross new bone formation around narrowed facet joints. There is marked bony encroachment upon the exit foramina, especially the left. Gas is seen in the disk (vacuum phenomenon).

anterior and posterior *spina bifida, hemivertebra, absent vertebra* or *diastematomyelia*. In some cases no vertebral deformity is demonstrable.

Scoliosis

This term describes a lateral curvature of the spine. Usually, but not always, there is a primary curve with a compensatory curve above and below, unless the primary curve is lumbar.

Classification of Scoliosis (after Cobb 1948)

1. Idiopathic
2. Osteogenic
   a. congenital, e.g. hemivertebra
   b. skeletal dysplasias, including neurofibromatosis
3. Neuropathic, e.g. polio, syringomyelia, Friedreich's ataxia
4. Hypopathic, e.g. muscular dystrophy
5. Thoracogenic, e.g. post-pneumonectomy or thoracoplasty.

Idiopathic Scoliosis is the most commonly seen form of scoliosis and may be further subdivided into the following groups:

- Infantile—age of onset 0–3 years
- Juvenile—age of onset 4–9 years
- Adolescent—age of onset 10 years, to the duration of growth.

In idiopathic scoliosis no other etiology can be discerned and the diagnosis is made by exclusion. The earlier the onset of disease, the more marked the curve at the time of spinal skeletal maturity, after which little further deterioration is to be expected. Spinal skeletal maturity is reached when the apophysis for the iliac crest turns down toward and reaches that for the posterior superior iliac

spine and, for this reason, films of the iliac crests are routinely obtained.

Idiopathic curves are associated with spinal rotation.

The curve can be measured by the method of Cobb (1948). The proximal and distal vertebrae at the margins of the curve do not show rotation of the spinous processes. Lines are drawn along the respective upper and lower end-plates at the margins of the curve and perpendiculars are drawn to these two lines. The angles at which they meet is the angle of the curve. Severe curves are 100° or more, mild curves less than 69°, and moderate between 70° and 99°.

DYSPLASIAS OF BONE

The diagnosis of these lesions is mainly radiological and often entirely so. The radiologist will observe such features as alteration in bone density and in the size and shape of the bones. He or she will also observe the distribution of the lesion and the parts of the bones affected.

Accurate diagnosis is now of prime importance and not merely an academic exercise. Genetic counseling is, of course, a well-established specialty depending on accurate diagnosis. In other fields, such as the *mucopolysaccharidoses*, new lines of therapy such as bone marrow transplants are being evaluated.

Cleidocranial Dysplasia (CCD) (synonym: *cleidocranial dysostosis*)

This is a benign hereditary condition which is inherited as an autosomal dominant and which is recognized during childhood. The disease has considerable variation of expression. Thirty per cent of cases are due to spontaneous mutation.

Radiological Features   Changes are widespread.

Clavicles   There may be total (in 10% of cases) or partial absence of the clavicle (Fig. 1.22A). The outer end is absent more frequently than the inner, but both to an extremely variable extent. Central defects also occur. The clavicles may also be normal. The scapulae tend to be small and high, and the glenoid fossae are small.

Thorax   The thorax is usually narrow, the ribs are short and directed obliquely downward. Respiratory distress may occur in the newborn. The sternum is incompletely ossified. Failure of fusion of neural arches occurs, with delay in maturation of vertebral bodies, which retain an infantile biconvex shape. Supernumerary or bifid ribs also occur.

Skull   In the newborn, mineralization is delayed. The facial bones are small but the mandible is normal in size. The fontanels remain open late and the sutures are widened. The bodies of the sphenoids are hypoplastic. Many Wormian bones are seen and frontal and parietal bossing may be present. Basilar invagination may also occur (Fig. 1.22B).

Pelvis   Delayed and imperfect ossification of the pubic bones is a recognized finding (Fig. 1.22C) and congenital coxa vara is frequently seen.

Teeth   See Chapter 50.

Hands   Anomalies of the hand are very common. The second and fifth metacarpals are long and have supernumerary ossification centers at their bases. The middle phalanges of the second and fifth phalanges are short. Cone epiphyses and distal phalangeal tapering are found.

   Short fibulae, congenital pseudarthrosis of the femur, genu valgum and *obliquity of the articular space of the ankle joint* are among many reported associations.

Pyknodysostosis

This condition has been confused with cleidocranial dysplasia (because of some similar clavicular and skull changes) and osteopetrosis (because of the generalized increase in diffuse bone density). It is inherited as an autosomal recessive disease, and parents may be closely related. The patients are short (below 150 cm), which is not a prominent feature of CCD. The skeleton is susceptible to fractures. The disease is rare and found in all races. The French painter Toulouse-Lautrec is believed to have suffered from this disease.

Radiographic Features

Skull   There is brachycephaly with wide sutures and persistence of open fontanels into adult life (Fig. 1.23A). Wormian bones are seen. The calvarium, base of skull and especially the orbital rims are very dense. The facial bones are small and the maxilla hypoplastic (Fig. 1.23A). The mandible has no angle—it is obtuse (see Ch. 50).

Limbs   Normal modeling of long bones is usually seen. The cortices are dense but the medullary canals not completely obliterated.

Thorax   Hypoplasia of the lateral ends of the clavicles is present to a varying degree The ribs are dense overall.

Spine   Failure of fusion of the neural arches and spondylolisthesis

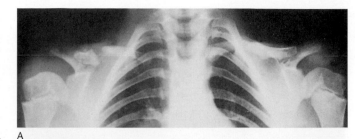
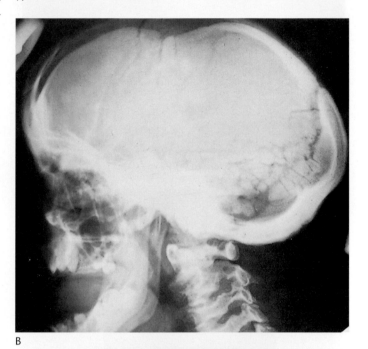
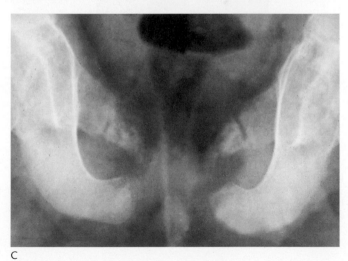

Fig. 1.22   Cleidocranial dysplasia. **A.** Clavicular defects are demonstrated, especially on the right side. **B.** Note delayed mineralization in the frontoparietal region and Wormian bones posteriorly. Facial bones are small but the mandible is normal. Delayed dentition is also seen. **C.** Failure of ossification of the symphysis pubis is demonstrated.

are found. In adults the vertebral bodies resemble spools, with large anterior and posterior defects. The bones are uniformly dense (Fig. 1.23B).

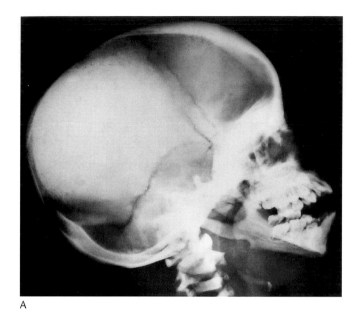

A

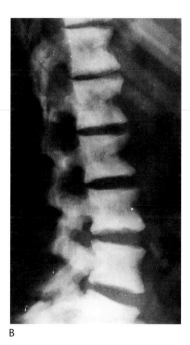

B

Fig. 1.23   Pyknodysostosis. **A.** The skull shows failure of sutural fusion and sclerosis of the base. The angle of the mandible is obtuse and the maxilla hypoplastic (see Ch. 50). **B.** The lumbar vertebral bodies show a spool shape with quite prominent anterior defects. Overall there is sclerosis.

Hands   Acro-osteolysis occurs, often with irregular distal fragments of the distal phalanges.

Acro-osteolysis (eponym: *Hajdu–Cheney syndrome*)

Acro-osteolysis means disintegration of bone of the tips of the fingers and toes. This specific syndrome is inherited as an autosomal dominant. Other features include spinal osteoporosis, Wormian bones in children and basilar invagination causing

Table 1.1   Atrophic Changes in Distal Phalanges

Atrophy of distal phalanges may be seen in disorders due to many causes:

Congenital	Many forms of phalangeal agenesis may be found as congenital familial disorders
Dysplastic	Cleidocranial dysplasia Pyknodysostosis Acro-osteolysis
Infective	In acute infection usually only one digit affected—diagnosis obvious Leprosy—neurotrophic factors contributory Sarcoid
Trauma	Frostbite. Electrical injuries
Poisons	Ergot—peripheral arterial spasm and gangrene Polyvinyl tank cleaners
Metabolic	Hyperparathyroidism
Vascular	Scleroderma with secondary Raynaud's phenomenon Occlusive vascular disease Pseudoxanthoma elasticum
Neurotrophic	Tabes syringomyelia Diabetes—vascular and infective changes may be contributory
Neoplastic	Kaposi sarcoma, where diffuse cutaneous and visual lesions are seen
Miscellaneous	Psoriasis, pityriasis rubra, epidermolysis bullosa, reticulohistiocytosis Ainhum Neurofibromatosis Progeria

posterior fossa symptoms. Other types of inherited phalangeal resorption exist.

There are many *other causes* of resorption of distal phalanges (Table 1.1). In some, resorption has a characteristic pattern and is accompanied by other features of the disease. Thus, in hyperparathyroidism, tuft resorption is accompanied by subperiosteal bone resorption around the cortices of middle phalanges.

Some patients have neurological lesions, e.g. in *syphilis*, *syringomyelia* and *diabetes*. In some conditions, such as *rheumatoid arthritis* and *psoriasis*, peripheral vascular deficiency has been shown to occur in the region of tuft resorption.

Osteogenesis Imperfecta (synonym: *fragilitas ossium;* eponyms: *Vrolik = congenital recessive form, Lobstein = dominant form*)

This is a relatively rare disorder manifested by increased fragility of bones and osteoporosis, as well as dental abnormalities (see Ch. 50), lax joints and thin skin. This disorder is due to an abnormality of Type I collagen, so that the sclera, cornea, joints and skin are also abnormal.

The original classification distinguished a severe recessive form and a milder and more common dominant type.

The current classification (Sillence et al 1979) divides the disease into four basic types with further subtypes.

Type 1   This is the most common type; over 70% of cases of osteogenesis imperfecta fit into this category. It has *autosomal dominant* inheritance. Sclerae are blue. Bone fragility is mild. Stature is only mildly reduced. Deafness occurs in adult life.

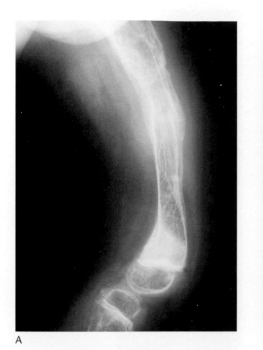
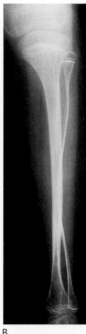

A   B

Fig. 1.24 Osteogenesis imperfecta **A**. There is osteopenia. A fracture has resulted in bowing and a periostitis. **B**. The long bones are gracile and bowed. Marked osteopenia is also present.

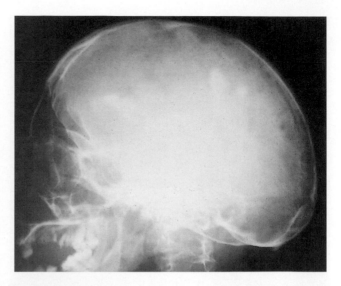

Fig. 1.25 Osteogenesis imperfecta. Persistence of Wormian bones and basilar invagination are shown.

This group is further divided into *Type 1A*—normal teeth, minor skeletal change—and *Type 1B*—dentinogenesis imperfecta (q.v.) and more severe skeletal change (Fig. 1.24A).

Osteoporosis occurs with cortical thinning with bowed, thin and gracile long bones (Fig. 1.24B). In 10% fractures are seen at birth and in 10% fractures never occur. Most fractures occur in young children. Wormian bones are seen in the skull (Fig. 1.25).

Type 2   Ten per cent of cases of osteogenesis imperfecta are due to this *spontaneous dominant* new mutation which is usually lethal in utero or early infancy. The sclerae are dark blue.

Overall the bones are grossly demineralized with thin cortices. Numerous healed or healing rib fractures are seen at birth despite the protection of amniotic fluid. Fractures also occur during delivery.

This group is further divided into:

Type 2A. The long bones are bowed, short and *broad*. Numerous fractures are seen. The ribs are *broad* with continuous beading (Fig. 1.26).

Type 2B. The long bones are as in Type 2A, but the ribs show less or no beading.

Type 2C. The long bones are *thinned*, show numerous fractures and the ribs too are *thin* and beaded.

Fairbank (1951) had already distinguished between a 'thick bone type' and a 'thin bone type'. Gross callus formation may be seen, but non-union may be present. Mineralization in the skull may be severely retarded. Only the petrous bones may be clearly seen. The skull is enlarged and numerous Wormian bones are seen.

Type 3   This occurs in 15% of patients, is a severe and progressively deforming type and is usually due to a new mutation. Sclerae may be blue at birth but are usually normal in adolescence.

Overall the bones are demineralized. Vertebral compression is seen and a kyphoscoliosis results. The long bones are osteoporotic and thin. Multiple fractures in childhood result in bowing (Fig. 1.27).

In the skull, ossification is again poor, sutures are wide and Wormian bones persist. This type has associated dentinogenesis imperfecta.

Type 4   Again, there are two subtypes—4A with no dental lesion, 4B with dentinogenesis imperfecta. This group constitutes 5%. Sclerae are usually normal. Fractures are seen at birth in 30% and bony fragility is mild.

Patients with a benign form of the disease may not present till adult life. Multiple fractures occur over a few years; eventually the diagnosis is made. Healing may be with excessive callus, so that a sarcoma is simulated. Sarcomatous degeneration is indeed described, but is rare. Occasionally, pseudarthroses are seen as in neurofibromatosis. Deafness is found in adults and may be due to ankylosis of ossicles and osteosclerosis.

The pelvis shows protrusio acetabuli, and further compression hinders childbirth. The ribs are so soft and thin that the downward pull of the intercostal muscles makes their posterior portion convex *downward*.

Differential Diagnosis

Battered Baby Syndrome   In osteogenesis imperfecta the fractures are often diaphyseal rather than metaphyseal, and the urinary hydroxyproline is often elevated. The differentiation is often of medico-legal significance.

Idiopathic juvenile osteoporosis starts just before puberty and is usually self-limiting. Vertebral compression (Fig. 1.28) and characteristically *metaphyseal* fractures, especially of the lower limb long bones, occur (Fig. 1.29). The calcium balance is

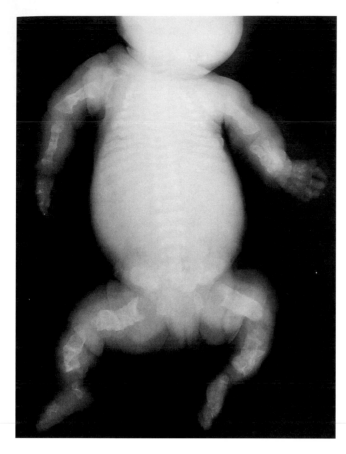

Fig. 1.26 Osteogenesis imperfecta. The child is stillborn. Multiple fractures are demonstrated in the short and broad long bones, which are cystic in appearance. Numerous rib fractures are seen.

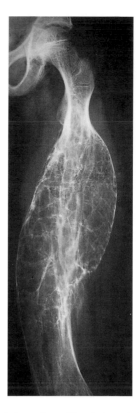

Fig. 1.27 Osteogenesis imperfecta. The skeleton is immature. The femur is expanded and bowed at the site of previous fractures. The midshaft has a cystic, or soap-bubble, appearance.

negative only in severe cases, otherwise the biochemical findings are normal.

Fibrogenesis Imperfecta Ossium

This is a rare condition which affects elderly patients and usually presents with pathological fractures. Radiologically, a gross coarsening of trabeculae is present so that the disease looks like Paget's disease (Fig. 1.30). All the bones are affected except the skull. Unlike Paget's disease, the bones retain their usual contour.

Osteopetrosis (synonym: *marble bones;* eponym: *Albers–Schönberg disease*)

As with osteogenesis imperfecta and many other dysplasias, there are many forms of this disease.

1. A severe, often fatal, early form, manifest in infancy or childhood and inherited in an autosomal recessive form. This has been diagnosed in utero (Figs 1.31, 1.32).

2. A more benign, tarda form, later in onset, inherited as a dominant. This autosomal dominant form can be further subdivided into:

- Type I. Marked thickening of the sclerotic skull *vault* but with an almost normal spine
- Type II. A sclerotic skull *base* and a 'rugger jersey' spine. Patients with Type II have a high risk of fracture; those with Type I do not.

3. An intermediate form with recessive inheritance.

4. A syndrome of *carbonic anhydrase 2 deficiency* associated with *renal tubular acidosis.*

Histologically, there is failure of resorption of the primary primitive fetal spongiosa by the vascular mesenchyme. This primitive bone has a higher calcium content on ashing, and appears denser on radiology. The bone is brittle and fractures easily, but heals normally.

Normal bone may be laid down in episodes so that zones of normal and of denser bone may be seen, but the marrow is encroached upon and extramedullary hemopoiesis occurs (Fig. 1.31).

In the severe forms of the disease, anemia and hepatosplenomegaly are found within months of birth and life expectancy is poor.

In the tarda form of the disease, the diagnosis is often made fortuitously when 2–3 fractures occur, perhaps in the space of a year, in an adult patient. The bones may be slightly dense. Modeling abnormalities are seen with metaphyseal undertubulation.

Dental disease is common (see Ch. 51) with osteomyelitis occurring in the rather compact bone.

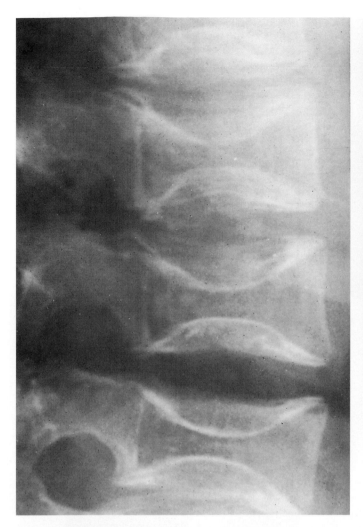

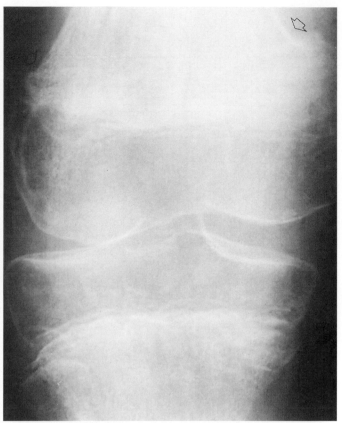

Fig. 1.29 Metaphyseal fractures around the knee in idiopathic juvenile osteoporosis distinguish this condition from osteogenesis imperfecta.

Fig. 1.28 Idiopathic juvenile osteoporosis. Gross vertebral compression affects mainly the central portions of the vertebral bodies.

Radiological Features Increased density and thickening of long bones, especially metaphyses, can be seen in utero. The presence of a 'bone within a bone' differentiates osteopetrosis from the other sclerosing dysplasias. This is due to the cyclic nature of the disease, so that the dense shadow of, say, the tibia at the time of formation of abnormal bone is seen within the outline of the current normal or abnormal shadow. The timing of intrauterine onset of disease can thus be assessed. This 'bone within a bone' may be vertical in the long bone shafts and digits, transverse at the metaphyses or arcuate beneath the iliac crests.

Long Bones Besides the '*Erlenmeyer flask*' deformity due to failure of metaphyseal remodeling, giving gross distal under-tubulation, and the presence of dense bone, vertical fine lucencies extending to the metaphyses are also present (Fig. 1.32), probably due to vascular channels being better seen against dense bone.

Fractures are usually transverse (Fig. 1.33) and heal with normal callus. Residual varus results from proximal femoral fractures. Some diaphyseal remodeling is to be expected. Skeletal maturation is normal.

Skull (For dental abnormalities, see Ch. 51.) The bones of the skull base are initially affected with sclerosis and thickening,

prominent in the floor of the anterior cranial fossa. The cranium is affected to a lesser degree. The sphenoid and frontal sinuses and mastoids are underpneumatized or not at all. Neural foramina are encroached upon and blindness results in serious cases. Bone softening with hydrocephalus does not appear to be a problem.

Spine Platyspondyly does not seem to occur, but spondylolisthesis does. In vertebral bodies, an appearance like a 'rugger jersey' spine may be seen due to the inserted shadow of an earlier, more dense body (Fig. 1.34), especially in Type 2-II.

In the adult form of the disease, the bones are roughly normal in shape. The medulla in the proximal skeleton is primarily involved and the periphery spared. Mild, uniform increase in density may be seen.

There is an association with renal tubular acidosis and dense cerebral calcification in patients with carbonic anhydrase 2 deficiency.

Melorheostosis (eponym: *Léri's disease*)

This is a very rare lesion affecting both sexes; no familial trend has been reported. Though the condition has not been observed in a child under the age of 3 years, there is strong presumptive evidence that it is present at birth.

Patients may complain of pain and of restricted movements of joints but the condition is often asymptomatic. Some cases are associated with skin lesions, such as scleroderma, and with vascular anomalies; joint contractures may be found in some patients.

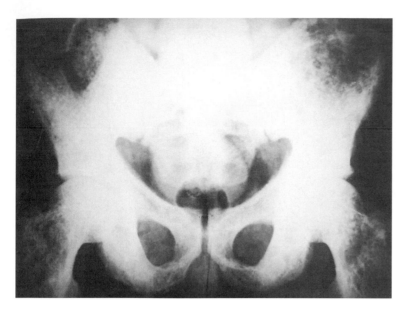

Fig. 1.30 Fibrogenesis imperfecta. Marked coarsening of trabeculation occurs throughout the skeleton but the bones retain their contour.

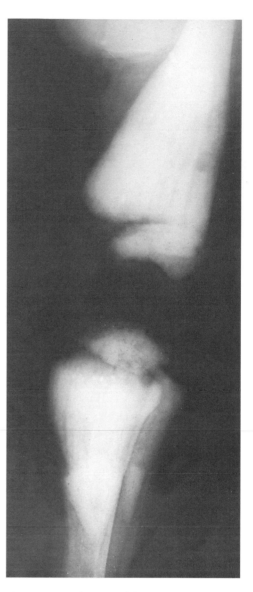

Fig. 1.32 Osteopetrosis—fine vertical lucencies are seen extending to the metaphyses, together with a 'bone within a bone' appearance at the tibial and fibular diaphyses.

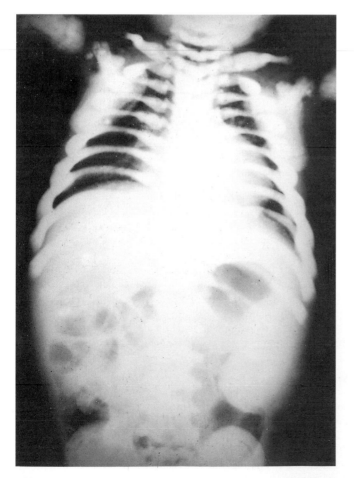

Fig. 1.31 Osteopetrosis. Bone density is uniformly increased apart from a small curved zone of normal bone at the iliac crest metaphysis. The spleen is the site of extramedullary hemopoiesis.

The condition is characterized by the presence of dense irregular bone running down the cortex of a long bone. Both the internal and external aspects of the cortex may be affected. Dense areas tend to be overgrown and bowing may result. Murray and McCredie (1979) have pointed out that the distribution of the new bone corresponds to a sclerotome, the segmental root nerve innervation of a bone.

The new bone has been likened to molten wax running down the side of a burning candle (Fig. 1.35). The lesions tend to be segmental and unilateral, though both limbs on one side may be affected. Occasionally the condition is bilateral but never symmetric. Some lesions are progressive. The lower limbs are most commonly affected. Premature epiphyseal fusion may result, so that an affected limb may be larger or smaller than normal.

The skull, spine and ribs are rarely affected. Ectopic bone may be found in soft tissues around joints between affected bones.

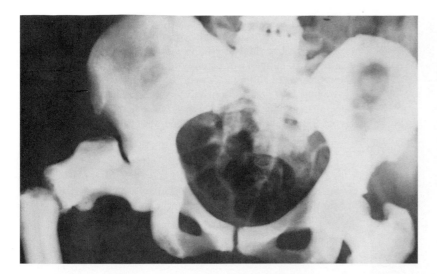

Fig. 1.33 Osteopetrosis—spontaneous fracture of upper end of right femur.

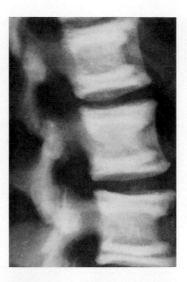

Fig. 1.34 Osteopetrosis—note inset of an earlier vertebra within each vertebral body.

Osteopoikylosis (synonym: *osteopathia condensans disseminata*)

This is usually an incidental radiological finding but some patients have associated skin nodules. The lesions are familial. It affects both sexes equally and is characterized by the presence of multiple, dense, radiopaque spots which are round, oval or lanceolate, and tend to be situated parallel to the axis of the affected bone. They are usually uniform in density but may have relatively clear central zones. Any bone may be affected. They occur especially frequently in the ends of long bones and around joints, in the carpus and tarsus, and in the pelvis (Fig. 1.36). This lesion must be differentiated from serious conditions such as tuberous sclerosis and metastases, but their distributions around joints, and the fact that the nodules rarely increase in size or number under observation, distinguish this benign condition from metastases.

Osteopathia Striata (eponym: *Voorhoeve's disease*)

In this asymptomatic disorder sclerotic striations are found in the long bones, especially of the lower limbs, affecting both bone ends and diaphyses (Fig. 1.37).

Fibrous Dysplasia

This is a disease of unknown etiology. It is probably more common in women. The disease is found in two forms, monostotic and polyostotic. With polyostotic disease, over 50% of the skeleton may be involved, but symmetry is unusual and the lesions tend to be unilaterally distributed. The lesions are usually found incidentally or following pathological fracture. Deformity may occasionally be marked. The alkaline phosphatase is elevated but does not correlate with the extent of the disease. The age of onset is usually between 10 and 30, but polyostotic disease may present in the first decade. The lesions often cease growing with skeletal maturity but may be seen in old age. Monostotic lesions are more likely to enlarge in adult life. Prognosis is worse when the lesions occur early in life.

Pathologically, medullary bone is replaced by well-defined areas of fibrous tissue, and cysts containing blood or serous fluid. These appear similar on radiographs (Fig. 1.38). The fibrous tissue then undergoes varying degrees of abnormal ossification so that some of the lesions show an increase in density, dependent on the extent of ossification. This increase in density may thus be patchy, giving a cottonwool appearance, or homogeneous giving a ground-glass appearance.

Radiologically, the lesions have a smooth dense margin of varying width, often so wide as to resemble the rind of an orange. The bone is expanded and the cortex scalloped and thinned but intact. Lesions tend to be multilocular and expand down the medulla rather than cause great cortical expansion (Fig. 1.39). Unlike Paget's disease, the bone ends are not necessarily affected and lesions tend to be diametaphyseal. Bone ends may be involved after fusion, and epiphyses may be involved in the child.

Any bone may be affected, though involvement of the spine is uncommon and vertebral collapse is unusual. Lesions do not really need to be diagnosed by biopsy as the appearances are usually characteristic.

The pelvis (Fig. 1.40), femur and ribs are commonly involved. In the skull, the frontal, sphenoid, parietal and maxillary bones and mandible are often affected (Fig. 1.41).

In the *femur*, deformity due to softening, expansion and fracture give an appearance likened to a 'shepherd's crook' (Fig. 1.42) and discrepancies in limb length result. Lesions are well-defined and may be expanded with well-defined margins. These may be lucent, dense or a mixture of the two, with small flecks of density due to ossification (Fig. 1.43).

In the *skull*, a grossly expanded sclerotic hyperostosis of the sphenoid may resemble a meningioma. Orbital fissures may be encroached upon and proptosis may result. Obliteration and bony expansion of the facial sinuses make the face appear grotesque and mask-like. In the vault, lesions tend to be grossly expansile, sclerotic, but localized (blister lesion).

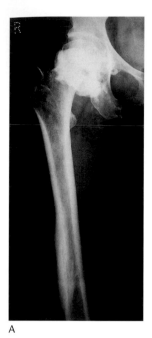
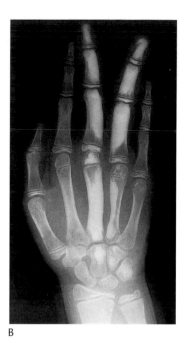

A   B

Fig. 1.35 Melorheostosis. **A**. Marked new bone formation is seen on the lateral aspect of the midshaft femoral cortex and around the femoral neck. The proximal lesion resembles an osteoma. **B**. In this patient, the abnormal bone shows an increase in size which expands the bone cortically and obliterates the medulla. The third and fourth fingers are separated because of the position of the overgrowth of new bone.

The lesions show increased uptake on *radionuclide scanning*. The degree of increase depends on the nature of the underlying lesion—whether fluid-filled cysts, non-mineralized matrix, or sclerotic, ground-glass or patchily mineralized. On *MRI* cysts will show features of fluid, i.e. gray on T_1-weighted images, bright on T_2-weighted or STIR sequences. The greater the degree of mineralization, the lower the signal, either homogeneous or spotty. Hypocellular fibrous tissue is generally of low signal on T_2-weighted images (Fig. 1.44).

Complications

a. Fractures, deformity and irregularity of limb length have been mentioned. Nerve palsies may occur in the skull.

b. Endocrine complications. *Albright syndrome* consists of skin pigmentation, usually on the side of the bone lesions, fibrous

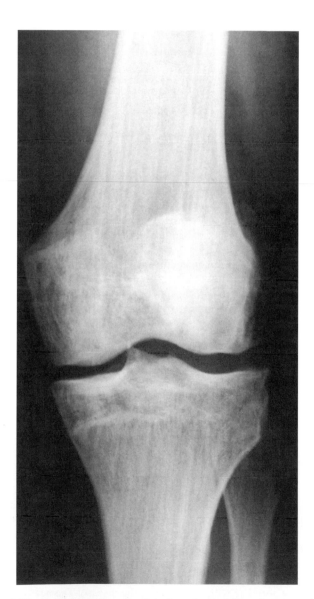

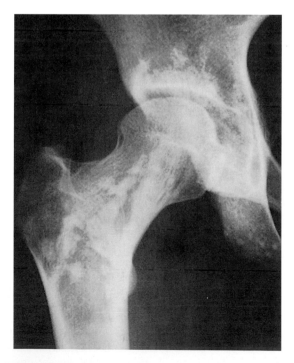

Fig. 1.36 Osteopoikylosis.

Fig. 1.37 Vertical striation extends to the articular surfaces in osteopathia striata.

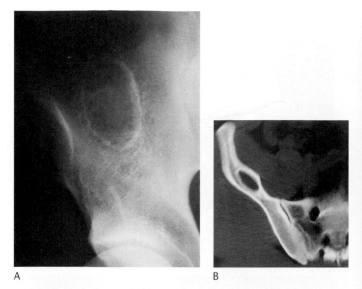

Fig. 1.38 A. Fibrous dysplasia. A well-defined relatively lytic lesion demonstrated in the iliac crest is shown at CT scanning **B.** to be cystic.

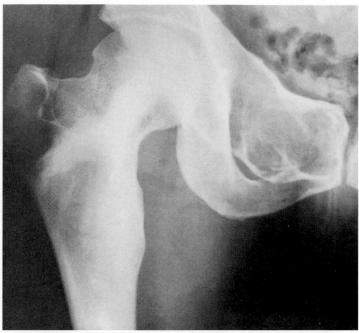

Fig. 1.40 Fibrous dysplasia—large expanding lesion in superior pubic ramus and sclerosis in upper end of the femur.

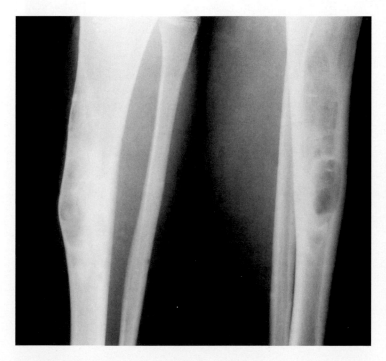

Fig. 1.39 Fibrous dysplasia. A multilocular, partly cystic, expansile lesion of the midshaft femur is surrounded by a thick rim of reactive sclerosis.

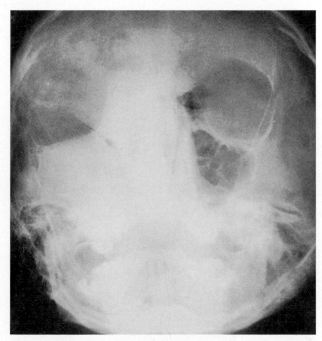

Fig. 1.41 Fibrous dysplasia—involvement of maxilla and facial bones on right side.

dysplasia (usually polyostotic) and precocious puberty. This occurs usually in girls, and only rarely in boys. Most patients with skin pigmentation and polyostotic disease do not have associated endocrine disease and, in girls, only 50% have precocious puberty. *Hyperthyroidism, acromegaly, Cushing syndrome, gynecomastia* and *parathyroid enlargement* have all been reported in association with polyostotic fibrous dysplasia.

c. Sarcomatous degeneration occurs in less than 1% of patients, usually to *fibrosarcoma* (Fig. 1.45). Some, but not all, of these patients give a history of previous irradiation.

Chondrodystrophia Calcificans Congenita
(synonyms: *chondrodysplasia punctata, dysplasia epiphysealis punctata, stippled epiphyses*)

This disease exists in at least three types, inherited differently.

1. *Rhizomelic* type (recessive)—usually lethal; the most common fatal type
2. *Non-rhizomelic* types (Conradi–Hünermann)
   a. Dominant—common, usually mild
   b. X-linked dominant—lethal in males.

These have similar radiographic changes. Ichthyosis may be seen in the rhizomelic and X-linked forms.

The less severe Conradi form of the condition is characterized in infancy by stippling or punctate calcification of the tarsus and carpus, long bone epiphyses, vertebral transverse processes and the pubic bones. The resulting epiphyses in later life are often misshapen, and deformities with asymmetric limb shortening result. The spine often ends up scoliotic but, if the infants survive, life expectancy is normal but with an appearance resembling multiple epiphyseal dysplasia (q.v.).

The more severe forms usually result in death in the first year; survivors are likely to be mentally defective. Stippling is present as above but is, if anything, more gross, also occurring in the

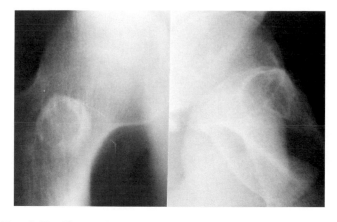

Fig. 1.43 Fibrous dysplasia. A relatively common and very typical appearance of a lesion at the femoral neck with a well-defined 'rind' of sclerotic bone.

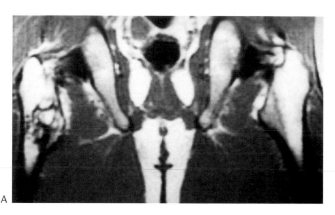

A

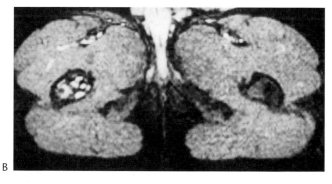

B

Fig. 1.44 Fibrous dysplasia, right femur: MR scans. **A**. There is a localized well-defined expansile lesion with an intact cortex showing areas of mixed signal on the T$_1$-weighted coronal image. **B**. The axial fat suppression study confirms the expansion of the bone and shows fluid within well-loculated cysts in the lesion.

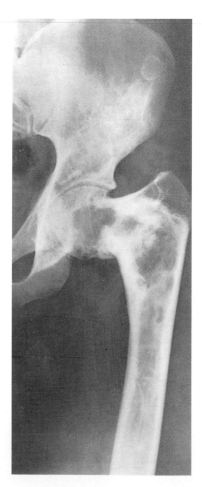

Fig. 1.42. Fibrous dysplasia—marked coxa vara secondary to cystic changes in the femoral neck. Sclerotic changes also in left ilium.

trachea. Long bones show gross symmetric shortening and metaphyseal irregularity. In this form the vertebral bodies show a vertical radiolucency on the lateral view which does not occur in the dominant type (Fig. 1.46). In survivors, there is marked retardation of epiphyseal development.

Multiple Epiphyseal Dysplasia (synonym: *dysplasia epiphysealis multiplex*)

This condition, which is transmitted as an autosomal dominant, primarily affects the epiphyses. Dwarfism of the short-limb type may be seen. The condition may express itself in various ways, so much so that some writers subdivide the disease into a severe form (*Fairbank*) characterized by small epiphyses, and a mild type (*Ribbing*) characterized by flat epiphyses.

In order of frequency, the epiphyses affected are those of the hips, shoulders, ankles, knees, wrists and elbows. Epiphyses tend to appear late and are fragmented and flattened (Figs 1.47–50); the deformities persist throughout life and cause premature osteoarthritis. The femoral capital epiphyses show symmetric flattening and fragmentation in the immature skeleton, the symmetry distinguishing this from bilateral Perthes' disease. Symmetric fragmentation is also seen in *myxedema* in association with skeletal retardation.

No characteristic changes are found in the metaphyses but they may be widened to conform to the deformed contiguous epiphyses. Secondary changes in contour are often seen in glenoid and acetabular fossae. The carpal and tarsal bones may be affected and digits and toes may be 'stubby'. The skull is not affected. Some features may be characteristic but none is constant.

a. *Lower tibial epiphysis*—the lateral part of the lower tibial epiphysis is thinner than the medial part; the trochlear part of the talus is shaped to conform to the abnormal mortice. A tibiotalar slant results (Fig. 1.48).

b. *The double-layered patella* (Fig. 1.49) is characteristic but is found in few cases.

c. *The femoral and tibial condyles* may be hypoplastic and the intercondylar notch shallow (Fig. 1.50). Flattening of the femoral and tibial condyles makes the joint look widened.

Spinal changes are seldom pronounced and may be absent. The appearances in the spine, if present, resemble *osteochondritis*.

Some cases of *chondrodystrophia calcificans congenita* may survive and their pattern may later resemble that of multiple epiphyseal dysplasia.

Dysplasia Epiphysealis Hemimelica (synonym: *tarsoepiphyseal aclasis*; eponym: *Trevor's disease*)

In this rare condition, irregular overgrowth of part of an epiphysis or epiphyses lying on one side of a single limb is seen (Fig. 1.51). The epiphysis is enlarged and an irregularly ossifying cartilage mass further arises on it. The leg is commonly affected but the arm may be. Sometimes both an arm and a leg may be involved and bilateral lesions have been recorded. If more than one epiphysis is affected, then the same parts, i.e. the medial or lateral, of the other epiphyses are abnormal.

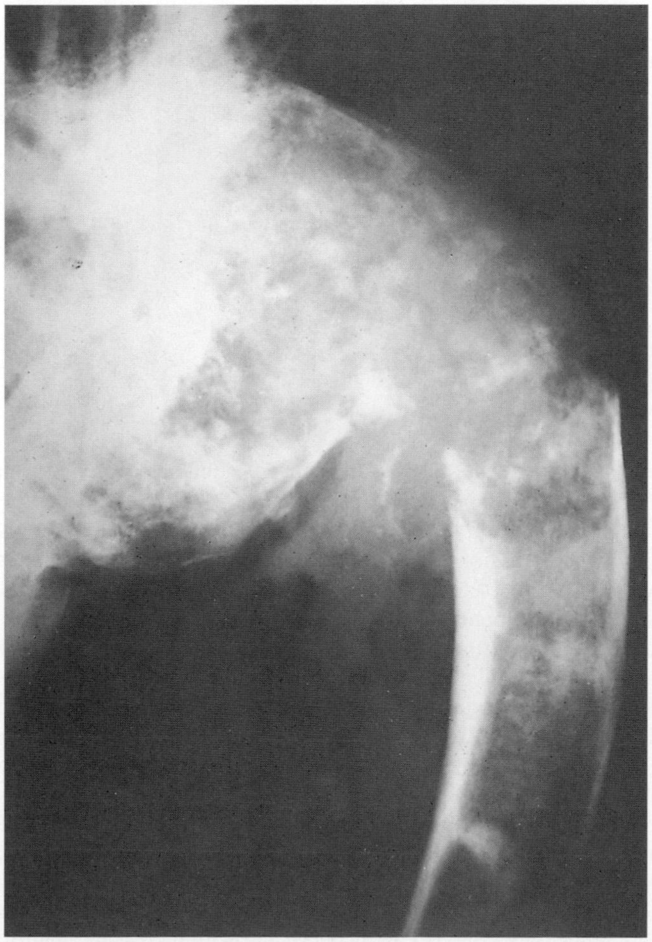

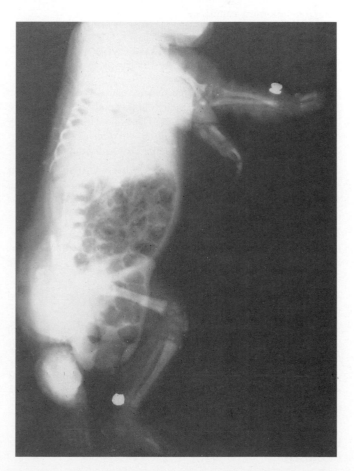

Fig. 1.45   A pathological fracture with irregular bone destruction due to malignant degeneration is superimposed upon fibrous dysplasia.

Fig. 1.46   Chondrodystrophia calcificans congenita. Clefts of the vertebral bodies are prominent in this case, together with stippled epiphyses and punctate calcifications around the joints and in the tracheal cartilages.

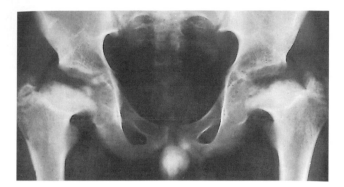

Fig. 1.47   Dysplasia epiphysealis multiplex. Both femoral heads are hypoplastic and fragmented. The femoral necks are irregular and broad. Similar changes are seen at the greater trochanteric apophyses. Dysplastic acetabula are demonstrated.

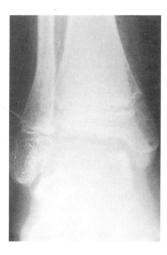

Fig. 1.48   Dysplasia epiphysealis multiplex, showing thinning of the outer part of the lower tibial epiphysis; this is seen in about half of all cases.

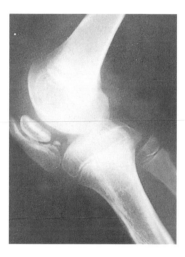

Fig. 1.49   Knee of same patient as Fig. 1-48. Marked fragmentation of the patella.

Hyperplasia of the affected epiphysis may lead to a lesion that is indistinguishable radiologically and histologically from an osteochondroma. The lesions may be easily palpable. Such a feature is relatively common in the lower end of the fibula and adjacent talus (Fig. 1.52). All the epiphyses around the ankle enlarge, even those not affected by a superimposed osteochondroma, and abnormalities of fusion of growth plates occur; a 'chevron' deformity can result.

Metaphyseal Chondrodysplasia (synonyms: *metaphyseal dysplasia, metaphyseal dysostosis*)

1. *Schmid* described a mild type that is relatively common (Fig. 1.53). Metaphyses of long bones are cupped and resemble rickets. No biochemical changes are found. The patient may be wrongly diagnosed as suffering from *vitamin D-resistant rickets* and consequently and injudiciously given large doses of vitamin D.

2. *Jansen's metaphyseal chondrodysplasia.* Grossly irregular mineralization is seen in the metaphyses of tubular bones (Fig. 1.54). A large gap is also seen between the epiphyses and disordered metaphyses.

3. Other types named after *Pena* and *Vaandrager* show intermediate involvement of metaphyses, less than in the Jansen type but more than in the Schmid type. Such lesions may resemble *Ollier's disease.*

4. Some cases of metaphyseal chondrodysplasia are associated with *pancreatic insufficiency* and *neutropenia.*

5. *McKusick* described a syndrome of sparse hair, metaphyseal lesions and dwarfism in Amish families—*cartilage–hair hypoplasia.*

6. Sometimes metaphyseal changes are associated with lesions of the spine—such conditions should be designated *spondylometaphyseal dysostosis.*

Diaphyseal Aclasis (synonym: *hereditary multiple exostoses*)

This disease is inherited and familial. Sixty per cent of those affected have an involved parent. The remainder are presumably mutants to the gene. The sex incidence is equal and lesions within the family are not necessarily of the same severity.

The bones chiefly affected are the long bones, especially in the *metaphyseal* regions of the shoulders, hips, knees and ankles, which become irregularly expanded and club-shaped. Upon these local enlargements of the shaft are projected osseous excrescences—*exostoses*—which are round or pointed. Their cortex merges with that of the shaft and their cancellous bone merges with the cancellous bone of the shaft, that is, they do not lie upon the cortex. Exostoses are also found on the vertebral bodies and on the medial border of the scapula. The epiphyses are not involved.

Exostoses may be seen as small metaphyseal projections in infants and their growth may be observed. With growth, they come to point away from the adjacent joint (Fig. 1.55). During skeletal growth, the bony exostoses are covered by a cartilage cap which undergoes spotty calcification, and with increasing maturity the cartilaginous mass becomes increasingly dense and a smooth margin can be discerned. By the time growth ceases, the cartilage

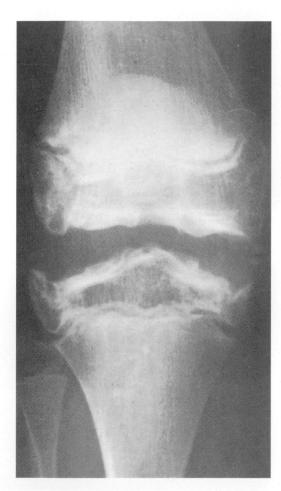

Fig. 1.50 Dysplasia epiphysealis multiplex—angular condyles and flat intercondylar notch. This is a characteristic appearance though not always present.

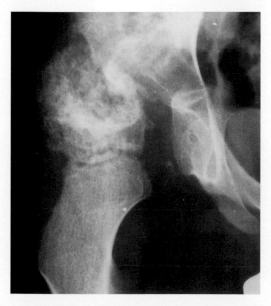

Fig. 1.51 Dysplasia epiphysealis hemimelica. Marked overgrowth of the femoral head. It is subluxed laterally. The superior portion resembles a partially calcified cartilaginous tumor.

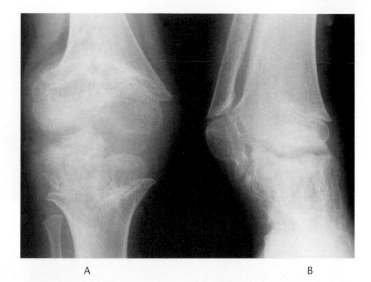

Fig. 1.52 A. At the knee there is overgrowth of the epiphyses with premature fusion centrally resulting in a chevron deformity. There is a large osteochondromatous growth on top of the proximal tibial epiphysis laterally and also affecting the lateral femoral condyle. **B.** Premature fusion is demonstrated at the distal tibial growth plate laterally and osteochondromatous overgrowth is demonstrated at the epiphysis and also at the adjacent talus. The distal fibular epiphysis is abnormal in shape and quite markedly overgrown.

has usually completely ossified. The exostoses and the metaphyseal clubbing are separate lesions though the former may be superimposed on the latter.

Increase in transverse width is often accompanied by shortening so that deformities result. These changes are especially common at the radius and ulna, resulting in Madelung's deformity (Fig. 1.56). Metacarpal bowing, radio-ulnar synostosis and radial head dislocation may also be found. *Ollier's disease* gives a similar appearance.

Lesions may be apparent early in life, especially if it is known that one parent is affected, or a lesion may affect a subcutaneous bone such as the tibia. Nerve compression may occur and paraplegia may result if the vertebral column is affected (Fig. 1.57). Some lesions may present with a dull ache, but pain and rapid growth raise the possibility of malignant degeneration. The incidence of *chondrosarcoma* in diaphyseal aclasis is said to be about 10%, and these are often around the hip.

Achondroplasia

This is the most common type of disproportionate dwarfism. In sufferers, one part of a limb shows relatively greater shortening. If proximal, *rhizomelia* is present; if medial, *mesomelia*; if distal, *acromelia*. In recent years many conditions, such as *thanatophoric dwarfism*, have been split off from achondroplasia so that a truly homogeneous picture now emerges. Inheritance is autosomal dominant, but most cases (85%) seem to be due to mutation of the gene, probably in older fathers. The patients have normal intelligence though a lack of muscle tone at birth suggests retardation.

The children have characteristic features at birth. *Trident hands* with short, stubby fingers, a *depressed nasal bridge* with a

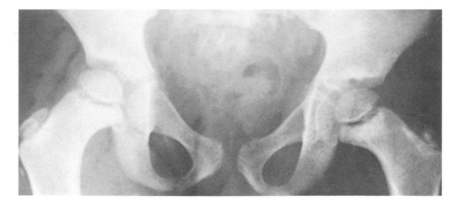

Fig. 1.53 Metaphyseal chondrodysplasia, type Schmid; mild changes only in upper femoral metaphyses. Other metaphyses were similarly affected.

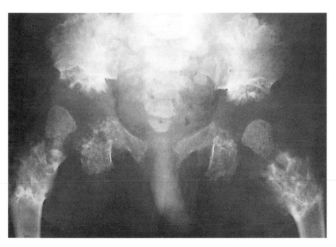

Fig. 1.54 Metaphyseal chondrodysplasia, type Jansen.

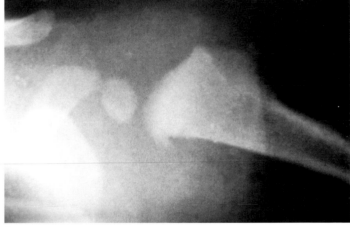

A

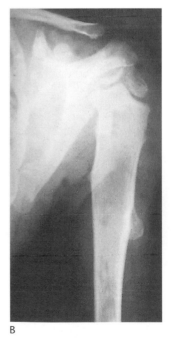

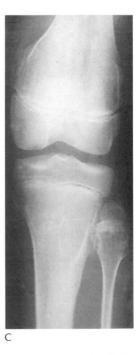

B   C

prominent forehead and a disproportionately *large skull*, and *prominent buttocks* due to lumbar lordosis are all seen. The large head can obstruct labor. Limb bones are short with a rhizomelic pattern.

Radiological Findings

Long Bones The tubular bones are short, appear relatively widened and have prominent muscle insertions. The humeri and femora are affected more than distal bones (rhizomelia). The fibulae are long and bowed. The epiphyses are deformed by their insertion into V-shaped defects at the metaphyses. The epiphyses themselves have V-shaped distal ends with deep intercondylar notches—the 'chevron' sign. The appearances are similar to those seen with local premature fusion after infection, trauma or irradiation. The joint spaces appear widened owing to the proximity of epiphyses and metaphyses.

Retardation of ossification and a reduced anteroposterior diameter cause the upper ends of the femora of babies to appear relatively radiolucent. A defect is present in older children at the site of the epiphysis of the tibial tubercle due to an excess of uncalcified cartilage at this age.

Pelvis The pelvis is small and its diameters reduced. The iliac blades are particularly small and rather square—the 'tombstone'

Fig. 1.55 Growing lesions in multiple exostoses (diaphyseal aclasis). **A**. Initial radiograph taken at 3 months of age shows small metaphyseal spurs. **B**. Left humerus at three and a half years. **C**. Left knee at 10 years of the same child.

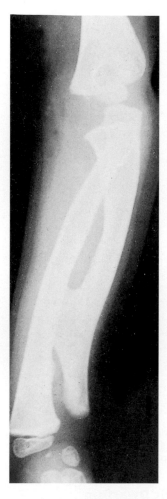

Fig. 1.56 Diaphyseal aclasis—typical deformity of bones of the forearm.

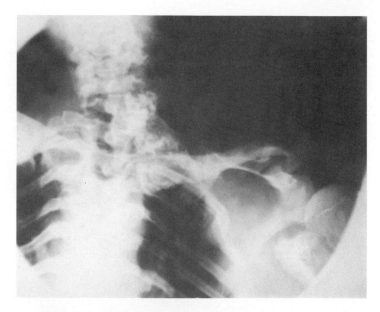

Fig. 1.57 Diaphyseal aclasis. Exostoses are seen associated with the spine in this patient who developed paraplegia.

Chest The ribs are short, the anterior ends widened and the sternum short and broad. The scapulae have peculiar shapes, losing their sharp angles; the glenoid fossae are small in relation to the humeral heads.

Hands and Feet Tubular bones of the hands and feet appear short and wide, but carpal and tarsal bones are little affected (Fig. 1.60). The *trident hand*, in which all the fingers are almost of equal length and diverge from one another in two pairs plus the thumb, is often found.

Hypochondroplasia

This is a condition which has been separated from classic achondroplasia, though there are some features in common. The skull is never affected, and the patients are either normal or mildly reduced in height. The disease is inherited as a dominant. The abdomen and buttocks are prominent, as in achondroplasia, and the legs are bowed in childhood.

Radiologically, there is rhizomelia with a short, broad femoral neck. The distal fibula is overgrown compared with the distal tibia (Fig. 1.61). The iliac bones are smaller than normal but not as markedly reduced as in achondroplasia. The interpedicular distances narrow from L1 to L5 and the pedicles are short, so that spinal stenosis results (Fig. 1.62). The lumbar lordosis is increased.

Pseudoachondroplasia

This condition is a short-limbed dwarfism occurring in both recessive and dominant forms of mild or marked severity, so that some patients are barely affected and some are grossly deformed. In all patients, however, the skull is normal, distinguishing this condition from achondroplasia. Also, no changes are seen in the first year of life.

appearance. The acetabula are set posteriorly and the acetabular roofs are horizontal (Fig. 1.58). L5 is deeply set and excessive pelvic tilt causes prominence of the buttocks and an illusion of lordosis. The sacrosciatic notch is narrow, with a prominent medially directed spur. The pelvic inlet resembles a champagne glass.

Spine The anteroposterior diameters of vertebral bodies are often short but the height of vertebral bodies is insignificantly reduced. In the thoracolumbar region a vertebral body or two may appear wedged or bullet-nosed. In some, a thoracolumbar vertebral body may resemble that found in Hurler syndrome. Scalloping at the back of vertebrae may be seen (Fig. 1.59).

The spinal canal in the lumbar region tapers caudally so that the interpedicular distances decrease from L1 to L5 (Figs 1.58, 1.59). The lateral view will also show the small spinal canal. Severe symptoms from disk protrusions are liable to develop in later life—the spinal stenosis in the lumbosacral region is an important predisposing factor and can be confirmed by radiculography, CT or MRI.

Skull changes are mandatory to the diagnosis of achondroplasia. The calvarium is large but the base is shortened. The sella may be small. The foramen magnum is characteristically small and funnel-shaped; hydrocephalus may occur and has been attributed to this mechanical cause.

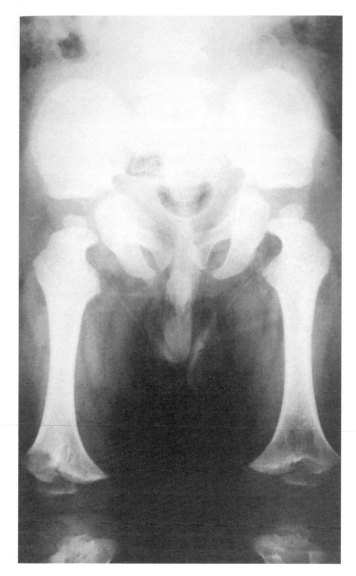

Fig. 1.58 Achondroplasia. Square iliac blades with horizontal acetabular roofs. Note also the narrow interpedicular distances in the lumbosacral region and the defects at the distal femoral metaphyses into which the epiphyses insert.

Spine   Vertebral bodies may be flat and irregular with central anterior 'tongues' (Fig. 1.63A). In adult life, appearances vary from near normal to platyspondyly and scoliosis. The spine in multiple epiphyseal dysplasia is barely affected.

Long Bones   The epiphyses are delayed in appearance and markedly irregular (Fig. 1.63B), again differing from achondroplasia. Metaphyses are broad and spurred. After fusion, epiphyseal dysplasia of varying degrees of severity is found.

Pelvis   The acetabulum is irregular and premature osteoarthritis of the hips occurs. The ilia are large and the pubes and ischia short.

Hands   In severe cases, the tubular bones are short and stubby with delay in ossification of irregular epiphyses and carpal bones (Fig. 1.63C). In the adult, the metacarpals end up shortened. Shortening of radius and ulna may be marked and both bones at the wrist may be hypoplastic centrally, giving a 'V' appearance.

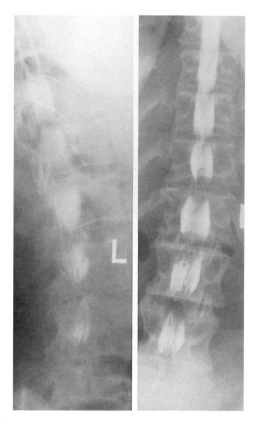

Fig. 1.59 Achondroplasia. Canal stenosis is demonstrated at radiculography. Posterior scalloping of vertebral bodies is shown between areas of diskal indentation upon the opacified theca.

Thanatophoric Dwarfism

This has relatively recently been separated from achondroplasia and is the commonest fatal neonatal dysplasia.

Radiological Findings

Limbs   There is rhizomelic dwarfism but the long bones are bowed. The metaphyses are irregular. Epiphyses of the knee are absent at birth. Short, wide metacarpals and phalanges are shown.

Axial Skeleton   There is marked platyspondyly but the posterior vertebral elements are normal so that, on an anterior view, the vertebral bodies resemble the letter H (Fig. 1.64). The pelvis shows poor mineralization of ischium and pubis, and small square iliac blades. The skull often shows lateral temporal bulging ('cloverleaf skull') due to craniostenosis.

The ribs are short and flared anteriorly.

The infants are stillborn or die shortly after birth.

Asphyxiating Thoracic Dystrophy (eponym: *Jeune disease*)

Most, but not all, patients with the disease die in infancy from respiratory distress. In contradistinction to thanatophoric dwarfism, the spine is normal and the long bones are not curved and only a little shortened.

The thorax is stenotic. The ribs are short and horizontal and the clavicles highly placed (Fig. 1.65).

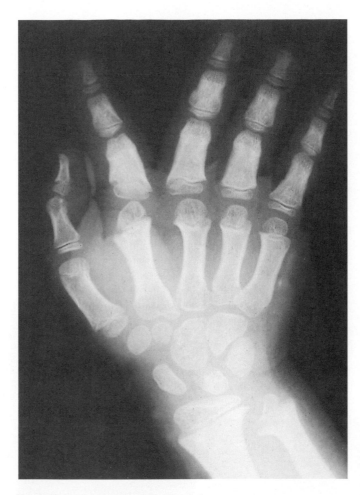

Fig. 1.60   Trident hand in achondroplasia.

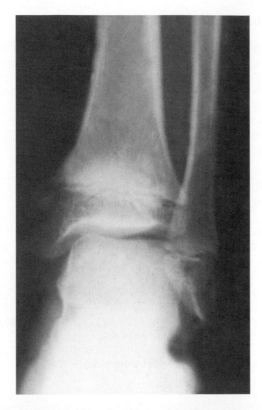

Fig. 1.61   Overgrowth of the distal fibula in hypochondroplasia.

Polydactyly is present in many cases and epiphyses are present at the knee.

Inheritance is autosomal recessive. In those patients who survive, renal failure may result, even if bone changes revert to normal.

Chondroectodermal Dysplasia (eponym: *Ellis–van Creveld syndrome*)

Fifty per cent of patients have congenital cardiac defects which may be fatal. The inheritance is autosomal recessive.

Radiographic Features

Limbs   In the limbs, the paired long bones are short and the metaphyses dome-shaped (Fig. 1.66); the dwarfism is mesomelic. At the proximal tibia the developing epiphysis is situated over the abnormal medial tibial plateau and is defective laterally, so that valgus deformity results. Postaxial polysyndactyly is also present (Fig. 1.67). Carpal development is delayed and carpal fusions are seen, especially between capitate and hamate.

Axial Skeleton   The skull and spine are normal. The rib cage resembles that seen in asphyxiating thoracic dystrophy. The acetabulum has a medial spur in the region of the triradiate cartilage.

The ectodermal dysplasia, with partial or total absence of teeth, and abnormal hair and nails, is not seen in asphyxiating thoracic dystrophy.

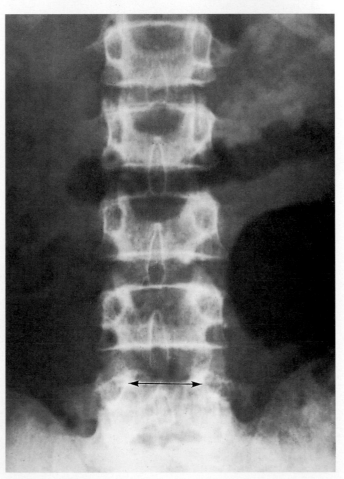

Fig. 1.62   Hypochondroplasia. A narrowed interpedicular distance at L5 in the same patient as Fig. 1.61.

Dyschondrosteosis (eponym: *Léri–Weill syndrome*)

This is inherited as an autosomal dominant. The patients are often female, short in stature with a mesomeric type of dwarfism. There is hypoplasia of the inner aspect of the distal radius; the ulna is therefore prominent and is subluxated dorsally (Madelung's deformity). The carpal bones herniate proximally into the deficiency caused by the hypoplastic radius (Fig. 1.68).

The medial aspect of the proximal/distal tibia is similarly defective, and the fibula may be hypoplastic.

THE MUCOPOLYSACCHARIDOSES AND MUCOLIPIDOSES

The above terms embrace an extremely complex group of disorders. All members of the group are associated with an abnormality in mucopolysaccharide or glycoprotein metabolism. The most that can be expected of the radiologist is to suggest a diagnosis of mucopolysaccharidosis (MPS), and niceties of nosology are the province of the clinician, geneticist and biochemist. The same considerations apply to the mucolipidoses.

Types of mucopolysaccharidoses are:

1. MPS I-H (Hurler syndrome; gargoylism)
2. MPS II (Hunter syndrome)
3. MPS III (Sanfilippo syndrome)
4. MPS IV (Morquio–Brailsford syndrome)
5. MPS I-S (Scheie syndrome)
6. MPS VI (Maroteaux–Lamy syndrome).

The *Hunter* type is inherited as an X-linked recessive, the rest as autosomal recessives. Some are severe, others relatively mild. Sufferers have various degrees of mental retardation, corneal clouding and skeletal changes.

MPS I-H (synonym: *gargoylism*; eponym: *Hurler syndrome*)

Radiological Features   Changes include macrocephaly, J-shaped sella, thickened calvaria, oar-shaped ribs and hook-shaped vertebral bodies (Fig. 1.69). The ilia are widely flared, the femoral ossific nuclei fragmented, and coxa valga is usual. The proximal ends of the metacarpals taper and in older children the distal ends of the radius and especially the ulna slope toward each other (Fig. 1.70).

MPS IV (eponym: *Morquio–Brailsford syndrome*)

This condition presents with dwarfism, due mainly to shortness of the spine and to a marked kyphosis. The tubular bones are also

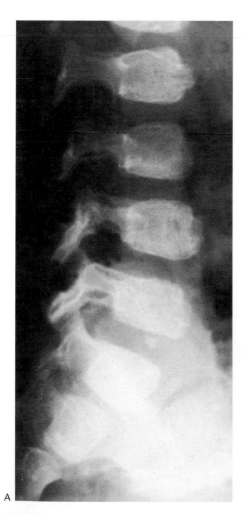

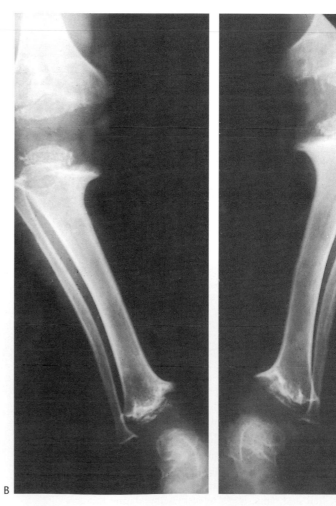

Fig. 1.63   Pseudoachondroplasia. **A**. Tongue-like projections of the vertebral bodies with superior and inferior defects. **B**. Long bones—irregular epiphyses and metaphyses with tilt deformities.

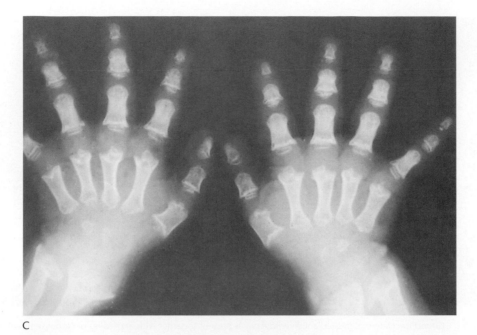

C

Fig. 1.63   C. Hands—the radius and ulna are flared at the metaphyses, the carpal bone epiphyses delayed and irregular, and the metacarpals short. The phalanges are stubby and the epiphyses angular and irregular.

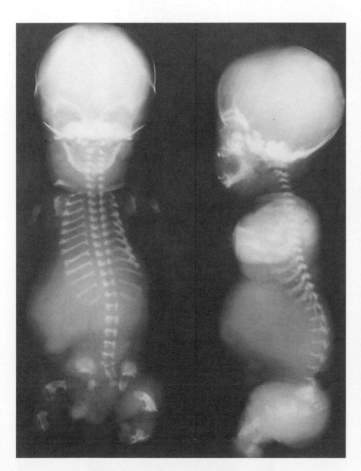

Fig. 1.64   Thanatophoric dwarfism. A cloverleaf skull is present. The scapulae are hypoplastic and the clavicles high. Platyspondyly is shown, resulting in H-shaped vertebral bodies. The bones are short and bowed.

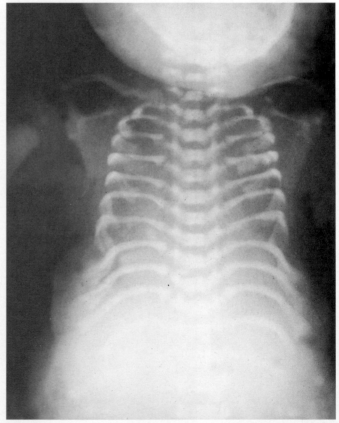

Fig. 1.65   Asphyxiating thoracic dystrophy—short horizontal ribs with high clavicles but a normal spine. The scapulae are hypoplastic.

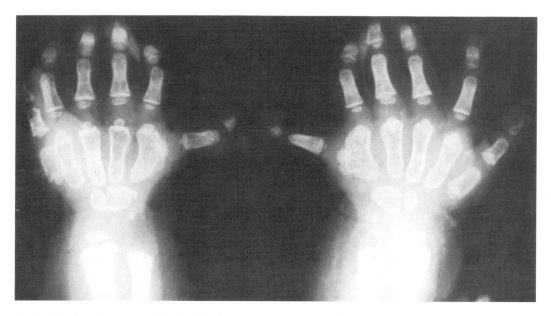

Fig. 1.67 Chondroectodermal dysplasia. Polysyndactyly is present together with anomalies of carpal segmentation.

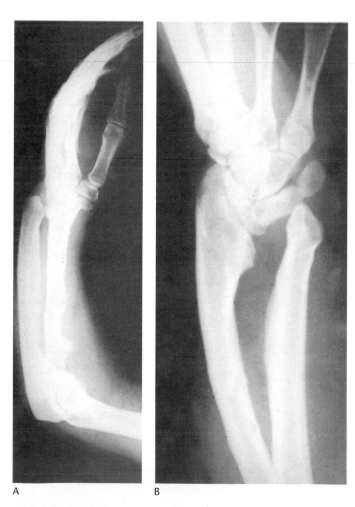

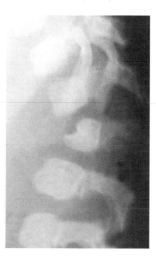

Fig. 1.69 MPS I-H (Hurler syndrome). Hypoplasia of L2 body with a pronounced inferior beak and a resulting angular kyphosis.

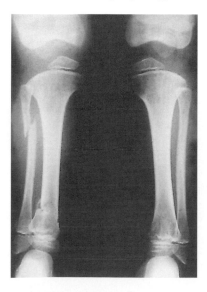

A   B

Fig. 1.68 Dyschondrosteosis. **A.** There is separation of the hypoplastic distal radius and ulna with proximal herniation of the carpus. **B.** The lateral view shows the posterior situation of the ulna and hypoplasia of the proximal radius.

Fig. 1.66 Chondroectodermal dysplasia. Hypoplasia of the lateral portion of the upper tibial epiphysis is present and the metaphysis is dome-shaped. Incidental fractures are demonstrated.

widely affected. The lesion may be familial. Intelligence is unimpaired.

Radiographic Features   Spinal changes are the dominant feature. The vertebrae are flat, and in childhood tend to have a characteristic form. The upper and lower surfaces of the vertebral body are defective and a central tongue of bone protrudes forward (Fig. 1.71). This appearance is best seen in the lower thoracic and upper lumbar region. Later, as growth proceeds, the defect becomes repaired. One thoracolumbar vertebra may be smaller than its fellows and displaced posteriorly, causing a marked kyphosis.

As a rule, tubular bones are not markedly affected but may be short and rather wide with somewhat irregular metaphyses. The epiphyses are markedly irregular and fragmented, notably those of the femoral heads. The joint spaces are increased and the joint surfaces, e.g. of the acetabulum and glenoid, are shallow and irregular.

The pelvis tends to be narrow, or shaped like that of an ape (Fig. 1.72). In the hands and feet the tubular bones are short and stubby, and some irregularity of the carpal and tarsal bones is also found.

Spondyloepiphyseal Dysplasia

The term 'spondyloepiphyseal dysplasia' (SED) is used to embrace a group of conditions characterized by platyspondyly and dysplasia of other bones. The degrees of spinal and tubular bone involvement and the amount of dwarfism vary between the different groups.

1. *X-linked variety—SED tarda*. This type has a distinctive spinal lesion. Mounds of dense bone are found on the superior and inferior surfaces of the posterior parts of the vertebral end-plates (Fig. 1.73). The tubular bones are not much affected and may resemble those in mild cases of dysplasia epiphysealis multiplex. The iliac wings are characteristically small. Hip degeneration frequently occurs prematurely (Fig. 1.74).

2. *Dominant variety—SED congenita*. In these patients the platyspondyly is maximal in the thoracic spine. Lesions of tubular bones are severe and early osteoarthritis may be expected. The hands are unaffected. Retinal detachment is common.

3. *Recessive variety*. The platyspondyly is generalized and the severe wedging of the dominant form is not found.

Hypophosphatasia

This is a genetically determined metabolic disease, included in this section on account of its manifestations. Several subgroups have been described, dependent on the age of onset and severity of symptoms. They are characterized by: 1. low or absent serum alkaline phosphatase; 2. phosphoethanolamine in the urine and plasma; 3. hypercalcemia in severe forms.

In the severe type, gross general failure of ossification of the skeleton is seen (Fig. 1.75). These babies do not survive. Some less severe forms present as severe rickets. If they survive, the radiographic picture may resemble that of Ollier's disease. An adult form of this condition is characterized by osteoporosis and a tendency to fractures.

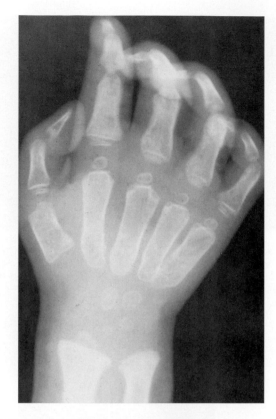

Fig. 1.70   MPS I-H (Hurler syndrome). Undertubulation is associated with demineralization. The metacarpals are pointed proximally. The distal radius and ulna are angulated.

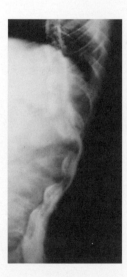

Fig. 1.71   MPS IV (Morquio–Brailsford syndrome). At radiculography, multiple stenotic levels are demonstrated in the lower thoracic and lumbar regions, with scalloping of the posterior aspects of the vertebral bodies. Hypoplasia of an upper lumbar vertebral body is demonstrated. The 'beak' is central; a kyphos results.

Arachnodactyly (eponym: *Marfan syndrome*)

This condition is inherited as an autosomal dominant. Clinically, the long bones are lengthened and muscle weakness, hypermobility and lens dislocations are found. A high arched palate,

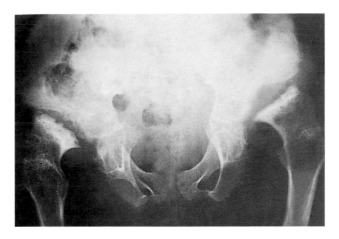

Fig. 1.72 MPS IV. Simian pelvis, fragmented, maldeveloped femoral capital epiphyses with associated metaphyseal irregularity. Shallow acetabula with dislocation of both femoral heads shown also—a feature sometimes seen in this condition.

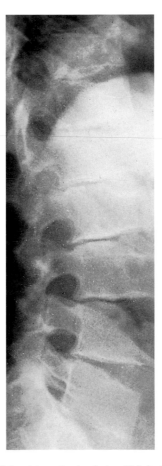

Fig. 1.73 Spondyloepiphyseal dysplasia (X-linked recessive form) showing characteristic platyspondyly. Mounds of bone are seen on the superior and inferior parts of the posterior parts of the vertebral bodies. Gas is seen in the prematurely degenerate disks.

depressed sternum and scoliosis also occur. Cardiovascular lesions include aortic dissections, atrial septal defects and mitral valve lesions.

Radiographic Features   The tubular bones are elongated and slender, the distal bones being much more affected than the proximal ones. The hands and feet are especially elongated (Fig. 1.76) and occasionally their bones have extra epiphyses. Kyphosis and scoliosis are frequent findings. Some scalloping of the back of vertebral bodies may be seen.

The diagnosis is usually straightforward. Estimation of the *metacarpal index* will aid the diagnosis in doubtful cases. This index is estimated by measuring the lengths of the second, third, fourth and fifth metacarpals and dividing their breadths taken at the exact midpoint. The resulting figures, from each of the four metacarpals, are added together and divided by four. In normal adult subjects the metacarpal index varies from 5.4 to 7.9; in arachnodactyly the range varies from 8.4 to 10.4.

Homocystinuria

This lesion has some similarity to Marfan's syndrome but is inherited as an autosomal recessive. A definite biochemical abnormality has been demonstrated. Absence of the enzyme cystathionine β-synthase results in an excess of urinary homocystine. The most important feature is that thrombosis of arteries and veins is liable to occur, especially after catheterization, and fatalities have been reported.

Osteoporosis in the spine, with posterior scalloping of the vertebral bodies (Fig. 1.77), differentiates this condition radiologically from Marfan's syndrome. Epiphyses and carpal bones tend to be enlarged and metaphyses broadened (Fig. 1.78), but arachnodactyly is less marked. Also these patients tend to have pes cavus and grosser sternal lesions than in Marfan's syndrome. Cardiac and aortic lesions are less common.

Achondrogenesis

This is an uncommon lethal form of infantile dysplasia characterized by a large deformed head with gross underdevelopment of the limbs and a large squat abdomen.

Radiologically, the long bones are extremely short, irregular and grossly undermineralized (Fig. 1.79). The pelvis is barely visualized at birth or in utero (Type I). In Type II, the limb bones are still short and metaphyses irregular, but slightly better mineralized. The vertebral bodies, however, may not be mineralized, especially caudally.

The diseases are both inherited as autosomal recessives.

Fibrodysplasia Ossificans Progressiva (synonym: *myositis ossificans progressiva;* eponym: *Munchmeyer's disease*)

The disease process primarily involves the connective tissues rather than muscle fibers. Soft-tissue swellings begin in utero or early in life. These painful swellings affect the neck and upper trunk. *Ossification* commences in the lumps within months and is aggravated by surgical biopsy. Large masses of bone form in voluntary muscles which may extend to the normal skeletal structures and resemble exostoses (Fig. 1.80). Movements become restricted.

A skeletal dysplasia is present at birth. Seventy-five per cent have involvement of the *great toe*, with fusion and microdactyly or hallux valgus (Fig. 1.81), and 50% have thumb hypoplasia and little finger clinodactyly. The femoral necks and mandibular

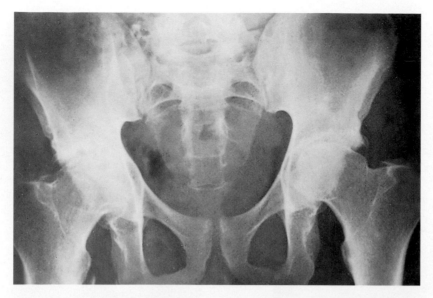

Fig. 1.74 Pelvis of patient in Fig. 1.73. Some (but not gross) osteoarthritis is seen, with some bilateral acetabular protrusion. The iliac wings are characteristically small in this condition.

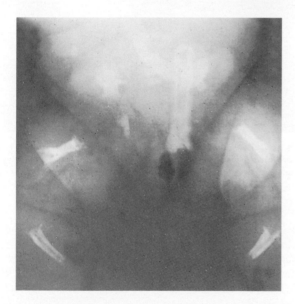

Fig. 1.75 Hypophosphatasia in newborn, gross failure of ossification of bones of the legs and of the pelvis.

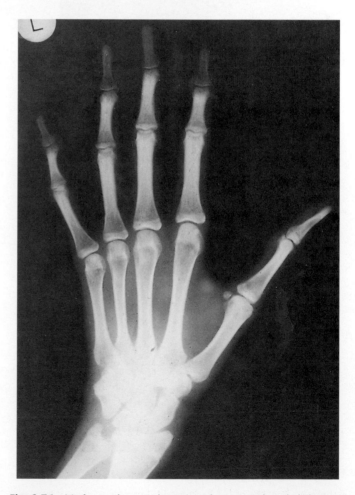

Fig. 1.76 Marfan syndrome—elongation of metacarpals and phalanges is demonstrated.

condyles are broad and the cervical vertebral bodies are hypoplastic and fused.

Inheritance is probably autosomal dominant but most cases are sporadic as few patients survive to reproductive age.

CHROMOSOMAL DISORDERS

Down's Syndrome (synonyms: *mongolism, trisomy 21*)

This condition is associated with an extra chromosome in the 21–22 group. The clinical diagnosis of older children suffering

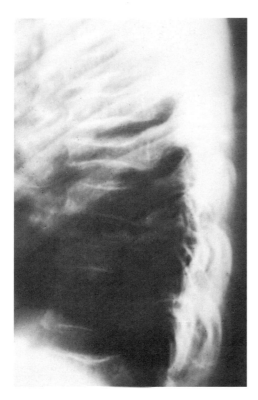

Fig. 1.77 Homocystinuria. Osteoporosis is associated with platyspondyly of the thoracic spine.

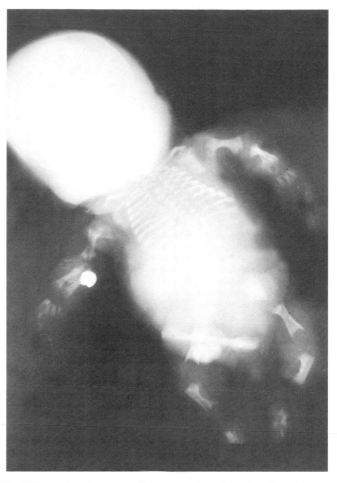

Fig. 1.79 Achondrogenesis. Gross shortening of the long bones is seen. The metaphyses are irregular and the epiphyses around the knee delayed in appearance. Poor mineralization of the caudal vertebral bodies, sacrum and pubic bones characterize Type II achondrogenesis.

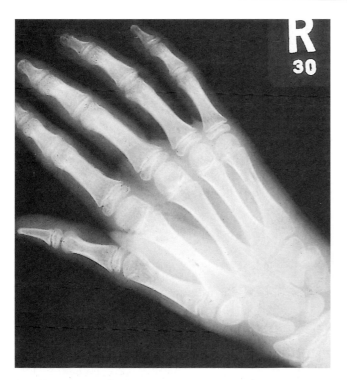

Fig. 1.78 Homocystinuria. Overgrowth of carpal epiphyses is present.

from mongolism is usually easy. In a baby the diagnosis may not be evident clinically but it is, of course, of great human importance. The newborn Down's syndrome baby has a large

ilium with a flat acetabular roof; an elongated tapering ischium develops after a few months.

Many other skeletal and visceral anomalies have been described in this disease, though none of them is invariably present. Some of the following anomalies have been recognized relatively recently:

1. Brachycephaly, hypoplasia of the nasal bones, maxillae and sphenoids, and absent frontal sinuses. Instability of the atlanto-axial joint and abnormalities in the upper cervical spine may be found in 20%.

2. The interorbital distance is decreased in most cases, indicating orbital hypotelorism.

3. Extra ossification centers for the manubrium sterni are found in 90% of cases between the ages of 1 and 4 years; this sign is seen in 20% of normal children of the same age group. The calcaneus may ossify in two centers.

4. Many Down's syndrome children have only eleven pairs of ribs.

5. The middle and distal phalanges of the fifth digits are often hypoplastic and curve inward—clinodactyly. The proximal phalanx of the thumb may be small and triangular or delta-shaped.

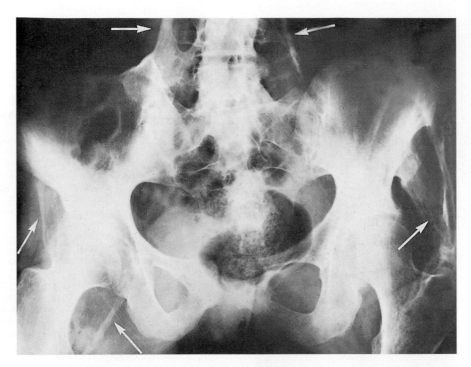

Fig. 1.80 Fibrodysplasia ossificans progressiva—soft-tissue ossification (arrows).

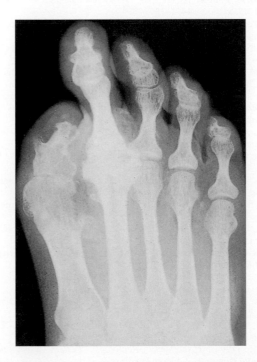

Fig. 1.81 Fibrodysplasia ossificans progressiva—developmental anomaly of the great toe. (Osteochondritis of the second metatarsal is also present.)

6. The lumbar vertebrae are often greater in height than in width, a reversal of the normal ratio, and they show concave anterior surfaces. Thus a lateral view of the lumbar spine may be of diagnostic help. This is not diagnostic of Down's syndrome but may be found in many children with delayed motor development.

7. Congenital heart disease is frequently found in Down's syndrome children, as is an aberrant right subclavian artery.

8. An increased incidence of duodenal stenosis and atresia and of Hirschsprung's disease may be found.

Turner's Syndrome

Not all patients with Turner's syndrome have an abnormal sex chromosome pattern, nor do all individuals with the characteristic chromosomal pattern have Turner's syndrome. The essential components of this condition are: *agenesis of the gonads*, *webbing of the neck* and *cubitus valgus*. The syndrome is confined to females. Mental deficiency, congenital cardiac and aortic lesions and anomalies of the kidneys such as malrotation are often associated. Sometimes males are found with a similar body configuration, *viz.* short stature and a webbed neck. However, these boys have a normal chromosomal pattern and they tend to get auricular septal defects and pulmonary stenosis rather than coarctation of the aorta which may be associated with Turner's syndrome.

Radiological Findings The skeletal features are inconstant and non-specific. Density of the skeleton, especially of the hands and feet, is reduced. General osteoporosis is frequent in older patients. The metacarpals may be short (Fig. 1.82) and accelerated fusion of the epiphysis may be found. The so-called 'metacarpal sign' is an expression of gross shortening of the fourth metacarpal. Minor shortening may be seen in some normal subjects.

The increase in the carrying angle of the elbow is better assessed clinically than radiologically. The medial tibial condyle is depressed and beak-like, and the medial femoral condyle may project downward (as in *Blount's disease*) (Fig. 1.83).

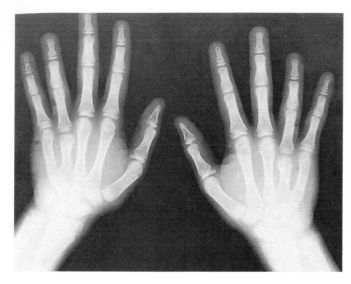

Fig. 1.82   Turner's syndrome—typical shortening of fourth metacarpals.

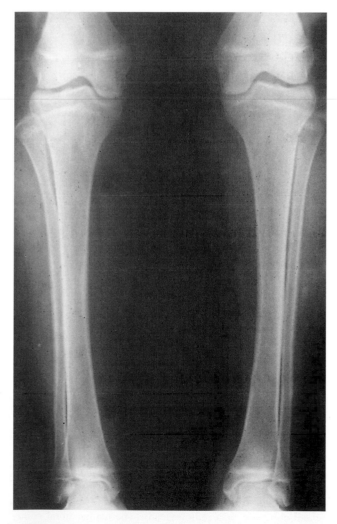

Fig. 1.83   Turner's syndrome. The medial tibial plateau is depressed and the adjacent femoral condyle enlarged.

Maldevelopment of the clavicles and slender ribs are often seen. Kyphosis and scoliosis are frequently found. Hypoplasia of the atlas and odontoid peg may be seen. In many females the pelvic inlet is android, the pubic arch narrowed and the sacrosciatic notches small.

REFERENCES AND SUGGESTIONS FOR FURTHER READING

Anderson, P. E. Jr., Bollerslev, J. (1987) Heterogeneity of autosomal dominant osteopetrosis. *Radiology*, **164**, 223–225.

Baker, S. L., Dent, C. E., Friedman, M., Watson, L. (1966) Fibrogenesis imperfecta ossium. *Journal of Bone and Joint Surgery*, **48B**, 804–825.

Beighton, P., Cremin, B. J. (1980) *Sclerosing Bone Dysplasias*. Berlin: Springer.

Bizarro, A. H. (1921) On the sesamoid and supernumerary bones of the limbs. *Journal of Anatomy (Cambridge)*, **55**, 256–268.

Blockley, N. J. (1969) Observations on infantile coxa vara. *Journal of Bone and Joint Surgery*, **51B**, 106–111.

Carty, H., Shaw, D., Brunelle, F., Kendall, B. (eds) (1994) *Imaging Children*. Edinburgh: Churchill Livingstone.

Clarke, N. M. P., Harcke, H. T., McHugh, P., Lee, M. S., Boruns, P., MacEwen, G. (1985) Real time ultrasound in the diagnosis of congenital dislocation of the hip. *Journal of Bone and Joint Surgery*, **67-B**, 406–412.

Cobb, J. R. (1948) *Outline for the Study of Scoliosis*. American Academy of Orthopedic Surgeons, Instructional Course Lectures, **5**, 261.

El-Tawil, T., Stoker, D. J. (1993) Benign osteopetrosis: a review of 42 cases showing two different patterns. *Skeletal Radiology*, **22**, 587–593.

Fairbank, T. (1951) *An Atlas of General Affections of the Skeleton*. Edinburgh: Livingstone.

Gibson, M. J., Middlemiss, H. (1971) Fibrous dysplasia of bone. *British Journal of Radiology*, **44**, 1–13.

Hernandez, R. J., Poznanski, A. K. (1985) CT evaluation of pediatric hip disorders. *Orthopedic Clinics of North America*, **16**, 513–541.

Heselson, N. G., Cremin, B. J., Beighton, P. (1978) Lethal chondrodysplasia punctata. *Clinical Radiology*, **29**, 679–684.

Houang, M. T., Brenton, D. P., Renton, P., Shaw, D. (1978) Idiopathic juvenile osteoporosis. *Skeletal Radiology*, **3**, 17–23.

James, J. I. P. (1959) Structural scoliosis. In: Nassim, R., Jackson Burrows, H. (eds) *Modern Trends in Diseases of the Vertebral Column*. London: Butterworth.

Jarvis, J. L., Keats, T. E. (1974) Cleidocranial dysostosis: a review of 40 new cases. *American Journal of Roentgenology*, **121**, 5–16.

Kaufmann, H. J. (1973) Progress in pediatric radiology. In: *Intrinsic Diseases of Bone*, Basel: Karger.

Langer, L. O. Jr., Baumann, P. A., Gorlin, R. J. (1967) Achondroplasia. *American Journal of Roentgenology*, **100**, 12–26.

Levinson, E. D., Ozonoff, M. B., Royen, P. M. (1977) Proximal femoral focal deficiency. *Radiology*, **125**, 197–203.

McCredie, J. (1975) Congenital fusion of bones—radiology, embryology and pathogenesis. *Clinical Radiology*, **26**, 47–75.

Murray, R. O., McCredie, J. (1979) Melorheostosis and the sclerotomes. *Skeletal Radiology*, **4**, 57–71.

Murray, R. O., Jacobson, H. G., Stoker, D. J. (1990) *The Radiology of Skeletal Disorders*, 3rd edn. Edinburgh: Churchill Livingstone.

Neuhauser, E. B. D., Wittenborg, M. H., Dehlinger, K. (1950) Diastematomyelia. *Radiology*, **54**, 659–664.

Poznanski, A. K. (1984) *The Hand in Radiologic Diagnosis*, 2nd edn. Philadelphia: Saunders.

Renton, P. (1990) *Orthopaedic Radiology: Pattern Recognition and Differential Diagnosis*. London: Dunitz.

Risser, J. C., Ferguson, A. B. (1936) Scoliosis: its prognosis. *Journal of Bone and Joint Surgery*, **18**, 667.

Sillence, D. O., Senn, A., Danks, D. M. (1979) Genetic heterogeneity in osteogenesis imperfecta. *Journal of Medical Genetics*, **16**, 101–116.

Solomon, L. (1963) Hereditary multiple exostoses. *Journal of Bone and Joint Surgery*, **45-B**, 292–304.

Spranger, J. (1976) The epiphyseal dysplasias. *Clinical Orthopaedics and Related Research*, **114**, 46–60.

Wynne-Davies, R., Hall, C. M., Apley, A. G. (1985) *Atlas of Skeletal Dysplasias*. Edinburgh: Churchill Livingstone.

2

PERIOSTEAL REACTION; BONE AND JOINT INFECTIONS; SARCOID

Peter Renton

PERIOSTEAL NEW BONE FORMATION (Periosteal Reaction)

New bone is laid down in many conditions with different etiologies (Table 2.1). In some the periosteum is physically elevated by tumor, hemorrhage or infection. Vascular abnormalities, viruses and auto-immune diseases may all cause new bone deposition. New bone may be deposited locally, around a solitary focus of disease, or may be generalized. In some systemic conditions, new bone is laid down in characteristic sites.

In its simplest form the new bone is seen as a linear density separated from the bony shaft by a clear zone, often later obliterated as the new bone merges with the cortex. Difficulty is caused by bones such as the fibula which have naturally irregular outlines. Insertions of interosseous membranes, ligaments and tendons in other bones also cause confusion.

There is a wide variety of types of periosteal reaction and often certain patterns can be discerned. However, the type of periosteal reaction cannot always be correlated with the underlying disease.

Tumors and Periosteal New Bone

Plain Film Appearances   A tumor, having broken through the cortex, elevates the periosteum and new bone forms beneath it. If the tumor grows slowly, the elevated periosteal new bone may remain intact and even take over the function of the destroyed cortex. If tumor growth is cyclic, as in Ewing sarcoma, successive layers of periosteal new bone are laid down, giving a lamellated or onion-skin appearance. If tumor growth is rapid, the periosteal new bone becomes disorganized and remains intact at the tumor margins only. Buttressing and elevation of periosteal new bone at tumor margins leads to a so-called Codman's triangle which is usually indicative of a malignant tumor, though in an aneurysmal bone cyst Codman's triangle really indicates rapidity of progression.

In Ewing sarcoma and in hypertrophic osteoarthropathy (see Ch. 4), the layers of new bone are characteristically fine, and thinner than the spaces between them. New bone in osteogenic sarcoma, parosteal osteosarcoma and secondary deposits tends to be coarser and less well-defined, so that the spicules are thicker than the intervening spaces. In osteogenic sarcoma, also, new bone may be perpendicular to the shaft and, originating from a finite focus of disease, resembles a sunray—so-called 'sunray spiculation'. This may also be found with angioma and thalassemia, but is then generally more orderly and better organized. Meningioma may resemble osteogenic sarcoma more closely, but the site is characteristic. Vertical spicules ('hair-on-end') are also found in Ewing sarcoma but, in keeping with the more diffuse nature of the underlying tumor, are not usually 'sunburst' but extend for a considerable distance along the bone and are more delicate. Vertical spiculation may result from bony deposition along the elevated and stretched fibers connecting periosteum to bone, the Sharpey's fibers.

Isotope Scans   Increase in uptake may be seen early, in the blood-pool phase, reflecting increased blood flow, and in the delayed scan, reflecting increase in bone turnover. Any displacement of cortex and periosteum and involvement of soft tissues further increases the size of the abnormal area of increase in uptake, which is seen superimposed on the pre-existing cortical image.

CT demonstrates cortical thickening. By altering the windows, changes within the periostitis may be better defined—lamellation, cloacae, stress fractures or tumor, e.g. osteoid osteoma.

MRI is generally not as good at showing cortical bone as is CT. Cortical signal is normally low because of the nature of compact bone. Periosteal new bone is seen as an accretion of low signal mass but edema, hemorrhage and tumor are especially bright on T_2-weighted and STIR sequences and better delineate the periosteal new bone and cortical changes.

Table 2.1   Causes of Periosteal New Bone Formation

Physiologic	In neonates, especially in prematurity
Congenital	Tuberous sclerosis
Dysplastic	Melorheostosis, Engelmann's disease
Traumatic	Local subperiosteal trauma; fracture, including march fracture Unrecognized skeletal trauma (Caffey's 'battered baby syndrome')
Infective	Acute: osteomyelitis—staphylococcal, streptococcal, pneumococcal, etc. Chronic: Brodie's abscess, tuberculosis, syphilis (congenital and acquired), yaws; also from nearby infection, e.g. varicose ulcer; ribs in pulmonary and pleural infections
Hypo- and hypervitaminosis	Rickets, scurvy, hypervitaminosis A
Endocrine	Thyroid acropachy, hyperparathyroidism in healing phase; secondary hyperparathyroidism in renal osteodystrophy
Vascular	Hemophilia and other bleeding disorders Myeloid metaplasia probably due to associated thrombocytopenia. Erythroblastic anemias. Leukemias. Varicose veins (before ulceration occurs) Hypertrophic pulmonary osteoarthropathy (probably of vascular etiology) and pachydermoperiostosis
Collagen diseases	Polyarteritis nodosa
Reticuloses	Hodgkin's disease, etc.
Neoplastic	Primary: *benign*—meningioma, angioma, osteoid osteoma; *malignant*—osteogenic sarcoma, fibrosarcoma, Ewing's sarcoma, etc. Secondary: any metastatic bony deposit may be associated with periosteal reaction
Primary joint lesions	Ankylosing spondylitis, juvenile chronic arthritis (Still's disease), Reiter syndrome, rheumatoid arthritis, osteoarthritis (femoral neck only)
Miscellaneous	Infantile cortical hyperostosis (Caffey), histiocytosis

Trauma and *inflammation* are the commonest causes of periosteal reaction both in adults and in children. *Primary malignant neoplasms* are rare but nearly always cause periosteal reaction. Periosteal reaction is occasionally seen in *metastases*. In adults, less common causes such as *reticuloses, hypertrophic pulmonary osteoarthropathy* and *varicose ulceration* may cause diagnostic difficulty. In neonates, *congenital syphilis* and *infantile cortical hyperostosis* must be remembered. Later, *scurvy, leukemia* and *erythroblastic anemias* (in immigrants) are possible causes. *Ewing's sarcoma* and *metastases from neuroblastoma* are other childhood causes which may prove diagnostically elusive.

Vascular Insufficiency and Periosteal New Bone

Venous stasis causes changes in the lower limb, especially at the diaphysis and distal metaphysis of the tibia and fibula. The periosteal new bone which is formed may be lamellar or irregular. Changes may be seen in the presence of chronic ulceration (Fig. 2.1), but also in its absence, so that an ulcer is not essential. Indeed, the periosteal new bone often extends far proximally from an ulcer. Phleboliths may be present and varicosities may also be seen in subcutaneous tissues, which appear thickened and edematous.

A florid and exuberant periosteal reaction occurs infrequently in *polyarteritis nodosa*. Arterial occlusion and skin ulceration are found and the periosteal reactions often occur around affected parts and in relation to skin lesions (Fig. 2.2).

Thyroid Acropachy

Literally, 'thickening of the extremities', this occurs in patients who have been treated for thyrotoxicosis and end up myxedematous.

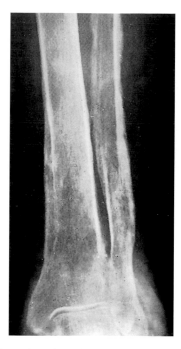

Fig. 2.1   Irregular periosteal new bone is demonstrated in a patient with varicose veins.

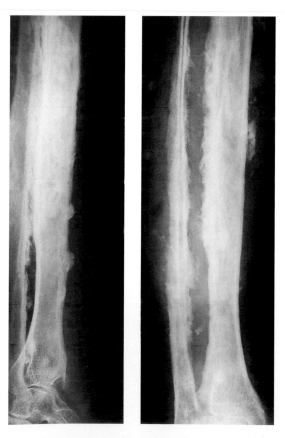

Fig. 2.2   Polyarteritis nodosa. An exuberant periostitis is seen along both tibia and fibula—much more florid than that seen in hypertrophic osteoarthropathy.

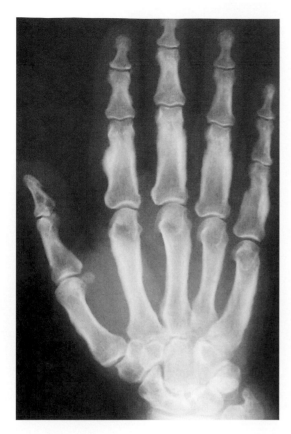

Fig. 2.3 Thyroid acropachy. Marked cortical thickening is demonstrated at the midshafts of the tubular bones of the hands (see Ch. 8).

The hands are more commonly affected than the feet. The distal ends of paired long bones are less often affected. The distribution is similar to that of hypertrophic osteoarthropathy but the new bone is more likely to be shaggy, spiculated and perpendicular to the shaft rather than lamellar. The overlying soft tissues are often grossly thickened (Fig. 2.3).

INFECTION

Osteomyelitis

An invading organism may attack bone by direct invasion from an infected wound, or from an infected joint, or it may gain access by hematogenous spread from distant foci, usually in the skin. Hematogenous osteomyelitis usually occurs during the period of growth, but all ages may be affected and cases are even found in old age. In infants, *Streptococcus* usually causes osteomyelitis. In adults, *Staphylococcus* is more common.

It is important to understand the blood supply to bone before describing blood-borne infection. The blood supply to a long bone is via:

1. *The nutrient artery.* This is the major source of blood supply throughout life. It supplies the marrow and most of the inner cortex.

2. *Periosteal vessels.* These supply the outer cortex.

3. *Metaphyseal and epiphyseal vessels.*

In the *infant*, vessels penetrate the epiphyseal plate in both directions. Metaphyseal infections can thus pass to the epiphysis and then the joint. Acute pyogenic arthritis is therefore a relatively common sequel of osteomyelitis in infants. The periosteum in infants is very loosely attached to underlying bone. Pus easily elevates periosteum and so can extend to the epiphyseal plate along the shaft. In situations where the metaphysis is intracapsular, such as the hip, metaphyseal infection also results in septic arthritis.

In *childhood*, between 2 and 16 years, few vessels cross the epiphyseal plate though the periosteum is still relatively loosely attached. The epiphysis and joint are thus less frequently infected. The metaphyseal vessels terminate instead in slow-flowing sinusoids which promote blood-borne infective change (Figs 2.4, 2.5).

In the *adult*, after the epiphyseal plate has fused, metaphyseal and epiphyseal vessels are again connected so that septic arthritis can recur. Periosteum, however, is well bound down and articular infections via a metaphyseal route are less likely.

The formation of pus in the bone deprives local cortex and medulla of its blood supply. Dead bone is resorbed by *granulation tissue*. Pieces of dead bone, especially if cortical or surrounded by

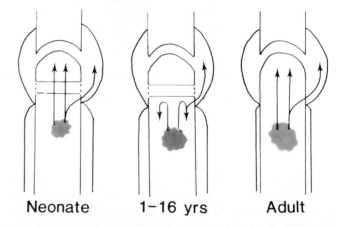

Fig. 2.4 Osteomyelitis. The three ages of infection and how change involves the joint.

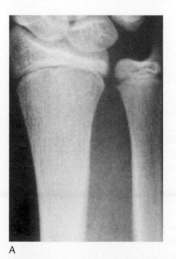 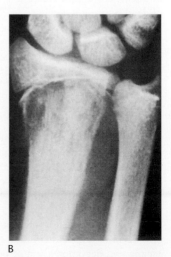

A   B

Fig. 2.5 **A.** Early metaphyseal infection. There is very minimal focal bone destruction at the distal radial metaphysis. **B.** With progressive bone destruction, metaphyseal abnormality is now very evident.

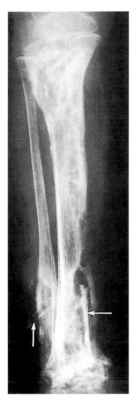

Fig. 2.6   Advanced osteomyelitis involving the whole of the right tibia and lower end of fibula. Note sequestrum in tibia (arrow) and further sequestrum being extruded from the fibula (arrow).

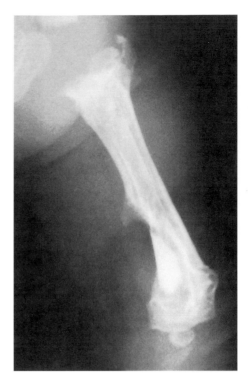

Fig. 2.7   Osteomyelitis of femur and septic arthritis of the hip in neonate. Note dislocation of hip, involucrum, cloaca and sequestrum.

pus, are not resorbed and remain as *sequestra* (Fig. 2.6). As sequestra are devitalized they remain denser than surrounding vital bone, which becomes demineralized due to hyperemia and immobilization. Absorption of sequestra is also facilitated by the presence of an *involucrum*. The involucrum forms beneath vital periosteum which has been elevated by pus. As periosteum is poorly attached in infants, involucrum formation is greater and so is the resorption of dead bone, and healing.

In areas of dead periosteum, defects in the involucrum occur. These *cloacae* allow pus and sequestra to escape, sometimes to the skin via a sinus. The track and its deep connection to bone can then be demonstrated by sinography using water-soluble contrast medium.

Radiological Findings   These depend to some extent on the age of the patient.

Soft-tissue changes may be immediately apparent, especially in infants. Swelling, with edema and blurring of fat planes is seen—in distinction to the soft-tissue masses around tumors, where the displaced fat planes are preserved. Osteoporosis may be visualized within 10–14 days of onset of symptoms. In children this is usually metaphyseal.

An involucrum is usually visualized after 3 weeks and is more prolific in infants and children than in adults (Fig. 2.7). The rapid escape and decompression of pus which results prevents vascular compression and infarction, and promotes healing. Computed and conventional tomography are invaluable in detecting sequestra. These are seen as fragments of dense bone within an area of local bone destruction. Treatment by antibiotics and/or surgical decompression affects the course of the disease so that often little apart from new bone may be found during the course of the disease.

With adequate treatment in infants and children, a return to more or less normal appearances with growth is to be expected unless the epiphyseal plate and epiphysis have been damaged, in which case growth abnormalities may result. In adults, the affected bone often remains sclerotic and irregular in outline (Fig. 2.8). Should chronic sepsis persist, tomography may reveal persistent cloacae and sequestra. The radiographic picture never returns completely to normal in cases discovered late (Table 2.2).

Table 2.2   Hematogenous Osteomyelitis of Tubular Bones

	Infant	*Child*	*Adult*
Localization	Metaphyseal with epiphyseal extension	Metaphyseal	Epiphyseal
Involucrum	Common	Common	Not common
Sequestration	Common	Common	Not common
Joint involvement	Common	Not common	Common
Soft-tissue abscess	Common	Common	Not common
Pathological fracture	Not common	Not common	Common*
Fistulae	Not common	Variable	Common

*In neglected cases
(Reproduced from *Diagnosis of Bone and Joint Disorders*, by courtesy of Drs D. Resnick and G. Niwayama, and W. B. Saunders, publishers.)

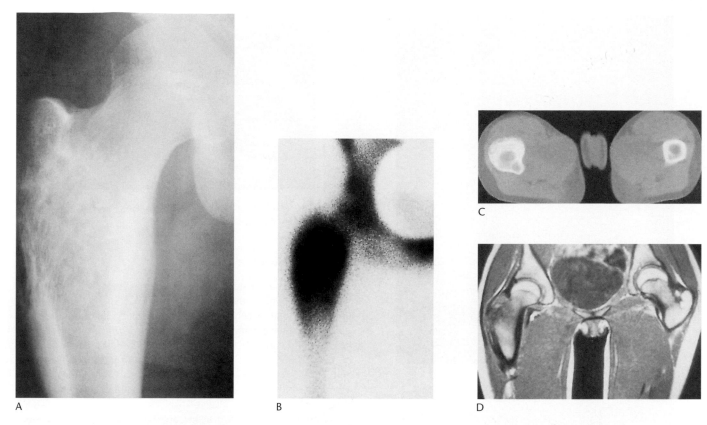

Fig. 2.8   Chronic osteomyelitis. **A.** The plain film shows mottled medullary destruction and a smooth periosteal reaction. **B.** The radionuclide bone scan shows gross increase in uptake locally. **C.** On CT scanning, gross periosteal reaction is demonstrated, causing considerable enlargement and sclerosis of bone. **D.** The MR scan shows the grossly altered signal in the affected femoral neck and greater trochanter, with replacement of the normal bright marrow signal on the T_1-weighted image. Cortical changes are demonstrated and a periostitis is seen.

Radionuclide Scanning in Bone Infection

Skeletal scintigraphy in suspected bone infection should rightly precede plain film examination. Plain radiographic changes cannot be seen for up to 10–14 days with simple infections, though in tuberculous disease changes are usually present at first presentation. Using scintigraphy, however, the diagnosis of osteomyelitis can be confirmed as early as 48 hours after the onset of the disease, even if clinical signs are equivocal. Early aggressive treatment may prevent gross bone destruction and, indeed, if given early enough on the basis of a positive scan, need never develop (Fig. 2.9).

Standard techniques involve the use of *technetium 99m-labeled phosphonate* and phosphate compounds. The accretion of radionuclide in bone is related to blood flow as well as to local bone turnover. This allows two separate sets of images to be obtained in osteomyelitis:

1. A 'blood-pool' image of the painful area immediately after injection. This shows increased local radioactivity, if positive, in areas of increased blood flow.

2. Delayed skeletal scintigraphic images at 3–4 hours. By this time the radionuclide has been absorbed onto bone crystal. This gives a skeletal image with local accentuation in areas of increased blood flow and bone turnover. This also differentiates osteomyelitis from cellulitis.

Using these techniques it can safely be said that not only is scanning more sensitive in detecting infective foci earlier, but it is nearly always accurate—positive or negative. It is however nonspecific, since tumors and infection may give similar appearances. Technetium uptake is limited if blood vessels are occluded in the infective process by tamponade or thrombus; thus, in neonates, up to 30% of scans may be negative because of this. Difficulty may also arise because the metaphysis is always the site of increased uptake in the growing skeleton. With metaphyseal infection, however, the depth of increase in uptake is greater.

Gallium 67-labeled citrate scans may be used when the technetium scan is negative in patients with clinical osteomyelitis, or even in conjunction with a technetium scan. Gallium concentrates avidly at the site of infection following local accumulation of leukocytes and proteins which are labeled in vivo. The radiation dose is higher however and the image poorer. Gallium scans are also probably more helpful in follow-up of active osteomyelitis, as such scans are negative earlier than technetium scans when disease becomes quiescent. Technetium scans remain positive for some time even in inactive disease, as the mode of uptake depends on a different physiologic process. Gallium scans cannot distinguish with accuracy between cellulitis and osteomyelitis.

Similar results may be obtained with in vitro *indium-labeled leukocytes* which are reinjected into the patient.

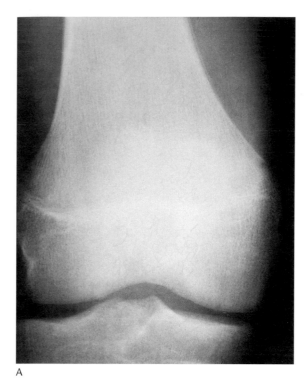

A

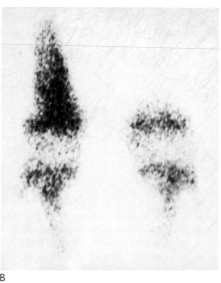

B

Fig. 2.9 Early osteomyelitis. **A.** There is a barely discernible radiolucency affecting the distal shaft of the femur, but an early periostitis is demonstrated medially and laterally. **B.** The radio-isotope bone scan shows the extent of the pathological change.

CT Scanning

Though of less value in the diagnosis of acute infection, CT demonstrates changes in subacute or chronic osteomyelitis well, especially those related to cortical bone or periosteum. Sequestra, as on conventional films, are shown as areas of dense or high attenuation spicules of bone lying in areas of osteolysis (Fig. 2.10). Cloacae, periostitis and local soft-tissue masses are shown. These may enhance with intravenous contrast medium.

CT-guided biopsy can be used to obtain material for culture.

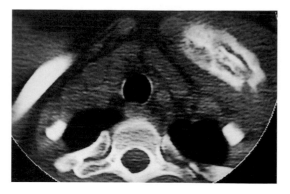

Fig. 2.10 Osteomyelitis of the clavicle with an involucrum and sequestrum, demonstrated at CT scanning.

Magnetic Resonance Imaging

MRI demonstrates osteomyelitis as early as isotope scanning and, where available, is the modality of choice in the diagnosis of musculoskeletal infection. Using appropriate weightings, or para-magnetic enhancement, changes of bone and soft-tissue edema may be identified early on, as may ischemia and destruction of cortex or marrow. Subsequent soft-tissue extension of pus through cloacae, and para-osseous abscesses may be seen. Central necrosis in abscesses may be shown. Images can be obtained in all planes (Fig. 2.8D).

Weightings in common usage are T_1, T_2 and fat suppression. Fatty marrow is bright in signal on T_1 studies, while the compact cortex, having less fluid, has a low signal. Edema and inflammatory changes increase signal dramatically on T_2-weighting and especially on STIR sequences (see Table 2.3).

Areas that become devitalized or necrotic will show loss of signal, and will not enhance after intravenous gadolinium.

Calcified tissues are generally better defined with CT but soft-tissue changes are better seen at MR scanning. While density changes in marrow infection can be assessed at CT, MR is much better at demonstrating the extent of pathology in bone and surrounding soft tissues and at least as sensitive as isotope scanning. The latter has the advantage of showing other possible foci of disease outside the area of interest.

Bone Biopsy in Infection

Bone biopsy by needle is performed in the diagnosis of both infections and tumors. In our radiological practise, the spine is the area most frequently biopsied; open biopsy for tissue and bacteriologic diagnosis is clearly a much more serious procedure and is generally not the first technique to be used.

Table 2.3   Signal Changes With Different Weightings

	T_1-weighting	T_2-weighting	STIR
Normal cortex	Low signal	Low signal	Low signal
Normal medulla	Very bright	Less bright	Low signal
Edematous cortex	Low signal	Bright	Very bright
Edematous medulla	Lowered signal enhancing with gadolinium	Bright	Very bright

As far as infection is concerned, the aims of biopsy are:

1. To confirm the presence of infection and exclude tumor or other causes of a radiological lesion
2. To distinguish the organism, both by direct microscopic examination of the aspirate and after culture
3. To allow correct antibiotic treatment after appropriate sensitivities have been established.

General anesthesia is unnecessary except in infancy or if non-cooperation is expected. Sedation and analgesia are adequate. Analgesia should be both intravenous and local, including infiltration of local anesthesia down to the periosteum.

Biopsy closed or open can be performed using for guidance fluoroscopy, ultrasound, CT or even MR scanners. Many types of biopsy needle are available. Some are of very large bore and consist of pointed trochars in a cannula which are used to enter bone, when the pointed trochar is replaced by a trephine with a cutting edge. Certainly, hard bone needs a rigid biopsy needle. Infected bone or disk, however, tends to be soft and, in practise, a fine aspiration needle is often all that is needed. Complications using a fine needle are usually minor. Pneumothorax and bleeding in the chest, or bleeding from abdominal organs, are not usually serious problems. The preference of the histologist governs the size of the sample the radiologist needs to obtain.

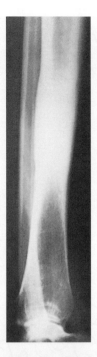

Fig. 2.11 Garré's type of osteomyelitis.

SPECIAL FORMS OF OSTEOMYELITIS

Sclerosing Osteomyelitis of Garré This condition is manifested by gross sclerosis in the absence of apparent bone destruction (Fig. 2.11). True examples of this condition are found occasionally, but some of the cases described in the past were probably examples of *osteoid osteoma*.

Brodie's Abscess This localized form of osteomyelitis is usually found in the cancellous tissue near the end of a long bone (Fig. 2.12). A well-circumscribed area of bone destruction has a surrounding zone of reactive sclerosis, sometimes accompanied by a periosteal reaction. It may have a finger-like extension into neighboring bone toward the epiphyseal plate, which, when present, is pathognomonic of infection ('tunneling') (Fig. 2.13). If a sequestrum is present an osteoid osteoma may be simulated.

Brodie's abscess typically enhances on the delayed isotope scan. An osteoid osteoma enhances centrally, both on the blood-pool and delayed scan due to its central vascularity. CT demonstrates central necrosis and sequestration of the Brodie's abscess, even in the presence of significant local surrounding sclerosis, much as would conventional linear tomography. At MR, it is to be expected that the central vascular material in the osteoid osteoma will exhibit brighter signal and enhancement, while necrotic tissue in the Brodie's abscess will not (Fig. 2.14).

OSTEOMYELITIS IN SPECIAL SITES

Skull Lesions occur secondary to scalp infection or frontal sinus suppuration (Fig. 2.15).

Mandible Infection may complicate a fracture into the mouth, or it may follow dental extraction. Infection via the pulp canal is probably most common and follows poor oral hygiene and dental decay.

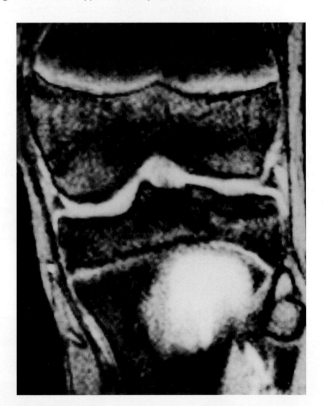

Fig. 2.12 Brodie's abscess demonstrated at MR. On this fat suppression image, the localized abscess is demonstrated as an area of extremely high signal.

Pelvis The sacroiliac joint is occasionally affected. It may be difficult radiologically to differentiate pyogenic from tuberculous lesions. Ankylosis of the sacroiliac joint may result from either cause.

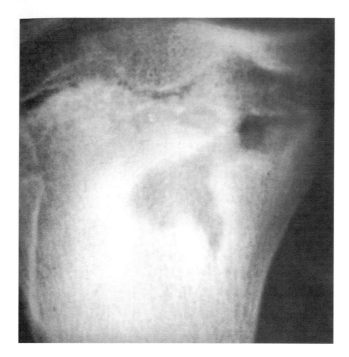

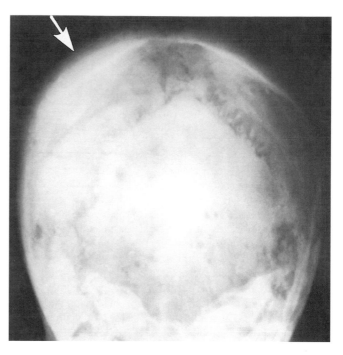

Fig. 2.13 A finger-like process of osteomyelitic bone destruction extends from the main focus. This is tunneling, which usually indicates the presence of chronic infection.

Fig. 2.15 Multiple areas of bone destruction and reactive sclerosis (arrow) are seen in a patient with chronic osteomyelitis.

Osteitis Pubis is a low-grade infection round the symphysis pubis which may complicate operations on the prostate and bladder or, occasionally, other pelvic operations.

Hands Bone infection may follow perforating injuries to the pulp space. The distal phalanx may be involved by osteomyelitis, or local pressure may cause ischemia and avascular necrosis.

A bizarre form of osteomyelitis, often due to oral organisms, follows bite wounds on hands or after punching the face and teeth, with resulting perforations and implantation (Fig. 2.16).

Feet Puncture wounds of the feet are common in children and in those societies where walking barefoot is common. Soft-tissue infections may lead to osteomyelitis, often with destruction of

joints. In the tropics, direct implantation by mycetoma results in 'Madura foot' (see below under Mycetoma). Implantation by thorns leads to a particular lesion.

Complications of Osteomyelitis

1. *Amyloid disease* infrequently complicates chronic osteomyelitis.
2. *Malignant changes* can follow longstanding suppurative osteomyelitis with draining sinuses. Increasing severity of symptoms with rapid osteolysis raises the possibility of a tumor, either an *epithelioma* of the sinus tract or, less frequently, an *osteosarcoma*.

Osteomyelitis of the Spine

Spinal osteomyelitis is not common, comprising less than 10% of bone infections (Epstein 1976), and can occur at any age. Patients often have a history of skin or pelvic infections. Spread of infection

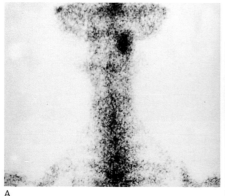

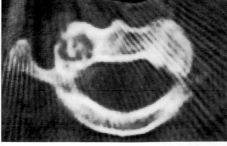

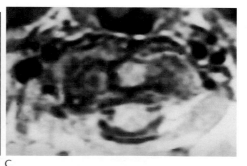

A   B   C

Fig. 2.14 Brodie's abscess. The plain film was not helpful. **A.** The radioisotope bone scan confirms the presence of a focal lesion in the upper cervical spine. **B.** The CT scan shows an appearance which could represent either an osteoid osteoma or a Brodie's abscess, that is, an area of osteolysis with central sclerosis and surrounding it a well-demarcated zone of reactive sclerosis. **C.** Changes at MR mirror those seen at CT in the lateral mass of C2.

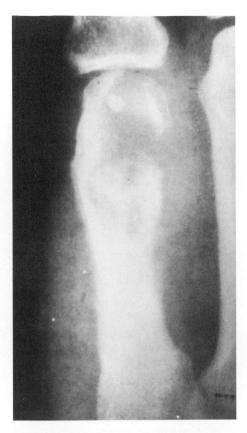

Fig. 2.16 Bone destruction, sequestrum formation and periostitis follow implantation of oral organisms after a bite.

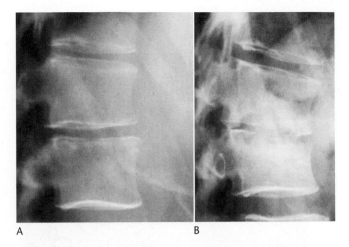

A   B

Fig. 2.17 Infective spondylitis. **A.** The initial film shows early bone destruction beneath the end-plates around a narrowed disk. **B.** The later film shows progressive destruction of disk and bone with surrounding reactive sclerosis.

is usually to the vertebral body rather than to appendages and is mainly blood-borne, though osteomyelitis may follow spinal surgery. Spread of disease from the pelvis is facilitated through Batson's vertebral venous plexus which is a valveless system of veins joining the pelvis with the rest of the axial skeleton via the spinal canal. Flow in this valveless system ebbs back and forth with changes in intra-abdominal pressure. Vertebral bodies are very vascular, especially below end-plates where large sinusoids with a sluggish blood flow potentiate infection. Spinal osteomyelitis is most common in the lumbar region and least common in the cervical and sacral spines.

Infective Diskitis   Perforating blood vessels still supply the disk in children and young adults so that in these age groups a primary infection of the disks can occur. Changes are most common in the lumbar spine.

Radiological Findings   Infection usually starts anteriorly beneath the end-plate. Plain film changes lag behind symptoms by 2–3 weeks, when a focus of osteolysis becomes visible and the cortex becomes blurred or vanishes. Infection may be beneath the anterior longitudinal ligament, facilitating vertical spread, or into the disk which is then rapidly destroyed and loses height (Figs 2.17, 2.18). The adjacent end-plate then also loses density and vertebral destruction begins in the body above or below. In most patients only two bodies are involved, and only rarely is the infection confined to one vertebral body.

Collapse of a vertebral body is accompanied by soft-tissue masses which are easily seen against air in the larynx, trachea or lung

(Fig. 2.19). Blurring or displacement of the psoas shadows also occurs. Kyphosis and cord compression may also follow.

Reparative processes can begin as early as 4–6 weeks after the onset of radiological change if treatment is effective. Sclerotic new bone is formed around the disk, in the bodies and at vertebral margins (Fig. 2.20). Dense spurs bridge disks peripherally. Ankylosis across disks may result in fusion of bodies. If this occurs after skeletal maturity, the sagittal diameters of vertebral bodies are not likely to be reduced. 'Ivory' vertebrae and soft-tissue calcification are occasionally found.

Isotope scanning here, as elsewhere, detects infection of bone and surrounding soft tissues before plain film changes are visible; further confirmation can be obtained with indium or gallium white-cell-labeled scans.

CT is of value in showing established disease and demonstrates trabecular destruction, soft-tissue masses and encroachment on the canal and cord. Intrathecal contrast may be used in conjunction with CT to show the relationship of a mass in the canal to the cord.

MRI is the most sensitive technique and is now the investigation of choice. Cortical destruction is seen on T_1-weighted studies; disk and marrow inflammation are well shown on T_2-weighted and STIR sequences (Fig. 2.18). Soft-tissue extension is particularly well demonstrated, as is abscess formation.

With treatment, the increase in signal on T_2-weighted studies seen early on declines so that, when the disease is inactive, the diskal remnant is seen as a narrowed dehydrated structure of low intensity. Persistence of increase in signal implies continuing inflammation.

OSTEOMYELITIS IN DIABETES

Infection occurs in both soft tissue and bone. Soft-tissue infection may follow a puncture through anesthetic skin and presents with swelling and loss of fat planes due to edema. In the presence of gas-producing organisms, spherical lucencies are seen extending proximally. Anesthetic ulcers show as soft-tissue defects, usually

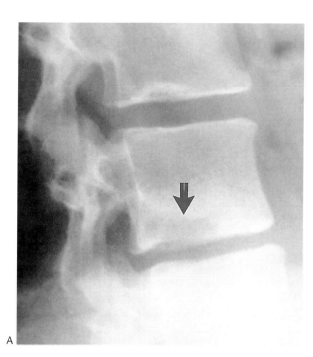

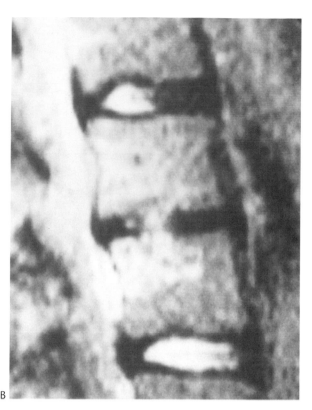

Fig. 2.18 Infective spondylitis. **A.** Another case showing destruction of disk and adjacent bone on the plain film. **B.** The MR scan shows disk narrowing, loss of the normal bright nuclear signal and its replacement by a rather diffuse abnormality involving the adjacent vertebral bodies due to infection.

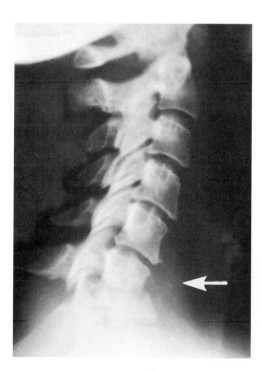

Fig. 2.19 End-plate destruction with diskal loss and a kyphosis is associated with facet subluxation and a large anterior soft-tissue mass (arrow).

over pressure points such as the metatarsal heads, and over the tips and proximal interphalangeal joints of the commonly associated claw toes. Initially painless, the ulcers involve underlying bones with the development of osteomyelitis. Sepsis may be superimposed on a neuropathic lesion, so that osteoporosis and destruction are accelerated (Fig. 2.21). If skin ulceration is absent, osteomyelitis is unlikely to be seen.

Chronic Granulomatous Disease of Childhood

This is a group of disorders in which the leukocytes are unable to respond normally to infections, especially to those organisms which cause chronic low-grade infections. Leukocytes are able to engulf bacilli but cannot destroy them so that toxins are still produced. A chronic inflammatory process results. Bones are commonly affected. Widespread small foci of osteolysis may be found, often abutting on to epiphyseal plates (Fig. 2.22). The lesions heal with florid formation of new bone, both endosteally and superficially, so that sclerosis and expansion result, often resembling malignant tumors (Fig. 2.23). The lesions are usually multifocal and isotope scans of the whole body are needed to show all the infective foci.

MRI demonstrates the inflammatory changes well on T_2-weighted and STIR sequences. Edema is shown to be extensive in the surrounding bone, including the epiphysis, and adjacent soft tissues. The destructive metaphyseal lesion is well demonstrated.

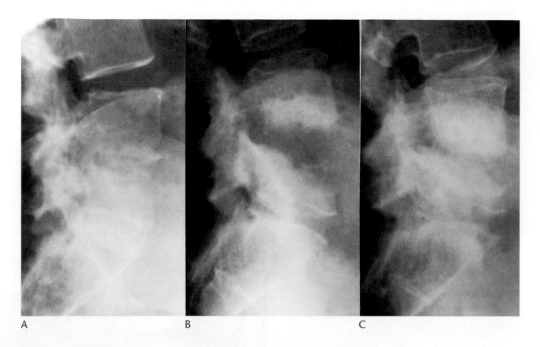

Fig. 2.20 Infective diskitis with progressive healing and reactive sclerotic change. **A.** September. **B.** October. **C.** Subsequent January.

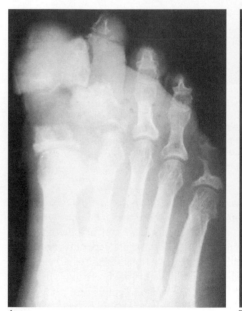
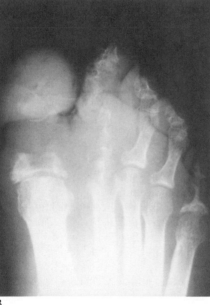

Fig. 2.21 A,B Osteomyelitis in diabetes. The changes at the little toe are those of neuropathic bone resorption. The cloudy resorption of bone with osteoporosis and soft-tissue swelling at the first and second toes indicate superimposed osteomyelitis.

Septic Arthritis

Joint infections occur at any age, but especially in children. *Staphylococci, Streptococci* and *Pneumococci* are common causative organisms. Usually only one joint is affected. If more than one joint is infected, an immune defect should be suspected or the possibility of steroid administration queried.

A joint may be contaminated by:

1. Direct intervention—following surgery, aspiration or perforating injury
2. Spread from adjacent bone (see above)
3. Hematogenous spread—direct infection of synovium by septic emboli.

Radiological Features   Initially synovial thickening and effusion distend the joint. Fat lines are displaced but may be blurred by

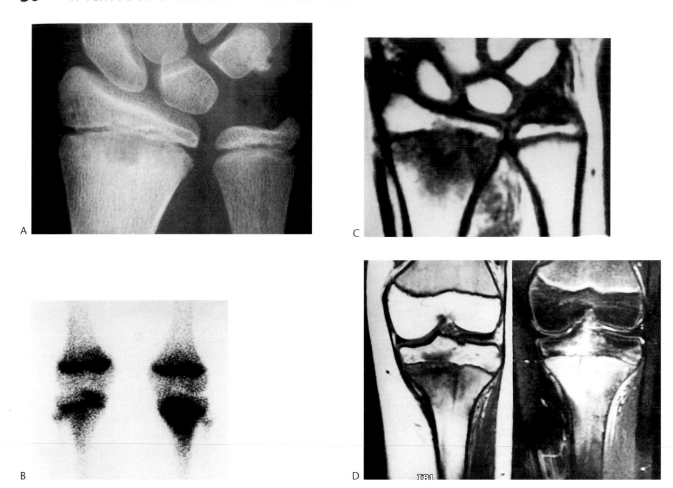

Fig. 2.22 Chronic granulomatous disease. **A.** There is a localized metaphyseal defect surrounded by sclerosis. These features are characteristic of chronic infection in a child. **B.** The MR scan confirms the presence of localized metaphyseal abnormality with replacement of the local fat. There is a mixture of destruction of bone, edema and reactive new bone formation at the margin of the lesion. **C.** Same patient. The radio-isotope bone scan shows increase in uptake in the proximal tibial metaphysis of the left knee. **D.** Coronal T_1 and STIR sequences confirm the presence of change, not merely in the metaphysis, as might be suggested on a plain film, but also in the epiphysis. Fluid replaces fat on both sequences. (Courtesy of Dr R. Phillips.)

edema. Demineralization follows hyperemia and immobilization. When infection begins to destroy cartilage, joint narrowing becomes apparent (Fig. 2.24). The articular cortex becomes blurred and then eroded, both peripherally and centrally, and subarticular bone is later destroyed. Severe cases are characterized by massive destruction, separation of bone ends, subluxation and dislocation.

During recovery, bones recalcify and in severe cases fibrous and bone ankylosis may result. Dystrophic calcification may be seen on occasion following pyogenic arthritis. Marginal erosions persist but their outlines become well demarcated and sclerotic.

Arthritis of the Hip in Infants (Tom Smith arthritis)
The hip joint in infants is especially susceptible to infection as explained above. In neonates sepsis may be transmitted via the umbilical vessels, often due to *Streptococcus*, but infection may be directly introduced following blood sampling at the groin. In infants, because of lax muscles around the hip and the cartilaginous nature of the acetabulum, an effusion may dislocate the hip (Fig. 2.25). This can be assessed even if the ossific nucleus has not appeared. Failure to recognize acute dislocation

may result in permanent deformity. In any case, gross metaphyseal destruction is soon apparent with cortical and medullary erosions. Gross sequestration rapidly occurs and an involucrum may involve the entire femur. The femoral shaft generally heals, but the femoral head and neck may be totally destroyed, never to appear. Deformity and shortening inevitably result. In older children, such change is less likely as the epiphyseal plate is not crossed by vessels. The femoral head, even if severely affected, then reconstitutes with a flattened mushroom-like appearance similar to old Perthes' disease or slipped epiphysis. Because of vascular compression, osteonecrosis may actually complicate infection.

Infection at major joints may show widening of the joint and distension of the capsule by effusion or pus. This can be assessed by plain film or ultrasound, which has the advantage that it can be followed by needle aspiration of fluid, microscopy and culture.

An isotope scan will be positive at an early stage. CT can be used for biopsy but patients should not be overinvestigated or treatment delayed because of a desire to use all imaging modalities. A diagnostic specimen should be obtained prior to instituting antibiotic therapy (Fig. 2.26).

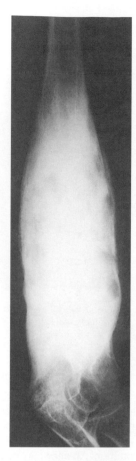

Fig. 2.23   Gross reactive sclerosis with new bone formation at multiple sites is found in chronic granulomatous disease.

MR is probably the investigation of choice in the early diagnosis of septic arthritis, where effusion and bone edema are clearly seen.

TUBERCULOSIS OF BONES AND JOINTS

Though the incidence of skeletal tuberculosis has fallen markedly in recent years, the disease has not yet been eradicated. One-third of our present-day patients are immigrants to Britain; they tend to produce unusual disease patterns which will be described later.

Hematogenous spread of infection to the skeleton is assumed to be from the lung and may occur at the time of primary infection or later from post-primary foci. Chest radiography, however, shows active disease in less than 50% of cases, the organism presumably having laid dormant and become active later. The bacillus lodges in the spongiosa of the metaphysis of a long bone, but the vertebral column is affected in 50% of cases. Lesions are usually single, though multifocal cystic osseous tuberculosis is described.

Certain features are relatively common. The tuberculous reaction is destructive and accompanied by pus which may later become calcified. Calcification of abscesses is rarely seen currently if antibiotic treatment is adequate. In contradistinction to pyogenic osteomyelitis, neither sequestration nor periostitis is a prominent feature. Abscesses often point to the skin and a sinus track may be demonstrated after injection of contrast medium.

Radiographic Appearances   The diagnosis is usually made after considerable delay and radiographic changes are seen at presentation, in contrast to pyogenic infections where radiographic changes occur 2–3 weeks after clinical presentation.

The *metaphysis* is the site of election; an oval or rounded focus will be found which soon crosses the epiphyseal line (Fig. 2.27). No surrounding sclerosis is to be expected. Sequestra are small and are absorbed by granulation tissue. Though slight periosteal reaction may be found if the local lesion is subcortical, this is not a prominent feature. The initial focus may sometimes be sited in the epiphysis.

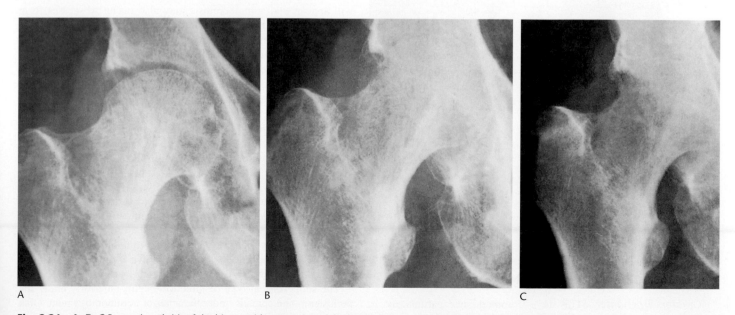

A   B   C

Fig. 2.24   **A, B, C** Pyogenic arthritis of the hip—rapid progression of the lesion during a period of one month.

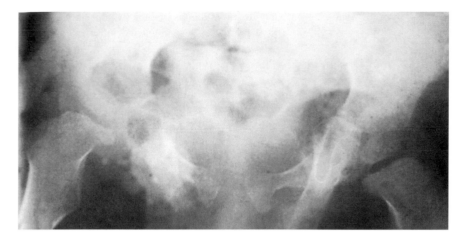

Fig. 2.25 Septic dislocation of the right hip.

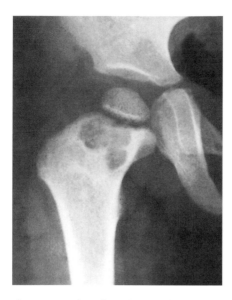

Fig. 2.27 Tuberculosis of femur—large metaphyseal focus.

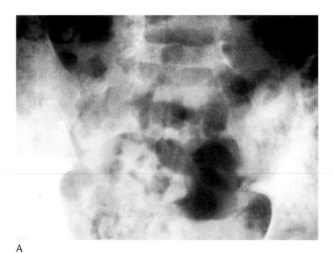

A

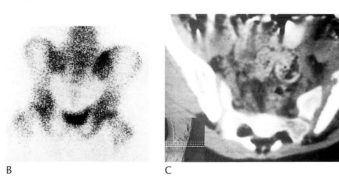

B   C

Fig. 2.26 Infective sacroiliitis. **A.** There is resorption of bone and sclerosis around the left sacroiliac joint. **B.** The radio-isotope bone scan shows the increase in uptake, and the CT scan **C.** shows the widened joint with areas of irregular bone destruction and soft-tissue swelling. (Courtesy of Dr H. Carty.)

Lesions of the diaphysis are rare, and even rarer is the multiple cystic type of lesion.

LESIONS OF INDIVIDUAL BONES

Greater Trochanter   This is a common site, particularly in adolescents and young adults. The lesion may start in the bone or

in the overlying bursa. The erosion may be deep, but often it is superficial and difficult to detect; sometimes it may be cystic (Fig. 2.28).

Spine   Roughly half the cases of osteoarticular tuberculosis seen in the UK occur in the spine. Most lesions occur in or below the mid-thoracic spine and involvement of the cervical and upper thoracic spine is uncommon. All ages may be affected.

Radiographic Appearances   (Fig. 2.29) Vertebral bodies may be first affected in three places—at the upper or lower disk margin, in the center, and anteriorly under the periosteum. The disk substance is often eroded. Two or more vertebrae may be attacked. Tomography may show the lesion to be more extensive than it appears from examination of plain films. Since the anterior parts of the vertebrae are most affected, a local *kyphos* or *gibbus* will appear, and some scoliosis may also occur. Abscesses form early and are easily seen in the thoracic region in contrast to the radiolucent lungs. In the lumbar region, lateral bulging of the psoas outlines may be demonstrable (Fig. 2.30). Abscesses may track widely and may become calcified. They may sometimes be intraosseous and subsequently calcify (Fig. 2.31). Rib crowding may be seen, even on a chest radiograph, if vertebral bodies collapse.

It is often difficult to differentiate between tuberculous and pyogenic spondylitis, especially if the patient is caucasian. Clearly, tuberculosis must always be suspected if the patient is of African or Asian origin. Reactive new bone formation is much less pronounced in tuberculous disease, so that sclerotic osteophytes are unusual. Disks are destroyed early with simple infections and later in tuberculosis. Calcification, where present, indicates tuberculosis.

The lesions generally respond rapidly to antibiotics, but before antibiotics were introduced, gross destructive lesions were common, and the affected vertebral bodies frequently became fused.

The subperiosteal type of infection begins anteriorly under the periosteum and spreads under the anterior common ligament. Disk destruction may be late and the anterior erosions difficult to detect.

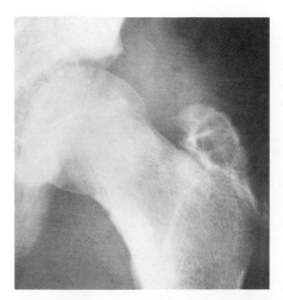

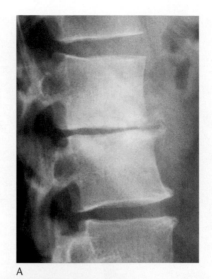

A

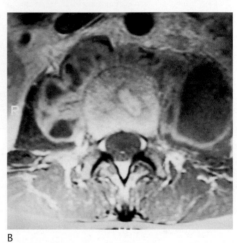

B

Fig. 2.28 Tuberculous focus in greater trochanter. This type is less common than a surface erosion.

Aortic pulsation, transmitted through an anterior paraspinal abscess between T4 and T10, may cause the vertebral bodies to become deeply concave anteriorly (Fig. 2.32). This process does not affect the intervertebral disks. An *aneurysm* causes similar changes by direct pulsation.

In black patients, tuberculous spondylitis has a somewhat different presentation. Often, only one vertebra is involved, with conspicuous preservation of adjacent disks, even if the body is totally destroyed or flattened. Occasionally, *vertebra plana* results (Fig. 2.33). Sclerosis and new bone formation is a feature of the disease in black patients, as in pyogenic spondylitis. More importantly, the posterior elements are frequently involved, especially in the lumbosacral and thoracolumbar junctions, often with huge abscesses (Fig. 2.34). The cervical spine is also more frequently involved than in white patients, with dysphagia or paraplegia as complications. Multiple lesions are also more common. Involvement of the spinal column also follows gibbus formation or extrusion of granulation tissue into the canal.

Tuberculous Dactylitis   This lesion is sometimes seen in the UK immigrant population. The affected phalanx is characteristically widened by medullary expansion (*spina ventosa*), whereas in syphilitic dactylitis the bone is widened by the production of cortical new bone (Fig. 2.35).

Skull   Tuberculous lesions are rare in the skull, except in UK immigrants. They may be localized and well-defined, resembling *eosinophilic granuloma*, or they may be more diffuse (Fig. 2.36). Overlying cold abscesses are generally associated.

Joint Lesions

Tuberculous arthritis usually affects major joints—the hip and knee especially. Multifocal infection is rare. Infection may be synovial or secondary to bony disease. The latter is facilitated as the epiphyseal plate apparently offers little resistance to tuberculosis.

Fig. 2.29 Tuberculous diskitis. **A.** The changes on the plain film are really quite similar to those that would be seen with a simple infection. There is diskal destruction associated with irregularity of the overlying end-plates and some reactive new bone formation. There is perhaps a suggestion on the plain film that a soft-tissue mass is demonstrated anterior to the vertebral bodies. **B.** The Mr T, W axial image shows the end-plate defect seen so well on the plain film but, in addition, psoas abscesses with central necrosis are demonstrated.

Early radiographic signs in synovial lesions are non-specific and will be manifested by capsular thickening, synovial effusion and surrounding osteoporosis. Later, continued hyperemia will cause accelerated maturation of bone ends and epiphyses if infection occurs in children. Bony trabeculae become blurred and the cortex thinned (Fig. 2.37).

The bone ends eventually become affected. Local marginal or surface erosions may appear (Fig. 2.38). Loss of joint space will ultimately occur, but this is not as prominent a feature as it is in pyogenic arthritis. Sometimes one-half of a joint will be affected and bony erosions seen on contiguous bony surfaces.

The advent of antibiotics has changed the picture considerably. Patients usually respond well to treatment so that only the earlier phases are now seen. Formerly such sequelae as subluxation and ankylosis of joints, severe bone atrophy and tracking abscesses were common.

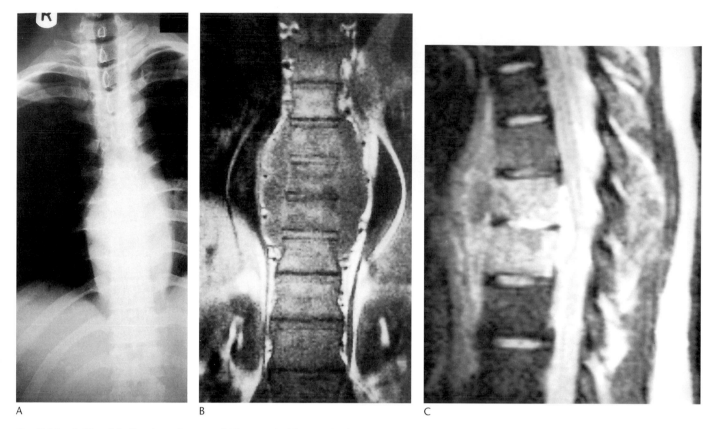

A B C

Fig. 2.30 **A.** The plain film shows features which are typical for spinal tuberculous disease. There is an extensive paraspinal soft-tissue mass. Detail in the underlying spine is poor but there is early crowding of ribs posteriorly, indicating early vertebral collapse. **B.** Coronal MR image of the lumbar spine demonstrates destruction of the intervertebral disk at the point where the paraspinal widening is maximal and this change is associated with alteration of signal from the vertebrae. **C.** The sagittal fat suppression image shows increase in signal in adjacent vertebral bodies together with anterior and posterior soft-tissue masses, the latter indenting the spinal canal and compressing the adjacent cord.

Joint tuberculosis is now rare in caucasian patients in the United Kingdom, but still occasionally seen in immigrant groups in whom a destructive lesion of bone and joints is more likely to be due to tuberculosis than simple infection. Diagnostic aspiration should be performed. In Africa and Asia, however, the lesions are treated immediately by chemotherapy as osteoarticular destruction is assumed to be tuberculous (Martini, 1988).

Hip This is a common site; lesions may arise in the acetabulum, synovium, femoral epiphysis or metaphysis. Sometimes infection spreads to the hip from foci in the greater trochanter or ischium. All degrees of bone loss of the femoral head and neck could be found. A frequent finding was the pointed 'bird's beak' appearance (Fig. 2.39) with intrapelvic protrusion.

Knee With synovial infection in childhood, effusion, osteoporosis and accelerated skeletal maturation are seen (Fig. 2.37). Overgrowth leads to modeling abnormalities, with big bulbous squared epiphyses, so that the appearance resembles that seen in *juvenile chronic arthritis* and *hemophilia*.

Shoulder The humeral head, the glenoid, or both may be affected (Fig. 2.40). Sometimes a lesion in the humeral head is large and cystic in appearance and may resemble an osteoclastoma.

Some tuberculous shoulder lesions run a relatively benign course without pus formation—*caries sicca.* In such cases a relatively small pitted erosion is seen on the humeral head. These may resemble degenerative changes.

Wrist and Carpus (Fig. 2.41) All carpal bones tend to be attacked in the adult, whereas more localized lesions are the tendency in children. This is possibly due to the relatively thicker articular cartilage in the latter. With cartilage destruction the carpal bones become crowded, and even if initially one bone is the focus of irregularity, the destructive process soon involves adjacent bones. Intense demineralization is found throughout the carpus and distal radius and ulna, within the confines of synovium. Demineralization is often also pronounced at distal small joints of the hand, with relative preservation of metacarpal and phalangeal shaft density. However, these joints are not eroded as in rheumatoid arthritis.

Sacroiliac Joints (Fig. 2.42) This joint is affected more often in young adults than in children. Only occasionally is the condition bilateral. Subarticular erosions cause widening of joint space. The infection is usually associated with abscess formation over the back of the joint and, later, pus may calcify. Tuberculous infection of the spine is a frequent accompaniment.

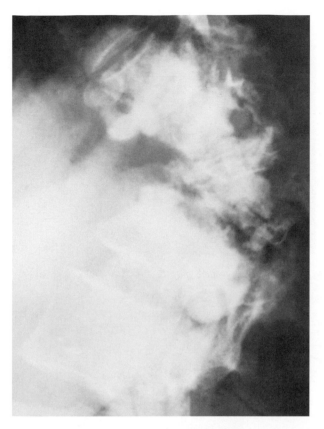

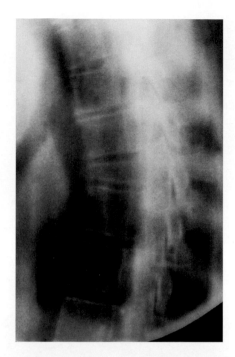

Fig. 2.33 Spinal osteomyelitis in a Saudi Arabian patient showing vertebra plana with preservation of the disk and end-plates.

Fig. 2.31 Tuberculous spondylitis has healed with calcifying psoas abscesses and angular kyphos.

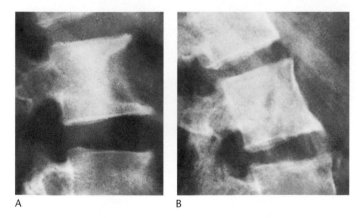

A   B

Fig. 2.32 **A, B** Anterior subperiosteal type of Pott's disease.

SYPHILIS OF BONES AND JOINTS

Very few cases of syphilis of bone are now seen in the UK. Yet up to the time of the Second World War it was a condition that merited serious consideration in the differential diagnosis of most conditions of bone. In this section merely a summary of the findings is presented and illustrations are selected with a view to emphasizing the protean pattern of the lesions.

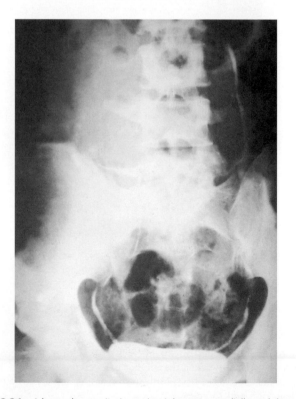

Fig. 2.34 A large abscess displaces the right ureter medially and destroys the right transverse process and adjacent part of the body of L5. Two and a half pints of tuberculous pus were removed at operation.

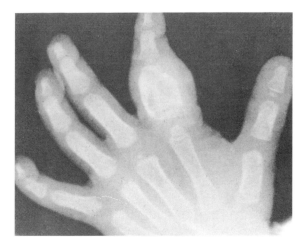

Fig. 2.35 Typical spina ventosa of the proximal phalanx of the forefinger. (Courtesy of Dr. D. J. Mitchell.)

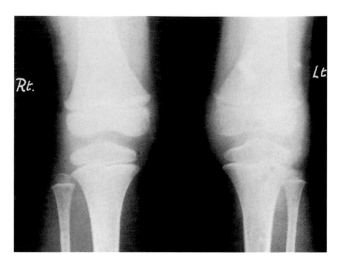

Fig. 2.37 Synovial tuberculosis of left knee—note synovial effusion, osteoporosis, blurring of trabeculae and accelerated maturation of bone ends (normal right knee for comparison).

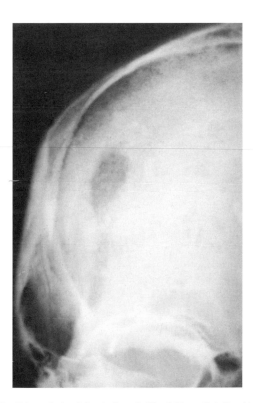

Fig. 2.36 Tuberculosis of the skull vault. The fairly well-defined lytic lesion was a solitary finding but these changes are often multiple. Note the gross tunneling.

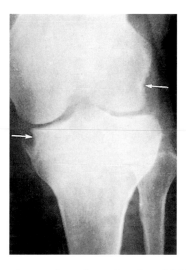

Fig. 2.38 Tuberculous erosions of margins of medial tibial condyle and lateral femoral condyle (arrows).

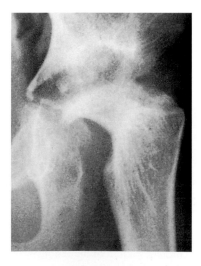

Fig. 2.39 Late tuberculosis of hip—'bird's beak' appearance.

Congenital Syphilis

Lesions may be found in infants whose serologic reactions are negative, especially when the mother is receiving treatment. They may appear early, i.e. from birth to 4 years, or later, i.e. between the ages of 5 and 15 years.

Radiographic Appearances The lesions may be widespread and usually symmetric. Generally they are best shown in the lower ends of the radius and ulna and around the knee. Changes are:

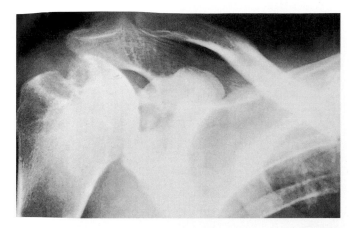

Fig. 2.40 Tuberculosis of shoulder—note lesions of humerus and glenoid and also lung.

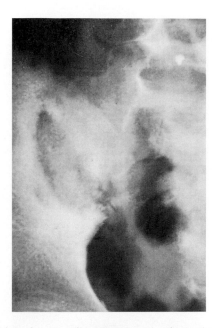

Fig. 2.42 Tuberculous sacroiliac joint—extensive destructive lesion.

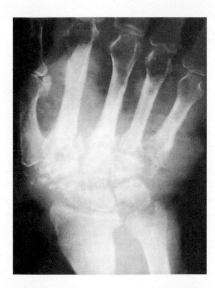

Fig. 2.41 There is soft-tissue swelling around the wrist with evidence of a widespread synovial abnormality. Bone and cartilage are destroyed. Osteoporosis is seen at the metacarpophalangeal joints. The metacarpal shafts however remain normal in density. The fifth metacarpal shaft has a periosteal reaction.

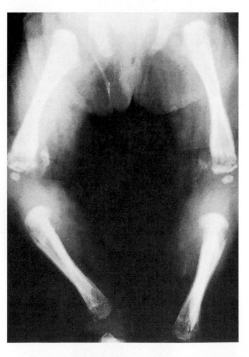

Fig. 2.43 Congenital syphilis—some increased density with subjacent translucent zones of lower ends of femora. Metaphyseal fractures are shown.

1. *Periostitis*. This is the commonest feature and is seen either as a thin layer or as more marked laminated layers. Marked thickening on the convexity of a diaphysis may be seen in later cases as, for example, in the so-called 'saber tibia'.

2. *Metaphysitis*. There may be irregularity of metaphyses, and metaphyseal fractures may occur (Fig. 2.43).

3. *Osteitis* or *osteomyelitis*. Erosions on the upper medial surfaces of the tibiae are very characteristic of congenital syphilis. Sometimes more diffuse osteomyelitis of single bones is seen. Syphilis is a productive lesion, so sclerosis will be found frequently in such lesions.

4. *Syphilitic dactylitis* is rare; it resembles tuberculous dactylitis.

5. *Skull lesions* may be purely sclerotic or may present as a combination of sclerosis and osteolysis. In purely sclerotic lesions, new bone may be laid down in the frontal and parietal regions, so producing the 'hot cross bun' skull.

Acquired Syphilis

Any bone may be affected by this condition. Radiological manifestations comprise periostitis and osteomyelitis.

Periostitis   This sign may be seen as a simple laminated periosteal reaction or as a more exuberant lace-like appearance. Bony spiculation at right angles to the shaft is rare but, when it occurs, may mimic a neoplastic lesion.

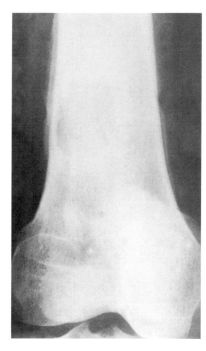

Fig. 2.44   Gumma of the lower femoral shaft. Note bone destruction and periosteal reaction.

Osteomyelitis   This may occur as a localized or as a diffuse lesion. The localized lesion is termed a *gumma* (Fig. 2.44), but a more diffuse lesion is often referred to as 'gummatous osteitis' (Figs 2.45, 2.46). Sclerosis is generally found; irregularity of bone trabeculation is often apparent. Syphilis causes a combination of destruction and proliferation of bone.

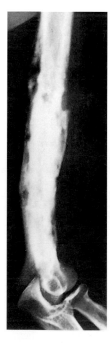

Fig. 2.45   Syphilitic osteomyelitis of the humerus. (Courtesy of Dr. W. Fowler.)

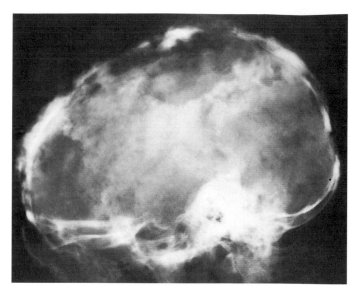

Fig. 2.46   Gummatous osteomyelitis of the skull.

It is important to remember the possibility of syphilis when presented with an atypical bone lesion.

SARCOIDOSIS

This disease is a non-caseating granulomatous disorder commoner in young adult males and especially in patients of black African descent. Changes in the skeleton are moderately common, occurring in up to 15% of cases. The hands and feet are far more commonly affected but any bone may be involved; lesions in the skull, vertebrae and long bones have all been described. Though the granulomata usually cause lysis of bone, often resembling tuberculosis, sclerosis occasionally results. Radionuclide scanning detects early bone lesions with greater sensitivity than plain radiographs.

Radiological Findings   The changes in the bones include:

1. Punched-out, well-defined areas of lucency in the phalanges. These are probably due to deposition of sarcoid tissue but, as in granulomatous *leprosy* (see below), the nutrient foramina are also said to be enlarged.

2. A more diffuse, reticular, lace-like pattern of resorption permeating the bone, described as a lattice-like appearance (Fig. 2.47).

3. Resorption of distal phalanges and of cortical bone along phalangeal shafts. Cortical resorption vaguely resembles that seen in *hyperparathyroidism*.

4. Sclerosis, which may be widely disseminated (Fig. 2.48).

5. Periosteal reaction.

6. Soft-tissue nodules—far commoner than bone changes.

7. Periarticular calcification due to hypercalcemia, which occurs in 20–45% of cases of sarcoid.

Sarcoid Arthritis   An arthritis is a common manifestation of sarcoid, occurring in up to 37% of patients, most commonly in females. In the acute form, joint destruction does not occur but, in

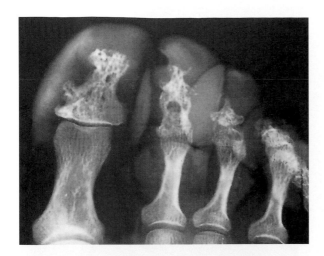

Fig. 2.47 Sarcoid—foot showing typical pseudocysts and absorption of tufts of distal phalanges.

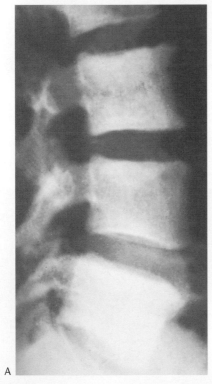

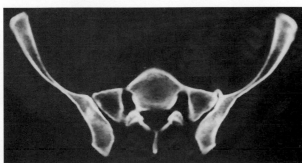

Fig. 2.48 Sarcoid. **A.** Multiple foci of sclerosis are a recognized, if uncommon, feature of sarcoid. **B.** Sclerotic change in sarcoidosis demonstrated at CT scanning.

chronic disease, a destructive arthropathy of large joints does rarely occur due to local granulomata.

RARE BONE INFECTIONS

Brucellosis (synonyms: *undulant fever, Malta fever*)

This disease is more prevalent in the UK than was once thought. Transmission is from unpasteurized milk or by direct contact with affected animals. *Brucellus melitensis* infects sheep, *Br. abortus* infects cattle and *Br. suis* pigs.

The bones are affected in 10% of cases, most often the spine and especially the lumbar region. Widespread granulomatous lesions may be present.

1. *Spinal lesions*. These bear a marked resemblance to other forms of osteomyelitis. Focal sclerosis develops to a marked degree around the end-plate (Fig. 2.49). The disk is rapidly destroyed and adjacent vertebrae rapidly affected. Healing is by the production of extremely large, coarse and shaggy bridging osteophytes.

2. *Changes in other bones*. The radiographic appearances resemble those of subacute osteomyelitis.

3. *Changes in joints*. These resemble the changes of *synovial tuberculosis*. In advanced cases erosive lesions may be seen.

In obscure and atypical bone infections, it is always advisable to test samples of the blood and of the synovial fluid of affected joints for agglutination reaction for brucellosis, and also for the typhoid and paratyphoid group of bacilli.

Actinomycosis

Bony lesions due to this disease are rarely seen. They usually result from direct extension of soft-tissue lesions. Manifestations may be seen in the following sites:

1. *Mandible*. Chronic osteomyelitis arises by direct spread from oral infections and infected cervical glands. The lesion appears to be irregularly destructive.

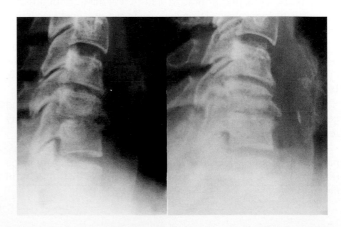

Fig. 2.49 Brucellosis. Vertebro-diskal destruction with florid new bone formation are characteristic features of this disease.

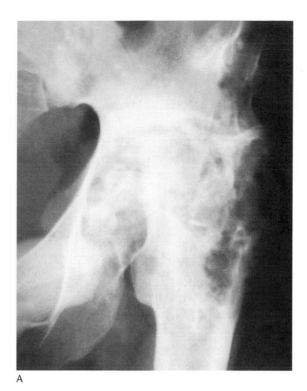

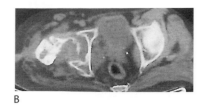

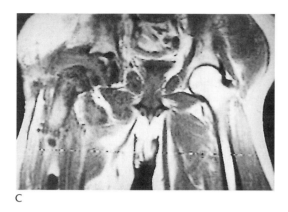

A   C

Fig. 2.50   Hydatid disease. **A.** Bone destruction with the formation of large cysts around both sides of the hip joint are a classic feature of osseous hydatid. Sequestra can be seen. At CT scanning **B.** and MR **C.** the cystic nature of the lesions is demonstrated, together with destruction of the hip joint from both sides.

---

2. *Ribs and thoracic spine.* Destructive foci and periosteal reaction in these bones arise from pleuropulmonary lesions.

3. *Right side of the pelvis and lumbar spine.* Infection spreads to these bones from ileocecal foci. Spinal lesions are usually accompanied by paravertebral abscesses. The disk is usually spared.

Very rarely, destructive metastatic foci are found in other bones.

Hydatid (Echinococcus) Disease

Hydatid disease is rare in the UK and in less than 2% of affected patients is bone involved. The pelvis, spine and proximal long bones are usually involved. The disease is found in sheep-farming areas.

The enlarging cysts in bone absorb trabeculae and spread along the medulla, thinning the cortex and expanding the bone. Later, the cystic lesions become well-defined, so that *fibrous dysplasia* may be simulated in long bones.

Around the hip joint, both the acetabulum and femoral head and neck are destroyed by large cystic lesions (Fig. 2.50). Fusion may result.

In the spine, the cysts break out of the cortex, forming large paraspinal masses which do not calcify but do cause paraplegia (Fig. 2.51). The appearance may resemble dumb-bell tumors in *neurofibromatosis.*

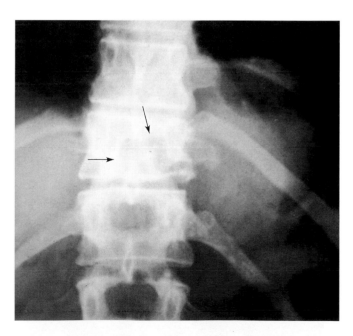

Fig. 2.51   This patient had never been outside England but had hydatid disease of the spine. Note the large paraspinal soft-tissue mass.

TROPICAL CONDITIONS

Yaws *(treponematosis)*

This disease, which has more or less been eradicated, may still be seen in chronic cases. It was prevalent in the Caribbean, Indonesia and parts of tropical Africa and South America, and is due to a non-venereal infection by *Treponema pertenue*. As the disease is not transmitted to the fetus, congenital yaws does not occur, but children become infected. Infection usually occurs through a cut or abrasion. Bony changes are seen in the secondary and tertiary stages; these are usually indistinguishable radiologically.

Any bone may be involved. The distribution may be random, but there is a tendency to symmetry. In the early stages, multiple, small, rarefied areas of bone destruction are shown with overlying periosteal new bone (Fig. 2.52). The hand may be especially affected. Larger areas of destruction occur in the skull and long bones, often with marked surrounding reactive sclerosis and new bone formation. Periostitis along the shaft, and softening of bone due to osteitis, lead to the sabre tibia deformity.

In the skull, gummatous lesions cause foci of osteolysis while slowly growing masses arising from the premaxilla produce a dense hyperostosis known as *goundou*. *Gangosa*, another manifestation of yaws, is an ulceration of the face causing severe necrosis of subjacent bone.

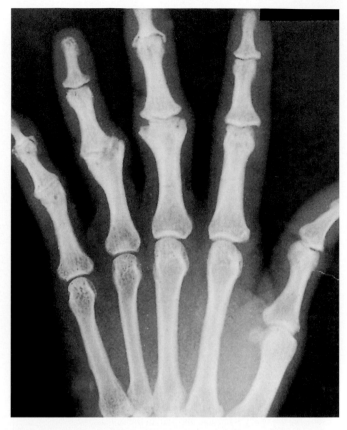

Fig. 2.53 Leprosy. Some small 'cysts' are seen, e.g. in the head of the proximal phalanx of the fifth finger—this condition is sometimes called 'osteitis multiplex cystica leprosa'. The end-results of lepra granulomata are seen in the heads of the proximal phalanges of the third and fourth fingers. (Courtesy of Dr. D. E. Paterson.)

Leprosy

This disease has a widespread geographic distribution, occurring in Egypt, Africa, Asia, the Caribbean and Pacific Islands. It is also seen in the UK's immigrant population. The lesions seen radiologically mostly affect the hands, feet and face, and are caused by infection by *M. leprae*. This bacillus is of low infectivity and prolonged exposure is needed. The nature of the disease depends on host resistance. The incidence of bony change in leprosy may be around 15%.

Three types of bony lesions are found:

1. *Specific changes of osteitis leprosa* (15%). Granulomata cause areas of focal cortical or medullary bone destruction. The lesions may be rounded or may infiltrate, giving a lacy pattern just as in sarcoid. In addition, medullary nutrient foramina enlarge (Fig. 2.53).

2. *Non-specific leprous osteitis* (50%). In these patients Hansen bacilli are rarely found in the marrow. Neuropathic resorption gives a 'licked candy stick' appearance with bone loss both longitudinally and circumferentially (Fig. 2.54). In addition, Charcot-like changes take place in the tarsus. These patients have abnormal, thickened nerves and arterial occlusions. Abnormal stance potentiates this bone resorption in the denervated weight-bearing foot.

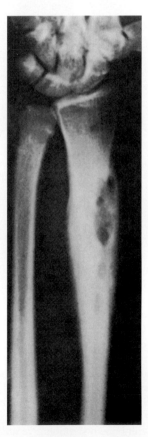

Fig. 2.52 Yaws—moderately early stage, showing destructive areas and much periosteal new bone formation. The appearances of the small destructive foci in yaws have been likened to the effects of a borer beetle. (Courtesy of Dr. A. G. Davies.)

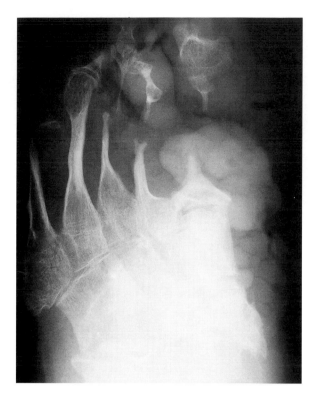

Fig. 2.54 Leprosy. 'Cup and pencil' or 'licked candy stick' appearances demonstrated associated with thickening and irregularity of the soft tissues, presumably the result of chronic infection in the soft tissues.

With anesthesia, plantar ulceration and bone and soft-tissue infections are superimposed, so that pyogenic osteomyelitis is common in these patients. These changes are superimposed upon those of the neuropathic osteopathy.

3. A *diffuse osteoporosis* is seen which is non-specific. Nerve calcification is occasionally seen.

Tropical Ulcer

This common lesion found throughout the tropics may also be seen in immigrants to the UK. Chronic indolent skin ulcers cause secondary bone changes, usually in the tibia or fibula. Periostitis is seen early in various forms, e.g. linear, onion-layer, lace-work and spicular. In very chronic cases, much dense cortical new bone is deposited and the final picture resembles that of an *ivory osteoma* (Fig. 2.55).

Coccidioidomycosis

This is a chronic granulomatous condition caused by a fungus and found in the south-western parts of the USA. The lesions are multiple and are most commonly found in the spine, pelvis, hands and feet. The bone lesions have the appearances of *acute* and *chronic osteomyelitis*; the joint lesions are similar to those found in *tuberculous arthritis*. The more frequent intrathoracic lesions of coccidioidomycosis are described in Chapter 15.

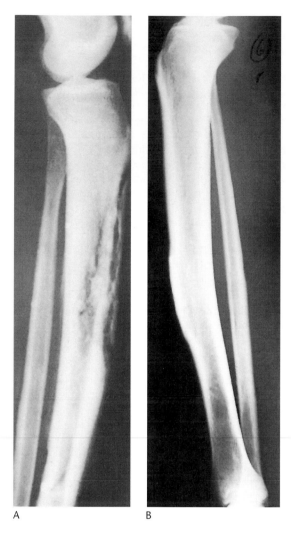

A   B

Fig. 2.55 Tropical ulcer. **A.** Extensive osteomyelitis is seen in the underlying tibia. **B.** Osteoma-like lesion on the front of the tibial shaft—a late sequel of tropical ulcer.

Mycetoma

Mycetoma implantation occurs mainly in the (bare) feet in semi-desert regions throughout the tropics. The skull and knees may also be implanted, usually by thorns. Different organisms are found in different regions—*M. mycetoma* in the Middle East, Africa and India, and *S. somaliensis* and *pelletieri* in the Sudan. Lesions due to *M. mycetoma* are usually localized as large, well-defined black fungus balls which can be seen on soft-tissue radiographs. These erode the cortices and cause cystic defects in the medulla. Madura foot results (the lesions were first described in that region of India). With superadded infection via the implantation track, gross bone destruction results (Fig. 2.56). Reactive sclerosis and a shaggy periostitis with bone resorption give an appearance likened to 'melting snow'. With *S. pelletieri*, diffuse infection occurs earlier but the end-stage appearances after secondary infection are usually similar.

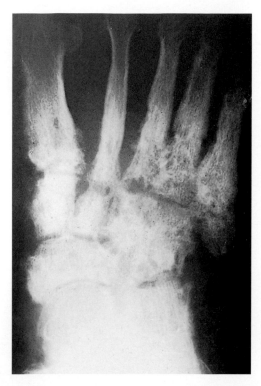

Fig. 2.56 Mycetoma (Madura foot)—diffuse infiltrating destruction affecting the whole tarsus and proximal ends of the metatarsals.

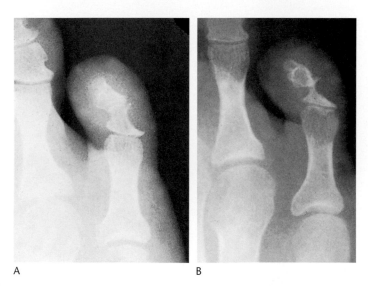

A   B

Fig. 2.57 Ainhum, showing progression of the lesion in an African immigrant. (**B**) was taken two years after (**A**).

Ainhum *(dactylosis spontanea)*

This is seen in 2% of the Nigerian population. The local word *ayan*, from which ainhum is derived, means to saw or file—and a pointed fifth or, less commonly, fourth toe is found (Fig. 2.57).

A groove begins on the medial side of the base of the toe which deepens. This can be identified radiologically. As the constriction deepens, autoamputation occurs, leaving a pointed proximal phalanx of the little toe.

Constriction Rings (Streeter's Bands) cause similar congenital lesions of hands and feet, often in association with club foot.

REFERENCES AND SUGGESTIONS FOR FURTHER READING

Chapman, M., Murray, R. O., Stoker, D. J. (1979) Tuberculosis of the bones and joints. *Seminars in Roentgenology*, **14** (4), 266–282.

Cockshott, P., Middlemiss, J. H. (1979) *Clinical Radiology in the Tropics*. Edinburgh: Churchill Livingstone.

Enna, C. D., Jacobson, R. R., Rausch, R. O. (1971) Bone changes in leprosy: correlation of clinical and radiographic features. *Radiology*, **100**, 295–306.

Epstein, B. S. (1976) *The Spine*, 4th edn. Philadelphia: Lea & Febiger.

Gohel, K., Dalinka, M. K., Edeiken, J. (1973) The serpiginous tract: a sign of subacute osteomyelitis. *Journal of the Canadian Association of Radiologists*, **24**, 337–339.

Golimbu, C., Firooznia, H., Ralii, M. (1984) CT osteomyelitis of the spine. *American Journal of Roentgenology*, **142**, 159–163.

Kolawole, T. M., Bohrer, S. P. (1970) Ulcer osteoma: bone response to tropical ulcer. *American Journal of Roentgenology*, **109**, 611–618.

Martini M (Ed) (1988) Tuberculosis of the bones and joints, Springer, Berlin.

Modic, M. T., Feiglin, D. H., Piraino, D. W., Boumphrey, I., Weinstein, M. A., Duchesneau, P. M., Rehm, S. (1985) Vertebral osteomyelitis: assessment using MR. *Radiology*, **157**, 157–166.

Murray, R. O., Jacobson, H. G., Stoker, D. J. (1990) *The Radiology of Skeletal Disorders,* 3rd edn. Edinburgh: Churchill Livingstone.

Renton, P. (1991) Radiology of the foot. In: Klenerman, L. (ed.), *The Foot and Its Disorders*, 3rd edn. Oxford: Blackwell Scientific.

Resnick, D. (1995) *Diagnosis of Bone and Joint Disorders*, 3rd edn. Philadelphia: Saunders.

Sharif, H. S., Aideyan, O. A., Clark, D. C., et al. (1989) Brucellar and tuberculous spondylitis: comparative imaging features. *Radiology*, **171**, 419–425.

Smith, A. S., Weinstein, M. A., Mizushima, A., Coughlin, B., Hayden, S. P., Lakin, M. M., Lanzieri, C. F. (1989) MR imaging characteristics of tuberculous spondylitis versus vertebral osteomyelitis. *American Journal of Roentgenology*, **153**, 399–405.

Unger, E., Moldofsky, P., Gatenby, R., Hartz, W., Broder, G. (1988) Diagnosis of osteomyelitis by MR imaging. *American Journal of Roentgenology*, **150**, 605–610.

Weaver, P., Lifeso, R. M. (1984) The radiological diagnosis of tuberculosis of the adult spine. *Skeletal Radiology*, **12**, 178–186.

3

AVASCULAR NECROSIS; OSTEOCHONDRITIS; MISCELLANEOUS BONE LESIONS

Peter Renton

OSTEONECROSIS (synonyms: *aseptic necrosis, avascular necrosis, bone infarction*)

The term 'osteonecrosis' implies that a segment of bone has lost its blood supply so that the cellular elements within it die. The phrase 'aseptic necrosis' indicates that infection generally plays no part in the process, though a sequestrum is also necrotic and avascular.

Pathology Ischemia of bone follows occlusion of arteries or veins and is therefore dependent on the anatomy of the blood supply to a given bone (a rise in venous pressure eventually arrests arterial supply). Ischemia results in death of hemopoietic tissue within 6–12 hours; of the osteoclasts, osteoblasts and osteocytes within 12–48 hours; and of marrow fat in 2–5 days. Empty osteocyte lacunae indicate death of bone. Dead bone at this stage is radiologically normal since the trabecular framework remains intact.

Revascularization is seen at the live marrow–dead marrow interface. The necrotic zone is invaded by capillaries, fibroblasts and macrophages. Fibrous tissue replaces dead marrow and in turn may calcify. New osteoblasts lay down fresh woven bone on the devitalized trabeculae. This advancing front of neovascularization and ossification has been termed 'creeping substitution' (Phemister).

At bone ends, cartilage receives nutrition from synovial fluid. Cartilage and subcartilaginous bone are not therefore necessarily affected.

Radiological Changes are thus:

Stage 1. No changes are visible.

Stage 2. Disuse, for instance following immobility, leads to osteoporosis, except in devitalized avascular bone which is now devoid of osteoclasts and osteocytes. Avascular areas are of normal or increased density, while immobile but vascular bone loses density. The avascular proximal pole of the scaphoid is dense after waist of scaphoid fractures.

Stage 3. At large joints—hips, shoulder, knee—a subcortical necrotic zone of transradiancy and trabecular loss beneath a thin and sclerotic cortex is shown (Fig. 3.1). This results in structural failure in subarticular bone at areas of maximal stress with cortical microfractures followed by collapse and trabecular compression (Fig. 3.2).

Stage 4. A flattened articular surface results with increased subarticular density as trabeculae are compressed into a smaller space (Fig. 3.3).

Stage 5. Osteoarthritis with joint space narrowing follows later.

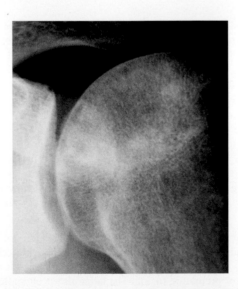

Fig. 3.1 Avascular necrosis. The cortex is thin and dense. There is a subcortical zone of demineralization. The head also shows a zone of creeping substitution, seen as a serpiginous area of increase in density around the infarcted area.

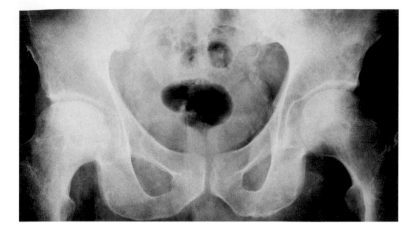

Fig. 3.2 Early collapse of the right femoral head is demonstrated. The superior contour shows flattening. Creeping substitution is also demonstrated here. Compare the contour of the right femoral head with that on the left side.

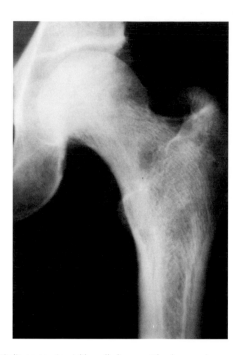

Fig. 3.4 Split cortex in sickle-cell disease. The bones show a generalized increase in density. The image of the old cortex is demonstrated within the upper femoral shaft.

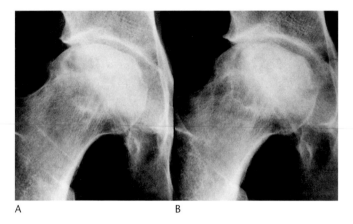

A   B

Fig. 3.3 Progressive collapse of the femoral head in association with subchondral cysts and sclerosis. **A**. February. **B**. September.

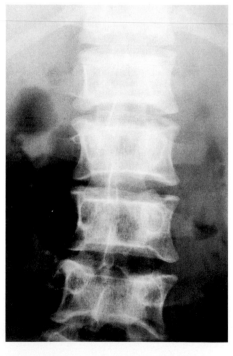

Fig. 3.5 End-plate infarcts in sickle-cell disease. The defects are extensive and flattened rather than more localized and rounded, as would be the case in Scheuermann's disease.

In the diametaphysis and subarticular regions, the infarcted area is surrounded by a serpiginous line of sclerosis, representing the advancing front of new bone laid down on the old trabecular framework. The central area within the infarct may look relatively lucent, or may actually be the site of osteoclastic resorption, but may also contain foci of added density representing dystrophic calcification in debris (Figs 3.2, 3.3).

In some diseases following infarction, a 'bone within a bone' or 'split cortex' is seen as a linear density lying within and parallel to the healthy cortex. This probably represents the old infarcted cortex left behind by processes of growth and remodeling beneath the vital periosteum. This change is seen in *Gaucher's* and *sickle-cell disease*, and following *osteomyelitis* (Fig. 3.4)

Epiphyseal Abnormalities Infarcts at growth plates, for instance, in the hands and at the vertebral end-plates in sickle-cell disease (Fig. 3.5), cause local arrest of growth or may result in 'cone' epiphyses or premature fusion. The latter also occurs after irradiation, infection or trauma.

Infarcted bone, e.g. following irradiation, is susceptible to fractures. This is seen in the ribs following irradiation for breast cancer and in the femoral necks after pelvic irradiation, though it is less common nowadays.

Isotope Scanning Changes in the isotope scan reflect the stages of the disease from photopenia in early avascular necrosis to

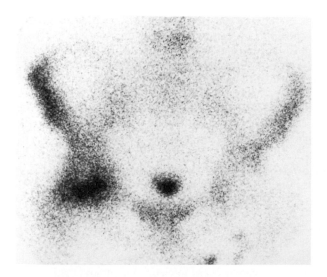

Fig. 3.6 Radio-isotope bone scan in avascular necrosis. Increase in uptake is demonstrated around the infarcted area, indicating healing at the margins of the infarct.

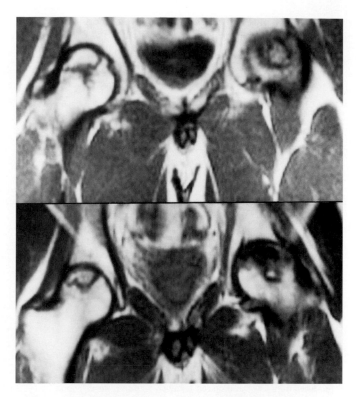

Fig. 3.7 Avascular necrosis. Coronal T_1-weighted images of the hip showing a serpiginous zone of low signal around the avascular areas.

increase in uptake when healing with vascular ingrowth takes place (Fig. 3.6).

MRI MR scanning is the most sensitive and accurate means of detecting changes in avascular necrosis. Sensitivity and specificity for avascular necrosis approach 100%, while false negative isotope scans occur early on in the disease.

Changes at MRI are usually seen in the anterosuperior segment of the femoral head. Initially, bright signal remains in the affected area but subsequently, after a week, this decreases corresponding to progressive lymphocytic infiltration and fibrosis. Radiographs remain normal.

A serpiginous zone of low signal on T_1- and T_2-weighted images develops around the avascular area, internal to which a zone of bright signal may be seen on T_2-weighted images; this represents edema or vascularity (Fig. 3.7). Hemorrhage, cyst formation, fibrosis and collapse of bone alter the shape and signal in the femoral head. Hemorrhage and cysts are of intermediate signal on T_1-weighting, but bright on T_2-weighted and STIR sequences. Sclerotic bone radiologically is of low signal on all sequences.

Anatomic changes of bone collapse and deformity may be seen on plain radiographs, CT and MR scans, but MRI is the most sensitive modality in the diagnosis of early disease. Sagittal, coronal and axial images allow optimal assessment of the extent of the disease. The vascular response in healing can also be assessed (Fig. 3.8).

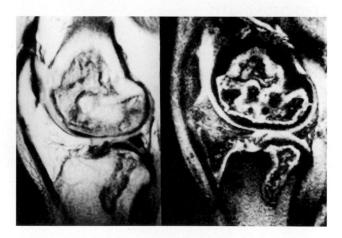

Fig. 3.8 Avascular necrosis. Changes are demonstrated on T_1- and T_2-weighted images on both sides of the joint. Areas of infarcted bone are demonstrated surrounded by fluid. There is also an effusion in the joint.

Causes of Osteonecrosis (Table 3.1)

Vascular insufficiency to bone is of three types.

1. *Interruption to the flow of blood* to bone most commonly follows trauma with tearing of blood vessels.

2. *Emboli or sludging.* This occurs in *sickle-cell disease* where abnormal red cells aggregate; in *pancreatitis* where fat emboli obstruct vessels; and in *decompression disease* where possibly gas bubbles occlude small vessels. Vasculitis, in collagen disorders and following irradiation, also occludes small vessels.

3. *Intraosseous compression of vessels* occurs in *Gaucher's disease*, where masses of Gaucher cells pack marrow spaces.

The Role of Drugs in Avascular Necrosis Steroids and non-steroidal anti-inflammatory drugs are associated with bone necrosis.

Pain relief and euphoria associated with prolonged dosage lead to overuse of often already damaged joints and a Charcot-type lesion results with bone less and eburnation. Similar changes may follow alcohol abuse. In addition, steroids cause vasculitis and marked subcortical osteoporosis which further potentiates bone collapse.

Table 3.1   Conditions Associated with Spontaneous Aseptic Bone Necrosis

**Alcoholism	**Hyperlipemia
Arthropathy	Hypertension
**Rheumatoid arthritis	**Hypertriglyceridemia
Psoriasis	**Hyperuricemia
Neuropathic	Immobilization
Osteoarthrosis	*Immunosuppressive therapy
Clotting defects	*Irradiation
Convulsive disorders	Microfractures
*Cushing syndrome	Mitral insufficiency
*Decompression syndrome	Myxedema
**Diabetes	Obesity
Endocarditis	**Pancreatitis
**Fat embolism	Peripheral neuropathy
Giant-cell arteritis	Peripheral vascular disease
**Gout	Periarteritis nodosa
*Hemoglobinopathy	Pregnancy
*Hemopoietic disorders	**Systemic lupus erythematosus
Hemophilia	*Thermal injuries
Gaucher's disease	Burns
Histiocytosis	Electrical
Polycythemia	Frostbite
*Hyperadrenocorticism	*Trauma
Hypercholesterolemia	

*Generally accepted contributory factor
**Commonly reported associated factor

(Reproduced from J. K. Davidson (ed.), *Aseptic Necrosis of Bone*, by kind permission of Excerpta Medica, Amsterdam.)

OSTEOCHONDRITIS (Osteochondrosis)

Osteochondritis is a disease of epiphyses, beginning as necrosis and followed by healing. The term 'osteochondritis' is used to describe the lesions but is a misnomer, as: 1. there is no inflammation; and 2. cartilage is not primarily involved. Over 40 sites have been described and all have eponyms which are too closely associated with the lesions to be currently abandoned (Table 3.2).

The mechanism of pathological change is not identical at all sites. Some changes, such as in Perthes' disease, are generally regarded as being due to vascular occlusion. The mechanism for this is not clearly understood, especially as in some patients an osteochondritis affects more than one epiphysis. At other sites— the tibial tubercle and the lower pole of patella—tendons avulse bone which subsequently necroses. Vertebra plana follows eosinophilic granuloma. Adolescent kyphosis may follow diskal herniation into end-plate defects.

Epiphyseal areas of necrosis eventually heal and are converted into normal bone. In some sites, especially at the femoral head, prominent metaphyseal changes are also present.

Osteochondritis of the Femoral Capital Epiphysis
(synonym: *coxa plana*; eponyms: *Waldenström* (1909), *Legg* (1910), *Calvé* (1910), *Perthes* (1910))

This condition is commoner in boys than girls (M:F = 4:1) and most cases present between 4 and 9 years of age. The age of onset is earlier in girls and the prognosis worse.

Bilateral disease is even more common in boys (M:F = 7:1) but the disease is rarely symmetric. If symmetry is present, *hypothyroidism* or *multiple epiphyseal dysplasia* should be excluded. There is no increased familial incidence, but parents of affected children are often elderly. Many of the affected children have a below-average birthweight and, at presentation, show skeletal growth retardation in the hands. This is especially seen in boys. There is an increased incidence of associated congenital anomalies, including congenital heart disease, pyloric stenosis, hernia, renal anomalies and undescended testes.

Following ischemia, the ossific nucleus of the epiphysis necroses, causing growth arrest. The overlying cartilage, which is supplied by synovial fluid, survives and thickens, especially in the non-weight-bearing regions, medially and laterally. Creeping substitution eventually occurs in the ossific nucleus which thus becomes denser, the process usually reaching the dome from the peripheral and deep parts of the epiphysis.

The Irritable Hip Syndrome   A few patients with this syndrome (up to 7%) develop changes of Perthes' disease. The affected children present with acute hip pain and often fever and a raised ESR. Most cases resolve with simple bed rest, but prolonged immobilization and traction may be necessary. Other causes of acute hip pain— infection or juvenile arthritis—must be excluded.

Table 3.2   Types of Eponymous Osteochondritis

Disease	Cause	Site
Legg–Calvé–Perthes	Primary aseptic necrosis	Femoral head
Köhler	? Primary aseptic necrosis ? Necrosis following fracture	Tarsal navicular
Freiberg	? Primary aseptic necrosis ? Necrosis following fracture	Metatarsal head
Kienböck	? Necrosis following fracture ? Primary aseptic necrosis	Lunate
Osgood–Schlatter	Necrosis following partial avulsion of patellar tendon	Tibial tubercle
Sinding–Larsen	Necrosis following partial avulsion of patellar tendon	Lower pole of patella
Sever	Necrosis following partial avulsion of tendo Achilles	Calcaneal apophysis
Calvé	Eosinophilic granuloma	Vertebral body epiphysis
Scheuermann	Disk herniation through defective end-plate	Ring-like epiphysis of vertebra

(Reproduced from J. K. Davidson (ed.), *Aseptic Necrosis of Bone,* by kind permission of Dr Mary Catto, and Excerpta Medica, Amsterdam)

Radiological Features

1. *Lateral displacement of the femoral head.* Early on, and in the irritable hip syndrome, displacement of the femoral head (Waldenström's sign) is seen (Fig. 3.9), possibly due to effusion or to thickening of the ligamentum teres. Later, the superior part of the joint may also be widened. These changes may be seen on ultrasound.

2. *A subcortical fissure in the femoral ossific nucleus.* This sign is seen early in the disease but is transient. It is best seen in the 'frog' lateral view.

3. *Reduction in size of the ossific nucleus of the epiphysis.* This is found in some 50% of cases and is due to growth retardation. The medial joint space then seems wider.

4. *Increase in density of the femoral ossific nucleus.* This is due to trabecular compression, dystrophic calcification in debris and creeping substitution (see above) (Fig. 3.10).

Catterall (1971) has grouped Perthes' disease according to the degree of epiphyseal involvement as assessed radiologically (Fig. 3.11). Prognosis depends on the degree of radiological involvement.

Stages of the Disease occur within each group.

There is an *initial* phase of onset, with widening of the joint space and increased density of all or part of the ossific nucleus, which is followed by collapse of part or all of the nucleus, according to group. *Repair* removes the fragmented, crushed necrotic bone. *Healing* shows as an increase in size and re-ossification (Fig. 3.10). *Remodeling* then occurs and is aided when the femoral head is completely contained within the acetabulum. Uncovering of the lateral margin of the femoral head has a bad prognosis.

The metaphyseal lesion leads to an abnormal femoral neck. The most severely involved cases have a broad, short neck, that is, the neck length/width ratio is lower than normal (Fig. 3.10).

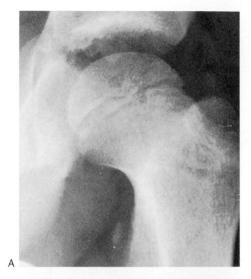

A

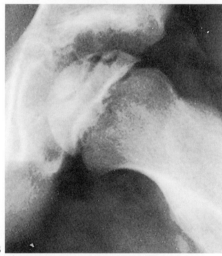

B

Fig. 3.9 A. Perthes' disease, showing increased joint space in AP view. **B.** Fissures in the femoral head are shown well in the frog view.

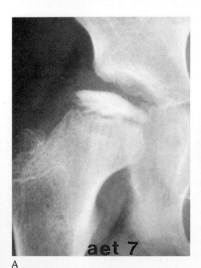

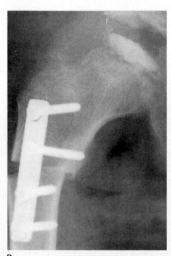

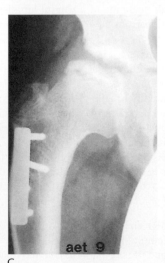

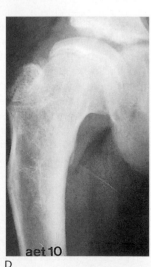

A B C D

Fig. 3.10 Perthes' disease. A series of radiographs showing the stages of healing. **A.** The initial radiograph shows a flattened, sclerotic femoral head. **B.** An osteotomy is performed. **C, D.** Later films show resorption of the sclerotic dead bone and its replacement with vital bone, resulting in a mushroom-shaped femoral head.

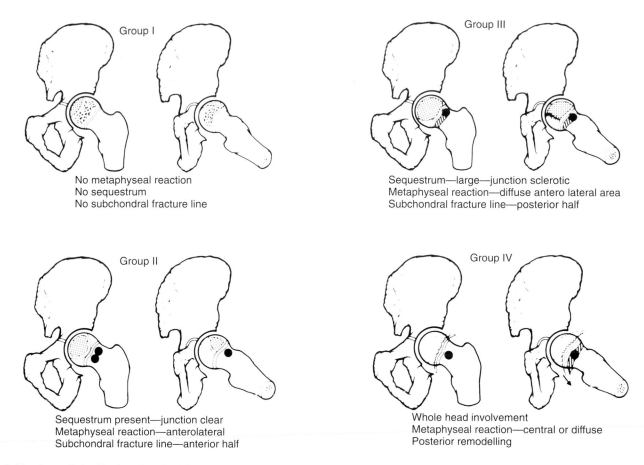

Group I

No metaphyseal reaction
No sequestrum
No subchondral fracture line

Group II

Sequestrum present—junction clear
Metaphyseal reaction—anterolateral
Subchondral fracture line—anterior half

Group III

Sequestrum—large—junction sclerotic
Metaphyseal reaction—diffuse antero lateral area
Subchondral fracture line—posterior half

Group IV

Whole head involvement
Metaphyseal reaction—central or diffuse
Posterior remodelling

Fig. 3.11 Catterall classification of Perthes' disease. (Reproduced by courtesy of Mr. A. Catterall, F.R.C.S.; see list of Further Reading).

Prognosis The prognosis in untreated disease is proportional to the degree of epiphyseal involvement. Thus, Group I and Group II patients have a good prognosis.

Radionuclide Bone Scanning Technetium scan images of bone depend in part on blood flow to bone. Avascular areas therefore are seen as scan *defects*. Nuclide scanning of a painful hip distinguishes a 'cold' area in infarction from an area of increased uptake in infective or inflammatory disease. It seems logical to scan all children with acutely painful hips.

In the early stage, when no radiological abnormality is yet visible in the child with an avascular lesion, a defect is seen in the femoral head image on radionuclide scanning. In the early case, the size of the defect on the scan correlates well with the eventual size of the defect on radiography, which only becomes assessable some 6–9 months after the initial nuclide scan (Fig. 3.12).

In cases of established disease, correlation of the scan defect with radiological change is less helpful, as revascularization gives a local increase in activity, so that the defect size is underestimated.

MRI in Perthes' Disease MRI changes are seen in bone and cartilaginous structures of the femoral head and acetabulum.

The ossific nucleus flattens and the normal bright signal related to marrow fat diminishes following loss of the normal circulation. The signal seen from this region varies with the stage of disease and healing, and may range from low early on in the disease to a mixture of high and low when revascularization occurs or if cysts are present. The bone deformity is visualized. Metaphyseal irregularity is seen and an abnormal relationship of the entire head to the acetabulum shown (Fig. 3.13).

MRI also shows thickening of the non-ossified cartilage of the femoral head, especially laterally, and of the acetabulum, especially the labrum. This change of cartilaginous hypertrophy is reproducible experimentally after ligation of the epiphyseal arterial supply, and is seen at arthrography, which is invasive, as well as at MRI. The degree of acetabular covering of the developing femoral head, as well as articular congruity, is seen both at MRI and arthrography, though arthrography allows the relationship between the head and socket to be assessed dynamically as a precursor to surgery.

Osteochondritis of the Tibial Tubercle (eponyms: *Osgood's disease, Schlatter's disease*)

The diagnosis is essentially clinical and is confirmed radiologically by a soft-tissue lateral film of the area. This demonstrates local soft-tissue swelling over an often fragmented and dense tuberosity (Fig. 3.14). The other knee should also be examined radiologically, especially to compare the soft tissues. The condition is usually self-limiting and rest brings relief of symptoms.

The tubercle fuses to the shaft at 15 years, but occasionally remains unfused and fragmented. Examination of soft tissues will rule out ongoing disease.

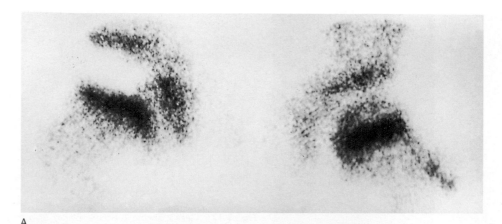

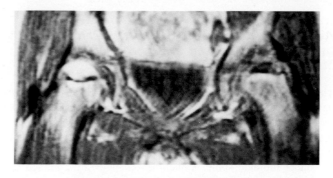

Fig. 3.12 Perthes' disease. **A**. The lateral aspect of the right femoral head does not show up on radionuclide scanning. **B**. On X-ray, the involved area looks smaller than on the scan.

Fig. 3.13 Perthes' disease. A T₁-weighted MR scan showing collapse of the left femoral head with avascular changes. The head is subluxated laterally in addition, and is uncovered laterally. Note the movement artefact.

Osteochondritis of the Metatarsal Head (eponyms: *Freiberg's infraction, Köhler's disease*)

The second metatarsal head is most frequently involved. The condition is commoner in girls. Its usual incidence is between 10 and 15 years. There is a history of chronic trauma, e.g. girls wearing high heels for the first time.

Radiographic Appearances Condensation, increased density (Fig. 3.15) and fragmentation of the epiphysis are seen. The joint

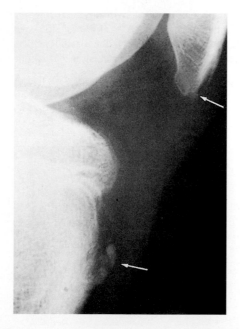

Fig. 3.14 Osgood–Schlatter disease. Note also some osteochondritis of the epiphysis of the lower pole of the patella.

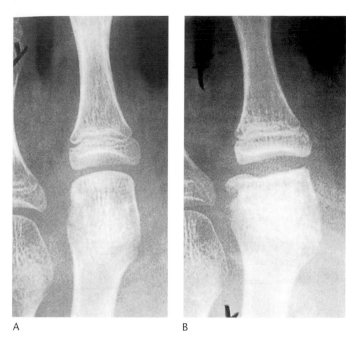

A   B

Fig. 3.15 Osteochondritis of the second metatarsal head. **A**. Minimal change of increased density of the epiphysis. **B**. Later stage of flattening of the epiphysis, increased joint space and loose body separation.

space may be increased in size and the opposing bone surfaces greatly splayed. Gradual thickening of the metatarsal neck and shaft occurs.

Osteochondritis of the Tarsal Navicular (eponym: *Köhler's disease*)

As in Osgood–Schlatter disease, the combination of pain and radiological change is needed for the diagnosis to be made. The disease is much more common in boys. Age incidence is 3–10 years, with the peak between 5 and 6 years, and the disease appears earlier in girls—as does the ossific nucleus itself. The process is thought to be ischemic in origin. 15–20% are bilateral.

Radiographic Appearances Irregularity of the outline of the navicular and fissure formation are early signs. The bone may appear later as a mere dense disk (Fig. 3.16). No loss of cartilage

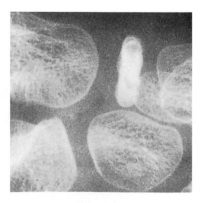

Fig. 3.16 Osteochondritis of the tarsal navicular.

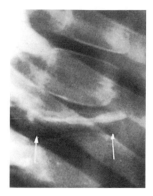

Fig. 3.17 Calvé's disease (vertebra plana) of a mid thoracic vertebral body. Complete regeneration occurred. No evidence of histiocytosis was found on biopsy.

on either side of the bone occurs. The onset of regeneration is shown by the production of new bone round the compression disk.

Osteochondritis of the Vertebral Body (synonym: *vertebra plana*; eponym: *Calvé's disease*)

This condition is manifested by collapse and increased density of a vertebral body; the adjacent disk spaces are normal or increased in width (Fig. 3.17). Recovery to normal shape follows, but it may be incomplete.

Most cases may be shown to be a manifestation of *histiocytosis*. Regeneration is expected but histiocytosis may be associated with paraplegia. *Leukemia*, *Ewing sarcoma*, *metastases*, *tuberculosis*, etc. may cause similar appearances and should always be excluded before a diagnosis of Calvé's disease is accepted.

Adolescent Kyphosis (synonyms: *vertebral epiphysitis, osteochondritis of vertebral epiphyseal plates;* eponym: *Scheuermann's disease*)

The condition affects both sexes; it usually begins at puberty, having peak incidence from 15 to 16 years. The mid and lower thoracic spine is the region most commonly affected and usually several adjacent vertebrae are involved (Fig. 3.18). Less frequently, the lesion may be found in the lumbar spine (Fig.3.19) and in the upper thoracic spine. Sometimes changes are confined to a single vertebra.

Radiographic Appearances Irregularity is seen affecting the superior and inferior parts of the vertebral bodies. Later, wedging of vertebral bodies and kyphosis appear. Some scoliosis may also be present. Schmorl's nodes are seen and disk spaces become narrowed. Sometimes a small paraspinal bulge is observed at the level of the lesion.

The radiographic picture tends to remain static for a while. Improvement is slow and consolidation may take several years. Radiographic recovery is often incomplete: various degrees of irregularity and wedging of thoracolumbar vertebrae may be permanent. Indeed, evidence of old adolescent kyphosis is one of the most frequent abnormalities seen in spinal radiographs.

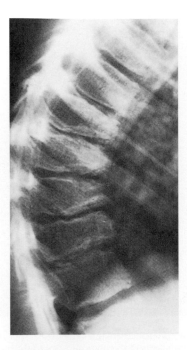

Fig. 3.18   Adolescent kyphosis (advanced case).

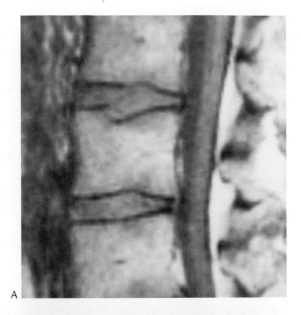

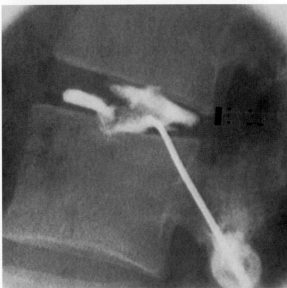

Fig. 3.20   A. T$_1$-weighted sagittal MR scan of the lumbar spine showing rounded, fairly central end-plate defects into which diskal material is herniated. **B.** The diskogram of the same patient shows the diskal herniation into the defects.

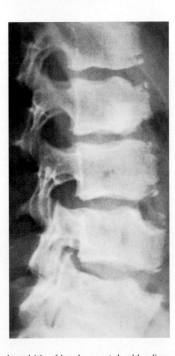

Fig. 3.19   Osteochondritis of lumbar vertebral bodies.

No constitutional effects are found in adolescent kyphosis and the vertebral defects are bounded by sclerotic rims, which are not seen in tuberculous lesions.

Residual wedging in late cases may be indistinguishable from that caused by a previous compression fracture. The ring apophysis may be displaced by diskal herniation, never to unite. It is then seen as a triangular fragment of bone adjacent to the end-plate. Diskography shows a disk filled with contrast medium which extends between the vertebral body and the detached fragment of bone.

Changes at MR imaging reflect changes seen on the plain film (and at diskography) (Fig. 3.20). The affected disk is narrowed and usually shows a loss of signal, indicating dehydration. The disk is seen to herniate into the end-plate defect and beneath the non-fused ring apophysis.

Osteochondritis at Other Sites

Most osteochondritis is found in the hip or spine. Other sites include:

1. *Capitellum.*
2. *Patella—primary center* (Köhler's disease).

3. *Patella—secondary center* (Sinding–Larsen disease). Some cases are associated with Osgood–Schlatter disease. This condition is also almost always due to an avulsion strain by the patellar ligament (Fig. 3.21).

4. *Tibia vara* (osteochondritis of the medial tibial condyle—Blount's disease). This change may be seen from the first to the 12th year of age, but is most common in the earlier age group. As the name implies, the abnormality is usually to be seen on the medial aspect of the knee joint. An irregular defect is often present on the medial aspect of the proximal tibial metaphysis beneath which a large and prominent spur sticks out, almost at right angles (Fig. 3.22). The adjacent aspect of the tibial epiphysis may be defective, and a local femoral spur may also be seen. The overall effect is a varus deformity. The lateral aspect of the proximal tibial metaphysis is straight, and not bowed as in physiologic bow-legs. The changes are possibly related to early onset of walking.

Osteochondritis in Adult Bones

Often a closer link with trauma is seen in adult osteochondritis than in juvenile cases, but this is not always so. Sites subject to trauma include the *scaphoid*, the *carpal lunate* (Kienböck's disease) (Fig. 3.23), the *tarsal navicular* and the *medial sesamoid bone of the great toe*, as well as the *os trigonum*. Fragmentation, collapse and sclerosis, perhaps with cyst formation, are seen on the plain film. CT demonstrates these changes and allows reconstruction in any plane. MR scans show the changes in anatomy and a mixture of low signal indicating collapse, bone condensation and sclerosis as seen on the plain film, as well as the bright signal of fluid or cyst formation and vascularity indicating healing.

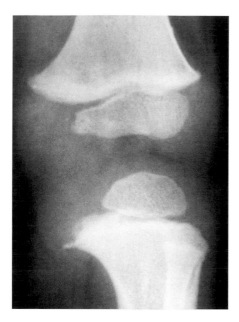

Fig. 3.22   Blount's disease. There is a large medial spur at the upper tibial metaphysis with irregularity of the bone adjacent to the growth plate.

Osteochondritis Dissecans

In this condition fragments of articular cartilage, with or without subchondral bone, become partially or completely detached at characteristic sites. The separated fragment is avascular, in contradistinction to that at an osteochondral fracture, and the 'bed' of the defect remains vital, in contradistinction to avascular necrosis.

Sites of election are the medial femoral condyle, the capitellum of the humerus and the trochlear surface of the talus. The lesion is twice as common in males as females and about one-third of all cases are bilateral. In some patients several epiphyses are affected. The condition is not always symptomatic. The lesion characteristically occurs in adolescence and early adult life. It is the commonest cause of a loose body in the joint of a young adult. The present tendency is to emphasize the role of trauma in the etiology of this lesion.

Radiographic Features   In early cases it may be necessary to take several views of the joint in different degrees of obliquity in order to demonstrate the lesion adequately. Conventional topography is often helpful, and arthrography is sometimes useful.

When separation of the fragment is being established, one will see a radiolucent ring surrounding the bony fragment when viewed from the front; the loosening fragment may be seen opposite a pit in the bone when viewed in profile (Figs 3.24, 3.25). The loose fragments are usually small and ovoid in shape though they may be larger and irregular.

The fragment may become completely separated and form an intra-articular loose body. If entirely cartilaginous in content, the image of the loose body will not be seen on routine radiographs but it may be demonstrable by arthrography. If not removed surgically, the loose body may grow and calcify later; it is able to obtain adequate nourishment from synovial fluid even when it is completely detached from its parent bone. On the other hand, the

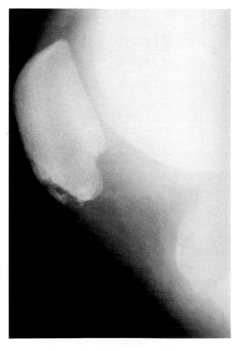

Fig. 3.21   Sinding–Larsen disease. A good plain film will demonstrate thickening of the ligamentum patellae origin, together with irregularity of the bone from which it originates. The lower pole seems irregular and lengthened. In later life, elongation of the patella inferiorly is probably the result of this disease in adolescence.

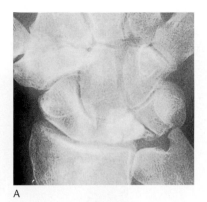
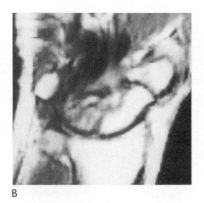

A   B

Fig. 3.23   A. Osteochondritis of the lunate bone (Kienbock's disease). **B.** Avascular necrosis of the lunate. On MR scanning the lunate shows a mixed signal, with patchy areas of low and high density. Compare with the normal signal coming from the scaphoid.

fragment may not become free, but may become absorbed leaving a residual gap in the underlying bone.

CT is, as elsewhere, a good imaging modality for showing cortical defects and loose bodies. The defects can thus be seen in the axial plane at the elbow and knee, and the appropriate coronal or sagittal reconstruction views obtained.

MR images are obtained in all planes. The vitality of the underlying bone can be confirmed, as well as the integrity of the overlying cartilage. A thin film of fluid, bright on T_2-weighted images, separates the dissected fragment from the underlying bone. STIR sequences will also show this feature as well as any bone edema.

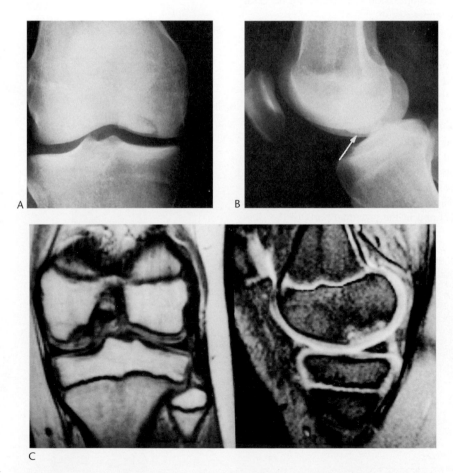

A   B

C

Fig. 3.24   A,B Osteochondritis dissecans of the medial femoral condyle. **C** T_1 coronal and sagittal fat suppression images of the knee demonstrating osteochondritis dissecans at a typical site. On the latter image, the defect is seen to contain fluid.

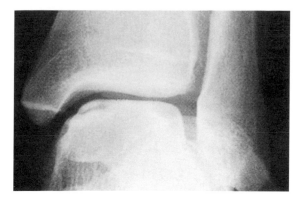

Fig. 3.25 Osteochondritis dissecans of the medial part of the articular surface of the talus.

Caisson Disease (synonym: *dysbaric osteonecrosis*)

Exposure to a hyperbaric atmosphere may result in decompression sickness—'the bends'—and in the late complication of osteonecrosis. The lesions are liable to appear if the worker is too rapidly decompressed. It is thought that nitrogen becomes liberated from bone marrow and causes bone infarcts by occluding small blood vessels.

A history of previous decompression sickness is not necessary for the occurrence of osteonecrosis.

Radiographic Findings

1. *Juxta-articular lesions*. They are recognized as:

   a. a transradiant subcortical band that may underlie as much as two-thirds of the articular cortex (Fig. 3.26)

   b. collapse of part of the articular cortex

   c. sequestration of part of the cortex

   d. secondary osteoarthritis.

2. *Neck and shaft lesions*. They cause the following appearances:

   a. Dense areas—small, multiple, bilateral, ill-defined opacities resembling bone islands in the upper ends of the femoral and humeral shafts and in the femoral neck.

   b. Irregular calcified areas—typically in the distal part of the femoral shafts (Fig. 3.27) and in the proximal parts of the shafts of the humeri and tibiae.

c. Malignant changes have occasionally been reported in such infarcts, usually in the form of *malignant fibrous histiocytoma* (Fig. 3.28).

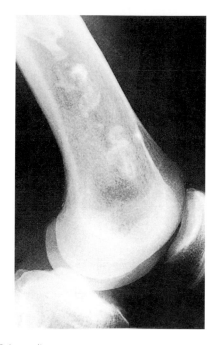

Fig. 3.27   Caisson disease.

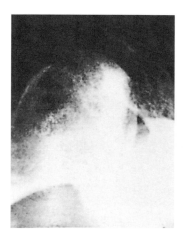

Fig. 3.26   Caisson disease. The humeral head shows a subcortical band of radiolucency with underlying sclerosis. The articular surface is collapsing.

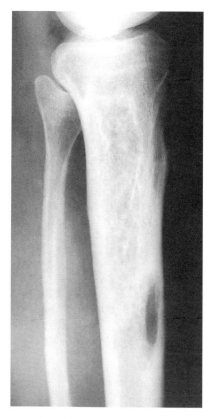

Fig. 3.28   Changes of medullary infarction are associated with an area of osteolysis due to fibrosarcoma.

Infantile Cortical Hyperostosis (eponym: *Caffey's disease*)

The cause of this disease is unknown. Many affected children have high fever, most have raised sedimentation rates and occasionally pleural exudates are found. However, an infective agent has never been identified. Occasionally, the disease has been reported in siblings, cousins and twins.

The condition has been diagnosed in utero. Usually, however, the babies are well for several weeks before the onset. The average age of onset is 9 weeks, and cases do not apparently start after the age of 5 months.

Three features common to all these patients are hyperirritability, soft-tissue swelling and bony cortical thickening. The soft-tissue swellings may be very painful, but are deeply situated and not accompanied by surface warmth or discoloration. Such swellings appear before bony changes are demonstrable and they disappear long before the bone lesions resolve. Sometimes the swellings may recur at their original site or new swellings may appear at other sites. The disease is characterized by the patchy distribution of the lesions and by remissions and relapses.

Bones commonly affected are the *mandible, ribs* (Fig. 3.29), *clavicle, scapula* and the *ulna*, but any tubular bones except the phalanges may be affected. The condition may also be found in the *skull* and *pelvis*, but not in the spine. Lesions are confined to the shafts of the bones, and the epiphyses and metaphyses are not affected. This distribution affords a ready differentiation from rickets, scurvy and congenital syphilis.

Radiologically, marked periosteal proliferation and cortical thickening are seen in bones beneath the soft-tissue swellings. The cortical hyperostosis may be massive. Patients usually recover after several weeks or months; in about 12 months, bones will usually have returned to normal.

Paget's Disease (synonym: *osteitis deformans*)

Sir James Paget first described this disease in 1876. Its origin is not definitely known. Nonetheless, current thinking is that a 'slow' virus may be the initiating factor. Though no virus has been isolated, histologic changes are seen that are present in viral infections.

There is variation in the distribution of the disease. It is common in the United Kingdom, parts of the United States, Australia and New Zealand, but uncommon in the Far and Middle East and Scandinavia. Within Britain, there appear to be some regional differences in the incidence.

The incidence of the disease as judged by pathological and radiological surveys is 3–4% of the population. Slightly more men are affected than women. Paget's disease is predominantly found in the elderly. Monostotic disease is not common (10–20%). Overall, the condition is found most commonly in the *sacrum* and *lumbar spine*, followed by the *skull*, *pelvis* and *femur*. Apart from the skull, the weight-bearing and persisting red marrow areas are most commonly involved, though multiple rib and upper limb lesions are uncommon. No bone is exempt. Lesions of the fibula are very rare.

The radiographic appearances are explained by the underlying pathological processes.

1. An initial phase of increased osteoclastic activity results in bone resorption. This early phase is osteolytic and is not commonly seen radiologically, still less in established disease. It may persist in the skull, as *osteoporosis circumscripta* (Fig. 3.30).

2. Mixed phase (spongy type with coarse, irregular trabeculation). Increased resorption of bone is followed by increased formation

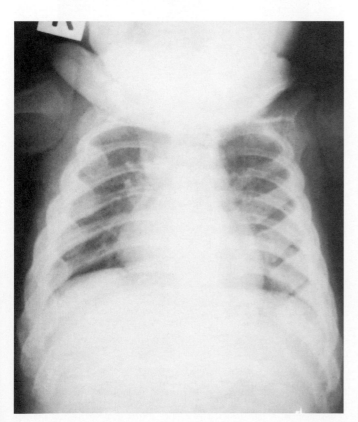

Fig. 3.29 Caffey's disease. Gross periostitis affects the ribs and the mandible is also thickened. (Courtesy of Dr Ann Barrington, Sheffield.)

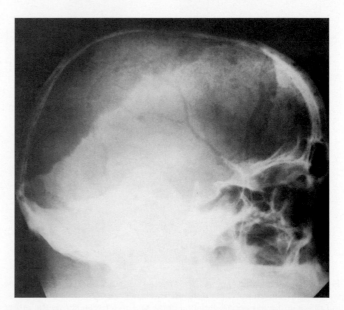

Fig. 3.30 Osteoporosis circumscripta. A well-defined osteolytic lesion affects most of the skull vault.

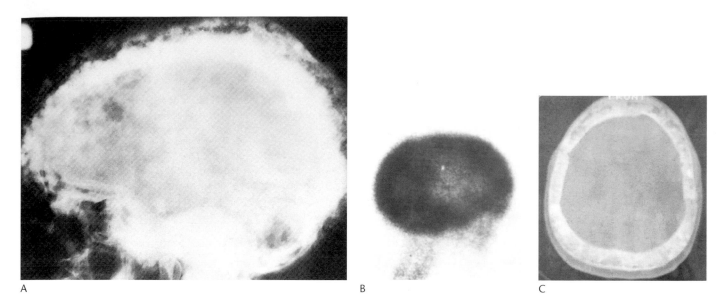

A   B   C

Fig. 3.31   Paget's disease of the skull. **A** Marked thickening of calvarium. Note the well-demarcated intracranial border of the inner table. Marked sclerosis of the base of the skull is also present. **B,C** Paget's disease demonstrated by radionuclide and CT scanning. The vault is thickened and there is increased isotope uptake.

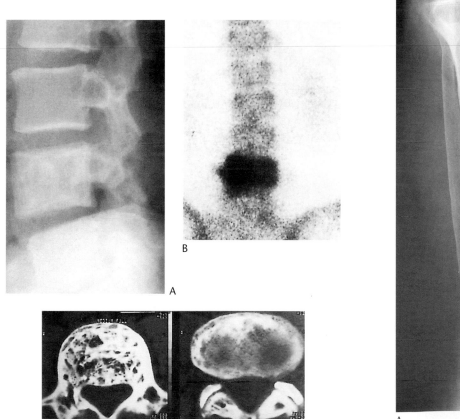

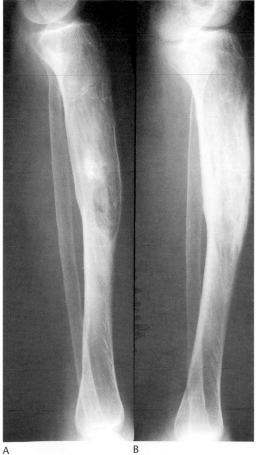

A   B

Fig. 3.32   Paget's disease. **A**. The affected vertebral body is expanded as well as showing abnormal texture. **B**. The bone scan confirms the increase in uptake in the expanded vertebral body. **C**. The CT scan shows the rather spongy texture of the abnormal body, extending into the pedicles and laminae.

Fig. 3.33   Paget's disease. **A**. The initial radiograph shows a zone of resorption due to active disease. The distal end of the process has a flame- or V-shape. **B**. A film taken a year later shows a mixed phase, perhaps proceeding on to quiescence in the same area. The lesion does not apparently reach the proximal articular surface of the tibia but, in this long bone, it does not always do so. It seems in this patient to be related to the fused growth plate for the tibial tuberosity.

of abnormally coarsened trabeculae of increased volume (Figs 3.31, 3.32). Haversian systems are destroyed and replaced by new bone with a characteristic mosaic pattern. The margin between cortex and medulla is lost.

3. Sclerotic phase (amorphous appearance). Osteoclastic activity declines and osteoblastic activity proceeds, so that disorganized new bone of increased density replaces lytic areas. Eventually the disease becomes quiescent.

Radiological Features

Long Bones Paget's disease starts at a bone end and, as it extends to the other bone end, it is demarcated from normal bone by a V-shaped zone of transition (Fig. 3.33).

Long bones increase in cortical width and the femur and tibia may be bowed. Bones also increase in length; this may result in bowing if only one of a pair of long bones is affected. Paget's disease may cause more bony enlargement than is seen in any other disease.

Pelvis In the early stages loss of some trabeculae with coarsening of those remaining may be seen. Thickening and loss of clarity of the ileopectineal line and the teardrop also indicate the disease. Narrowing of the hip joint space, especially in a medial direction, leads to protrusio with deformity of the pelvic brim. Secondary osteoarthritis then develops (Fig. 3.34).

Vertebrae All three forms of the disease may be found in the vertebrae. The neural arch and pedicles may be involved as well as the vertebral body, and all parts are enlarged. The width of the body is increased so that the interpedicular distance is also increased, even if the pedicles are enlarged. A characteristic, if infrequent, finding is a 'picture-frame' appearance with condensed, thickened end-plates and vertebral margins enclosing a cystic spongiosa (Fig. 3.35). The condensed end-plates are not seen with hemangiomas and involvement of posterior elements is also less common. Enlargement is unusual in both hemangiomas and metastatic disease.

Collapse is common and may cause spinal nerve compression. Vertebral enlargement distinguishes this from osteoporotic or malignant disease.

Skull In the skull, the disease begins as a destructive process affecting the outer table and sparing the inner table (Fig. 3.30). The full picture of osteoporosis circumscripta is rarely seen. In the reparative stage, sclerosis of the inner table is pronounced, and later the diploic spaces and the outer table become thickened. A classic, widespread 'cottonwool' effect results (Fig 3.31A). The cranial cavity is not encroached upon.

Dental abnormalities include loss of lamina dura and hypercementosis (see Ch. 50).

Radionuclide Bone Scanning is of value during early activity, when it will pick up lesions which may not be radiologically detectable, while in the quiescent phase the presence of disease is best shown by conventional means. The total body scan detects disease in sites not routinely examined, such as the foot, but such sites are not commonly affected. The scan does however provide a quick overview of the skeleton and is useful in assessing change or malignant degeneration, so that follow-up is probably best performed by scanning (Fig. 3.36).

Computed Tomography Because changes are in mineralized tissue, they are well reflected at CT scanning. Bone resorption, expansion, cysts or sclerosis are seen. Lesions in long bones are more easily imaged on plain films, but lesions of the skull involving optic foramina and the middle ear are well shown on CT scans. 3-D reconstruction in particular can show skull deformity, but is generally of value only if reconstructive surgery is contemplated.

MRI Because the changes of Paget's disease vary with the stage of the disease, and because these are so well recognized on plain films, MRI is probably better used to assess the complications of Paget's disease related to bone expansion (Fig. 3.37) and subsequent relation to compromised soft tissues, e.g. nerves, and fractures.

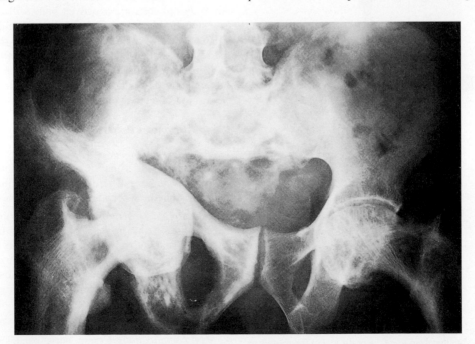

Fig. 3.34 Pelvis in Paget's disease. There is a combination of spongy and amorphous bone. Note the striated appearance of the left femoral head and neck. Marked deformity of the pelvic inlet and acetabular protrusion on the right are shown. There is enlargement of the right pubis and ischium.

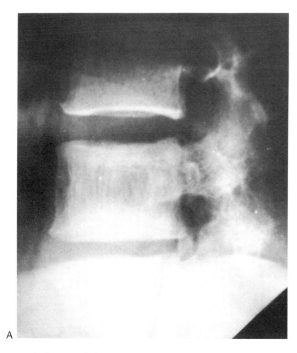

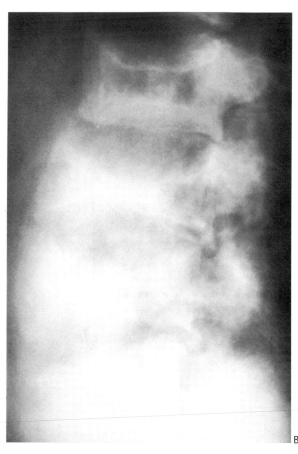

Fig. 3.35 Paget's disease of the spine. **A**. Picture-frame appearance in a vertebral body. The appendages are also enlarged. **B**. Vertebral collapse and *expansion* together with abnormal bone texture in another patient.

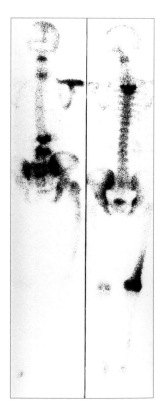

Fig. 3.36 Radio-isotope bone scan (anterior and posterior scans) in Paget's disease showing multifocal areas of increase in uptake related to active disease.

Malignant degeneration and expansion into soft tissues are especially well demonstrated.

With uncomplicated disease, the bone is seen to be expanded. An excess of sclerotic or woven bone will be seen as an area of low signal with thickened, irregular trabeculae interspersed with fat. Cortical thickening is especially well shown. Hypervascular tissue in expanded bone might suggest malignant change in this age group. Soft-tissue change would occur with fractures or sarcomatous degeneration. Correlation with plain films is thus always indicated to avoid erroneous diagnosis.

Complications of Paget's Disease

1. *Marginal (incremental) or incomplete transverse fractures.* These fractures are usually found on the thickened convex surface of the bowed bone where they may be multiple. Occasionally, such a fracture may become complete (see below).

2. *Pathological fractures* are the commonest complication of Paget's disease and are most often seen in the early stages of the disease. Usually transverse, they are more common in women. Often multiple, they are most common in the upper femur and upper tibia. Healing is poorer in Paget's disease than in normal bone. Sarcoma may follow a pathological fracture. Bone may also be avulsed at sites of muscle insertions.

3. *Osteoarthritis* occurs at major joints (see above).

4. *Skull complications.* Cranial nerve palsies result when foramina are encroached upon. Vascular compromise also causes blindness.

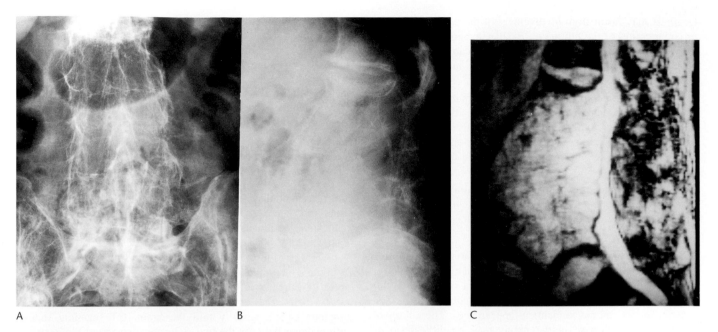

A   B   C

Fig. 3.37 Paget's disease. **A,B** The radiographs show three expanded and apparently fused vertebral bodies in the lumbar spine. They are demineralized. The appearances are those of a highly vascular form of Paget's disease in an active phase. **C**. The MR scan confirms the presence of expansion and fusion with encroachment upon the canal, and confirms the presence of vascularity.

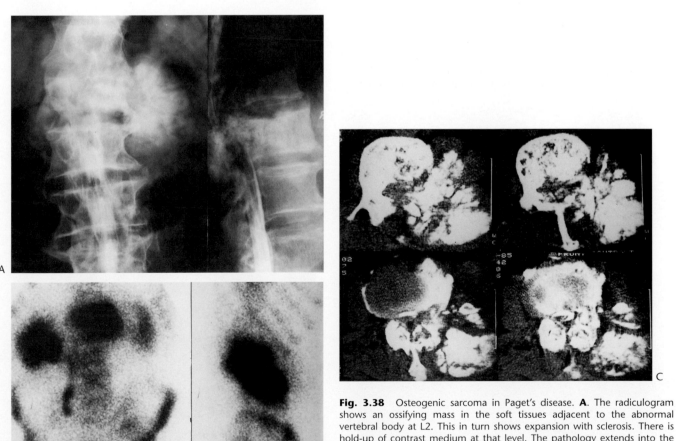

Fig. 3.38 Osteogenic sarcoma in Paget's disease. **A**. The radiculogram shows an ossifying mass in the soft tissues adjacent to the abnormal vertebral body at L2. This in turn shows expansion with sclerosis. There is hold-up of contrast medium at that level. The pathology extends into the neural arch. **B**. The radio-isotope bone scan confirms the presence of change at this level and also shows ureteric obstruction, presumably by pathologically enlarged lymph nodes in the pelvis. **C**. The CT scan confirms the presence of sclerotic Paget's disease within the vertebral body but also demonstrates the ossifying sarcomatous mass in the soft tissues. The canal is encroached upon. (Courtesy of Dr K. Walmsley.)

Deafness may result from involvement of the ossicles or cochlea or compression of the 8th nerve. Basilar invagination may cause brainstem compression. CSF obstruction can lead to hydrocephalus. Stretching of vertebral arteries may give rise to vertebrobasilar insufficiency.

5. *Cardiovascular complications.* Cardiac output is increased and, if much of the skeleton is actively involved, cardiomegaly, cardiac ischemia and high output failure may result. Systemic hypertension and calcification of the media of the arteries also result, not purely due to age but related to the extent of the disease and its activity.

6. *Malignant degeneration.* Osteogenic sarcoma and, to a lesser extent, fibrosarcoma, chondrosarcoma and malignant fibrous histiocytoma may arise as complications of Paget's disease (Fig. 3.38) (see Ch. 5).

Differential Diagnosis   Most difficulties arise in monostotic cases. Sometimes a full bone survey will reveal evidence of Paget's disease elsewhere. A solitary dense vertebra or *vertebra nigra* may cause diagnostic difficulties because *osteoblastic metastases* and *reticuloses* can cause identical appearances. The amorphous type of Paget's disease in the pelvis may be difficult to differentiate from *prostatic secondaries*, especially if little bone enlargement is evident. Elevation of the serum acid phosphatase will be found in the latter lesion.

An *angioma* of a vertebral body may resemble Paget's disease, but an angioma will not produce the typical widening of the bone seen in Paget's disease. The remaining trabeculae in an angioma are well-defined and are surrounded by (vascular) marrow. Angiomas, especially affecting only part of the body, are commonly seen at MRI and should not be confused with malignant tumors.

Leontiasis Ossea

This term is used in two senses: *specifically* for an isolated progressive sclerosing hyperostosis of the skull, and *descriptively* when diseases such as Paget's disease and fibrous dysplasia affect the skull and facial bones. Whether or not the condition is ever a specific entity is debatable. It could well be that the isolated lesion is really a form of fibrous dysplasia.

Tuberous Sclerosis (synonym: *epiloia*; eponyms: *von Recklinghausen* (1862), *Bourneville* (1880))

The classic clinical manifestations are a triad of epilepsy, mental retardation and adenoma sebaceum. The disease is inherited as an autosomal dominant condition but most cases are sporadic. Pathologically, hamartomas are formed in many of the body tissues —brain, eyes, lungs, kidneys and gastrointestinal tract.

In the skeleton, the commonest finding is that of poorly defined areas of sclerosis, affecting the skull, spine and pelvis. In the *skull*, woolly areas of density may be due to osteosclerosis, or to tuberous calcifications within the brain. CT scanning rapidly differentiates between the two. Sclerosis also affects the *vertebral*

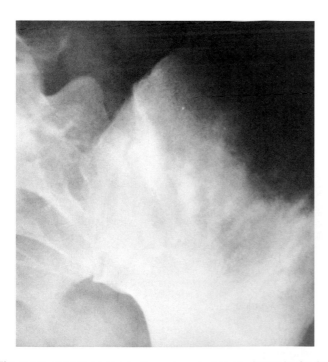

Fig. 3.39   Tuberous sclerosis. Flame-shaped areas of sclerosis in the iliac blades.

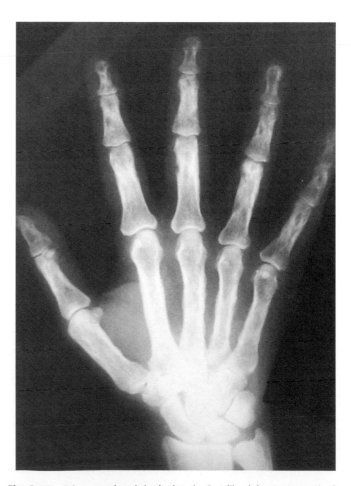

Fig. 3.40   Tuberous sclerosis in the hands. Cyst-like defects are seen in the bones, both beneath the fingernails and more proximally. Cortical defects and periostitis are also present.

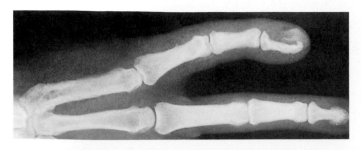

bodies. In the *pelvis*, the iliac blades are the sites of flame-shaped densities which do not resemble metastases (Fig. 3.39), or more nodular densities which do simulate malignancy.

Periostitis may be found on long bones, metatarsals and, to a lesser extent, metacarpals. In the *hands*, rather than the feet, cysts occur in phalanges (Fig. 3.40). These may be related to subungual fibromas and are well demarcated (Fig. 3.41).

Fig. 3.41 Tuberous sclerosis. Note periosteal thickening of fifth metacarpal, cysts in head of proximal phalanx and pressure erosion of distal phalanx by subungual tumor. (Courtesy of Dr L. Langton.)

REFERENCES AND SUGGESTIONS FOR FURTHER READING

Aichroth, P. (1971) Osteochondritis dissecans of the knee—a clinical survey. *Journal of Bone and Joint Surgery*, **55B**, 440–447.

Berquist, T. H. (ed.) (1995) *MRI of the musculoskeletal system*, 3rd edn. New York: Raven Press.

Bush, B. H., Bramson, R. T., Ogden, J. A. (1988) Legg–Calvé–Perthes' disease: detection of cartilaginous and synovial changes with MR imaging. *Radiology*, **167**, 473–476.

Catterall, A. (1971) The natural history of Perthes' disease. *Journal of Bone and Joint Surgery*, **53B**, 37–53.

Catterall, A. (1982) *Legg–Calvé–Perthes' Disease*. Edinburgh: Churchill Livingstone.

Davidson, J. K. (ed.) (1975) *Aseptic Necrosis of Bone*. Amsterdam: Excerpta Medica.

Ficat, R. F. (1983) Treatment of avascular necrosis of the femoral head. *Hip*, **2**, 279–295.

Fisher, R. L., Roderique, J. W., Brown, D. C., Danigelis, J. A., Ozonoff, M. B.,

Sziklas, J. J. (1980) The relationship of isotopic bone imaging guiding the prognosis in Legg–Perthes' disease. *Clinical Orthopaedics*, **150**, 23–29.

Hamdy, R. C. (1981) *Paget's Disease of Bone*. New York: Praeger.

Markisz, J. A., Knowles, R. J. R, Altchek, D. W., Schneider, R., Whalen, J. P., Cahill, P. T. (1987) Segmental patterns of avascular necrosis of the femoral heads: early detection with MR imaging. *Radiology*, **162**, 717–720.

Mitchell, M. D., Kunkel, H. L., Steinberg, M. E., Kressel, H. Y., Alavi, A., Axel, L. (1986) Avascular necrosis of the hip: comparison of MR, CT and scintigraphy. *American Journal of Roentgenology*, **147**, 67–71.

Murray, R. O., Jacobson, H. G., Stoker, D. J. (1990) *The Radiology of Skeletal Disorders*, 3rd edn. Edinburgh: Churchill Livingstone.

Resnick, D., Niwayama, G. (1995) *Diagnosis of Bone and Joint Disorders*, 3rd edn. Philadelphia: Saunders.

Ryan, P. J., Fogelman, I. (1994) The role of nuclear medicine in orthopaedics. *Nuclear Medicine Communications*, **15**, 341–360.

4

DISEASES OF JOINTS

Peter Renton

RHEUMATOID ARTHRITIS

This disease is seen at all ages, but especially from 20–55 years, with smaller peaks in childhood and in the elderly. Women are more commonly affected (M:F = 1:3).

The joints most typically involved are the small joints, especially the metatarsophalangeal and metacarpophalangeal and carpal joints, but any joint, including the temporomandibular and cricoarytenoid, may be affected. The axial skeleton is later and less often affected, with the exception of the cervical spine. Sites of ligamentous and tendinous insertions (entheses) are also infrequently involved. The tendency at the peripheral joints is to symmetry, and often identical digits on either side of the body are affected. Asymmetry of distribution may follow unilateral paralysis or weakness, when under-utilization of a limb may prevent the onset of rheumatoid disease in that limb. Conversely, asymmetry may follow overuse of a limb which often is more severely involved. This is seen especially in men and in those performing heavy manual work. In general, excess physical activity leads to more severe forms of joint disease.

Radiological Findings

The Plain Film

Joint changes may be summarized as follows:

1. Soft-tissue changes
2. Osteoporosis
3. Joint space changes and alignment deformities
4. Periostitis
5. Erosions
6. Secondary osteoarthritis.

Changes 1, 2, 4 and 5 may be seen at entheses, that is, metabolically active sites of ligamentous and tendinous insertions into bone. Rheumatoid arthritis is a systemic disease, and other body systems may be involved, e.g. lung parenchyma and pleura.

1. Soft-tissue Changes These changes are best assessed clinically but may also be shown radiologically in the hand (Fig. 4.1), knee or foot and other joints. Soft-tissue swelling is due to edema of periarticular tissues and to synovial inflammation in bursae, joint spaces and along tendon sheaths. Joint distension also follows an increase in synovial fluid.

In the hand, fusiform swelling due to capsular distension and local edema may be seen over interphalangeal and metacarpophalangeal joints, especially the first, second and fifth. Soft-tissue swelling over the third and fourth metacarpophalangeal joints is seen as a local increase in density and occasionally as a soft-tissue projection into adjacent web spaces. Soft-tissue swelling over the ulnar styloid can be due to local involvement of the extensor carpi ulnaris tendon sheath. Changes at the radial styloid are related to local radiocarpal joint synovial hypertrophy.

Soft-tissue changes are less well demonstrated in the foot. Changes over the first and fifth metacarpophalangeal joints reflect synovitis in the bursae over the first and fifth metatarsal heads, but swelling over the remaining metatarsophalangeal joints may be seen as fusiform increases in density.

The Achilles tendon inserts into the back of the calcaneus below its upper margin. It is sharply demarcated anteriorly by the pre-Achilles fat pad and, more inferiorly, by the retrocalcaneal bursa. Local synovitis thickens the bursa and edema obliterates the fat and blurs out the tendon, which also thickens (Fig. 4.2). Similar changes occur inferiorly, at the plantar fascial origin at the base of the calcaneus.

Distension of the capsule of the knee joint is shown on the anteroposterior radiograph as a lateral bulging of the normally poorly seen fat lines over the distal femur. On a lateral view of the knee the suprapatellar pouch is distended and its surrounding fat lines blurred. Posteriorly, a distended joint capsule may give a local increase in density and in this way a Baker cyst is often identified. This can be confirmed by ultrasound or arthrography.

On the lateral view of the elbow, the anterior and posterior fat planes are displaced in a direction vertical to the long axis of the joint, but may be obliterated by local edema.

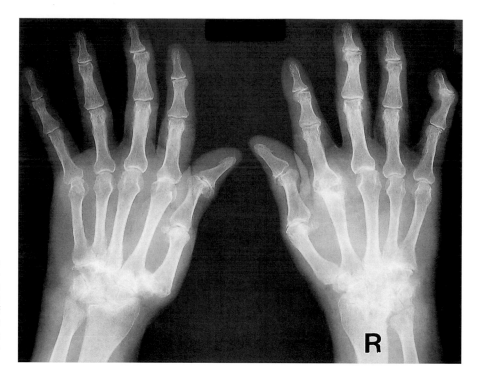

Fig. 4.1 Rheumatoid arthritis. Bilateral changes are fairly symmetric. Soft-tissue swelling is demonstrated, especially over the ulnar styloids. Erosions are demonstrated at the carpus, distal radius and ulna, with joint space narrowing and collapse of bone. Metacarpophalangeal erosions are also seen associated with joint space narrowing. There is a swan-neck deformity of the right fifth distal interphalangeal joint.

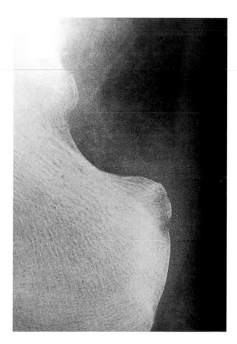

Fig. 4.2 Retrocalcaneal bursitis in association with thickening of the tendo Achilles and a retrocalcaneal erosion. A soft-tissue mass is demonstrated in the angle normally filled by fat between the insertion of the tendon and the upper calcaneus.

Swelling around an affected joint is symmetric, while in gout the swelling is eccentric. In rheumatoid arthritis, however, a rheumatoid nodule may cause a localized eccentric swelling, and these often occur at pressure points.

2. Osteoporosis   Assessment of osteoporosis depends in part on film quality, and comparison between normal and abnormal joints

in the same patient may be helpful. Interpretation is subjective and changes are seen only after loss of 25–50% of mineral. Differences in assessment of osteoporosis may exist, both between different observers and between the same observer at different times.

Osteoporosis in rheumatoid arthritis is of two types:

Generalized   This may be due to steroids or limitation of movement due to pain, or muscle wasting. This type is uncommon and occurs late in the course of the disease. It may also reflect coincidental bone loss in post-menopausal women, commonly affected by this disorder.

Local osteoporosis around joints occurs earlier and is due to synovial inflammation and hyperemia.

Osteoporosis increases in incidence with the duration of the disease and the age of the patient. Some 30% of patients show it at presentation but, two years after, 80% are affected.

Osteoporosis is a precursor of erosive disease and may mask early erosions. Generalized or solitary *sclerosis* of one or more distal phalanges (terminal phalangeal sclerosis) is often rendered more prominent because of osteoporosis elsewhere. This occurs in some 35% of patients with rheumatoid arthritis and other arthropathies and may be present before any other abnormality. In a woman, especially, it may prognosticate future disease, but is seen in some normal patients.

3. Joint Space Changes and Alignment Deformities   In the early stage a joint space may be widened by synovial hypertrophy and an effusion. Later in the disease, joint spaces narrow due to cartilage destruction by pannus (Fig. 4.3). Narrowing of joint spaces may, however, be apparent rather than real in the presence of flexion deformities, so that an oblique view is needed to assess the space. Alignment abnormalities at joints may result from local synovitis weakening the capsule and tendinitis preventing normal

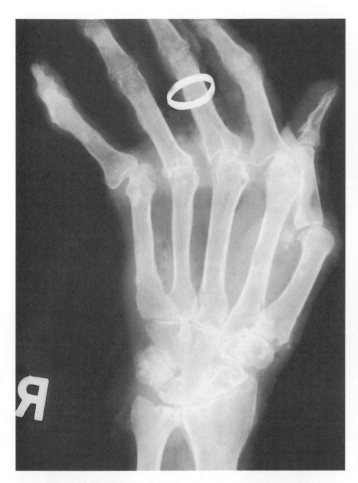

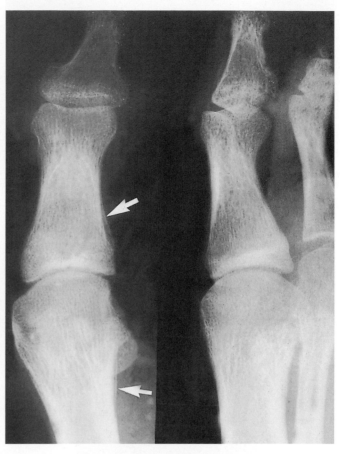

Fig. 4.3 Gross rheumatoid arthritis at the carpus with ulnar deviation, subluxation and joint narrowing at the metacarpophalangeal joints. Boutonnière deformities are present at the index and little fingers.

Fig. 4.4 Rheumatoid arthritis with narrowing of the metatarsophalangeal joint of the great toe and a fine periostitis on the adjacent shafts (arrows).

musculotendinous action. Tendons may also rupture in the region of roughened bone. Thus, rotator cuff tears allow upward subluxation of the eroded humeral head.

The classic changes of alignment in the rheumatoid hand are irreversible. Subluxations at metacarpophalangeal joints lead to ulnar deviation (Fig. 4.3) which occurs in up to 50% of those with chronic disease. This is also associated with increasing palmar flexion. This change may result from ulnar deviation of extensor tendons.

The boutonnière deformity (Fig. 4.3) results from proximal interphalangeal joint flexion and distal interphalangeal joint extension, and the swan-neck deformity from the reverse (proximal interphalangeal joint extension and distal interphalangeal joint flexion). The boutonnière deformity is the more common.

Similarly, lateral deviation of the toes may be found. Hallux valgus is especially common. The hallux sesamoids sublux between the first and second metatarsal heads and the transverse arch flattens as local inflammation causes ligamentous laxity.

4. Periostitis Local periosteal reactions occur either along the midshaft of a phalanx of metacarpal as a reaction to local tendinitis, or at the metaphysis near a joint affected by synovitis. Such changes are less common in rheumatoid arthritis than in the seronegative arthropathies. They are difficult to identify, may be

mistaken for lumbrical impressions, and are commoner in the feet (Fig. 4.4). Periostitis in the form of fluffy calcaneal spurs, plantar and posterior, is also less common in rheumatoid arthritis than in the seronegative arthropathies (Fig. 4.5). When present, they are larger and more irregular than the normal small well-corticated spurs of the elderly. Spurs may arise ab initio or may follow healing of erosions.

5. Erosions These are the most important diagnostic change but are not necessarily present when the patient first attends. Their incidence rises from less than 40% of patients at three months to up to 90% or 95% at ten years.

Classic periarticular erosions occur at the so-called 'bare areas' of bone between the edge of the articular cartilage and the attachment of the joint capsule (Fig. 4.6).

Erosions in rheumatoid arthritis should be sought for at the common sites. Supplementary views, such as the Norgaard 'ball-catcher' (supine 25° oblique view), may be needed. Erosions appear earlier and are more often seen in the feet, 90% of which will eventually be affected, than in the hands (75%), and most often at the fifth metacarpophalangeal joint. The hallux metacarpophalangeal is the least often involved. Erosions affect typically the lateral side of the fifth metatarsal but the medial side of the others.

The metatarsal head erodes before the base of the distal phalanx.

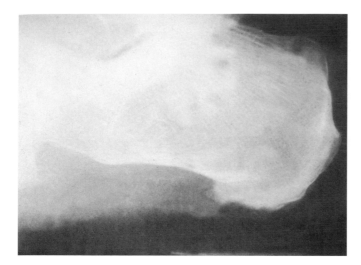

Fig. 4.5 Irregularity and erosion in the region of the plantar spur distinguishes this painful lesion from the normal benign spur, which is seen in around 20% of the population.

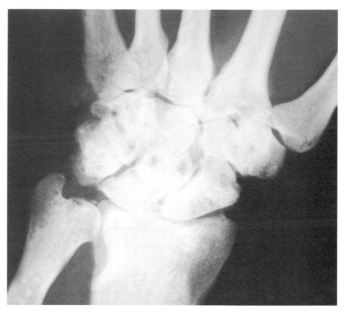

Fig. 4.7 Rheumatoid arthritis. Apart from the carpal changes, there are also erosions at the distal radio-ulnar joint, proximal to the triangular cartilage at the distal ulna, and at the ulnar styloid tip.

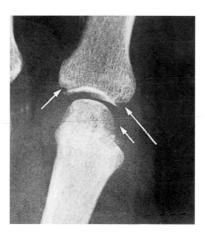

Fig. 4.6 Early rheumatoid arthritis showing marginal erosions (arrows).

In the hand, the second and third metacarpophalangeal joints are the earliest affected, initially on the radial aspects. More distal erosions are inconstant. Erosions occur at the ulnar styloid, at the radial styloid and at the proximal compartment of the distal radio-ulnar joint (Fig. 4.7). Carpal erosions occur throughout the wrist. An erosion is, for example, commonly seen on the lateral scaphoid at its waist. Carpal disease may be followed by fusion, but this is uncommon elsewhere in adult rheumatoid arthritis. On occasion, massive carpal destruction may be found in the presence of virtually normal peripheral joints.

Tarsal erosions, other than at the posterior and inferior surfaces of the calcaneus, are uncommon and are also less common in rheumatoid arthritis than in the seronegative spondyloarthropathies (Fig. 4.8). In rheumatoid arthritis, erosions are usually seen at or above the insertion of the tendo-Achilles into the back of the calcaneus.

Erosions are first seen as an area of local demineralization beneath the cortex which eventually vanishes, leaving irregular underlying trabeculae. The destroyed area increases in size and, as pannus spreads over articular surfaces, the entire articular

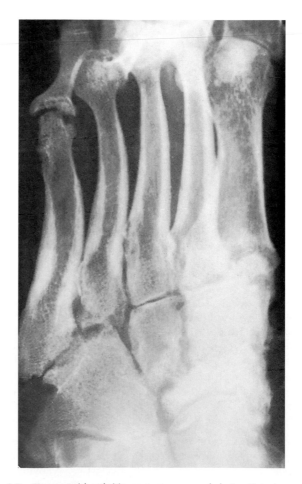

Fig. 4.8 Rheumatoid arthritis—very pronounced destructive changes in the tarsus and in metatarsal heads.

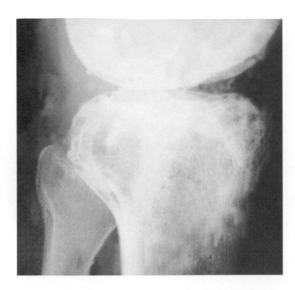

Fig. 4.9 A large cyst is seen beneath the articular surface of the tibia—rheumatoid arthritis.

eroded (as opposed to the superior in osteoarthritis). Muscle pull on adjacent irregular articular surfaces leads to medial migration of the femoral head and acetabular resorption, causing protrusio acetabuli. This is classic, but not pathognomonic of rheumatoid arthritis, as it also occurs in osteoarthritis, in conditions with bone softening, and in an idiopathic inherited form. Gross loss of bone, especially at the femoral head, may result in a 'bird's beak' appearance (Fig. 4.10). Marked loss of bone around articular surfaces is also common at the elbow (Fig. 4.11) and shoulder, and deformities of alignment follow. Bone loss at the acromioclavicular joint may often be seen on a chest radiograph, with pointing of adjacent bone ends and scalloping of the under-surface of the acromion (Fig. 4.12). Erosions of the superior aspects of the upper ribs are seen in patients with longstanding disease and muscle wasting, and are probably due to the adjacent scapula rubbing on the rib.

cortex may be destroyed, leaving a pointed bone end. Chronic trauma, in weight-bearing or due to abnormal tendon alignment, may further collapse articular surfaces. Steroids and analgesics also modify the disease so that neuropathic-type destructive changes may result. Healing rarely reverses erosions and so it is not often that a normal appearance returns. Usually the margins of healed erosions become corticated and they do not enlarge on follow-up.

Erosive change is less common at the larger joints but often bone destruction is greater owing to the greater stresses placed on knees, elbows and shoulders. On occasion, intraosseous defects—*cysts* or *geodes*—up to 2–3 cm in diameter, may be seen beneath joint surfaces (Fig. 4.9). An alternative form of change at large articular surfaces is a superficial surface irregularity with a little reactive sclerosis in the presence of much joint narrowing. This change is seen at the elbow, knee and hip. In the hip joint it is characteristically the medial joint space which is narrowed and

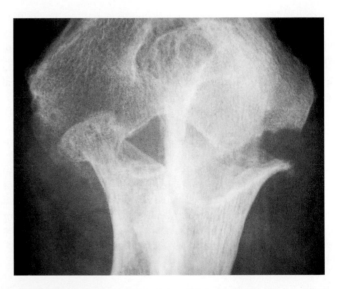

Fig. 4.11 Rheumatoid arthritis of the elbow showing marked resorption of all the articular surfaces with marginal erosions, especially well seen at the radial neck and trochlea.

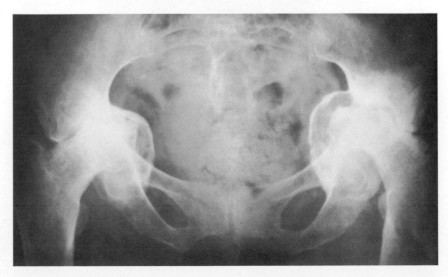

Fig. 4.10 Rheumatoid arthritis—extreme protrusio with medial migration and erosion of the femoral heads. Compare this film with Fig. 4.50B (protrusio in osteoarthritis).

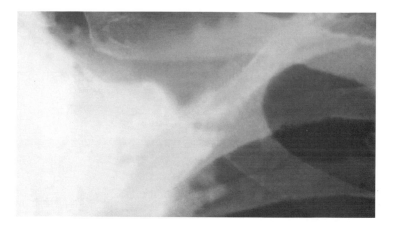

Fig. 4.12 Widening of the right acromioclavicular joint with well-demarcated margins distinguishes rheumatoid arthritis from hyperparathyroidism. The erosion of the third and fourth ribs superiorly may be seen in both conditions.

Rheumatoid Changes in the Axial Skeleton

Sacroiliac Joints   Changes are less common and less severe than in seronegative disease but may be seen in up to 30% of those with longstanding disease. The changes are more common in women (cf. ankylosing spondylitis) and rarely end in fusion.

Spinal Changes   Rheumatoid changes are common in the cervical spine but uncommon in the thoracic and lumbar regions.

Osteoporosis, disk narrowing and end-plate irregularity are seen with only a little reactive new bone formation at the *upper* cervical vertebrae. Osteoarthritis, in distinction, is seen more inferiorly. Facet joint erosions may result in subluxation (Fig. 4.13), so that nerve entrapment follows. Subluxation and erosion also occur at the synovial joint between the odontoid peg and arch of atlas (Fig. 4.14), and are potentiated by laxity of ligaments around the peg. Separation in flexion of more than 2.5 mm in adults or 5 mm in children is held to be abnormal. This instability can be seen in up to 30% of patients with chronic rheumatoid arthritis. The eroded odontoid may also fracture.

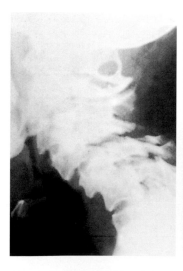
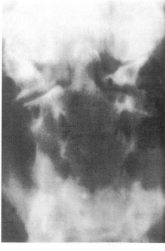

Fig. 4.13 Rheumatoid arthritis of the cervical spine—gross bizarre destruction. Subluxation of C4 on C5 and of C5 on C6 is seen. Note gross destruction in the spinous processes and posterior arches.

Fig. 4.14 Rheumatoid arthritis of cervical spine—tomographic section showing erosions of the left atlanto-axial articulation. Similar changes affect the right side and also the occipito-atlanto joints and the odontoid peg.

Resorption of bone at non-articular surfaces occurs in the cervical spine at the spinous processes, which become short, sharp and tapered in patients with chronic disease (Fig. 4.13).

6. Secondary Osteoarthritis   Weight-bearing joints affected by rheumatoid arthritis often develop secondary osteoarthritis. Indeed, at the hips, osteoarthritic change may be superimposed on a previously unrecognized rheumatoid arthritis. Reactive sclerosis and new bone formation in osteoarthritis is not marked in those whose underlying disease has characteristic features of osteoporosis and bone destruction.

Arthrography

Following joint aspiration a single or double air-contrast technique can be used to demonstrate the status of synovium, cartilage and bone. Synovial proliferation and irregularity may be present in a distended capsule. Marginal and articular cartilage loss can be confirmed. Loose bodies are shown in the joint. Cysts or geodes may fill with contrast (Fig. 4.15).

The technique is now infrequently employed, but rupture of the capsule or a Baker cyst shows leak of contrast into adjacent muscles. Here, the pain may simulate a deep vein thrombosis. Arthrography confirms the leak; ultrasound can be used to show either a deep vein thrombosis or a normal vein which may be displaced by a large cyst. MRI of course shows the cyst and leak (Fig. 4.16).

CT Scanning

In the axial plane CT can be used to demonstrate erosions with considerable clarity, especially in the carpus and tarsus, and to show joint space narrowing and erosive change. New bone around joints and disks is especially well shown with CT, as is joint fusion.

Radionuclide Scanning

^{99m}Tc phosphate images show increased blood flow to synovium in the early or blood-pool phase of the scan; on delayed image obtained at 3 hours, increased uptake is shown at sites of increased bone turnover. Isotope scanning is highly sensitive in the arthritides but shows poor specificity for individual diseases, relying on distribution of abnormal foci to make a specific diagnosis (Fig. 4.17). In rheumatoid disease, isotopes are at least 70% more sensitive than conventional films and also are a good

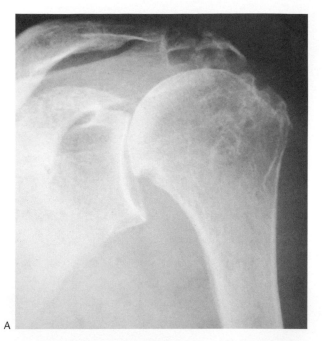
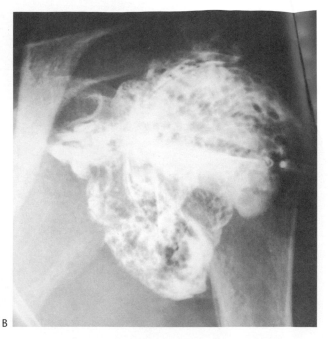

A B

Fig. 4.15 Rheumatoid arthritis. **A**. Erosions and upward subluxation of the humeral head. **B**. Arthrogram showing numerous 'millet seeds' floating freely within the joint. There is also a rotator cuff tear.

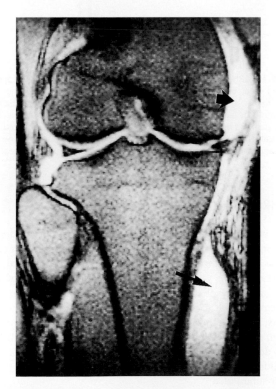

Fig. 4.16 A large effusion is demonstrated in the joint as well as a medially directed cyst which extends down distally to the upper midshaft tibia (arrows). There is in addition extensive edema in the soft tissues external to the joint.

prognosticator for subsequent erosions. Inactive erosions may be negative at phosphate scanning. Spatial discrimination is improved by the use of SPECT (single photon emission computed tomography).

Periosteal reactions show up as a generalized increase in uptake and thickening of the cortical image.

Ultrasound

Bone is refractory to sound waves, and structures deep in joints cannot be imaged. Synovial margins can be seen, as can superficial tendons and ligaments. Ultrasound can be used to show:

- The capsule, synovium, effusions and loose bodies
- Surrounding ligaments and tendons
- Leaks of synovium into muscles, e.g. a ruptured Baker cyst
- Tears and tumors in muscle.

Magnetic Resonance Imaging

Using MRI, synovium, synovial fluid, cartilage, ligaments, tendon and bone can all be identified.

Erosions are seen earlier and more often at MRI than on plain films and are seen as marginal low-signal defects in bone. Pannus is seen as a soft-tissue signal mass adjacent to the erosion. When synovial proliferation is vascular, it is even better demonstrated after the use of intravenous gadolinium.

MR is not only sensitive (as is isotope scanning) but also specific (unlike scanning). MR is superior in showing not only erosions but also subarticular cysts and bone edema. Effusions and tendinous change as well as extra-articular collections of fluid are seen with MR so that, where available, this is the investigation of choice in the initial diagnosis of disease and its progression (Fig. 4.18). MRI is also superior to any other modality in demonstrating cartilage loss in both osteoarthritis and rheumatoid disease.

Changes in the tendo Achilles and its insertion into the hind foot are better seen at MR than on plain films (Fig. 4.2). The

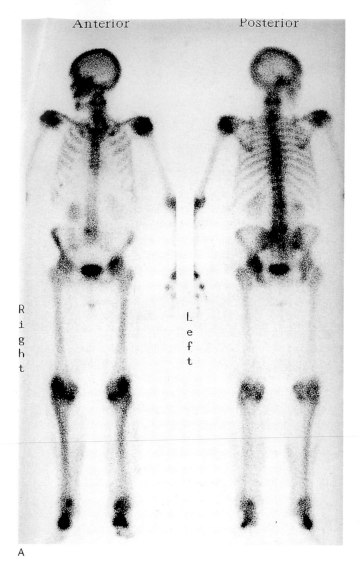

A

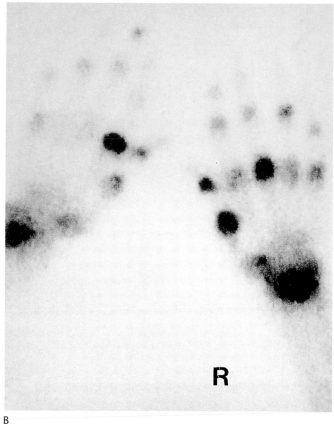

B

Fig. 4.17 Rheumatoid arthritis. **A**. Whole body radio-isotope scan showing areas of increase in uptake in the neck, both shoulder joints, the elbow joints, the left hip, both knees and ankles in a patient with rheumatoid disease. The distribution of disease is shown, but the changes on this scan are not specific. (Courtesy of Dr A. Hilson.) **B**. Localized images of the hands showing changes of a more specific distribution. (Courtesy of Dr A. Saifuddin.)

tendon is of low signal and stands out clearly against the fat which surrounds it. In tendinitis, the tendon is thickened, often grossly so, and is surrounded by (bright-signaled) edema. Central areas of cystic necrosis in this or any other tendon are always bright on T_2-weighted or STIR sequence images. Erosions in the insertion are seen as cortical defects, often with surrounding local edema. The enlarged retrocalcaneal bursa is also clearly demonstrated at MRI (Fig. 4.19).

C1/C2 Lesions

Changes at C1 and C2 were better shown by linear tomography than on conventional plain films and, subsequently, by CT in both the axial plane and with sagittal and coronal reconstruction. Opacification of the CSF renders both the cord and soft-tissue masses visible and allows change in flexion and extension to be visualized during the examination (Fig. 4.20).

MRI is now the investigation of choice for imaging the craniocervical junction, and the status of the cord can be assessed simultaneously (Fig. 4.21). Bone, pannus, cord and CSF are all simultaneously imaged. Changes in flexion and extension also assessed, but are equally well seen on a plain film.

ARTHRITIS IN CHILDREN

There are many causes of polyarthritis in children, the most common being viral infections. It is now recognized that chronic childhood polyarthritis is a heterogeneous group of disorders, the generic term for which is '*juvenile chronic polyarthritis*' (Table 4.1). Some 10% of the total eventually have a *seropositive* form of disease similar to, or identical with, adult rheumatoid arthritis, that is, an essentially peripheral erosive polyarthritis. The remaining patients have *seronegative* juvenile chronic arthritis for which definite clinical and histologic diagnostic criteria exist.

Children with seronegative juvenile chronic arthritis may be further subdivided:

1. *Acute systemic onset type* (true Still's disease) with constitutional symptoms and hepatosplenomegaly, but little or no joint involvement.

2. *Pauci-articular* (not more than four joints involved) affecting especially the knees, wrists and ankles. This usually ends up as:

3. *Polyarticular disease*, which may also present at the onset. Radiological changes are late and the disease is non-erosive.

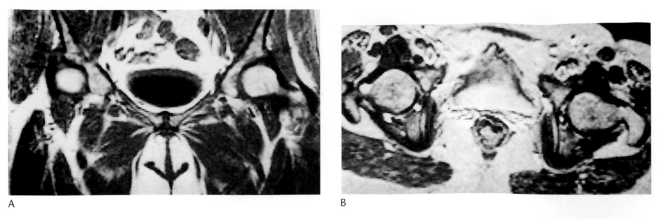

A   B

Fig. 4.18   Rheumatoid arthritis. **A**. Coronal T$_1$-weighted image. Erosive change at the acetabular margin, especially superiorly on the right, with synovial thickening seen as an intermediate signal soft-tissue mass with adjacent bony erosion. **B**. The axial image shows a small effusion in the joint.

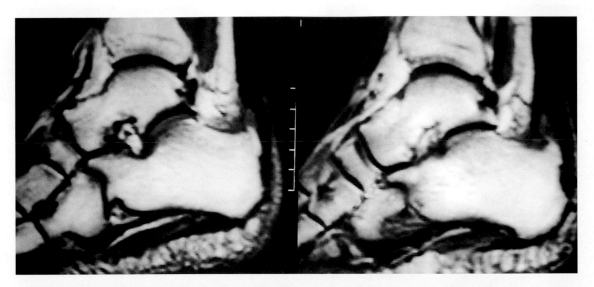

Fig. 4.19   Retrocalcaneal bursitis with an erosion. The tendo-Achilles is thickened distally; the bone is eroded at its insertion and there is also an erosion on the upper aspect of the calcaneus associated with a local bursitis.

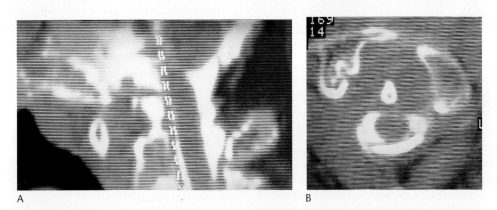

A   B

Fig. 4.20 A   Sagittal CT reconstruction showing odontoid peg erosion and separation of the space between the peg and arch. There is a soft-tissue mass interposed between the two structures. The peg is upwardly subluxated. (Courtesy of Dr. J. Stevens.) **B**. CT radiculography in rheumatoid arthritis. The odontoid peg is eroded and separated from the arch of the atlas by a soft-tissue mass. (Courtesy of Dr J. Stevens.)

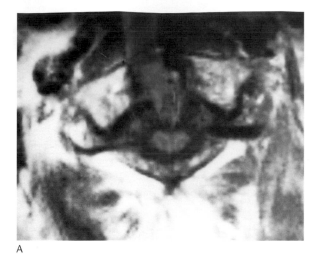

A

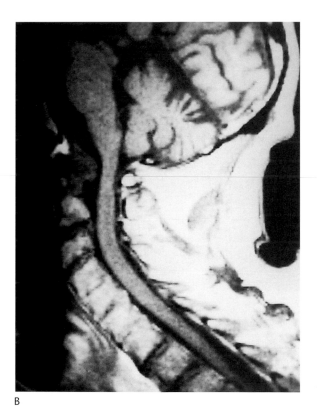

B

Fig. 4.21 Rheumatoid arthritis at MR scanning. **A**. T$_1$-weighted axial image. **B**. T$_1$-weighted sagittal image. A soft-tissue mass is seen in the region of the eroded odontoid peg and this indents the cord. Note diskal changes at all levels in the cervical spine.

In the carpus and tarsus the bones show accelerated maturation due to hyperemia, crowding of bones with joint space narrowing and an abnormal angular shape (Fig. 4.22). In general, early overgrowth of epiphyseal centers (Fig. 4.23) with squaring or angulation (Fig. 4.24) leads to premature fusion and eventual hypoplasia. This occurs at metacarpal and metatarsal epiphyses and around the knees, hips, elbows and shoulders. The abnormally modeled bone ends cannot be easily distinguished from the similar changes of synovial tuberculosis or hemophilia. Osteoporosis may result

Table 4.1 Classification of Juvenile Chronic Arthritis

1. Adult-type rheumatoid arthritis (with IgM rheumatoid factor)
2. Polyarthritis with ankylosing spondylitis-type sacroiliitis
3. Still's disease
   a. systemic
   b. polyarticular
   c. pauciarticular, with or without chronic iridocyclitis
4. Psoriatic arthropathy
5. Arthritis associated with ulcerative colitis or regional enteritis (as in adults)
6. Polyarthropathies associated with other disorders, such as systemic lupus erythematosus or familial Mediterranean fever, etc.

(Reproduced by kind permission of Dr. B. M. Ansell.)

from hyperemia or steroid administration which, in large doses, also causes undergrowth. Pathological fractures may result. Residual trabeculae along lines of stress are rendered very prominent. At the elbow, marked radial head enlargement may be seen and the paired long bones may bow. The cervical spine is often affected and indeed is the cause of presentation in 2% of cases. Diminution of neck movement is followed by apophyseal joint changes, maximal at C2–3, where erosions lead to ankylosis. The associated vertebral bodies fail to develop. Atlanto-axial subluxation is said to occur only rarely in those patients with seronegative disease, and neurocentral joint lesions do not occur in seronegative disease.

Juvenile Ankylosing Spondylitis has a characteristic onset at about 10 years of age. It is five times more common in boys and presents initially with an asymmetric peripheral arthropathy. Sacroiliac changes develop some 5–15 years later.

SERONEGATIVE SPONDYLOARTHROPATHIES

This is a group of non-rheumatoid seronegative disorders which have clinical, radiological and familial interrelationships. There are definite criteria for their diagnosis. These features include:

1. Absence of rheumatoid factors
2. Peripheral arthropathy
3. Sacroiliitis with or without ankylosing spondylitis
4. Clinical overlap, including two or more of the following features—psoriatic skin or nail lesions; conjunctivitis; ulceration of mouth, intestines or genitals; genitourinary infections; erythema nodosum
5. Increased incidence of the same or any other of these diseases in families.

The diseases which fit into these categories are:

1. Ankylosing spondylitis
2. Psoriatic arthritis
3. Reiter syndrome
4. Ulcerative colitis
5. Crohn's disease
6. Whipple's disease
7. Behçet syndrome.

The interrelationships between the diseases are seen in Figure 4.25. Chronic inflammatory bowel disease can, for instance, be seen to be linked to spondylitis and uveitis, while spondylitis is further linked to aortitis, seronegative arthritis and psoriasis.

This genetic and clinical overlap accounts for the marked radiological overlap of these syndromes, so that spondylitis is seen in many of these conditions. Nonetheless, differences in the type of spondylitis seen in these diseases also exist.

Psoriatic Arthritis

An association between psoriasis and arthritis was described as long ago as 1822. Some 10% of patients develop arthritis before the skin lesions appear, in 25% the two develop simultaneously and, in 65%, psoriasis precedes arthritis, often by up to 35 years. It seems that about 5% of patients with psoriasis develop an arthritis, but 15–30% of these are seropositive and have a radiological appearance identical with that of rheumatoid disease. The remainder have a 'pure' pattern of psoriatic arthropathy, or a mixture of the two types. Normal bone mineralization is regarded as a solid diagnostic criterion for psoriatic arthritis, but is not in fact particularly common, especially in chronic or severe disease.

The hands are as frequently affected by erosive change as are the feet in psoriatic arthropathy, in contradistinction to the patterns of Reiter syndrome. Nail changes are related to resorption of the distal phalanges but no definite correlation exists between nail lesions and interphalangeal joints erosions. Erosions have a predilection for the distal interphalangeal joints (Fig. 4.26), and especially the interphalangeal joint of the great toe. Erosive changes are asymmetric, even late in the disease, unlike rheumatoid arthritis,

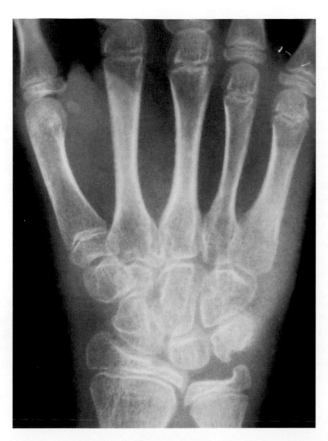

Fig. 4.22 Juvenile chronic arthritis. Accelerated skeletal maturity with modeling abnormalities of the carpal bones and osteoporosis.

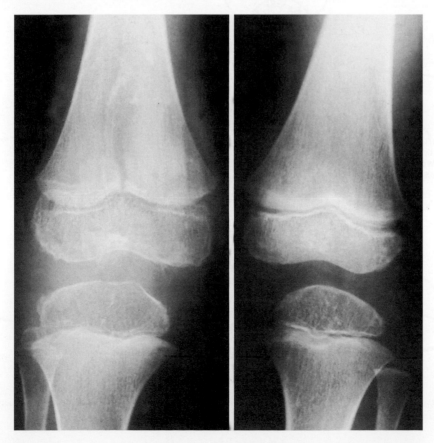

Fig. 4.23 Juvenile chronic arthritis. Monarticular arthritis with soft-tissue swelling and overgrowth of the epiphyses at the right knee. Normal left knee.

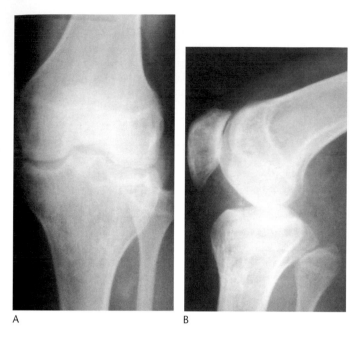

A   B

Fig. 4.24 Juvenile chronic arthritis. After five years, modeling abnormalities and osteoporosis are seen, but erosive change is not present.

and especially if the metacarpophalangeal joints are involved. Joint narrowing may never occur.

Erosions are modified by proliferation of adjacent new bone at the interphalangeal joints and especially around erosions on the calcaneus, where large, irregular fluffy painful spurs form both posteriorly and inferiorly. Such erosions are not found as often as in Reiter syndrome (these changes are uncommon in rheumatoid arthritis). Late changes in the hands include osseous fusion of the interphalangeal joints, and a 'cup-and-pencil' appearance at affected joints, leading to arthritis mutilans, but not ulnar deviation.

Periostitis in psoriatic arthritis occurs along the shafts of the tubular bones on hands and feet, which become sclerotic and expanded and, in association with soft-tissue swelling, gives a 'sausage digit' (Fig. 4.27).

Involvement of the larger joints is not common, but *sacroiliitis* may be seen in up to 50% of those with psoriatic arthritis. Usually symmetric, erosions, joint widening and sclerosis are seen but fusion is less common than in ankylosing spondylitis.

Paravertebral ossification may be the only feature of an osteopathy, even occurring in the absence of sacroiliac or digital disease. These *syndesmophytes*, which may be vertically directed and are not always attached to vertebral margins, should be distinguished from the more horizontally directed degenerative osteophytes. Vertebral squaring is uncommon in psoriatic spondylitis (Fig. 4.28).

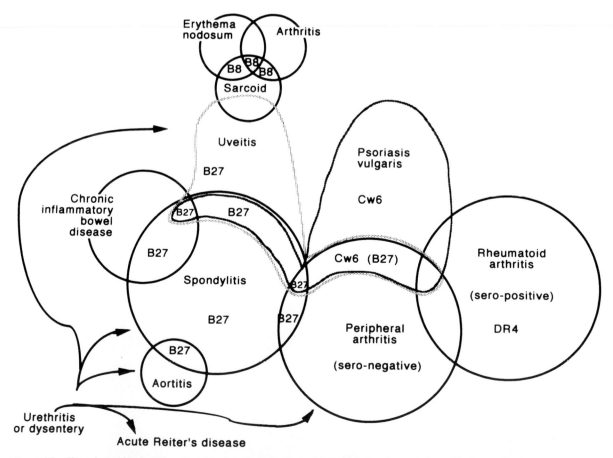

Fig. 4.25 The relationship between the different manifestations of arthritis is shown, together with the appropriate tissue markers. (Courtesy of Dr D. A. Brewerton.)

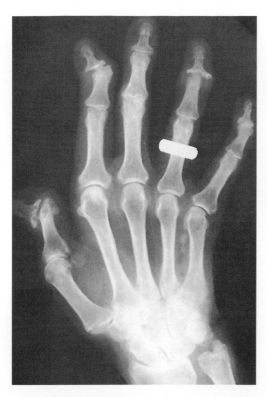

Fig. 4.26 Psoriasis. Erosive changes with overlying soft-tissue swelling are found predominantly at the distal interphalangeal joints. The erosions are initially peripheral, and splaying of the distal phalangeal bases results.

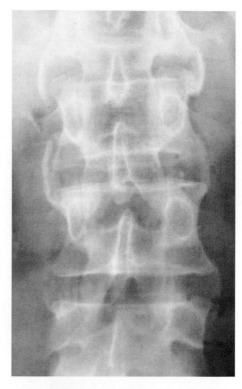

Fig. 4.28 Psoriatic spondylitis. Non-marginal vertical floating syndesmophytes are more typical of psoriasis and are less often seen in ankylosing spondylitis. (Courtesy of Dr J. T. Patton.)

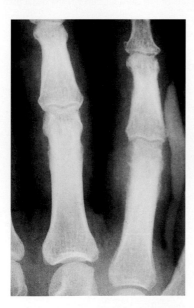

Fig. 4.27 A 'sausage digit' in psoriatic arthritis. There is soft-tissue swelling. Periostitis is demonstrated. The bone shows an apparent increase in density.

Reiter Syndrome

This occurs most commonly in young men and is usually sexually transmitted. The classic triad in the UK consists of a male patient with arthritis, urethritis and conjunctivitis. Gonococcal arthritis may thus cause confusion, especially if the classic three features

of Reiter syndrome are not all present. In continental Europe, the similar syndrome, originally described by Reiter in 1916, occurs in association with bacillary dysentery in both sexes.

Skeletal abnormalities will eventually be found in up to 80% of patients. Initial attacks of pain subside, but later recur, leaving progressive change at joints and entheses (the sites of musculotendinous insertion into bone). Reiter syndrome affects the feet rather than the hands, and also in a more severe form. In the foot, erosions occur at the metatarsophalangeal joints and the interphalangeal joint of the great toe. Osteoporosis is not a prominent feature of the disorder. It can be asymmetric, unlike rheumatoid arthritis.

Irregular erosions occur at entheses. Periostitis may be fine and lamellar in acute cases (Fig. 4.29), or fluffy and irregular in chronic disease. Painful erosions (Fig. 4.30) and reactive spurs are very common around the calcaneus, probably more so than in any other arthropathy, occurring in 20% of patients. In contrast to ankylosing spondylitis, the feet are severely affected. Sacroiliitis develops late in Reiter syndrome but may be seen in about half of all cases (Fig. 4.31). The changes are often asymmetric. Fusion is also less frequent than in ankylosing spondylitis. Spinal non-marginal syndesmophytes, identical to those seen in psoriatic arthritis, occur, especially around the thoracolumbar junction, but less frequently than in psoriatic arthritis.

Ankylosing Spondylitis

Ankylosing spondylitis (Marie Strumpell arthritis, Bechterew disease) is a seronegative spondyloarthropathy. Some 90% of

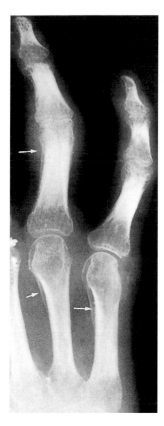

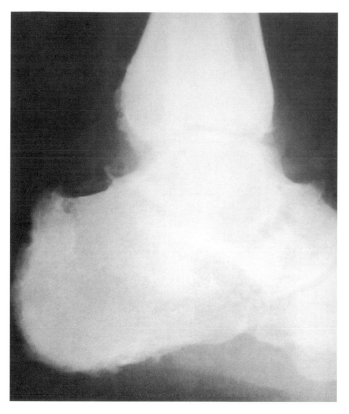

Fig. 4.29   Reiter syndrome—acute form, showing marked osteoporosis and periosteal reaction (arrows).

Fig. 4.30   Reiter syndrome. Periostitis and erosive changes on the plantar and posterior aspects of the calcaneus and of the distal tibia.

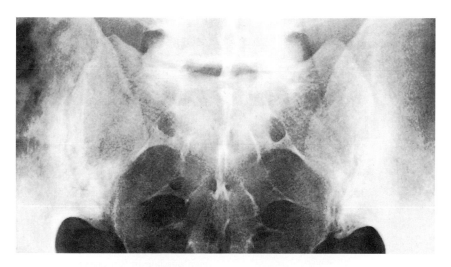

Fig. 4.31   Sacroiliitis in Reiter syndrome.

patients with this disease have the HLA-B27 antigen or, to put it another way, an individual with this antigen is 300 times as likely to have ankylosing spondylitis as is a person without the antigen. Sixty-five per cent of patients with psoriasis and spondylitis, or inflammatory bowel disease and spondylitis, have HLA-B27 but in psoriasis with a peripheral arthropathy there is only a weak association if spondylitis or sacroiliitis are not present. Thus the antigen is essentially related to the presence of spinal changes.

Histologically, the synovitis of ankylosing spondylitis is identical with that of rheumatoid arthritis; the enthesopathy consists of destruction of ligaments and local bone with subjacent inflammatory infiltrates. The destructive lesion heals by deposition of new bone which joins the eroded ligament, causing healing with bone proliferation at non-articular sites, syndesmophytes at vertebral margins and ossification of joint capsules.

Though the disease may affect children, it is said to occur more often in young men in their late teens and twenties, but recently it has been realized that women may be affected in equal numbers. The onset is often insidious so that sacroiliitis is usually seen at presentation. Spondylitis need not be present but develops subsequently, often at the thoracolumbar region initially, but sometimes affecting the cervical spine in females. Spinal changes without sacroiliac changes are very rare in this disease.

Sacroiliac Joints

Symmetric change is almost inevitable (Fig. 4.32A). Erosions, often worse on the iliac side, widen the joint and its hazy margins may resemble the normal adolescent joint. The erosions later show considerable sclerosis, and the joint narrows as irregular new bone bridges the joint space, so that fusion eventually occurs.

Joint changes are assessed using the *prone* view of the sacroiliac joint, though oblique views are helpful. Linear tomography gives good images of the sacroiliac joints, but was superseded by CT scanning, which defines cortical bone well (Fig. 4.32B). Images are free of overlying gut shadows. Small and early erosions can be visualized. This is probably the examination of choice.

Radionuclide scanning shows non-specific increase in uptake unilaterally or bilaterally. Bilateral change may be more difficult to assess if increase in uptake is symmetric. An increase in the ratio of counts between sacroiliac joints and the sacrum of more than 1.4:1 was held to indicate the presence of sacroiliitis (Fig. 4.33).

Spinal Changes

Erosions of vertebral margins heal by proliferation of sclerotic bone, which stands out in marked contrast to the rest of the vertebral body (Fig. 4.34). These healed erosions of vertebral margins may account for vertebral 'squaring'; an alternative cause is the laying down of new bone anteriorly beneath the longitudinal ligament. Both mechanisms may be operative (Fig. 4.35).

Further bony outgrowths in a later stage of healing lead to neat,

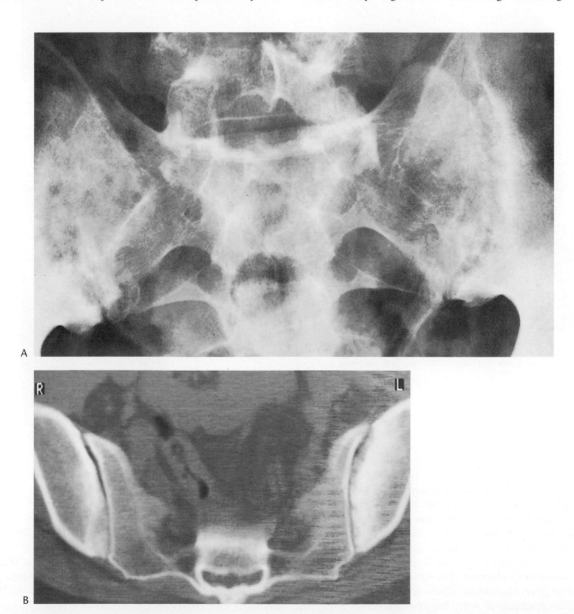

Fig. 4.32 Ankylosing spondylitis—early. **A**. Serrated margins of sacroiliac joints and periarticular sclerosis. **B**. CT scanning demonstrates bilateral sacroiliitis.

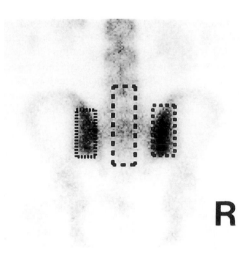

Fig. 4.33 Ankylosing spondylitis. Increase in uptake is demonstrated at both sacroiliac joints, greater on the right, in this posterior scan. (Courtesy of Dr A. Hilson.)

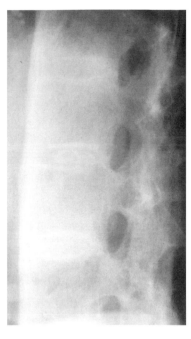

Fig. 4.35 Ankylosing spondylitis. Squaring of vertebral bodies is demonstrated, much of which is due to ossification in the line of the anterior longitudinal ligament. Longstanding fusion has resulted in calcification of the diskal nucleus. There is also quite marked ankylosis of the posterior spinal elements.

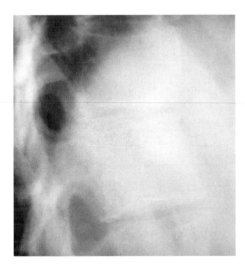

Fig. 4.34 Ankylosing spondylitis. Diskal narrowing and adjacent erosions heal with prolific new bone formation. Sclerosis and vertebral squaring result.

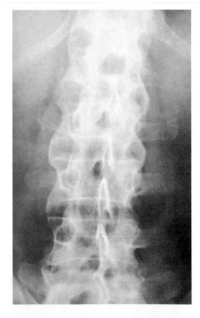

Fig. 4.36 Ankylosing spondylitis—'bamboo spine' with marginal syndesmophytes.

vertically disposed marginal syndesmophytes which may extend all the way up the spine (Fig. 4.36). The ossification lies in the annulus. Similar well-defined bands of ossification may be seen in the interspinous ligaments and around minor and major joints. If the intervertebral disk is intact at the time of syndesmophyte formation, it often never narrows, but may undergo central calcification. This phenomenon often follows vertebral fusion from any cause. Should the disk bulge, the syndesmophytes may be displaced. Syndesmophytes give the spine a knobbly appearance (Fig. 4.36), likened to a bamboo stick. Erosions at costotransverse and apophyseal joints also end in fusion. A cauda equina syndrome may result from arachnoiditis when large posterior dural diverticula are occasionally seen at radiculography, with osseous defects in the laminae.

If the patient falls forward onto the head or chest, the rigid spine may snap, often through the porotic bone just beneath the end-plate. Hypermobility may be demonstrated on fluoroscopy. Fractures may also occur through disks (Fig. 4.37).

Occasionally, localized destructive lesions of adjacent end-plates are seen, with disk narrowing and marked reactive sclerosis

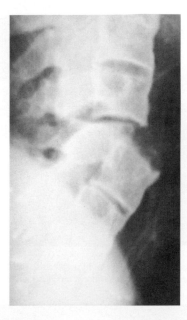

Fig. 4.37 Cervical spine in ankylosing spondylitis, with fractures through the C4/5 and C5/6 disks.

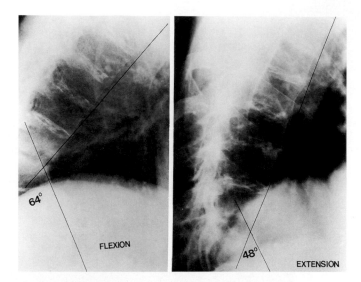

Fig. 4.38 Ankylosing spondylitis (Romanus lesion). End-plate irregularity is demonstrated together with reactive sclerosis in the underlying bone in this patient with ankylosing spondylitis. There is also instability at this level.

(Fig. 4.38). This lesion resembles infective diskitis or neuropathy but is probably post-traumatic. An associated pseudarthrosis is usually present at the neural arch at the same level.

Peripheral Joints Osteoporosis, erosions and joint space narrowing are less prominent than in rheumatoid arthritis, but shaggy periostitis and ankylosis are more common. At the hip, a prominent fringe of new bone may form at the capsule–bone junction. Bony ankylosis may precede or follow prosthetic joint replacement (Fig. 4.39).

Enthesopathies at iliac, ischial and calcaneal sites of ligamentous and tendinous insertions cause erosions followed by marked sclerotic periostitis.

Enteropathic Spondyloarthropathies

Ulcerative colitis, regional enteritis and Whipple's disease may be associated with joint disease of two distinct types.

Peripheral Arthropathy Episodes of fleeting asymmetric peripheral arthritis follow the cyclic course of the gut disease and its severity is also proportional to the extent of the lesion. Radiographic change is usually confined to soft-tissue swelling and local periostitis. These patients are seronegative and HLA-B27 negative.

Sacroiliitis and Spondylitis Pelvic and spinal changes identical to those of ankylosing spondylitis are seen. These do not correlate with gut disease activity but may precede its onset and continue to worsen even if, for instance, the colon is totally removed. These patients (usually male) have a high level of HLA-B27 antigen.

Diffuse Idiopathic Skeletal Hyperostosis (DISH)
(Forestier's disease, senile ankylosing spondylitis)

This condition was originally thought to affect the spine only. The current title clearly indicates that the condition is a generalized

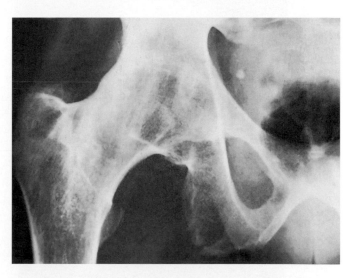

Fig. 4.39 Ankylosing spondylitis—note bony ankylosis across joint cartilage. Irregularity of the surface of the ischium is also shown.

one, in which extensive ossification is found at many sites. It is usually seen in elderly men (M:F = 3:1). Some studies show an increased incidence of HLA-B27 in patients with DISH.

In the spine, dense ossification is found in the cervical (Fig. 4.40) and especially lower thoracic regions. Bone is laid down often in continuity anteriorly and, in the thoracic region, on the right side, as the left-sided aortic pulsation prevents its deposition. The thick, flowing, corticated plaques may indent the esophagus. This florid exuberance is grosser than that seen in degenerative change. While continuity might also be seen following spinal infections, in DISH it is superimposed on a background of normal vertebrae and disks. On the other hand, osteoarthritis shows underlying bone and disk disease.

The sacroiliac joints may appear symmetrically fused on a plain film of the pelvis (Fig. 4.41). CT scanning demonstrates ligamentous and osteophytic ankylosis around the joint in the

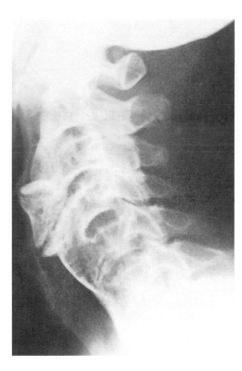

Fig. 4.40 Senile ankylosing hyperostosis—this is an extreme example of this common lesion. A tremendous amount of new bone has formed. The outlines of the original vertebral bodies and disk spaces are preserved.

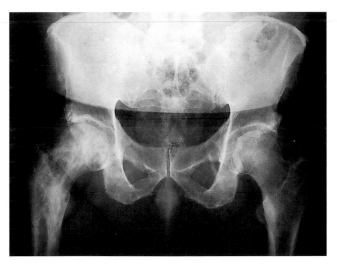

Fig. 4.41 Diffuse idiopathic skeletal hyperostosis. The plain radiograph of this patient demonstrates new bone formation at the iliac crests and ischia as well as fusion of the sacroiliac joints superiorly. There is also Paget's disease in the right femur.

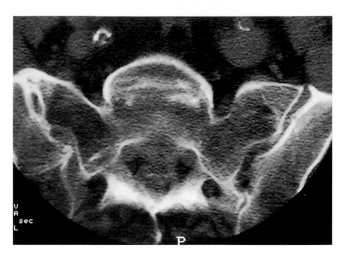

Fig. 4.42 Diffuse idiopathic skeletal hyperostosis. The CT scan shows that the joint spaces are still patent but there is ankylosis anteriorly.

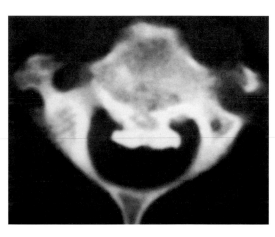

Fig. 4.43 Diffuse idiopathic skeletal hyperostosis with ossification of the posterior longitudinal ligament. New bone is seen anteriorly on this cervical vertebral body and posteriorly in the canal along the line of the posterior longitudinal ligament.

Rarely, posterior ligamentous ossification (OPLL) encroaches on the theca and produces cord compression (Fig. 4.43).

Ossification of the Posterior Longitudinal Ligament (OPLL)

New bone formation is seen in the posterior longitudinal ligament as an isolated phenomenon, often in Japanese, or in diffuse idiopathic skeletal hyperostosis (DISH) or ankylosing spondylitis. The new bone is well shown on CT or MR scans (Fig. 4.43). Radio-isotope scans show an increase in uptake in the spine if enough new bone is present in ankylosing spondylitis or DISH.

OSTEOARTHRITIS (Osteoarthrosis, degenerative arthritis, hypertrophic arthritis)

Osteoarthritis is a degenerative condition affecting articulations, especially those which bear weight or those subjected to much 'wear and tear'. The disease may be considered *primary* when no

absence of erosions (Fig. 4.42). The patients may complain of spinal stiffness and low back pain. Florid neo-ossification is also seen at extraspinal sites, around the iliac crests, ischia and above the acetabulum, and at the sites of ligamentous or tendinous insertions into bone.

Similar changes are found in the foot, especially on the calcaneus, where florid spur formation is sometimes seen. The new bone is generally well-defined and not related to local erosive or degenerative change. Fusion between the paired long bones may occasionally occur.

underlying cause can be discerned, or *secondary* if the joint is abnormal in form ab initio or is subjected to unusual stresses. In terms of end-stage appearances and treatment, the difference is probably academic.

Though there may be differences in the radiological appearances of osteoarthritis at different joints, degenerative disease has a number of specific features wherever it occurs.

Joint Space Narrowing

The width of a joint space seen radiologically is due to the radiolucent cartilage; joint space narrowing is therefore the result of cartilage destruction. Often in a given joint a predictable pattern of joint narrowing may be expected. This change characteristically occurs in areas of excessive weight-bearing.

Joint Space Remodeling

Joint narrowing due to cartilage destruction is followed by loss of underlying bone in stressed areas, and formation of new bone and cartilage in non-stressed area and at joint margins, so that joint alignment alters (Fig. 4.44).

Beneath areas of cartilage destruction, eburnation results (Figs 4.44, 4.45). Localized increase in density is presumably due to: 1. stress-induced new bone formation; and 2. trabecular collapse. Flattening and sclerosis result. New bone is formed in areas of low stress, at joint margins—peripheral osteophytosis, or within the joint—central osteophytosis. Osteophytic new bone is formed in response to new lines of force and prevents further malalignment. Buttressing osteophytes may thus be seen on the narrower side of a degenerate disk.

Cyst or geode formation in subarticular regions occurs in osteoarthritis as well as in rheumatoid arthritis and is found in the weight-bearing areas, often associated with joint narrowing, eburnation and collapse of bone (Fig. 4.46).

Loose Bodies

These are formed by detachment of osteophytes, crumbling of articular surfaces or ossification of cartilage debris (Fig. 4.47). Osteoporosis and bony ankylosis are not manifestations of degenerative disease. Indeed, hypertrophic new bone is seldom seen in patients who are osteoporotic. Osteoporotic patients often fracture their femoral necks, but do not form masses of new bone about their hips. Conversely, patients with florid osteophytosis tend to have good bone density and fewer femoral neck fractures. When osteoarthritis results in pain and immobility, osteoporosis and soft-tissue wasting may result secondarily.

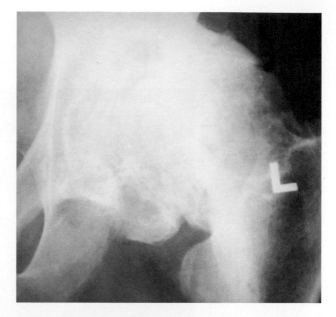

Fig. 4.44 Osteoarthritis of the hip. Lateral migration of the femoral head with loss of bone superiorly and marked new bone formation, both on the medial aspect of the head and at the adjacent part of the acetabulum. A superior acetabular cyst is present.

As so many of the changes in osteoarthritis relate to cortical bone, they are well imaged on plain films and CT scans, the latter showing osteophytes, erosions and cysts especially well. MR is, however, the preferred imaging modality for osteoarthritis in the major joints. As in rheumatoid arthritis, changes of cartilage loss and subcartilaginous bone, edema, cysts and necrosis are well demonstrated, together with loose bodies in the joint space and

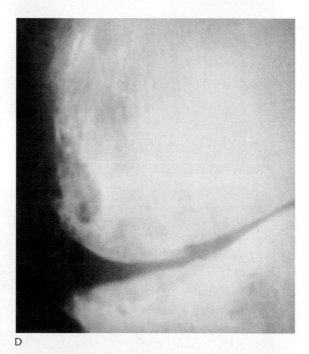

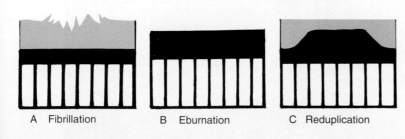

Fig. 4.45 **A,B,C** Patterns of degeneration (see text). Key: gray = cartilage; black = cortex; stripes = medulla. **D**. Reduplication with new bone laid down on the articular surface.

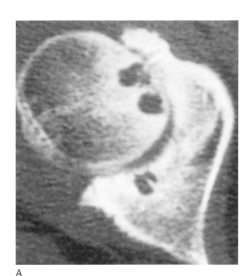

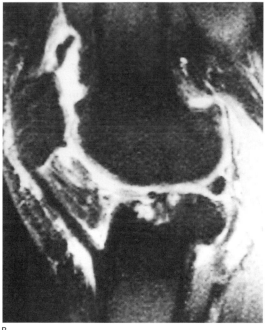

A

B

Fig. 4.46 A CT scan of osteoarthritis showing new bone formation within the acetabulum and cyst formation at the articular surface. **B**. Osteoarthritis demonstrated at MRI: sagittal STIR (fat suppression) sequence showing loss of joint space, subarticular cyst formation in the tibia with edema of the periarticular soft tissues, as well as an effusion in the joint.

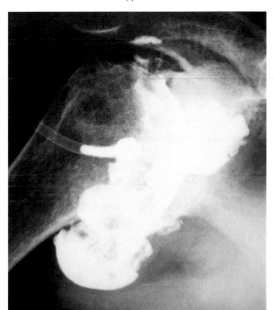

A

Fig. 4.47 Osteoarthritis. **A**. Right shoulder arthrogram. There is irregularity of the synovium and numerous loose bodies are demonstrated within the joint space. There is also a small rotator cuff tear. **B**. MRI demonstrates degenerative changes of the knee with an effusion, loss of the medial meniscus, marginal osteophytosis and a large loose body lying medially within the joint.

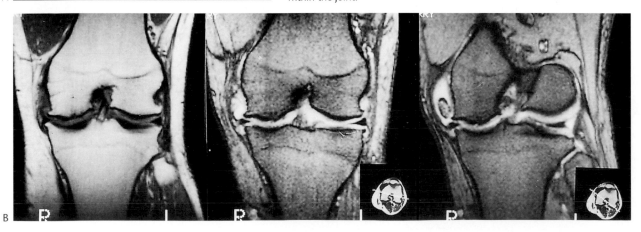

B

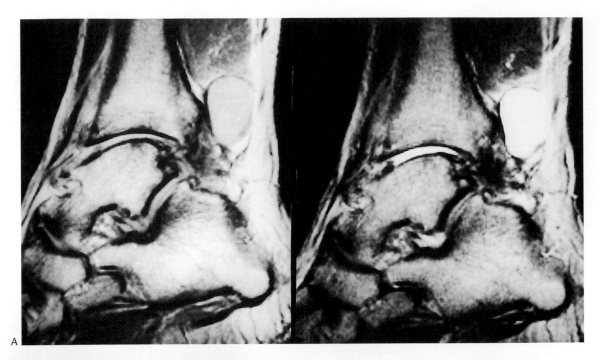

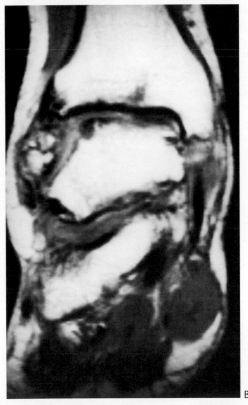

Fig. 4.48 A,B Osteoarthritis of the ankle. Articular irregularity with synovial thickening and effusions as well as synovial diverticula are demonstrated. Loss of articular cartilage is seen and erosive changes are demonstrated, especially on the upper surface of the talus. Osteophytes are demonstrated at the malleoli. There is a very large anterior talar osteophyte associated with local synovial proliferation, seen on the sagittal images.

Osteoarthritis in Particular Joints

The Hip Joint

Murray (1965) has shown that only 35% of cases have no underlying radiologically determinable abnormality. Many patients who develop premature osteoarthritis—in their 40s—are found to have a pre-existing abnormality. Some result from childhood—congenital dysplasias, congenital dislocation of the hip, acetabular dysplasia, Perthes disease or slipped epiphysis. The underlying cause is often recognizable. Others occur later—Paget's disease, scoliosis, rheumatoid arthritis and variants and aseptic necrosis from any cause.

There is no 'typical' appearance for osteoarthritis of the hip; rather, groups of different patterns may be defined. The appearances are complicated by analgesic therapy which may result in a neuropathic-type appearance with eburnation and rapid loss of bone (Fig. 4.49).

Patterns of Osteoarthritis of the Hip

These depend on the direction of migration of the femoral head which may be displaced superiorly (78%) (Fig. 4.50A), or medially (22%) (Fig. 4.50B). Superior migration may occur laterally (Fig. 4.44), medially, or in an intermediate direction with narrowing of the appropriate segments of the joint.

Medial migration may lead to protrusio acetabuli (Fig. 4.50B), lateral migration to lateral acetabular restraining osteophytes and new bone within the medial aspect of the acetabulum (Fig. 4.44).

effusions. Osteophytes are especially well shown. Capsular thickening and plicae, and extracapsular changes in collateral ligaments and tendons are all probably better seen than by any other means (Fig. 4.48).

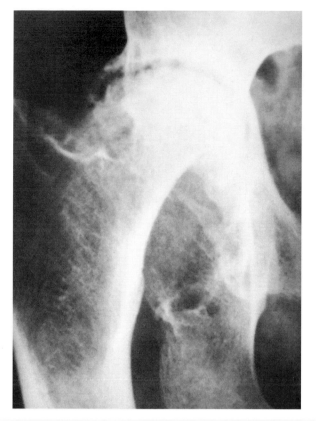

Fig. 4.49 Loss of the femoral head and deepening of the acetabulum may be the end-stage of osteoarthritis.

Capsular traction leads to buttressing new bone formation, usually on the medial, rather than the lateral, aspect of the femoral neck (Fig. 4.44).

The end result is often a femoral head which shows bone loss in weight-bearing areas and bone proliferation in non-weight-bearing areas (Fig. 4.44). The acetabulum may be deepened following medial migration or show new bone medially and superolaterally following lateral migration of the femoral head.

The Shoulder Joint

Osteoarthritis does not usually occur at the glenohumeral articulation in the absence of a predisposing factor, e.g. the use of crutches, or secondary to acromegaly, or with the malalignment that follows a chronic rotator cuff tear. Golding (1962) has shown that degenerative changes in the shoulder joint are closely linked with soft-tissue degeneration. Radiological manifestations include erosion, cysts and sclerosis of the greater tuberosity, cysts or irregular sclerosis along the anatomic neck (at the site of the capsular insertion) (Fig. 4.51); later atrophy of the tuberosities and upward subluxation of the humeral head occur. Occasionally, however, examples of the more classic type of osteoarthritis are seen in the shoulder, manifested by osteophytosis, sclerosis and marked loss of cartilage space (Fig. 4.52). Changes are commonly seen at the acromioclavicular joint, with irregularity, sclerosis and cyst formation at the articular surfaces.

The Knee Joint

This is the most commonly affected joint found in clinical practice. It consists of three compartments—a medial and lateral tibio-femoral, and the patellofemoral. The bone most commonly involved

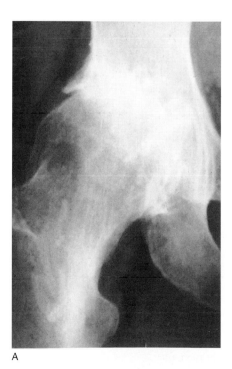
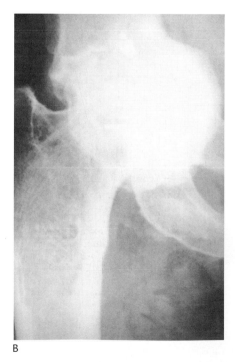
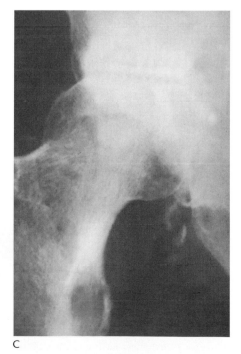

A   B   C

Fig. 4.50 Patterns of osteoarthritis. **A**. Superior migration of the femoral head. There is new bone on the medial aspect of the acetabulum. **B**. Osteoarthritis associated with protrusio acetabuli. **C**. Migration of the femoral head is in a superomedial direction.

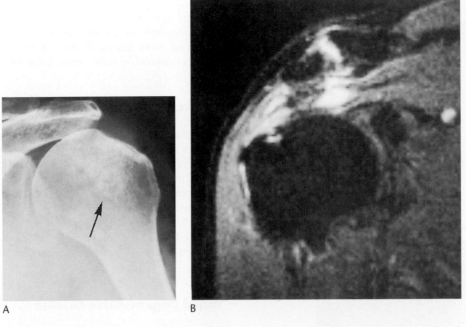

A   B

Fig. 4.51 A. Osteoarthritis of the shoulder—note excavation of the upper part of the anatomical neck with local sclerosis, and cysts seen en face (arrow). **B**. Widespread abnormalities are present on this coronal image of the shoulder. There is degeneration with an effusion around the acromioclavicular joint, a subacromial bursitis and considerable thickening of the rotator cuff, which shows a cyst in its body. In addition, there is a distal tendinitis associated with an erosion of the greater tuberosity.

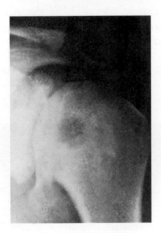

Fig. 4.52 Osteoarthritis of the shoulder, classic type—loss of joint space, eburnation, cyst formation and osteophytosis shown.

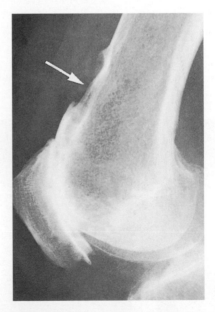

Fig. 4.53 Osteoarthritis of patellofemoral joint. There is a groove on the lower anterior part of the femoral shaft (arrow).

in osteoarthritic change is the *patella*, which is especially subjected to large loads when the knee is flexed in a squatting position. Joint narrowing, osteophytosis and articular irregularity can be seen at the patellofemoral compartment on the lateral and skyline views, especially at the lateral facet of the patella, and the patella often migrates outward. The lateral view also shows a scalloped defect of the anterior distal femur, especially in severely affected women (Fig. 4.53).

Spiking of the tibial spines and osteophytes on the articular margins are seen in early disease. Joint narrowing affecting one or other compartment results in valgus or varus deformity, best seen

in erect anteroposterior views, with gross buttressing osteophytosis on the side of the narrowing. The opposite compartment may then be widened. Varus deformity is more common and is possibly related to the more common medial meniscus abnormalities (Fig. 4.54). Osteoarthritis of the knees is also more common in the obese. The *fabella* may also be enlarged and irregular in osteoarthritis.

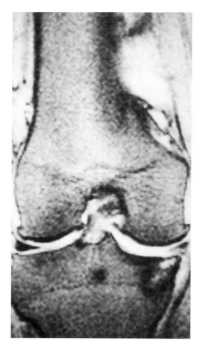

Fig. 4.54 Osteoarthritis. A degenerate and torn medial meniscus is associated with marginal osteophytosis and a subarticular cyst in the tibia. In addition, there is spiking of the tibial spines and at the intercondylar notch. An effusion is also present.

The Hands

The carpometacarpal joint of the thumb and the trapezioscaphoid joint are commonly affected, especially in women (Fig. 4.55). These joints are seldom involved in rheumatoid arthritis. In osteoarthritis, in contrast to the changes in rheumatoid arthritis,

the distal interphalangeal joints are most commonly affected, but any joint may be involved. Narrowing may affect all, or a few, distal interphalangeal joints, with large osteophytes on the distal phalangeal bases and overlying soft-tissue swelling. There may be small periarticular ossicles in the adjacent soft tissues (Fig. 4.56).

Erosive Osteoarthritis

Patients are typically seronegative and complain of episodic pain due to a symmetric arthritis of the interphalangeal joints and, less commonly, metacarpophalangeal and carpometacarpal joints. Bone density remains good but the joints show a mixture of marked joint narrowing and erosion with florid base-of-phalanx new bone formation. The erosions spread across the entire joint surface, which then collapses (Fig. 4.57). Fusion at interphalangeal joints or marked deformity may result. Pathologically, the synovium is inflamed and some patients seem to develop rheumatoid arthritis later.

Spinal Degenerative Disease

Though the structure of a disk and its surrounding vertebral endplates differs anatomically from that at a synovial articulation, the radiological appearance of degeneration at both sites is similar. The space between two opposing bones becomes narrowed and marginal new bone formation, 'articular' irregularity and sclerosis appear. Later, malalignment may result. In the spine the marginal new bone results from elevation of the paraspinal ligaments following disk narrowing. New bone forms beneath the displaced and elevated ligaments. The outgrowths—osteophytes—are generally laterally directed. Osteophytes also develop on the concavity of a scoliosis, no doubt also secondary to ligamentous

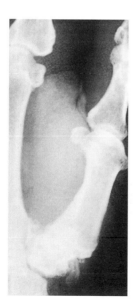

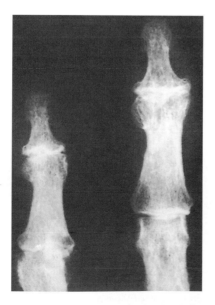

Fig. 4.55 Severe osteoarthritis of the carpometacarpal joint of the thumb.

Fig. 4.56 Osteoarthritis. Joint narrowing and osteophyte formation, with broadening of the joint underlying the Heberden's nodes.

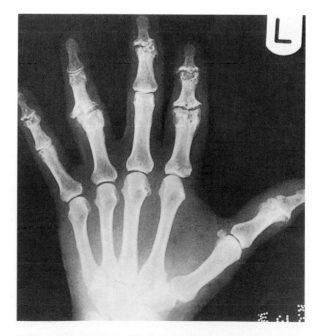

Fig. 4.57 Erosive osteoarthritis of the interphalangeal joints. Appearance of destruction around some proximal and distal interphalangeal joints.

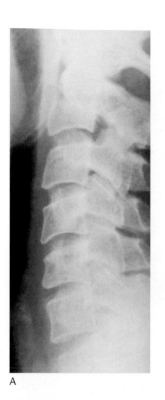

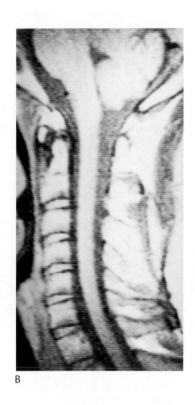

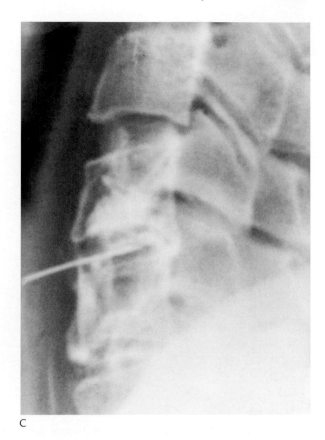

A

B

C

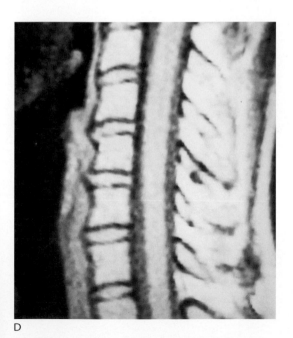

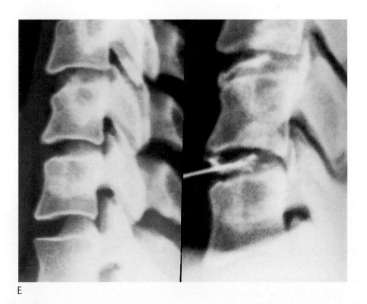

D

E

Fig. 4.58 Early cervical spondylosis. **A**. The plain film shows slight loss of the normal curve centered around the C5/6 disk which is also minimally narrowed. There are no osteophytes as yet. **B**. The MR scan confirms the minimal loss of height of this disk. There is no loss of signal and no dorsal protrusion of diskal material. **C**. A diskogram confirms the presence of an annular tear with substantial leak of contrast. **D**. Cervical spondylosis in a more advanced form. The MR scan is abnormal with anterior diskal bulging and marginal osteophytosis at C4/5 and C5/6 levels. **E**. In the diskogram of the same patient anterior and posterior annular tears are demonstrated with dorsal bulging. The anterior annular tears are shown to extend to the osteophytes.

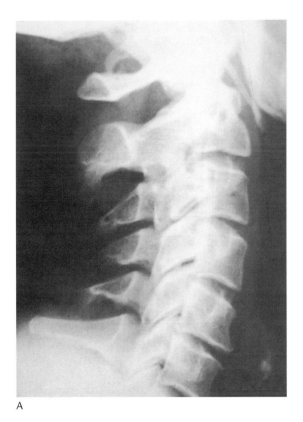
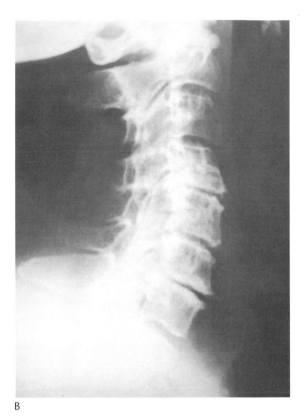

A   B

Fig. 4.59   Cervical spondylosis. **A**. There is early narrowing of the C5/6 disk and the beginnings of anterior osteophytosis. **B**. Disk degeneration is now pronounced, with both anterior and posterior osteophytes.

redundancy, but act as a buttress, similar to the restraining osteophytes in hip degeneration.

Disk degeneration alters mobility at the apophyseal joints, where degenerative changes become manifest by joint space narrowing and sclerosis. Facet slip at these joints results in encroachment on exit foramina, and new bone around them may narrow the spinal canal. Compressive symptoms result. Degenerative instability, scoliosis and spondylolysis may also result.

Cervical Spine   Additional synovial joints, the uncovertebral or neurocentral joints of Luschka, are found from C3 down and are easily recognized on the anteroposterior view. As elsewhere, disk degeneration results in narrowing of these joints with osteophytic lipping. In the adult, maximal movement between flexion and extension occurs around the level of the disk between the fifth and sixth cervical vertebral bodies and it is here that the earliest and also most severe degenerative changes are to be found. The next most common site of changes is around the C6/7 disk, but degeneration is less common superiorly (Fig. 4.58).

In established osteoarthritis, spinal movement is restricted between flexion and extension. The normal lordosis is lost and the spine is straightened in affected segments. A lateral view in flexion demonstrates functional change with lack of movement at affected levels.

Oblique views confirm the level of degeneration, and show encroachment on exit foramina at levels affected by disk narrowing (Figs 4.59, 4.60).

Posterior vertebral body osteophytosis, disk narrowing and longitudinal ligament laxity may all cause cord compression.

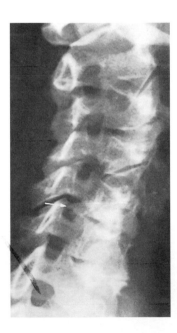

Fig. 4.60   Oblique projection of cervical spine showing large-osteophytic protrusions into the C5/6 intervertebral foramen (arrow).

Thoracic Spine   Degeneration in the thoracic spine is not usually severe or significant, though girdle type pain may result, or even long tract signs if disk material herniates posteriorly.

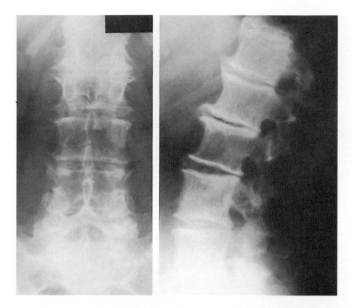

Fig. 4.61 Lumbar spondylosis. There is diskal narrowing and a vacuum phenomenon is present in the degenerative disks. Marginal osteophytes are present. Inferiorly the facet joints show features of degeneration and, with the increase in lordosis, the spinous processes are in contact.

Minor disk narrowing and osteophytosis is usually present anteriorly, especially in the elderly, often in association with a smooth kyphos.

Lumbar Spine Disk narrowing most commonly affects the L4/5 and L5/S1 disks. When the radiograph is initially inspected the number of lumbar type vertebral bodies should be noted. The first sacral body may be totally or partially lumbarized, with a narrow disk between S1 and S2, but L5 may be sacralized. In this case, the lowest free disk is 'high' with respect to the iliac crest, is subjected to greater stress and is more liable to degeneration. Any departure from normal anatomy alters the distribution of stresses and renders the local disk liable to premature degeneration. A unilateral pseudarthrosis between S1 transverse process and the iliac crest may be the seat of local degeneration. Facet joint degeneration may cause osteophytic encroachment into the spinal canal and exit foramina (trophism). Slip at the facets narrows the exit foramina further. Disk degeneration may result in fissuring and gas is seen in the disk space—a 'vacuum' phenomenon—as well as calcification on occasion.

Facet and disk degeneration may result in vertebral slip without pars defects. With an excessive lordosis, contact between 'kissing' spinous processes may result in soft-tissue entrapment and local pain (Fig. 4.61). As in the cervical spine, degeneration results in loss of the curve, rigidity and loss of movement between flexion and extension.

Diskography—the insertion of opaque contrast medium into the nucleus of the disk—is used to demonstrate the integrity of the nucleus and annulus. Pain reproduction during injection confirms the level of abnormality prior to surgery (Fig. 4.62) and can demonstrate that a disk which is abnormal at MR may be pain-free. Conversely, a disk which is normal at MR may be abnormal at diskography (Fig. 4.58).

MR in Diskal Disease Possibly the earliest change in degeneration is circumferential fissuring and radial tearing of the annulus. These changes, occurring in the third and fourth decades, are associated with an abnormal diskogram. The MRI scan, however, may be normal, as loss of disk height and dehydration

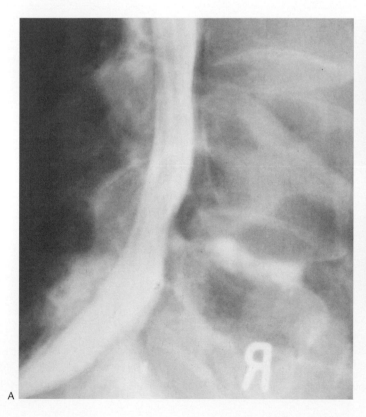

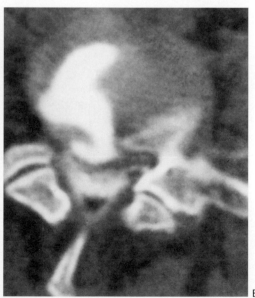

Fig. 4.62 A. Simultaneous diskography and radiculography demonstrate a torn annulus, through which contrast medium escapes and impinges upon the opacified theca. **B**. The CT scan shows, in the axial plane, the site of the annular tear and the displacement of the nucleus. Indentation of the opacified thecal sac is demonstrated.

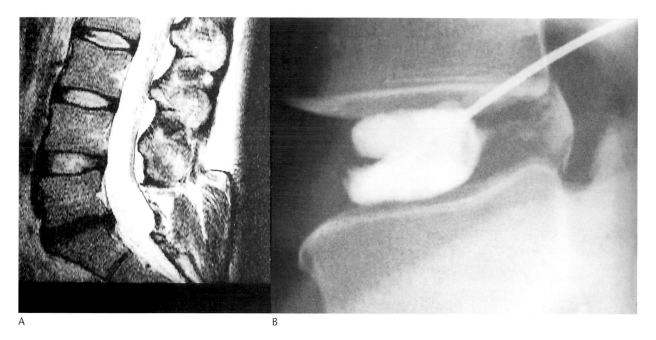

A   B

Fig. 4.63 Lumbar degeneration. **A**. The L5/S1 disk is clearly grossly abnormal showing loss of height and signal, together with a dorsal diskal protrusion. At L4/5 there is early loss of signal. **B**. The diskogram shows an essentially normal nucleus, but there is a fine annular tear which is associated with a bulge. No extraneous leak. This injection was extremely painful.

have not yet occurred (Fig. 4.63). Subsequent dehydration and fissuring in the disk are associated with loss of signal, so that the disk is no longer bright on T_2-weighted images. Loss of disk height and of the lordosis occurs. Osteophytes develop. In the underlying vertebral body, edema, cysts or reactive new bone formation are seen. Posterior and anterior annular fissures, which are intrinsically painful, extend to the diskal margins which in turn tear. Disk material herniates into the canal, centrally or peripherally, or into the exit foramina, or laterally. At all these sites compression results in a radiculopathy (Fig. 4.64).

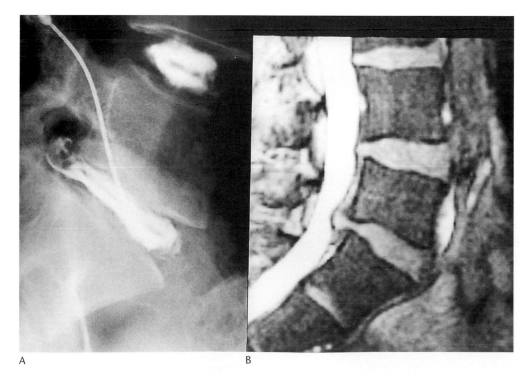

A   B

Fig. 4.64 **A,B** MR and diskography demonstrate a dorsal diskal protrusion with narrowing of the canal at that level.

MRI demonstrates disk degeneration and protrusion well. Often multiple areas of unsuspected disease may be seen. Not all, however, will be symptomatic. Almost all elderly patients will have evidence of spondylosis at one or more levels, but few are symptomatic.

Gout

Radiographic Findings

1. *Erosions*. These are caused by deposition of *sodium biurate* and are typically punched out in appearance. They tend to appear near joint margins. As they enlarge, they tend to involve more of the cortex of the shaft rather than the articular surface (Fig. 4.65). Large erosions extend to the articular cortex and diffusely in the shafts (Fig. 4.66). Cartilage destruction is a relatively late mani-

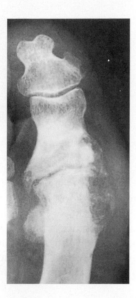

festation. Usually much bony destruction is seen before cartilage loss supervenes. In the hand, gout tends to attack the distal and proximal interphalangeal joints, whereas rheumatoid arthritis affects the metacarpophalangeal and proximal interphalangeal joints.

2. *Osteoporosis* is not seen except in advanced cases which have been immobilized.

3. *Tophi*. These are shown as soft-tissue swellings eccentric in distribution, in contradistinction to the fusiform soft-tissue swellings of rheumatoid arthritis (Fig. 4.66). Eventually, both soft-tissue and intraosseous tophi may become calcified (Fig. 4.67), but this is uncommon.

Differential Diagnosis   Differentiation between gout and *multiple enchondromas* may be difficult radiographically. The tendency of multiple enchondromas to spare bone ends is an important diagnostic point. The clinical findings and history readily differentiate the two conditions.

In practice, the most frequent difficulty is in differentiating gout from *rheumatoid arthritis*. Important points are: the longer latent period of gout; its eccentric, often gross soft-tissue swellings; and tendency to attack distal interphalangeal joints. Osteoporosis is found much more frequently in rheumatoid arthritis. Rheumatoid erosions are not so sharply defined as those of gout. Calcified tophi are, of course, diagnostic of gout. In difficult cases, differentiation will be made by laboratory tests revealing a raised uric acid level in blood.

Hypertrophic (Pulmonary) Osteoarthropathy

This condition was originally thought to be associated solely with intrathoracic disease, but it is now known to be associated with intra-abdominal and other diseases. The word 'pulmonary' is best avoided in the title. The vast majority of cases are associated with intrathoracic neoplasms, mainly bronchogenic carcinoma, up to

Fig. 4.65 Gout—erosion on medial part of first metacarpal extends away from the joint surface.

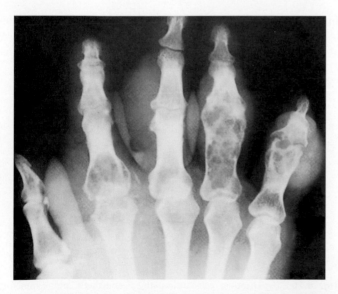

Fig. 4.66 Very advanced gout. Note eccentric soft-tissue swellings, intraosseous tophi extending to bone ends and lack of osteoporosis.

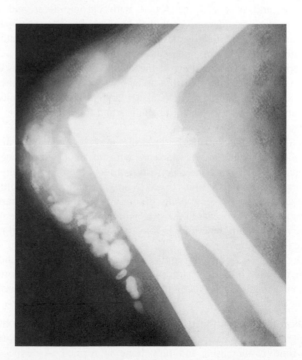

Fig. 4.67 Gout—large calcified tophi in olecranon bursa.

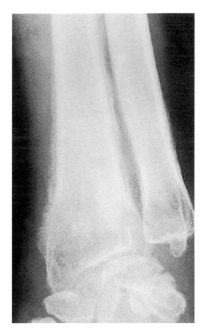

Fig. 4.68 Hypertrophic osteoarthropathy—exuberant periosteal reaction of the radius and ulna. In this patient, changes in the bones of the hands were minimal.

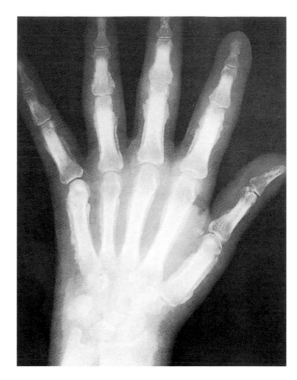

Fig. 4.69 Hypertrophic osteoarthropathy secondary to pulmonary neoplasm.

12% of which have hypertrophic osteoarthropathy, with the exception of oat-cell carcinomas. Hypertrophic osteoarthropathy is also associated with secondary lung tumors. Its highest incidence is found with fibrous mesothelioma of the pleura. Hypertrophic osteoarthropathy is more common with peripherally seated tumors.

Hypertrophic osteoarthropathy is also observed with bronchiectasis, rarely with tuberculosis, and congenital cyanotic heart disease, and may also be found with chronic liver and gut inflammatory disorders. Even though hypertrophic osteoarthropathy is usually accompanied by clubbing, the latter should be separated on clinical, radiological and pathological grounds.

Periostitis is seen earliest at the distal third of the radius and ulna (Fig. 4.68), then the tibia and fibula, and then the humerus and femur, metacarpals, metatarsals and proximal and middle phalanges (Fig. 4.69). Distal phalanges and the axial skeleton are rarely affected.

Radiologically, soft-tissue swelling may be seen over distal phalanges if clubbing is present, but the underlying bone is normal. In the long bones, periostitis affects the distal diaphyses but the bone ends are uninvolved. A single fine layer, or multiple layers, of periosteal new bone, giving an onion-skin appearance, may be seen. On occasion the periostitis may be shaggy. The new bone merges with the cortex in longstanding cases. Endosteal new bone is not seen.

Occasionally joint pain and swelling are related to an underlying arthritis, usually of larger joints. Radiologically, osteoporosis and effusions may be recognized but erosions do not apparently occur.

Radionuclide Scanning in Hypertrophic Osteoarthropathy
Hypertrophic osteoarthropathy is a disease in which blood flow to the limb is increased and new bone is formed. As expected, scanning is an accurate and sensitive means of detecting disease, and the changes are seen before those on the plain films. Increased uptake is seen symmetrically along the shafts of affected long bones paralleling the cortices and thus differing from focal or widespread metastatic foci. With treatment of the underlying condition, the changes evident on both film and scan regress. Increased uptake on scan is also seen around affected joints (Fig. 4.70).

Pachydermoperiostosis

In this condition radiological changes identical with those seen in hypertrophic osteoarthropathy present early in life, often after

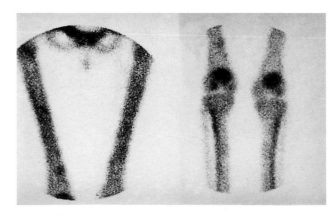

Fig. 4.70 Hypertrophic osteoarthropathy. Generalized and symmetric diffuse increase in uptake is associated with thickening of the bony image at isotope scanning.

puberty. Though the periosteal new bone is similar to that seen in hypertrophic osteoarthropathy, it is often coarser and may extend further along the shafts to the epiphyses. A familial history is present in over 50% of cases and males are said to be more commonly affected. No related chest disease is found. The skin of the face, especially the forehead, becomes thickened and greasy with acne and hyperhydrosis.

Systemic Lupus Erythematosus

This disorder is more common in young females and in black Africans. It is associated with a 'butterfly' skin rash over the cheeks, with pleurisy, pericarditis, glomerulonephritis and psychiatric disorders. It may be precipitated by drugs.

Systemic lupus erythematosus may present with a symmetric peripheral arthropathy in which erosive change is infrequent. Soft-tissue swelling and osteoporosis are seen, but erosive change is minimal and uncommon. Soft-tissue calcification also occurs around the joints and in blood vessels. Alignment deformities of the hands are more typical, so that ulnar deviation and swan-neck deformites are seen, which are reversible, voluntarily and involuntarily.

Avascular necrosis is common, being found in the hips, knees and shoulder joints. It probably follows steroid therapy but, in view of the high incidence (10%), may be due to the disease alone. C1/C2 subluxation may be found.

Progressive Systemic Sclerosis

This is a widespread disorder of connective tissue which often presents with Raynaud's phenomenon due to small vessel occlusion. Fibrosis of the skin, especially over distal phalanges, leads to resorption of the distal phalanges and then progressively of the middle and proximal phalanges. Soft-tissue calcification is seen, especially over distal phalanges and around joints. Fibrosis may lead to contractures (Fig. 4.71). These changes may be preceded or accompanied by a polyarthritis similar to rheumatoid arthritis in at least 10% of patients. Osteoporosis, joint space narrowing, erosions and subluxations may be seen. Changes of an erosive arthropathy in association with calcification should suggest the presence of progressive systemic sclerosis.

Jaccoud's Arthropathy

This arthropathy does not involve synovium but causes capsular fibrosis. Deformities of the hands and feet, that are initially reversible, occur. Lateral deviation of the hands and feet may be seen when these parts are examined without weight-bearing. When pressed down into the cassette surface, the deformities vanish. The joint spaces are mainly preserved. True erosions are not found, but so-called 'hook' erosions of the metacarpal heads are produced, possibly because of local capsular pressure (see Fig. 4.71). The patients are seronegative for rheumatoid arthritis.

Mixed Connective Tissue Disease

This is a so-called 'overlap syndrome' comprising a mixture of features of rheumatoid arthritis, dermatomyositis, systemic lupus erythematosus and progressive systemic sclerosis.

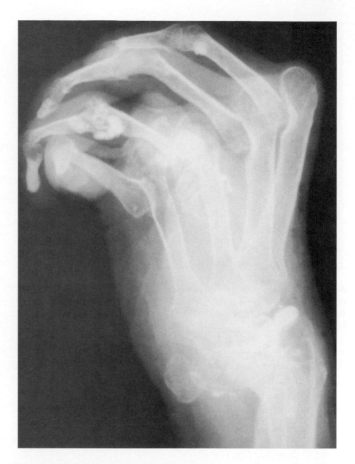

Fig. 4.71   Scleroderma. Contractures result in pressure resorption of bone at metacarpal necks. Para-articular calcification is prominent, as is distal phalangeal sclerosis.

Osteoporosis, soft-tissue swelling and joint space narrowing are found at affected joints. The distribution also may mimic rheumatoid arthritis, but distal interphalangeal joints may be affected and the peripheral arthropathy may be asymmetric. Erosive change is not inevitably present at these sites, which are a mixture of the sites of rheumatoid arthritis and psoriasis. The distal phalanges show soft-tissue loss, distal tuft bone resorption and calcification suggesting progressive systemic sclerosis. Ulnar drift, as in systemic lupus erythematosus or rheumatoid arthritis, is also seen. Pericardial and pleural effusions may be shown by chest radiography.

IMAGING OF JOINTS

Arthrography involves the injection of iodine-based water-soluble contrast media, or air, or both, into a joint. It has become less commonly used for two main reasons.

1. *Arthroscopy* is used as a primary diagnostic modality by the surgeon who can proceed directly on to surgery. The knee, shoulder and temporomandibular joints are all routinely examined by this mode. Arthrography was as accurate in the diagnosis of meniscal lesions as arthroscopy, but far less accurate for diagnosis of cruciate ligament change as well as abnormalities of cartilage.

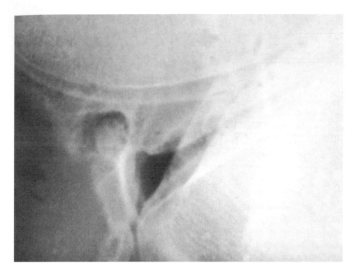

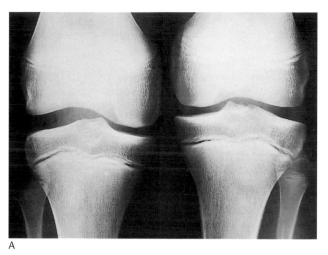

Fig. 4.72 Posterior horn of the lateral meniscus shows a peripheral defect through which runs the popliteus tendon sheath. The superior and inferior struts around the defect are intact.

2. *MRI* is becoming more generally available. Changes can be seen both in the joint, e.g. the menisci, cruciate ligaments and cartilage at the knee, and also in the subarticular bone and in the extrasynovial tissues. Changes of bone marrow, e.g. edema or hemorrhage, or in the adjacent ligaments and tendons can be assessed. Where MRI is available, the use of arthrography has declined dramatically.

Knee Joint

Arthrography The normal meniscus is triangular in cross-section. The lateral meniscus has a posterior peripheral defect for a synovial tunnel in which runs the popliteus tendon (Fig. 4.72). In utero, the menisci are larger, bisecting the joint. Rarely, this large bulbous fetal structure persists into adult life as a diskoid meniscus, usually on the lateral side, well seen at arthrography and MRI, and on the plain film by widening of the lateral compartment (Fig. 4.73).

Tears are seen as fissures containing air or contrast. They are more common in the medial meniscus, especially posteriorly. They may be partial, or extend from the top to the bottom of the meniscus, which may be partially or totally peripherally detached.

Loose bodies may be seen, and the state of the articular cartilage in the region of the meniscal section under examination fairly well assessed. Baker cysts can be seen (Fig. 4.74).

Optimal arthrography needs an experienced operator. It is advantageous to have a fine-focus tube in the fluoroscopy unit. Only the superficial surfaces of the internal structures of the joint are well seen. Cruciate ligaments are not consistently well seen.

MRI MRI shows not only the surfaces of the intra-articular structures but also shows change *within* the menisci and cruciate and other ligaments, and in adjacent structures—bone and muscle.

Changes in the menisci have been graded 0–3 (Fig. 4.75). Fluid or myxoid degeneration in the meniscus is seen as a band of increased signal on T_2-weighted and STIR images in the body of the meniscus (Grades 1–2) (Fig. 4.73). If the signal extends to the

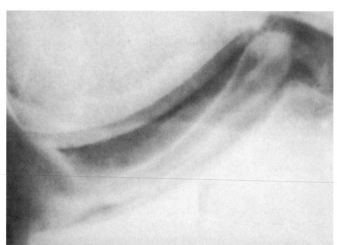

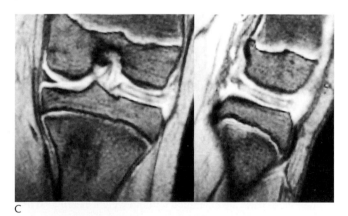

Fig. 4.73 Diskoid meniscus. **A**. The plain film shows dishing of the lateral tibial plateau. **B**. Arthrography. The meniscus extends medially to the midline of the joint and has a bulbous internal aspect. **C**. The MR scan shows the same external contour of the meniscus as the arthrogram but shows cystic degeneration within the structure of the meniscus. Note also the increase in signal at the metaphysis—a normal feature.

meniscal surface (Grade 3), a tear is present (Fig. 4.76). Grade 1–2 changes do, with time, become Grade 3 lesions. Recurrent tears post-meniscectomy are also easily diagnosed. Cysts at the

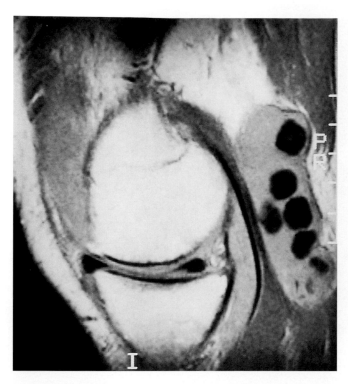

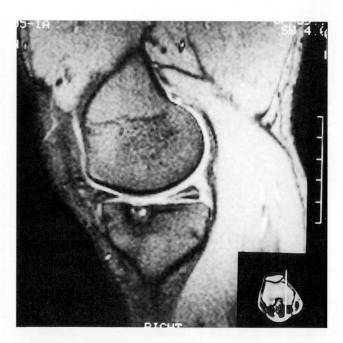

Fig. 4.76 Tear of the posterior horn of the medial meniscus associated with a tibial cyst. Peripheral meniscal cysts originating from degenerate menisci are seen on sagittal, axial and coronal images at MR scanning.

Fig. 4.74 Sagittal T$_1$-weighted image of the knee. The medial meniscus is torn. There is a large Baker cyst which contains loose bodies.

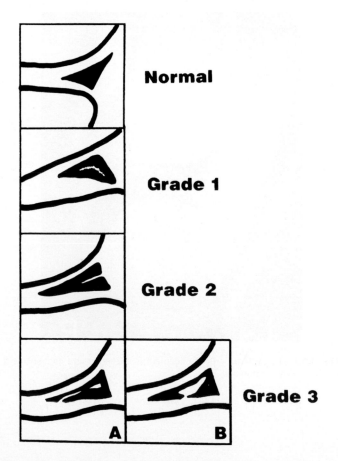

Fig. 4.75 Classification of meniscal change at MR from normal to tear, according to Mink et al (1993).

periphery of the meniscus extend into the adjacent soft tissues as adventitial bursae (Fig. 4.77).

The cruciate ligaments are especially well shown. The posterior is thick and easily seen and it is not often damaged (Fig. 4.78). The anterior is thinner, runs obliquely to the sagittal plane and is less well seen, but is more easily damaged, often in association with a medial meniscal tear. Fluid may be seen in the ligament following acute injury (Fig. 4.79) or there may be total retraction. Chronic changes are of fibrosis and deformity.

The collateral ligaments are well seen on coronal images and tears, especially of the medial, can be identified following injury (Fig. 4.80).

STIR weightings show edema in the articular cartilage and edema, bruising or cysts in the underlying bone (Fig. 4.81). Degenerative changes are best seen at MRI, often in the presence of local meniscal abnormalities.

Baker cysts may rupture, causing symptoms similar to those of a deep vein thrombosis. These cysts can be seen on occasion on a plain film, but are well shown with ultrasound, arthrography (Fig. 4.82) or MRI (see Figs 4.16, 4.74), as is the leak. A negative venogram rules out a deep vein thrombosis, but the popliteal vein may be displaced by the cyst.

Ultrasound is of limited practical value in the knee, as the vulnerable structures are contained deep in the joint. The sound waves cannot pass through bone and so deep structures cannot be visualized. Nonetheless, superficial soft tissues can be seen, including the patellar tendon, collateral ligaments and superficial meniscal parts, as well as effusions (Fig. 4.83).

Radio-isotope Scanning Single photon emission computed tomography (SPECT) can be used to show meniscal abnormalities by demonstrating increase in uptake in the condyles and tibial plateau. Changes at SPECT are said to have both high sensitivity and specificity (Fig. 4.84).

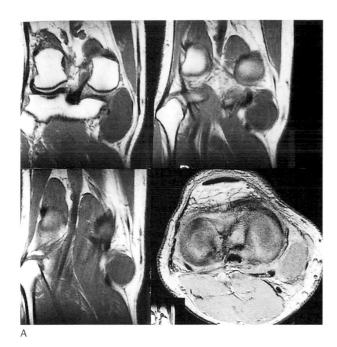

A

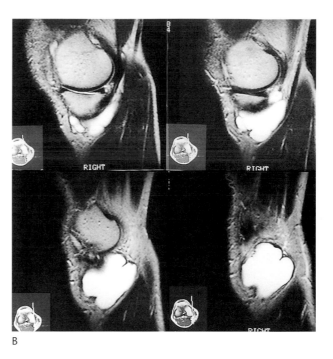

B

Fig. 4.77 A medially directed cyst related to an abnormal posterior horn is shown in coronal, axial and sagittal images. The cyst is palpable beneath the skin and serial images track its communication to the interior of the joint.

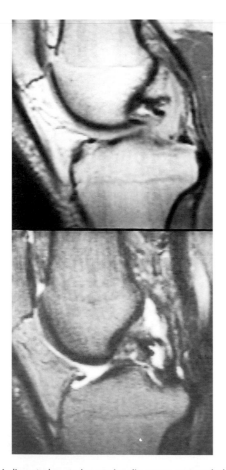

Fig. 4.78 A disrupted posterior cruciate ligament surrounded by effusion.

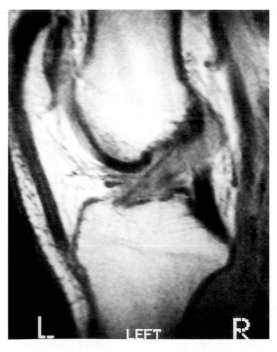

Fig. 4.79 The anterior cruciate ligament is thickened and contains fluid on this T_1-weighted image.

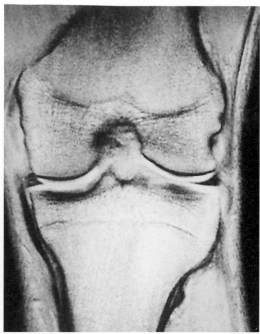

Fig. 4.80   Coronal T$_2$-weighted image of the knee demonstrates a tear of the medial collateral ligament.

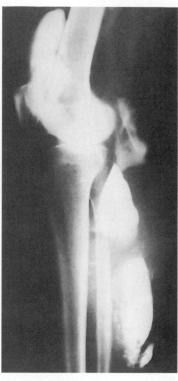

Fig. 4.82   Rupture of a Baker cyst is demonstrated. This is probably chronic, as the cavity in the calf has a smooth margin. (Courtesy of Dr A. R. Taylor.)

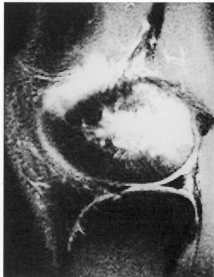

Fig. 4.81   Bone bruising in the medial femoral condyle well demonstrated on a sagittal fat suppression image of the knee.

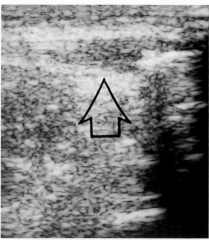

Fig. 4.83   Grade I patellar tendinitis. A focal area of hypoechogenicity (arrow) at the proximal pole of the tendon indicates a mild to moderate tendinitis. (Courtesy of Dr S. Burnett.)

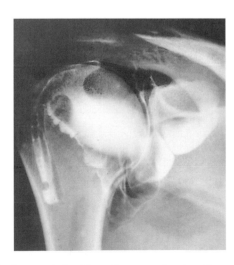

Fig. 4.84 Radio-isotope bone scan (SPECT) of the knee shows focal areas of increase in uptake (arrowed) at sites of proven abnormality of the menisci. (Courtesy of Dr I. Fogelman.)

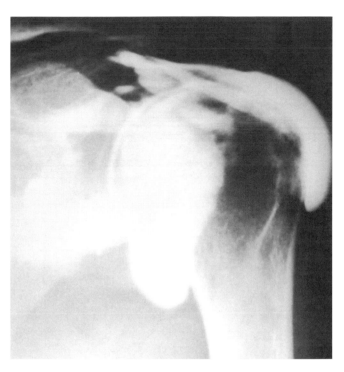

Fig. 4.86 A rupture of the rotator cuff is seen at shoulder arthrography, with contrast medium filling the subacromial space.

Shoulder Joint

Arthrography is used especially to demonstrate tears of the rotator cuff and the long head of biceps, but also to demonstrate loose bodies and to assess joint volumes in restrictive capsulitis.

The normal shoulder has an intact Mahoney's line (cf. Shenton's line) and a space of 1–1.5 cm between the humeral head and the acromion. This space consists (from above downward) of the subacromial bursa, the rotator cuff, the long head of biceps and the shoulder joint space proper. The two synovial spaces are thus separate (Fig. 4.85). With chronic rotator cuff tears, the defect in the tendon allows the humeral head to sublux upward and contrast medium fills the subacromial bursa from the glenohumeral joint, that is, it comes to lie beneath the acromion,

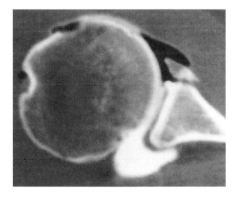

Fig. 4.87 CT arthrotomography showing a labral and glenoid fracture.

which may be scalloped by the elevated humeral head (Fig. 4.86) (see also Fig. 9.35A).

On an axial view, contrast medium is shown to extend inferiorly, below the line of the anatomic neck. The normal joint also shows a normal subcoracoid recess and an axillary recess.

Double-contrast arthrography may be combined with axial tomography. This especially demonstrates the presence or absence of articular cartilage at the glenoid labrum and humeral head, as well as showing the presence or absence of a hatchet defect following recurrent dislocation (Fig. 4.87). In addition, the long head of biceps tendon is well demonstrated in its sheath. Foreign bodies are especially easily shown in the shoulder.

Here again, however, where available, MRI has largely superseded arthrography and CT arthrography, largely because it is non-invasive.

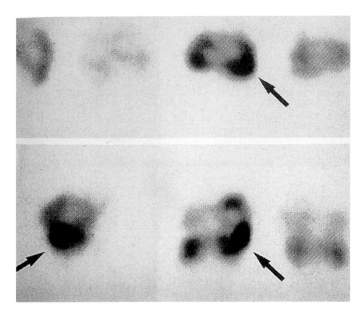

Fig. 4.85 A normal shoulder arthrogram showing the extent of the glenohumeral synovium. There is no contrast beneath the acromion. The synovial reflection around the long head of biceps tendon is shown.

MRI shows changes within the tendons. Attention should be directed to the acromioclavicular joint on coronal images as bone and soft-tissue hypertrophy cause compression and edema of the underlying supraspinatus muscle.

The presence of a subacromial osteophyte has been shown to lead to changes in the underlying rotator cuff tendon. This important spur of bone causes first pressure atrophy and subsequent rupture of the tendon (Fig. 4.88). Tendinitis is seen as an increase of signal in the normally low signal of the tendon. Tears may be partial and superior or inferior, or total (Fig. 4.89). Tendon retraction occurs, and the humeral head subluxes upward. Degenerative cysts are often seen at the rotator cuff insertion, and are well seen on STIR or T_2-weighted images.

Axial scans show the long head of biceps tendon in its sheath; tenosynovitis may be present with a distended sheath.

The labrum is usually seen as a triangular structure arising from the anterior and posterior glenoid margins on axial scans, and the upper and lower margins on coronal images. Tears or detachments are shown on T_2 or STIR weightings, giving an appearance similar to those seen after the introduction of contrast medium into the joint and CT scanning (Fig. 4.90).

Ultrasound is more useful in the shoulder than in the knee as the important soft tissues—the supraspinatus muscle and tendon and the long head of biceps—are more accessible, but overall MRI gives more detail.

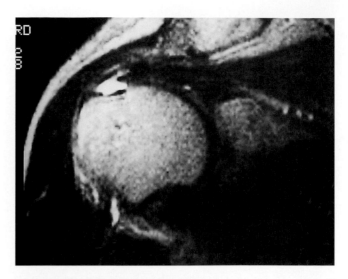

Fig. 4.89 Total rotator cuff tear with retraction. Axial CT of the shoulder demonstrates an anterior labral tear.

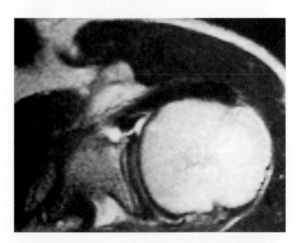

Fig. 4.90 A tear of the labrum glenoidale anteriorly shown at MR scanning. Fluid provides the contrast medium on the T_2-weighted image.

Ankle Joint

Investigation of ligamentous injuries is the main indication, but *arthrography* is seldom used in practice in studying this joint. In the normal arthrogram, contrast medium may extend upward for 1 cm into the inferior tibiofibular joint. In ligamentous and capsular ruptures, contrast medium will seep into adjacent tissues and into tendon sheaths.

MRI has proved to be of great value in the ankle. Effusions are seen, as in other joints. Tendons around the joint are assessed. Thickening, loss of clarity and increase in signal are especially well seen in the tendons behind the malleoli, with distension of the sheaths (Fig. 4.91). *Tenosynography* need no longer be performed.

The Achilles tendon is especially well shown. Tendinous thickening and central necrosis may be followed by rupture. These changes are all seen in ultrasound scans too (Fig. 4.92).

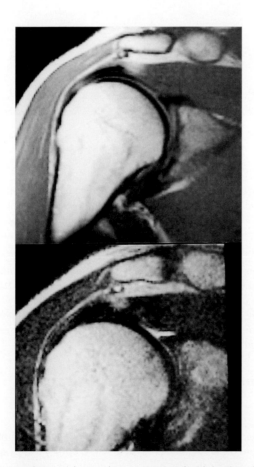

Fig. 4.88 A subacromial osteophyte is associated with local tendinitis (T_1- and T_2-weightings).

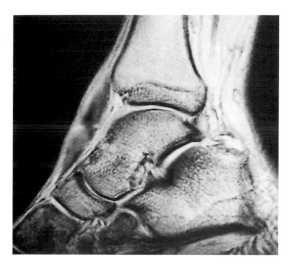

Fig. 4.91 Thickening of the tibialis anterior tendon demonstrated at MR.

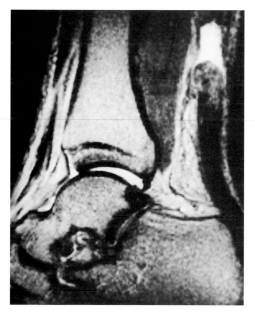

Fig. 4.92 Total rupture of a thickened tendo Achilles demonstrated at MR. Fluid fills the space between the retracted parts.

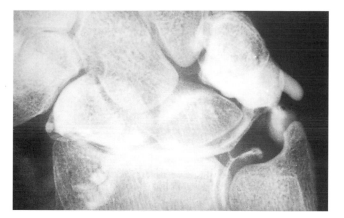

Fig. 4.93 Injection of the radiocarpal joint space has demonstrated a tear of the triangular cartilage and filling of the distal radio-ulnar joint at arthrography.

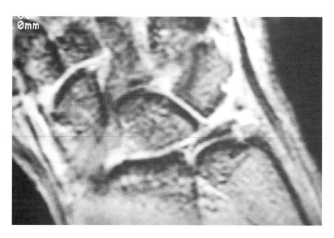

Fig. 4.94 MRI of the triangular cartilage. There is bright signal within the bulk of the triangular cartilage extending to its distal surface.

Changes in bone—avascular necrosis, osteochondritis, stress fractures, degeneration and bruising—are all well shown by MRI.

Elbow Joint

Arthrography of the elbow is usually performed in the search for loose bodies. Capsular ruptures are shown by spreading of contrast medium into adjacent soft tissues. Intra-articular loose bodies are outlined by contrast medium.

Wrist Joint

Arthrography has been used to demonstrate the integrity of the triangular cartilage. Injection of the radiocarpal joint at fluoroscopy shows a torn cartilage and filling of the distal radio-ulnar joint (Fig. 4.93). Unfortunately this can occur as a normal variant in up to 15%. The joint spaces around the proximal row of carpal bones fill during this injection, but the distal intercarpal joint spaces should not, if the local ligaments are intact.

MRI demonstrates the triangular cartilage in coronal images and edema or tears, as well as detachments, are seen (Fig. 4.94).

Axial images of the wrist are also used in the *carpal tunnel syndrome*. Bowing of the flexor retinaculum and compression of the intermediate signal median nerve in the tunnel are associated with local edema.

Hip Joint

Indications for investigation include:

1. Evaluation of hip dysplasias—congenital dislocation of the hip, proximal focal femoral deficiency, epiphyseal dysplasias
2. Evaluation of Perthes disease
3. Assessment of synovial infection, inflammation or tumors

4. Localization of loose bodies

5. Assessment of pain following total hip replacement.

Anatomy of the Infant Hip   The plain radiograph may show a shallow acetabulum and a small, or no, ossific nucleus for the proximal femoral epiphysis. The rest of the 'lucent' joint space is, of course, taken up by articular cartilage, and this is demonstrated after contrast medium has been injected. The ossific nucleus lies centrally within the spherical cartilage (Fig. 4.95).

The acetabular cartilaginous labrum deepens the acetabulum and has a triangular, sharply pointed prominence on its superolateral aspect, the *limbus*. This is covered by synovium and is lax. If medially displaced into the joint, it prevents normal location of the femoral head.

The cartilage of the head should fit congruously within that of the acetabulum; contrast medium should be parallel with and evenly distributed between them, indicating that the joint space is even throughout (Fig. 4.95).

Hip arthrography in children should be performed under fluoroscopic control and, if possible, videotape recordings should be made during manipulation of the hip, as well as taking static films. The head should be contained at all times within the congruous acetabulum and its movement not restricted.

Congenital Dislocation of the Hip   With partial dislocation, or subluxation, movement is excessive and the lateral aspect of the head is uncovered. The limbus and 'rose thorn' are elevated and laterally displaced. Contrast medium pools medially with distension of the medial joint space. Manipulation of the hip under screen control in congenital dislocation of the hip shows the positions in which the femoral head and acetabular fossa are congruous (Fig. 4.96A) and incongruous (Fig. 4.96B). This information aids the surgeon in planning the operation required to facilitate joint development.

With total dislocation, the cartilaginous femoral head is totally uncovered; the limbus is medially and posteriorly displaced and may prevent reduction. Contrast medium again pools medially.

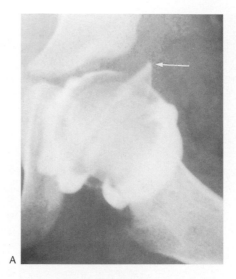

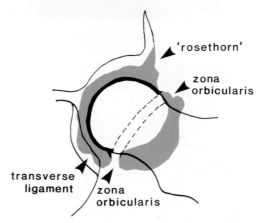

Fig. 4.95   **A**. Arthrogram of the hip showing 'rose thorn' appearance of the normal limbus (arrow). The 'rose thorn' is larger than usual. **B**. Diagramatic representation of the normal hip arthrogram (see text).

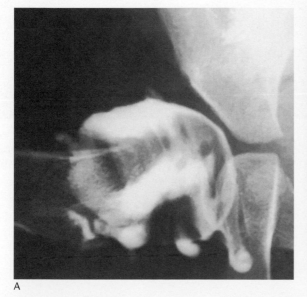

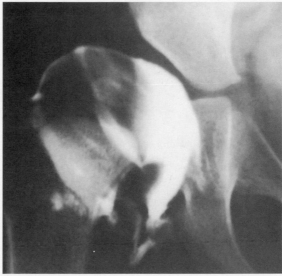

Fig. 4.96   Hip arthrogram in a child. The acetabulum is dysplastic. The ossific nucleus is seen within the largely cartilaginous head. **A**. In abduction the femoral head is congruous with the acetabular cartilage. **B**. In the neutral position the femoral head is incongruous, with pooling of contrast agent medially.

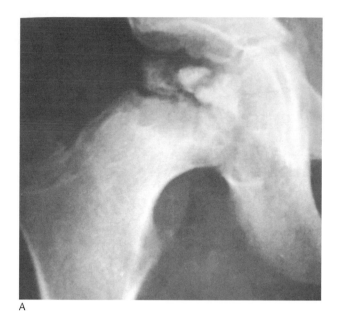

A

Lateral subluxation of the head and medial displacement of the limbus narrows the capsule, giving a so-called 'hour-glass' constriction.

Perthes Disease It must be understood that the ossific nucleus is not the entire femoral head and, in Perthes disease, the cartilaginous outine of the femoral head is essentially normal and not flat, irregular and fragmented, as the ossific nucleus may be. Arthrography does not diagnose Perthes disease but determines: 1. the size and shape of articular cartilage; 2. the presence or absence of congruity (Fig. 4.97).

Hip Arthrography in Adults.

Indications Most adult hip arthrograms are performed to assess either loosening or infection of a prosthesis. These patients complain of pain of increasing severity, often years after hip replacement. Such complications arise in up to 20% of patients, and 5% are infected.

Methyl methacrylate cement causes thermal necrosis of bone. A 1 mm zone of lucency is thus to be expected at the cement–bone interface, especially around the cup of the acetabular prosthesis.

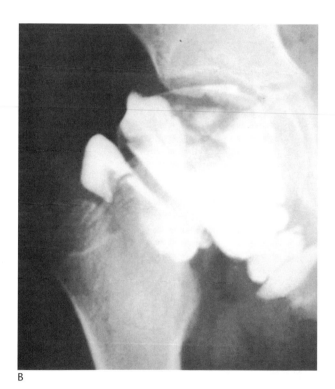

B

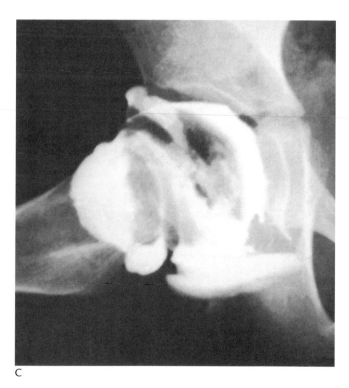

C

Fig. 4.97 **A**. Gross Perthes disease of the femoral head. **B**. The outline of the cartilaginous epiphysis is somewhat dome-shaped with slight flattening and broadening laterally. The lateral aspect of the femoral head is uncovered but in the neutral position is in congruity. **C**. In abduction there is pooling of contrast agent medially within the joint.

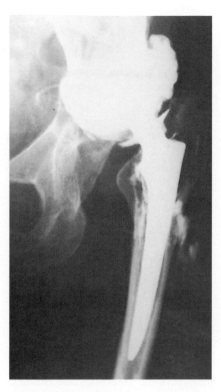

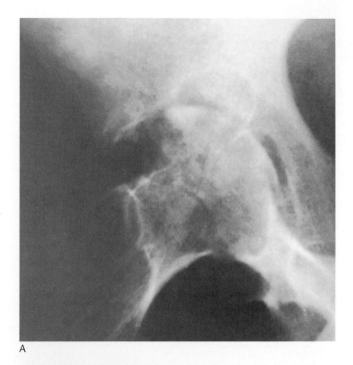

A

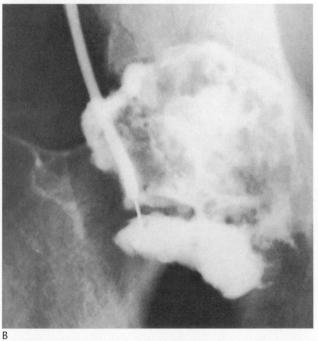

B

Fig. 4.98 Loosening of the hip prosthesis is demonstrated at arthrography. Contrast medium surrounds the acetabular component and tracks down the femoral stem. There is also a defect in the bone through which contrast medium escapes into the soft tissues.

Lucency between cement and metal is less prominent and may result from movement during insertion of the prosthesis, pressure on weight-bearing or osteoclastic stimulation. Excessive or progressive widening of the interface lucency, or settling of the prosthesis into bone or cement, may indicate loosening or infection with resorption of bone.

Loosening is shown at arthrography by tracking of contrast medium between interfaces (Fig. 4.98). This is especially seen at the femoral component, but a thin (less than 1 mm) smear of contrast medium around the cup does not necessarily indicate loosening, especially if it covers the entire cup.

Infection also causes bone resorption at interfaces, but occasionally sinuses develop. Sinograms then show a connection with the prosthesis. Bone resorption is usually more severe and focal.

Synovial lesions or loose bodies may also be demonstrated by arthrography (Fig. 4.99). The needle is again inserted vertically over the central part of the femoral neck.

Fig. 4.99 Synovial tuberculosis. **A**. The plain film shows bone and cartilage destruction on both sides of the joint. **B**. The arthrogram shows gross irregular synovial hypertrophy. The geode does not fill.

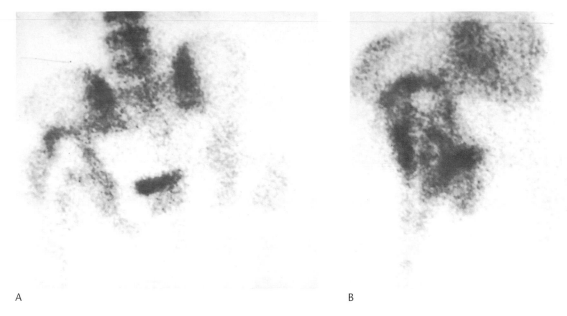

A   B

Fig. 4.100 Technetium bone scan. **A**. Anterior scan of pelvis. **B**. Oblique scan of right hip. The prosthesis can be seen as a defect on the scan and there is increased uptake around it, especially at the femoral component.

Radionuclide Bone Scanning and Prosthetic Loosening
Following insertion of a prosthesis, increased uptake of tracer is to be expected in the surrounding bone. This is uniformly distributed and lasts for up to one year, after which no increase is seen. No conclusion as to abnormality can be drawn in this early stage. After this time, *focal* increase in uptake using ^{99m}Tc-labeled phosphate tracers can be assumed to represent infection or loosening or both. Such uptake is most commonly found at the tip of the femoral prosthetic stem and along its lateral margin (Fig. 4.100).

Differentiation between loosening and infection cannot be made using ^{99m}Tc scans, though a negative technetium scan probably rules out these factors as a cause of hip pain. Differential scanning using ^{67}Ga citrate in addition to technetium is said to differentiate between loosening and infection. Gallium localizes well in leukocytes at the site of infection. This change is best seen 24 hours after injection, when the vascular phase of increased local uptake is over. A positive technetium but negative gallium scan indicates loosening alone; if both are positive, infection is probably present.

REFERENCES AND SUGGESTIONS FOR FURTHER READING

Aisen, A. M., Martel, W., Ellis, J. H., McCune, W. J. (1987) Cervical spine involvement in rheumatoid arthritis. *Radiology*, **165**, 159–163.

Ansell, B. M. (1990) *Rheumatic Disorders in Childhood*. London: Butterworths.

Ansell, B. M., Kent, P. A. (1977) Radiological changes in juvenile chronic polyarthritis. *Skeletal Radiology*, **1**, 129–144.

Borlaza, G. S., Seigel, R., Kuhns, L. R., Good, A. E., Rapp, R., Martel, W. (1981) CT Computed tomography in the evaluation of sacroiliac arthritis. *Radiology*, **139**, 437–440.

Burk, D. L. Jr., Karasick, D., Mitchell, D. G., Rifkin, M. D. (1990) MR imaging of the shoulder: correlation with plain radiography. *American Journal of Roentgenology*, **154**, 549–553.

Freiberger, R. H., Kaye, J. J. (1979) *Arthrography*. New York: Appleton-Century-Croft.

Golding, F. C. (1962) The shoulder—the forgotten joint. *British Journal of Radiology*, **35**, 149–158.

Golimbu, C. N., Firooznia, H., Melone, C. P., Rafii, M., Weinreb, J., Leber, C. (1989) Tears of the triangular fibrocartilage of the wrist: MR imaging. *Radiology*, **173**, 731–733.

Goodman, N. (1967) The significance of terminal phalangeal sclerosis. *Radiology*, **69**, 709–712.

Greenfield, G. B., Schorsch, H., Shkolnick, A. (1967). The various roentgen appearances of pulmonary hypertrophic osteoarthropathy. *American Journal of Roentgenology*, **101**, 927–931.

Grenier, N., Gréselle, J. F., Douws, C., Vital, J. M., Sénégas, J., Broussin, J., Caillé, J. M. (1990) MR imaging of foraminal and extraforaminal lumbar disk herniations. *Journal of Computer Assisted Tomography*, **14**, 243–249.

Hall, F. M. (1989) Sonography of the shoulder. *Radiology*, **113**, 113–130.

Kieft, G. J., Dijkmans, B. A. C., Bloem, J. L., Kroon, H. L. (1990) Magnetic resonance imaging of the shoulder in patients with rheumatoid arthritis. *Annals of Rheumatic Disorders*, **49**, 7–11.

Lazarus, J. H., Galloway, J. K. (1973) Pachydermoperiostosis. *American Journal of Roentgenology*, **118**, 308–313.

Lee, B. C. P., Kazam, E., Newman, A. D. (1987) Computed tomography of the spine and the spinal cord. *Radiology*, **128**, 95–102.

Maddison, P. J., Isenberg, D. A., Woo, P., Glass, D. N. (eds) (1993) *Oxford Textbook of Rheumatology*. Oxford: Oxford University Press.

Martel, W., Stuck, K. J., Dworin, A. M., Hyland, R. G. (1980) Erosive osteoarthritis and psoriatic arthritis: a radiologic comparison in the hand, wrist and foot. *American Journal of Roentgenology*, **134**, 125–135.

Mesgarzadeh, M., Schneck, C. D., Bonakdarpour, A., Mitra, A., Conaway, D. (1989) Carpal tunnel: MR imaging. Part II. Carpal tunnel syndrome. *Radiology*, **171**, 749–754.

Middleton, W. D., Kneeland, J. B., Carrera, G. F. et al (1987) High resolution MR imaging of the normal rotator cuff. *American Journal of Roentgenology*, **148**, 559–564.

Mink, J. H., Reicher, M. A., Crues, J. V. (1993) *MRI of the Knee*, pp. 100–103, 2nd edn. New York: Raven Press.

Modic, M. T., Steinberg, P. M., Ross, J. S., Masaryk, T. J., Carter, J. R. (1988) Degenerative disk disease: assessment of changes in vertebral body marrow with MR imaging. *Radiology*, **166**, 193–199.

Murphey, M. D., Wetzel, L. H., Bramble, J. M., Levine, E., Simpson, K. M., Lindlsey, H. B. (1991) Sacroiliitis: MR imaging findings. *Radiology*, **180**, 239–244.

Murray, R. O. (1965) The aetiology of primary osteoarthritis of the hip. *British Journal of Radiology*, **38**, 810–824.

Neer, C. S. (1983) Impingement lesions. *Clinical Orthopaedics*, **173**, 70–77.

Park, W. M., O'Neill, M., McCall, I. W. (1979) The radiology of rheumatoid involvement of the cervical spine. *Skeletal Radiology*, **4**, 1–7.

Patton, J. T. (1976) Differential diagnosis of inflammatory spondylitis. *Skeletal Radiology*, **1**, 77–85.

Peter, J. P., Pearson, C. M., Marmor, L. (1966) Erosive osteoarthritis of the hands. *Arthritis and Rheumatism*, **9**, 365–387.

Resnick, D. (1995) *Diagnosis of Bone and Joint Disorders*, 3rd edn. Philadelphia: Saunders.

Resnick, D., Shaul, R., Robins, J. M. (1975) Diffuse idiopathic skeletal hyperostosis: Forestier's disease with extraspinal manifestations. *Radiology*, **115**, 513–524.

Reynolds, H., Carter, S. W., Murtagh, F. R., Rechtine, G. R. (1987) Cervical rheumatoid arthritis: value of flexion and extension views in imaging. *Radiology*, **164**, 215–218.

Ryan, P. J., Taylor, M., Grevitt, M., Allen, P., Shields, J., Clarke, S. E. M., Fogelman, I. (1993) Bone single-photon emission tomography in recent meniscal tears: an assessment of diagnostic criteria. *European Journal of Nuclear Medicine*, **20**, 703–707.

Sholkoff, S. D., Glickman, M. G., Steinbach, H. L. (1970) Roentgenology of Reiter's syndrome. *Radiology*, **97**, 497–503.

Yulish, B. S., Lieberman, J. M., Newman, A. J., Bryan, P. J., Mulopulos, G. P., Modic, M. T. (1987) Juvenile rheumatoid arthritis: assessment with MR imaging. *Radiology*, **165**, 149–152.

Zinberg, E. M., Palmer, A. K., Coren, A. B., Levinsohn, E. M. (1988) The triple injection wrist arthrogram. *Journal of Hand Surgery (Am)*, **13**, 803–809.

5

TUMORS AND TUMOR-LIKE CONDITIONS OF BONE (1)

Iain Watt and Mark Cobby

Bone tumors present problems which vary from simple to impossible. Whilst benign and innocuous lesions such as fibrous cortical defects arc common, and may occur in up to 30% of normal children, primary malignant tumors of bone are relatively rare and are responsible for only 1% of all deaths from neoplasia. Consequently most radiologists will see comparatively few cases and, even in referral centres, considerable difficulty often arises in making a diagnosis.

When presented with a lesion in a bone, three important questions require to be answered:

- Is the lesion neoplastic or infective?
- Is it benign or malignant?
- Is it a primary or secondary neoplasm?

In many cases these problems can be resolved without hesitation. In others, notably those in which cartilaginous tissue is involved, great difficulty may be experienced. It must never be forgotten that it is much more common for malignancy in bones to be metastatic rather than primary. It is important that a radiological diagnosis should be made prior to biopsy. An apparently simple radiological diagnosis may not be confirmed histologically and vice versa. Biopsy itself may significantly alter radiological features. It is also important to remember that although the pathologist may be regarded as the final arbiter, fully representative material must be available for opinion, and this may require sectioning the whole lesion. In some benign conditions, such as non-ossifying fibroma or an osteochondroma, it may be considered unnecessary to resort to pathological confirmation, and a conservative attitude or treatment by a minor surgical procedure may be adopted. On the other hand, if a more radical course is being considered, radiology serves not only to provide a diagnosis but also to delineate soft-tissue and bony involvement, thereby permitting procedural planning. Inadequate investigations have occasionally been responsible for erroneous diagnoses of benign lesions as malignant, resulting in unnecessary surgical procedures, including such iatrogenic disasters as amputation.

Many different types of bone tumor are now recognized, varying greatly in their mode of clinical presentation, pathology and behavior. Their etiology remains obscure. Some appear to be superimposed upon a pre-existing disease such as Paget's disease or bone infarction. An increased incidence of both benign and malignant neoplasms is known to follow radiation therapy.

Classification of Bone Tumors

It would be convenient to classify bone tumors according to their cell of origin or histogenesis. However, histologically the exact cell of origin of a tumor is not always certain and typing may depend only on the cell or cells which predominate in the developed lesion. In some cases a single tumor may produce several major different types of cell line (for example, osteosarcoma); in others, undifferentiated small round cells may be a predominant histologic feature, permitting only a broad collective diagnosis of malignant round-cell tumor. A number of interrelated connective tissue cells are present in bone, and from this skeletal connective tissue the majority of bone tumors appear to arise. Other bone tumors are related to non-osseous components of the skeleton, including blood vessels and nerves. Those associated with hematopoietic and lymphoreticular elements are discussed elsewhere (Ch. 7).

A classification of bone tumors is suggested in Table 5.1. Non-neoplastic tumors (the word tumor is literally synonymous with a swelling), abscess, hematoma and so forth, have been included since they must feature in the differential diagnosis. Never forget that a radiologically unusual metastasis is commoner, particularly in older patients, than a primary tumor.

Table 5.1   Classification of Primary Tumors of Bone

	Benign	Malignant
A. Presumed to arise from skeletal tissue		
Bony origin?	Bone island	Osteosarcoma
	Ivory osteoma	Parosteal osteosarcoma
	Osteoid osteoma	
	Osteoblastoma	
Cartilaginous?	Chondroma	Chondrosarcoma
	Chondroblastoma	Dedifferentiated
	Chondromyxoid fibroma	chondrosarcoma
		Mesenchymal
		chondrosarcoma
Fibrous?	Fibrous cortical defect	Fibrosarcoma
	Non-ossifying fibroma	
	Desmoplastic fibroma	Fibrous histiocytoma
	Fibromatosis	
	Atypical Paget's disease	Paget's sarcoma
Giant-cell	Giant-cell tumor	Malignant giant-cell
containing?	Aneurysmal bone cyst	tumor
	Hyperparathyroid brown	
	tumor	
B. Presumed to arise from other tissues in bones		
Blood vessels?	Hemangioma	Angiosarcoma
	Cystic angiomatosis	
	Hemangiomatosis	
	[Massive osteolysis/	
	vanishing bone	
	disease]	
	Glomus tumor	
	[Hemangiopericytoma]	
Nerves?	Neurofibroma	Neurofibrosarcoma
	Neurilemmoma	Neuroblastoma
Fat?	Lipoma	Liposarcoma
	[Intraosseous and	
	parosteal]	
Notochord?	—	Chordoma
Epithelium?	Implantation dermoid	Adamantinoma
Lymphoid/		Leukemias
hematopoietic?		Lymphomas
(see Ch. 7)		Plasmacytoma
		Myelomatosis
C. Presumed to arise from joints		
	Intraosseous ganglion	Synovioma
	Pigmented villonodular	
	synovitis	
	Synovial chondromatosis	
	[Differentiate from:	Synovioma
	Osteoarthritic cyst	
	Rheumatoid geode]	
D. No known origin		
	Solitary bone cyst	Malignant round-cell
		tumours
		(including Ewing's,
		neuroblastomas
		reticulosarcoma)
E. Non-neoplastic tumors		
(a tumor is a	Brodie's abscess	
swelling!)	Hydatid	
	Hematoma	
	Infarction	
	Histiocytosis	

GENERAL PRINCIPLES OF RADIOLOGICAL DIAGNOSIS OF BONE TUMORS

Before attempting to interpret the radiological features of a bone tumor, consider the age of the patient and the clinical history. Many tumors are found in fairly constant age groups. The history may be less useful, since many lesions present with non-specific features of pain, swelling or pathological fracture. However, lesions are not infrequently discovered by chance. The sex incidence in primary bone tumors is of little diagnostic value, although of relevance in skeletal metastasis.

The conventional radiograph is vital in establishing the diagnosis or differential diagnosis of a bone lesion and is supplemented where necessary by computerized tomography, scintigraphy, angiography and magnetic resonance imaging. Questions to consider include:

1. Is the Lesion Solitary or Multiple?   With the exception of multiple osteochondromas of diaphyseal aclasia and multiple cartilage tumors in dyschondroplasia, most primary bone tumors are solitary.

^{99m}Tc-HDP scintigraphy is commonly used to establish whether or not the lesion is unifocal (Fig. 5.1). Other abnormal foci may then be subjected to radiographic examination. Difficulties will be experienced in myelomatosis when most lesions are photon-

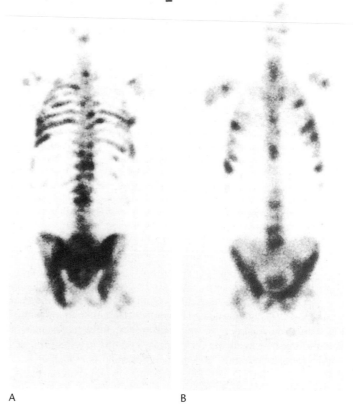

A   B

Fig. 5.1   Multiple skeletal metastases are demonstrated on a whole-body radionuclide bone scan. The primary tumor was carcinoma of the breast in a middle-aged woman. Note the predominantly axial distribution of the lesions, many of which were not apparent on conventional radiographs. **A.** PA view. **B.** AP view.

deficient, or with metastasis from some primary carcinomas, such as cholangiocarcinoma or primary pelvic lesions, including cervix uteri. The high false-negative detection rate in these tumors may justify the more time-consuming and expensive radiographic skeletal survey. Never forget to take a radiograph of the chest, whether or not a skeletal survey has been undertaken. The diagnosis becomes easier if a bronchial carcinoma or an obvious metastasis can be detected.

2. What Type of Bone is Involved? It is of some value to differentiate between flat bones and tubular bones since, for example, lesions in the axial skeleton or proximal ends of long bones are in the sites of persistent hematopoietic tissue and should always raise the possibility of a metastasis or lymphoma. Osteoid osteoma is very rare in membrane bone. A radiolucency in the mandible is more likely to be myeloma than metastasis. Although no part of the skeleton is exempt from involvement by a primary bone tumor, a large proportion are found in the pelvis and in the long bones, particularly around the hips and knees.

3. Where is the Lesion Within the Bone? Many benign tumors tend to appear in characteristic sites: for example, non-ossifying fibroma and fibrous cortical defects are by definition in the cortex, eccentrically toward the metadiaphysis of a long bone. Chondroblastoma occurs in an epiphysis or apophysis. Giant-cell tumor is almost invariably immediately subarticular and eccentric in location. Most tumors of cartilaginous origin, except those which are associated with an osteochondroma, have a medullary location.

4. Conventional Radiographic Features. Never settle for anything less than perfect plain films. It is important that soft-tissue detail is not lost on an overexposed film, because soft-tissue tumor extension typically presents a well-defined margin, whereas soft-tissue swelling associated with inflammation has ill-defined margins. Similarly, soft-tissue calcification or ossification may be overlooked. Do not settle for underpenetrated films since the inner texture of a tumor, for example the ground-glass quality of fibrous dysplasia, may be overlooked, or the radiolucent focus of an osteoid osteoma may not be visualized. Take films 'around the clock'. Simply because periosteal new bone cannot be visualized on a standard AP and lateral film does not mean that it will not be present on an oblique projection. Is the pattern of bone change destructive, proliferative or both? Correlating the size of the lesion with the length of history may be a guide as to its rapidity of growth, and similarly, follow-up films permit an assessment of its aggressive potential or malignancy. Tumors of osteoblastic origin are commonly, but not always, bone-producing. Consequently areas of increased density and/or surrounding new bone formation extending into soft tissue are likely to be evident. Cartilaginous tumors are mainly radiolucent but small foci of calcification represent an important hallmark.

5. What Do the Margins of the Lesion Look Like? Is there a narrow or wide zone of transition between apparent tumor and normal bone? A wide zone of transition suggests a lesion that is rapidly growing such as an aggressive tumor or infection. Is the zone of transition marked with bone reaction or not? A thin rim of sclerosis is present characteristically around a non-ossifying fibroma, whereas extensive sclerosis is typical of a cortical osteoid osteoma. These findings are, of course, not constant and ill-defined sclerosis with a widened zone of transition may occur in such benign con-

ditions as histiocytosis. Examine the cortex; is it resorbed from within, indicating medullary lesions such as cartilaginous tumors or myelomatosis? Peripheral cortical lesions are more commonly caused by pressure or direct invasion from abnormalities in adjacent soft tissues. Exceptions to this are the 'saucerization' of Ewing sarcoma and metastasis. If the margins of such a cortical defect are smooth the lesion is usually benign, e.g. a neurofibroma, or non-neoplastic, as in the case of anterior erosions of the vertebral bodies by an aortic aneurysm. Conversely an irregular margin may suggest invasion by a malignant soft-tissue lesion, e.g. metastasis, or direct invasion by carcinoma of the antrum or lymphoma. Finally, is there an associated soft-tissue mass? The presence of a soft-tissue mass can frequently be shown in relation to malignant bone tumors, although oblique views may be necessary to delineate the masses. An ill-defined soft-tissue mass is almost invariably associated with an inflammatory lesion. Examine the margin of the soft-tissue lesion to see whether or not there is a thin shell of bone as occurs in some aggressive types of aneurysmal bone cysts, particularly those arising in the spine.

Further Imaging Investigations

All further investigations are performed in order to delineate or elicit differential characteristics of a lesion already demonstrated on conventional radiographs, to precisely define the local extent of the lesion and to exclude the presence of metastasis. Where appropriate, imaging studies are also required to monitor preoperative (neoadjuvant) chemotherapy and to detect recurrent disease.

Tomography has been largely superseded by computerized tomography (CT) and magnetic resonance imaging (MR imaging). The object of a tomogram is either to delineate the characteristic radiological features summarized above or to assist demarcation of the intra- and extra-osseous extent of the abnormality.

Scintigraphy may be performed as the first additional investigation in most instances, depending on the availability of MR or CT. High-resolution gamma camera images using ^{99m}Tc-labeled diphosphonate compounds provide the optimal images. Two phases of the bone scan should be recorded. Firstly, by counting the first 300 000 events after the injection a blood-pool scan is obtained whilst the radiopharmaceutical is still largely in the intravascular or perivascular extracellular fluid space. Two to three hours later the skeleton is imaged, when the radiopharmaceutical has localized in bone and is in the delayed or bone-scan phase. The blood-pool phase is vital and should never be overlooked. Scintigraphy may be used to assess the primary presenting lesion and also to detect whether it is monostotic or accompanied by other skeletal lesions, such as metastasis.

Examine the blood-pool phase: is the lesion vascular, as in an aneurysmal bone cyst, or avascular, as in most cartilage tumors? Does the lesion itself accumulate radiopharmaceutical, suggesting that it is being bound into a fibrous, cartilaginous or bone-forming matrix, or is the lesion essentially photon-deficient with increased activity surrounding it, suggesting either a heterogeneous tumor or a host reaction? Does the lesion extend beyond the confines demonstrated by plain film, remembering that the apparent extent of intraosseous involvement can be slightly greater because the scan may not distinguish between bone-forming tumor and a rim of reactive host response? If the lesion is photon-rich, check the lungs since metastases from an osteosarcoma are occasionally detectable by bone scanning. Finally, are there any lesions elsewhere? If so, radiograph them.

Computerized tomography has an important part to play both in the assessment of the primary presenting lesion and in the detection of potential metastatic dissemination. CT will give an impression of the predominant variety of tissue present, particularly if there is fat or calcification. It will not, however, necessarily indicate whether or not those tissues are benign. Examine the intraosseous extent of the tumor, looking for subtle changes in medullary fat. Examine also extraosseous extent and soft-tissue relationships. Contrast-medium enhancement is of little value, since most tumors do not helpfully enhance. However, the vascular nature of a tumor may be detected and the relationship of the soft-tissue component of the tumor to blood vessels can be assessed. More pulmonary metastases are detected by CT than is possible with a conventional chest radiograph.

Angiography has been the subject of fashion but in recent years has fallen into disrepute. The initial hope that it would, in isolation, distinguish reliably between benign and malignant lesions has foundered. No characteristic angiographic feature of malignancy exists. However, two signs—encasement and tumor vessels—occur with much greater frequency in malignant tumors. Encasement results from the vessel being surrounded by tumor and hence is shown by a localized segment of narrowing. Tumor vessels are defined as structures pursuing a random course with an irregular branching pattern.

Angiography should be used in the differential, rather than in the absolute, diagnosis of a lesion, as for example to distinguish between tumor and infection. A malignant round-cell tumor has an intrinsically abnormal vascular pattern, whereas osteomyelitis is characterized by an increased number of normal arterial branches and enlarged periosteal veins. Similarly, angiography may be used to distinguish between tumors, since osteosarcomas are highly vascular, whereas most chondrosarcomas are hypovascular. It is arguable, however, whether angiography now contributes significantly to the assessment of primary tumors and their extent, since much of the information obtainable on angiogram may be obtained by scintigraphy, CT and MRI.

Angiography, however, may still be necessary in order to delineate involvement of major vessels by extension of a tumor into soft tissues when prosthetic or other limb conservation surgery is being considered. Interventional angiography has also enjoyed a vogue. Very vascular tumors may be infarcted prior to resection or intra-arterial chemotherapy given.

Magnetic Resonance Imaging Magnetic resonance images have come to be of prime importance in the assessment of bone and soft-tissue contrast, with the ability to distinguish between various soft tissues by altering pulse sequences. Not only is a superb delineation of intra and extra osseous extent of tumor possible but also the flexibility of imaging planes permits advantageous visualization for tumor staging and planning of surgery. Intraosseous edema and extra-osseous inflammatory response may also be demonstrated. The relationship between tumor masses, inflammatory response, blood vessels and other important structures such as joints may be demonstrated very accurately. This information is of prime importance in planning limb salvaging procedures and assessing whether or not soft-tissue compartments are breached.

Small foci of calcification and fine osseous detail may not, however, be visualized. CT remains valuable for this purpose. Similarly, current images of the lungs are not yet of high enough resolution to confidently detect the presence of a small metastasis. Again, CT is recommended for this purpose.

A measure of tumor aggressiveness may be obtained by measuring the rate of enhancement following intravenous contrast medium; well perfused, often cellular tumors, accumulate a high concentration of gadolinium, the rate at which this accumulates correlating well with biological activity. MR imaging is also invaluable in monitoring tumor response, such as osteogenic sarcoma, to neoadjuvant chemotherapy prior to limb salvage surgery, and will help determine the appropriate adjuvant (postoperative) chemotherapy. An indication of the tissue content of a lesion such as fat, hemorrhage, fibrosis or fluid may be evident from the MR images. Fluid—fluid levels characteristically are seen in aneurysmal bone cysts due to suspended solid old hemorrhagic material creating a layering effect within the fluid. Highly cellular tumors, such as those containing chondroid material, have a particularly high signal intensity on T_2-weighted images and may have a lobulated appearance. By comparison, relatively acellular tumors with a high collagen content will show a low signal intensity on all sequences, including T_2-weighted and STIR sequences. Gadolinium-enhanced images can help to differentiate between viable tumor, reactive edema and necrosis, and can be used to guide the biopsy site.

METASTATIC TUMOR INVOLVEMENT OF BONE

The later stages of many malignant neoplasms are associated almost inevitably with metastasis, and the skeleton is very commonly affected. The radiographic presence of such lesions very often lags behind their detectability by scintigraphy, CT or MR (Fig. 5.2). Bony metastases are present in approximately 25% of all deaths from malignant disease. Any primary tumor may metastasize to bone, but in women the most important carcinoma is breast, from which secondary deposits develop in about two-thirds of cases. In men, approximately 80% of cases of carcinoma of the prostate and a quarter of tumors of the lung and kidney may be expected to produce bone metastases. A metastasis, indeed, may be the presenting feature of the disease.

Whilst a bone metastasis may present as a pathological fracture, usually they produce only vague pain or are entirely occult. Biopsy of a metastasis may indicate the site of origin of a previously unsuspected primary tumor. Usually, the more malignant the primary tumor, the more rapidly does secondary spread occur. Some tumors, however, may present with a metastasis years before the primary lesion is clinically apparent and indeed the metastasis itself may remain virtually unchanged radiologically for a long time. This may be observed particularly with carcinoma of the thyroid. A latent period often separates the removal of a primary tumor, particularly from the breast, and the subsequent development of skeletal metastases.

The *spine*, *pelvis* and *ribs* are the most common sites of involvement together with the proximal ends of the *humeri* and *femora* and, less often, the *skull* (Fig. 5.1). These areas correspond to sites of persistent hematopoiesis in the adult, malignant spread usually occurring by a hematogenous route. Local spread to the lumbar spine and pelvis may be expected from tumors arising in the pelvis, notably carcinoma of the cervix. Some

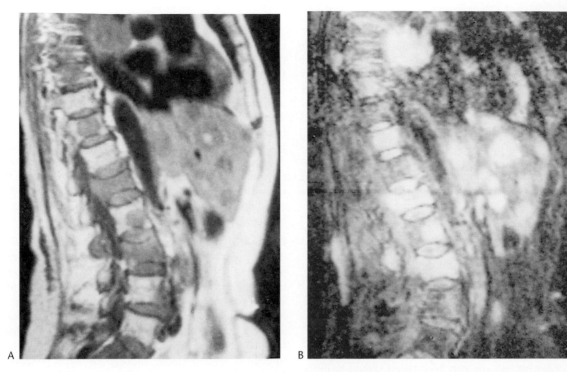

Fig. 5.2   Metastatic carcinoma of the bronchus. Sagittal T_1-weighted **A**. and STIR **B**. MRI sequences obtained in the body coil demonstrate extensive metastases throughout the thoracolumbar spine and liver. The primary bronchial carcinoma is also evident.

metastases have a predictable distribution, the majority of renal cell carcinoma metastases occurring in the lumbar spine and pelvis. They have a rather characteristic radiological appearance (see below). Metastasis distal to the knee and elbow is rare and usually arises from a primary tumor of the bronchus or pelvic organs, particularly colon and bladder.

Blood chemistry studies may be of some value. The *serum alkaline phosphatase* is always raised in the presence of multiple bony metastasis, but remains normal in myelomatosis. With widespread osteolytic destruction the *serum calcium* is usually elevated. In the case of carcinoma of the prostate a marked rise in the *serum acid phosphatase* and *prostate specific antigen* (PSA) levels is characteristic, the latter being now the marker of choice.

Some metastases respond to treatment with, for example, hormone therapy. Under these circumstances both radiography and scintigraphy are needed to monitor the progress of such lesions. Remember that it is inadequate simply to document the number and extent of metastases; it is a radiologist's duty to draw the clinician's attention to those which may be considered hazardous —for example, associated with significant vertebral body collapse (and the possible development of cord compression) or in long bones of the lower limb (with the potential for disabling fracture). In the latter circumstance prophylactic nailing of the femur or femoral neck will be considered if 50% or more of the cortex is destroyed.

Radiological Features   The majority of metastases are predominantly osteolytic. Typically they arise in the medulla and progressively extend in all directions, destroying the cortex, usually without the development of much periosteal reaction. Soft-tissue extension is relatively uncommon. Some metastases, particularly

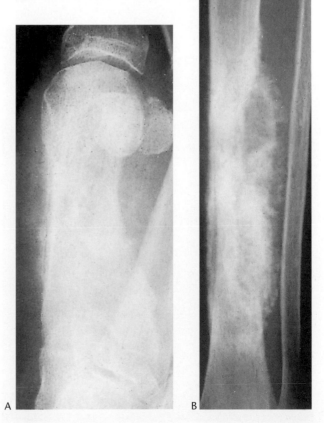

Fig. 5.3   Two examples of solitary metastases producing bone in the adjacent soft tissues. **A.** Carcinoma of the colon in a great toe metatarsal. **B.** Transitional cell carcinoma of the bladder in the mid tibia.

from bronchial carcinoma, may appear eccentric and primarily destroy cortex, especially in the femur. Others are predominantly osteoblastic, including those derived from the prostate, stomach and carcinoid. They produce dense and often well-circumscribed areas of increased radiopacity. Such lesions are less subject to pathological fracture. A small group of metastases is accompanied by tumor bone formation; this includes osteosarcoma, liposarcoma, transitional cell carcinoma (of either bladder or kidney) and some adenocarcinomas of the colon (Fig. 5.3).

The diagnosis of metastases is usually simplified by the multiplicity of lesions. Difficulty may arise when a lesion is apparently solitary. Unusual primary tumors are often responsible for unusual metastases and, further, a metastasis can simulate closely almost any known primary bone tumor!

Breast Not only is this the most common primary tumor in women but its metastases show an unusual affinity for bone. Bone scanning demonstrates a significant incidence of bone metastases at the time of diagnosis, roughly in proportion to the degree of malignancy. The lesions are usually osteolytic and commonly multiple. Diffuse infiltration, however, may cause an apparently coarse trabecular pattern without an obvious area of bone destruction. The condition should be suspected in the presence of vertebral compression fractures in older women. Differentiation of these from osteoporotic collapse may be difficult, although, in the latter, evidence of focal areas of bone destruction is usually lacking. MRI may be extremely helpful in the difficult case. Multiple lytic lesions also may resemble myelomatosis, but in that condition the margins of the lucencies are sharply defined with endosteal

scalloping and the serum alkaline phosphatase is usually normal.

About 10% of metastases from carcinoma of the breast produce osteoblastic lesions and in another 10% the lesions are mixed (Fig. 5.4). Sclerosis may occur in lytic lesions following successful hormone or radiation therapy.

Difficulty may be experienced in differentiating between intense disuse osteoporosis following radiotherapy and metastatic disease. This problem arises particularly around the shoulder where the bones inevitably have been included in the radiation field. The lesions of intense disuse osteoporosis, however, tend to be sharply defined and ellipsoid in the long axis of bone. Similarly, multiple rib fractures secondary to radiation therapy should not be mistaken for metastases. The fractures often occur at the edge of the radiation field and consequently tend to be in a line, a distribution observed also in osteomalacia.

Prostate This is the commonest secondary bone tumor in men and, in contrast to breast deposits, almost all these metastases are osteoblastic (Fig. 5.5). They appear as round or oval areas of increased density, particularly in the pelvis and spine, growing slowly and merging so that widespread and diffuse increase in bone density may ensue. Periosteal new bone formation and/or apparent expansion of bone may occur, so that the differentiation from Paget's disease may be difficult. The deposits may be shown to regress with hormone therapy. In some patients metastases

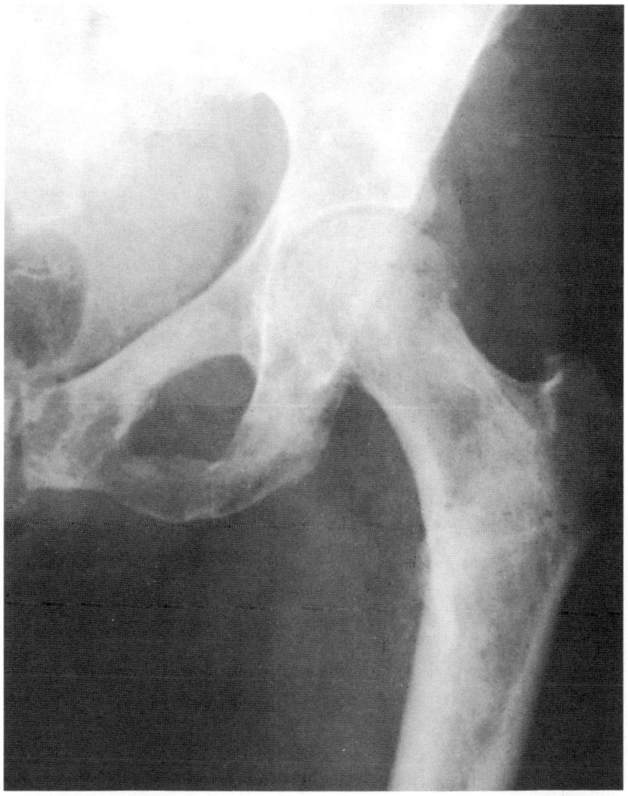

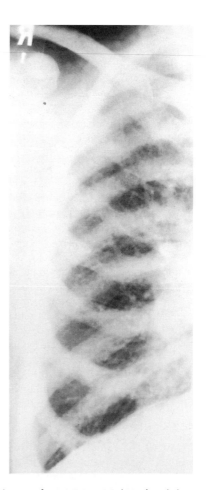

Fig. 5.4 Mixed skeletal metastases from carcinoma of the breast in a middle-aged woman.

Fig. 5.5 Carcinoma of prostate—extensive sclerosis is present in the ribs and clavicle due to widespread metastasis in an elderly man.

from the prostate may be osteolytic and expansile (Fig. 5.6). They may even be solitary. If the carcinoma involves the base of the bladder some metastases may be associated with new bone formation in the adjacent soft tissue, resembling an osteosarcoma.

Kidney   Renal cell carcinoma is characteristically responsible for solitary bone metastases, with a marked predilection for the pelvis and lumbar spine. Even when multiple their number seldom exceeds six. These lesions are typically expansile with a crenellated margin and usually have a typical radiological appearance (Fig. 5.7). They are richly vascular, as demonstrated scintigraphically or angiographically. These tumors are often slow growing and may have a relatively good prognosis, particularly following excision of the affected kidney and a solitary deposit. Transcatheter embolization may prove a useful addition to management.

Lung   In men this tumor is second only to the prostate in causing a high proportion of cases to develop skeletal metastases, such bone lesions occurring eventually in about a third. These metastases are almost always osteolytic and can be unusual, occurring in the small bones of the hand or eccentrically in the cortex of a long bone.

Alimentary Tract   Carcinoma of the stomach and colon, and carcinoid, may metastasize to bone in both sexes. Metastases from the stomach and carcinoid are often osteoblastic and may be multiple. The bone-forming characteristic of colonic metastases has been already emphasized.

Other primary tumors often produce bizarre and atypical radiological patterns. In particular the metastases from thyroid carcinoma are classically expansile, osteolytic and often solitary (Fig. 5.8).

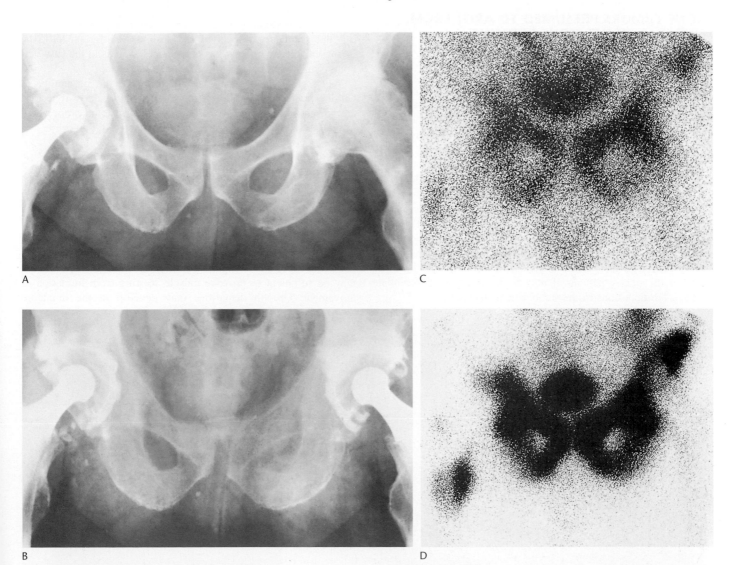

A

B

C

D

Fig. 5.6   Carcinoma of the prostate with expansile lytic metastases. **A.** A view of the pelvis before the onset of symptoms reveals no abnormality in the pubic rings. **B.** 5 years later the patient was complaining of severe pain in the groin. Note the ill-defined trabecular pattern, expansion of bone and ill-definition of cortex which has developed since the previous examination. **C.** Blood-pool phase of a bone scan and **D.** delayed image reveals a marked increase in activity. Note the abnormality in the lesser trochanter of the right femur. These features could not be distinguished from active aggressive Paget's disease on purely scintigraphic grounds except that the lesion in the right femur has not started at a joint. The diagnosis was established by biopsy and the presence of a very high acid phosphatase level in the blood.

INVASION AND DESTRUCTION OF BONE BY EXTRAOSSEOUS PRIMARY MALIGNANT TUMORS

Lesions of this type are rare compared with skeletal metastases, but may be observed in association with direct spread of such lesions as carcinoma of the cervix or bladder, and also from carcinoma of the paranasal sinuses. Malignant tumors adjacent to bone may cause resorption of the cortex with a permeative pattern, but lower-grade malignancies, including tendon sheath abnormalities, may produce well-defined cortical defects suggesting pressure erosion. Destruction of adjacent bones should suggest a lesion originating in soft tissues. An important example is involvement of the upper ribs by bronchial carcinoma (Pancoast tumor) in patients being assessed for neck, brachial plexus or shoulder pain (Fig. 5.9).

BONE TUMORS PRESUMED TO ARISE FROM SKELETAL TISSUE: BONE-FORMING

Bone Island (also known as *enostosis*)

Although no evidence exists to suggest that this is a true bony neoplasm, confusion may arise on occasions. The lesions may be single or multiple, are always medullary in location and consist of normal, compact lamellar bone. The lesion is uniformly dense, round or oval, and characteristically has radiating thorn-like spicules extending into the surrounding medullary cavity with a narrow zone of transition (Fig. 5.10). They usually measure less than 15 mm in diameter, but occasionally can be as large as 4 cm in size. Bone islands may grow up to the age of skeletal maturity and occasionally thereafter. Exceptionally they may regress. Periosteal new bone and cortical expansion do not occur. On a radionuclide bone scan they may show a slight increase in activity, the degree being related to their size. No blood-pool abnormality becomes evident. In elderly patients it may be necessary to differentiate these sclerotic lesions from osteoblastic metastases.

Osteoma

True osteomas are rather rare, arising principally from skull, paranasal sinuses and mandible (Fig. 5.11). They are benign, slow-growing tumors consisting entirely of well-differentiated bone. They have a broad base with a smooth well-defined margin. Two types are recognized: the dense variety, the so-called ivory osteoma; and the trabeculated or spongy variety more commonly occurring in the cranial vault. Whilst varying in size, few are larger than 2.5 cm in diameter. The tumor itself is asymptomatic, but growth from the inner table of the skull may produce raised intracranial pressure or other symptoms similar to those of a meningioma. Growth within the paranasal sinuses may interfere with nasal drainage, causing a mucocele. The rarer, spongy variety is shown histologically to contain moderate quantities of fibrous tissue and may be a variant of fibrous dysplasia.

Further investigation is rarely necessary apart from documenting the secondary effects of the lesion. Scintigraphically the increased activity reflects the size of the lesion as in the case of a bone island.

When craniofacial osteomas are detected, the possibility of Gardner syndrome should be considered, particularly if lesions are present in the mandible. The presence of osteomas elsewhere in the skeleton, soft-tissue tumors of connective tissue origin and polyposis coli establish the diagnosis.

Osteoid Osteoma

Unlike other bone tumors this lesion has a definite male preponderance of the order of three to one. The majority of cases present in the second and third decades. The typical history is of localized, intermittent bone pain of several weeks' or months' duration, occurring especially at night, with dramatic relief by aspirin. Pain may be sufficient to provoke muscle wasting from limitation of movement. Growth disparities may develop in the immature

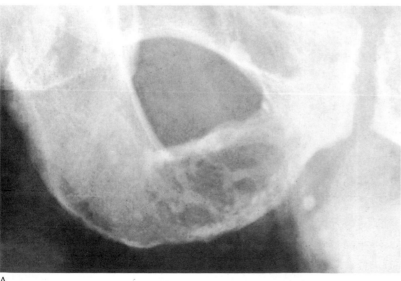

A

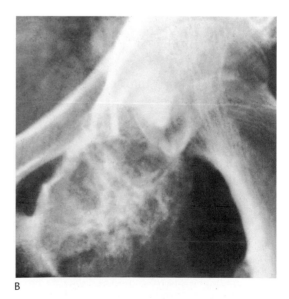

B

Fig. 5.7   A,B. Two examples of solitary metastases from renal cell carcinoma. In both cases these metastases were the presenting abnormality. Both are expansile and have crenellated margins, with trabeculation in the lesion.

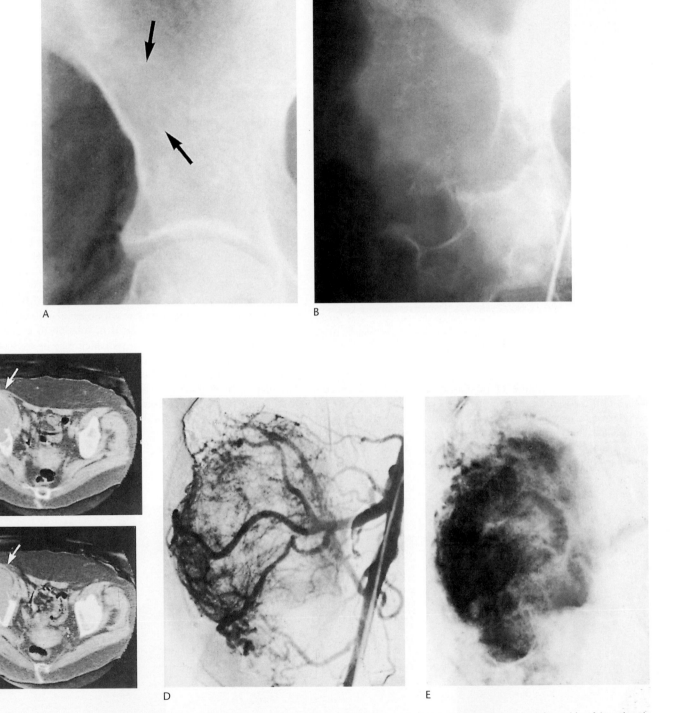

Fig. 5.8 Metastasis from carcinoma of thyroid. **A.** A localized view of the anterior inferior iliac crest shows a small radiolucent defect with a faint sclerotic margin (arrows). **B.** Five years later a very large destructive bone lesion is present with relatively well-defined margins and apparent strands of calcification within the lesion. **C.** CT confirms the very extensive nature of the tumor and shows the soft-tissue planes to be preserved (arrow). The strands of calcification are shown to be residual bone anteriorly and posteriorly and not new bone in the metastasis. **D** and **E.** Common iliac arteriography (subtraction images) demonstrates the very vascular nature of this metastasis. Note the increase in number of abnormal vessels with changing caliber, the dense tumor blush and early venous filling.

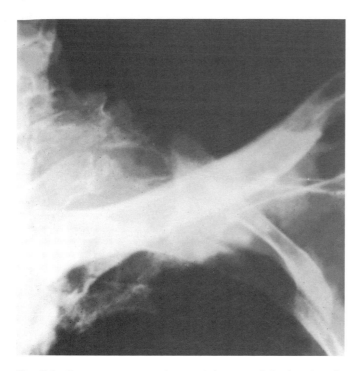

Fig. 5.9 Pancoast tumor—carcinoma of the apex of the lung invading and destroying the first and second ribs.

skeleton, including failure of tubulation and leg length discrepancy. Difficulty in diagnosis sometimes causes these patients to be referred to psychiatrists in the belief that their symptoms are functional. The natural history of this tumor is uncertain since most cases are treated by immediate surgical excision but it appears probable that untreated lesions eventually undergo spontaneous involution. The diaphyses of long bones are the sites of predilection with at least half of all cases occurring in the femur, especially its proximal end, and the tibia, although virtually any bone may be affected. When the spine is involved the tumor is almost always situated in the neural arch and not the vertebral body. The symptoms of spinal involvement may mimic those of an adolescent disk protrusion, and indeed painful scoliosis in a child or adolescent demands careful scrutiny of the neural arches at the apex of the concavity to exclude the presence of this tumor.

Radiological Features The lesion comprises a round or oval area or radiolucency with a sclerotic margin. This radiolucency usually contains a small dense opacity known, on this side of the Atlantic, as the *nidus* (Fig. 5.12). In North America the word nidus (meaning nest) is employed more correctly for the radiolucency itself. While the overall size of the lesion varies up to about 2.5 cm in diameter, the width of the central density rarely exceeds 1 cm. The lesion is surrounded by a variable degree of dense sclerosis. The extent of this density depends on the site of the tumor within the affected bone. It is minimal when the tumor lies in the spongy bone of the medulla, particularly close to joints (Figs 5.13, 5.14).

Occasionally no peripheral density may be evident and the small central opacity appears to lie within an area of radiolucency. More commonly, the lesion is sited in relation to cortical bone and is surrounded by dense sclerosis which may be extensive and extend into the medulla. When the lesion is adjacent to the periosteum in children new bone formation is particularly florid. The reactive new bone may be so dense that the lesion itself is obscured on conventional radiographs.

Provided that the essential features of the radiolucency and its central density are demonstrated, the diagnosis is usually established radiologically with little difficulty. Those arising in an intraarticular location (Fig. 5.14) or within the small bones of the hand

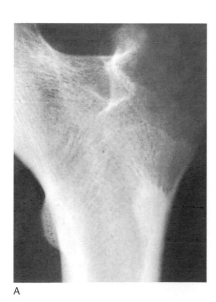

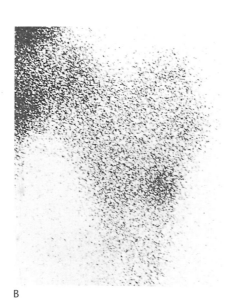

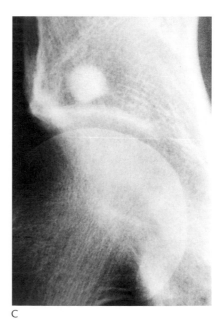

A   B   C

Fig. 5.10 Bone island—enostosis. **A.** A dense area of endosteal sclerosis present in the upper femoral shaft, discovered by chance following injury. **B.** A bone scan reveals slight increase in activity localized to the area of sclerosis. Biopsy confirmation. **C.** Enostosis, acetabular roof. Uniformly dense circular lesion with characteristic radiating spicules extending into the adjacent bone.

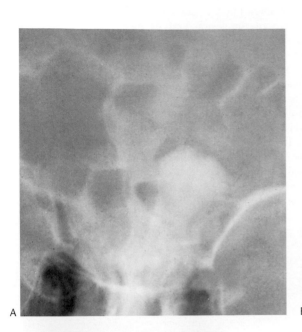

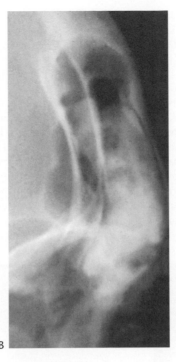

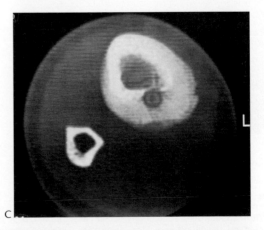

Fig. 5.11 Ivory osteomas of the frontal sinus. A typical, compact, rounded, dense opacity is demonstrated on **A.** the frontal view. **B.** In another patient a larger lesion has moulded to the shape of the sinus.

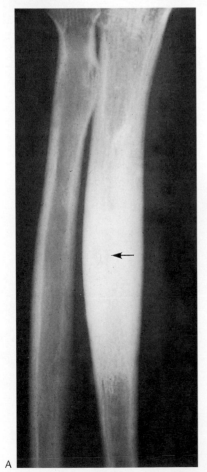

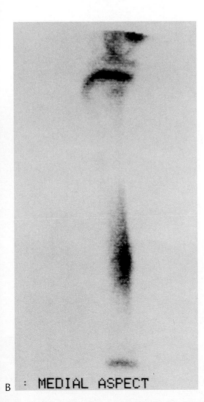

Fig. 5.12 Osteoid osteoma. **A.** Involving the ulna in a 13-year-old boy. The appearances are typical, with a well-defined area of radiolucency (arrow) containing a dense nidus. Extensive cortical sclerosis is present around the lesion. **B.** Radio-isotope bone scan in another patient demonstrating intense focal increased scintigraphic activity in the distal tibia surrounded by a more diffuse area of less intense activity, typical of an osteoid osteoma. **C.** CT section of the tibial lesion elegantly demonstrating the cortically located nidus.

and foot (Fig. 5.15) can have a very variable appearance, commonly resulting in a delayed diagnosis. When the lesion is surrounded by dense sclerosis further investigation is necessary, requiring overpenetrated films, tomography (either conventional or CT) and bone scintigraphy.

Because of the extensive sclerosis it is important not to overcount the bone scan which characteristically shows an intense focal area of increased activity due to the osteoid osteoma surrounded by less intense activity from the reactive sclerosis (Fig. 5.12). In the case of a medullary osteoid osteoma with little or no radiological abnormality on conventional films, bone scintigraphy remains the most important means of detecting the presence of a lesion. An intense focal abnormality is evident in the blood-pool image and intense activity persists in the delayed image. Scintigraphy should be undertaken in any young person with bone pain and apparently normal radiographs. These scinti-

graphic abnormalities correspond to the highly vascular nature of the neoplasm which may be demonstrated by angiography, particularly by the tumor blush evident in the late venous phase.

The presence of the lesion and its exact site may require localization with computerized tomography (Figs 5.12, 5.14). Extensive bone marrow edema may be seen on MR imaging although it is frequently difficult to identify the nidus unless contrast enhancement is used and sufficiently thin sections are obtained (Fig. 5.14).

The pain produced by these tumors is relieved immediately by surgical excision and the reactive new bone slowly undergoes remodeling. If, however, removal of the tumor is incomplete, not only will the pain persist but the lesion will recur. On rare occasions, osteoid osteoma may be multifocal, more than one opacity being contained within a single area of radiolucency. Some lesions near joints in childhood may be associated with synovitis, with

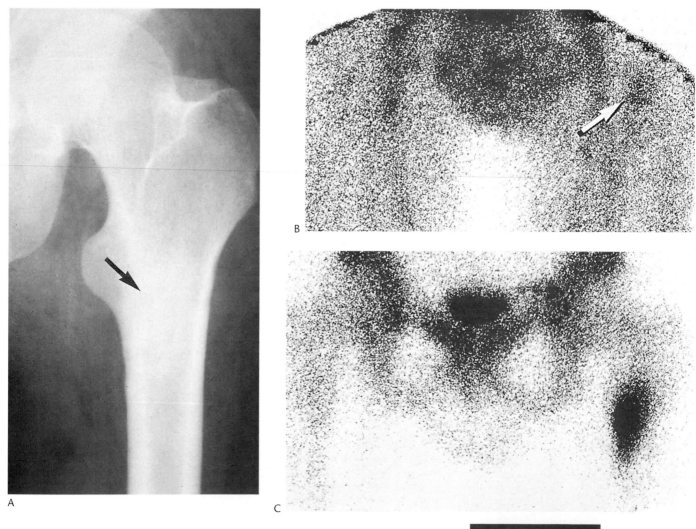

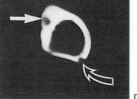

Fig. 5.13 Osteoid osteoma—a young man complaining of groin pain. **A.** Thought initially to have normal X-rays; however, in retrospect, a small radiolucency (arrow) is present. A bone scan was performed in order to detect any occult cause of pain. **B.** A localized focus of increased vascularity is shown on the blood-pool film (arrow). **C.** Extensive abnormality on the delayed film. **D.** Computerized tomography demonstrates the radiolucent defect anteriorly (closed arrow) with associated, consolidated periosteal new bone. A nutrient artery is shown posteriorly (open arrow) and is an incidental finding.

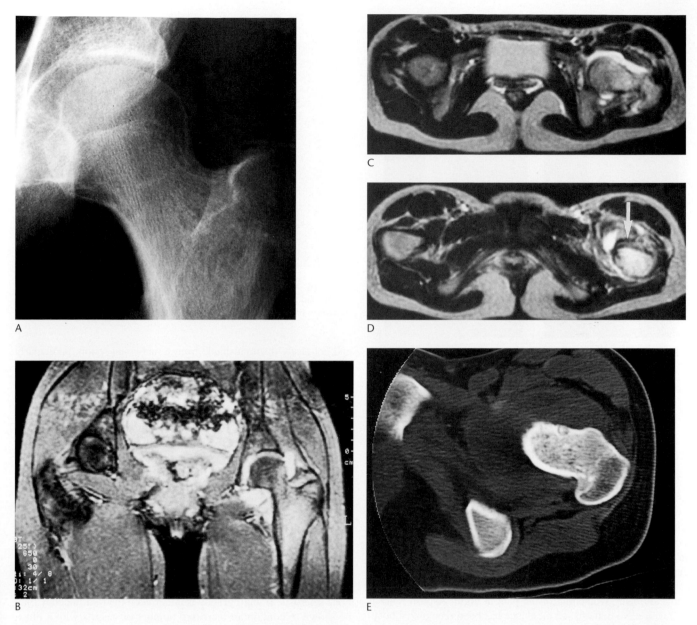

Fig. 5.14 Osteoid osteoma in a young girl complaining of left hip and knee pain, initially thought to be due to juvenile onset rheumatoid arthritis. **A.** A subtle radiolucency with a central density is shown in the basi-cervical region of the left femur. **B.** Coronal FFE-T$_2$* MR section demonstrating high signal intensity within the proximal left femur due to considerable bone marrow edema. A joint effusion is also evident together with some surrounding soft-tissue edema. **C.** Axial T$_2$-weighted **MR** image showing a prominent left hip joint effusion and bone marrow edema within the femoral neck. The nidus, however, is not evident. **D.** Axial T$_2$-weighted image through the proximal femur demonstrating more striking bone marrow edema distal to the joint capsule and level of the osteoid osteoma. Periosteal new bone formation is also shown anteriorly (arrow). **E.** Thin section CT showing the anteriorly located calcified nidus within the cortex of the femoral neck and the large joint effusion.

resulting diffuse hyaline cartilage thinning and disuse osteoporosis. Delay in establishing a diagnosis often results due to the atypical clinical presentation and lack of characteristic radiological appearances. Subsequent deformity of the joint and other growth disturbances may occur.

Osteoid osteoma must be differentiated from osteoblastoma (described below) and other causes of chronic cortical thickening. These include stress fracture, chronic sclerosing osteomyelitis, foreign body granulomas ('blackthorn'), polyarteritis nodosa and subperiosteal hematoma, particularly along the shin. In general

the distinction between osteoid osteoma and chronic osteomyelitis is straightforward. In osteomyelitis the area of radiolucency tends to be more irregular, although a sequestrum may be confused with a nidus. Whereas the central opacity of an osteoid osteoma is almost always round or slightly oval, the majority of osteomyelitic sequestra are irregular and often linear in shape. Scintigraphy shows a diffuse increase in activity both in the blood-pool and the delayed phases. MRI may demonstrate considerable bone edema in both cases but a fluid collection clearly indicates infection.

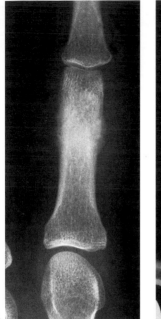
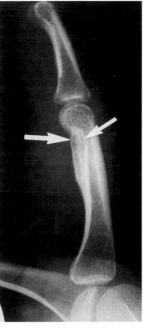

A   B

Fig. 5.15   Osteoid osteoma in the proximal phalanx of the index finger. **A.** The AP radiograph shows ill-defined periosteal new bone formation and some sclerosis involving the proximal phalanx. Marked soft-tissue edema is also evident. **B.** The lateral radiograph demonstrates apparent expansion and scalloping of the distal anterior cortex of the proximal phalanx with trabecular sclerosis distal to the radiolucent nidus (arrows).

Osteoblastoma

This tumor is now accepted as a distinct entity, although a considerable overlap undoubtedly exists with osteoid osteoma. Indeed the situation is confused by the occasional osteoid osteoma which is larger than usual and may be referred to as giant osteoid osteoma. Both osteoblastoma and osteoid osteoma superficially have similar histologic characteristics. The tumor is, in almost all circumstances, benign, but may be aggressive (see below). It is accompanied often by a long insidious history of pain, one in ten patients suffering worsening of the pain at night. Aspirin relief is not a feature. No definite sex incidence has been recognized but at least 80% of the patients are under the age of 30.

Whilst any bone may be involved, the majority of lesions occur in the spine and flat bones, particularly the vertebral appendages. Again, as in the case of osteoid osteoma, the last location may stimulate a scoliosis; indeed in one series as many as 50% of the patients had a scoliosis, some with positive neurologic signs.

Pathologically the lesion is larger than an osteoid osteoma, irregular in shape, friable and hemorrhagic. Abundant osteoid tissue is present with broad, widely spread trabeculae, in relation to which are numerous osteoblasts and osteoclasts. Many thin-walled capillaries account for the marked vascularity of the tumor.

Radiological Features   An area of radiolucency is typical, being considerably larger than that of an osteoid osteoma and of the order of 2–10 cm in diameter (Fig. 5.16). Difficulty may arise on occasions in distinguishing this appearance from an exceptionally large osteoid osteoma. The margins of the radiolucency show considerable irregularity, even though they are usually sharply demarcated. This margin, however, may sometimes be ill-defined

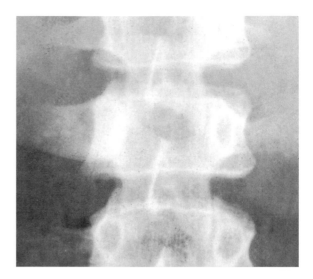

Fig. 5.16   Osteoblastoma of the right transverse process and pedicle of L3. An ill-defined radiolucency is shown within a sclerotic and expanded transverse process and pedicle.

and not easily distinguishable from a malignant lesion, particularly an osteosarcoma. A giant-cell tumor may be considered when the lesion is subarticular in location. Cortical expansion and exquisite thinning is common so that only a fine opaque shell may remain. This appearance simulates the cortical expansion caused by an aneurysmal bone cyst, but may be distinguished by the total absence of bone reaction and the poorly defined margin of the latter tumor.

The majority of osteoblastomas enlarge slowly, with consequent remodeling of bone around the lesion. The degree of associated bone sclerosis varies considerably but may be profound. Calcification or ossification of osteoid tissue within the tumor may cause a punctate or amorphous increase in density (Fig. 5.17), best appreciated on tomography or CT (Fig. 5.18). Calcification is never annular as in a cartilage tumor.

Scintigraphically these lesions are extremely active both in the blood-pool and delayed phases of a bone scan. On the delayed phase the lesion may seem very extensive, reflecting the secondary bone sclerosis. If angiography is undertaken the radiolucency may be shown to contain an increased number of vessels with a blush and small lakes of contrast medium, but encasement and other features suggestive of malignancy are not present. As with osteoid osteoma, *MRI* demonstrates considerable bone, and often soft-tissue, edema surrounding a lesion.

In the vast majority of patients the prognosis is excellent once total excision of the tumor has been achieved. On some occasions, however, an osteoblastoma behaves in an aggressive fashion, particularly after incomplete removal. Not only is the lesion radiographically aggressive, with soft-tissue masses containing ill-defined calcification and ossification, but a similar pattern of aggression is visible also under the microscope. On rare occasions the lesion behaves frankly as an osteosarcoma with pulmonary metastasis (Fig. 5.19).

Osteosarcoma

Osteosarcoma is the commonest primary malignant bone tumor, accounting for 25% of all primary bone tumors. Characteristically

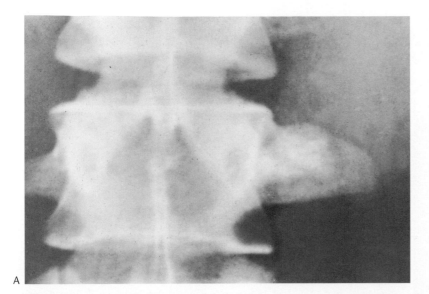
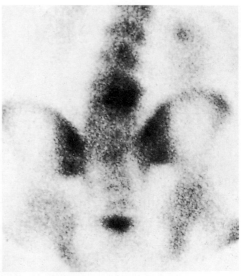

Fig. 5.17 Osteoblastoma of the left transverse process of L3. **A.** In this example the central area exhibits calcification. Expansion is present with diffuse sclerosis. **B.** Note on the bone scan (which has been reversed for ease of comparison) the extensive area of increased activity corresponding to the whole of the osteoblastoma on the plain film. Note also the scoliosis, with which these patients may present.

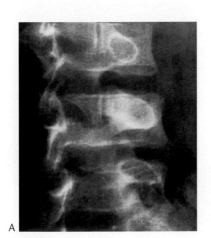
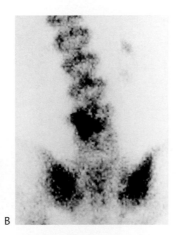
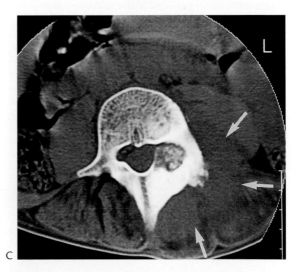

Fig. 5.18 Osteoblastoma of the left pedicle and lamina of L3. **A.** Conventional oblique radiograph showing expansion and sclerosis. **B.** Radio-isotope bone scan demonstrating extensive and marked increase in activity and a scoliosis. **C.** CT section showing punctate calcification of the lesion with expansion of the pedicle and lamina and prominent dense sclerosis. Considerable soft-tissue edema is also evident (arrows).

it is histologically pleomorphic, but two diagnostic features are: firstly, its ability to produce osteoid tissue, without necessarily the development of a cartilaginous precursor; and, secondly, the presence of abundant alkaline phosphatase histochemically within the tumor cells. The osteoid tissue may undergo some degree of ossification. However, because of the pleomorphic nature of the sarcoma a dominant cell line may modify the appearance. If osteoblasts predominate, tumor bone formation will result, whereas, if cells of cartilage origin are present, extensive calcification may be a presenting feature. Terms such as osteoblastic (Fig. 5.20), chondroblastic (Fig. 5.21), fibroblastic, and anaplastic or telangiectatic (Fig. 5.22) are often applied. No convincing evidence

has been established that these pathological subgroups have much influence on prognosis. Nonetheless, each has slightly different radiological characteristics. Osteosarcoma arising in relation to the periosteum and secondary to other conditions is considered below.

Osteosarcoma presents usually with localized pain or swelling, particularly around the knee, in an adolescent or young adult. Not infrequently the lesion may present with a pathological fracture (Fig. 5.23). A slight male preponderance exists, the peak incidence occurring between 10 and 25 years of age. Many of the tumors occurring in older age groups are associated with Paget's disease (see below). Although any bone may be involved, rather more than

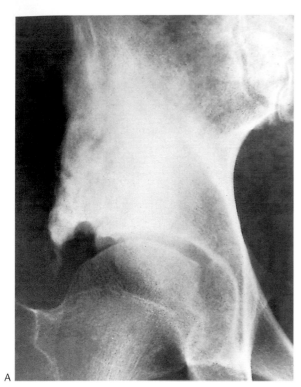

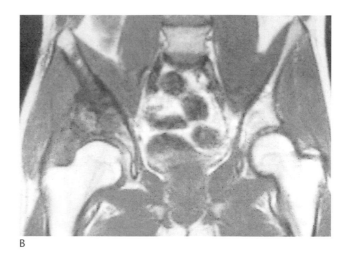

Fig. 5.19 Aggressive osteoblastoma. Conventional radiograph **A.** demonstrates a large area of ill-defined bone sclerosis extending into the soft tissues above the acetabular roof. This had been previously biopsied. A vague ill-defined zone of radiolucency is demonstrated within the proliferative new bone. A T$_1$-weighted coronal MR image **B.** demonstrates extensive low-signal abnormality throughout the whole of the right iliac blade down to the acetabular roof. A soft-tissue component is also evident. This scan also illustrates how difficult it can be to assess sclerotic lesions using MRI.

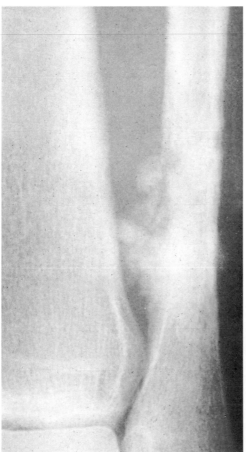

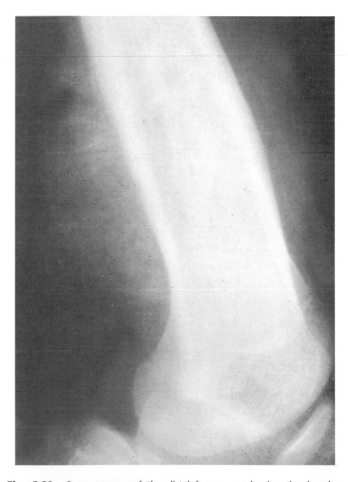

Fig. 5.20 Osteosarcoma of the distal fibula—predominantly osteoblastic. Amorphous calcification/ossification is present in the soft tissues with cortical destruction and a little periosteal new bone formation.

Fig. 5.21 Osteosarcoma of the distal femur—predominantly chondroblastic. Note the well-defined soft-tissue mass and radiating spiculation of calcification within it. Sclerosis and lysis are present within the medullary cavity which is slightly expanded.

half of all osteosarcomas are located around the knee, involving the metadiaphyses of the distal end of the femur and the proximal end of the tibia. Indeed the vast majority of osteosarcomas arise in those sites in long bones which are exhibiting the greatest longitudinal growth. Osteosarcomas are infrequently found in the pelvis and spine (Fig. 5.24). Involvement of the clavicle, ribs, scapula and the small bones of the hands and feet is rare. About 10% of tumors arise in the diaphysis. These have a similar age and sex incidence to ordinary osteosarcoma (see below). Orthodox teaching suggested that epiphyseal involvement occurs late, metaphyseal cartilage acting as a temporary barrier to spread of the tumor. Although this appears supported by the evidence of plain films, investigation by scintigraphy, angiography and MR has indicated that in many cases epiphyseal involvement occurs earlier.

The lesion commonly arises eccentrically in the medullary cavity, with ill-defined cortical destruction and soft-tissue involvement. The pleomorphic nature of the histology may cause misleading biopsy results, since if the sample is taken from areas rich in cartilaginous elements, a misdiagnosis of chondrosarcoma may occur. Metastatic spread occurs by the hematogenous route so that a search for pulmonary metastasis should be undertaken. Pulmonary metastasis is associated with an unusually high incidence of pneumothorax (Fig. 5.25). Any lung lesion arising in a patient with osteosarcoma should be regarded with suspicion (Fig. 5.26).

Lymphatic spread is relatively rare. In the later stages metastases may develop in bone; population surveys have suggested that these deposits are themselves metastatic from the pulmonary lesions.

Imaging Features   Typically, *conventional radiographs* will show an eccentric area of permeative bone destruction in the metadiaphysis adjacent to the knee joint, associated with cortical erosion and a well-defined soft-tissue mass. Elevation of the periosteum is associated with new bone formation, the so-called Codman's triangles. The epiphysis usually appears normal. The soft-tissue mass may contain calcification which may show either an amorphous or a spiculated appearance. A mixture of sclerosis and bone destruction is usually present within the bony lesion. Occasionally the lesion may be purely lytic.

Scintigraphically, increased vascularity is constant in the blood-pool phase of a bone scan with an extensive abnormality on the delayed images (Fig. 5.27). The extent of the tumor, as delineated by a bone scan, may be greater than that shown on conventional radiography, due to a surrounding rim of reactive bone. Scintigraphy may confirm epiphyseal spread of the tumor, but an apparent increase in activity in an adjacent joint should not be mistaken for synovial involvement. Scintigraphy also may detect the presence of lung metastasis, although this procedure is

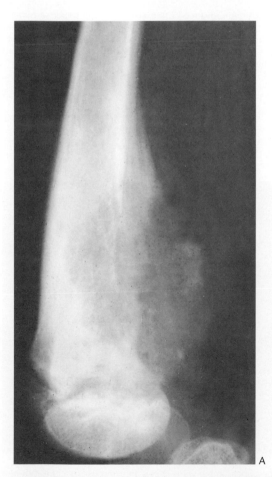

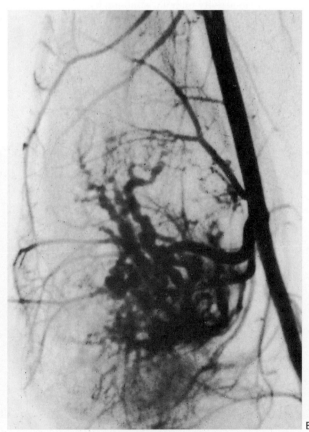

Fig. 5.22   Telangiectatic osteosarcoma of the distal femur. **A.** A predominantly radiolucent defect is shown on conventional radiograph which **B.** angiographically is shown to contain large, tortuous, pathological vessels. Well-marked Codman's triangles are present together with sclerosis in the shaft of the bone, surrounding the lesion.

not reliable if purely fibroblastic lesions are present or if the metastases have been treated.

Computerized tomography demonstrates to advantage those features evident on conventional radiographs and can also delineate the intra- and extra-osseous extent of tumor (Figs 5.27C, 5.28D). It is the most sensitive means of detecting pulmonary metastases (Fig. 5.26B). The *angiographic features* suggest an aggressive tumor and again may be used to establish the extent of tumor, if treatment by prosthetic replacement is being considered (Figs 5.28, 5.29).

Magnetic resonance imaging is the prime investigation of choice for osteosarcoma following conventional radiographs. An obvious heterogeneous tumor is demonstrated with surrounding bone and usually a soft-tissue mass. Areas of calcification and ossification are shown as low signal but even within the sclerotic component within the medullary canal there is usually high signal associated with tumor bulk. Careful delineation of the lesion and assessment of relationships between it and adjacent blood vessels and joints are essential in preoperative planning (Figs 5.30, 5.31, 5.32, 5.33). Marked enhancement is shown following contrast administration, particularly in non-ossified regions. Intramedullary skip lesions may also be identified.

Differential diagnosis is either from other neoplasms, including malignant round-cell tumors and metastases, or from chronic bone infections, including tuberculosis and mycetoma. In the case of infections the etiology may be suggested by diffuse ill-defined swelling of soft tissues, disproportionately extensive new bone formation and widespread activity on bone scintigraphy.

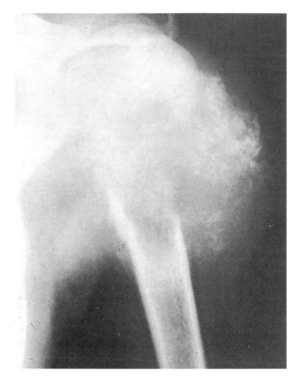

Fig. 5.23 An advanced osteosarcoma of the proximal humerus presents with a pathological fracture. A large well-defined soft-tissue mass contains calcification and ossification. Codman's triangles are present. Extensive tumor in the medulla has caused both bone destruction and bone formation.

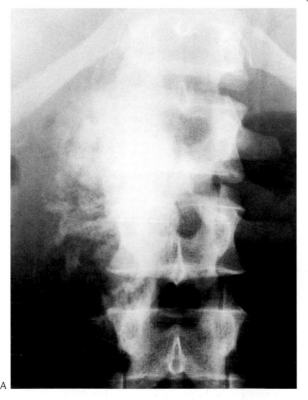

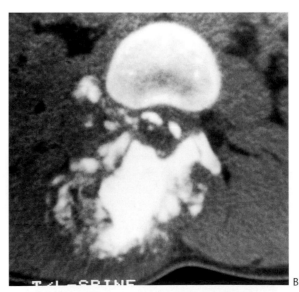

Fig. 5.24 Osteosarcoma of the spine. **A.** A conventional radiograph of the upper lumbar spine shows an extensive area of tumor new bone formation arising from the lamina of L1 and extending into the paravertebral soft tissues. **B.** The CT section demonstrates the origin and extent of the tumor. Marked compression of the dural sac results from extension onto the spinal canal.

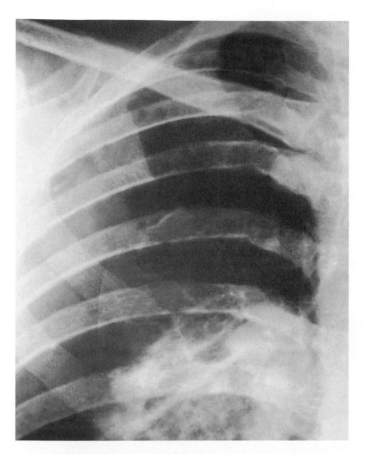

Fig. 5.25 Osteosarcoma—metastasis in the lungs presents with a pneumothorax.

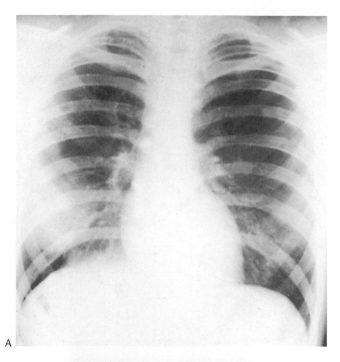

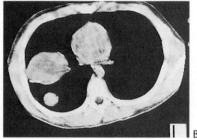

Fig. 5.26 Metastasis from osteosarcoma presents with **A.** an encysted pleural effusion on the right after several months apparently disease-free after amputation. **B.** A CT scan demonstrates the encysted effusion in the horizontal fissure with calcification dorsally due to metastasis. This feature had not been appreciated on conventional tomography. A second metastasis is shown in the right lower lobe, again not obvious on conventional radiographs.

Special Types of Osteosarcoma

Diaphyseal Approximately 10% of tumors arise in the diaphyses of long bones and may cause diagnostic confusion. Whilst most resemble those of osteosarcoma elsewhere (Fig. 5.34), others are purely lytic or indeed purely sclerotic (Fig. 5.35) and an accurate prebiopsy diagnosis may not be possible.

Central Osteosarcoma Similar difficulty may arise when a lesion presents in the metadiaphysis as an area of dense sclerosis which may be thought to represent a large bone island. Specific characteristics on plain films to suggest malignant disease are absent. Scintigraphy, MRI and angiography, however, will demonstrate much more aggressive features.

Multifocal Osteosarcoma is extremely rare and occurs only in childhood. The condition is rapidly fatal, with pulmonary metastases, and is characterized by a marked elevation of serum alkaline phosphatase. Radiologically symmetric and densely sclerotic lesions have a predilection for metaphyses and flat bones. Unlike ordinary osteosarcoma, epiphyseal and soft-tissue involvement occurs early.

Soft-tissue Osteosarcoma On rare occasions the tumor arises purely in soft tissue (Fig. 5.36). Various sites of origin have been described, including breast and kidney. Usually, however, the lesion is para-articular. The ill-defined amorphous nature of the soft-tissue opacification may suggest tumor bone rather than calcification. The differential diagnosis is from post-traumatic

myositis ossificans which can also produce markedly abnormal features with scintigraphy and angiography, particularly early in its evolution. Histologic examination of both entities can be fraught with diagnostic pitfalls in inexperienced hands.

Radiation-induced Sarcoma

Radiation Therapy Sarcomas arise in bone following radiation, typically when the total dose has exceeded 30 Gy (3000 rad), often after a latent interval of 7–10 years. Whilst most are fibrosarcomas, a few osteosarcomas occur. The diagnosis is not difficult radiologically but they often have a predominantly lytic nature and are markedly aggressive. They arise in predictable sites, based on radiation fields, for example in the pelvis following treatment of gynecological cancer (Fig. 5.37).

The Ingestion of Radioactive Material Radium and radiomesothorium were introduced in America in 1914 in the preparation of luminous paint. In applying this to watch dials, ingestion

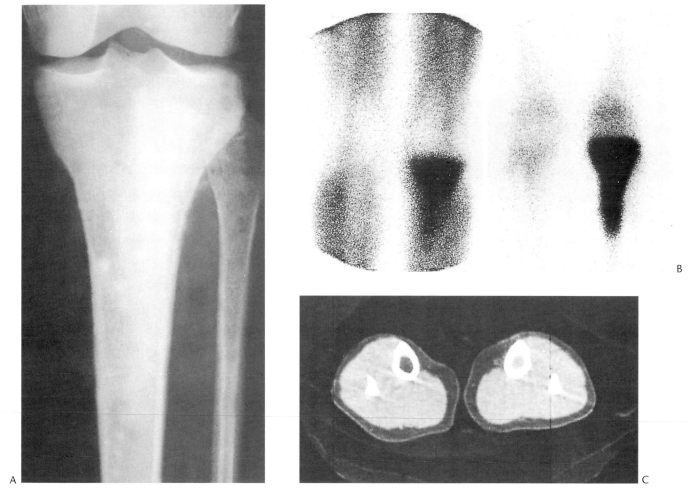

Fig. 5.27   Osteoblastic osteosarcoma of the proximal tibia. **A.** The conventional radiograph reveals patchy increased density in much of the upper tibia. Note a little new bone laterally. **B.** A scan in the early blood-pool (left) and delayed phases (right) demonstrates an extensive abnormality. Note the activity is more uniform and extensive than the apparent involvement shown on the plain film. The distal extent of the tumor is confirmed however by **C.** a CT scan which shows a subtle change in marrow attenuation below the level of the apparent tumor on plain film, an example of how CT may be used to gauge the extent of marrow involvement.

of the radioactive material occurred through pointing the paint brush with the lips. The subsequent development of osteosarcoma was first reported in 1931 although more usually areas of bone destruction and sclerosis are due to infarction. A long latent interval between ingestion and tumor development is typical. Thorium is, of course, associated with abdominal neoplasia (see Ch. 25).

Parosteal Osteosarcoma

Some confusion in nomenclature relates to osteosarcomas arising in or near the periosteum. For practical purposes these may be divided into two groups: parosteal osteosarcoma which will be described; and periosteal osteosarcoma which is similar in most ways to an ordinary osteosarcoma except that it arises close to the periosteum.

Parosteal osteosarcoma comprises some 1% of all malignant primary bone tumors and about 4% of osteosarcomas. Clinically it occurs in older patients, at least 50% being over the age of 30.

The tumor is slow-growing by comparison and has a much better prognosis. In low-grade lesions the histology may not immediately suggest a neoplasm at all. Parosteal osteosarcomas occur most commonly in the posterior distal femur and proximal humerus.

Radiological Features   Typically a dense tumor surrounds a long bone, particularly a femur or a tibia. The tumor bone may be extensive, ranging between 2 and 10 cm in length and as much as 5 cm in breadth. The margins are sharply defined but tend to undulate and the tumor is denser centrally and at the base than peripherally. Characteristically there is a radiolucent zone between the ossified outer margins of the tumor and adjacent host bone (Fig. 5.38). Penetrated films, tomography or CT may be required in order to demonstrate this sign, which may be obscured if the tumor is very large or has invaded the cortex. The tumor appears usually to be attached to the cortex by a broad pedicle. Endosteal sclerosis may occur. Marrow invasion is usually only seen in longstanding cases, following local recurrence or in high-grade lesions. Scintigraphically the blood-pool image is usually un-

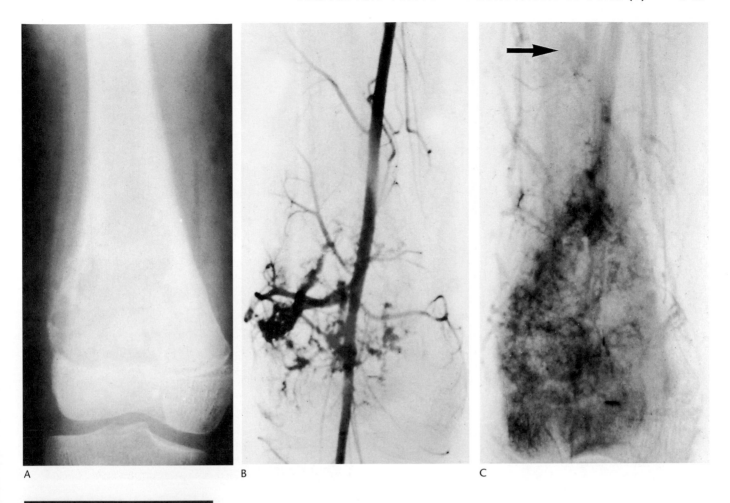

A   B   C

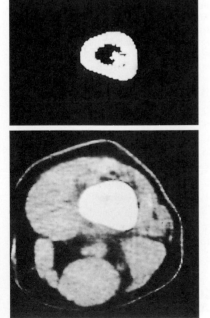

D

Fig. 5.28 Osteosarcoma of the distal femur of a young woman. **A.** The full intraosseous extent is difficult to assess on the plain film. **B.** An arteriogram demonstrates a very extensive pathological circulation and **C.** on the late capillary phase note that the tumor extends into the epiphysis, almost to the articular surface, and that there is a satellite or 'skip' lesion in the proximal femoral shaft (arrow). This latter lesion is confirmed by **D.** CT and is shown to be bone-forming (the upper image shows an attenuation of 188 HU in the lesion).

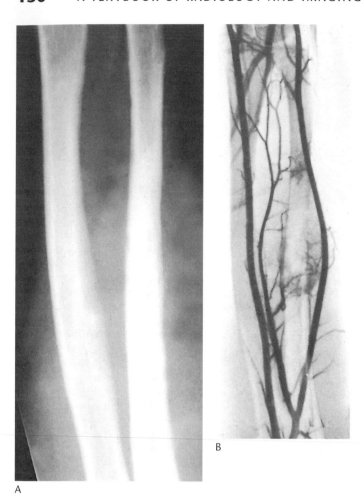

A

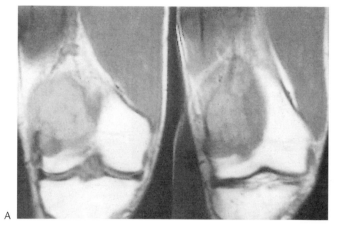

A

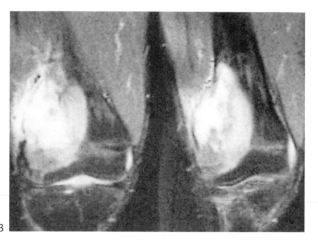

B

Fig. 5.29 Osteoblastic osteosarcoma. A middle-aged woman presented with pain and swelling in the midulna. **A.** A radiograph shows ill-defined sclerosis and cortical destruction. **B.** An angiogram demonstrates an egg-shaped soft-tissue mass with displacement of both the ulnar and interosseous arteries. The extraosseous extent of the tumor was thereby delineated.

Fig. 5.30 Osteosarcoma. Coronal T_1-weighted **A.** and STIR **B.** sequences demonstrate an extensive osteosarcoma of the lateral femoral condyle. The pleomorphic nature of the tumor can be appreciated by the more superficial main neoplasm with subadjacent marrow edema. Note the overlying abnormal vessels shown as a signal void and the joint effusion on the STIR sequence. Clear extension across the metaphysis is also shown. These features confirm an extracompartmental osteosarcoma.

remarkable although considerable increase in activity is evident in the delayed phase. Some evidence suggests that the malignancy of this tumor is reflected by the degree of abnormal vascularity on an angiogram (Fig. 5.39).

The condition must be differentiated from subperiosteal hematoma and other benign causes of periosteal new bone formation.

Sarcoma in Paget's Disease

Malignant tumors are said to arise in bone affected by Paget's disease in about 1% of cases. It is difficult to gauge the exact incidence, since many cases of Paget's disease are asymptomatic or diagnosed by chance. Clinically the possibility of a sarcoma arising in Paget's disease should be considered when alteration occurs in the character of bone pain, either an increase in severity or more precise localization; or if a pathological fracture develops. The presence of a soft-tissue mass and a further rise in the serum alkaline phosphatase may be observed. Sarcomas may occur in the polyostotic or monostotic disease, though there seems to be a particular predilection for the humerus in the latter. Overall the

skull, pelvis and long bones are typical sites (Fig. 5.40). Men are more commonly affected, even allowing for the increased male incidence of Paget's disease.

Histologically the tumors may be classified as osteosarcoma, fibrosarcoma and chondrosarcoma. However, the tumor is very aggressive and the outlook is very poor. Radiologically, in order of frequency, the lesion is lytic, mixed or sclerotic and the tumor grows rapidly with an extensive soft-tissue mass. The margins of the lesion within bone are usually ill-defined, frequently with extensive cortical destruction. Periosteal new bone formation is relatively uncommon.

BONE TUMORS PRESUMED TO ARISE FROM SKELETAL TISSUE: CARTILAGE-FORMING

Benign cartilage lesions divide into two main groups, central and peripheral. The former includes chondroma (with which must be considered the generalized dysplasia of bone—dyschondroplasia), benign chondroblastoma and chondromyxoid fibroma. The malig-

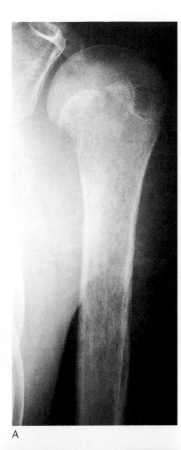

A

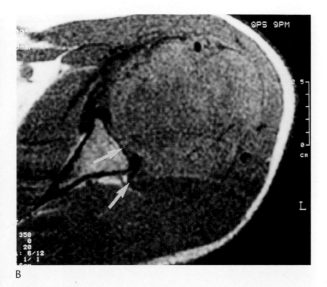

B

Fig. 5.31 Osteosarcoma of the proximal humerus. **A.** Conventional radiograph showing permeative bone destruction and focal areas of intramedullary sclerosis. A spiculated periosteal reaction is also evident. Axial T$_1$-weighted **B.** and **C.** coronal STIR images demonstrate the longitudinal extent of the tumor within the medullary canal and the extraosseous involvement, including extension into the shoulder joint (arrows).

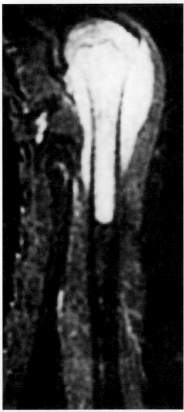

C

nant counterpart of chondroma is a central chondrosarcoma. There are no reports of the malignant transformation of chondroblastoma and chondromyxoid fibroma. The peripheral lesion to be considered is an osteochondroma, or cartilage-capped exostosis, which in its multiple form also constitutes a general bone dysplasia (diaphyseal aclasia). The cartilage cap of these lesions is a potential site for the development of chondrosarcoma. The majority of chondrosarcomas, however, arise without evidence of a pre-existing benign tumor.

Chondroma

Nearly all of these tumors are benign in their clinical presentation and in their radiological and histologic appearances, yet all must be regarded as the site of potential malignancy. It is very unusual for the common chondromatous lesions which occur in the hands and feet to become malignant but every flat or long bone cartilage tumor should be regarded as a potential risk if the patient survives long enough. The development of increasing pain, the demonstration, on serial films, of alteration in the radiological appearances or the late development of a pathological fracture are in themselves sufficient to justify anxiety. The transition from benign to malignant in the histologic spectrum may be very difficult and contentious.

These tumors are notoriously insensitive to therapy. Local recurrence is very high unless there is meticulous surgical removal, and cartilage tumors have the habit of becoming more aggressive with each subsequent episode of surgical or therapeutic interference. It must be emphasized that the exact time of change from benign to malignant is extremely hard to establish and it is possible that those tumors which are frankly malignant have been so since their inception. Whilst most cartilage tumors arise in

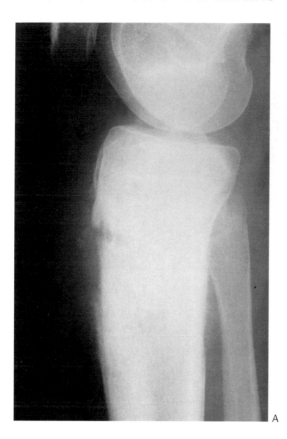

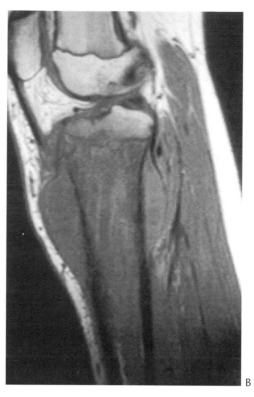

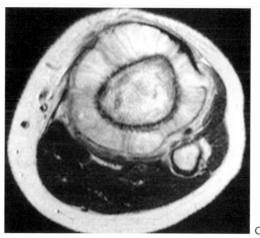

Fig. 5.32 Osteosarcoma of the proximal tibia. **A.** Conventional radiograph demonstrating an osteosclerotic lesion with Codman's triangles and a pretibial soft-tissue mass. **B.** Sagittal T₁-weighted image showing intramedullary involvement throughout the whole of the tibia included in the illustration and extension into the proximal epiphysis. Both posterior and anterior extraosseous involvement is evident. **C.** Axial turbo T₂-weighted image demonstrating circumferential soft-tissue involvement with radiating spicules of new bone within the soft-tissue component.

conjunction with bone it is important to note that they may occur in soft tissues, particularly tendon sheaths and in relation to synovium. They may even occur, intracranially and when present at the base of the skull should be considered in the differential diagnosis of chordoma.

Single tumors are common. Approximately half are found in the hands, in the medullary cavity of the phalanges, less common-ly in metacarpals. About 10% occur in the small bones of the feet. Long bones, particularly the femur, humerus and tibia, are involved in 20% of cases, the remainder occurring in flat bones, particu-larly the pelvis, scapula and vertebral bodies. It is in these areas that the potential danger of malignant transformation is greatest.

Clinical Features The age of onset is usually later than with bone-forming tumors. Since these lesions grow slowly, they are

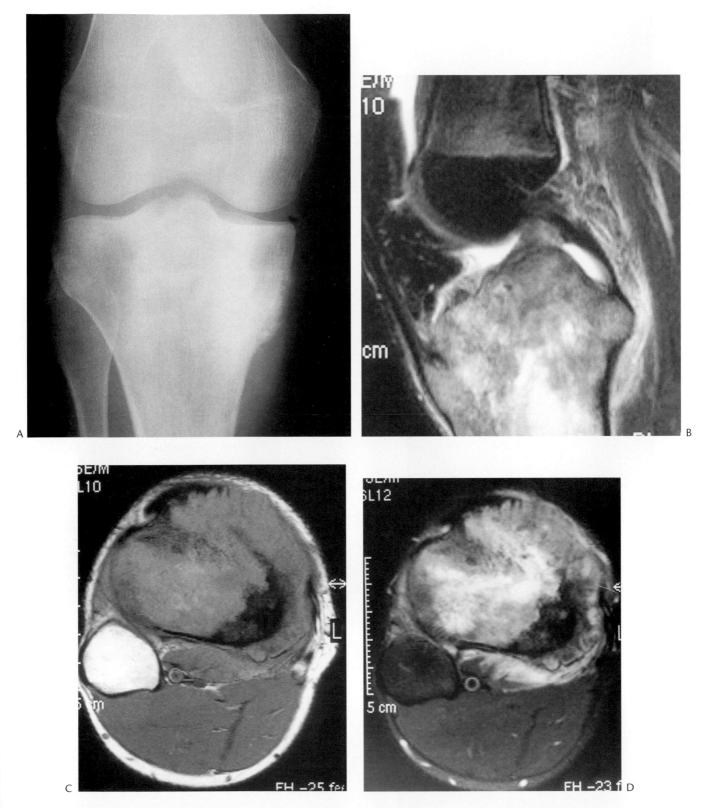

Fig. 5.33 Osteosarcoma of the proximal tibia. **A.** Conventional radiograph showing an osteoblastic lesion with periosteal new bone medially. **B.** Sagittal turbo T$_2$-weighted image with fat suppression, **C.** axial T$_1$-weighted image and **D.** axial turbo T$_2$-weighted image with fat suppression. The MR images elegantly demonstrate the heterogeneity of the tumour, the intramedullary involvement (note the normal fatty marrow within the distal femur and proximal fibula), periosteal new bone and involvement of the tibia origin of the patellar tendon. Perilesional edema and a joint effusion are also evident.

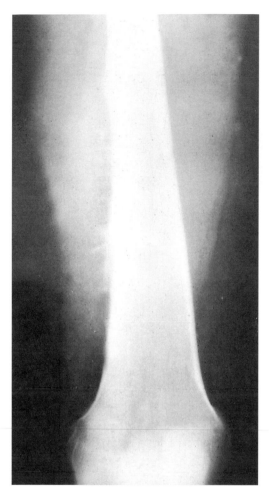

Fig. 5.34 Diaphyseal osteosarcoma of the midshaft of the femur. Note the radiating spiculation, of bone, Codman's triangles and well-defined soft-tissue mass.

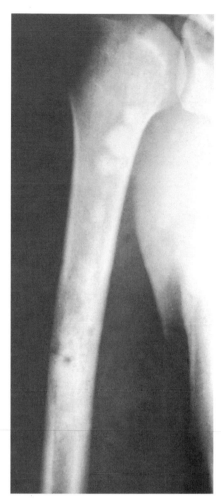

Fig. 5.35 Diaphyseal osteosarcoma. A pathological fracture is present in the mid humerus with extensive endosteal sclerosis and cortical destruction from the medullary aspect. Tumor is present to the neck of the humerus with areas of dense sclerosis and surrounding faint radiolucency. These 'skip' lesions do not represent isolated tumor; the shaft was involved continuously. This variety carries a poor prognosis.

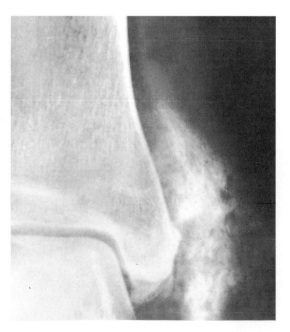

Fig. 5.36 Soft-tissue osteosarcoma. An elderly vicar complained of an enlarging soft-tissue mass adjacent to the medial malleolus of his right ankle. Note the amorphous soft-tissue ossification and calcification and normal bone underlying the lesion.

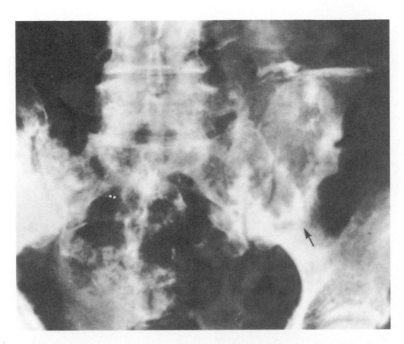

Fig. 5.37 Radiation sarcoma arising in the posterior iliac crest on the left, in an elderly woman treated 6 years previously for carcinoma of the cervix. The lesion is purely osteolytic with ill-defined surrounding sclerosis (arrows).

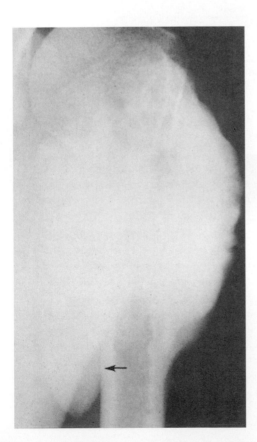

Fig. 5.38 Parosteal osteosarcoma of the proximal humerus. A well-defined mass of dense tumor bone surrounds the humeral shaft. A typical radiolucent line is present between the tumor bone and the proximal shaft inferomedially (arrow). The underlying bone appears normal.

rarely symptomatic and are often uncovered through examinations for other indications, particularly trauma. However, on direct questioning the patient may admit to having noted a localized hard swelling for many years. Pathological fracture is not uncommon. To restate, low-grade pain or swelling of recent onset should cause the possibility of chondrosarcoma to be considered.

Radiological Features Cartilaginous tissue is not radiopaque. The characteristic feature is of a single well-defined demarcated zone of radiolucency in the medulla. In the small bones of the hand and feet tumors are particularly likely to expand and thin the overlying cortex (Fig. 5.41), but without its destruction or the development of a periosteal reaction other than that following a fracture. The zone of transition is narrow and sclerotic. The endosteal margin may be scalloped. As in all neoplasms of cartilaginous origin, flecks of calcification are frequently present within the tumor, especially as they become more mature, and may assume a pathognomonic 'popcorn' or annular configuration. Calcification also may be observed, together with ossification, in healing callus following a pathological fracture. Lesions rarely extend to the ends of the affected bones and are often situated in the distal portions. Very few other osteolytic lesions in the bones of the hands are likely to cause diagnostic difficulty, apart from the rare implantation dermoid cyst in a terminal phalanx or perhaps fibrous dysplasia. These cartilaginous tumors are unremarkable scintigraphically, and angiographically their low vascularity is readily demonstrated; a marked increase of photon activity on a bone scan should raise the possibility of a pathological fracture or chondrosarcoma. The high water content of the hyaline cartilage matrix results in a particularly high signal intensity on T_2-weighted MR images which often have a lobulated contour. Magnetic resonance imaging, like other radiological techniques, can not distinguish between a benign enchondroma and a low-grade chondrosarcoma with certainty (Fig. 5.42).

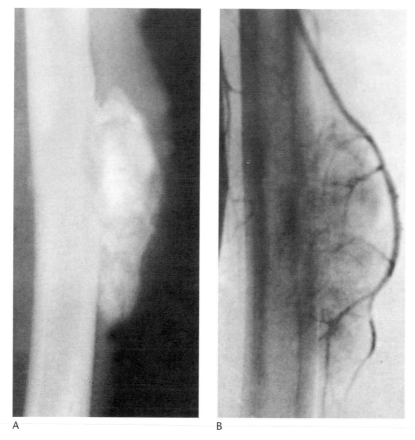

A   B

Fig. 5.39 Parosteal osteosarcoma arising from anterior aspect of the femur **A.** is shown **B.** angiographically to be unremarkable apart from a slight increase in number of branches going into the tumor. The lesion was found at biopsy to be of very low-grade malignancy.

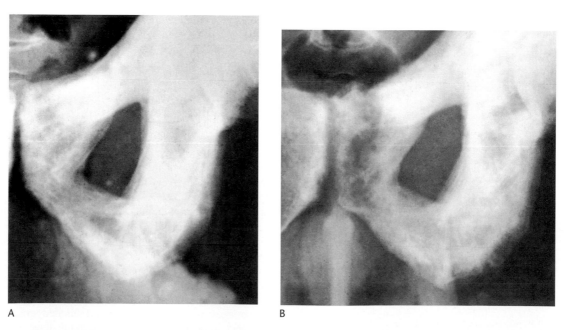

A   B

Fig. 5.40 Paget's sarcoma of the body of the pubis. **A.** No malignancy was seen in this man at initial presentation with polyostotic Paget's disease. **B.** Three years later, however, he complained of local pain with the development of a purely lytic destructive lesion involving the body of the pubis.

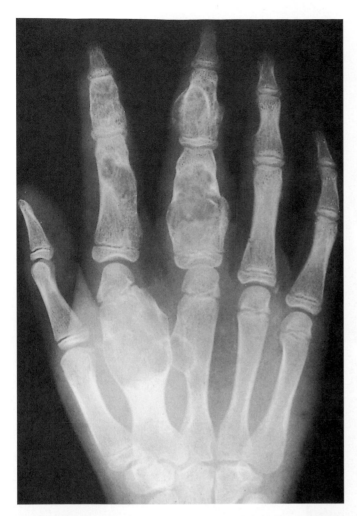

Fig. 5.41 Multiple chondromas in the hand. This child presented with painless swelling. Note the cortical expansion and thinning, well-defined defects, patchy amorphous calcification and moulding abnormalities indicating slow growth.

Less commonly chondromas develop in the medullary cavities of long bones and must be distinguished from other medullary osteolytic lesions. Here again the presence of calcification is a great help, but is not entirely specific. The tumor margin is usually sharply defined and accompanied by some evidence of sclerosis. The tumor erodes the cortex from within with a clear-cut edge. The cortex, however, remains intact and the development of an enlarging lesion may cause eccentric expansion of bone due to organized periosteal new bone. Most of these tumors are discovered in adult life and therefore differentiation from other osteolytic lesions, such as bone cysts and non-ossifying fibromas, offers less difficulty because of the patient's age. Evidence of extension of the lesion or irregularity of the margin (particularly in the presence of periosteal new bone formation or a soft-tissue mass) will immediately suggest a chondrosarcoma. Further investigation is unrewarding, although computerized tomography may identify or confirm cartilage calcification and both CT and MR may serve to delineate the extent of the intramedullary lesion.

It is necessary to distinguish the central variety of chondroma from unimportant areas of amorphous calcification arranged in a roughly linear fashion in the medullary canal, often described as 'cartilage rests'. The localized stippled nature of these opacities and the absence of any other radiological abnormality indicates the latter diagnosis. These lesions are scintigraphically inert. On the other hand, differentiation of a central chondroma from a medullary bone infarct may be more difficult. A helpful feature is the curvilinear peripheral calcification around the infarct rather than the annular calcification with a true cartilage tumor. Both lesions may be associated with subsequent malignant complications, differentiated chondrosarcoma from chondroma (see below) and fibrosarcoma or malignant fibrous histiocytoma from the wall of an infarct.

Special Types of Chondroma

Juxtacortical chondroma is a rare benign cartilage tumor usually arising in young adults and related to the cortex of a long bone, most commonly the humerus or femur. The presenting complaint is of a slowly enlarging hard mass which may not be tender (Fig. 5.43). Radiologically a well-defined soft-tissue mass may contain calcification and be bordered by a thin, but usually incomplete, shell of overlying bone. Pressure erosion produces scalloping of the underlying cortex and usually provokes a variable sclerotic reaction. The presence of calcification within the lesion makes the diagnosis of a cartilage-containing tumor relatively easy. On the other hand, if calcification is absent the mass may have to be distinguished from non-ossifying fibroma, periosteal lipoma or neurofibroma.

Multiple Enchondromas   The individual lesions of the bone dysplasia described by Ollier are now known as dyschondroplasia and are essentially neoplastic in type, corresponding to the descriptions already given. Cartilage tumors found in dysplasias may be extremely gross and cause complete destruction of the bones of the hand. In addition to the multiple cartilage tumors, columns of dysplastic cartilage frequently cause considerable tubulation anomalies and growth deformities of limbs. Although recognized in the literature to be subject to chondrosarcomatous change, this complication has been uncommon in the experience of the authors.

Maffucci Syndrome is the rare association of dyschondroplasia with cavernous hemangiomas in the soft tissues, the latter being characterized radiologically by soft-tissue masses containing phleboliths (Fig. 5.44). Chondrosarcomatous metaplasia is a recognized hazard of this entity and probably develops in about 20% of cases.

Chondroblastoma

This relatively rare tumor arises almost always in an epiphysis or apophysis, 50% occurring in the second decade of life. Presentation is of pain around the joint, usually of mild proportions, and of months' or even years' duration. Joint movement often is limited. Most of these tumors occur in epiphyses of long bones, especially around the hips, knees or shoulders, but some have been observed in apophyses. Histologically the appearances are distinctive, cartilage cells being interspersed with foci of calcification and giant cells. This lesion has been considered as a giant-cell tumor variant.

Radiologically a well-defined, radiolucent, oval lesion within an

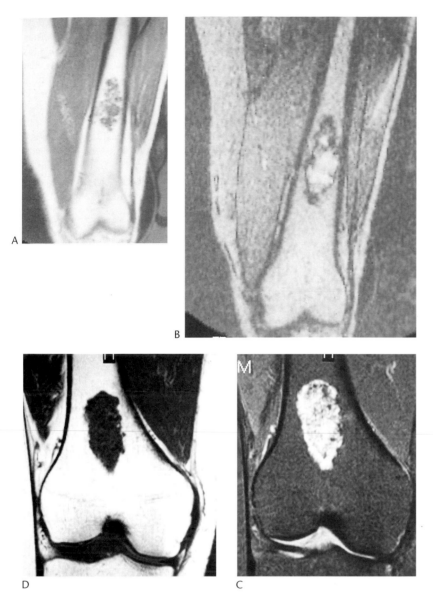

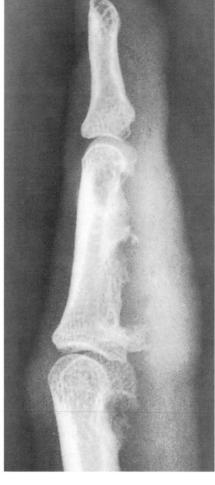

Fig. 5.43 Juxtacortical chondromas arising on the volar aspect of the proximal and middle phalanges of the index finger. Obvious pressure defects are present with new bone formation at the margins. Punctate calcification is present in the middle of the proximal lesion.

Fig. 5.42 Cartilage tumor. This patient presented with a longstanding ache in the thigh. Coronal T_1-weighted **A.** and STIR **B.** sequences demonstrate a mixed lesion within the femoral shaft. Note that the cartilage has high signal on the STIR sequence. A surrounding rim of sclerosis is shown by deficient signal on both images. Histologically, this tumor was considered benign, in spite of giving rise to symptoms and to increased activity on a radionuclide scan and showing a high water content on MRI. In a different patient, presenting with signs of internal derangement, a similar lesion is shown incidentally on **C.** coronal T_1-weighted and **D.** STIR images.

epiphysis is characteristic, often with a thin rim of sclerosis and cortical expansion (Fig. 5.45). The endosteal margin is well defined. Not infrequently the tumor extends into the metaphysis. Stippled calcification occurs in about a quarter of examples and in a smaller number an adjacent periosteal reaction may be present. The extreme vascularity of these lesions is confirmed by the blood-pool phase of the bone scan or by angiography. The delayed phase of a bone scan is not helpful. Computerized tomography or MR imaging may be of value in assessing the extent of those few lesions which expand rapidly into the soft tissues. No incidence of spontaneous malignant transformation, however, has been recorded (Fig. 5.46).

Chondromyxoid Fibroma

This tumor is predominantly chondroid, but contains myxomatous tissue and giant cells. Histologically it may be mistaken for a chondrosarcoma. The presenting complaints are non-specific, usually localized pain and swelling, often of many months' duration. The peak age incidence is between 20 and 30, with no particular sex incidence. Typically the lesion occurs around the knee joint in two-thirds of cases, with an especial affinity for the proximal end of the tibia. Flat bones and short bones have been affected.

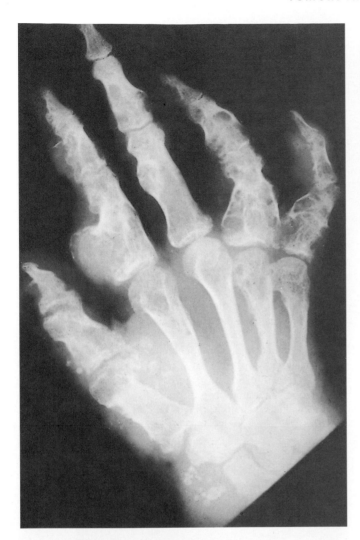

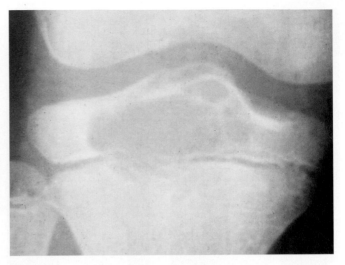

Fig. 5.45 Chondroblastoma in the proximal epiphysis of the tibia. The tumor has thinned the overlying cortex and extends across the growth plate into the upper metaphysis.

Fig. 5.44 Maffucci syndrome (woman aged 23). Numerous chondromas in this case of dyschondroplasia are accompanied by soft-tissue swelling which contains phleboliths indicating hemangiomas. These skeletal lesions are more liable than ordinary chondromas to undergo malignant transformation.

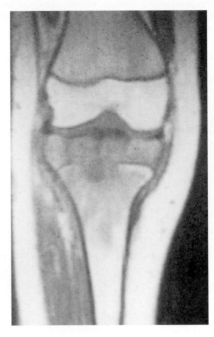

Fig. 5.46 Chondroblastoma. A chondroblastoma is demonstrated on a T_1-weighted coronal MR image rising in the upper tibial epiphysis and extending through the metaphysis. Persistent red marrow is present in the distal femoral and proximal tibial metaphysis.

Radiologically the predominant feature is a radiolucent, eccentric, space-occupying lesion which is situated in the metaphysis. The margin within bone is usually well defined, with surrounding sclerosis (Fig. 5.47). The sharpness of the margin between the lesion and the sclerosis contrasts with the rather ill-defined margin between the sclerosis and host bone. In many cases the cortex is expanded considerably (Fig. 5.48), the peripheral bony margin often becoming hazy and poorly defined. This aggressive appearance may be so marked that the possibility of malignant change may be considered. Unlike other cartilaginous neoplasms, calcification within the lesion is very uncommon.

Whilst *scintigraphy* in the blood-pool phase of a bone scan, or *angiography*, may reveal a slight increase in perfusion to the lesion, the vascular pattern is unremarkable. When the bone scan does show increased activity it is usually localized to the reactive sclerosis rather than to the lesion itself. *CT* may be necessary to delineate a cortical margin in the expanded soft-tissue mass.

This tumor is undoubtedly very closely related to benign chondroblastoma and indeed aneurysmal bone cyst, since all three contain giant cells. Histologic differentiation is usually easy, but unrepresentative biopsy material may create confusion. Radiologically, confusion will only occur when these lesions occur in childhood, although the typical location of a chondroblastoma and the ill-defined endosteal margin of an aneurysmal bone cyst will normally suggest the correct diagnosis.

Osteochondroma (cartilage-capped exostosis)

This lesion is essentially an osseous outgrowth arising from bony cortex. Usually it grows slowly during childhood and adolescence

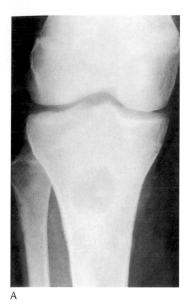
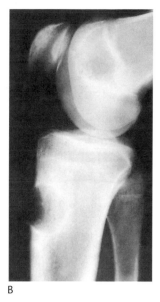

A　　　　　　　　　　B

Fig. 5.47 Chondromyxoid fibroma of the proximal tibia. Note the extremely well-defined radiolucent defect with a sclerotic margin on the endosteal aspect. **A.** AP view. **B.** Lateral view.

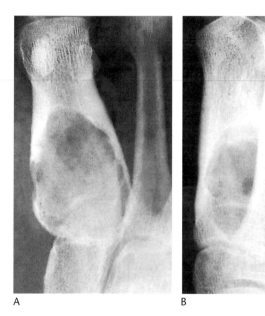

A　　　　　　　　　　B

Fig. 5.48 A,B. Chondromyxoid fibroma—great toe metatarsal. The tumor is eccentric in position with extreme cortical expansion and thinning. The endosteal margin is well-defined and faintly sclerotic. No calcification is present.

with endochondral ossification, the central spongiosa merging with that of the bone from which it is derived. Very occasionally the lesion involutes with increasing age and finally results only in a minor abnormality of tubulation. It is usual for growth to cease with skeletal maturity. Although commonly solitary the tumors may be multiple, when the condition is recognized as the deforming congenital bone dysplasia known as disphyseal aclasia (Ch. 1). The importance of this relatively common benign tumor, and its place among bone tumors, relates to the cartilage cap with which it is covered. This structure may be very prominent and in

this tissue lies the very small risk of malignancy in the form of chondrosarcoma. This risk is probably less than 1%, but may be significantly higher (of the order of 10%) in diaphyseal aclasia.

These tumors arise mainly in tubular bones near the metaphyses related to the sites of tendinous attachments. They are particularly common around the knee and the proximal end of the humerus. They may be either sessile or pedunculated. The latter type always grow away from the metaphysis, being directed toward the diaphysis. Flat bones also may be affected, the pelvis and scapula being equally involved. In the pelvis these lesions are almost invariably of the sessile type. Rare lesions related to the laminae of vertebral bodies may produce neurologic signs.

Both types occur equally in the sexes and may be entirely asymptomatic, apart from their cosmetic effect. Presentation usually follows minor trauma. They may interfere with footwear comfort and can cause localized neural or vascular compression. Such symptoms are unlikely to develop until the later stages of growth, at or around puberty. Surgical removal should be undertaken if any increase in pain or size of the lesion occurs, particularly after growth has ceased. Features of this type may indicate chondrosarcomatous change in the cartilage cap.

Radiological Features Osteochondromas have a characteristic appearance. With a pedunculated tumor it is particularly easy to identify the continuation of its cortex with that of the underlying bone from which it arises and the merging of its trabecular pattern into the medullary cavity through the cortical defect (Fig. 5.49).

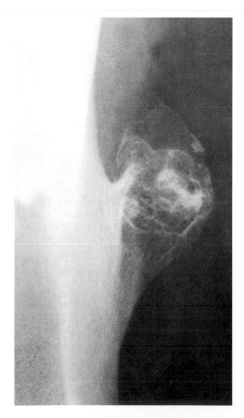

Fig. 5.49 Osteochondroma of the distal femur. The cortex is continuous with that of the underlying bone and trabecular bone merges with that of the femur. A well-defined cartilage cap contains calcification and is directed away from the joint.

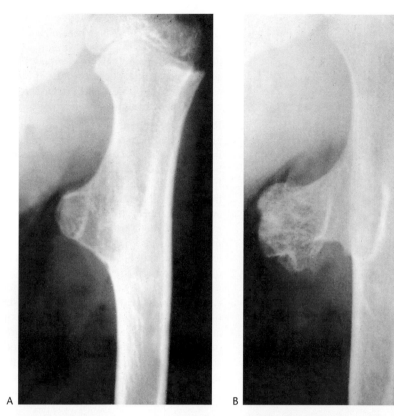

Fig. 5.50 A,B. A pedunculated osteochondroma exhibits growth over a 2-year period in the humerus of a child. Such growth is common and stops usually at, or soon after, puberty.

In young adults the cartilage cap may not be visualized on conventional radiographs, although seen clearly on CT and MRI. As age progresses calcification becomes apparent within the cartilaginous element of the tumor, causing an increase in punctate or curvilinear radiodensity. Thus the developed lesion in the adult is likely to show irregular calcification. Growth of osteochondromas usually occurs until skeletal maturation is complete (Fig. 5.50), ceasing thereafter. Rarely osteochondromas may be shown to regress (Fig. 5.51). Pedunculated tumors vary in size, but may be up to 8 or 10 cm in length and are typically directed away from the nearest joint. Flat and sessile types are more commonly related to flat bones, particularly the pelvis, and may grow to a substantial size, be of considerable irregularity and become very dense. In such cases the resemblance to a cauliflower may be striking! Provided that the sharply defined peripheral margin is preserved, and serial examinations reveal no increase in size, their benign nature may be assumed.

Any change in radiological appearance, particularly with the development of poor definition of the margin, even in one part of the lesion, is highly suggestive of chondrosarcoma, particularly if accompanied by a history of an insidious increase in local pain. Local resection and histologic studies then become essential because of the shortcomings of further radiological investigation in detecting chondrosarcoma (see below). *MR imaging* may be of assistance in suggesting the presence of sarcomatous change by showing the thickness of the cartilagious cap (greater than 1 cm should be viewed with suspicion), changes in the cartilage cap in an adult, and any infiltration of adjacent soft-tissue structures. The individual lesions of diaphyseal aclasia are those of any osteochondroma.

However, their multiplicity results in considerable moulding abnormality and deformity (Fig. 5.52).

Chondrosarcoma

Differentiation of this malignant member of the group of cartilage-forming tumors is to be made from osteosarcoma, with which it may be confused. Chondrosarcoma forms a spectrum of malignancy, but usually develops later in life than osteosarcoma and carries a much better prospect of survival because metastases often occur very late. A high-grade (aggressively malignant) chondrosarcoma, however, behaves in a fashion very similar to an osteosarcoma.

The **clinical problem**, therefore, is not so much that of metastatic dissemination but of local recurrence. Failure to provide adequate and early excision is attended by the subsequent necessity of further and more difficult surgical procedures. Some evidence exists that each surgical insult causes the tumor to become even more aggressive. Certain pleomorphic osteosarcomas demonstrate cartilage formation, but the established chondrosarcoma is associated with cartilage which is mature in its development. Although some of this cartilaginous tissue may ossify, no direct ossification (unlike an osteosarcoma) takes place in the absence of a chondroid precursor. In addition these cells are histochemically negative for the production of alkaline phosphatase.

Chondrosarcomas may develop in a cartilaginous lesion previously thought to be benign. Malignancy may arise in the cartilage cap of an osteochondroma or in a long or flat bone (Fig. 5.53). Chondrosarcoma of the hand or foot is distinctly unusual.

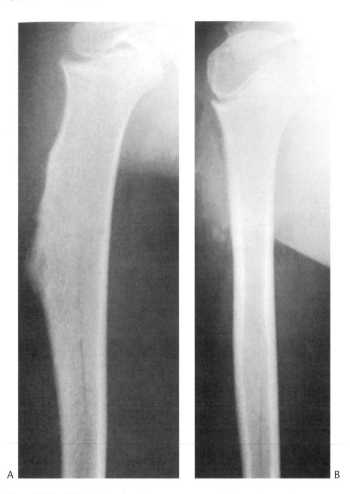

A   B

Fig. 5.51 A,B. Osteochondromas may rarely be shown to regress, remodeling resulting in normal appearances. Here an osteochondroma of the proximal humerus cannot be visualized 6 years later.

The lesions of dyschondroplasia, particularly if associated with the hemangiomas of Maffucci syndrome, are also subject to malignant change. Nonetheless the incidence of what might be called secondary chondrosarcoma is far less common than those apparently arising de novo. Indeed only 10% of these neoplasms arise from a recognizable precursor, usually the cartilage cap of an osteochondroma, especially in patients suffering from diaphyseal aclasia.

Primary chondrosarcoma occurs mainly between the ages of 30 and 70 years and is relatively rare distal to the elbow and knee joints, the pelvis and ribs being the most common sites, followed closely by the proximal end of the femur. Because of this distribution, virtually all chondromas arising in flat and long bones should be regarded as potentially malignant ab initio. Diagnosis may be delayed on account of slow growth or relatively mild symptomatology. The tumor, therefore, may be very large when it is first recognized.

Prognosis for chondrosarcoma is relatively good if complete surgical excision is possible before dissemination, metastases only occurring in the later stages by the hematogenous route. Because of the risks of local recurrence, it may be necessary to undertake amputation. The histologic spectrum of chondrosarcoma varies widely. Difficulties with differentiation arise, at the benign end of the spectrum, from a benign chondroma and, at the aggressive end, from an osteosarcoma. In consequence, interpretation by a highly skilled pathologist is essential. Particularly in a case of less aggressive chondrosarcoma, situated in a site of easy access, such as the proximal end of the femur, prosthetic replacement is an effective and cosmetic surgical treatment.

Radiological Features   When a chondrosarcoma arises from a previous cartilaginous lesion the diagnosis is usually straightforward. In the case of osteochondroma particular attention should be paid to areas of local cortical destruction with ill-defined margins. In addition, it may be possible to demonstrate an associated soft-tissue mass representing abnormal cartilage growth. These features are demonstrated more clearly by MR imaging. The conventional radiological demonstration of cartilage within such a mass by punctuate or curvilinear calcification may be absent, as this characteristic feature tends to occur in the more mature parts of these tumors. Similarly the central chondroma which becomes malignant tends clinically to grow silently, spreading within the medullary cavity to produce irregular medullary destruction. Uneven infiltration makes it difficult to determine the margin between normal and abnormal tissue. Irregular calcification is likely to be present in the older and central parts of the tumor. These more organized zones may be destroyed by newer malignant infiltration, indicating the dedifferentiated form of chondrosarcoma.

As growth proceeds slowly, the tumor causes smooth, scalloped erosions on the endosteal aspect of the cortex. An overlying lamellar periosteal reaction is not rare, especially if the malignancy is low-grade. In consequence, the ultimate thickness of the cortex around the tumor may exceed that in the unaffected portion of the bone, the appearance then being that of a localized fusiform expansion (Fig. 5.54). Pathological fractures are quite common and may draw initial attention to these tumors.

The malignant nature of the lesion is unequivocally established when penetration of the cortex is shown together with an associated and clearly defined soft-tissue mass, within which calcification, or even ossification, may occur (Fig. 5.55).

Primary Chondrosarcoma, particularly in its early stages, presents difficult diagnostic problems as the presenting symptoms of minor pain or discomfort may be accompanied by only minimal radiological change. This may be a poorly defined area of medullary translucency with possibly a little periosteal reaction or the presence of an abnormal soft-tissue mass. The acetabulum is sometimes the site of the development of these rather nebulous and difficult lesions (Figs 5.56, 5.57). The first radiological evidence of its presence may be a soft-tissue mass projecting into the pelvic cavity. The cortex of flat bones tends to be thinner than that of long bones, and chondrosarcomas of the ribs or the pelvis penetrate it at an early stage. This feature may be demonstrated more clearly by CT. Hence these tumors are especially liable to grow to a substantial size over a prolonged period, particularly if in a clinically occult area. Rapid growth naturally indicates a more aggressive type of malignancy.

As may be expected, the more mature cartilage elements frequently progress to calcification and ossification, and larger tumors often have a lobulated or cauliflower appearance. Very rarely a chondrosarcoma may arise in soft tissues, including tendon sheath and meninges. Cranial lesions also can arise from the sphenoid

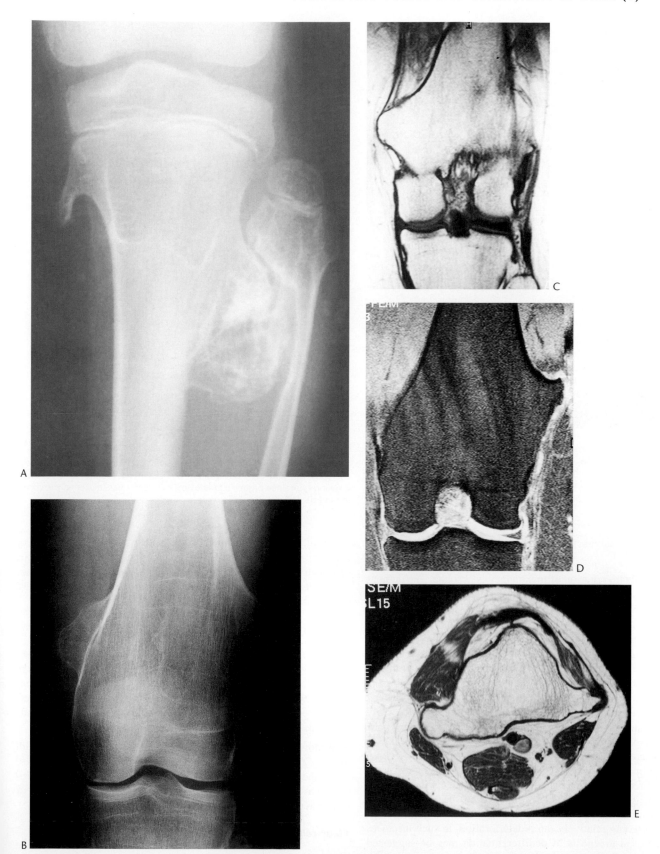

Fig. 5.52 Diaphyseal aclasia. **A.** Multiple osteochondromas are present in the proximal tibia and fibula. A large sessile lesion of the proximal tibia has caused widening of the interosseous space and secondary moulding abnormalities of both the tibia and fibula. In another patient **B**, similar modeling abnormalities are shown. On MR imaging, following ligamentous injury, only a minimal cartilage cap can be identified on the medial osteochondroma, and a slightly thicker cap on the laterally projecting osteochondroma: **C** coronal T₁-weighted, **D** coronal FFE-T₂ and **E** axial T₁-weighted images.

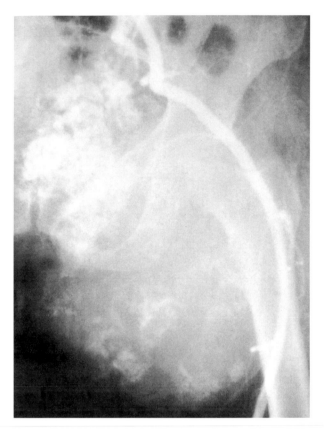

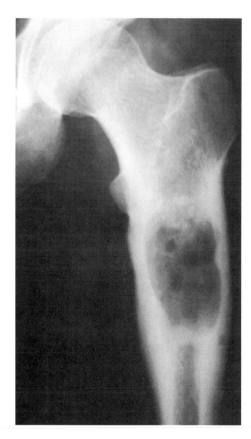

Fig. 5.53 Chondrosarcoma arising from the superior public ramus on the left. A huge mass is present containing extensive calcification. The femoral artery is displaced by the mass but note the absence of any pathological circulation. This is typical of a low-grade chondrosarcoma.

Fig. 5.54 Central chondrosarcoma. The destructive lesion in the femoral shaft has smooth well-defined margins, but in the upper portion some characteristic punctate calcification is visible. The tumor is of a slow-growing type since organized periosteal new bone has thickened the cortex around the lesion.

(Fig. 5.58) and clivus where they require differentiation from chordoma.

Radiologically no criterion of malignancy is absolute. The demonstration of increase in size and ill-defined margins on plain film is highly suggestive. Destruction of organized existing cartilage calcification is indicative also of local infiltration. The demonstration of cortical disruption is helpful.

Scintigraphically most of these neoplams tend to have a slight increase in activity only on the delayed phase of a bone scan, but high-grade chondrosarcomas may demonstrate an increase in the blood-pool image. *Angiographically*, minor vascular displacement is usually evident, with scanty new vessels in the majority. Only when the tumor is of particularly high-grade malignancy is the type of increased perfusion and new vessel formation similar to that associated with an osteosarcoma. Whilst *MRI* may infer a cartilage tumor, by virtue of the high water content of cartilage, only the direct infiltration of adjacent soft tissues will definitely suggest malignancy (Fig. 5.57). Reference has been made above to malignant cartilaginous tumors of relatively low-grade malignancy undergoing relatively rapid deterioration. In such instances the radiological diagnosis of dedifferentiation may be suggested when an area of osteolytic destruction develops adjacent to the original tumor (Fig. 5.59) and which may destroy part of the pre-existing calcified portion of the tumor. These dedifferentiated

forms may exhibit the microscopic appearance of a frank osteosarcoma, fibrosarcoma or, not uncommonly, malignant fibrous histiocytoma with its characteristic storiform pattern of the tumor cells (see below). The age, sex and clinical features otherwise are comparable to those of an orthodox chondrosarcoma.

Mesenchymal Chondrosarcoma

This malignant cartilage tumor is rare. Histologically it is characterized by the presence of more or less differentiated cartilage together with highly vascular spindle-cell or round-cell mesenchymal tissue. About a third of these tumors arise in the soft tissues, especially in the extremities (thigh and calf). The soft-tissue mass frequently shows irregular calcification (Fig. 5.60).

Radiologically this lesion shows a rapid increase in size with highly aggressive features and the early detection of metastases. The condition affects adults at an earlier age than most chondrosarcomas although in general the age group is older than that of osteosarcoma.

Clear-cell Chondrosarcoma

This is an uncommon variant of chondrosarcoma which is typically located within the epiphysis, usually occurring within the proximal humerus, femur or tibia.

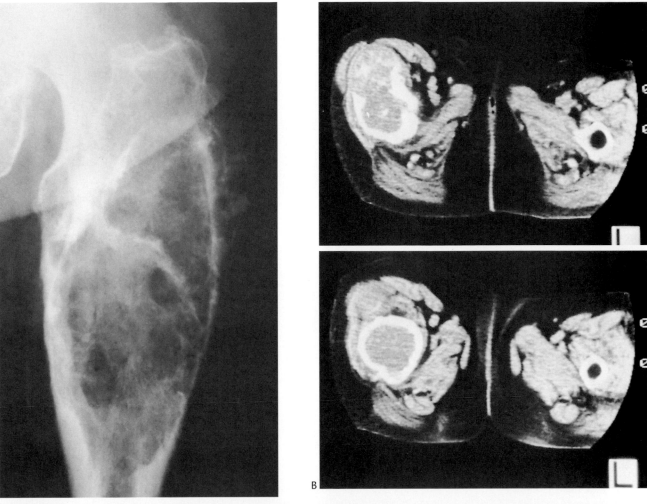

A

B

Fig. 5.55   A,B Central chondrosarcoma. **A.** The tumor is more aggressive than that in Fig. 5.54, and has extended into soft tissues. This is confirmed by CT **B** showing extension anterior to the femoral shaft (W200, L25). Calcification is present both in the soft-tissue mass and within the shaft lesion.

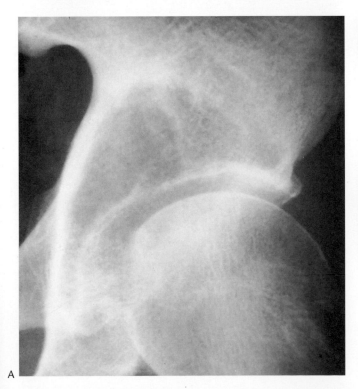

A

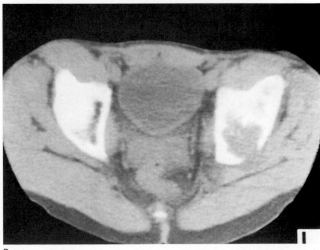

B

Fig. 5.56 Chondrosarcoma arising in the acetabulum of a 45-year-old man. **A.** The tumor is purely lytic. Cortical thickening is shown medially. **B.** CT demonstrates disruption of the cortex posteriorly, with a localized soft-tissue mass beneath the glutei and faint calcification within the lesion.

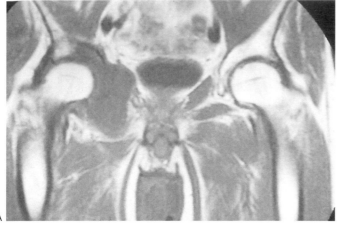

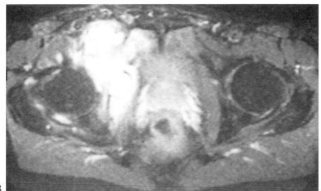

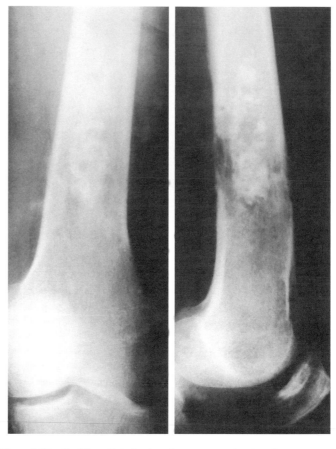

Fig. 5.57 Chondrosarcoma. A chondrosarcoma arising primarily in the region of the acetabulum. A coronal T$_1$-weighted **A** and axial STIR sequence **B** demonstrate a large lobulated mass occupying the floor of the acetabulum and extending through into the pelvis and the obturator foramen. Note the high signal on STIR, suggesting aggressive tumor, with also some increased signal surrounding the lesion due to edema (secondary response). There is clear involvement of the hip joint.

Fig. 5.59 Dedifferentiated chondrosarcoma. A chondrosarcoma is present centrally within the distal femoral shaft, characterized by slight expansion and amorphous calcification. In addition an area of osteolysis is present with cortical destruction around the lower half of the tumor. The latter represents a high-grade malignancy arising in conjunction with a pre-existing relatively low-grade tumor.

Radiologically clear-cell chondrosarcoma resembles chondro-blastoma, resulting in a well-defined osteolytic lesion in the epiphysis which may have a sclerotic border. A periosteal reaction is not seen although calcification within the lesion may occur.

REFERENCES AND SUGGESTIONS FOR FURTHER READING

See end of Chapter 7

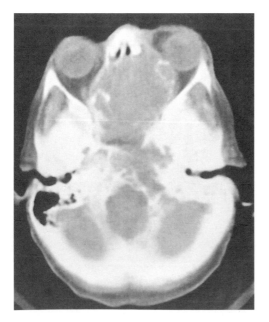

Fig. 5.58 Chondrosarcoma arising in the sphenoid bone of an adult woman. A large soft-tissue tumor extends from the nasal cavity to the middle fossa. A thin sclerotic margin outlines the mass, which contains faint punctate calcification. Note the displacement of the globe.

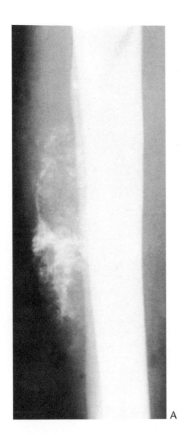

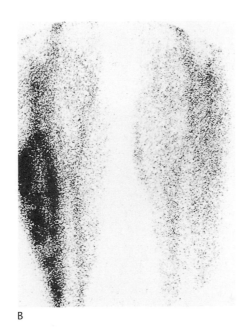

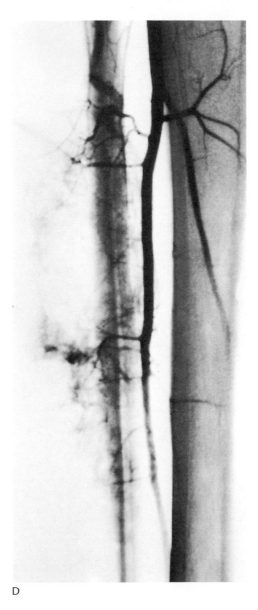

A

B

C

D

Fig. 5-60. Mesenchymal chondrosarcoma. A hard mass had been present in this middle-aged man's calf for 8 years. Recently it had increased in size. A soft-tissue radiograph **A** shows extensive calcification in a well-defined tumor mass. **B.** The blood-pool phase of a bone scan reveals a marked increase in vascularity throughout the lesion which is intensely active on **C** the delayed images (top right). Note also the presence of multiple metastases, particularly in vertebrae and the pelvis. **D.** A femoral arteriogram confirms the markedly abnormal vascularity with pathological vessels throughout the tumor mass. The similarity between the extent of the abnormality shown angiographically and on the blood-pool phase of the bone scan is striking.

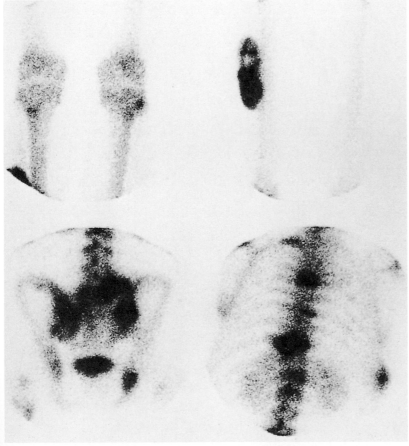

6

TUMORS AND TUMOR-LIKE CONDITIONS OF BONE (2)

Iain Watt and Mark Cobby

BONE TUMORS PRESUMED TO ARISE FROM SKELETAL TISSUE—FIBROUS TUMORS

1. Fibrous Cortical Defect

Fibrous cortical defects are extremely common, occurring in up to a third of normal children between the ages of 2 and 15 years. Characteristically they occur around the knee, especially in the distal posteromedial femoral cortex. They are almost always discovered by chance and are not known to be symptomatic.

Radiologically they are blister-like expansions of the cortex with a thin shell of overlying bone (Fig. 6.1). They may be slightly lobulated, but are always sharply defined (Fig. 6.2) and have a fine sclerotic margin, particularly when seen in profile. Because of their characteristic site they are radiolucent when observed in a frontal view of the knee. An oblique projection will always show the cortical location. With increasing skeletal maturity the lesion may appear to migrate toward the diaphysis before becoming progressively sclerotic and involuting completely. *Bone scans* are unremarkable, revealing only a minimal increase in activity on the delayed phase in proportion to the size of the lesion.

The differential diagnosis, when the lesion occurs in its typical site, is from a cortical desmoid or cortical avulsion syndrome which occurs at the insertion of the adductor magnus muscle or the origin of the medial head of the gastrocnemius muscle. This abnormality is attributed to chronic low-grade traction resulting in irregularity of the femoral cortex, sometimes with a radiolucency, but often with irregular calcification. Because these lesions are almost certainly of traumatic origin, an abnormal increase in activity is evident on a bone scan and a slight increase in vascularity is seen on an angiogram. The typical site and lack of endosteal abnormality should prevent the misdiagnosis of a sarcoma.

2. Non-ossifying Fibroma

This lesion is similar to a fibrous cortical defect except that it is much larger and characteristically occurs in a slightly older age group, between 10 and 20 years. The vast majority are found around the knee joint, the distal end of the femur being the most common location. The lesion occasionally presents with a pathological fracture (Fig. 6.3). Usually it is asymptomatic.

The Radiological Findings reveal an area of increased radiolucency which is sharply defined in the metadiaphysis, the margins are smooth and sharp, with a rather lobulated appearance, and are defined by a thin zone of reactive sclerosis. In larger bones such as the tibia and fibula the lesion may be eccentric and appropriate oblique views will show its relationship to one of the cortices. However, in more slender bones, such as the fibula, the whole width of the bone may be involved. On the outer margin the cortex is usually slightly expanded but remains intact and thinned. Scintigraphically only a minimal increase in activity can be detected on the delayed phase scan, the degree of increased activity solely reflecting the size of the lesion, unless there has been a pathological fracture. As in fibrous cortical defect, the natural history is for the lesion to regress, initially by an increase in the surrounding zone of sclerosis and latterly by replacement with normal bone (Fig. 6.4). There is a debatable association of multiple non-ossifying fibromas with neurofibromatosis.

The differential diagnosis, particularly when the whole width of the bone is involved, is from a solitary bone cyst or monostotic fibrous dysplasia. Differentiation from the former may be very difficult on all radiological grounds whereas distinction from monostotic fibrous dysplasia is relatively straightforward, due to the avidity of the latter for bone-seeking radiopharmaceuticals.

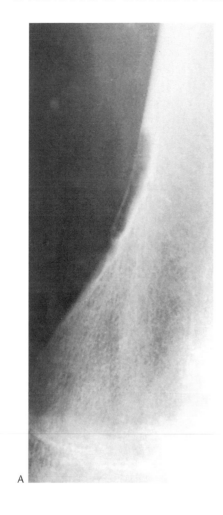

A

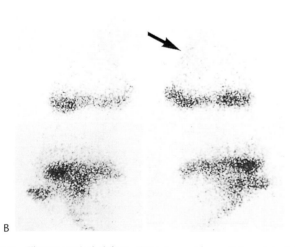

B

Fig. 6.1 Fibrous cortical defect arising in posteromedial aspect of the distal medial femur. **A.** The abnormality is confined to the cortex with very fine shell of overlying bone and a sharply defined endosteal margin. **B.** A bone scan demonstrates a slight increase in activity (arrow) at the site of the lesion.

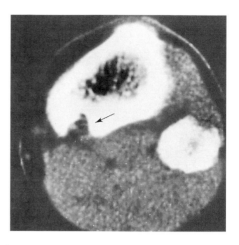

Fig. 6.2 Fibrous cortical defect in the upper medial tibia is shown on CT. Note the purely cortical position of the defect and its sharply defined margin. The thin shell of overlying bone is not seen completely because of the partial volume effect.

3. Desmoplastic Fibroma

This rare tumor exhibits dense fibrous tissue, simulating desmoid tumors of the abdominal wall. Relatively few occur in bone and then usually in young adults. Pain is a constant presenting feature. The lesion is often tender. The majority arise in the metadiaphysis of long bones (Fig. 6.5), although the pelvis and spine are other sites of predilection.

Radiologically they tend to be large, solitary and destructive, with an expanded and irregular sclerotic margin and often with a trabeculated pattern. There may be a slight increase in density within the lesion, so that superficially it may resemble monostotic fibrous dysplasia. Slight irregularity of the margin may suggest an aneurysmal bone cyst when the lesion is purely osteolytic.

Multiple fibromatous tumors are present in **congenital multiple fibromatosis**, in which half the patients have associated bony abnormalities. This rare childhood condition demonstrates multiple, rounded, corticated, cystic metaphyseal lesions, often with sharply defined sclerotic margins. These fibromatous foci tend to regress with increasing age and have an excellent prognosis. In **infantile myofibromatosis (congenital generalized fibromatosis)** similar multiple nodular fibroblastic lesions of the soft tissues, frequently associated with multiple lytic bone lesions, occur with disseminated involvement of muscle, heart and lungs; the outlook in this group is poor.

4. Fibrosarcoma

Although this is the least common of the malignant primary tumors arising in skeletal connective tissue, representing about 5% of all, individual lesions vary widely in their appearances and to this extent can create diagnostic difficulties. This variation corresponds to a wide range of histologic characteristics, but the degree of malignancy and the radiological features correlate reasonably well. Many of the characteristics lie between those of osteosarcoma and chondrosarcoma.

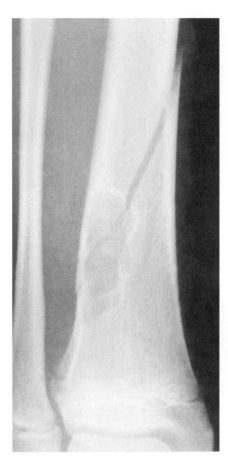

Fig. 6.3 Non-ossifying fibroma of the distal tibia presenting with a fracture. The well-defined outline and eccentric position of the tumor are demonstrated together with sharply defined sclerotic margins.

Fibrosarcoma occurs most commonly in the third to sixth decades, with no sex difference. Presentation is usually due to low-grade pain, sometimes swelling, usually present for less than a year. In many the precipitating factor may be a pathological fracture (Fig. 6.6). Whilst a few of these tumors arise primarily in soft tissue and cause secondary bony changes, the majority develop primarily in bone and may be either medullary or periosteal in location. A medullary lesion is considerably more common and usually arises in the metaphyseal area. Approximately 80% occur around the knee. It is less usual for a flat bone to be involved. The rarer periosteal type has a more widespread distribution, but still has a predilection for long bones, where any portion of the shaft may be affected. This type tends to develop a clinically palpable mass in the earlier stages.

Radiological Features The tumor is essentially osteolytic, provokes little new bone formation and usually lacks calcification or ossification. The medullary variety is characterized usually by an irregular area of radiolucency. The zone of transition may vary from being relatively narrow, indicating a well-differentiated tumor, to being diffuse and permeative, suggesting a highly aggressive tumor (Fig. 6.7). With very low grade tumors a minimal degree of sclerosis may surround the radiolucency. Slowly growing tumors may thin and expand the cortex, but with a diffuse infiltrative pattern it is more usual for cortical destruction to occur. The subsequent soft-tissue extensions are without calcification or ossification, and periosteal new bone formation is unremarkable. This feature may differentiate the tumor from osteosarcoma or chondrosarcoma.

Periosteal tumors, on the other hand, frequently exhibit shaggy ill-defined periosteal new bone formation. Destruction of the outer side of the cortex frequently takes place, but the erosion is usually clearly defined, almost as though a piece of bone has been removed surgically. In this respect considerable variance is shown from the poor definition of the edge of most malignant tumors. Consequently

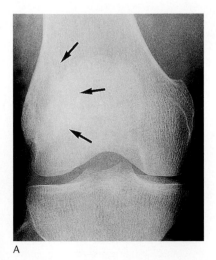

A

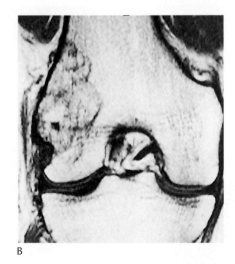

B

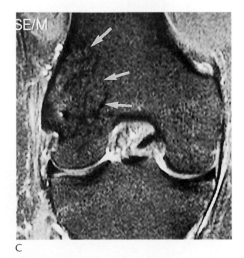

C

Fig. 6.4 Sclerosis of a non-ossifying fibroma. Incidental finding following multiple ligamentous injuries to the knee. **A.** Conventional radiograph. Only a faint band of sclerosis is shown around the margins of the fibroma (arrows). **B.** Coronal T_1-weighted and (**C**) STIR MR images showing mixed fibrous and normal marrow replacement (arrows) within the involuted lesion. Tears of the anterior cruciate and medial collateral ligaments are also evident.

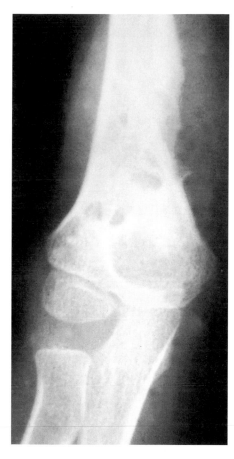

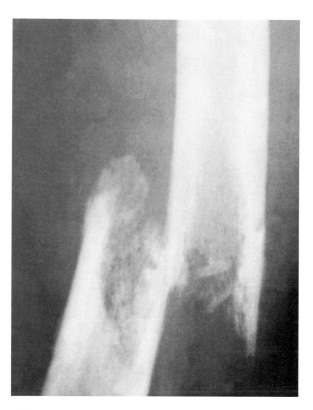

Fig. 6.6 Fibrosarcoma—presenting with pathological fracture of the femur in a woman of 50. Ill-defined bone destruction, particularly of the medulla, is associated with very minor periosteal new bone formation and no sclerosis. The cortex has been thinned on the endosteal surface.

Fig. 6.5 Desmoplastic fibroma. A destructive, lobulated lesion is present in the distal metadiaphysis of the humerus. Bone expansion is present with sclerotic margins around the tumor. A soft-tissue component has caused consolidated periosteal new bone formation.

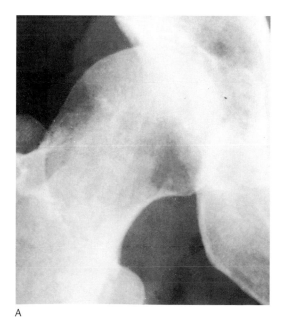

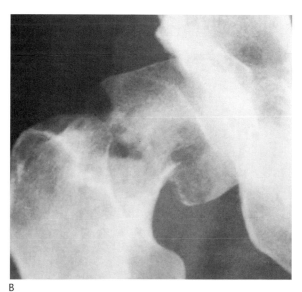

A   B

Fig. 6.7 Fibrosarcoma arising in the medulla of the femoral head and neck. This 35-year-old man presented with poorly localized pain in the hip. **A.** At presentation an ill-defined area of bone destruction on the medial aspect of the femoral head and neck. The cortex is preserved with no new bone formation. **B.** Three months later a pathological fracture has occurred through the destructive lesion.

the impression may be gained of a benign periosteally related tumor, such as a lipoma. Secondary involvement of bone may result also from a fibrosarcoma arising in soft tissue.

As with the conventional radiographic appearances, angiography roughly mirrors the degree of malignancy of the tumor. CT and MRI will define the extent of the tumor and its relationship to neurovascular structures. The success of a bone scan is variable, as it depends on the degree of bone response and the amount of periosteal new bone formation. Metastatic dissemination from fibrosarcoma is not usually detectable with a bone-seeking agent.

Fibrosarcoma may also arise in the fibrous wall of a medullary infarct, following irradiation or secondary to chronic osteomyelitis and is one of the histologic patterns associated with Paget's sarcoma. To differentiate fibrosarcoma of bone from other malignancies is by no means straightforward. The major differential is from osteo-sarcoma and chondrosarcoma. Moreover, the more aggressive, ill-defined varieties may be indistinguishable from malignant round-cell tumors, particularly non-Hodgkin's lymphoma.

5. Malignant Fibrous Histiocytoma

A group of tumors have been separated, mainly from fibrosarcomas, on the basis of histologic and clinical findings. These aggressive, often metastasizing, tumors are probably of histiocytic origin. They occur in an older population, usually around 55 years of age, affected individuals complaining chiefly of pain, swelling or of a slowly enlarging mass. The majority develop in soft tissues. The relatively small number arising in bone have a predilection for the femur and the ends of the tibia and humerus. Others arise in the pelvis and ribs.

The Radiological Features are primarily those of an ill-defined, purely osteolytic lesion with early cortical destruction, frequently in a permeative fashion, often with some expansion. To this extent they resemble fibrosarcomas of an aggressive type. Occasionally punctate, soft-tissue calcification is present and a small proportion exhibit periosteal reaction and endosteal sclerosis (Fig. 6.8). A soft-tissue mass often develops early. Angiographically, areas of avascularity and hypervascularity are typical, including the demon-stration of new vessels and encasement. Scintigraphy is not usually informative. Many cases present with multiple skeletal lesions and the initial impression is of skeletal metastases rather than of a primary or multifocal bone tumor. As with fibrosarcoma, malignant round-cell tumors require consideration in the differential diagnosis.

6. Adamantinoma of Long Bone

This rather unusual neoplasm is almost invariably located in the tibial shaft. **Clinically**, localized pain and swelling have usually been present for several years. The age range varies from 15 to 55 years. On examination a soft-tissue, possibly cystic, swelling is palpated. Histologically, difficulty may arise in differentiating this lesion from metastatic adenocarcinoma or squamous-cell carcinoma, since the glandular and fibrous component of the tumor may suggest an epithelial derivation.

Radiologically an eccentric area of destruction usually involves the anterior portion of the tibial shaft. Slight expansion and cortical thinning, with a cystic or multiloculated appearance, are usual (Fig. 6.9). Periosteal reaction is not marked, but cortical destruction may be extensive. The margin of the tumor varies from being sharply and clearly defined, with a slight sclerotic margin, to a hazy zone of transition several millimeters in width, comparable to that observed in giant-cell tumors. Some of these tumors may be 15 cm long or more, with satellite lesions.

Adamantinoma probably has a relationship to ossifying fibroma, which may be itself a localized form of fibrous dysplasia, in which it has been observed to develop as a late complication. Whilst the

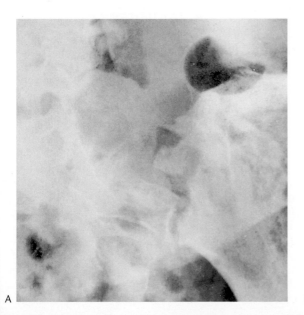 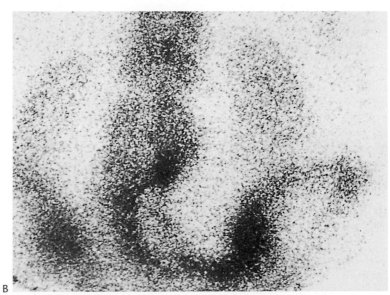

A   B

Fig. 6.8   Malignant fibrous histiocytoma arising in the sacral ala of a 60-year-old woman. **A.** A purely destructive, lytic lesion is present with slight sclerosis around its margins. Note that the lower border of L5 has also been destroyed together with part of the iliac wing. **B.** A radionuclide bone scan shows the tumor to be photon-deficient but a rim of increased activity corresponds to reactive bone sclerosis.

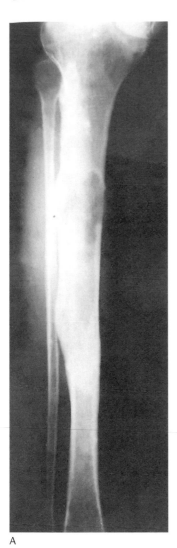

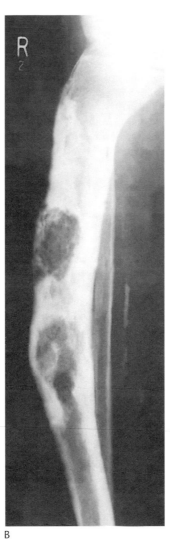

A   B

Fig. 6.9 Adamantinoma of the tibia. Eccentric areas of bone destruction are present anteriorly with thinning of the cortex. The cortex is expanded. In addition to this abnormality, sclerosis and ill-defined cortical thickening are present throughout the whole of the tibia, which is also bowed. These features are due to associated fibrous dysplasia (or a close variety sometimes known as ossifying fibroma which occurs only at this site). **A.** AP view. **B.** Lateral view.

radiological appearances of adamantinoma are not pathognomonic, the location and the clinical history suggest the diagnosis. The tumor continues to grow at a slow rate, but is characterized by local recurrence and eventual metastasis to lung. Extensive local resection is the usual form of treatment.

BONE TUMORS PRESUMED TO ARISE FROM SKELETAL TISSUE: GIANT-CELL-CONTAINING

A group of tumors rich in giant cells, formerly confused in the literature, has now been subdivided, on histological and radiological grounds, into giant-cell tumor ('osteoclastoma') and the giant-cell tumor variants. The latter include chondroblastoma (Ch. 5), chondromyxoid fibroma (Ch. 5) and aneurysmal bone cyst (see below). However, all these variants exhibit some areas which are histo-

logically identical. In consequence, whilst broadly clear-cut radiological and histologic categorization is possible, a definite overlap exists. The 'brown' tumors of hyperparathyroidism have also been included in this category.

1. Giant-cell Tumor (*Osteoclastoma*)

These tumors conform to a fairly constant clinical and radiological pattern. As with many other tumors, the initial presentation is of localized pain and swelling, some presenting following trauma or as an incidental finding. Histologically, richly vascular tissue contains plump spindle cells and numerous giant cells containing 50 to 100 nuclei. The tumor forms neither bone nor cartilage.

It is locally aggressive and likely in more than half of instances to recur in spite of extensive curettage or excision with or without radiotherapy.

A small proportion are malignant. Malignancy may be mistaken in those which are initially extremely aggressive and others that become so following surgical or therapeutic intervention. Sometimes confusion arises because the extreme aggressiveness of the tumor, histologically and radiologically, does not correlate with the subsequent development of distant metastases to the lung. A small group of undoubtedly malignant, metastatic giant-cell tumors has been recognized, often with a dominant fibrosarcomatous stroma. Attempts at histologic and radiological grading have had only limited prognostic value.

The majority of patients present between the ages of 20 and 40 years. Only about 3% of cases develop in immature skeletons, distinguishing these patients from those with aneurysmal bone cysts, in whom the tumor maximally occurs prior to epiphyseal fusion. Giant-cell tumors are multifocal in about 0.5% of cases, often in the hands. The solitary lesion shows a predilection for bones adjacent to the knee joint and the distal end of the radius. Histologic review of a number of cases in which spinal lesions have been detected has indicated that the correct diagnosis is much more commonly an aneurysmal bone cyst. Facial bones appear to be exempt.

Radiological Features A zone of radiolucency is typically situated immediately beneath the articular cortex, sited eccentrically at the end of a long bone (Fig. 6.10). The exception to this rule is when the lesion arises in a former apophysis, notably the greater trochanter. Unless complicated by a fracture, the lesion does not contain calcification or ossification, although in about 40% of cases it is characterized by a 'soap-bubble' pattern of trabeculation. The margins are purely osteolytic; a sclerotic margin is rarely evident. Characteristically, therefore, the margin is hazy and ill-defined with no bone reaction (Fig. 6.11).

More aggressive lesions are associated with widening of the zone of transition. The overlying cortex may be expanded and exquisitely thinned, without the development of periosteal new bone formation, except as a response to a pathological fracture (Fig. 6.12). The tumor may produce a well-defined extension into the adjacent soft tissues, without evidence of calcification or new bone formation. The presence of such a soft-tissue mass does not, of necessity, indicate a sarcoma. This complication is inferred by a rapid change in size or character of the tumor on sequential radiographs.

Angiographically, and on the blood-pool phase of a bone scan, vascularity is markedly increased, typically with an increased

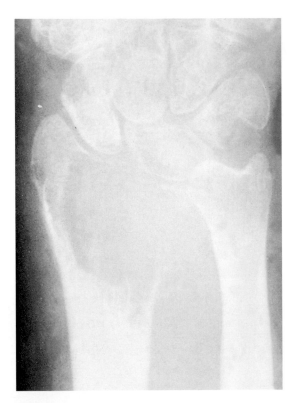

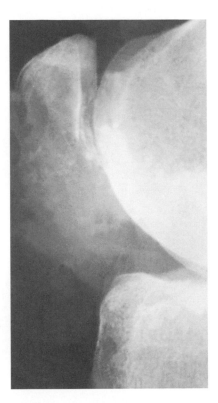

Fig. 6.10 Giant-cell tumor arising in the distal radius of an adult man. A characteristic, eccentric, immediately subarticular position makes this diagnosis very probable. The margins are ill defined with no sclerotic reaction.

Fig. 6.11 Giant-cell tumor of the patella. Giant-cell tumors can arise in almost any bone but those around the knee are particularly affected. Note the immediately subarticular, eccentric position of the tumor which is purely osteolytic with no sclerotic reaction. The epiphyses have fused.

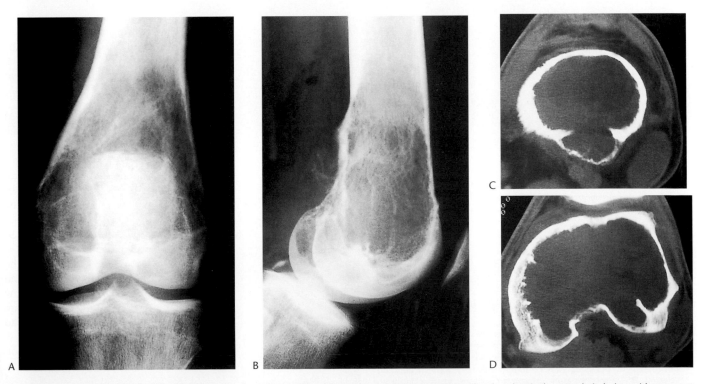

Fig. 6.12 Giant-cell tumor of the distal femur AP **A.** and lateral **B.** radiographs showing a large immediately subarticular osteolytic lesion with apparent trabeculation and a wide zone of transition proximally. A localized area of cortical expansion is demonstrated posteriorly with a thin overlying shell of bone. **C** and **D.** CT sections through the lesion demonstrating the localized dorsal expansion and intact overlying cortex. The apparent trabeculation demonstrated on the conventional radiographs is shown to be due to unresorbed ridges of cortical or trabecular bone at the margins of the lesion.

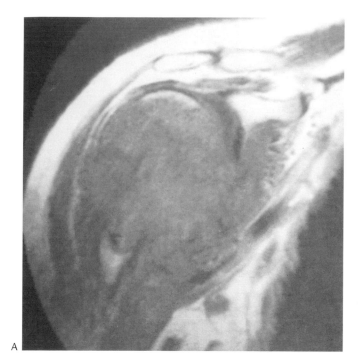

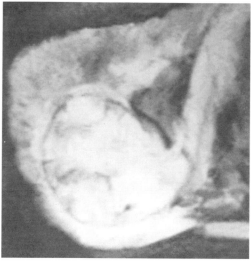

Fig. 6.13 A giant-cell tumor of humerus. Coronal T_1-weighted **A.** and axial STIR sequence **B.** demonstrate a large lobulated mass in the humeral head and neck replacing all normal bone structures. Note the close approximation both to the articular surface and the displaced axillary vessels.

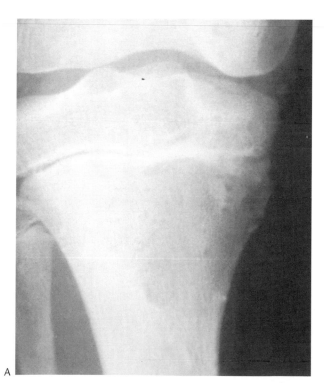

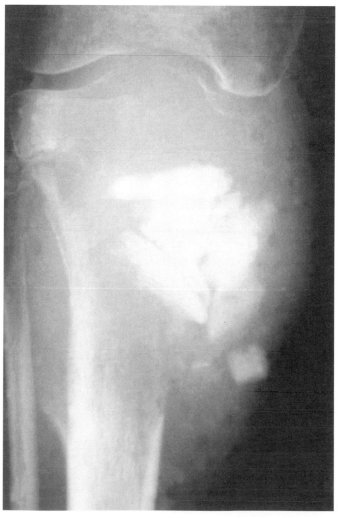

Fig. 6.14 Giant-cell-rich osteosarcoma. **A.** A radiograph of this boy at presentation demonstrates an eccentric, purely osteolytic lesion in the upper tibial metaphysis. The cortex has been breached but there is no periosteal new bone and only very faint surrounding sclerosis. **B.** Six months later, following curettage and packing with bone chips, the flagrantly aggressive nature of this tumor is obvious. Note now the Codman's triangle on the lateral aspect of the tibial shaft and a substantial soft-tissue mass that contains ossification.

number of vessels, arteriovenous shunting and tumor staining. Many exhibit encasement. These features do not correlate with either clinical aggressiveness or sarcomatous change and may be extremely difficult to distinguish from those observed in other giant-cell-containing tumors, particularly aneurysmal bone cysts. The delayed phase of a bone scan is usually normal. CT or MRI (Fig. 6.13) may be necessary to delineate fully the soft-tissue extent of the tumor.

Many of the rather more aggressive giant-cell-containing tumors in the younger age group may in fact be giant-cell-rich osteosarcomas (Fig. 6.14). It is possible that some of the reported metastasizing malignant giant-cell tumors may be of this type. Usually, however, little difficulty arises in differential diagnosis, the eccentric, purely lytic and subarticular location of the tumor being characteristic. Differential diagnosis includes aneurysmal bone cysts and chondroblastoma. The 'brown' tumors of hyperparathyroidism and monostotic fibrous dysplasia require consideration (Fig. 6.15). Occasionally an intraosseous ganglion or large subarticular geode may cause confusion (Fig. 6.16).

In spite of apparently successful curettage and packing with bone chips, these tumors have a tendency to recur, even years after initial treatment. Intraosseous recurrence results in osteolysis adjacent to the previous surgery. Occasionally soft-tissue deposits implanted at the time of surgery will appear as enlarging ossified masses. Secondary sarcomatous change may also occur following radiotherapy after intervals of several years. On rare occasions the tumor may cross a joint or extend from one bone to another.

2. Aneurysmal Bone Cyst

The exact etiology of this tumor is unknown, but the descriptive name is derived from the macroscopic appearances of a blood-filled, expansile, sponge-like tumor containing numerous giant cells.

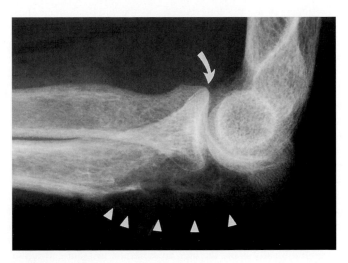

Fig. 6.15 Brown tumor of hyperparathyroidism simulating the appearance of a giant-cell tumor. An osteolytic lesion in the proximal ulna is shown extending to the immediate subarticular region. The margins are poorly defined and there is marked thinning and expansion of the dorsal cortex (arrowheads). A clue to the correct diagnosis, however, is provided by the subtle chondrocalcinosis of the articular surface radial head (curved arrow).

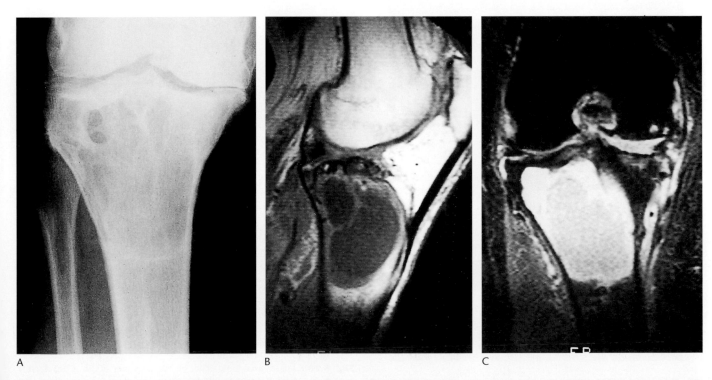

A   B   C

Fig. 6.16 Large subarticular geode mimicking a giant-cell tumor. **A.** Conventional AP radiograph showing a large subarticular osteolucency with well-defined distal margins in the proximal tibia. Prominent medial compartment osteoarthritis is shown. **B.** Sagittal T$_1$-weighted and **C.** coronal STIR MR images showing the multiloculated cystic nature of the tibial geode and the well-marked knee joint osteoarthritis.

Aneurysmal bone cyst has been shown to arise in association with other abnormalities of the skeleton, particularly non-ossifying fibroma, fibrous dysplasia and chondromyxoid fibroma. Such lesions have been described as 'secondary' aneurysmal bone cysts. They have also been recorded following a fracture.

These tumors present in childhood or early adolescent life, with a predilection for the long bones and the lumbar spine. Those arising in the spine occur slightly later, between 10 and 20 years of age. The neural arch is more commonly involved than the body, half of these cases involving more than one vertebra. The prognosis is entirely benign apart from secondary neurologic lesions due to spinal canal compression.

Radiological Features Typically an area of bone resorption occurs with slight or marked expansion (Fig. 6.17), the size of the lesion varying between 2 and, in gross examples, as much as 20 cm in diameter. The overlying cortex is thinned and may be expanded (Fig. 6.18) to such a degree that in places it can be identified only by tomography or CT. The endosteal margin is relatively well-defined against cortex, and an ill-defined zone of transition is usual between the lesion and medullary bone, occasionally with slight sclerosis. A margin of this type is similar to that observed in giant-cell tumor. Sometimes it is scalloped or irregular (Fig. 6.19). Angiographically many features are common to giant-cell tumor, in particular a rich increase in vessels with diffuse opacification and early venous filling. This appearance may be shown in the blood-pool phase of a bone scan. Both CT and MRI may show fluid levels in the vascular spaces.

Most lesions evolve slowly. However a few show a highly aggressive radiological pattern and may increase alarmingly in size, even doubling in a few weeks. The possibility of a very malignant vascular tumor such as an angiosarcoma may then be entertained.

Differentiation from giant-cell tumor is aided by the age of the patient, as three-quarters of aneurysmal bone cysts occur before epiphyseal fusion has occurred, and their widespread anatomic distribution contrasts with the majority of giant-cell tumors occurring around the knee and wrist. Therefore difficulty is likely to arise only when the abnormality occurs after epiphyseal closure or when it is situated at the end of a long bone. Aneurysmal bone cyst rarely extends to the articular surface and is often central, compared to the subarticular eccentric nature of giant-cell tumor. The spinal lesions need to be differentiated from osteoblastoma and osteoid osteoma. The bone-forming nature of these latter two tumors, together with their associated sclerotic reactions, provides valuable differential diagnostic signs.

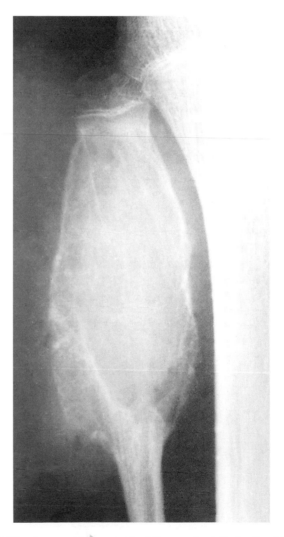

Fig. 6.18 Aneurysmal bone cyst of the proximal fibula. Considerably greater expansion has occurred in this example. The cortex is now very thin though apparently intact. The zone of transition between the lesion and adjacent bone is narrow but ill defined. Note apparent multiple septa within the lesion.

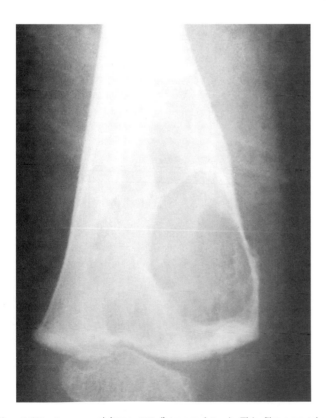

Fig. 6.17 Aneurysmal bone cyst (boy aged two). This film was taken because of an asymptomatic swelling and shows the characteristic features of metaphyseal involvement, cortical expansion and thinning, with a relatively well-defined endosteal margin.

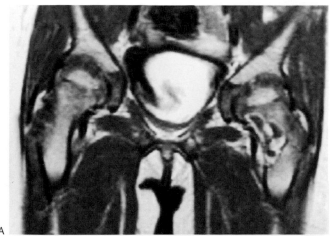

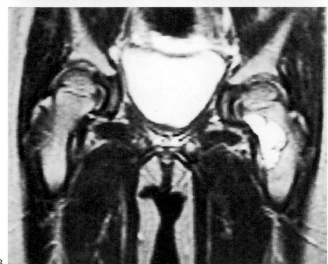

Aneurysmal bone cysts are treated by curettage or radiotherapy, the latter being particularly valuable in spinal lesions where surgery may be considered hazardous. An increasing role, however, has developed for transcatheter embolization in the management of these tumors. Aneurysmal bone cyst is a particularly good example of the importance of radiological investigation being complete before biopsy is undertaken, since these lesions, not surprisingly, bleed considerably and the preoperative demonstration of the vascular nature of this tumor may save some embarrassment!

TUMORS PRESUMED TO ARISE FROM OTHER TISSUES IN BONE: BLOOD VESSELS

1. Hemangioma

Intraosseous hemangiomas are benign and slow-growing. Malignancy is virtually unknown. Many of these benign vascular neoplasms are asymptomatic, their presence being detected incidentally.

They are not infrequently shown on MR studies of the spine, particularly lumbar (Fig. 6.20). The autopsy incidence is about 10%. A few cause swelling and mild pain. Occasionally, significant neurologic deficits may occur secondary to the collapse of an involved vertebral body with or without an extraosseous soft-tissue tumor component. The age of presentation is between 10 and 45 years.

Hemangiomas are either cavernous, with large thin-walled vessels occurring particularly in vertebrae and the skull, or capillary, tending to spread in a sunburst pattern. Typically the tumor is solitary, the commonest site being a thoracic or lumbar vertebral body.

Radiologically, conventional radiographs show increased translucency with a characteristic fine vertical striation (Fig. 6.21). Half the lesions involve purely the vertebral body, the other half

Fig. 6.19 Aneurysmal bone cyst of the left femoral neck. **A.** Coronal gadolinium enhanced T$_1$-weighted and **B.** coronal T$_2$-weighted MR images showing an apparently multiloculated metaphyseal lesion with marked enhancement particularly around the rim of the lesion.

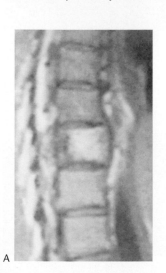

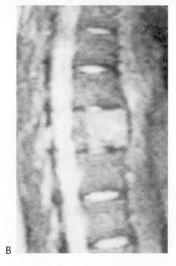

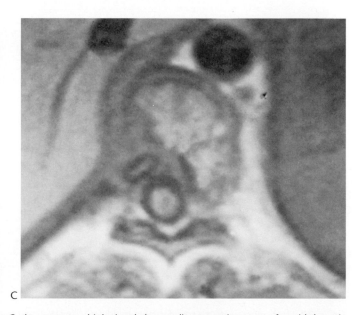

Fig. 6.20 Sagittal T$_1$-weighted **A.**, T$_2$MAST **B.** and T$_1$-weighted axial images **C.** demonstrate a high-signal abnormality occupying most of a mid-thoracic vertebral body extending back into the posterior elements on the left. High-signal lesions both on T$_1$ and T$_2$ are usually benign in the spine. This particular case subsequently required surgery because of compression fracture. Note expansion of the vertebral body which is relatively unusual in benign hemangioma.

extending into the posterior elements. A small proportion have an associated soft-tissue mass. The overall size of the vertebral body is often within normal limits, a helpful differential feature from Paget's disease.

The remainder of the skeleton is affected in approximately half of cases, the skull and long bones being sites of predilection, although other areas may uncommonly be involved (Figs 6.22 and 6.23). Although these tumors may present a striated appearance in long bones and ribs, as in the vertebral lesions, the radiological changes in these other areas are usually very different, tending to be osteolytic with sclerotic margins and often causing some cortical expansion. The osteolytic component has a soap-bubble appearance within which a sunburst or stippled radiodensity may be evident, possibly extending into the soft tissues with radiating spicules of bone. This pattern may be encountered with a capillary hemangioma, particularly in the skull and pelvis (Fig. 6.24). In some cases localized cortical thickening, from which peripheral bone spicules may extend, simulates an osteosarcoma. However, closer scrutiny and appropriate further investigation resolves any difficulty.

Soft-tissue cavernous hemangiomas may be recognized by well-defined circular calcifications due to phleboliths (Fig. 6.25). This is one component of Maffucci syndrome, the other being multiple chondromas (see Fig. 5.44).

Scintigraphically, the bone lesion shows increased activity on the delayed phase of a bone scan (Fig. 6.26). Both bone and soft-tissue lesions may be detected by a blood-pool scan (Fig. 6.27). The appearance of increased activity in a vertebral tumor cannot therefore be used to distinguish between Paget's disease, a sclerotic metastasis or a hemangioma. MRI will demonstrate any soft-tissue mass arising from a vertebral lesion. It may be important to demonstrate the artery of Adamkiewicz with spinal arteriography to avoid paraplegia if surgical excision or transcatheter embolization is required. Some lesions respond well to radiotherapy, particularly those in vertebrae.

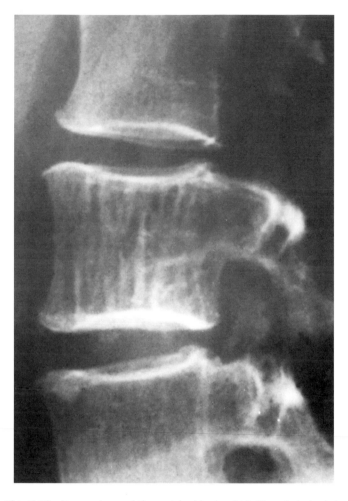

Fig. 6.21 Hemangioma of the vertebral body of L3. The whole body is marked by the characteristic vertical striation, which in this example does not extend into the pedicles.

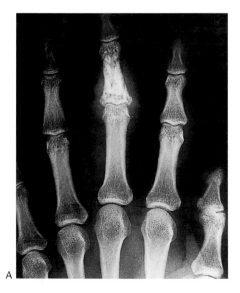
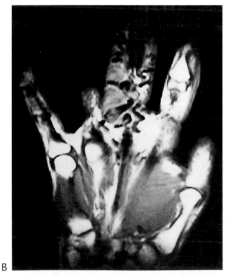
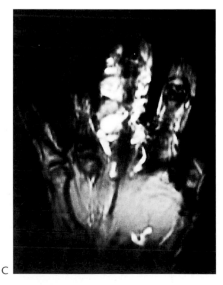

A   B   C

Fig. 6.22 Hemangioma of the middle finger middle phalanx with associated prominent soft-tissue component. **A.** Conventional radiograph showing sclerotic striated phalanx of the middle finger and soft-tissue swelling. **B.** Coronal T_1-weighted and **C.** gradient echo MR images showing the extensive soft-tissue component of the cavernous hemangioma. The dilated abnormal vessels and vascular spaces appear as characteristic low-signal serpiginous channels on the T_1-weighted sequence but have a high signal intensity on the gradient echo image.

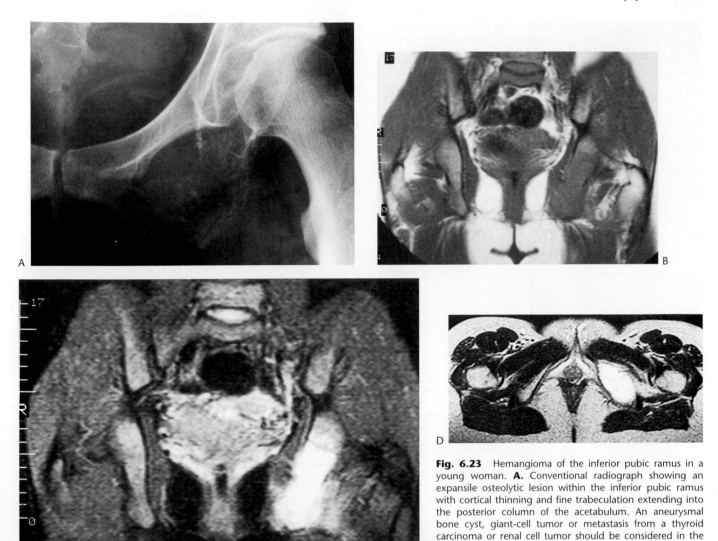

Fig. 6.23 Hemangioma of the inferior pubic ramus in a young woman. **A.** Conventional radiograph showing an expansile osteolytic lesion within the inferior pubic ramus with cortical thinning and fine trabeculation extending into the posterior column of the acetabulum. An aneurysmal bone cyst, giant-cell tumor or metastasis from a thyroid carcinoma or renal cell tumor should be considered in the differential diagnosis. **B.** Coronal T_1-weighted, **C.** STIR and **D.** axial T_2-weighted MR images of the pelvis showing the extent of the expansile lesion within the inferior pubic ramus and posterior acetabulum. Marked bony expansion is evident but there is no soft-tissue component to the tumor.

2. Vanishing Bone Disease (Gorham's disease)

This relatively rare syndrome is a variant of angiomatosis of bone in which vascular proliferation predominates. Its origin is unknown. It is recognized usually in childhood, but more than one-third of patients are over the age of 35. Progressive weakness and limitation of movement of the affected area characterize the onset. Pain is not an early feature, although obviously occurring with a pathological fracture. After a period of months or years the limb becomes useless or flail. The course is unpredictable, either stabilizing or progressing fatally with the development of chylothorax.

Radiologically an ill-defined area of radiolucency may be observed in a single bone, but this destructive process progresses slowly to involve adjacent bones without respect for intervening joints (Fig. 6.28). Symptoms, however, may be so insidious that extensive absorption of many adjacent bony structures may be revealed at the initial examination. Arteriography and lymphography

Fig. 6.24 Hemangioma of the skull is shown on a localized view of the temporal fossa. Note the purely osteolytic lesion with stippled radio-densities.

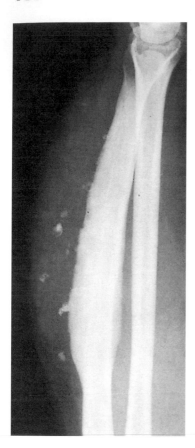

Fig. 6.25 Cavernous hemangioma of the soft tissues of the forearm is diagnosed by the presence of soft-tissue swelling within which there are phleboliths. The presence of extensive consolidated periosteal new bone and bowing of the ulna suggest an intimate relationship with the periosteum.

Fig. 6.26 Vertebral hemangioma was detected initially **A.** on a whole-body radionuclide bone scan in this middle-aged woman with carcinoma of the breast. A marked increase in activity is present throughout the whole of L3. **B.** A radiograph demonstrates fine striation within an enlarged vertebral body. The pedicles, particularly that on the right, are enlarged. **C.** Computerized tomography confirms multiple radiolucencies throughout the vertebral body. This patient remained free of metastasis on annual follow-up for 5 years.

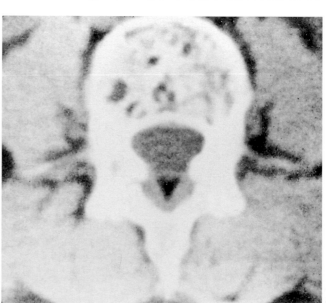

A

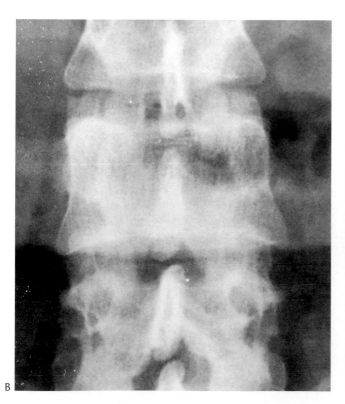

B

C

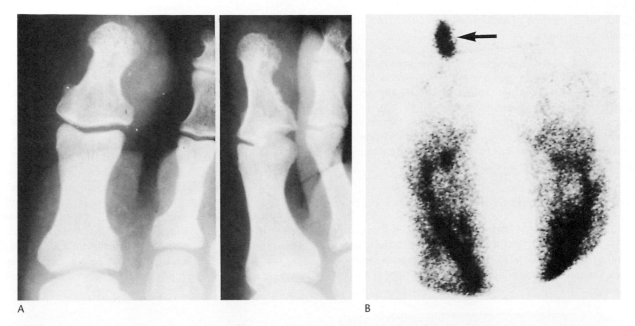

Fig. 6.27 Soft-tissue hemangioma of the great toe. This patient complained of a swollen great toe with a purple area of discoloration. **A.** A plain film reveals soft-tissue swelling and pressure erosion of the plantar aspect of the distal phalanx. **B.** A blood-pool scan confirms an intense focus of activity (arrow) corresponding to the cavernous hemangioma.

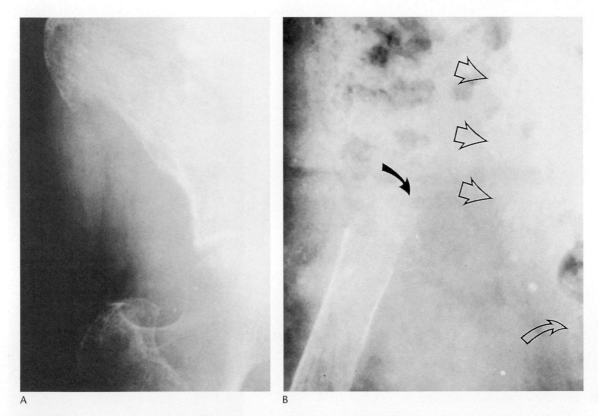

Fig. 6.28 Vanishing bone disease. A 70-year-old woman presented with poorly localized pain in her right hip. **A.** A radiograph at presentation reveals ill-defined destruction at the anterior inferior iliac spine. **B.** Nine months later there is total destruction of the whole of the hemipelvis and hip joint. Note the faint outline of the residual femoral head (arrow), pathological fracture of the femoral neck and the articular surfaces of the sacrum and symphysis pubis which no longer articulate with bone (open arrows).

have shown no connection of these lesions to either the vascular or lymphatic circulations.

The radiological appearance is consequently that of a diffuse increase in translucency with progressive absorption of the affected structures. In the course of the process, deformity is likely to develop and may be crippling. Although local recurrence is a major hazard, slow progression is the rule.

Similar massive osteolysis may occur with tumorous masses of lymphatic origin (*lymphangiomatosis*). Histologic differentiation of the cavernous spaces that are found may be difficult and the radiological features are virtually identical.

3. Cystic Angiomatosis of Bone

This rare entity is probably due to a hamartomatous malformation of primitive vessels. It may be difficult to distinguish the tissue of origin. Some lesions are clearly related to blood vessels, others to lymphatics. Among numerous synonyms, cystic angiomatosis is the most descriptive.

The condition may be recognized in childhood or adolescence in the virtual absence of symptoms, other than mild bony swellings or, occasionally, a pathological fracture. The diagnostic radiological abnormalities may be discovered incidentally. Broadly, two groups of patients are affected, those with and those without visceral and/or cutaneous involvement. The former have multiple angiomatous lesions in abdominal viscera, brain, muscle, lungs and lymph nodes, and although these lesions are histologically innocent, death may be caused from anemia or bleeding. The prognosis in the latter group is excellent.

Radiologically, multiple sharply defined radiolucent lesions surrounded by a narrow sclerotic margin involve both cortex and medulla (Fig. 6.29). An initial impression of myeloma may be given. The skull, flat bones and proximal ends of long bones are affected particularly. Scintigraphically, activity may be increased around the lesions. Angiography is usually normal, but in those cases which have differentiated more closely along lymphatic lines a connection with deep lymphatics may be demonstrated by lymphography.

4. Glomus Tumor

This rare, highly differentiated, benign vascular tumor affects soft tissues more than bone. It creates, however, pressure erosion, usually of a terminal phalanx, particularly the subungual portion (Fig. 6.30). A few lesions may originally arise in bone. Typically an extremely sharp margin is associated with a well-marked sclerotic rim.

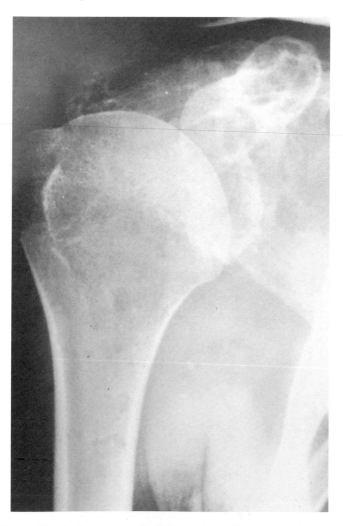

Fig. 6.29 Cystic angiomatosis of bone. Shortly before taking his university entrance examination this young man complained of a vague discomfort in his right shoulder. Note multiple well-defined radiolucencies involving the acromion, coracoid, glenoid and upper humeral shaft. The latter has a rather 'woodworm'-like appearance. Lesions were present elsewhere in the skeleton but he had no soft-tissue abnormality.

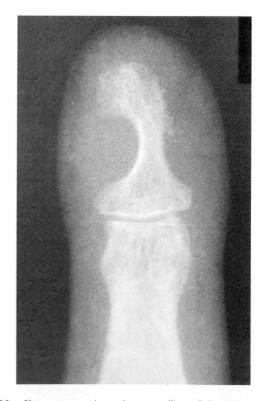

Fig. 6.30 Glomus tumor. Intermittent swelling of the index finger had been present for many years and had, intermittently, been exquisitely painful. A discrete soft-tissue mass caused a pressure erosion on the radial side of the terminal phalanx.

Clinically the tumors are exquisitely tender and have many episodes of stabbing pain, particularly with the rarer and less differentiated hemangiopericytoma. Angiographically, the lesion is richly vascular, and so may be detected on a blood-pool scan or on the early phase of a bone scan. The correct clinical diagnosis is usually established with little difficulty by the classic triad of pain, tenderness and sensitivity to cold.

5. Angiosarcoma *(Hemangioendothelial sarcoma)*

Primary malignant vascular tumors in bone are rare. None has been observed to arise from a benign precursor.

Radiologically the lesions are purely lytic and rapidly fatal, with metastatic spread to the lungs often being present at the time the diagnosis is made. The destructive areas have irregular endosteal margins with slight expansion or coarse loculation occasionally giving a rather soap-bubble appearance. Distinction of this lesion from a highly vascular (telangiectatic) osteosarcoma may be very difficult. A clue may be derived from the sometimes multifocal nature of angiosarcoma, occurring in about one-third of cases.

TUMORS PRESUMED TO ARISE FROM OTHER TISSUES IN BONE: NERVE TISSUE

1. Neurofibroma and Neurilemmoma

There is no clear distinction between these two tumors. It is thought that neurilemmoma or schwannoma arises from a specific cell, the Schwann cell, whereas neurofibromas come from non-specific cells in nerve sheath. When these lesions enlarge in intimate relation to bone, the latter undergoes pressure erosion resulting in an osseous defect. Radiological differentiation between such lesions is not possible. However there is some histologic importance since neurilemmomas are usually solitary and never undergo malignant change, whereas neurofibromas are often multiple and may become sarcomatous. Tumors arise at any age, and in either sex, usually giving rise to symptoms only as the result of nerve pressure or occasionally pathological fracture. Nerve pressure arises typically when the tumor is located within an osseous canal. Neurilemmomas have a predilection for the mandible whereas neurofibromas are more closely related to the spinal canal.

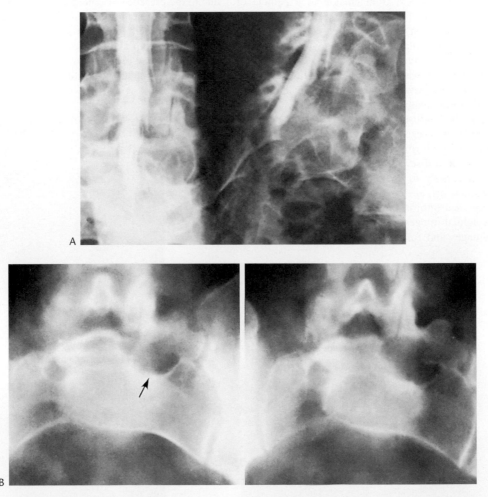

Fig. 6.31 Neurofibroma arising in the exit foramen of the first sacral segment. The patient presented with sciatic pain and **A.** two views from a water-soluble radiculogram reveal amputation of the S1 nerve root sheath, displacement of the S1 and S2 roots and a large well-defined rounded radiolucency with sclerotic margins in the exit foramen. **B.** Frontal tomograms confirm a large bony defect (arrow), compared with the normal right foramen.

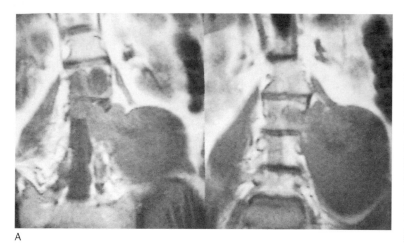

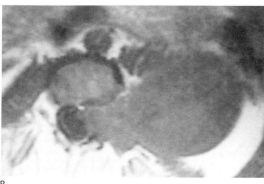

A   B

Fig. 6.32 Neurofibroma demonstrated by MRI coronal T$_1$-weighted **A.** and axial **B.** images. A typical dumb-bell tumor is shown with large extra neural component. Note, however, there is extension into the exit foramen and also intrathecal abnormalities.

Radiological Features The presence of a benign lesion within the spinal canal may be evident from erosion of a pedicle or widening of an exit foramen (Figs 6.31 and 6.32). The width of the interpedicular distance may also be increased. A soft-tissue mass projecting through the enlarged foramen is typical of the so-called *dumb-bell tumor*. Discrete pressure erosions on the surface of bone may be observed elsewhere in the skeleton (Fig. 6.33), but as these tumors are able to grow away from bone they are usually not symptomatic. Neurofibromas cause notches at the inferior surface of ribs but should not be confused with those in coarctation of the aorta, since they vary both in size and in distribution, not principally affecting the fourth to eighth ribs. All erosive lesions are rounded and clearly defined with a discrete sclerotic margin. CT or MRI, however, may be necessary to demonstrate that they have predominantly a soft-tissue origin.

On MR imaging neurofibromas have an intermediate signal intensity on T$_1$-weighted images, and a very high signal intensity on T$_2$-weighted images and following gadolinium enhancement.

Sometimes areas of lower signal intensity centrally may be seen due to the presence of collagen and fibrous tissue. Because of the predilection of neurofibromas to arise in nerve roots, many appear in the lumbosacral area and are detected during the investigation of low back pain and sciatica (Figs 6.34 and 6.35). MR imaging also allows easy recognition of plexiform neurofibromas as they extend in a lobulated infiltrating pattern along neural bundles.

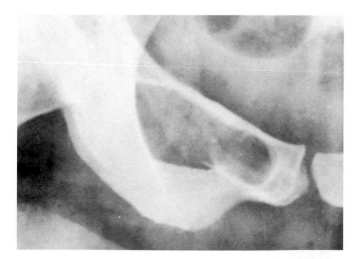

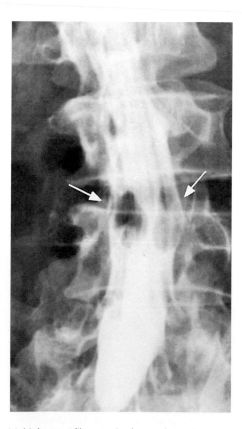

Fig. 6.33 Neurofibroma arising in the obturator ring has caused considerable pressure erosion of both right pubic rami, particularly the superior one. The margins of the pressure defect are sharply defined.

Fig. 6.34 Multiple neurofibromas in the cauda equina. This middle-aged patient was investigated for low back pain by radiculography. Two large ovoid neurofibromas are shown in close relationship to the L4 and L5 roots.

2. Neurofibromatosis

Neurofibromatosis is often noticed at birth or soon after. Typical clinical manifestations are *cafe-au-lait spots* and *multiple cutaneous tumors*. Larger soft-tissue masses or growth disparities may also become apparent. These include scoliosis, pseudoarthrosis of long bones (particularly the tibia) and hemihypertrophy. Scoliosis, usually of short segment distribution, often occurs in the thoracic spine. In addition numerous abnormalities arise related to the neural canal, including generalized dilatation (dural ectasia) with scalloping of vertebral bodies (Fig. 6.35), internal meningoceles and dysraphic anomalies (see Ch. 55). Abnormal rib tubulation results in a 'ribbon-shaped' appearance. A particularly common abnormality is defective ossification of the posterior superior wall of the orbit. Pseudarthrosis of the tibia is characterized by marked absorption of the fracture margins, so that they become pointed (Fig. 6.36). Similar lesions may occur in the radius or clavicle. A number of published reports suggest that malignant sarcomatous change is relatively common, of the order of 5–12% of affected patients. The radiological appearances then become those of an infiltrating diffuse destructive process.

Many extraskeletal manifestations of neurofibromatosis occur because of the neuroectodermal and mesodermal derivation of the tissue (Fig. 6.37). Gliomas of the optic nerves, pheochromocytomas, aneurysms of cerebral and renal arteries, and acoustic neurilemmomas are well recognized. Similarly the incidence of fibrous tumor of bone is increased, particularly around the knee where radiologically

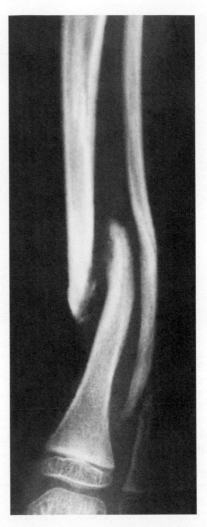

Fig. 6.36 Neurofibromatosis. Pseudarthroses of the tibia and fibula shown in an infant. Bowing of bone and absence of any evidence of bone repair are typical.

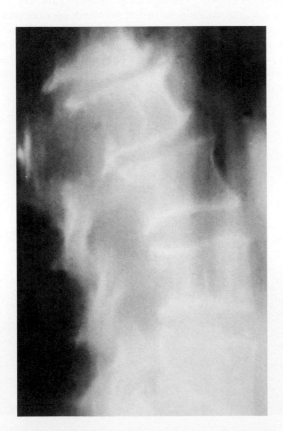

Fig. 6.35 Neurofibromatosis. A lateral tomogram of the lumbar spine demonstrates typical posterior scalloping, part of the general dysplasia of the neural canal and its contents found in this condition.

they seem identical to non-ossifying fibromas and fibrous cortical defects.

TUMORS PRESUMED TO ARISE FROM OTHER TISSUES IN BONE: FATTY TISSUE

Lipoma and Liposarcoma

Although fat represents one of the normal connective tissue elements within bone, intraosseous lipomas are exceedingly rare. The few that have been observed usually cause an oval lytic lesion within a long bone of the lower limb or the calcaneus. In a long bone the appearances may bear a distinct resemblance to non-ossifying fibroma. A sharply defined discrete sclerotic margin is associated with bone expansion and trabeculation. Periosteal new bone formation is not a feature. Within the calcaneus an intraosseus lipoma has a characteristic appearance, presenting as an osteolytic lesion with a central focus of ossification and sclerotic margins (Fig. 6.38). It invariably occurs in the same location as a simple

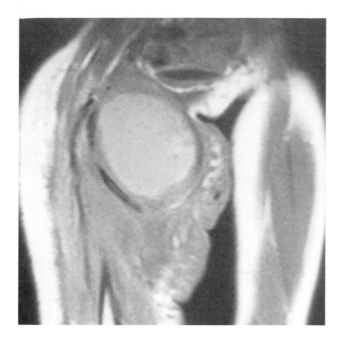

Fig. 6.37 A coronal T$_1$-weighted sequence of the thighs demonstrates an obvious abnormality on the right. In addition to a solitary neurofibroma displacing the femoral vessels (shown by a signal void), there is clear mesenchymal dysplasia, with extensive abnormalities of subcutaneous tissue and hemihypertrophy.

bone cyst within the triangular radiolucent zone between the major trabecular groups

Parosteal Lipomas on the other hand present a much more characteristic appearance with strands of ossification forming around the radiolucent fatty lobules of this rare tumor (Fig. 6.39). They tend to be very slow in growth and produce minor symptoms. Marked

periosteal new bone formation does occur, with an obvious, but well-defined, soft-tissue mass.

A more aggressive nature, however, must be considered when the soft-tissue element fails to contain fatty lucencies, possibly indicating the presence of a **parosteal liposarcoma. Intraosseous liposarcoma** has been described but is exceedingly rare and produces an ill-defined lytic area, usually in the femur or tibia, which is extremely vascular. Rapid extension into the soft tissues, and early pulmonary metastasis, is usual.

The characteristic radiolucencies of soft-tissue lipomas are discussed in Chapter 52, and **lipomas in the lumbar canal** are considered in Chapter 55. **Macrodystrophia lipomatosa** is a rare form of localized gigantism of a hand or foot accompanied by an overgrowth of the associated mesenchymal elements, particularly fat.

TUMORS PRESUMED TO ARISE FROM OTHER TISSUES IN BONE: NOTOCHORD

Chordoma

The notochord extends, during embryologic development, from the coccyx to the buccopharyngeal membrane and is the precursor of the vertebrae and intervertebral disks. Chordoma is a destructive bone tumor believed to arise from notochord cell rests. All are locally malignant with a strong tendency to recur after attempted excision. The lesions are slow growing and become apparent due to pressure symptoms, with or without localized pain. The extreme ends of the axial skeleton are mainly involved, approximately half the lesions arising in the sacrum and/or coccyx, the others in the basioccipital and basisphenoid regions of the skull. A vertebral origin is found only in 15% of patients. Adjacent vertebrae may be involved. A fatal outcome results from a local extension, metastatic spread being unusual.

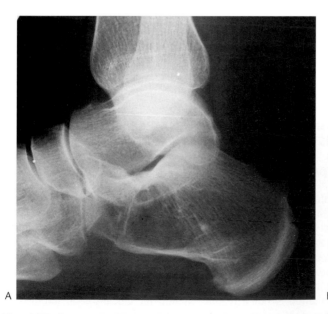
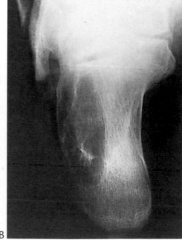
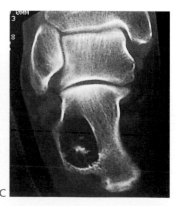

Fig. 6.38 Intraosseous lipoma within the calcaneus. **A.** Lateral and **B.** axial conventional radiographs showing an osteolytic lesion characteristically located between the major trabecular groups of the bone. A thin sclerotic margin surrounds the lesion which contains an eccentric stellate calcified focus. **C.** Coronal CT of the hind foot establishing the fat content of the lesion.

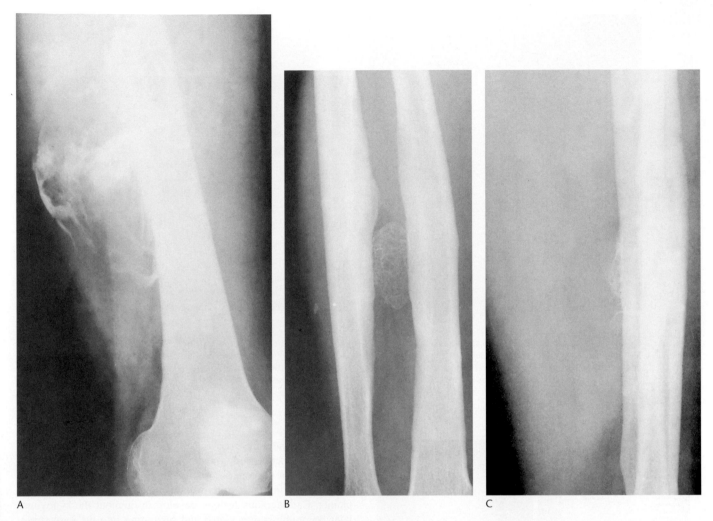

A   B   C

Fig. 6.39   Parosteal lipoma. Two examples are shown of parosteal lipomas arising in middle-aged patients. Both presented with a painless, rather firm mass, apparently attached to bone. **A.** A large lesion arising on the lateral aspect of the femur. Note the strands of ossification surrounding the radiolucent areas of fat. **B** and **C.** A more discrete tumor arises from the interosseous membrane of the forearm. A fatty radiolucency is present, together with ossification in the soft tissues and some periosteal new bone formation.

The usual clinical presentation is of a man between 40 and 70, the clinical symptoms and signs depending on the site of obstruction. Constipation is often a feature of those arising from the sacrum.

Radiological Features   In the sacral area the tumor typically arises in the midline and involves the fourth or fifth sacral vertebra (Fig. 6.40). The lesion is purely lytic, relatively well-defined, usually being oval or slightly lobulated. It may contain areas of calcification. The sacral margins may occasionally be sclerotic. The soft-tissue structures within the pelvis are displaced anteriorly. Tumors arising at the basioccipital or hypophyseal regions are accompanied by erosion and destruction of the dorsum sellae and clivus. Once again a lobulated or rounded area of bone destruction is associated with a large soft-tissue mass displacing nasopharynx anteriorly and sometimes containing amorphous calcification. Here the differential diagnosis is from chondrosarcoma, whereas in the sacrum the possibility of plasmacytoma or a giant-cell tumor should be considered.

TUMORS PRESUMED TO ARISE FROM OTHER TISSUES IN BONE: EPITHELIAL ORIGIN

Implantation Dermoid Cysts

These rare lesions almost always follow a penetrating wound associated with a crush fracture, when it is assumed that epithelial cells are carried into the underlying bony structure. Typically they arise in distal phalanges of adolescents or young adults, the left middle finger being the single commonest site. The lesion grows slowly over many years.

Radiologically a well-defined translucency results, with slight expansion and sharply defined margins around which a minimal sclerotic reaction may be visible (Fig. 6.41). Subungual fibromas represent the only serious differential diagnostic possibility. A glomus tumor is almost invariably extraosseous.

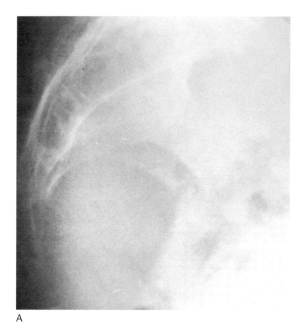

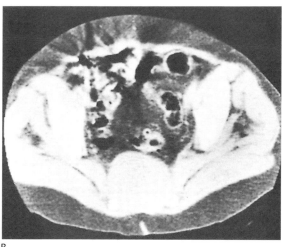

A   B

Fig. 6.40   Chordoma of the distal sacrum. **A.** A lateral film demonstrates a large soft-tissue mass displacing bowel anteriorly. The anterior cortex of the distal sacral vertebrae are ill defined and the coccyx is not seen. **B.** Computerized tomography demonstrates the typical well-defined soft-tissue mass extending anteriorly from the sacrum. The anterior cortex of the sacrum has been destroyed. Chordomas usually exhibit an apparent disproportion between the size of the soft-tissue mass and the extent of the bony involvement.

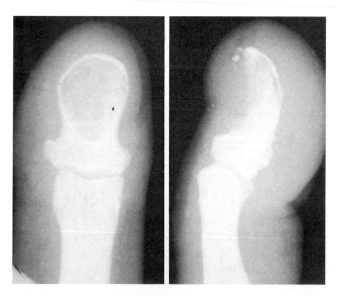

Fig. 6.41   Implantation dermoid cyst. A cystic lesion in the terminal phalanx of the thumb was found in an elderly woman many years after a penetrating injury. The sharp definition of its margins and the location of the lesion are characteristic.

TUMORS RELATED TO JOINTS

1. Synovial Chondromatosis *(Osteochondromatosis)*

This is a relatively unusual synovial disease, commonly regarded as a benign neoplasm, in which metaplastic cartilage formation occurs throughout the synovium. Typically young and middle-aged adults are affected, with a male preponderance and an affinity for large joints, in particular the knee, hip and elbow. Minimal pain, swelling and limitation of movement are the usual presenting complaints. Cartilaginous lesions develop throughout the synovium, later becoming pedunculated and separating into the joint space. When large enough they undergo ossification. This condition undoubtedly progresses in phases, with episodes of synovitis and the shedding of loose bodies (Fig. 6.42).

In the early stages the only abnormality which may be detected on conventional radiographs is an apparent joint effusion. This may be delineated by CT, when a slight increase in density may be observed.

Arthrography, however, demonstrates not only an irregular, nodular synovium (Fig. 6.43) but also cartilaginous loose bodies. The unenhanced MRI appearances may be non-specific, particularly in the absence of cartilage calcification, demonstrating only homogeneous high signal intensity on T_2-weighted images, mimicking a joint effusion. However, the mass and proliferative effects of the lesion may be evident with erosion of bone, hyaline cartilage and normal intra-articular structures, such as the pulvinar fat pad within the acetabular fossa. Calcification and ossification of the cartilaginous masses result in numerous oval or rounded opacities, often of similar size, demonstrated on conventional radiographs. Serial examination may show these to be fairly constant in position. Scintigraphy using a bone-seeking radiopharmaceutical often demonstrates an appreciable increase in activity localized particularly in the larger masses, suggesting that active ossification and calcification are occurring. Eventually extensive capsular distension may result in marginal bony erosions occurring characteristically at the insertion of joint capsule, with clearly defined margins. Synovial

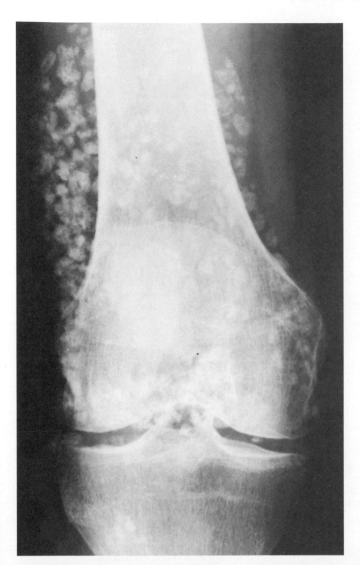

Fig. 6.42 Synovial chondromatosis. Hundreds of calcified lesions are shown in relation to the synovium, all of them approximately the same size. Nearly all were loose bodies.

chondromatosis also occurs in tendon sheaths, usually in the hand, wrist or foot, and bursae. Chondrosarcoma is an extremely rare complication.

2. Pigmented Villonodular Synovitis

The etiology of this disorder of synovium is not known. It is generally regarded as a benign neoplasm. The disease may be mono-articular or polyarticular, the latter being very rare. Adolescents and young adults are affected, usually complaining of local pain and swelling, occasionally with cystic masses related to a large joint, usually the knee or hip. Histologically the appearances show considerable variation, with proliferation of villonodular masses of synovial tissue associated with the deposition of hemosiderin, a feature which may be detected by increased tissue attenuation on CT and low signal intensity masses on MRI due to the para-magnetic effect of hemosiderin.

Radiologically, synovial thickening is usually evident, particularly with soft-tissue exposures. Features which suggest the diagnosis are sharply defined para-articular erosions with sclerotic margins, particularly if these lesions are present on both sides of the affected joint (Figs 6.44, 6.45). As in gout, integrity of the articular surfaces and preservation of the width of the joint space are maintained until relatively late in the disease. Disuse osteoporosis is not an initial feature. Calcification within the synovial mass is exceedingly rare, unlike malignant synovioma. Arthrographically, the thickening of the synovium is confirmed, usually being diffuse in larger joints, such as the knee, whereas in small joints, particularly metacarpophalangeal joints, the thickening is nodular (Fig. 6.46).

Characteristic appearances on MR imaging are often seen with a diffuse heterogeneous signal intensity mass, traversed by low signal intensity septae, containing clumps of tissue with a variable signal intensity. The exact appearances will depend on the relative proportions of fat, hemosiderin, fibrous stroma, synovitis and cellular elements making up the lesion (Fig. 6.47). Bone erosions are also well demonstrated. The synovium of tendon sheaths and bursae may also be affected by this disease (also called giant-cell tumor of tendon sheath) (Fig. 6.48).

3. Lipoma Arborescens

This condition occurs most commonly in the knee and is charac-terized by a mass of numerous fat-laden synovial villous projections (lipomatosis of the synovium). On conventional radiographs the radiolucent arborizing fatty projections may be evident as a soft-tissue mass originating from the joint. The lesion can be elegantly demonstrated on MR imaging which will confirm the fatty nature of the tumor (Fig. 6.49).

4. Dialysis Related Amyloidosis

This is a relatively recently recognized complication of long-term hemodialysis. It is due to the deposition of a unique form of amyloid derived from circulating Beta 2-microglobulin. The con-dition is characterized by painful stiff joints, usually first involving the shoulders and less often the hands, wrists and other large joints. The carpal tunnel syndrome is a common presentation. The disease is seldom seen before five years of treatment.

Radiologically the conventional radiographic findings may mimic pigmented villonodular synovitis with well-defined pressure-like erosions, often with sclerotic margins, involving both sides of the joint (Fig. 6.50). On MR imaging a characteristic appearance is demonstrated with bony erosions and synovial masses exhibiting a predominately low signal intensity on both T_1- and T_2-weighted images (Fig. 6.51).

5. Synovioma

This is a highly malignant tumor growing rapidly with early metastases to lymph nodes, unlike most other musculoskeletal tumors. Young adults are most commonly affected, the mean age being 35. The lesion arises in soft tissue adjacent to synovial structures of joints, tendon sheaths and bursae. Seventy per cent of cases involve the lower extremities, particularly around the knee. Clinically, a soft-tissue mass or ill-defined swelling is present in nearly three-quarters of patients, associated with local pain.

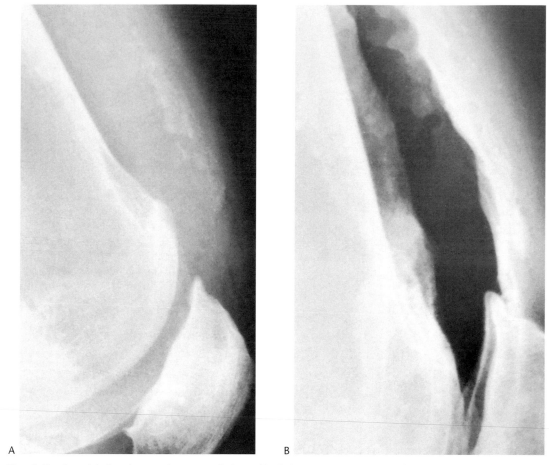

A   B

Fig. 6.43 Synovial chondromatosis. **A.** A preliminary film before knee arthrography demonstrates calcification in the thickened suprapatellar pouch. **B.** A localized view of the knee arthrogram demonstrates both nodular synovial thickening and intrasynovial calcification.

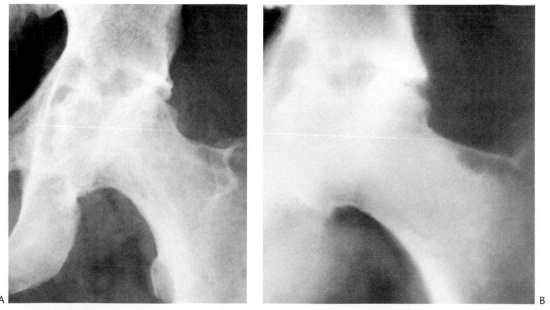

A   B

Fig. 6.44 Pigmented villonodular synovitis of the hip. **A.** The conventional radiograph illustrates sharply defined radiolucent defects involving the acetabulum and the femoral head and neck. **B.** The sharply defined nature of the lesions confirmed on tomography. Note the sclerotic margins. This patient has relatively advanced disease and joint space narrowing is present.

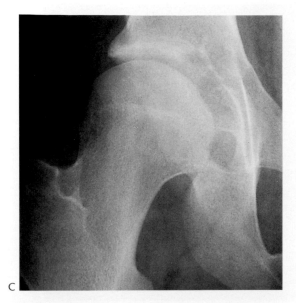

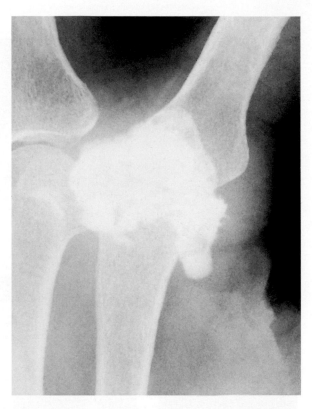

Fig. 6.44 C. In another patient the well-defined radiolucencies are confined to the acetabular side of the joint and the joint space is preserved or widened.

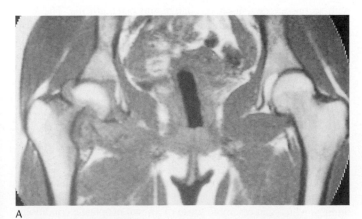

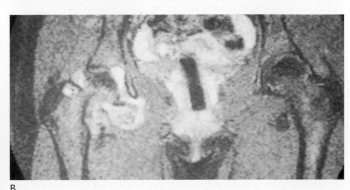

Fig. 6.45 Pigmented villonodular synovitis of the hip. Coronal T_1-weighted **A.** and STIR sequence **B.** demonstrate a lobulated synovial mass on the right with modestly high signal on the STIR sequence, though less so than the joint effusion associated with it. Note the replacement of the pulvina on the T_1-weighted sequence by tumor. A tampon is present in the vagina.

Fig. 6.46 Pigmented villonodular synovitis of the index finger metacarpophalangeal joint. An arthrogram confirms an enlarged joint space and thickened nodular synovium.

Radiologically, a soft-tissue mass is shown associated with a joint, about one patient in five demonstrating calcification of an amorphous nature. Ossification does not occur, unlike the later stages of synovial chondromatosis. About 10% of cases are associated with bone involvement, shown radiologically by irregular bone destruction, particularly at capsular attachments (Fig. 6.52).

This tumor may occasionally arise in the synovial lining of tendon sheaths, producing a similar soft-tissue mass. Secondary involvement of adjacent bone has been observed, particularly in the feet.

5. Intraosseous Ganglion

This is a relatively uncommon lesion, representing ganglion material within a long tubular bone, the origin of which is unclear. Direct communication with a joint is demonstrated rarely. It may, on occasion, be shown to extend from an extraosseous lesion. Patients are between 30 and 60 years of age and two-thirds complain of local joint pain, often related to exercise. Most commonly the lesion occurs around the knee or ankle; hips and carpus are also common sites.

Radiologically, an oval or circular eccentric osteolytic lesion is shown, which is often expansile, with a thin sclerotic rim. These may appear multilocular, varying between 1 and 5 cm in size (Fig. 6.53).

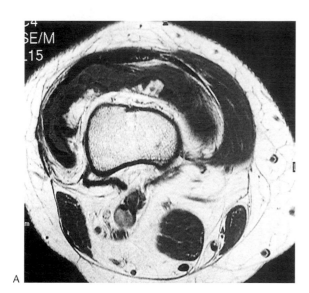
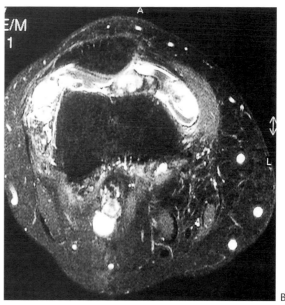

Fig. 6.47   Pigmented villonodular synovitis of the knee joint. **A.** Axial T_1-weighted and **B.** T_2-weighted fat-suppressed MR images through the patella and suprapatellar recess showing a heterogeneous mass within the joint made up of fat, hemosiderin, fibrous tissue and cellular elements.

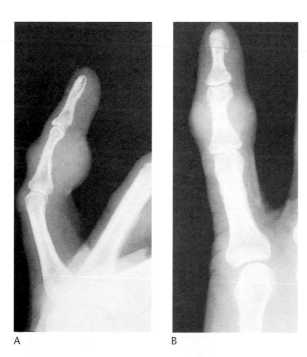

Fig. 6.48   **A,B** Pigmented villonodular synovitis of the flexor tendon sheath of the middle finger. A sharply circumscribed soft-tissue mass has caused slight pressure erosion of the middle phalanx.

6. Subarticular Arthritic Cyst and Geode

Though not neoplasms, these space-occupying lesions may occasionally cause confusion. Described in detail elsewhere (Ch. 4),

they most usually accompany rheumatoid disease, particularly with secondary degenerative change and osteoarthritis. The knee and hip are classic sites; the latter may present with a pathological fracture. The historical and radiological features of a pre-existing arthropathy should assist the diagnosis, together with the discrete sclerotic margins and close relationship with a joint (Fig. 6.54).

TUMORS OF NO KNOWN ORIGIN

1. Solitary Bone Cyst (Unicameral bone cyst)

This entirely benign lesion is unlikely to be a true neoplasm, but is considered here since its diagnosis depends largely on radiological findings which can resemble those of known neoplastic conditions, and because of its predilection to recur after treatment.

Solitary bone cysts are always unilocular. The site of origin depends on the patient's age: prior to epiphyseal fusion the majority occur in the proximal humeri and femora (Figs 6.55, 6.56) the former being the most usual site. Following skeletal maturation some lesions occur in such bones as the calcaneus (Fig. 6.57). Solitary bone cysts are commoner in males and develop during skeletal growth. Childhood and early adolescence is therefore the usual time for them to be discovered. More than half present due to a pathological fracture, a few may produce minor discomfort, others are found incidentally.

During the stage of skeletal development the lesion lies close to the metaphysis and is often situated in the midline, extending across the whole shaft. With further skeletal growth normal bone develops between the cyst and metaphysis so that the lesion is seen to be carried toward the diaphysis. Hence those which develop early eventually lie in the middle of the shaft of a bone. The cyst contains clear liquid unless there has been contamination by bleeding following a fracture. It is lined by a thin layer of connective tissue.

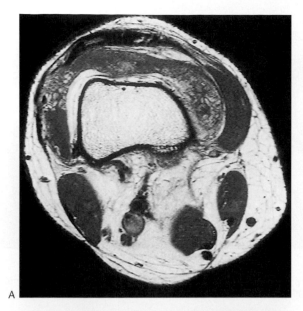

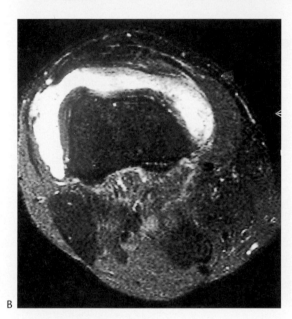

Fig. 6.49 Lipoma arborescens of the knee joint. **A.** Axial T$_1$-weighted and **B.** T$_2$-weighted fat-suppressed MR images through the suprapatellar recess showing numerous fatty fronds of synovium and a large joint effusion. Note how the high signal intensity villous projections on the T$_1$-weighted image are suppressed on the T$_2$-weighted fat-suppressed sequence.

Radiologically, an area of translucency in the metadiaphysis is characteristic. The overlying cortex is often thinned and slightly expanded with no periosteal reaction unless a fracture has occurred. The lesion may develop in relation to an apophysis, particularly the greater trochanter of the femur. In the earlier stages of growth, metaphyseal cysts tend to have a continuous rounded, sharply defined margin on the metaphyseal side but perhaps slightly less demarcation on the diaphyseal side. Sclerotic reaction is usually present around the margin but may be quite discrete. A serpiginous margin may cause the cyst to appear multilocular. As normal bone

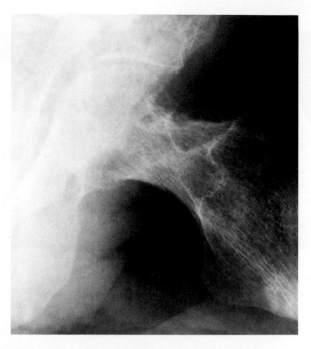

Fig. 6.50 Dialysis related amyloidosis of the hip resulting in pressure-like erosions of the femoral neck. Note the coarsened quality of the trabecular bone due to secondary hyperparathyroidism.

grows in the metaphysis, subsequent examination demonstrates the apparent migration of the lesion along the shaft of the affected bone, with an increasing sclerotic reaction around its margins. On bone scanning no abnormality develops in the blood-pool phase, in contrast to aneurysmal bone cysts. The delayed image demonstrates increased activity only around the margins of the lesion, unlike fibrous dysplasia (Fig. 6.58). The only serious differential diagnostic possibility is a chondroma, but no calcification occurs in a simple bone cyst unless callus has formed from a fracture.

The prognosis depends partly on the patient's age. Before the age of 10 recurrences are frequent, whereas after that age primary healing usually occurs even after fractures. Because of the risk of pathological fracture the majority of patients are treated by curettage and packing with bone chips. Some lesions have been reported to regress satisfactorily after injection with steroids.

2. Ewing Sarcoma: Malignant Round-cell Tumors

A group of highly malignant tumors involving bone is characterized histologically by numerous small round cells. Within this group are included Ewing sarcoma, metastatic neuroblastoma, non-Hodgkin's lymphoma and undifferentiated tumors. Pathological distinction may be extremely difficult, even with the benefit of electron microscopy and histochemical techniques. Whilst it is clear that these entities show considerable overlap, Ewing sarcoma is sufficiently distinctive to require definitive description.

Clinically, pain of several weeks' or months' duration is accompanied by localized tender swelling. The majority of patients are between 5 and 30 years of age. This rapidly progressive

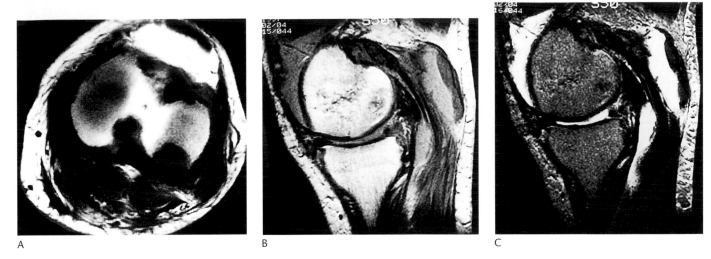

Fig. 6.51   Dialysis related amyloidosis of the knee. **A.** Axial T_1-weighted, sagittal proton density **B.** and T_2-weighted **C.** MR images showing numerous erosions of the margin of the tibia and characteristic low signal intensity masses within the synovium, most evident posteriorly within the popliteal cyst. A large joint effusion is also present.

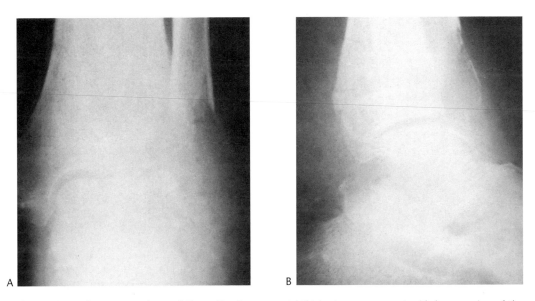

Fig. 6.52   Malignant synovioma of the ankle. Gross synovial thickening was present with hazy erosion of the capsular attachment. **A.** AP view. **B.** Lateral view.

malignant tumor is characterized by pyrexia, anemia and a raised ESR. These clinical symptoms and signs may closely simulate osteomyelitis but occur also in non-Hodgkin's lymphoma. It should be emphasized that the child with a Ewing's tumor is ill, in contrast to those with such benign lesions as eosinophilic granuloma which may cause similar radiological appearances.

Histologically the malignant round cells typically contain glycogen granules. The lesion is most often found in a long bone, the diaphysis being more commonly affected than a metaphysis. In about 40% of cases, however, the axial skeleton is involved, particularly the pelvis and ribs. Metastatic spread occurs early to lungs and to other bones where the radiological and histologic findings are virtually identical. The time delay between the discovery of the primary lesion and the development of secondary deposits suggest that this tumor does indeed originate in bone, unlike some other malignant round-cell tumors.

Radiologically the appearances are inconclusive. The lesion is essentially destructive, ill defined and principally involves the medullary cavity. Cortical erosions and overlying periosteal reactions occur early; indeed a periosteal reaction may be the only sign of abnormality (Figs 6.59, 6.60). Although the onion-peel lamellar type of periosteal reaction is classically associated with this lesion, it is observed only infrequently. Onion-peel periosteal reaction occurs in many other lesions, including osteosarcoma and infection. Elevation of periosteal new bone at the margins of cortical erosions (Codman's triangles) may emphasize the shallow cortical erosions;

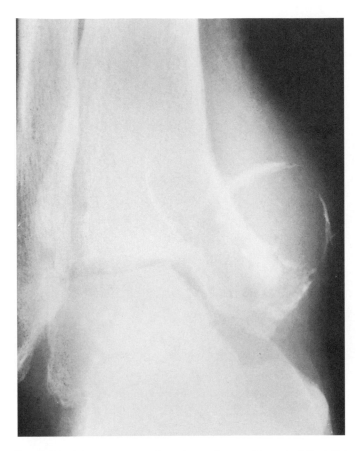

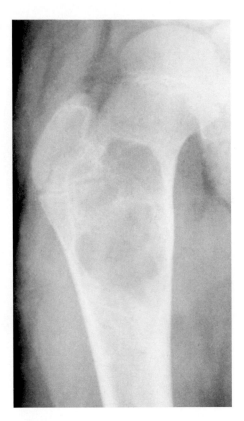

Fig. 6.53 Intraosseous ganglion. An oval, eccentric, osteolytic lesion arises from the medial malleolus with a thin sclerotic margin.

Fig. 6.55 Solitary bone cyst of the proximal femur showing expansion and thinning of the cortex, clearly defined endosteal margins but no calcification or periosteal new bone formation.

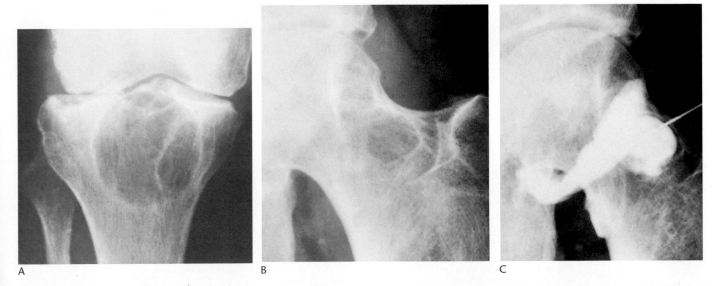

A   B   C

Fig. 6.54 Subarticular geodes. **A.** An elderly lady with rheumatoid arthritis and secondary degenerative arthritis has a typical, large geode immediately beneath the articular surface of the tibia. **B.** A younger man with rheumatoid disease has an oval, well-defined defect in the upper femoral neck. This too has a sclerotic margin. **C.** Aspiration of the defect yielded synovial fluid, and injection of contrast medium confirmed communication between the subarticular geode and the joint cavity.

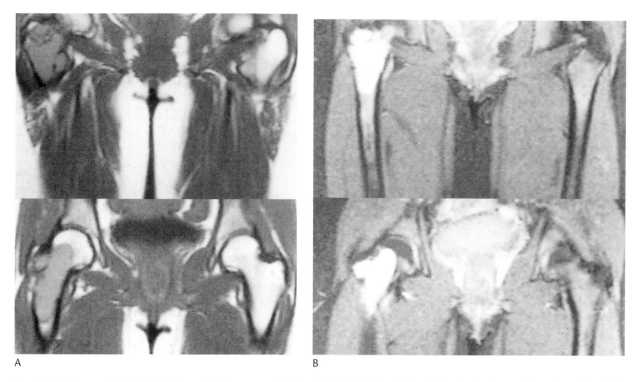

A   B

Fig. 6.56   A coronal T$_1$-weighted **A.** and STIR sequence **B.** with a typical liquid-containing lesion in the intertrochanteric region of the right femur. The relatively classic characteristics of a liquid-containing well-defined structure permit a confident diagnosis of a simple cyst.

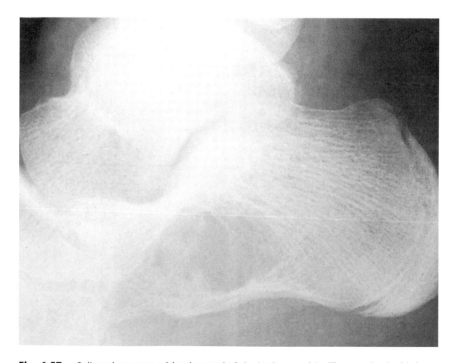

Fig. 6.57.   Solitary bone cyst arising in a typical site in the os calcis. The margins in this bone tend to be less well defined.

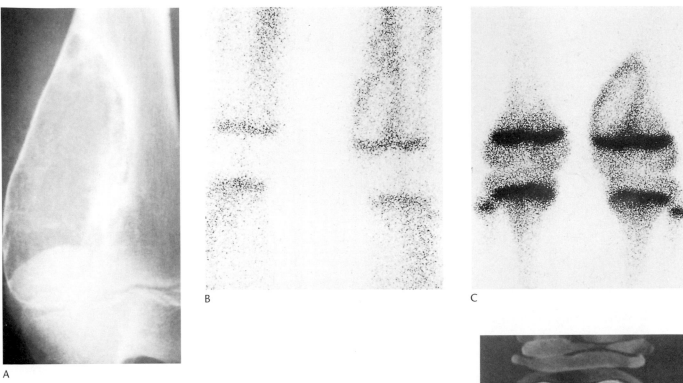

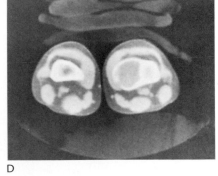

Fig. 6.58 Solitary bone cyst of the distal femur. The lesion is rather atypical **A.** and plain film diagnosis is not easy. However, it illustrates how further investigations can help in differential diagnosis. A bone scan, **B.** in the blood-pool phase and **C.** in the delayed phase, shows increased activity around the margin of the lesion corresponding to sclerosis on plain film. **D.** A CT scan demonstrates a soft-tissue density expansile lesion with no calcification. The differential diagnosis includes aneurysmal bone cyst, fibrous dysplasia (monostotic) and a chondroma. Aneurysmal bone cyst is vascular in the blood-pool phase of a bone scan, fibrous dysplasia markedly so on the delayed scan. Calcification may be expected on CT in a chondroma.

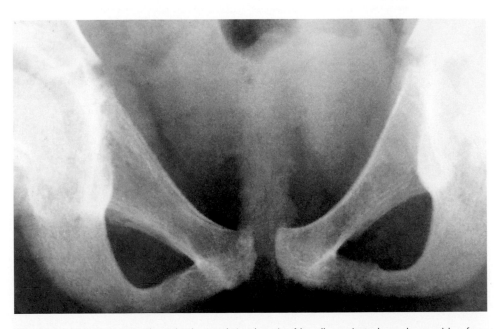

Fig. 6.59 Ewing sarcoma. The only abnormal sign here is of lamellar periosteal new bone arising from the superior pubic ramus on the right.

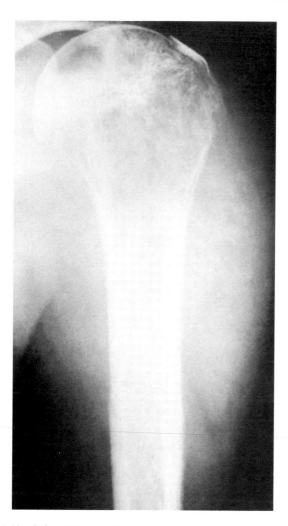

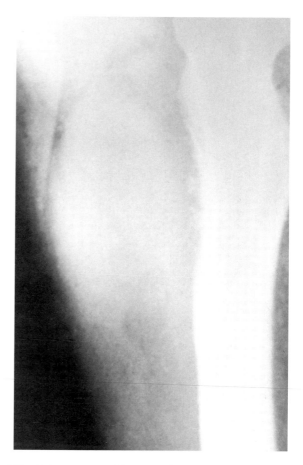

Fig. 6.60 Ewing sarcoma. This tumor is much more advanced, with a well-defined soft-tissue mass, Codman's triangles, ossification and calcification in the soft tissues and ill-defined bony destruction. The radiological distinction from osteosarcoma is difficult.

Fig. 6.61 Ewing sarcoma arising primarily in the soft tissues of the thigh. A well-marked erosion ('saucerization') defect has been caused with periosteal new bone formation.

known as 'saucerization' defects, they offer a highly suspicious diagnostic feature (Fig. 6.61). The tumor is highly vascular and grows rapidly.

Angiographically, the extensive soft-tissue component and abnormal circulation is obvious (Fig. 6.62). The blood-pool phase of a bone scan also demonstrates increased vascularity, but, in the delayed phase, an increase in activity is evident only at the margins of the tumor within bone and in periosteal new bone.

CT or MRI will optimally delineate the osseous and soft-tissue extent of the tumor, which is often much greater than may be appreciated on conventional radiographs (Figs 6.63, 6.64). A whole-body radionuclide bone scan is also of value in detecting recurrences and metastasis. The differential diagnosis may be difficult. Osteosarcoma may present almost identical radiological features, and non-malignant conditions such as histiocytosis and aggressive osteomyelitis (particularly from *Staphylococcus*) require consideration.

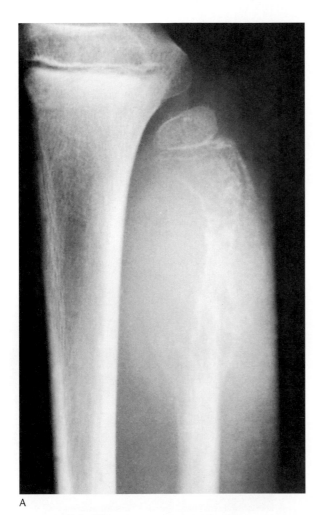

A

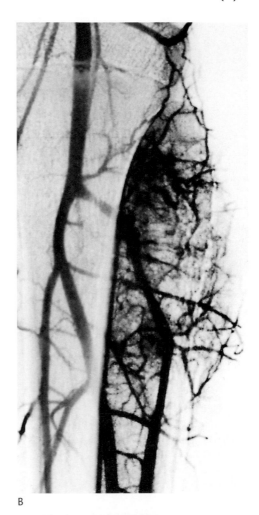

B

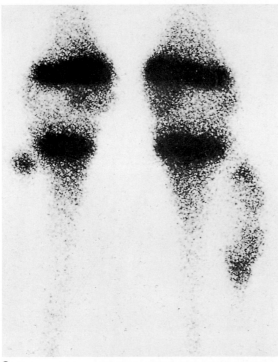

C

Fig. 6.62 Ewing sarcoma of bone arising in the proximal fibula of an 8-year-old. **A.** An advanced tumor is shown on plain films, with Codman's triangles, a soft-tissue mass and ill-defined bone destruction. **B.** The subtraction print of femoral arteriogram demonstrates a very abnormal circulation with a large soft-tissue mass. **C.** A bone scan, in the delayed phase, demonstrates increased activity where new bone formation is present on plain films. The lesion itself is photon-deficient. Osteosarcoma may present similar appearances.

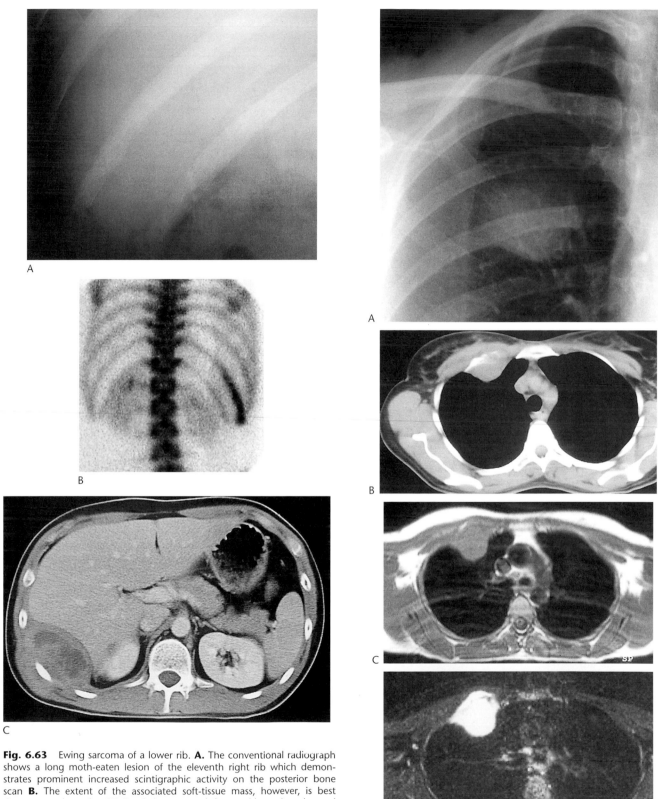

Fig. 6.63 Ewing sarcoma of a lower rib. **A.** The conventional radiograph shows a long moth-eaten lesion of the eleventh right rib which demonstrates prominent increased scintigraphic activity on the posterior bone scan **B.** The extent of the associated soft-tissue mass, however, is best demonstrated on the CT **C.** of the upper abdomen (dynamic enhanced scan).

REFERENCES AND SUGGESTIONS FOR FURTHER READING

See end of Chapter 7

Fig. 6.64 Ewing sarcoma of the anterior aspect of the right second rib. **A.** On the conventional radiograph the appearances simulate an intrapulmonary lesion. **B.** CT section showing destruction of the second rib and associated soft-tissue mass. **C.** On the axial T_1-weighted image the soft-tissue component of the lesion has an intermediate signal intensity and with the STIR sequence **D.** an extremely high signal intensity.

7

DISORDERS OF THE LYMPHORETICULAR SYSTEM AND OTHER HEMOPOIETIC DISORDERS

Iain Watt and Mark Cobby

This important group of disorders is responsible for some of the most bizarre radiological abnormalities encountered in the skeleton and may be subdivided conveniently into diseases affecting:

1. Red blood cells
2. White blood cells
3. Lymphoreticular system
4. Coagulation mechanism.

DISEASES PRIMARILY INVOLVING RED BLOOD CELLS

In the infant, red marrow extends throughout the medullary cavities of the whole skeleton. During the first few months of life red blood cells are also produced by the spleen and liver, this function being described as extramedullary erythropoiesis. As the physiological requirement for erythrocyte production diminishes progressively during the years of growth, a cessation of this function occurs in the liver and spleen and later by regression of the red marrow areas in the peripheral skeleton. By the age of 20 years red marrow is normally confined to the proximal ends of the femora and humeri and to the axial skeleton. Residual areas of fatty non-hematopoietic marrow in the appendicular skeleton, as well as the liver and spleen, may be reactivated should the need arise. Such a response occurs normally after a severe hemorrhage. These episodes are insufficiently prolonged to cause conventional radiographic changes although this reconversion from fatty to red marrow is readily identified on MR imaging.

Chronic hemolytic anemias, however, in which red blood cells suffer extensive destruction, are followed in many instances by such a degree of marrow hyperplasia that striking skeletal abnormalities result. The great majority of these diseases are congenital and hereditary in origin. The red blood cells are abnormal in shape, in fragility and in the type of hemoglobin which they contain. The clinical picture is that of any chronic anemia. Dyspnea, pallor, fatigue and weakness are often accompanied by jaundice due to erythrocyte destruction. If extramedullary hematopoiesis occurs, the liver and spleen may be enlarged, particularly the latter, especially when the anemia is profound. Cardiac enlargement and failure may occur, many of the more severely affected patients dying before puberty.

Radiological changes in the skeleton, resulting from marrow hyperplasia, vary greatly with disease severity. In children, the changes are widespread and are usually demonstrated most easily in the extremities and the skull. To some degree, marrow hyperplasia causes destruction of many of the medullary trabeculae. This is followed by thinning and expansion and even perforation of the overlying cortex. In many patients this hyperplasia achieves its compensatory object, so that a state of erythrocytic balance is reached. The areas of bone destruction show features of repair, by formation of fibrous tissue and the development of reactive bone sclerosis. The latter thickens the remaining trabeculae and, in some, the endosteal aspect of the cortex, to produce an overall increase in bone density. As age advances, the peripheral bones, now in a state of balance, tend to revert to a normal appearance, but some residual increase of density may remain. Evidence of continued erythropoiesis to a greater degree than normal is then confined to the physiological red marrow areas.

Extramedullary hematopoiesis, in addition to producing evidence of hepatosplenomegaly, may be revealed by the presence of

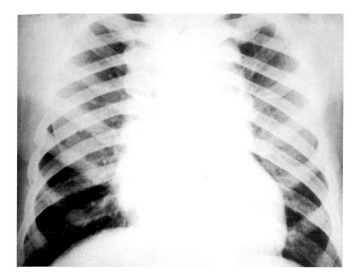

Fig. 7.1 Thalassemia. Lobulated soft-tissue masses due to extramedullary hematopoiesis are present adjacent to the thoracic spine.

sharply defined paravertebral soft-tissue masses of hematopoietic tissue, especially around the thoracic spine (Fig. 7.1).

THALASSEMIA (*Cooley's anemia*)

Described by Cooley in 1927, this condition, known also as Mediterranean anemia, is by no means confined to Mediterranean countries or races. Geographical distribution extends eastward in a broad band through Asia and West Africa. In such areas it is commonplace. It may be encountered anywhere in the world in individuals having a heredity originating from these areas.

The disease is due to abnormalities of the hemoglobin molecule, of which many have been established. Homozygous subjects, who have inherited the trait from both parents, develop the more severe form of the disease, known clinically as thalassemia major, whereas heterozygous subjects develop a minor form. Both may vary greatly in severity, so that distinction between them and other hematological variants is of relatively little radiological importance. Severe forms usually become manifest in the first two years of life. Although the majority of these patients die before puberty, some survive to early adult life. Those with less severe disease live correspondingly longer and minimal manifestations may be found only by examination of the blood of individuals who otherwise appear entirely normal. The important clinical features, in addition to those of other anemias, are dwarfing, delay in development of secondary sexual characteristics, and either 'mongoloid' or 'rodent' facies due to expansion of the underlying facial bones as a consequence of erythroblastic hypertrophy.

Radiological Changes Hyperplasia of the marrow destroys many of the medullary trabeculae and expands and thins the overlying cortex. In children this is evident especially in the hands, when the shafts of the phalanges and metacarpals become biconvex instead of being biconcave (Fig. 7.2). The feet are affected in the same way. Similar abnormalities in the ribs (Fig. 7.3) and long bones (Fig. 7.4) may produce apparent failure of modeling with, for example, flask-shaped femora (Fig. 7.5). In the skull the

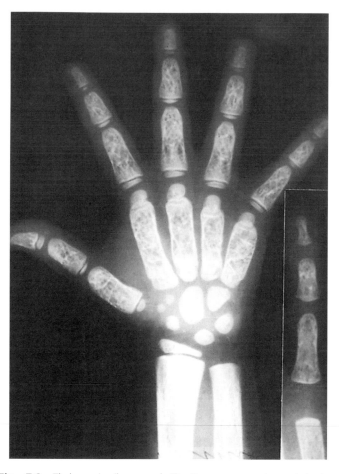

Fig. 7.2 Thalassemia (boy aged 7). Gross marrow hyperplasia has expanded and thinned overlying cortical bone. Medullary trabeculae have been destroyed and the residual ones are coarsened. Inset—early changes of the same type in a finger of a child aged 4.

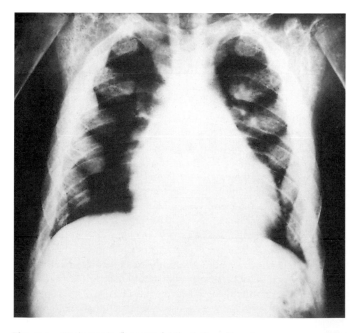

Fig. 7.3 Thalassemia (boy aged 15). A chest film shows gross expansion of bone structures due to marrow hyperplasia. Note particularly involvement of the ribs and scapulae.

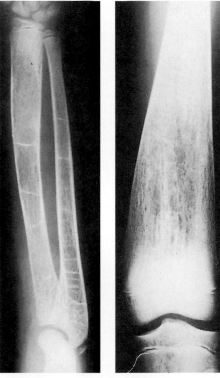

Fig. 7.4   Fig. 7.5

Fig. 7.4 Thalassemia. Considerable bone expansion, cortical thinning and simplification of trabecular pattern is demonstrated in the forearm of a boy of 15.

Fig. 7.5 Thalassemia. Considerable marrow expansion has produced a flask shape of the distal femur. The coarsened trabecular pattern and cortical thinning are obvious.

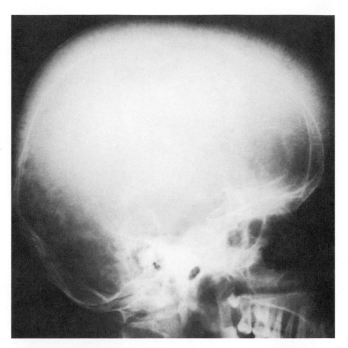

Fig. 7.6 Thalassemia. Thickening of the outer table of the skull in the frontal area with perpendicular striation—'hairbrush sign'.

diploic space is widened and gross thinning of the outer table may be followed by marked diploic thickening, starting in the frontal region, but usually exempting the occipital bone in which the marrow content is minimal (Fig. 7.6). The 'classic' appearance of the 'hairbrush' spicules is relatively uncommon. These changes appear considerably later than those in the short bones of the extremities. Development of the air spaces of the skull, especially the maxillary antra and the mastoids, is impaired as a result of hyperplasia of the marrow, accounting for the clinical manifestation of 'rodent' facies, with malocclusion. The spine shows only diffuse demineralization with the same generalized coarsened trabecular pattern as that observed in the appendicular skeleton. Vertebral collapse is uncommon.

Osseous abnormalities of this type may be observed also in a number of lesser forms of thalassemia and its variants, including those associated with other abnormal hemoglobins and the sickle-cell trait. In all these conditions, however, the changes tend to be very much less prominent than in thalassemia major.

Sickle-cell Disease

This chronic hemolytic anemia is also congenital and hereditary in origin. The erythrocytes, when hypoxic, become abnormal in shape, being unusually long and slender. The abnormal hemoglobin

which they contain has a reduced oxygen-carrying capacity. The disease occurs almost exclusively in black races, especially those in Central Africa or their descendants, who are homozygous for the sickling trait. This trait may be crossed with normal or abnormal hemoglobins, including thalassemia. In these crossed types, the patient is less severely affected, both clinically and radiologically. Differentiation of the true homozygous state from the variants (of which combination with hemoglobin C is the most common) is of some importance. The former group rarely survive after the age of 30, whereas the latter may have a normal lifespan. The former are characterized clinically by early onset of the severe anemic picture, with frequent skeletal and abdominal crises. These acutely painful episodes, lasting for several days, are due essentially to infarction, attributed to vascular blockage by collections of erythrocytes which have undergone sickling in areas of capillary stasis with resultant hypoxia.

Infarcts may affect many systems. The fundamental skeletal abnormalities consist of hyperplasia of marrow with superimposition of areas of bone necrosis due to infarction and subsequent growth disparities. A further clinical complication is the development of infection within these infarcts, particularly in lesions developing in the long bones of children.

Radiological Changes   The chronic hemolytic state is reflected by the development of characteristic and diagnostic radiological abnormalities, affecting primarily the erythropoietic skeleton, and also the soft tissues involved by extramedullary hematopoiesis. The frequency with which abnormalities are discovered increases with age. All variants of sickle-cell disease produce essentially similar radiological abnormalities.

1. **Marrow hyperplasia** is fundamental. In this disease, however, the effects on the skeleton, which are so prominent in thalassemia major, occur in modified form, even in its worst clinical manifes-

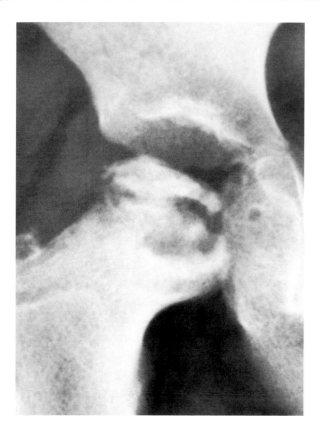

Fig. 7.7 Sickle-cell disease. Infarction in the proximal femoral metaphysis has produced a large defect with avascular necrosis of the femoral head. These features are similar to those of Perthes disease.

thalassemia, in which infarction is virtually unknown, this type of involvement of the skeleton is common. The consequent radiological abnormalities are comparable to those observed in other systemic disorders such as dysbaric osteonecrosis (caisson disease) and Gaucher's disease. Such infarcts are usually multiple and most commonly affect the femoral and humeral heads (Fig. 7.7), and, in particular, medullary bone. Medullary infarcts may be of two varieties, either with sharply defined margins or producing diffuse sclerosis. In their mildest form they may be recognized in an asymptomatic patient. The classic 'snowcap' sign refers to the subarticular area of increased density, particularly in a humeral head, which reflects the revascularization of an area of bone which has been necrotic (Fig. 7.8). At this phase of development bone scans are usually abnormal with increased activity. However, in acute infarction a photon deficiency is often present within 24 hours of the insult (Fig. 7.9). Repairing bone is brittle, however, and fractures easily—varying from 'osteochondritis dissecans' to complete collapse.

Femoral heads affected in childhood present an appearance exactly comparable to Perthes disease (Fig. 7.7). In young black children the areas of predilection for infarctions are the small tubular bones of the hands and feet (Figs 7.10, 7.11), causing destructive changes accompanied by massive and painful soft-

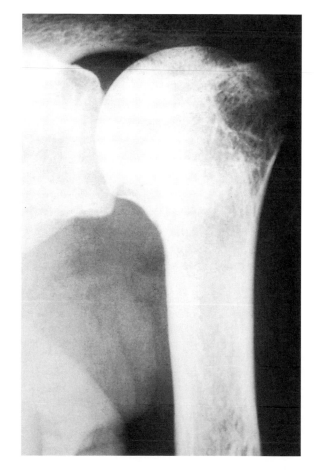

Fig. 7.8 Sickle-cell disease. Endosteal bone deposition has resulted in diffuse sclerosis beneath the articular surface (the 'snow-cap' sign) due to medullary infarction. Note the lack of distinction between cortical and medullary bone in the upper humeral shaft, again due to endosteal deposition of bone.

tations being less severe. A generalized osteoporotic appearance is evident throughout the hematopoietic areas of the skeleton, but even in infants and children it is recognized more easily in the axial than the peripheral skeleton. This feature is not diagnostic, but in a black child should arouse suspicion. Unlike severe thalassemia, significant modeling abnormalities are uncommon so that the air spaces of the paranasal sinuses are rarely affected. The diploic space of the skull may be widened, with consequent bossing. If a state of erythrocytic balance is achieved, diffuse trabecular thickening is likely to develop.

Such an appearance may be shown incidentally in an asymptomatic adult sickle-cell trait carrier. In more advanced cases, a coarse medullary pattern is associated with enlarged vascular channels in bone, especially in proximal or middle phalanges.

2. Endosteal Apposition of Bone Inward cortical thickening is separated occasionally by a thin zone of translucency, to result in the appearance in the long bones of 'a bone within a bone'. This sign may be observed in other conditions, including Gaucher's disease (see below). The medullary cavities, in severe cases, may ultimately be grossly narrowed and almost obliterated, so that a diffuse and generalized increase in bone density results. This does not occur in the axial skeleton, which is a persistent red marrow area, and this provides an important diagnostic feature, even in the absence of other signs.

3. Infarction of bone provides the diagnostic hallmark of this disease. Infarction of various tissues is considered to be the cause of the classic clinical episodes of sickle-cell crises. Unlike

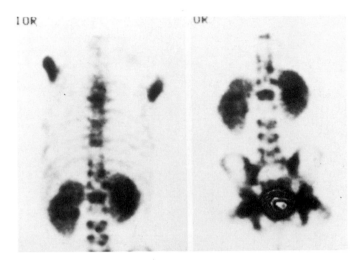

Fig. 7.9 Sickle-cell disease. A bone scan performed 16 hours after the onset of severe pain in a boy with known sickle-cell disease. Acute infarction of L2 has resulted in a relative photon deficiency in this area. Previous infarctions, in varying phases of evolution, are shown as areas of increased activity (see particularly L1 and mid-thoracic vertebrae).

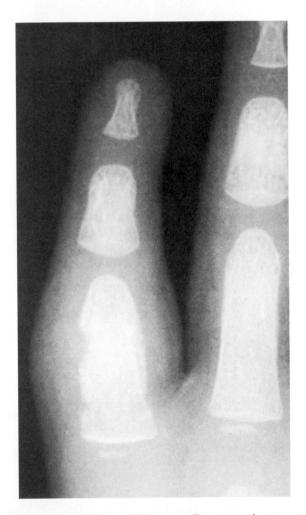

Fig. 7.10 Sickle-cell disease. Soft-tissue swelling surrounds an expanded proximal phalanx. Medullary expansion is present with simplification of trabecular pattern and penetration of the cortex. The distinction between these changes and osteomyelitis is extremely difficult.

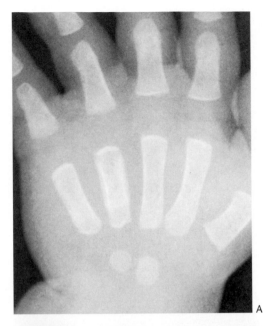

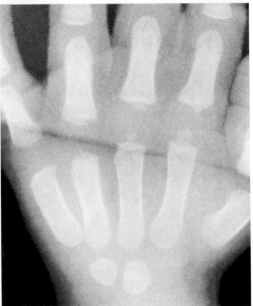

Fig. 7.11 Sickle-cell disease, infarction in childhood. **A.** At presentation, periosteal new bone formation surrounds the diaphysis of the fourth finger metacarpal. **B.** Ten months later resolution has occurred and growth has proceeded normally. The distinction between infarction and infection may be very difficult. In this case no specific treatment was given.

tissue swellings and periosteal reactions which may be florid and reflect associated infarction of cortical bone (sickle-cell dactylitis or 'hand–foot' syndrome). These findings may indicate the correct diagnosis, but other causes of infantile periosteal reactions such as cortical hyperostosis of both the infantile or traumatic types, tuberculous dactylitis, or possibly hypervitaminosis A, may require consideration. The formation of perpendicular bony spicules on the skull, uncommon even in thalassemia, is distinctly unusual. More important is the possibility of superadded infection, discussed below.

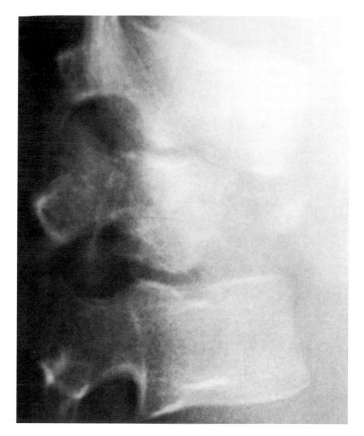

Fig. 7.12 Sickle-cell disease. Flat depressions within the vertebral bodies with sloping sides typify metaphyseal infarct ('the vertebral step sign' or H-shaped vertebra). Frank destruction of the vertebral body with narrowing of the contiguous disk spaces is due to associated salmonella osteomyelitis.

Infarcts of vertebral bodies are another characteristic radiological stigma. Generalized depressions of the central portions of the vertebral end-plates are common, and may be demonstrated in an asymptomatic patient. The depressions are often concave and rounded, initially, simulating an ordinary nucleus pulposus impression on a bone which is already porotic. Infarction may be diagnosed when the centre of the depression is flat and the sides slope obliquely, producing characteristic H-shaped vertebrae (Fig. 7.12).

The diaphyses of the long bones, especially in the older child and the adolescent, are sites of predilection for infarction. Typically they involve the zones between the mid diaphysis and the metaphyses, the so-called 'intermediate fifths'. When the metaphysis is involved significant deformity may occur due to growth arrest. *Central metaphyseal defects* and lucencies are typical. These in turn may produce fragmentation and deformity of the epiphyses. They may also be the site of pathological fractures. Infarcts may be massive, causing bone destruction, sequestration, reactive sclerosis and even the formation of involucrum. The pattern may suggest acute pyogenic osteomyelitis.

4. Superadded Infection The areas of bone necrosis caused by infarction are especially susceptible to infection, classically by salmonella organisms of the paratyphoid B group. Differentiation between the pure infarct and those which have been infected in this way may be extremely difficult (Fig. 7.13) both radiologically

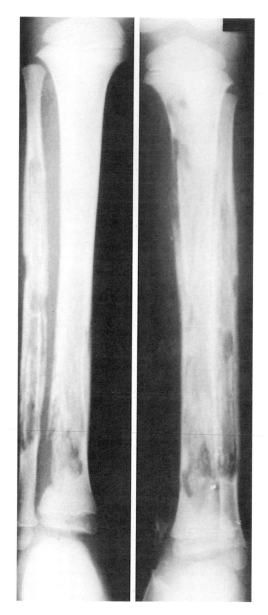

Fig. 7.13 Sickle-cell disease with salmonella osteomyelitis. (Nigerian boy aged 4). Extreme destructive changes in the long bones have been caused by infection superimposed upon infarction. Numerous sequestra are present. (Courtesy of Mr Geoffrey Walker.)

and pathologically, since cultures are often sterile. Such lesions are liable to occur especially in the tubular bones of the hands and feet in infants and in the long bones and the spine of older children (Fig. 7.12). In the adult, septic arthritis may be superimposed on an adjacent infarct. With appropriate treatment, either by conservative antibiotic therapy or by active surgical measures, including sequestrectomy, healing usually takes place with remarkable rapidity.

5. Soft-tissue involvement, as in the other chronic hemolytic anemias, and such disorders of the marrow as Gaucher's disease, is shown by hepatosplenomegaly caused by extramedullary hematopoiesis. Heterotopic masses of hematopoietic tissue may develop in the dorsal paravertebral areas. Release of iron pigments by accelerated destruction of erythrocytes may precipitate the formation of biliary calculi.

Erythroblastosis Fetalis (*Hemolytic disease of the newborn*)

Hemolytic anemia occurring in the fetus and newborn results from immunological incompatibility between the blood of the mother and the fetus, most commonly due to Rh factor, although other hematological errors of this type are known. The severity of the affection of the infant may vary widely, from a mild anemia to icterus neonatorum and fetal hydrops.

The Rh-positive erythrocytes of the fetus, crossing the placental barrier in a mother without Rh antigen, stimulate maternal formation of anti-Rh antibodies which traverse the placenta to enter the fetal circulation, there to hemolyze the fetal red blood cells. The danger of infants being affected by this incompatibility increases with the number of conceptions, but early recognition of the disorder and the adoption of prophylactic measures has greatly reduced its incidence.

Radiological Changes The only skeletal abnormality is the development of transverse metaphyseal translucencies in the long bones. These translucencies are non-specific, since they may occur also with other severe maternal illnesses during pregnancy and also in congenital syphilis. With successful treatment the translucent areas ossify with residual growth lines. In the spine, such growth lines often cause 'ghost shadows' within the vertebral bodies. Fetal hydrops may be diagnosed sonographically (Ch. 44) by the detection of growth retardation, effusions and subcutaneous edema. The fetus is displaced by enlargement of the placenta.

Other Chronic Anemias

The anemia of infants suffering from **iron deficiency** may produce radiological changes in the skull due to marrow hyperplasia similar to those of the less severe congenital anemias. An inadequate diet is the usual cause, but malabsorption or abnormal loss of iron may be important factors. The widening of the diploic space and the subsequent bossing of the skull vault are again characteristic, but the disease has never been reported to cause changes sufficiently severe to involve the long bones and facial bones.

Hereditary spherocytosis is an inherited defect in which the red blood cells are of an abnormal round shape. The anemia which results may produce mild changes comparable to the other congenital anemias. Removal of the spleen permits the bone structures to revert to a normal appearance.

Fanconi syndrome, of congenital aplastic anemia with multiple congenital anomalies (not to be confused with the other syndrome described by the same author and concerned with osteomalacia and an abnormal renal tubular mechanism), is of interest in that the hematological changes are unlikely to appear before the age of 2 years. These consist of hypoplastic anemia, marrow hypoplasia and skin pigmentation. The defect is inherited and congenital abnormalities of the skeleton are associated, such as deficient formation of the bones of the thumb, first metacarpal and radius; other abnormalities, including congenital dislocation of the hip and club foot also have been observed. These are evident long before the hematological abnormalities become apparent, and the latter are not responsible for any skeletal abnormalities. Some cases have terminated in leukemia.

Polycythemia

This condition is due to overproduction of red cells. Although occasionally responsible for bone infarction, it produces no characteristic radiological changes in the skeleton. Transition to myeloid metaplasia is common. Pulmonary abnormalities in polycythemia may occur in the form of increased reticulation or fine mottling.

DISEASES PRIMARILY INVOLVING WHITE BLOOD CELLS

Leukemia

Children are most commonly affected, almost invariably by an acute form. In adults the disease may also be acute, but it is more commonly chronic. Hematopoietic tissue is widely distributed throughout the skeleton of a child but is confined in the adult to the 'red marrow' areas of the axial skeleton and the proximal ends of the humeri and femora. Thus radiological changes in the bones are commonly in the younger age groups. More than half the children affected show skeletal abnormalities, while in adults these are found in fewer than 10% of cases. While the diagnosis is usually confirmed by examination of the blood and sternal marrow, bone changes may precede the development of a grossly pathological blood picture, especially in the so-called *aleukemic* type.

Differentiation between myeloid and lymphatic types of leukemia cannot be made by radiological examination.

Radiological changes are observed mainly in **children** and consist of the following:

1. *Metaphyseal translucencies.* In children the most characteristic sign, occurring in 90% of cases, is the presence of bands of translucency running transversely across the metaphyses (Figs 7.14, 7.15). Such bands may be narrow and incomplete in the early stages of the disease, but in the course of a few weeks they may be found to traverse the metaphysis completely and be as much as 5 mm in width. The most rapidly growing areas—knees, wrists and ankles—are commonly affected first, but later the metaphyses of the shoulders, hips and vertebral bodies also may be involved. With treatment, remission may occur, and the bands of translucency resolve.

2. *Metaphyseal cortical erosions* on the medial side of the proximal ends of the humeral (Fig. 7.16A) and tibial shafts sometimes occur as an early feature. They are usually bilateral.

3. *Osteolytic lesions* develop in over half the cases. Usually they are punctuate and diffusely scattered, though solitary and larger lesions may occur. While any portion of the skeleton may be involved by such leukemic deposits, they are commonest in the shafts of the long bones (Fig. 7.17). When the vertebral bodies are involved, collapse often takes place before specific areas of rarefaction can be identified (Fig. 7.16B).

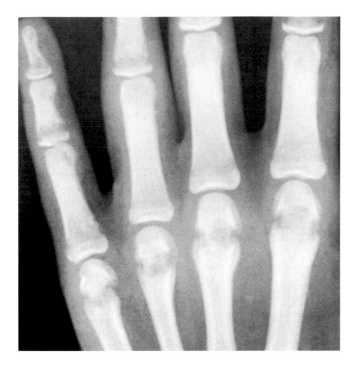

Fig. 7.14 Acute leukemia. Extensive metaphyseal radiolucencies are present with adjacent periosteal new bone formation.

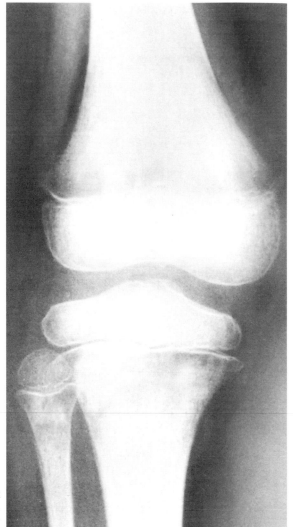

Fig. 7.15 Lymphatic leukemia. Metaphyseal radiolucencies are present around the knee. Endosteal sclerosis is present adjacent to these lesions, obscuring the corticomedullary junction. Minor periosteal new bone formation is present in the upper tibia and fibula.

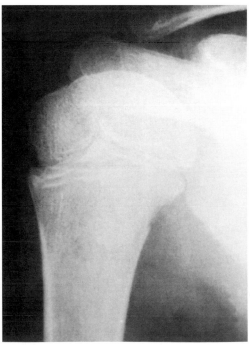

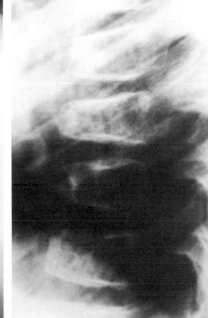

Fig. 7.16 Lymphatic leukemia. **A.** Erosions of the medial side of the proximal metaphyses of both humeri were present in this 8-year-old. The disease was in an aleukemic phase, not an uncommon finding even when skeletal changes are present. **B.** The same child complained of back pain. Multiple vertebral collapse is shown with the preservation of disk-space height. Overall bone density is reduced with a simplified trabecular pattern.

A

B

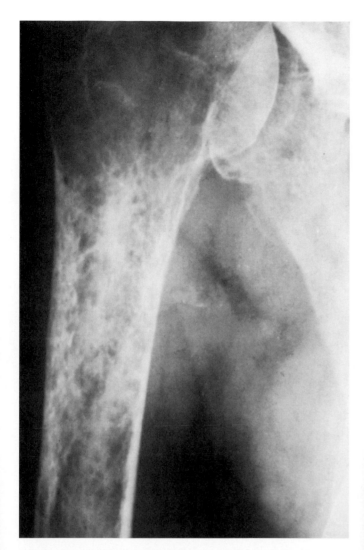

Fig. 7.17 Chronic lymphatic leukemia—adult type. Diffuse medullary infiltration is shown in the humerus and scapula with cortical erosion.

4. *Periosteal reactions* are usually associated with underlying bony lesions.

5. *Osteosclerosis of the metaphysis* is a rare but well-recognized primary manifestation. It may develop during treatment.

In *metastatic neuroblastoma* skeletal changes take place which may be indistinguishable from leukemia. Separation of the sutures of the skull in the former condition is a helpful differentiating sign.

In **adults** skeletal lesions are rare. As has been stressed before, the deposits occur essentially in red marrow areas. Changes include *porosis, translucent areas* of leukemic bone destruction (which tend to be oval with the long axis parallel to the shaft), and *vertebral destruction and collapse*. Periosteal reactions are unusual. Occasionally, generalized *osteosclerosis* of the marrow area is evident. This is likely to be caused by trabecular thickening during periods of remission and may be patchy in type. In some instances, however, the leukemic changes may be a secondary and terminal process in myeloid metaplasia.

Myeloid Metaplasia (*Myelofibrosis and myelosclerosis*)

This syndrome is characterized by the triad of myelofibrosis, myeloid metaplasia and features in the peripheral blood film which simulate leukemia. The relationship between myeloid metaplasia, myelosclerosis and other diseases, including polycythemia rubra vera and chronic myeloid leukemia, is intimate. The typical patient is a middle-aged or elderly adult, the primary disorder being metaplasia of the marrow cells to fibrous tissue. The usual presenting complaints are fatigue and abdominal fullness due to hepatosplenomegaly. Obliteration of the hematopoietic tissue results in progressive anemia, the appearance of immature red and white cells in the peripheral blood and compensatory splenomegaly. In the later stages of the disease, the fibrous tissue becomes converted to bone, and endosteal cortical thickening develops. Polycythemia may be followed by myeloid metaplasia and it appears probable that nearly half of the developed cases of myeloid metaplasia previously had some form of this blood disorder. Purine hypermetabolism may manifest itself as secondary gout.

Radiological Changes In the sclerotic stage of the disease increased density of the bones may be diffuse or patchy in nature. Areas of relative translucency due to fibrosis may persist (Fig. 7.18). The increased density is due to new bone deposition on the

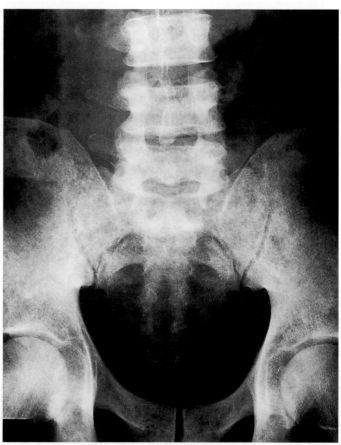

Fig. 7.18 Myeloid metaplasia. Widespread but patchy areas of sclerosis are shown throughout the pelvis and lumbar spine.

trabeculae and also to the endosteal cortical thickening with loss of the normal cortico-medullary distinction. Narrowing of the medullary space becomes clearly visible and resembles, in the long bones, the later stages of sickle-cell anemia. Irregular periosteal reactions, particularly near the ends of long bones, may occur. These may be well organized and continuous with the cortex or separated from it by a zone of translucency. While the red marrow areas (particularly the pelvis) are especially subject to these pathological changes, the whole skeleton may be affected. Density of the skull is associated with obliteration of the diploic space, though some persistent areas of fibrosis may remain translucent. Splenomegaly is almost invariably evident (Fig. 7.19).

Differentiation must be made from other conditions causing a generalized increase of bone density. The congenital sclerosing dysplasias, including osteopetrosis, are likely to be encountered in adult life only as an incidental finding or in association with a pathological fracture. Fluorosis is likely to occur in an endemic area. Mastocytosis may cause some confusion, but the lesions are usually less diffuse and are accompanied by urticaria pigmentosa. Sclerosing and widespread metastasis, particularly prostatic, should not be forgotten.

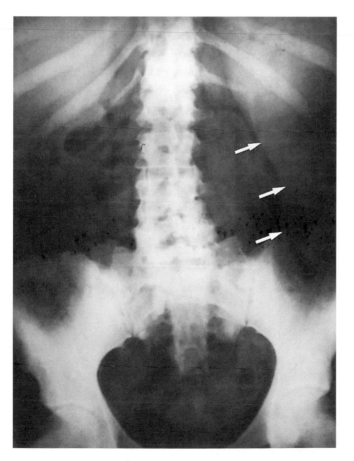

Fig. 7.19 Myeloid metaplasia (woman aged 63). All the bones are diffusely dense with lack of distinction between cortical and medullary bone. The spleen is grossly enlarged (arrows).

DISORDERS OF THE LYMPHORETICULAR SYSTEM

Four main groups of disorder will be considered, divided for convenience as follows:

A. Lymphomas: including Hodgkin's and non-Hodgkin's lymphomas
B. Plasma-cell disease: plasmacytoma and multiple myeloma
C. Histiocytosis
D. Storage disorders: Gaucher's disease and Niemann–Pick disease.

THE LYMPHOMAS

The classification of the proliferative disorders of the lymphoreticular system is changing constantly and is based essentially upon histologic features detected in lymph nodes. Consequently caution is necessary in extending such classifications to bone or bowel lymphoma. Malignant lymphoma is a generic term embracing all previously named tumors, including Hodgkin's disease, lymphadenoma, lymphosarcoma, reticulum-cell sarcoma and others.

Malignant lymphomas may be subdivided into two groups: Hodgkin's disease and a group of non-Hodgkin's lymphomas.

Hodgkin's Disease

This defined tumor has an agreed classification on histologic grounds, named after Rye. This comprises nodular sclerosing Hodgkin's disease, a complaint of young women involving intrathoracic lymph nodes, and three others: lymphocyte-predominant Hodgkin's disease, mixed cellularity Hodgkin's disease and lymphocyte-depleted Hodgkin's disease. The last three comprise a spectrum with, in order listed, worsening outlook. Bone involvement always implies a less favorable prognosis. It is a feature of widespread disease and has been found at postmortem in more than half of cases. Skeletal lesions at presentation are far less common. Primary Hodgkin's disease of bone probably does not occur. There is no correlation between the variety of Hodgkin's disease and the nature of the individual bony lesions it produces.

The age of onset varies widely from childhood to old age but the diagnosis is most commonly made in young adults. The red marrow areas are the most frequent sites of presentation, the majority of lesions being found in the spine, thoracic cage and pelvis. Bone pain may precede, by several months, the development of these lesions and the importance of serial radiological examination, either radiographic or scintigraphic, must be stressed.

Radiological changes in the skeleton. The majority of early bone lesions are destructive and often large at the time they are first observed, either from direct involvement from affected soft tissues, particularly lymph nodes, or from infiltration of bone marrow. About a third are essentially osteolytic in type (Fig. 7.20). The majority are however of mixed type with patchy sclerosis and destruction (Fig. 7.21). Diffuse trabecular thickening causes sclerotic lesions in the remainder (Fig. 7.22). Such an appearance may develop in a few months, being preceded by bone pain, and may well show no preliminary bone destruction. It may also

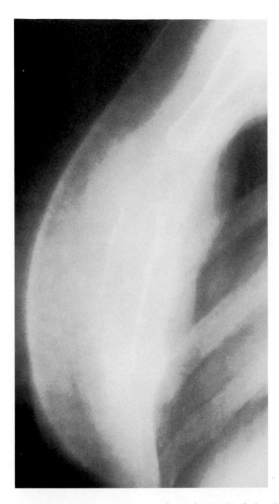

Fig. 7.20 Hodgkin's disease. An expanding, destructive lesion involves the body of the sternum, with anterior and posterior soft-tissue masses. Bizarre changes in this bone should always arouse suspicion of a lymphoma.

disk space does become narrowed, preservation of density of the vertebral end-plates usually permits differentiation from an infective diskitis where loss of this density is an early diagnostic sign. Lesions in the ribs may be found by themselves, sometimes being observed in a chest radiograph. They are usually osteolytic and expanding in type.

The sternum is also a not-infrequent site for a lesion to appear, again usually osteolytic, but sometimes mixed in type with perpendicular spicules of new bone. Presternal and retrosternal soft-tissue swelling is not uncommon (Fig. 7.20). In the pelvis, mixed or sclerosing types tend to predominate. The medial portions of the innominate bones are often dense. Osteolytic lesions, rather non-specific in appearance, are not uncommon in the ischia and change from either type to the mixed pattern may be observed in serial examinations.

In the long bones the sites of predilection are the red marrow areas in the proximal portions of the femora and humeri. These are much more often of the osteolytic type and many small translucencies, oval in the long axis of the bone, may extend throughout the marrow cavity and may cause endosteal scalloping of the cortex. While such an appearance is a feature of this disease, it may be observed also in non-Hodgkin's lymphoma, leukemia and Gaucher's disease. Fusion of such areas may produce a honeycomb pattern, with coarse residual trabeculation, very like the medullary changes of Gaucher's disease. Organized periosteal reactions are not infrequent. Such a feature is rare in Gaucher's disease.

The skull, clavicles and scapulae are sometimes affected. Pathological fractures are uncommon. With sclerosing lesions in elderly individuals, confusion with Paget's disease may easily arise, but the characteristic enlargement of the affected bone in that disease will probably be absent. Differentiation, in all these lesions, must be made from metastasis. Intrathoracic disease may present with hypertrophic osteoarthropathy.

Non-Hodgkin's Lymphoma

This forms a much more difficult spectrum of disease with a continually evolving classification. That commonly used is based on lymph-node histology and cytoimmunochemistry. As a simplification, non-Hodgkin's lymphomas (NHL) are categorized according to the histologic architecture of the tumor into follicular or diffuse forms, and according to their cell type into B-cell and T-cell tumors. As a working formulation the tumor is then classified as low, medium or high grade. In general, low-grade tumors tend to be follicular B-cell lymphomas and high-grade tumors tend to be diffuse T-cell lymphomas.

It is difficult to assess how many patients actually present with primary skeletal non-Hodgkin's lymphoma; the proportion is probably less than one-third, the majority of patients having diffuse disease at diagnosis. Experience suggests that low-grade NHL may present as a primary bone tumor, although in older patients particularly it can be multifocal and systemic. It is unlikely that high-grade NHL ever presents primarily in the skeleton.

Low-Grade Non-Hodgkin's Lymphoma

Skeletal involvement by low-grade NHL may be with localized pain and swelling, often over a protracted period. The tumor may

follow treatment of a formerly osteolytic lesion. Conversely, some sclerotic lesions may be observed to become osteolytic or normal following treatment (Fig. 7.22). Whereas the osteolytic lesions may thin, displace and erode the overlying cortex and develop associated soft-tissue masses, the primary sclerotic lesion does not cause enlargement of the affected bone. Skeletal scintigraphy is a sensitive means of detecting the presence of bony lesions, particularly when sclerotic deposits have developed. The method is less reliable when purely lytic lesions are present. MRI is extremely sensitive (Fig. 7.23).

The spine is by far the most frequently involved area. A feature which is almost diagnostic is anterior erosion of a vertebral body (Fig. 7.24). This may or may not present reactive sclerosis in its margin and is attributed to involvement of adjacent paravertebral lymph nodes. Several vertebrae may be affected and the osteolytic lesions are likely to collapse. Soft-tissue masses will stimulate paravertebral abscesses. The sclerotic type shows a diffuse increase of density, possibly also with some anterior erosion but without increase in size of the affected body. A solitary dense vertebra, especially in young adults, is suggestive of this disease. In all these types the intervertebral disks are usually spared, aiding differentiation from an infection. Even in the rare cases where a

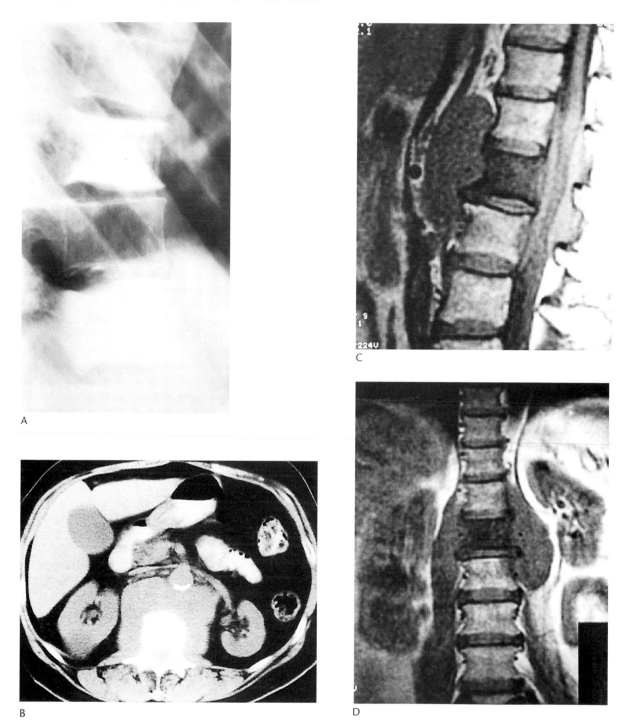

Fig. 7.21   Hodgkin's disease. **A.** The common pattern of endosteal sclerosis and patchy bone destruction is shown in the vertebral body of T9 in an adult man. Similar changes are also present at T11. These features are virtually diagnostic. **B.** In another patient, an intravenous enhanced CT section of the abdomen demonstrates a densely sclerotic lumbar vertebral body associated with a large paravertebral soft-tissue mass. **C.** Sagittal and **D.** coronal T_1-weighted images show low signal intensity within the upper lumbar vertebral body due to diffuse sclerosis and the extent of the soft-tissue mass. This extends into the central spinal canal and circumferentially around the thecal sac.

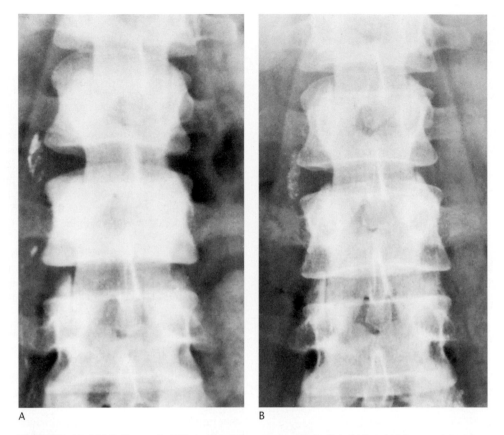

A   B

Fig. 7.22 Hodgkin's disease. **A.** Diffuse sclerosis is present in the bodies of L2 and L3 in a young woman at presentation with the disease. **B.** Two years later, following treatment, the appearances have reverted to normal. (Lymphographic contrast medium is present in para-aortic nodes.)

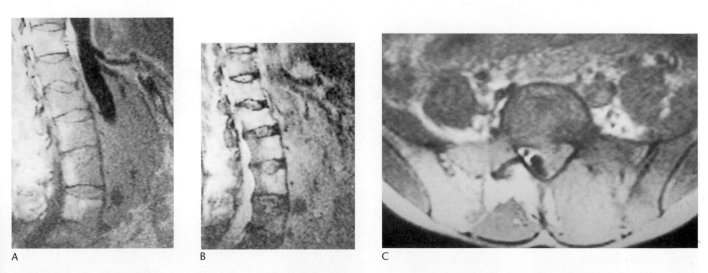

A   B   C

Fig. 7.23 Hodgkin's lymphoma. T_1-weighted **A.** and STIR **B.** sagittal images demonstrate extensive abnormality of the marrow of the lumbar spine. In addition a huge mass of lymph nodes is demonstrated anteriorly, wrapped around the abdominal aorta and displacing the superior mesenteric artery. An axial image **C.** demonstrates not only body and left ala involvement of the sacrum but also subcutaneous and spinal canal extension of the tumor. The thecal sac is displaced to the right.

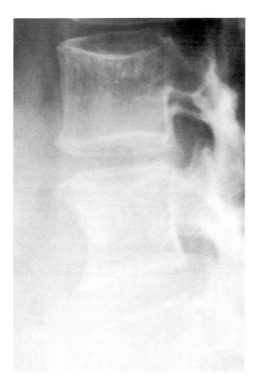

Fig. 7.24 Hodgkin's disease. A typical anterior scalloping of L4 is due to pressure erosion from enlarged lymph nodes. The cortex is preserved, as are the disk spaces.

malignancies including *osteosarcoma, metastasis* and *malignant round-cell tumors.* Indeed differentiation between these tumors in a young adult may be extremely difficult, not only on clinical and radiological grounds, but also histologically.

The lesion may arise as an apparently primary tumor within bone marrow tending to remain confined to the skeleton, although it may spread to other bones and only at a later stage to lymph nodes and viscera.

In its primary form the condition is localized to a single bone with a marked predilection for the long bones (Fig. 7.25). Nearly half the cases occur in the vicinity of the knee (Fig. 7.26) often with an associated synovial effusion. The proximal end of the humerus is another common site and about a third of cases are found in the flat bones of the axial skeleton. Spinal, rib and pelvic involvement tends to occur with the extraskeletal form, and in the older age group.

The tumor may be extremely radiosensitive, and radiotherapy alone or combined with amputation has resulted in many long survivals (Fig. 7.27). Even though a primary lesion may have regressed entirely with radiotherapy, generalized skeletal dissemination is likely to occur eventually.

Radiological Changes The earliest evidence of the tumor is diffuse medullary destruction of a patchy nature with very poorly defined margins (Fig. 7.25, 7.28). At this stage it may be impossible to differentiate the lesion radiologically from any other aggressive neoplasm. In particular, an osteolytic metastasis is likely to present the greatest difficulty. The lesion may resemble other primary malignant neoplasms stimulating little or no reactive bone formation such as Ewing's tumor, fibrosarcoma or malignant fibrous histiocytoma. Radiological confusion with osteomyelitis may also arise, particularly as overlying periosteal reaction is present in half the cases (Fig. 7.26). Indeed periosteal reaction may be present before medullary changes become evident. Scintigraphically the features are unremarkable. Usually increased activity

be asymptomatic, lesions presenting with pathological fracture. Males are affected twice as commonly as females. The majority are observed in the third and fourth decades although presentation during later years is not unusual. The lesions may be multifocal in the older age group. These tumors may be confused with other

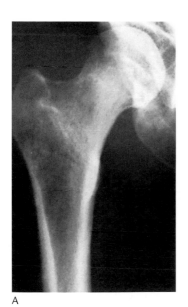

A

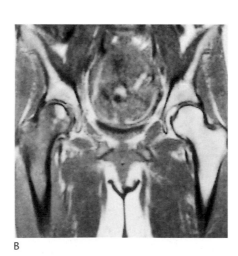

B

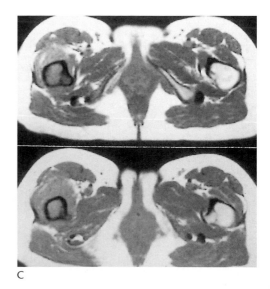

C

Fig. 7.25 Non-Hodgkin's lymphoma. Conventional radiograph **A.** is virtually normal save for the slight suggestion of patchy ill-defined bone destruction. Subsequent T_1-weighted coronal **B.** and axial **C.** MR images demonstrate not only extensive marrow replacement but also a substantial enveloping soft-tissue mass. The degree and extent of tumor involvement of bone was virtually impossible to appreciate from the radiographic examinations.

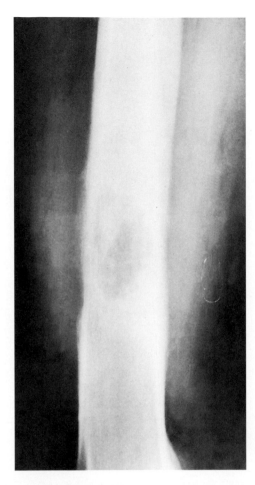

Fig. 7.26 Non-Hodgkin's lymphoma. A purely destructive lesion is present in the distal femur of a woman patient. The margins are ill defined with cortical destruction. Periosteal new bone formation is present adjacent to this destruction. These appearances resemble metastasis and osteosarcoma.

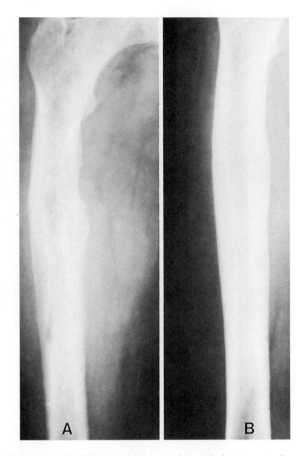

Fig. 7.27 Non-Hodgkin's lymphoma. Advanced changes are shown in the femoral shaft, with dramatic resolution 11 months later following local radiotherapy.

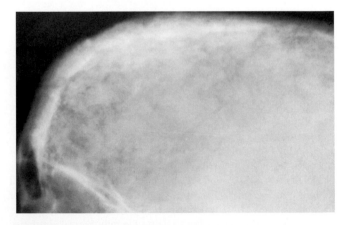

Fig. 7.28 Non-Hodgkin's lymphoma. Extensive patchy destruction of the cranium was present in this adult patient with generalized disease.

is detected. Multifocal lesions may be found. Radiologically the area of destruction spreads widely through the marrow cavity and remains patchy in nature. Much of the adjacent cortex undergoes resorption with the development of well-defined soft-tissue swelling from soft-tissue tumor extension. Cortical thickening and reactive sclerosis are not prominent features, although they may occur exceptionally.

In the generalized form of the disease, lesions may be detected throughout the skeleton and each present the same characteristics as a solitary focus (Fig. 7.29). The patient is likely to be over the age of 40. The ultimate degree of osseous destruction may be extreme.

High-Grade Non-Hodgkin's Lymphoma

This malignant tumor is rarer than Hodgkin's disease and mainly affects an older age group: patients in the fifth and sixth decades. Nonetheless a number of cases have been observed in children and in these a male sex preponderance has been found. A proportion of these patients develop frank *lymphocytic leukemia*.

The incidence of bone lesions is of the order of 10–20%, although more are detected at postmortem. Prognostically bone

lesions imply a poor outcome. Primary skeletal involvement is probably extremely rare.

Radiological changes in the skeleton resemble very closely those of Hodgkin's disease; other lesions grow more rapidly and are almost always osteolytic in type. Areas of destruction, commonly

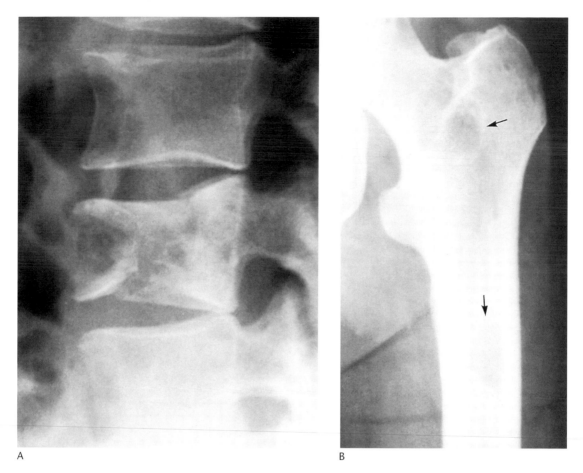

A   B

Fig. 7.29 A,B Non-Hodgkin's lymphoma. Multifocal disease was found at presentation in an elderly patient with low back pain. In addition to a pathological fracture of a lumbar vertebral body, ill-defined endosteal defects are present in the femoral shaft (arrows).

in red marrow areas, may be large with diffuse and irregular margins, and with scalloping of the inner aspects of the cortex. They may be solitary or multiple and, because of their osteolytic nature, pathological fractures are common. The latter affect especially the femoral and humeral necks and may cause collapse of vertebral bodies. When the lesions are multiple they all tend to be of the same osteolytic type, unlike Hodgkin's disease when all the different types of bone change may be present. Erosion of the cortex is likely to be followed by the formation of large associated soft-tissue masses with relatively little periosteal reaction. Such erosions usually take place through an area of cortex which has already been thinned and expanded by under-lying pathological process, emphasizing the radiological similarity of the individual lesions to Ewing sarcoma.

Burkitt's Tumor

An exceptional and particularly aggressive form of non-Hodgkin's lymphoma is common in African children and has been reported in other parts of the world. Large, destructive lesions develop especially in the mandible and maxilla (Fig. 7.30).

Radiologically these lesions are purely osteolytic and grow

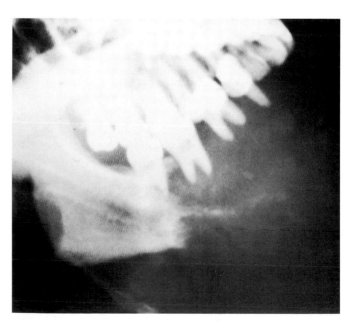

Fig. 7.30 Burkitt's tumor. A large destructive lesion in the mandible of this African child is typical of this form of lymphoma.

rapidly. The jaw lesions are characterized by the resorption of the lamina dura with multiple lytic foci which eventually coalesce with radiating spicules of bone. Spinal lesions are characterized by lytic, ill-defined destructive foci with paravertebral masses. In long bones the permeative lytic nature of the tumor, particularly with cortical erosions, may resemble a Ewing sarcoma. Foci develop in soft tissues, particularly the kidneys, ovaries and abdominal lymph nodes.

The disease is associated with a virus (Epstein–Barr) and is especially prevalent in endemic malarial areas. Regression can occur following the use of cytotoxic drugs.

Mastocytosis

The rare condition of urticaria pigmentosa is associated with enlargement of the liver, spleen and lymph nodes due to the proliferation of mast cells. The disease is relatively benign, but a few instances of leukemic termination have been recorded. Bone changes are usually identified in early adult life.

Radiological Changes   In probably a third of cases, generalized skeletal changes are present. These are diffuse or circumscribed areas of increased density, apparently due to thickening of the medullary trabeculae (Fig. 7.31). It may be difficult to identify the endosteal margin of the cortex. The absorption of some trabeculae and the thickening of others may cause the osseous structures to have a coarse pattern (Fig. 7.32) but the generalized increase in density usually predominates. Any bone may be affected. At this stage it is possible to demonstrate only a few mast cells in the bone marrow. The appearance may closely resemble *myelosclerosis*,

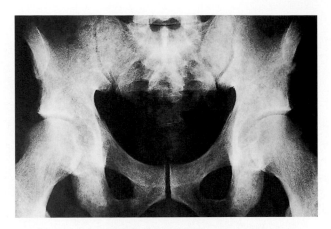

Fig. 7.32   Mastocytosis. A coarse pattern of generalized sclerosis is shown.

the *sclerosing types of leukemia*, *chronic anemias* and *osteopetrosis*. Occasionally the dense areas are sharply defined, of considerable size and localized to a few areas. Particularly in young adults, differentiation from Hodgkin's disease must be made.

PLASMA-CELL DISEASES

Plasma cells represent the end-product of B-lymphocyte maturation. Pathological proliferation produces either a local tumor (plasmacytoma) or disseminated disease (myelomatosis).

Plasmacytoma

This condition is unifocal, causing a localized destructive lesion in the skeleton, in a red marrow area. Many other descriptive terms, such as solitary myeloma, for this localized lesion have been used. Although for many years it may remain localized, and without health disturbance, ultimately it undergoes transition to generalized myelomatosis. A latent interval of 5–10 years is usual. Consequently the outlook is better than multiple myelomatosis. In comparison with the latter these lesions are uncommon. The exact incidence is difficult to assess since they are frequently asymptomatic. For example, a plasmacytoma in a rib may be noted incidentally on a routine examination of the chest.

When symptoms occur they are commonly those of bone pain, particularly backache. The vertebral bodies, especially in the thoracolumbar and lumbar regions, are the most common sites for these lesions and are likely to undergo partial collapse. The pelvis, especially the ilium, femur and humerus are the next most commonly involved sites.

The vast majority of affected individuals are between 30 and 60 years of age so that this is almost entirely a disease of late middle age. The differential diagnosis always includes a solitary osteolytic metastasis.

Radiological Changes   These lesions arise in areas of red marrow function. Bone expansion, which may be considerable with thinning of the overlying cortex, is common but, when a vertebral body is affected, collapse may precede such apparent expansions. The margins are usually well defined and sharply demarcated and

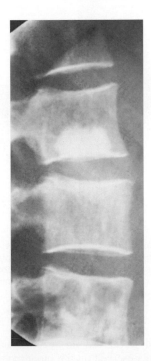

Fig. 7.31   Mastocytosis (man aged 34). A localized area of endosteal sclerosis is present in the body of L1. In addition, ill-defined thinning of trabeculae is demonstrated in L2 and patchier changes in the upper surface of L3.

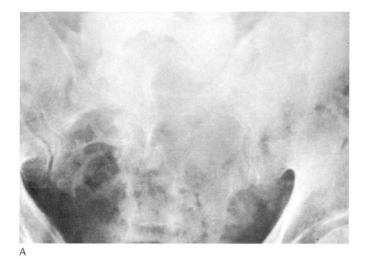

A

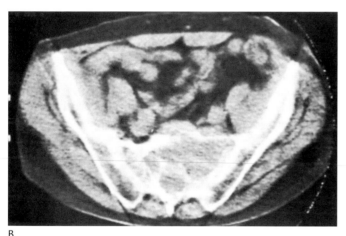

B

Fig. 7.33 Plasmacytoma of sacrum. **A.** An adult man exhibits a well-defined radiolucent defect involving the left sacral ala. **B.** CT scan demonstrated extensive destructive nature of the tumor, seen clearly to cross the midline. Note the marked cortical thinning with absence of sclerosis or periosteal new bone formation.

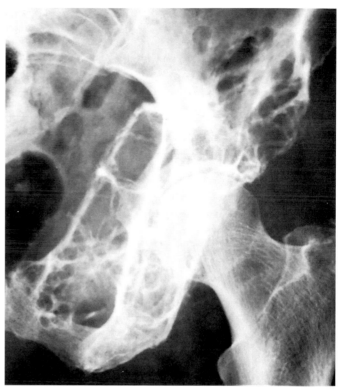

Fig. 7.34 Plasmacytoma of pelvis. This very extensive lesion was unaccompanied by any systemic abnormality. Bone expansion is associated with coarse trabeculation, producing a soap-bubble appearance.

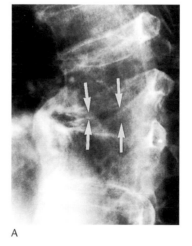

A

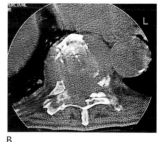

B

Fig. 7.35 Plasmacytoma presenting with paraparesis. **A.** Conventional radiograph of the thoracic spine showing vertebra plana (arrows). **B.** CT demonstrating the degree of bony destruction, associated paravertebral mass and marked posterior extension into the spinal canal resulting in severe cord compression.

characteristically without a sclerotic reaction (Fig. 7.33). Coarse trabecular strands of increased density may give a network appearance in the area of destruction, and exceptionally the lesion may be entirely sclerotic. Large lesions in flat bones may assume a soap-bubble appearance (Fig. 7.34).

Differential diagnosis of these tumors may be difficult. In view of the age group concerned the most important is an osteolytic *metastasis*. In vertebrae, such metastases are likely to involve the pedicles more commonly. Metastatic disease apart, the development of a solitary osteolytic lesion in a vertebral body in a patient in late middle age should always be considered as a plasmacytoma (Figs 7.35, 7.36). *Chordoma* may produce similar features. Other differential diagnoses to be considered, especially with an expanding lytic focus in a rib, are *fibrous dysplasia*, a 'brown' tumor of *hyperparathyroidism* and, particularly when the lesion is adjacent to an articular surface, a *giant-cell tumor*. Resemblance to a giant-cell tumor may be close; however, these lesions are found in early adult life and furthermore have a different distribution, commonly affecting the appendicular skeleton, whereas plasmacytoma is more likely to be axial.

Scintigraphy and *CT* afford no specific diagnostic features. Increased activity is observed on the blood-pool phase of a bone scan, while the delayed phase shows increased activity around the margins. CT confirms the extent of these tumors but does not afford tissue-specific information.

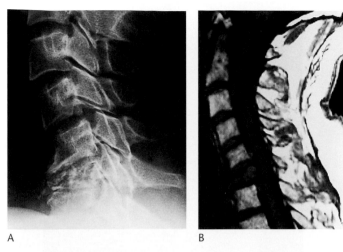

A   B

Fig. 7.36 Plasmacytoma. **A.** Conventional cervical spine radiograph showing osteolytic destruction of C6 with pathological collapse of the vertebral body. **B.** Sagittal T_1-weighted MR image showing the intermediate signal intensity lesion of C6 resulting in focal extradural compression of the spinal cord.

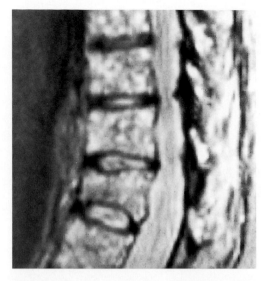

Fig. 7.37 Multiple myeloma. Sagittal T_2-weighted image of the thoracolumbar junction showing multiple foci of high signal intensity within the vertebral bodies.

Multiple Myelomatosis

The disseminated or generalized form of plasma-cell infiltration of bone marrow is known as multiple myelomatosis. This entity may be preceded by a solitary plasmacytoma or arise de novo.

It is much more common for the widespread form to present radiologically as a fully developed entity in the over-40 age group. Men are affected twice as often as women. Persistent bone pain or a pathological fracture are usually the first complaints.

Plasma-cell proliferation causes elevation of the total serum proteins, due to the production of abnormal immunoglobulins. Such proliferation eventually takes place at the expense of all other marrow functions so that a non-specific leukopenia and secondary anemia develop. In about half of cases, presence of an abnormal urinary protein constituent, Bence Jones proteose, may be demonstrated. Abnormal proteinuria causes cast formation in the renal tubules with impairment of renal function. Hypercalcemia, hypercalcuria and amyloidosis occur, the last in about 10% of all cases and resembles the distribution of primary amyloidosis. The hypercalcemia and hypercalcuria are unassociated with an elevation of either the serum alkaline phosphatase or phosphate levels.

The pattern of bone destruction may vary from diffuse osteoporosis, through small and almost insignificant areas of translucency, to rounded or oval defects with sharply defined margins. The last, regarded as characteristic, develops relatively late. Frequently the defects coalesce to produce even larger areas of osteolysis.

Radiological Changes The two cardinal features are generalized reduction in bone density and localized areas of radiolucency in red marrow areas. The axial skeleton, therefore, is affected predominantly. Lesions may be observed also in the shafts of long bones and in the skull. In spite of positive bone marrow aspiration, radiological features may be absent in as many as one-third of cases, at least at initial presentation. This group of patients tend to develop generalized osteoporosis.

Since the detection of skeletal lesions is important in management, radiology plays a large part in assessing the extent of disease. Generally speaking a radiographic skeletal survey is superior to scintigraphic investigation using a bone-scanning agent, because the lesions are essentially osteolytic with no bone reaction. A bone scan is superior, however, in detecting lesions in the ribs because the associated fractures are demonstrated more easily.

Diffuse osteoporosis alone can cause suspicion of the disease in an elderly patient. Even though senile osteoporosis may be expected, the possibility of myelomatosis always merits consideration, particularly when symptomatic bone pain is present (Fig 7.37). The smaller areas of radiolucency are poorly demarcated and appear to be irregular accentuations of the generalized osteoporotic process (Fig. 7.38). The rounded and oval defects that develop are characterized by the sharp definition of their edges. Reactive marginal sclerosis is absent. Typically the cortex is eroded from within sharply defined margins (Fig. 7.39).

Exceptionally, however, sclerosing changes have been reported. These have varied, some resembling focal lesions of prostatic metastases, some the spiculation of osteosarcoma and some a generalized diffuse increase in density. This very rare form of multiple myelomatosis occurs in probably 2% of cases, and is frequently accompanied by a peripheral neuropathy.

Treatment, as in other conditions, may alter these appearances and, during its course, it is common to observe some lesions resolving whilst others evolve.

The **distribution of lesions** is very widespread and destructive foci are commonly located in the long bones in addition to the axial skeleton. Involvement of the skull is variable. Diffuse and irregular translucencies with generalized osteoporosis are not uncommon. Such changes eventually become pronounced and extensive. The disease will not always be evident by the presence of the classic 'raindrop' lesions, circular defects varying in diameter from a few millimeters to 2 or 3 cm. Indeed, the skull may be normal, even in the presence of many lesions elsewhere in

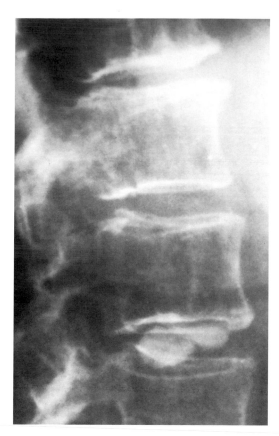

Fig. 7.38 Myelomatosis. Diffuse marrow involvement has resulted in an overall reduction in bone density similar to that seen in osteoporosis. However the rather patchy nature of radiolucencies should raise the possibility of myeloma.

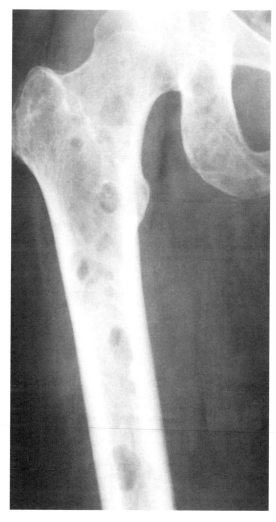

Fig. 7.39 Typical localized lesions of myeloma are demonstrated in the upper femur of an adult woman. The sharply defined rounded defects with endosteal erosion of the cortex are characteristic.

the skeleton. Areas of osteolysis may be observed also in the mandible, a site only rarely affected by metastasis. Myelomatous lesions may erode the cortex and extend into the adjacent soft tissues. The resulting soft-tissue masses are helpful in differentiating the advanced forms of the disease from the lesions of metastatic carcinoma which much less commonly produce extension into the soft tissues. The spine is often merely osteoporotic, but as the disease advances, multiple foci of destruction, almost invariably accompanied by some degree of collapse of the affected bodies, are likely to be present. With such collapse, paravertebral soft-tissue shadows are common. Differentiation from inflammatory lesions can be made, as the intervertebral disk spaces and the articular surfaces are not affected. The pedicles and posterior elements are involved less frequently and at a later stage than occurs with metastases. In the thorax a destructive rib lesion with a large associated soft-tissue mass is much more suggestive of myelomatosis than of a plasmacytoma. Diffuse involvement, however, is more usual, numerous cystic foci of characteristic appearance being visible. The clavicles and scapulae may also show these destructive changes.

The long bones are affected most commonly in the persistent red marrow areas of the proximal ends of the humeri and femora. Lesions, however, are by no means found only in such areas, and irregular or punched-out translucencies in the shafts of other bones may be the first radiological manifestation of disease. In some

advanced cases lytic defects may be due also to secondary amyloidosis, which can complicate many chronic disorders such as rheumatoid disease and longstanding infections.

Pathological fractures are very often the initiating factor in the diagnosis of the disease. These fractures heal remarkably quickly and soundly with massive callus and new bone formation. This response is somewhat surprising in view of the numerous cystic lesions and widespread osteoporosis which are likely to be present without any evidence of reactive sclerosis.

POEMS Syndrome

An uncommon condition with the acronym POEMS is characterized by a chronic progressive Polyneuropathy, Organomegaly (hepatosplenomegaly), Endocrinopathy (commonly diabetes mellitus), M-proteins (plasma-cell dyscrasia), and Skin changes (hirsutism, pigmentation, edema). It is usually seen in young men and radiologically presents with multiple sclerotic lesions, most commonly in the spine and pelvis.

HISTIOCYTOSIS

The basic pathological abnormality in this group of diseases is a proliferation of histiocytic cells occurring particularly in the bone marrow, the spleen, the liver, the lymphatic glands and the lungs. In the more chronic forms these cells become swollen with lipid deposits, essentially cholesterol (though the blood cholesterol level remains normal) and they present the pathological appearances of 'foam cells'. Some of these become necrotic and are replaced by fibrous tissue.

Various forms of the condition have been regarded in the past as separate entities. These forms are outlined below but it must be emphasized that this subdivision is entirely arbitrary since histiocytosis essentially presents a spectrum of disease.

Eosinophilic Granuloma

This is the most mild expression of histiocytosis. Pathological changes are predominantly bony, although occasionally pulmonary involvement may occur. Children, especially boys, between 3 and 12 years are most commonly affected, although these lesions may be observed in adolescents, young adults and exceptionally the middle-aged. Any bone may be affected. A quarter of cases occur in the skull. The skull, pelvis and femora between them account for nearly two-thirds of all cases.

Clinically pain and swelling may be accompanied by mild fever. Histologically the eosinophilic infiltration is found around collections of histiocytes. In this relatively mild form necrosis and fibrosis are rare and the appearance of foam cells suggests a more serious variety.

Radiological Changes Translucent areas of bone destruction,

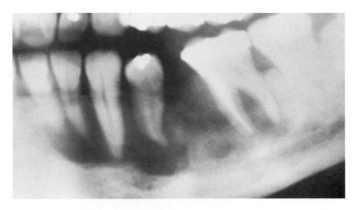

Fig. 7.40 Histiocytosis. A purely osteolytic lesion is present in the mandible, with well-defined, slightly scalloped margins. The lamina dura has been destroyed. The teeth seem to 'float in air'.

with sharply defined margins and often of considerable size, are characteristic. The round or oval defects may have scalloped margins (Fig. 7.40). Although in the active phase they provoke no sclerotic margin, the healing phase, which usually develops by spontaneous regression, is marked by peripheral sclerosis round the lesion and slow reconstitution of the bony structure (Fig. 7.41). This healing phase may be accelerated by biopsy, radiotherapy or steroid injection. True expansion is uncommon except in ribs and vertebra bodies. Apparent expansion may result from thickening of the overlying periosteum, especially if the cortex has been partially eroded (Fig. 7.42) or infarction has occurred. In approximately two-thirds of patients the lesions are *solitary*.

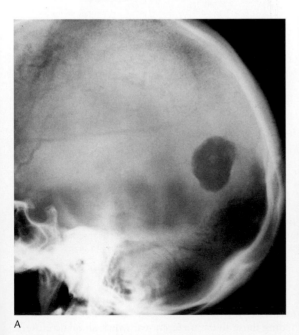
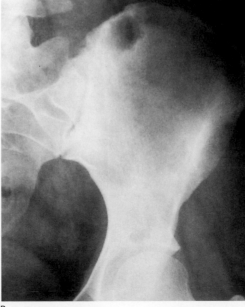
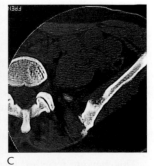

A   B   C

Fig. 7.41 Histiocytosis. **A.** Lateral skull radiograph showing a well-defined osteolytic lesion with a narrow zone of transition and no sclerosis in the posterior parietal region. **B.** Osteolytic lesion of the innominate bone with ill-defined peripheral sclerosis. **C.** CT of the innominate lesion showing destruction of the anterior cortex of the iliac wing and the ill-defined surrounding sclerosis of this healing lesion.

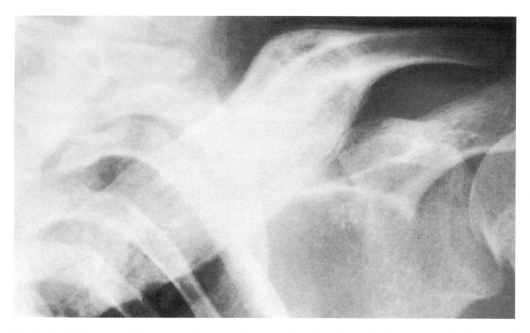

Fig. 7.42 Histiocytosis. Extensive involvement of a bone, here the clavicle, is often associated with layered periosteal new bone causing bony expansion. Ill-defined areas of resorption may be visualized in the lesion. This was the only abnormality found in a young girl over several years' follow-up.

Differential diagnosis of a solitary lesion of this type may be extremely difficult and is either from osteomyelitis or Ewing's tumor, which has a similar age incidence. Skeletal survey may disclose the presence of other asymptomatic lesions, facilitating the diagnosis. *Multiple* eosinophilic granulomas are usually found to be in different phases of evolution (Fig. 7.41). As one lesion resolves another may appear in a different part of the skeleton. In the skull particularly, new lesions several centimeters in diameter may appear in as many weeks. Button sequestra may be observed. Skeletal scintigraphy is a sensitive means of detecting the lesions, particularly in the healing phase, and may be used in follow-up studies.

Solitary lesions in the spine may collapse, partially or completely, the latter presenting the classic appearance of *vertebra plana* (Fig. 7.43). The most commonly affected site is the thoracic spine. The lesions at one time were considered to represent an 'osteochondritis' and were named *Calvé's disease*. During the phase of collapse, the walls of the affected vertebral body tend to bulge laterally and paravertebral soft-tissue shadows may be evident. The disk spaces on either side remain intact and may even be widened. As healing occurs, remarkably good reconstitution of these vertebral bodies may take place if sufficient years of growth remain. The vast majority of vertebral plana lesions, especially in a relatively healthy child, are caused by an eosinophilic granuloma, and confirmatory biopsy is usually unnecessary. The differential diagnosis of collapse of a single vertebral body includes the relative rarities of Ewing's tumor, metastasis from a neuroblastoma, benign osteoblastoma or, most exceptionally, a bizarre and atypical tuberculous focus.

This benign form of histiocytosis occasionally affects long bones and initially has a predilection for the diaphysis (Fig. 7.44). However, metaphyseal involvement may occur again causing confusion with a pyogenic infection. A rare entity, *chronic*

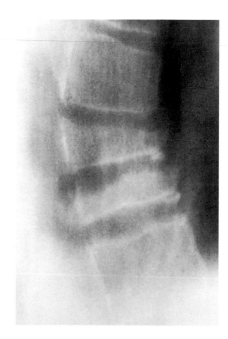

Fig. 7.43 Histiocytosis. Vertebral lesions in the thoracic spine are shown on a lateral tomogram. The bodies of T7 and 8 have collapsed with a slight increase in bone density. Note the relative preservation of the disk spaces.

granulomatous (Landing–Shirkey) disease, tends to cause skeletal lesions, including those in the metaphyses, which simulate closely the radiological appearance of multiple eosinophilic granulomas. This condition is usually due to inherited and inadequate responses of leukocytes to infection.

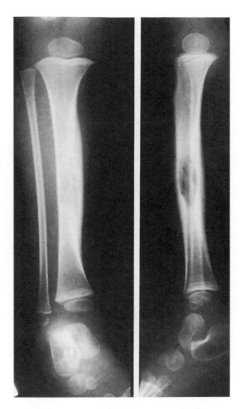

Fig. 7.44 Histiocytosis. A healing diaphyseal lesion exhibits periosteal new bone formation and minimal sclerosis around the margins of the radiolucency.

Hand–Schüller–Christian Disease

This is a more chronic form of the disease, with dissemination of lesions in the lungs, lymph nodes, liver and spleen, in addition to virtually constant and early involvement of the skeleton.

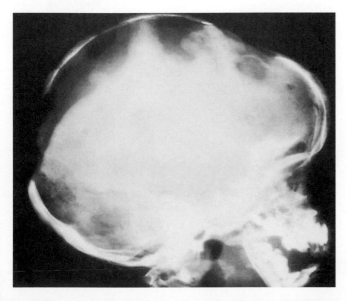

Fig. 7.45 Histiocytosis. Extensive skull involvement in a child with the Hand–Schüller–Christian type of lesion. The areas of destruction in the flat bones of the skull have a map-like configuration.

The early case reports drew attention to a syndrome consisting of skull defects, exophthalmos and diabetes insipidus, the last two being associated with lesions round the orbit and the hypophysis respectively. Children below the age of 5 years are most frequently affected, though sporadic cases occur at later ages up to middle life. The course of the disease is chronic, often extending over 10 or more years. It is characterized by soreness of the mouth and loose teeth, due to deposits in the gums and jaws, and skin lesions. Abnormalities in the temporal bone are common, with an associated otitis media. The eventual prognosis is good, since spontaneous remission, possibly initiated or accelerated by radiotherapy, takes place in the majority of cases. Over 10%, however, terminate fatally.

Radiological Changes The bone defects are essentially the same as those of eosinophilic granulomas. They are, however, very much more numerous and particularly affect the flat bones. In the skull they frequently coalesce to produce widespread irregular defects usually likened to a map and described as the 'geographical skull', both tables often suffering extensive osteolysis (Fig. 7.45). Lesions in the mandible and maxilla begin

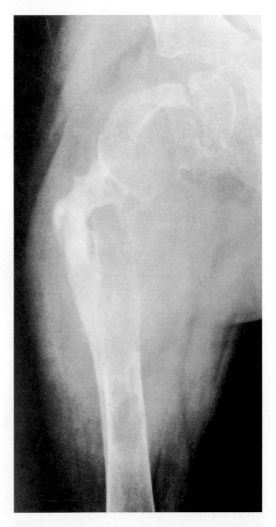

Fig. 7.46 Histiocytosis. Hand–Schüller–Christian type. Very extensive radiolucencies are present both in the metaphysis and diaphysis of this child's femur. A healed pathological fracture is present. Histiocytosis should always be considered in the differential diagnosis of bizarre bone lesions.

round the tooth roots, so that the teeth, which are never affected, remain dense and appear to 'float in air' (Fig. 7.40). Several vertebrae may be completely or partially collapsed and extensive lesions may develop in the scapulae, ribs and pelvis. Osteolytic pelvic lesions or vertebral collapse in a child are suggestive of this disease. Long bone involvement is less common (Fig. 7.46).

In a relatively early stage, sclerotic reaction round the sharply defined margins of these lesions will be absent. When healing does occur the lesions fill in by sclerosis in the same way as eosinophilic granulomas. New lesions may appear after the original ones have begun to heal, emphasizing again the wide spectrum of radiological change in histiocytosis.

The lungs show a fine nodular infiltration in the acute phase. With healing, these fibrose and persist as linear strands of increased density, but the presence of pulmonary changes in histiocytosis indicates a worse prognosis (Fig. 7.47).

Letterer–Siwe Disease

This is an acute or sub-acute disseminated form of the disease, occurring very rarely in infants below the age of 2 years and presenting a much more severe clinical picture. It is characterized by a pyrexia, with a rash and mouth sores, bleeding gums, respiratory symptoms and failure to thrive. Particular involvement of the extraskeletal tissues occurs with enlargement of the liver, spleen and lymph nodes. The disease usually ends fatally, often in a few months and at the most in 2 years. In those cases with a rapidly fatal outcome, skeletal lesions are unlikely to be demonstrated radiologically, having insufficient time to develop. Nevertheless, histologic change may be present in the bone

marrow, with widespread masses of histiocytes and eosinophilic infiltration, comparable with the early histologic picture of the benign eosinophilic granuloma. Only in the rare cases that survive do fibrosis and cholesterol-containing foam cells become apparent.

Radiological Changes   Bone lesions, when they occur, are indistinguishable from those of Hand–Schüller–Christian disease, but tend to be even more widely spread, both in the flat bones and even more in the metadiaphyseal areas of the long bones (Fig. 7.48). They show no trace of the sclerotic reaction round their sharply defined, punched-out margins. Diffuse pulmonary infiltration is common. This may closely resemble miliary tuberculosis and is a variety of honeycomb lung.

In summary, histiocytosis is a disease primarily of childhood, although exceptionally its more benign manifestations may be observed in early adult life. The older the child, and the more the lesions are confined to the skeleton rather than other tissues, the better the prognosis. It must be appreciated that the benign eosinophilic granuloma may deteriorate to a chronic, multifocal form of the spectrum, and rarely vice versa.

STORAGE DISORDERS OF THE LYMPHORETICULAR SYSTEM

A number of conditions have been described in which the lymphoreticular system is the site of abnormal deposition of lipoproteins, usually as a result of inborn errors of metabolism. The commonest of these rare disorders are Gaucher's disease and Niemann–Pick disease.

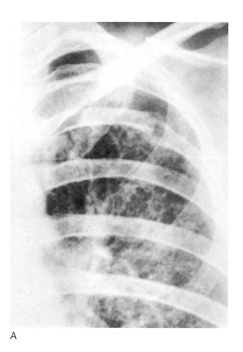
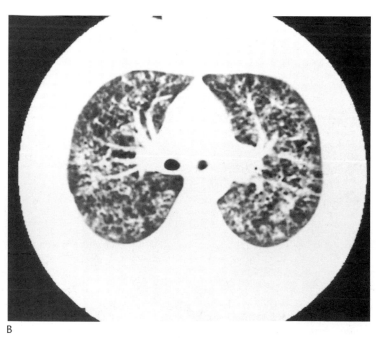

A   B

Fig. 7.47   Histiocytosis. Adult pulmonary involvement (man aged 20). **A.** A localized view from a chest radiograph demonstrates a coarse interstitial pulmonary fibrosis. Note also a pathological fracture of the left fourth rib due to a bony deposit. **B.** A CT scan demonstrates peripheral interstitial pulmonary fibrosis with thickened interlobular septa and irregular honeycombing.

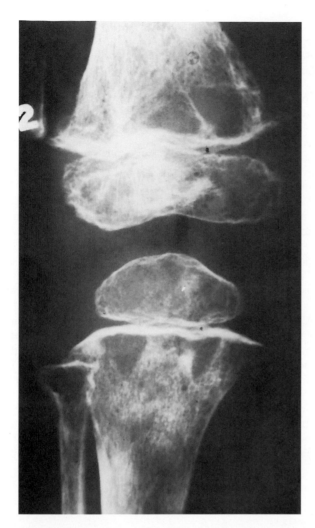

Fig. 7.48 Histiocytosis, Letterer–Siwe type. Massive destructive lesions are present throughout the skeleton, but affect particularly the metadiaphyseal areas of the long bones. A similar appearance could be produced by metastases from a neuroblastoma or the advanced stages of leukemia.

Gaucher's Disease

Young Jewish females are particularly susceptible to this hereditary condition caused by deficiency of β-glucosidase. It is not confined to this ethnic group or sex. Although manifestations of the condition commonly become apparent in the later years of childhood and in early adult life, the disease may be so chronic, and of such insidious onset, that it may be recognized for the first time only in middle age or even later life. In infancy the rapidly fatal course of this systemic disease is characterized by gross neurological changes and pulmonary infiltration.

In the juvenile and young adult variety, the principal complaint is of weakness and fatigue with progressive dementia. On clinical examination splenic enlargement is detected in 95% of cases. Bone pain may be present, sometimes severe. In the chronic form of the disease characteristic and diagnostic bone changes may be expected. Histologic examination reveals numerous large histiocytes within which an abnormal lipoprotein, kerasin, is present. These

cells are disseminated throughout the marrow of the hematopoietic skeleton, in addition to the spleen and liver.

Radiological Changes Diffuse infiltration of the bone marrow causes widespread and irregular medullary radiolucency. When collections of the abnormal histiocytes occur destructive medullary lesions become visible and abnormal modeling of the long bones may be evident. Expansion of the distal ends of the femora begins with a loss of the normal concavity of the medial sides. Eventually this justifies the classic description of 'flask-shaped', on the analogy of the contour of the Erlenmeyer flask (Fig. 7.49). This feature is, however, not diagnostic of Gaucher's disease and may be seen in other conditions including hemolytic anemias (thalassemia), leukemia, and osteopetrosis. Other bones, notably the tibia and humerus, may be similarly affected.

Destructive lesions cause localized endosteal cortical erosions, with sharply defined scalloped borders. As these lesions increase in size and coalesce, the areas of bone abnormality may become exceedingly widespread, both in the individual bone and in the skeleton as a whole. *Infarction of bone* is not uncommon (Fig. 7.50). The femoral and humeral heads, especially the former, are often involved in this way. In a child such infarction may simulate Perthes disease. In an adult the destructive changes in the femoral head that develop cannot be differentiated from avascular necrosis of other origin. *Bone scintigraphy* may be helpful in the assessment of acute bone pain in order to detect early infarction (Fig.

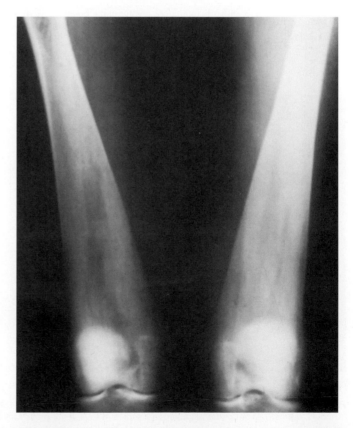

Fig. 7.49 Gaucher's disease (woman aged 20). Abnormal modeling of the distal ends of the femora has resulted in typical flask-shaped appearance. An osteolytic lesion with a coarse trabecular pattern is present in the right femur.

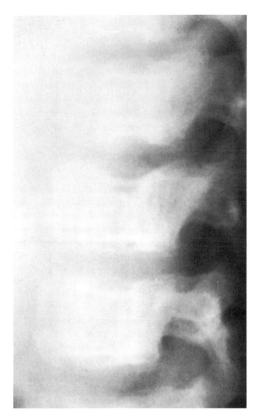

Fig. 7.50 Gaucher's disease. Infarctions in vertebral bodies have produced the 'bone within a bone' appearance throughout the lumbar spine in this child.

7.51). Subsequent disruption of articular surfaces promotes osteoarthritis (Fig. 7.52).

Pathological fractures may follow relatively minor trauma. While fractures may occur through any affected bone, compression of a vertebral body is the usual lesion. As in many other conditions, these compression fractures are most likely to be found in the lower dorsal or lumbar regions, the areas of greatest stress. Frank zones of osteolysis in the spine are rare in Gaucher's disease, but generalized osteoporosis is common. Pathological fractures also occur in the femoral neck causing coxa vara, and in sites where no concomitant radiological abnormality can be identified.

Usually bone trabeculae are destroyed, but the chronic form of the disease may be characterized by sclerotic reaction within the bone. A coarse network of dense medullary strands results which may give the appearance of a honeycomb. In addition, endosteal thickening may develop, as in the later stages of sickle-cell disease and myelosclerosis, the appearances again being suggestive of a 'bone within a bone'. On the outer surface, diffuse periosteal reactions may develop, usually overlying an intact cortex.

As a result of these reactive changes in the later stages of the disease, the radiological picture may be confusing. It is particularly important for differentiation from chronic osteomyelitis to be made, as misguided surgical intervention has sometimes been followed by chronic and resistant infection with persistent discharging sinuses.

Unlike some of the other diseases in this group, notably the chronic hemolytic anemias, the distribution of these lesions tends to be peripheral rather than central. The chronic form of the disease may cause characteristic changes in the first decade; the

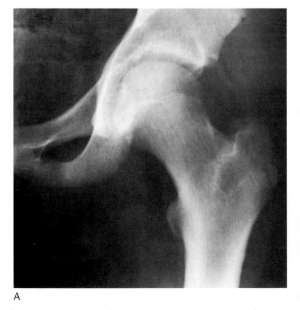

A

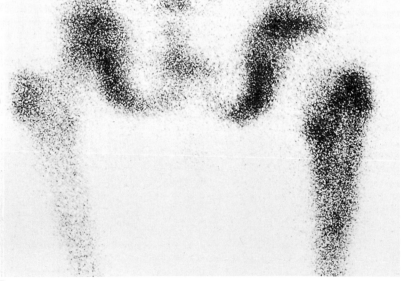

B

Fig. 7.51 Gaucher's disease—acute bone infarction. **A.** A radiograph of a 13-year-old girl, with known Gaucher's disease, presenting with acute hip pain of 12 hours, duration. Slight endosteal sclerosis is shown in the inferior pubic ramus and an area of ill-defined radiolucency in the intertrochanteric region. **B.** The delayed phase of a bone scan reveals the femoral head and neck to be markedly photon-deficient consistent with acute infarction. Abnormally increased activity is present also at site of previous disease.

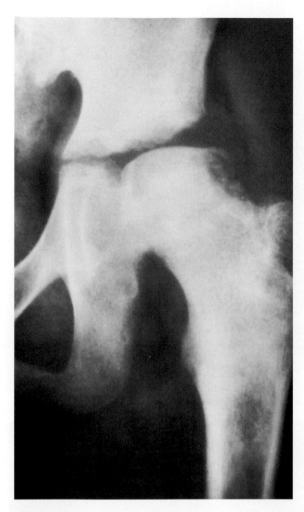

Fig. 7.52 Gaucher's disease. This adolescent has considerable deformity of the femoral head and acetabulum secondary to episodes of infarction. Evidence of degenerative arthritis is already present.

diffuse medullary osteoporosis and abnormality of modeling in the distal ends of the femora are likely to be the first radiological manifestations. The changes may be widespread and may resemble thalassemia, except that the bones of the hands and feet are usually completely or relatively exempt.

In the adult, the long tubular bones are usually the site of lesions, destructive processes in the pelvis and thoracic cage being rarely evident. Nevertheless involvement of the axial skeleton does occur, as shown by the frequency of spinal osteoporosis and occasional vertebral collapse, which may be apparent even in the absence of other radiological evidence of this disease. No characteristic lesions are recognized in the skull, but diffuse osteoporosis has been reported. Frank cystic areas of destruction have been noted round the tooth roots in the mandible.

In the radiological assessment of any skeletal abnormality, appreciation of associated abnormalities of soft tissue is important. In this instance the combination of the changes described above, with a patient with an appropriate ethnic background and with splenomegaly, provides a strong diagnostic triad. Enlargement of the spleen, and often the liver, is almost constant in this disease. Pulmonary involvement is unusual, but an appearance

suggestive of interstitial fibrosis may be observed, particularly in young children, even in the absence of skeletal involvement.

Niemann–Pick Disease

This rare disorder of the lymphoreticular system, of a type similar to Gaucher's disease, has, in its classic form, a predilection for Jewish girls under the age of 2 years. The abnormal lipoprotein in the 'foam cells' in this instance is *sphingomyelin*. Osseous changes are less severe than in Gaucher's disease. Nevertheless, careful study may disclose generalized osteoporosis, minor coarsening of the trabeculae and minor modeling abnormalities.

Overt areas of osteolysis do occur, but are unusual and may resemble the lesions of histiocytosis. On the other hand interstitial pulmonary infiltration, causing a 'honeycomb' lung appearance, and hepatosplenomegaly are common in classic cases, for which the prognosis is grave. Other types of the condition have been recognized in older children.

DISORDERS OF THE COAGULATION MECHANISM

HEMOPHILIA AND ITS VARIANTS

The normal process of blood coagulation depends on a number of factors. Many of these have been recognized and their individual deficiencies have led to descriptions of several disease entities within the hemophiliac group.

From the radiological aspect the most important of these disorders are classic **hemophilia**, due to deficiency of factor VIII, and the rarer **Christmas disease**, due to deficiency of factor IX. These hereditary diseases primarily affect males, being X-linked, usually recessive disorders. The degree of affliction is related to the level of deficiency.

The bleeding tendency is usually observed during the first year of life and may affect any tissue system. Christmas disease is usually less severe. Bleeding is considered to result from trauma, possibly very slight, rather than being spontaneous. Bleeding into joints is characteristic. Such episodes commonly become more frequent during the later years of childhood and adolescence. Milder forms of the disease may cause formation of large, soft-tissue hematomas without significant joint involvement. This is true of **von Willebrand's disease**, which affects both sexes equally and is transmitted in an autosomal dominant manner. If, however, the factor VIII level is low, bleeding into joints can occur in this condition.

Radiological changes in the skeleton are caused by bleeding into joints, within bony structures and beneath the periosteum. Frequent repetition of such episodes, particularly at an early age, increases their severity.

Intra-articular hemorrhage   In the early stages of the disease, the soft-tissue distension of a joint due to a hemarthrosis cannot be distinguished radiologically from a frank traumatic or inflammatory synovial effusion. Frequent repetition of hemorrhagic incidents results in synovial thickening and articular erosions. Initially these erosions tend to be marginal in distribution. At the same time the bony structures in the vicinity of an affected joint are likely to become porotic, partly through disuse, but even more through persistent hyperemia associated with organization of the

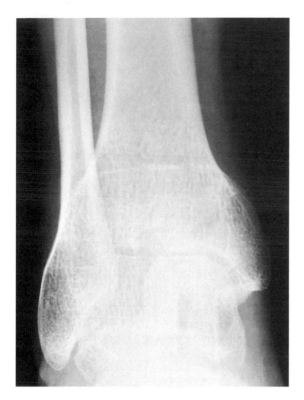

Fig. 7.53 Hemophilia. The former epiphyses are disproportionately large, presenting a 'squared' appearance. Hyaline cartilage thickness at the ankle joint is reduced.

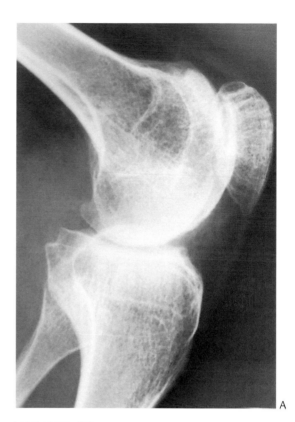

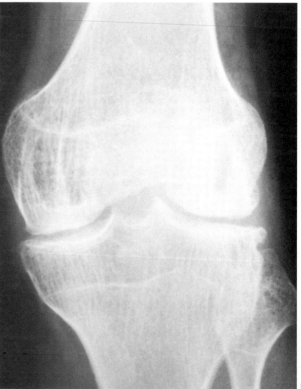

hemarthroses. This latter factor, as with hyperemia of any other cause, commonly causes enlargement of the growing epiphyses (Fig. 7.53). Such epiphyses may also become abnormal in shape and often fuse prematurely. Differentiation from a chronic inflammatory synovitis, particularly tuberculous, may present radiological difficulty. The trabecular pattern of the bone becomes coarse and often has a lattice appearance. Secondary degenerative changes develop prematurely (Fig. 7.54).

The knee is affected almost invariably, involvement being frequently bilateral. The intercondylar notch becomes wide and deep. The patella may develop an unusually rectangular shape and its proximal articular surface is a common site of an erosion.

The elbows and ankles also are commonly affected. A characteristic abnormality in the former joint is an enlarged and deformed radial head. The shoulders and wrists are less frequently involved. Bleeding into the hip is unusual, but when this does occur avascular necrosis of the femoral head causes an appearance comparable to Perthes disease. Distended joint capsules, particularly those of the elbows, may become radiologically dense by deposition within them of hemosiderin (Fig. 7.55).

Intraosseous hemorrhage   Juxta-articular cystic lesions may be observed in the later stages of the disease, with a peculiar predilection for the proximal humeral epiphyses and the olecranon processes. While many are comparable to the post-traumatic subarticular cysts of degenerative joint disease, the fact that some of these cysts are remote from the articular surfaces has led to the belief that they may be caused by hemorrhage within the bone itself.

Fig. 7.54 A, B. Hemophilia. Typical appearances in an adult patient subject to recurrent hemarthroses since childhood. As well as the enlarged, squared appearance of the former epiphyses, hyaline cartilage width is reduced, and osteophytes are present due to secondary osteoarthritis. Areas of radiolucency within medullary bone probably represent old intraosseous hemorrhages.

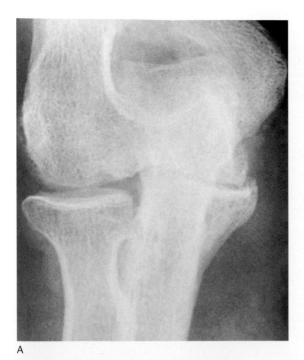

A

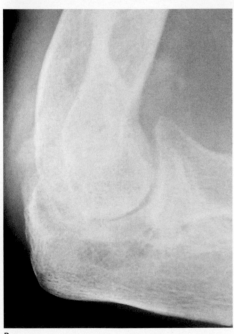

B

Fig. 7.55 A,B. Hemophilia. Repeated intra-articular hemorrhages have caused overgrowth of the epiphyses, particularly the head of the radius. The joint capsule is distended and the synovium is amorphously dense due to the deposition of hemosiderin from recurrent hemarthroses. A sub-articular cyst is present in the olecranon fossa, and degenerative changes, in the form of hyaline cartilage thinning and osteophyte formation, are present.

Subperiosteal hemorrhage Large osteolytic lesions known as hemophiliac pseudotumors occur in about 1 or 2% of severely affected patients. They have been observed especially in the iliac wings and in the shafts of the long bones of the lower limb,

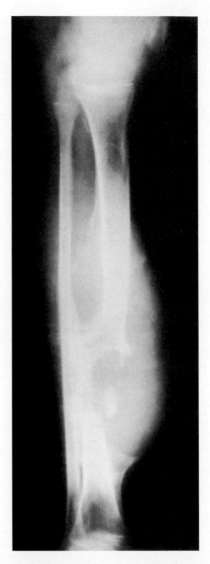

Fig. 7.56 Hemophiliac pseudotumor. A huge destructive lesion in the tibia, with relatively well-defined margins, is associated with some periosteal reaction. Although an initial impression may be of a malignant tumor, changes of hemophilic arthropathy can be seen in the knee and ankle.

although other bones, including the calcaneus, have been involved (Fig. 7.56). These destructive lesions have been attributed to bleeding below the periosteum and often are accompanied by large swellings, sometimes relatively painless, of the soft tissues. Relation to a former traumatic incident may occasionally be established. Absorption of the underlying cortex and medulla with elevation of the periosteal margins results in an appearance which may be highly suggestive of a malignant bone tumor. Calcification is not uncommon within the space-occupying lesions. A diagnostic clue, however, may be provided by evidence in an adjacent joint of a hemophiliac arthropathy. Failure to appreciate the nature of this entity, nevertheless, has resulted in iatrogenic disasters by unnecessary amputation.

The diagnosis of hemophilia is likely to be made clinically, but the radiologist must be aware of its skeletal manifestations, including not only the typical arthropathies and bone cysts, but also and importantly the rare hemophiliac pseudotumors.

REFERENCES AND SUGGESTIONS FOR FURTHER READING (CHAPTERS 5–7)

Bullough, P. G., Vigorita, V. J. (1984) *Atlas of Orthopaedic Pathology*. New York: Gower Medical.

Dahlin, D. C., Krishnan, K. U. (1986) *Bone Tumors*, 4th edn. Springfield: C. C. Thomas.

Galasko, C. S. B., Isherwood, I. (eds) (1989) *Imaging Techniques in Orthopaedics*. Berlin: Springer.

Resnick, D., Niwayama, G. (1995) *Diagnosis of Bone and Joint Disorders*, 3rd edn. Philadelphia: W.B. Saunders.

Murray, R. O., Jacobson, H. G., Stoker D. (1989) *The Radiology of Skeletal Disorders*, 3rd edn. Edinburgh: Churchill Livingstone.

Wilner, D. (1982) *Radiology of Bone Tumors and Allied Disorders*. Philadelphia: W.B. Saunders.

Yaghmai, T. (1979) *Angiography of Bone and Soft Tissue Lesions*. Berlin: Springer.

8

METABOLIC AND ENDOCRINE DISORDERS AFFECTING BONE

Jeremy W. R. Young

In general, metabolic bone disease affects the skeleton in one of two ways; there is either too much or too little calcified bone. The latter change, which comprises the majority of metabolic bone disease, is due either to a decrease in the amount of bone formed, or to excessive resorption of bone. In turn this may be due to a variety of causes but most commonly to abnormalities of vitamin D and calcium metabolism, which in turn arise from abnormality of diet or renal function, endocrine abnormalities (particularly of the parathyroid gland), drug therapy or poisoning.

For the most part metabolic processes involve the skeleton as a whole. The radiographic changes of metabolic bone diseases are therefore predominantly diffuse or at least multifocal, involving many areas of the skeleton, although on occasion isolated lesions may be found, such as brown tumors in hyperparathyroidism. Another feature of metabolic bone disease is the tendency to involve specific locations, and to be symmetric in the body, as seen in the 'Looser's zones' of osteomalacia (see below). Radiographic evaluation of metabolic disease, and in particular the evaluation of changes in bone density, is difficult, as up to 40% of bone mass may be lost before it becomes apparent radiographically. Various techniques have been devised for the measurement of bone density. The more important ones are described below.

BONE DENSITY MEASUREMENTS

Radiogrammetry This measures the cortical thickness of metacarpals and other tubular bones from standard radiographs (Fig. 8.1). It is particularly useful in serial studies, and comparison with a large normal population can be made. Although inexpensive and easy to perform, it does not reliably reflect bone mineral content.

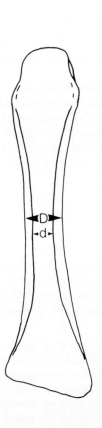

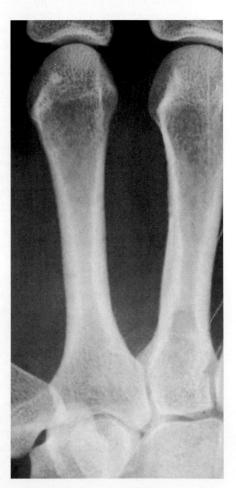

Fig. 8.1 Measurement of the cortical thickness, particularly of the right second metacarpal shaft, has been used widely in assessing bone mass. The measurement D − d = total thickness of cortical bone and is probably the most satisfactory of the simple indices that have been proposed. (Reproduced from C.R. Paterson (1974) *Metabolic Disorders of Bone*, by kind permission of Blackwell, Oxford.)

Single Photon Absorption This couples a monoenergetic photon source such as iodine-125 with a sodium iodide scintillation counter. The mineral content in the scan path is calculated from the difference in photon absorption between bone and soft tissue. The major criticism is that this measures mineral content in the appendicular skeleton, and that cortical bone measurements in the peripheries correlate poorly with dual photon absorptiometry in the spine.

Dual Photon Absorptiometry As a photon source this uses gadolinium-153 which emits photons at two different energy levels. This allows scanning of the spine and femur, as it is independent of variation in soft-tissue thickness. Because of the need to normalize the results due to different bone thickness, the technique cannot measure absolute bone mineral content, but is useful in quantitating mineral content changes. Nevertheless good correlation with CT mineral density evaluation has been obtained.

Neutron Activation Analysis This technique uses high energy neutrons to activate calcium-48 to calcium-49. The decay back to ^{48}Ca can then be measured with a gamma counter. As approximately 98% of body calcium is in the bones, this gives a reasonably accurate determination of total body calcium. With modifications, assessment of regional calcium can also be made. However, the technique is only available in a few specialized centers.

Quantitative Computed Tomography CT is very effective for bone mineral content measurements, and has the advantage of being able to measure small volumes of bone, thus enabling measurement of both cortical and cancellous bone. In practice the mid portion of a vertebral body is used. A mineral reference phantom such as potassium phosphate solution is needed for calibration. Either single or dual-energy techniques may be used, although the accuracy of single-energy CT is variable and depends upon the amount of fat in the bone marrow.

Single-slice techniques are not suitable for bone mineral density readings in the femur, due to the complex trabecular architecture in this region. However this can be obtained by a complex multislice three-dimensional technique with sophisticated computer-generated histograms. At present CT analysis would appear to be the most reliable and adaptable technique for bone density measurements.

Other Techniques The above techniques are those most widely known and used at this time. Other techniques however are also in use or are being developed.

Dual Energy Projection Radiography uses a CT scanner, with the patient scanned during longitudinal motion, multiple readings being obtained through the region of interest. Calibration with a multichamber phantom is again used, and a 'mineral equivalent' value is expressed in g/dl of potassium phosphate. The technique is again only available in specialized centers.

Magnetic Resonance Imaging has been suggested as another technique by virtue of the fact that T_1 and T_2 relaxation times for lumbar vertebral marrow have shown a decrease with increasing age, except for T_2 in women. This is explained by the replacement of active with fatty marrow. More rapid loss of bone mineral content in elderly women may explain the fact that T_1 and T_2 values are greater than in men of the same age. Calibration phantoms will have to be designed, however, to compensate for variations in signal sensitivity and magnetic field variations, if the technique is to become an accurate method for the determination of bone mineral content.

Broad Band Ultrasound Attenuation This technique is not generally available, but measures the attenuation of ultrasound at various frequencies, and calculates the attenuation index. This is based on the fact that attenuation is greater at higher frequencies, and bone therefore acts as a frequency sensitive filter for ultrasound waves. The attenuation, which is expressed in decibels, is an almost linear function of frequency, and the slope of the function is defined as the broad band ultrasound attenuation index. Results suggest that this technique can be used to help differentiate between patients with osteoporosis and healthy patients and is comparable to dual X-ray absorptiometry.

Dual X-ray Absorptiometry This technique uses X-rays, with a collimated beam, scanning over the region of interest in a rectilinear fashion, while the tube potential is switched rapidly between two different kvps (usually 70 and 140 kvp). The bone mineral density is calculated by determining the amount of mineral content related to the projected area of the region of interest.

BIOCHEMISTRY

Biochemical findings in metabolic and endocrine disease of the bone are variable, but can be extremely helpful in making the diagnosis. They are summarized in Table 8.1.

CHANGES DUE TO VITAMIN D ABNORMALITIES

Vitamin D is derived either from the diet, or via the action of ultraviolet light on the skin. After hydroxylation of cholecalciferol in the liver, further hydroxylation occurs in the kidney to generate the active form of vitamin D, 1,25-dihydroxycholecalciferol (1,25 DHCC), which has several modes of action. In bone, homeostasis is maintained as 1,25 DHCC has two actions: mobilization of calcium and phosphorus, and promotion of mineralization and maturation. The former requires the presence of both 1,25 DHCC and parathormone. Also, 1,25 DHCC absorption of calcium and phosphorus is promoted in the intestines. In addition, it affects the kidney, both directly, on proximal renal tubular function, and indirectly, by stimulating production of relatively inert 24,25-dihydroxycholecalciferol, which has a negative feedback effect, limiting 1,25 DHCC production. Finally, there are receptors in other organs, particularly the pituitary, placenta and breast, which are thought to reflect the increased demand for calcium during growth, pregnancy and lactation.

Rickets and Osteomalacia (Vitamin D deficiency)

Rickets and osteomalacia are the same basic disorder, occurring in children and adults respectively. The pathological changes result from an interruption of development and, in particular, mineralization of the growth plate in the developing skeleton, or from lack of mineralization of osteoid in the mature skeleton. They occur as a result of a lack of the actions of vitamin D which in turn may be due to dietary lack, lack of production by the body, failure of absorption, or defective metabolism. In practice, as the body can normally generate sufficient vitamin D when there is adequate

Table 8.1 Laboratory Changes in Metabolic Bone Disease

	Serum Levels				Urine Levels	
	Calcium	Phosphorus	Alkaline phosphatase	Urea or creatinine	Calcium	Hydroxy proline
Osteoporosis	N	N	N	N	N	N or ↑
Hyperparathyroidism						
Primary	↑	↓	N or ↑	N or ↑	N or ↑	↑
Secondary	N or ↓	↑	↑	↑	↓	↑
Tertiary	↑	N or ↓	N or ↑	↑	N or ↑	N or ↑
Hypoparathyroidism	↓	↑	N	N	↓	N
Pseudohypoparathyroidism	↓	↑	N	N	↓	N
Hyperthyroidism	N or ↑	N	N	N	↑	↑
Rickets/osteomalacia						
Vitamin D deficiency	↓	↓	↑	N	↓	N
Vitamin D refractory	N	↓	↑	N or ↑	↓	N
Hypophosphatasia	N or ↑	N	↓	N	N or ↑	↓

N = normal   ↑ = elevated   ↓ = lowered

ultraviolet light, nutritional deficiency only occurs when there is a dietary lack together with too little exposure to ultraviolet light. This is most commonly seen in black immigrants who make their homes in colder and less sunny areas. It may also occur in the neglected elderly, particularly in larger cities in the higher latitudes.

Malabsorption states, including Crohn's disease and scleroderma, can result in osteomalacia (see Table 8.2). Liver disease, whether ductal or hepatocellular, is also a cause of osteomalacia, although osteoporosis is also found histologically. The osteomalacia of liver disease is multi-factorial, but appears largely due to malabsorption of vitamin D, as bile salts are necessary for vitamin D absorption in micelle form. In celiac disease, the small bowel is less responsive to the action of vitamin D in calcium transport.

Drug therapy may produce osteomalacia, particularly long-term anticonvulsant therapy (phenytoin/dilantin). A similar effect has also been reported with rifampicin and glutethimide.

Finally, many toxins have been found to cause osteomalacia by causing tubular damage and phosphate deficiency. These include aluminum hydroxide, magnesium sulfate, and cadmium, the latter being associated with alkaline battery manufacture, or the painful condition of 'itai-itai' (ouch, ouch) reported in Japan in patients drinking cadmium-polluted water.

RICKETS

There are many causes of rickets in childhood. In general, however, the radiological features are similar, although varying in severity and location. The skeletal effects are due to a lack of calcification of osteoid. Consequently the most obvious changes are at the metaphysis, where the most rapid growth is occurring. The initial abnormality is a loss of the normal 'zone of provisional calcification' adjacent to the metaphysis, although usually, by the time radiographs are obtained, significant metaphyseal abnormality is seen. This begins as an indistinctness of the metaphyseal margin, progressing to a 'frayed' appearance with a widening of the growth plate, due to lack of calcification of metaphyseal bone Fig. 8.2). Weight-bearing and stress on the uncalcified bone give rise to splaying and cupping of the metaphysis (Fig. 8.3).

A similar but less marked effect occurs in the subperiosteal layer, which may cause lack of distinctness of the cortical margin.

Table 8.2 Malabsorption States Causing Osteomalacia

Crohn's disease
Celiac disease
Lymphoma
Amyloidosis
Small bowel fistula
Postoperative states (bowel resection)
Hepatobiliary disease

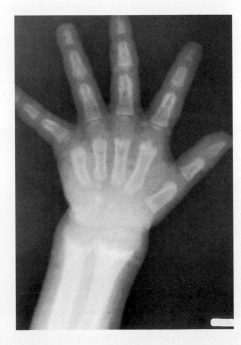

Fig. 8.2 Rickets. There is obvious 'fraying' of the metaphyseal margin, with a wide growth plate seen at the distal radius and metacarpals.

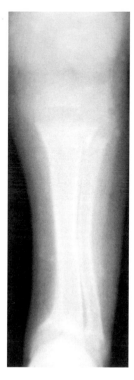

Fig. 8.3 Rickets. There is splaying of all the visible metaphyses with, in addition, some characteristic S-shaped bowing of the bones of the lower leg.

Eventually a generalized reduction in bone density is seen, and in longstanding cases fractures may occur. Looser's zones are not seen as often as in osteomalacia (see below). In the epiphysis there may be some haziness of the cortical margins.

With treatment mineralization occurs, giving rise to a dense white line at the zone of provisional calcification adjacent to the metaphysis, but becoming contiguous with the metaphysis during the healing process. In cases of intermittent dietary vitamin deficiency, or inadequate treatment, the metaphysis will show patchy sclerosis. In severe cases of rickets additional deformities of the bones occur, with bowing of the long bones (particularly of the lower limbs—(Fig. 8.3), thoracic kyphosis with a 'pigeon chest', enlargement of the anterior ribs causing the 'rickety rosary' (Fig. 8.4), and bossing of the skull. Rickets may be seen in low-birthweight and premature infants, and may be severe, causing spontaneous fractures and respiratory difficulty. Affected infants are usually below 1000 g in weight, or less than 28 weeks' gestation.

Vitamin D-resistant rickets (Familial hypophosphatasia)

This condition is usually inherited in a dominant sex-linked fashion. Affected women pass the disease on to half of their sons and daughters, whilst affected men pass the disease on to none of their sons and half of their daughters. The disease is similar to rickets in radiographic appearance, but it is refractory to vitamin D therapy, and growth retardation may be marked. The radiographic changes are variable from mild to severe, and may be similar to the metaphyseal dysplasia of the Schmid variety (see Ch. 1).

Acquired Hypophosphatemic Rickets

Rarely, hypophosphatemia has been seen in association with tumors of bone or soft tissues, frequently fibrous in origin. It has also been reported in association with prostatic carcinoma and oat-cell carcinoma of the lung; a similar condition has also been reported with other conditions, e.g. neurofibromatosis, fibrous dysplasia.

Vitamin D-Resistant Rickets Associated with Renal Tubular Disorders

A variety of renal dysfunction syndromes produce rickets and osteomalacia. These include hypercalcemia, renal phosphate loss and secondary hypophosphatemia, aminoaciduria and renal tubular acidosis. In renal tubular acidosis affected patients demonstrate retarded growth and short stature. As well as the changes of osteomalacia, nephrocalcinosis and nephrolithiasis are seen (Fig. 8.5).

Osteomalacia

This refers to the changes resulting from vitamin D deficiency in the mature skeleton. Bone pain is a frequent complaint. Serum

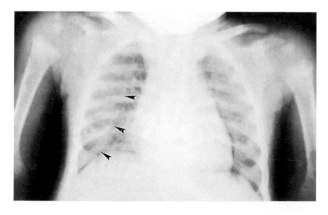

Fig. 8.4 Rickety rosary. Widening of the anterior ribs is clearly demonstrated. The classic metaphyseal changes of rickets are also seen in the proximal humeri.

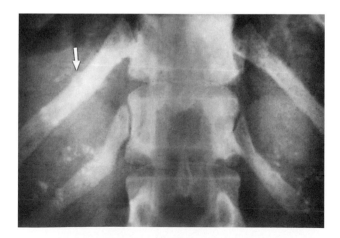

Fig. 8.5 Renal tubular acidosis. The combination of nephrocalcinosis and osteomalacia (Looser's zone—arrow) in the right 11th rib is characteristic, although symptomatic bone disease affects only a minority of patients. (Courtesy of Dr D.J. Stoker and Institute of Orthopaedics.)

alkaline phosphatase is elevated, and serum phosphorus is low. The hallmark of osteomalacia is the pseudofracture or 'Looser's zone'. This is a narrow zone of lucency, usually running perpendicular or nearly perpendicular to the bone cortex. Initially poorly defined, these zones become progressively more prominent, with sclerotic margins (Fig. 8.6). They are generally accepted as occurring at sites of stress as subclinical stress fractures that are repaired by unossified osteoid. They are frequently bilateral and symmetric, and occur at regular sites (Fig. 8.7) such as the pubic rami, proximal femur (Fig. 8.8), scapula (Fig. 8.6), lower ribs, and ulna (Fig. 8.9). Osteopenia develops with 'pencilling-in' of the vertebral bodies, and loss of vertebral height in a characteristic 'codfish vertebra' pattern (Fig. 8.10).

Bowing of the long bones may occur. Compression wedge fractures of the vertebrae are less common than in osteoporosis. The histopathology of osteomalacia is characteristic, with excessive osteoid and/or failure of ossification of new bone.

Hypophosphatasia

Inherited as an autosomal recessive trait, this rare disorder presents with a radiographic picture which varies from a mild to a very severe form of rickets, depending upon the age of onset, the neonatal variety being most severe and generally lethal. There is a low serum alkaline phosphatase, and increased urinary phosphoethanolamine. In severe cases an exaggerated fraying of the metaphysis is seen, with uncalcified osteoid extending into the metaphysis (Fig. 8.11). Craniostenosis and nephrocalcinosis may occur, and deformities, particularly of the distal phalanges and tibia, are seen.

Familial Hyperphosphatemia

An extremely rare condition of autosomal recessive inheritance, this presents in early infancy. The radiographic appearance is

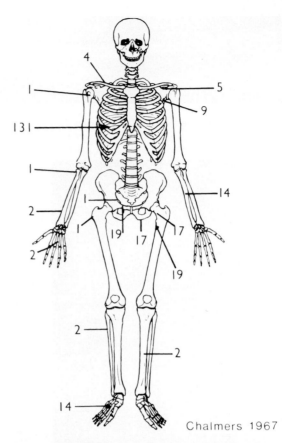

Chalmers 1967

Fig. 8.7   Sites of incidence of Looser's zones in osteomalacia in a group of middle-aged and elderly patients with dietetic osteomalacia. (Courtesy of Dr D.J. Stoker and Institute of Orthopaedics.)

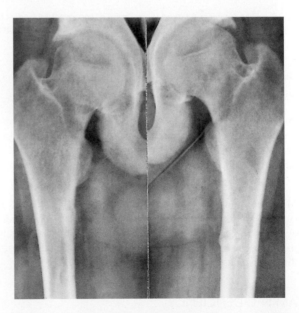

Fig. 8.8   Looser's zones. Symmetric lucencies are seen involving the medial cortex of the proximal femur bilaterally—another characteristic site.

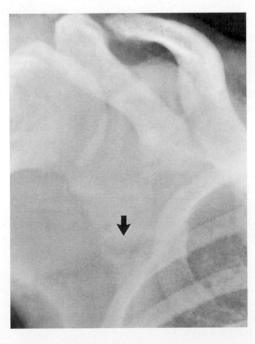

Fig. 8.6   Looser's zone. There is lucency with surrounding sclerosis in the lateral border of the scapula—a common site.

similar to that of Paget's disease, but occurring in infancy and demonstrating more symmetry; the conditions however are unrelated. The skull vault is thickened and the long bones are

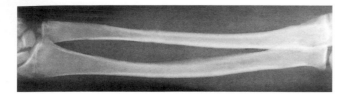

Fig. 8.9 Looser's zone. The characteristic lucency of the mid ulna is seen.

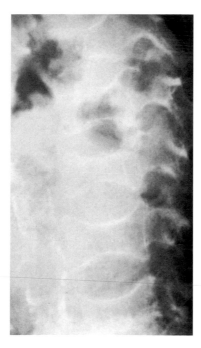

Fig. 8.10 Osteomalacia. Marked biconcavity of the vertebral bodies (codfish vertebrae). (Courtesy of Dr D.J. Stoker and Institute of Orthopaedics.)

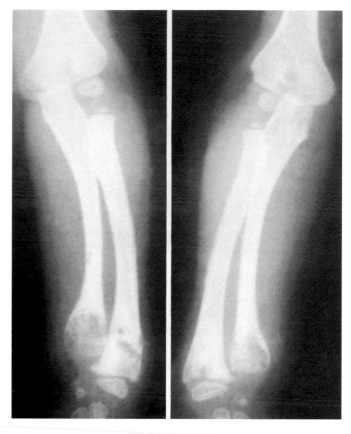

Fig. 8.11 Hypophosphatasia. In this child metaphyseal ossification is delayed in the ulnae whilst the distal radii contain islands of non-ossified tissue. (Courtesy of Dr D.J. Stoker and Institute of Orthopaedics.)

tubular, enlarged and bowed, but with cortical irregularity (Fig. 8.12). Serum alkaline phosphatase is elevated.

Fibrogenesis Imperfecta Ossium   This rare disorder presents with coarsening of the trabecular pattern of the bones, and in particular the ends of the long bones. Multiple fractures are seen. Serum alkaline phosphatase is elevated.

Axial Osteomalacia   This rare condition is characterized by a coarsening of the bony trabeculae, similar to that seen in fibrogenesis imperfecta ossium, but only involving the vertebrae, pelvis and ribs. Histologically osteomalacia is found, but serum alkaline phosphatase levels are normal.

VITAMIN C DEFICIENCY

Vitamin C deficiency leads to a deficiency in the formation of bone matrix, as it is necessary for the formation of hydroxyproline, which is vital for collagen. About 90% of the matrix of mature bone is collagen, and hence a lack of collagen will have a severe effect on bone formation. In childhood, this gives rise to scurvy. The adult counterpart is osteoporosis.

Scurvy

Scurvy is rare before six months of age since the storage of vitamin C in the neonate is generally adequate. Children present with limb pain and irritability. Radiographically, four characteristic signs are seen.

1. The epiphysis is small, and sharply marginated by a sclerotic rim (Wimberger sign) (Fig. 8.13).
2. The zone of provisional calcification at the growing metaphysis is dense, giving a white line (Fränkel's line) (Fig. 8.13).
3. Beneath this is a lucent zone, due to lack of mineralization of osteoid (Trumerfeld zone).
4. Finally, as this area is weakened, it is prone to fractures which manifest themselves at the cortical margin, giving rise to (Pelkan's) spurs.

In addition, due to capillary fragility, subperiosteal hemorrhages occur (Fig. 8.14) which may give rise to periosteal elevation and subsequent new bone formation, particularly following treatment. This dense periosteal new bone should be differentiated from that found in battered infants.

Following treatment, dense bands of bone may be left, resembling growth arrest lines.

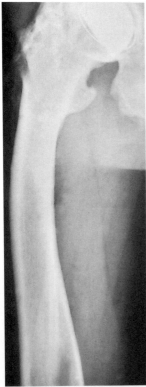

Fig. 8.12 Familial hyperphosphatemia. **A**. The femur is abnormal with some bowing, increased width, and prominent but irregular cortex, somewhat resembling Paget's disease (Courtesy of Dr C.S. Resnik). **B**. The radiological appearances in this child are diagnostic. The bones are widened with loss of differentiation of cortex and medulla. A coarse trabecular pattern and bowing are also evident. These features resemble those of Paget's disease. (Courtesy of Dr D.J. Stoker and Institute of Orthopaedics.)

A

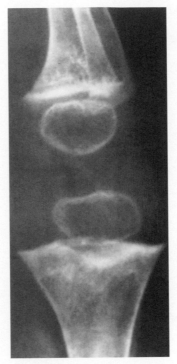

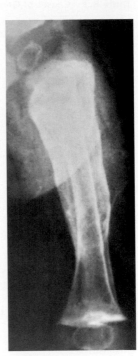

Fig. 8.13   *Fig. 8.14*

Fig. 8.13 Scurvy. The margins of the epiphyses are sclerotic (Wimberger sign). There is a narrow epiphyseal plate, with increased density of the zone of provisional calcification (Fränkel's line). The lucent zone beneath this is due to lack of mineralized osteoid (Trumerfeld zone).

Fig. 8.14 Scurvy. Subperiosteal hemorrhage has elevated the periosteum. The healing stage shows marked periosteal new bone formation. (Courtesy of Dr C.S. Resnik.)

OSTEOPOROSIS

Osteoporosis is the most frequent metabolic bone disease, and is due to a decrease in bone mass. It is the result of many underlying causes (Table 8.3). In general, the loss of bone mass gives rise to increased incidence of fractures, particularly in the femoral neck, spine (compression fractures), distal radius, and pubic symphysis. In osteoporosis the microstructure of the bone is normal, but the quantity of bone is diminished. This eventually gives rise to a clear loss of bone density, radiographically best described as osteopenia. This radiographic appearance of generalized osteopenia however is not specific to osteoporosis and can be seen in a variety of conditions (Table 8.4).

In addition there are many conditions that can give rise to localized osteopenia (Table 8.5).

In osteoporosis trabecular loss is most evident radiographically in the spine where there is a loss of density, which may be appreciated as 'pencilling in' of the vertebra by the more radiographically dense end-plates (Fig. 8.15). Biconcave vertebral bodies (codfish vertebrae) may occur. In the femoral neck the osteopenia is manifested by an apparent increase in density of the residual trabeculae (Fig. 8.16). Endosteal and intracortical resorption of bone is prominent, producing cortical thinning most evident in the appendicular skeleton.

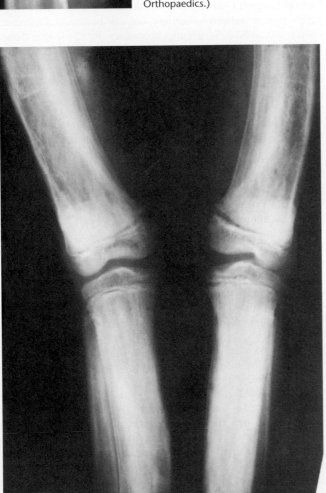

B

Table 8.3   Causes of Generalized Osteoporosis

Age-related conditions (senile and post-menopausal states)
Deficiency states
Malnutrition
Calcium deficiency
Scurvy
Drugs
Steroids
Heparin
Metabolic
Hyperthyroidism
Hyperparathyroidism
Cushing's disease
Acromegaly
Pregnancy
Diabetes mellitus
Hypogonadism
Alcoholism
Chronic liver disease
Anemias
Idiopathic

Table 8.4   Major Causes of Diffuse Osteopenia

Osteoporosis
Osteomalacia
Hyperparathyroidism
Neoplasia (particularly multiple myeloma)

Table 8.5   Major Causes of Localized Osteoporosis

Immobilization
Post-fracture
Sudeck's atrophy
Arthritis
Infection

Post-Menopausal and Senile Osteoporosis *(Involutional Osteoporosis)*   Post-menopausal osteoporosis occurs in women typically aged 50–65. There is a disproportionate loss of trabecular bone, giving rise to rapid bone loss, and a proportionate increase in fractures, particularly of the vertebrae and distal radius. In the vertebrae, loss of height and anterior wedging occur, which may lead to a marked kyphotic deformity (Fig. 8.15). The changes of osteoporosis have been linked to reduced estrogen levels, although additional factors such as skeletal size, level of activity, nutritional status and genetic determinants have been proposed. In general, once osteoporosis is established, estrogen therapy does not affect the radiographic density of the bone. Blood chemistry is usually normal, although urinary hydroxyproline levels may be elevated in the acute stage.

Senile osteoporosis differs from post-menopausal osteoporosis in that there is proportionate loss of cortical and trabecular bone. Fractures occur most commonly in the femoral neck, proximal humerus, tibia and pelvis. There is no dramatic increase in bone loss in the post-menopausal stage, and patients tend to be older. The ratio of affected women to men is approximately 2:1. The etiology is uncertain, but reduced intestinal absorption, diminished adrenal function and secondary hyperparathyroidism may play a role.

Idiopathic Juvenile Osteoporosis   This disorder is a rare self-limiting disease that affects both sexes and occurs typically before puberty. Patients present with bone pain, backache or limp related to fractures, characteristically of the metaphysis of the long bones with minimal trauma. Compressions of the vertebrae with kyphosis may result. The diagnosis is one of exclusion, particularly from leukemia, lymphoma and hypercorticosteroid states. Another radiographic diagnostic consideration is osteogenesis imperfecta, as this also presents with diffuse osteoporosis and multiple fractures (Fig. 8.17). Blood chemistry is normal.

Idiopathic Male Osteoporosis   A number of male patients present with generalized osteopenia before the age of 60. No definite predisposing factors have been found. Hypercalciuria and increased calcium absorption seem to be constant findings, and the condition may be an acquired defect in bone metabolism. Again, this is a diagnosis of exclusion.

Endocrine-induced Osteoporosis

Abnormality of function of the adrenal, pituitary and thyroid glands, hyperfunction of the parathyroids and hypofunction of the pancreas and gonads have all been linked with osteoporosis. As well as osteoporosis, other skeletal abnormalities are associated with particular endocrine disorders.

Steroid-induced Osteoporosis *(Cushing's disease)*   Glucocortical excess may be related to therapy, but can be due to a number of causes although it is usually secondary to Cushing's disease. Histologic studies have revealed decreased bone formation and increased resorption. Biochemically there is a negative calcium balance and hypercalciuria. Exuberant callus formation at fractures is seen, particularly in long bones, ribs (Fig. 8.18) and vertebral bodies. In the latter case, a characteristic increased density of the end-plates occurs (Fig. 8.19). Avascular necrosis may occur, particularly of the femoral head. In children, growth may be retarded. Rib fractures may be multiple, painless and unsuspected.

Hypogonadism   In boys, this results in delayed closure of the epiphyseal plates. As a result, the patients have long limbs in relation to their trunks. A similar hypogonadal disorder in girls (Turner syndrome), results in short stature, increased carrying angle at the elbow, a short fourth metacarpal and changes of Blount's disease at the knee. Congenital cardiovascular anomalies also occur, most commonly coarctation of the aorta.

The thyroid gland

Hyperthyroidism   In hyperthyroidism, a generalized osteoporosis may be seen. There is an increased metabolic ratio, with an increase in both bone formation and resorption. Increased cortical striations of the long bones are seen. Thyroid therapy acropachy is a rare condition which usually follows therapy for previous hyperthyroidism or occurs in patients who have been on thyroid therapy for many years. There is a characteristic periosteal thickening in the extremities and particularly in the hands (Fig. 8.20). It must be distinguished from hypertrophic osteoarthropathy which is also found in the extremities (Figs 8.21, 8.22) but is usually exquisitely painful. Exophthalmos and pretibial myxedema are frequently present. Rarely, hyperthyroidism appears in childhood, when accelerated skeletal maturation occurs.

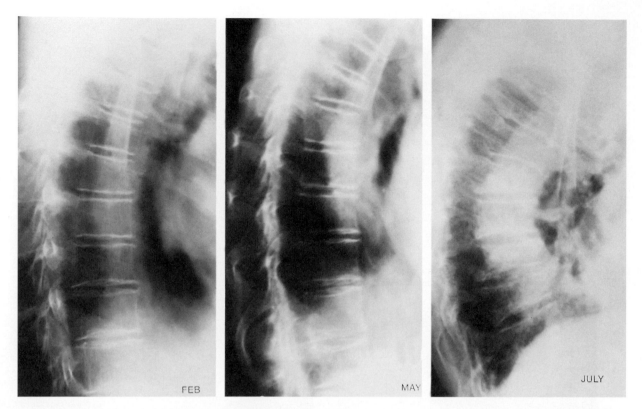

Fig. 8.15   Post-menopausal osteoporosis. Serial films in this patient show the progressive development of kyphosis as a result of anterior wedging of the thoracic vertebral bodies during the course of six months. (Courtesy of Dr D.J. Stoker and Institute of Orthopaedics.)

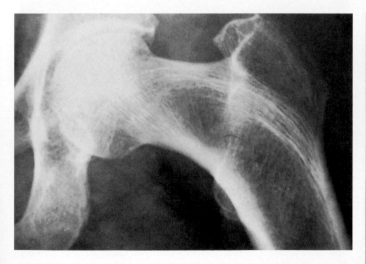

Fig. 8.16   Osteoporosis. In this patient, resorption of the secondary trabeculae has left the primary trabeculae to delineate the lines of stress within the femoral neck.

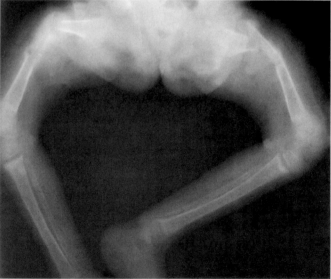

Fig. 8.17   Osteogenesis imperfecta. There is diffuse osteoporosis, with fractures of both femora. These are already showing marked callus formation.

Hypothyroidism   Although it is not associated with osteoporosis, it is appropriate to discuss this condition at this point. In children, skeletal maturation is delayed and growth is retarded. Epiphyses are late in appearing (Fig. 8.23) and fragmented, although when they do appear the sequence is normal. This may cause an appearance in the hip that must be differentiated from Perthes disease. Wormian bones are seen in the skull, and the sella is either small and bowl-shaped (young children), or of large rounded 'cherry sella' configuration (older children). The paranasal sinuses are underdeveloped. In the spine, bullet-shaped vertebral bodies are seen, especially at the thoracolumbar junction, where kyphosis may develop. All the long bones are

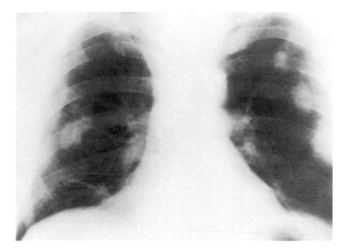

Fig. 8.18 Cushing's disease. Excessive callus formation is seen at multiple fracture sites in the ribs. The patient had functional adrenal carcinoma.

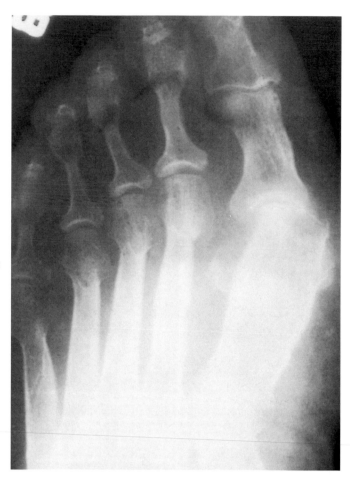

Fig. 8.20 Thyroid acropachy. A dense periosteal reaction is seen along the first metatarsal. Although this can occur in any of the digits, the first is a characteristic site.

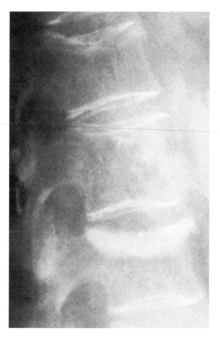

Fig. 8.19 Cushing's disease. Generalized reduction in bone density simulates post-menopausal osteoporosis in this patient. The compression fracture of the superior border of the body of L4 has characteristically produced dense callus. This feature is almost, but not entirely, pathognomonic of glucocorticosteroid excess. (Courtesy of Dr D.J. Stoker and Institute of Orthopaedics.)

short. In the pelvis the incidence of slipped capital femoral epiphysis is increased, and the pelvis itself is often narrow, with coxa vara deformities. In the adult the changes are exaggerated (Fig. 8.24).

Hyperpituitarism *(Acromegaly)*

It is questionable whether acromegaly is a cause for true osteoporosis. It will however be included in this section. Gigantism in the immature skeleton, and acromegaly in the adult,

result from excessive growth hormone production by an eosinophilic adenoma. The radiographic features of acromegaly include enlarged mastoid air cells and sinuses, frontal bossing and prognathism (Fig. 8.25). Pituitary fossa enlargement may be seen on the plain film (Fig. 8.25), although CT and MRI are more helpful in evaluating for a pituitary adenoma (see Ch. 57). In the spine, enlargement of the vertebral bodies with posterior scalloping is seen (Fig. 8.26). The hands show characteristic enlargement of the bones and soft tissues with spade-like terminal tufts, or arrowhead distal phalanges (Fig. 8.27). Widening of the joint spaces due to overgrowth of articular cartilage may be seen (Fig. 8.27). The feet show evidence of increased thickness of the heel pads although this is no longer regarded as an infallible sign of acromegaly (Fig. 8.28). The long bones of the feet are elongated, although the feet usually remain slender. Prominence of muscle attachments, and premature or exaggerated degenerative change may be seen (Fig. 8.29). Calcification of the pinna of the ear occurs. Chondrocalcinosis has been reported as a rare variation, although crystal arthropathy has been suggested as the underlying cause by some authors.

The parathyroid glands

Hypoparathyroidism Rarely, osteoporosis is seen in patients

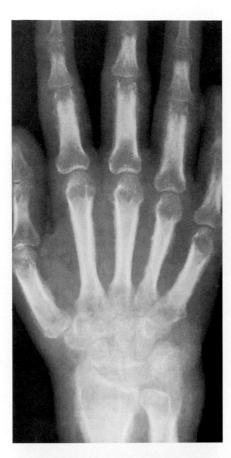

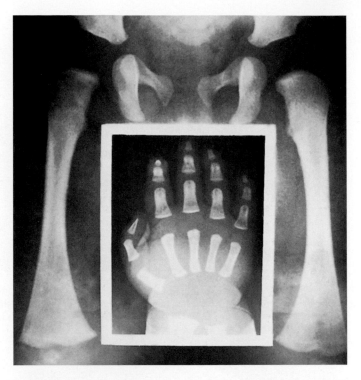

Fig. 8.23 Cretinism. Marked skeletal retardation was present in this 12-month-old child. Note that the carpal and proximal femoral centers have not yet appeared. (Courtesy of Dr D.J. Stoker and Institute of Orthopaedics.)

Fig. 8.21 Hypertrophic (pulmonary) osteoarthropathy. There is marked periosteal reaction along most of the visualized bones.

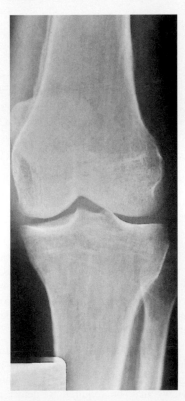

Fig. 8.22 Hypertrophic osteoarthropathy: periosteal reaction is identified along the medial aspect of the distal femur.

with hypoparathyroidism. The most common cause for hypoparathyroidism is parathyroid gland removal at thyroid surgery, or ^{131}I thyroid therapy. Rarely it can result from excessive therapeutic radiation, hemorrhage, infection, tumor deposition in the thyroid gland, or iron deposition in iron overload conditions. Idiopathic hypoparathyroidism, either autoimmune or familial, can occur without atrophy of the glands. It is associated with a variety of endocrine and immune deficiency states including Addison's disease, ovarian dysgenesis, hypothyroidism and chronic mucocutaneous candidiasis. Circulating antibodies to the parathyroid, thyroid and adrenal glands have been found. Calcium deposition in the basal ganglia occurs and osteosclerosis, particularly of the pelvis, inner table of the skull, proximal femur, and vertebral bodies can be seen, as well as abnormal tooth development. Serum calcium is low, and phosphate diuresis follows parathormone administration.

Pseudohypoparathyroidism This is inherited in a dominant fashion and is characterized by hypocalcemia and hyperphosphatemia which are unresponsive to parathormone. The parathyroid glands are normal, but there is 'end-organ' resistance to parathormone. This may be due to a defect in the adenyl cyclase cyclic AMP system in the renal tubules and bones. Basal ganglia calcification is more common than in idiopathic hypoparathyroidism. Short metacarpals are seen, particularly the fourth and fifth (Fig. 8.30). Abnormal dentition is also seen, with hypoplasia and cranial defects, and there may be calcification in the connective tissues of the skin, ligaments, tendons and fascial planes. Coxa vara, coxa valga, cone-shaped epiphyses, and bowing of long bones are also reported. Secondary hyperparathyroidism is a feature of this disorder.

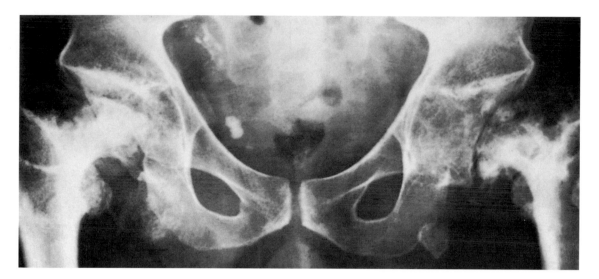

Fig. 8.24 Adult cretinism. This 39-year-old man received no therapy until four years before this film was obtained. Coxa vara is present, whilst the femoral heads are deformed and irregularly ossified in the absence of thyroid hormone during development. (Courtesy of Dr D.J. Stoker and Institute of Orthopaedics.)

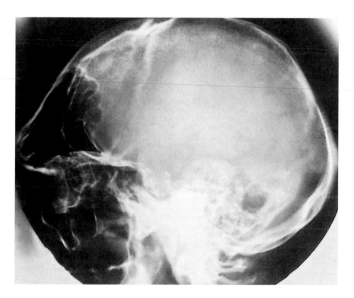

Fig. 8.25 Acromegaly. The frontal sinuses are markedly enlarged, and there is frontal bossing. A double floor is seen in the pituitary fossa with 'ballooning'.

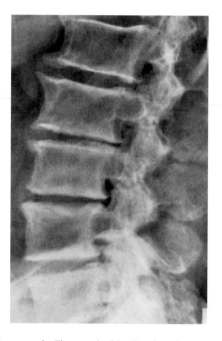

Fig. 8.26 Acromegaly. The vertebral bodies show bony overgrowth. Mild posterior scalloping is also seen at several levels. (Courtesy of Dr C.S. Resnik.)

Pseudopseudohypoparathyroidism This condition presents with the same clinical and radiographic appearances as pseudohypoparathyroidism, but with normal blood chemistry.

Hyperparathyroidism

This condition is divided into the primary, secondary and tertiary forms. In the **primary** form, increased hormone production occurs as a result of parathyroid adenomas (75%), hyperplasia or carcinoma. It occurs most commonly in middle-aged and elderly people, and is more common in women (2:1). Symptoms include weakness, lassitude, constipation, polydypsia, polyuria, peptic ulceration, renal calculi and psychiatric problems. Radiographically, bone resorption is seen, and although frank osteopenia is difficult to detect radiographically in early cases, bone mineral content measurements confirm bone mineral loss in approximately 50% of cases. More advanced cases demonstrate bone density loss, and sometimes ground-glass appearance.

Subperiosteal erosion of bone, particularly along the radial aspect of the middle phalanx of the middle and index finger is virtually pathognomonic (Fig. 8.31), although fine-grain film or magnification views may be required to detect it. Other sites include the medial aspect of the proximal tibia (Fig. 8.32), femur

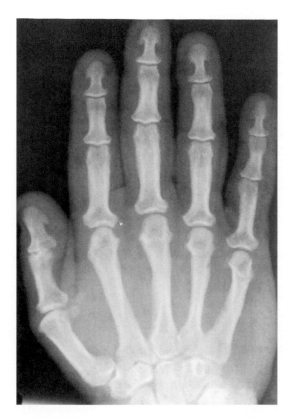

Fig. 8.27   Acromegaly. There is obvious enlargement of the soft tissues and phalanges with prominent joint spaces due to increased cartilage thickness. The distal phalanges show the characteristic 'arrowhead' configuration.

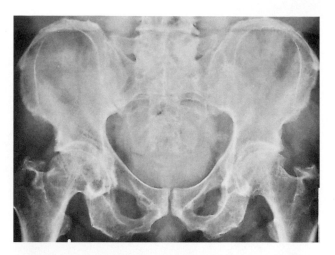

Fig. 8.29   Acromegaly. There is overgrowth of the bone in the iliac crests and irregular bony prominence of the sites of muscle attachments throughout the pelvis.

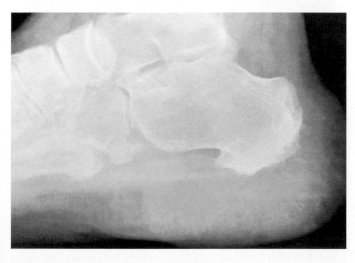

Fig. 8.28   Acromegaly. There is marked prominence of the soft tissues of the heel pad which measures approximately 35 mm.

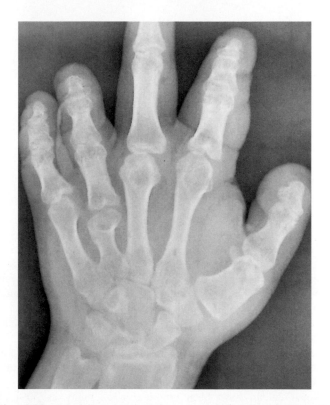

Fig. 8.30   Pseudohypoparathyroidism. A markedly short fourth metacarpal bone is seen. Although not specific for pseudohypoparathyroidism, this is a characteristic finding. (Courtesy of Dr C.S. Resnik.)

and humerus, and the ribs. Loss of the lamina dura around the teeth occurs, although this is not specific for hyperparathyroidism.

Subchondral bone resorption is another common occurrence, being found at the distal, and sometimes proximal end of the clavicle (Fig. 8.33), symphysis pubis and sacroiliac joints. This may also occur at the vertebral end-plates, which may permit disk herniation (Schmorl's nodes).

Intracortical bone resorption is another feature of hyperparathyroidism, resulting from osteoclastic activity within the Haversian canals. This gives rise to small (2–5 mm) oval or cigar-shaped lucencies within the cortex (Fig. 8.34). This is a feature of rapid bone turnover, and is also seen in other conditions, such as *hyperthyroidism*, *osteomalacia* and *acute (focal) osteoporosis* (Fig. 8.35). Loss of the corticomedullary junction may occur with a 'basket-work' appearance to the cortex. In the skull, a characteristic

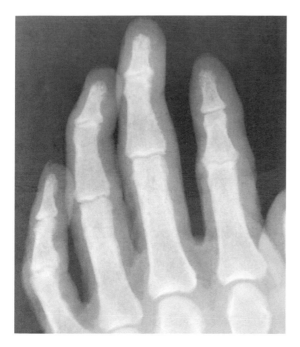

Fig. 8.31 Hyperparathyroidism. There is marked subperiosteal resorption of the radial aspect of many of the phalanges and erosion of the tufts. (Courtesy of Dr D.J. Stoker and Institute of Orthopaedics.)

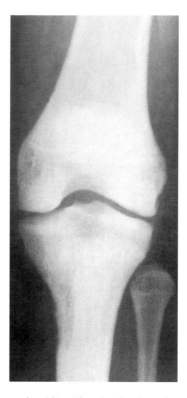

Fig. 8.32 Hyperparathyroidism. There is subperiosteal erosion of the medial side of the proximal tibia.

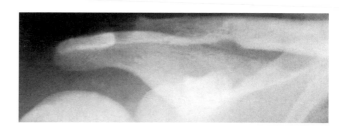

Fig. 8.33 Hyperparathyroidism. There is subperiosteal erosion of the distal end of the clavicle, as well as on the inferior surface at the site of the attachment of the coracoclavicular ligament.

granular or mottled appearance may occur, giving rise to the so-called 'pepper-pot' or 'salt-and-pepper' (USA) skull (Fig. 8.36).

Subligamentous resorption occurs at sites of ligament or tendon insertions, and is seen in the ischial tuberosity, greater and lesser trochanters, inferior calcaneus and inferior surface of the distal clavicle (Fig. 8.33).

Brown tumors are locally destructive areas of intense osteoclastic activity. They present as a lytic lesion which may be expansive (Fig. 8.37), and may destroy the overlying cortex. Pathological fractures may occur (Fig. 8.38). The lesions are generally well defined, and may be multilocular. Following treatment, they may resolve, but can persist for many years.

Rarely, an erosive arthropathy may also occur. This usually involves the hands, wrists and shoulders. It may simulate the appearance of rheumatoid arthritis, but subperiosteal resorption is usually a concurrent feature, and the distal interphalangeal joints are often involved, unlike rheumatoid arthritis.

Renal calculi have been reported in as many as 50% of patients. The majority are calcium oxalate, although a minority are uric acid stones. Nephrocalcinosis also occurs, but is less common.

Secondary hyperparathyroidism Parathyroid hyperplasia involving all of the glands occurs in response to persistent hypocalcemia. This can be seen in *rickets, osteomalacia* and *chronic renal failure*. The skeletal changes are similar to those of primary hyperparathyroidism although brown tumors are less frequently seen. Nevertheless, as secondary hyperparathyroidism is so much more common than primary hyperparathyroidism, in practice brown tumors are more commonly seen as a result of the former. Calcification of arteries and soft tissues occurs, but is most common in the secondary hyperparathyroidism of renal osteodystrophy.

Chronic renal failure can result from numerous diseases, the most common of which is glomerulonephritis. Musculoskeletal manifestations are increasingly recognized, due to improving long-term patient survival secondary to hemodialysis. The radiographic appearances fall into two distinct categories: those associated with renal osteodystrophy itself, and those relating to aluminum toxicity, amyloid deposition, crystal deposition, infection, and avascular necrosis.

Renal osteodystrophy is of particular interest as it combines the findings of osteomalacia, hyperparathyroidism and bone sclerosis. As in hyperparathyroidism, the commonest finding in secondary hyperparathyroidism of renal osteodystrophy is subperiosteal absorption, although all manifestations may be seen. The reported prevalence of osseous resorption has been shown to increase from 10% in the early stages of disease, to 50–70% of patients after 3–9 years of dialysis. With improving techniques of hemodialysis, however, and the use of parathyroidectomy, bone resorption (ex-

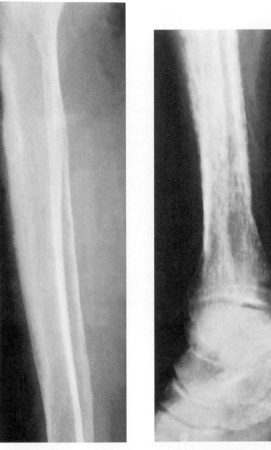

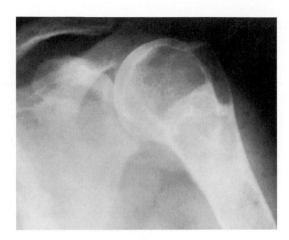

Fig. 8.37 Brown tumor of hyperparathyroidism. There is a well-defined, lytic, mildly expansive lesion of the proximal humerus.

Fig. 8.34   Fig. 8.35

Fig. 8.34 Hyperparathyroidism. Intracortical bone resorption is seen, with multiple small oval lucencies within the cortical bone.

Fig. 8.35 Severe disuse osteoporosis. There is marked intracortical bone resorption, particularly evident in the tibia.

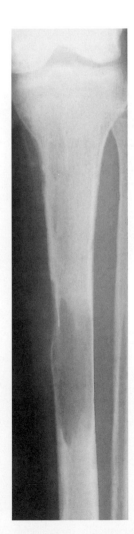

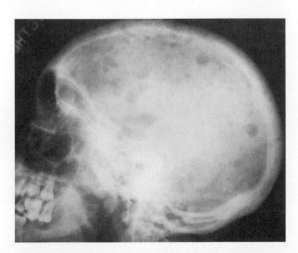

Fig. 8.36 Hyperparathyroidism. 'Salt-and-pepper' or 'pepper-pot' skull. There are multiple characteristic lucencies throughout the skull.

Fig. 8.38 Brown tumor of the mid tibia. The patient was found to have a parathyroid adenoma.

cluding subchondral resorption in the hands) often shows resolution. Calcification of arteries, articular cartilage and periarticular tissues also occurs in renal osteodystrophy.

Osteomalacia is identified predominantly by the presence of Looser's zones. Osteosclerosis occurs in 9–34% of patients, and may occasionally be the only manifestation of renal osteo-dystrophy. It has a predilection for the axial skeleton, favoring the vertebral end-plates (rugger jersey spine—Fig. 8.39), the pelvis, ribs and clavicles. It also involves the metaphyses (rarely epiphyses) of long bones, and the skull.

Osteopenia has been reported in up to 85% of patients, and is the end result of the effects of osteomalacia, bone resorption, and a decrease in bone quantity (osteoporosis). This is due to a combination of factors including chronic metabolic acidosis, poor nutrition, azotemia, steroid use, hyperparathyroidism and low levels of vitamin D.

In children, metaphyseal changes resembling rickets are seen, which together with cortical erosions can give rise to the so-called 'rotting fence-post' appearance, particularly at the femoral neck (Fig. 8.40). Slipped capital epiphyses are also seen as a complication, most commonly involving the proximal femur.

Other Manifestations A form of *arthropathy* has been associated with chronic renal failure, and is seen in patients on long-term hemodialysis. This consists of changes resembling Charcot joints, but without the extensive bone debris. The most common sites are the shoulder and spine (Fig. 8.41). The etiology is most likely *crystal deposition* and *amyloidosis*.

Aluminum accumulation occurs in long-term hemodialysis patients, resulting most commonly from the ingestion of aluminum salts in phosphate-binding antacids used to control hyper-phosphatemia. The effects are mostly cerebral and musculoskeletal. Many of the changes are identical to those of osteomalacia, but the characteristics of aluminum toxicity are lack of osteosclerosis, less evidence of subperiosteal resorption, avascular necrosis, and more than three fractures not associated with trauma. The ribs, vertebrae, hips and pelvis are the commonest sites, although the extremities, particularly the long bones, may be involved.

Crystal deposition also occurs in chronic renal failure patients. The crystals involved are calcium hydroxyapatite (CPPD), monosodium urate, and calcium oxalate. These can induce synovitis and bursitis. Interestingly, however, the typical arthritic changes of CPPD are unusual.

Osteomyelitis and *septic arthritis* with bacteria or fungi are well-recognized complications, particularly after long-term hemodialysis, and transplantation. Predisposing fractures are immunosuppressive therapy, long-term debilitation, and dialysis arteriovenous fistulae, providing an entry site for the organisms.

Avascular necrosis, most likely resulting from steroid therapy, is common, occurring in up to 40% of patients after renal trans-plantation. This most commonly involves the femoral head, although the humeral head, knee, and talus are frequently involved.

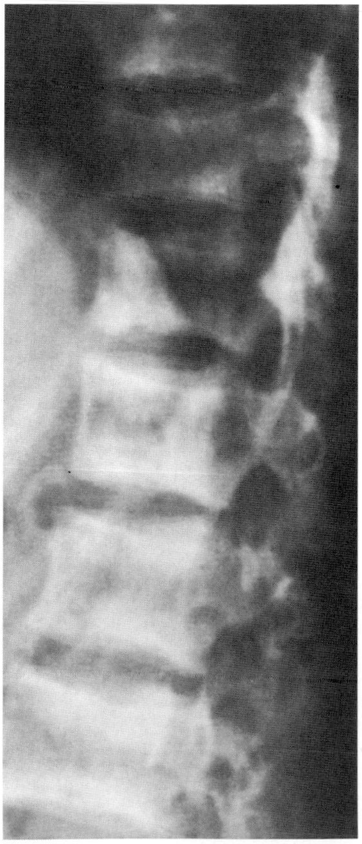

Fig. 8.39 Renal osteodystrophy: 'rugger jersey' spine. Typical end-plate sclerosis is seen with alternating bands of lucency. (Courtesy of Dr D.J. Stoker and Institute of Orthopaedics.)

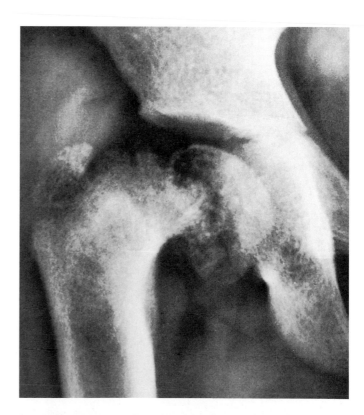

Fig. 8.40 Uremic osteodystrophy in childhood. In this child with chronic renal failure, the combination of rickets and secondary hyperparathyroidism affects the skeleton. The femoral metaphysis is irregular and the capital epiphysis shows considerable displacement. This has been likened to a 'rotting fence-post'.

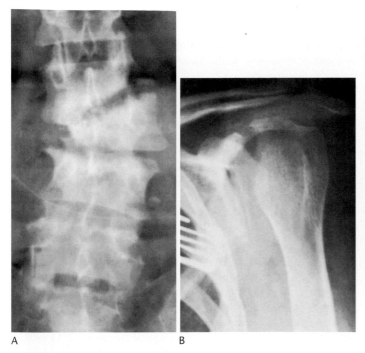

A   B

Fig. 8.41 Chronic renal failure: hemodialysis patient. **A**. There is an appearance resembling a Charcot spine, or even infection. **B**. A destructive arthropathy of the shoulder is also seen, without evidence of infection or neuropathy.

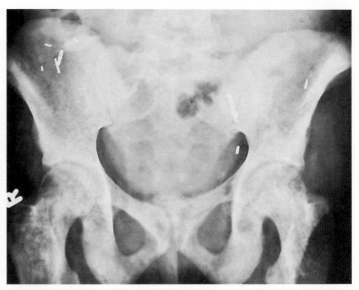

Fig. 8.42 Oxalosis. There is a generalized but slightly patchy increase in density of much of the visualized skeleton, due to calcium oxalate deposition.

Tertiary Hyperparathyroidism This term applies to cases in which secondary hyperparathyroidism gives rise to autonomous hyperparathyroidism. Treatment of the underlying disorder fails to control the hyperparathyroidism. Surgical removal of the autonomous parathyroid tissue is necessary.

Drug- and Toxin-induced Osteoporosis

Heparin, immunosuppressants, and alcohol, as well as corticosteroids, have all been implicated in osteoporosis. The development of osteoporosis has been reported in patients who receive large doses of heparin (usually greater than 15 000 units per day) although the mechanism is uncertain. The activity of mast cells may be an important factor.

In alcoholics the cause is not known, but it may well be, at least in part, dietary or due to concurrent osteomalacia secondary to associated liver disease.

Pregnancy and Related Conditions

Rarely, osteoporosis may be observed during pregnancy, although the cause for this has not been determined.

Other Causes of Osteoporosis

Other causes of generalized osteoporosis include multiple myeloma, glycogen storage diseases, marrow packing disorders such as Gaucher's disease, chronic liver disease, nutritional deficiency states, and chronic anemias. Osteogenesis imperfecta exhibits marked osteoporosis, Wormian bones, and fractures which heal with marked callus formation (Fig. 8.17). Blue sclerae and deafness are also found. Homocystinuria is another cause of osteoporosis.

Oxalosis Primary hyperoxaluria is inherited as an autosomal recessive trait. The main feature is recurrent urinary calculi, progressing to renal failure. Calcium oxalate deposition in bone and soft tissues occurs in those who survive with dialysis (Fig. 8.42).

Ochronosis (*Alkaptonuria*) This rare hereditary disorder of tyrosine metabolism is inherited as an autosomal recessive trait. Due to a lack of homogentisic acid oxalate, homogentisic acid accumulates in the tissues, particularly connective tissue. The radiographic features are mainly those of degenerative disease of the peripheral joints (Fig. 8.43) and calcification of spinal disk spaces (Fig. 8.44). In the spine, advanced changes may lead to an appearance resembling ankylosing spondylitis. Although kyphoscoliosis may occur in the spine, in the major joints there may be considerable joint space narrowing without marked osteophyte formation or sclerosis until the later stages.

Miscellaneous Conditions *Wilson's disease* (hepatolenticular degeneration) is a rare autosomal recessive disorder of copper metabolism that produces skeletal changes of osteomalacia and a form of arthritis. Other metabolic disorders, such as hemochromatosis and calcium pyrophosphate dihydrate deposition disease, also mainly produce joint disease.

Hemochromatosis may also give rise to a generalized osteopenia.

Copper deficiency in infants is rare, but is reported in severely malnourished infants, and in infants on long-term parenteral nutrition. There is reduction in bone density, cortical thinning and metaphyseal irregularity, with delayed maturation. However, unlike rickets, the zone of provisional calcification is preserved.

Homocystinuria This is a rare disorder inherited in an autosomal recessive manner and due to a deficiency in the activity of the enzyme cystathiamine synthetase, which converts homocysteine

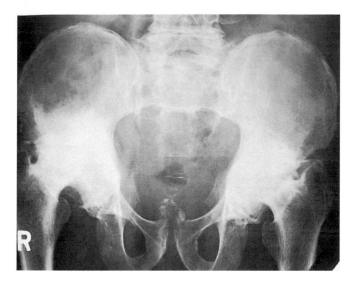

Fig. 8.43   Ochronosis. Gross narrowing of the joint spaces of both hips is associated with other evidence of severe degenerative disease. The intervertebral disk spaces are calcified and narrowed. (Courtesy of Dr D.J. Stoker and Institute of Orthopaedics.)

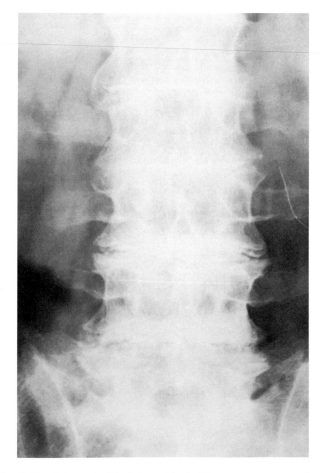

Fig. 8.44   Ochronosis. The intervertebral disk spaces are narrowed and calcified. Such widespread change is uncommon in uncomplicated degenerative spondylosis. (Courtesy of Dr D.J. Stoker and Institute of Orthopaedics.)

to cystathionine and cysteine. In one form of the disease (pyridoxine-resistant), changes in the skeleton include osteoporosis, arachnodactyly, epiphyseal enlargement, scoliosis, sternal deformity, and valgus deformity of the knees and hips. Being pyridoxine-resistant, this requires a low methionine diet. The other form of the disease is responsive to pyridoxine, and normal skeletal development follows.

Localized Osteoporosis

On occasion a localized osteoporosis may occur. The commonest cause for this is disuse osteoporosis, which may result from pain following trauma, severe vascular disease, infection or enforced immobilization. A rapid, aggressive-looking resorption of bone occurs, most marked in the cortical and subarticular areas of the bones (Fig. 8.35).

Reflex Sympathetic Dystrophy Syndrome (*Sudeck's atrophy, algodystrophy, reflex neurovascular dystrophy*)   This is regarded as a distinct entity, including terms such as causalgia, Sudeck's atrophy, shoulder–hand syndrome and reflex sympathetic dystrophy. The condition has been reported in association with prior trauma, surgery or infectious states, as well as vasculitis, calcific tendonitis, neoplasia, disk herniation, myocardial infarction, degenerative cervical spine disease and cardiovascular disorders. Symptoms usually include pain, swelling, stiffness, and weakness, but may be associated with hyperesthesia, vasomotor changes and disability. It is thought to be related to abnormal neural reflexes. Endosteal bone resorption is the most prevalent form of demineralization in this condition, although subperiosteal resorption, periarticular porosis, intracortical resorption and subchondral erosions are also seen (see Fig. 9.27). Despite the superficial similarities of pain and osteoporosis seen with transient osteoporosis and regional migratory osteoporosis (see below), the pattern of bone marrow edema seen in these conditions is not identified in patients with reflex sympathetic dystrophy.

Transient (Regional) Osteoporosis   This is a rare condition of large joints where gross focal osteoporosis and pain occur. The femoral head is the commonest site. It occurs typically in young and middle-aged adults, and is more common in men. Interestingly, when it occurs in women, the left hip is almost exclusively affected, and the disease occurs in the third trimester of pregnancy. There is no history of trauma or infection. Some authors believe that it is a form of Sudeck's atrophy. Synovial biopsy may show mild chronic inflammation. Symptoms resolve spontaneously in 4–10 months.

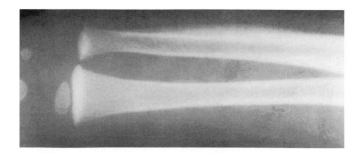

Fig. 8.45   Hypervitaminosis A. There is increased cortical density, most marked in the ulna.

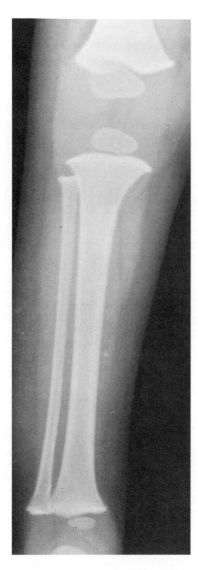

Fig. 8.46   Lead lines: metaphyseal bands of increased density.

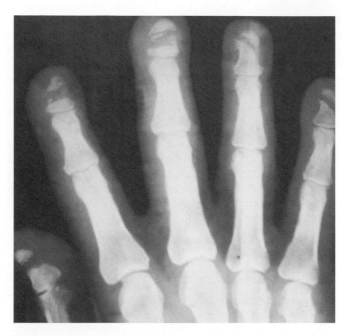

Fig. 8.47 Vinyl chloride poisoning. Inhalation or ingestion of vinyl chloride may produce this characteristic resorption of the central portions of the terminal phalanges. (Courtesy of Dr D.J. Stoker and Institute of Orthopaedics.)

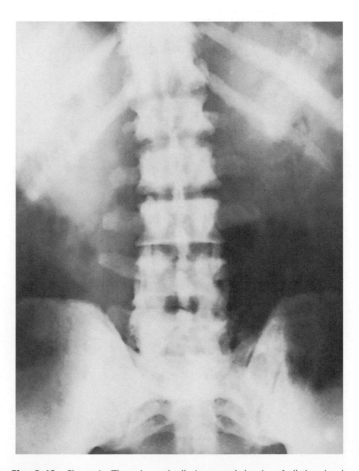

Fig. 8.48   Fluorosis. There is markedly increased density of all the visualized bones. (Courtesy of Dr D.J. Stoker and Institute of Orthopaedics.)

Regional Migratory Osteoporosis   This condition is migratory in nature, and the hip is involved less frequently than other areas, such as the knee, ankle and foot. It is commoner in men than in women, and is most evident between 30 and 50. Clinically it is similar to transient osteoporosis of the hip, the involvement of each joint lasting approximately nine months. Recurrences in other bones may occur successively, or be separated by up to two years or more.

Idiopathic chondrolysis of the hip is a rare disorder of unknown etiology. It affects predominantly adolescent girls and young women, particularly blacks, and gives rise to localized pain and marked osteoporosis. Early degenerative change results.

TOXIC EFFECTS ON THE SKELETON

Many toxins and poisons may affect the skeleton. Some common conditions are discussed below.

Hypervitaminosis A Overdosage of vitamin A may occur in children, but is rare in adults. It gives rise to hypercalcemia and an increase in periosteal new bone. Tender swellings of the limbs may occur. Radiographically, dense periosteal new bone is identified (Fig. 8.45), which, in contrast to infantile cortical hyperostosis, is not seen usually until after the first year of life. Withdrawal of vitamin A supplements results in remodeling of the bone.

Lead poisoning occurs in children who ingest lead-containing paint or water from lead-containing pipes and leads to lead deposition in the growing metaphyseal regions. This may cause modeling deformities and increased bone density, although most of this is due to reactive change (Fig. 8.46). Lead encephalopathy is a serious complication.

Bismuth intoxication (often following treatment for syphilis in the past) causes a similar appearance.

Vinyl chloride poisoning, found in workers in PVC manufacture, causes Raynaud's phenomenon and a characteristic form of acro-osteolysis (Fig. 8.47). Sacroiliitis is also seen, and hemangiosarcoma of the liver has been reported.

Fluorosis, due to chronic fluoride poisoning, is endemic in some parts of the Middle and Far East, but may also occur in aluminum smelting industries, and from drinking wine when fluorine is used as a preservative. A generalized increased bone density is seen (Fig. 8.48), which is again due to osteoclastic response to the fluorine rather than to fluorine deposition per se. Cortical thickening occurs, causing encroachment upon the medullary cavity, and ossification of ligamentous and musculotendinous attachments is seen. Endemic fluorosis is rare in children unless there are exceptionally high levels of fluorine; it may be associated with crippling stiffness and pain.

REFERENCES AND SUGGESTIONS FOR FURTHER READING

General
Fogelman, I., Carr, D. (1980) A comparison of bone scanning and radiology in the evaluation of patients with metabolic bone disease. *Clinical Radiology*, **31**, 321–326.

Genant, H. K., et al (1980) Computed tomography of the musculoskeletal system. *Journal of Bone and Joint Surgery*, **62-A**, 1088–1101.

Lenchik L., Sartoris D. J., (1997) Current concepts in osteoporisis. *American Journal of Roentgenology*, **168**, 905–

Pitt, M. J. (1981) Ricketic and osteomalacia syndromes. *Radiologic Clinics of North America*, **19**, 581–599.

Resnick, D. (ed) (1989) *Bone and Joint Imaging*. Philadelphia: W. B. Saunders.

Bone Density
Dequeker, J., Johnston, C. C. Jr. (eds) (1982) *Non-invasive Bone Measurements: Methodological Problems*. Oxford: I.R.L. Press.

Funke, M., Kopka, L., Vosshenrich R. et al (1995) Broad band ultrasound attenuation in the diagnosis of osteoporosis: correlation with osteodensitometry and fracture. *Radiology*, **194**, 77–81.

Genant, H. K., Black, J. E., Steigler, P. et al (1987) Quantitative computed tomography in assessment of osteoporosis. *Seminars in Nuclear Medicine*, **17**, 316–323.

Herd, R. J., Blake, G. M., Ramalingham, T. et al (1993) Measurements of postmenopausal bone loss with a new contact ultrasound system. *Calcified Tissue International*, **53**, 153–157.

Pacifici, R., Rupich, R., Griffin, N. et al (1990) Dual energy radiography versus quantitative computer tomography for the diagnosis of osteoporosis. *Journal of Clinical Endocrinology and Metabolism*, **70**, 705–710.

Endocrine Disorders
Genant, H. K., Baron, J. M., Strauss, F. H., II, Paloyan, E., Jowsey, J. (1975) Osteosclerosis in primary hyperparathyroidism. *American Journal of Medicine*, **59**, 104–109.

Kho, K. M., Wright, A. D., Doyle, F. H. (1970) Heel pad thickness in acromegaly. *British Journal of Radiology*, **43**, 119–125.

Meema, H. E., Schatz, D. L. (1970) Simple radiologic demonstration of cortical bone loss in thyrotoxicosis. *Radiology*, **97**, 9–15.

Osteomalacia and Rickets
Callenbach, J. C., Shennan, M. B., Abramson, S. J., Hall, R. T. (1981) Etiologic factors in rickets of very low-birth-weight infants. *Journal of Pediatrics*, **98**, 800–805.

Swischuk, L. E., Hayden, C. K., Jr. (1979) Rickets: a roentgenographic scheme for diagnosis. *Pediatric Radiology*, **8**, 203–208.

Poisons and Toxins
Betts, P. R., Watson, S. M., Astley, R. (1973) A suggested role of radiology in lead poisoning. *Annales de Radiologie*, **16**, 183–187.

Caffey, J. (1951) Chronic poisoning due to excess of vitamin A. *American Journal of Roentgenology*, **65**, 12–26.

Christie, D. V. (1980) The spectrum of radiographic bone changes in children with fluorosis. *Radiology*, **136**, 85–90.

Harris, D. K., Adams, W. G. F. (1967) Acro-osteolysis occurring in polymerization of vinyl chloride. *British Medical Journal*, **iii**, 712–714.

Renal Failure/Hemodialysis
Griffin, C. N. (1986) Severe erosive arthritis of large joints in chronic renal failure. *Skeletal Radiology*, **12**, 24–33.

Kaplan, P., Resnick, D., Murphey, M. et al (1986) Destructive noninfectious spondyloarthropathy in hemodialysis patients: a report of four cases. *Radiology*, **162**, 241–247.

Murphy, M. D., Sartoris, D. J., Quale, J. L. et al (1993) Musculoskeletal manifestations of chronic renal insufficiency. *Radiographics*, **13(2)**, 357–379.

Naidich, J. B., Massey, R. T., McHeffey-Atkinson, B. et al (1988) Spondyloarthropathy from long-term hemodialysis. *Radiology*, **167**, 761–766.

Miscellaneous
Caffey, J. (1972) Familial hyperphosphatasaemia with ateliosis and hypermetabolism of growing membranous bone. *Bulletin of the Hospital for Joint Diseases*, **33**, 81–110.

Houang, M. T. D., Brenton, D. P., Renton, P., Shaw, D. G. (1978) Idiopathic juvenile osteoporosis. *Skeletal Radiology*, **3**, 17–23.

Kozlowski, K. et al (1976) Hypophosphatasia. Review of 25 cases. *Pediatric Radiology*, **5**, 103–117.

Moule, N. J., Golding, J. S. R. (1976) Idiopathic chondrolysis of the hip. *Clinical Radiology*, **25**, 247–251.

Schwatzmon, R. J., McLellan, T. L. (1987) Reflex sympathetic dystrophy: a review. *Archives of Neurology*, **44**, 555–561.

Steinbach, H. L., Young, D. A. (1966) The roentgen appearances of pseudo-hypoparathyroidism and pseudo-pseudohypoparathyroidism. *American Journal of Roentgenology*, **97**, 49–66.

9

SKELETAL TRAUMA: GENERAL CONSIDERATIONS

Jeremy W.R. Young

Skeletal trauma is one of the most important aspects of orthopedic radiology, being by far the commonest problem presented to the musculoskeletal radiologist. Despite this fact, however, trauma radiology continues to be the most neglected aspect of this sub-specialty, particularly in teaching institutions. This may reflect an illogical approach to skeletal trauma in the past, whereby fractures and dislocations were presented as a confusing list of unassociated injuries, often better known by eponyms. More recently there has been a trend toward classifying fractures by the force of injury causing them. This allows a more logical and thoughtful approach, and enhances understanding of fracture patterns, and associated injuries.

A fracture of a bone occurs when there is a break in the continuity of bone, which may be either complete or incomplete. When a loading force is applied to bone, it initially deforms elastically, i.e. as the load is removed the deformity of the bone is reversed and the bone returns to normal. As the loading force is increased, the elasticity of the bone is overcome, and a plastic 'fracture' occurs, with the bone remaining deformed after cessation of the load. Finally, complete failure of the bone will occur, giving rise to a fracture. Repetitive loading of a bone at 'sub-fracture' levels may lead to the development of stress fracture (see below). Fractures are described in many different ways, as discussed below.

Terminology

The descriptive terms *open* or *closed* refer to whether the bone fragments communicate with the outside environment or not. If bone fragments penetrate the skin, the fracture is 'open' (Fig. 9.1). If the fracture remains covered with intact skin, it is called 'closed'. Although apparent on clinical inspection, various radiographic signs will also suggest an open fracture (Table 9.1).

The nature of the fracture lines also describes the fracture. Generally a single fracture line follows one of three major types—*transverse*, *oblique* or *spiral*—although a combination of these is often present. In addition, if the injury produces more

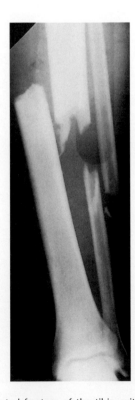

Fig. 9.1 A comminuted fracture of the tibia, with medial displacement and overriding of the distal fragment. Because of the proximity of the skin surface to the anteromedial aspect of the tibia, penetration of the skin is likely; in fact, air is seen in the soft tissues, indicating that penetration has occurred. There is lateral angulation of the distal fragment. A segmental fibula fracture is noted.

Table 9.1   Radiographic Signs of Open Fracture

Obvious protrusion of bone fragments beyond the soft-tissue margins
Absence of portions of the bone
Gross soft-tissue disruption extending to the bone surface
Subcutaneous gas
Foreign material within the fracture

than one fracture line, the fracture is said to be *comminuted*. Comminuted fractures will often produce what is known as a *'butterfly'* fragment (Fig. 9.2). A segmental fracture is one in which a segment of bone is isolated by fractures at each end (Fig. 9.3).

Fractures may also be termed *'incomplete'* or *'complete'*. Incomplete fractures occur most commonly in children, when bone resilience is greater, and are of three types: *plastic* fractures occur when there is bending of the bone without cortical disruption, or acute angulation; a *'torus'* or *buckle* fracture is the term applied to a fracture of the cortex on the 'compressive' side of the bone with an intact cortex on the tension side (Fig. 9.4): *greenstick* fracture is the converse of the torus fracture, occurring only on the tension side.

Fractures should be evaluated for continuity and proximity of the fracture fragments.

Apposition refers to the position of the major fragments with respect to each other. Fragments which are not apposed are

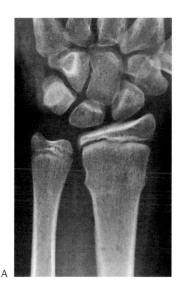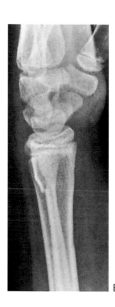

Fig. 9.4   A,B Torus fracture of the radius. The cortex is buckled on the dorsal surface. Apart from minor plastic deformity, the volar surface is intact.

described as being *distracted* if the displacement is along the long axis of the bone, or displaced out of the long axis. In such cases, the fracture should be described according to the direction of displacement of the distal fragment relative to the proximal bone.

Alignment refers to the relationship along the axis of major fragments. Abnormality of alignment may be described in two ways. The most logical refers to the alignment of the distal fragment with respect to the proximal (Fig. 9.1). This has the additional advantage of following the same 'rules' as apply to displacement. The alternative method, commonly used by orthopedic surgeons, is to describe the angulation as the direction of the apex of the angle at the fracture site.

'Varus' and *'valgus angulation'* are terms that are commonly used, particularly by orthopedic surgeons—they refer to the alignment of the distal fragment with respect to the midline of the body, with varus indicating angulation of the distal fragment toward the midline and valgus the reverse.

Impaction is the descriptive term for fractures in which the bone fragments are driven into each other.

Abnormality of *rotation* of the distal fragment is an important finding and should always be assessed. This requires visualization of both ends of the bone on the same radiograph, so that the orientation of the proximal and distal joints can be assessed.

Associated Soft-tissue Abnormalities

Although the majority of fractures are readily identified, on occasion they may be difficult or impossible to see on initial radiographs. Additional clues may be helpful in such cases.

For example, fractures around a joint may provide evidence of a joint effusion or hemarthrosis, providing the joint capsule remains intact. This can be particularly useful at the elbow, where elevation of the fat pads, either anterior or posterior, is good evidence of injury (Fig. 9.5). Lack of obvious bone injury should be regarded with caution, and delayed views after immobilization will often reveal a fracture.

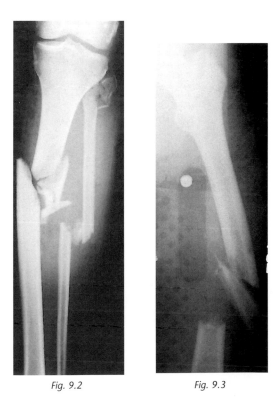

Fig. 9.2   *Fig. 9.3*

Fig. 9.2   A comminuted fracture of the tibia, with a triangular 'butterfly' fragment.

Fig. 9.3   Segmental fracture of the femur: by definition a comminuted fracture. In this case the isolated segment is clearly malaligned.

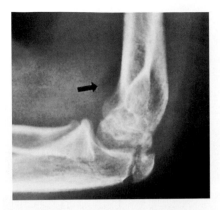

Fig. 9.5 Elbow effusion: elevation of the anterior fat pad (arrow). Although not pathognomonic for fracture, anterior fat pad elevation indicates significant effusion, and is frequently associated with a fracture. Careful inspection of the unfused radial head shows a minor cortical step-off of the metaphysis, indicating a fracture.

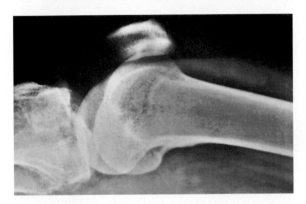

Fig. 9.6 A fat–fluid level (lipohemarthrosis) is seen in the knee joint on this cross-table lateral view. This indicates intra-articular bone injury.

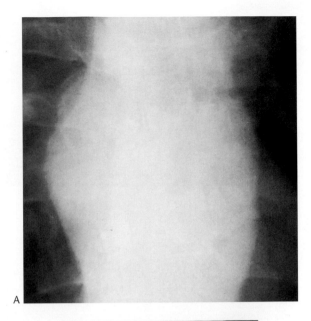

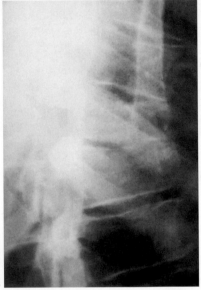

Fig. 9.7 **A,B** Compression fractures of the vertebral bodies of T7, T8 and T9 with large paraspinal hematoma which took many months to absorb, still being visible after the fracture had consolidated. (Courtesy of Dr D.J. Stoker and Institute of Orthopaedics.)

A fat–fluid level (*lipohemarthrosis*) within a joint, most commonly seen in the knee with the radiograph made with a horizontal beam, is also firm presumptive evidence of an intra-articular fracture, the fat being derived from the bone marrow (Fig. 9.6). In the thoracic spine, a hemorrhage from a vertebral fracture can be seen as a localized paravertebral soft-tissue mass, giving an appearance similar to that seen in an abscess (Fig. 9.7).

Soft-tissue swelling in the retropharyngeal space has also been cited as being a reliable sign of cervical spine trauma, although more recently the value of this sign has been questioned.

Fracture Healing

After a fracture has occurred, the process of healing begins. Initially, a hematoma forms between the bone ends, occasionally causing periosteal elevation. Granulation tissue then forms between the fracture fragments, with immature osteoid (callus) laid down on the bone surface acting as an early bridge. This first becomes calcified, but eventually woven bone is laid down, leading to firm bone union.

The early stages of bone formation are not visible radiographically, but in a healthy person new bone formation is visible within 4–6 weeks, with the healing process complete in 4–6 months for a single fracture in a large tubular bone. Delay in union, however, may be evident by a delay in the appearance of new bone, and can occur from a variety of causes (see below).

EVALUATION OF SKELETAL TRAUMA

The vast majority of injuries can be adequately visualized by **plain radiographs**. On occasion, however, other methods may be needed. **Tomography** has traditionally been used to assess fractures which are not visible or are poorly seen on plain radiographs. **Computed tomography (CT)** is vastly superior to tomography, with the additional advantage of imaging surrounding soft tissues. If CT is available, there are very limited indications for tomography, although this may be useful in cervical spine trauma (see Ch. 10),

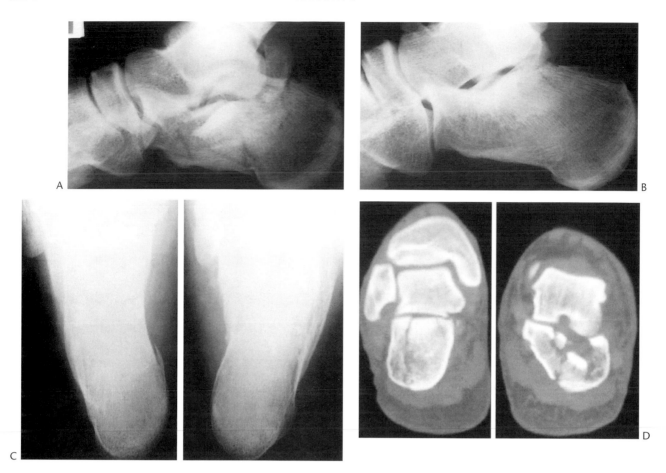

Fig. 9.8 There are comminuted fractures of both calcanea. The extent of the injury, and in particular of the articular involvement, is poorly displayed by the plain radiographs **A–C.** particularly on the right. **D.** CT images, however, demonstrate that there is an obvious disorganization of fragments at the articular surface on the left, and a mildly depressed segment on the right.

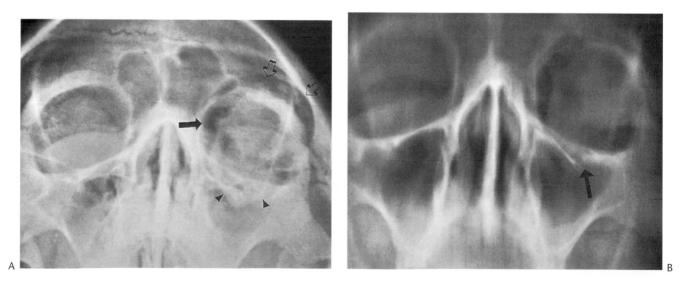

Fig. 9.9 **A.** Note orbital emphysema on the left, with air surrounding the eyeball (arrow) and beneath the eyelid (open arrows). This is highly suggestive of a blow-out fracture. In this case there is irregularity of the inferior orbital rim (arrowheads), with an apparent soft-tissue density projecting into the maxillary sinus. **B.** Tomography confirms the fracture of the orbital floor (arrow).

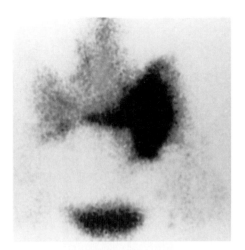

Fig. 9.10 Stress fractures of the sacrum. This elderly patient underwent radio-isotope bone scan for pain in the lower back. A characteristic pattern of increased tracer uptake indicates a stress fracture in the osteoporotic sacrum.

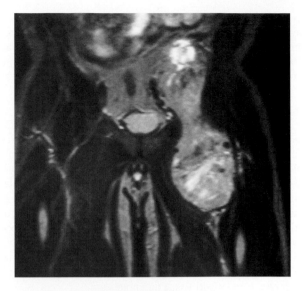

Fig. 9.11 Coronal MRI image (T_2-weighted) of the pelvis and thighs of a young gymnast who complained of pain and swelling in the groin. A well-defined lesion of mixed signal intensity occupies the region of the iliopsoas. The mixed signal pattern is common in hematoma, indicating the complexity of the hematoma and variations in hemoglobin, deoxyhemoglobin, methemoglobin and hemosiderin levels.

or in assessing the growth plate for early growth arrest following Salter–Harris fractures in children. In addition, tomography may be used to evaluate depression of bone fragments in tibial plateau fractures, or to determine the position of fragments in fractures of the tibial plafond, talus and calcaneus. In these cases, however, it can be argued that CT provides information that is at least as good, if not better (Fig. 9.8). Tomography may also be helpful in suspected blow-out fractures of the orbit (Fig. 9.9) as, in theory, CT may miss fractures of the floor of the orbit if obtained only in the axial plane. High-quality coronal CT however avoids this problem.

Nuclear medicine can be helpful in detecting occult fractures, e.g. of the scaphoid or femoral neck, although a positive scan may not be seen for 24 hours following injury, especially in older patients. Nuclear medicine can also delineate stress fractures of bone, often with a characteristic appearance (Fig. 9.10).

Magnetic resonance imaging (MRI) in many centers has become the method of choice for evaluating injuries of joints and surrounding tissues. It has the ability to detect not only injury to the surrounding soft tissues, but also occult injury to the bones themselves, such as 'bone bruising', subchondral fractures, and post-traumatic avascular necrosis. Amongst its advantages are its ability to demonstrate soft-tissue detail, its capability of multiplanar imaging, and its lack of ionizing radiation. These features

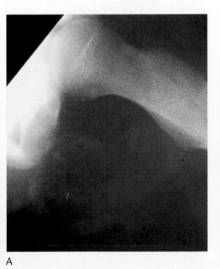

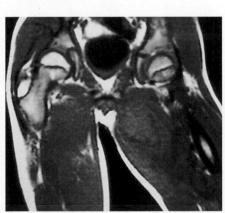

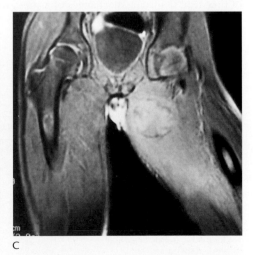

A   B   C

Fig. 9.12 **A.** A calcified 'mass' in the thigh of this 16-year-old was investigated to exclude tumor. **B.** T_1 coronal MRI images demonstrate a mass of low signal intensity, with surrounding low signal intensity edema, with **C.**, increased signal intensity on T_2 images. There is also a well-defined, low signal intensity 'ring' of calcification. There appearances are characteristic of post-traumatic myositis ossificans.

are responsible for the rapidly increasing use of MRI in musculo-skeletal radiology. Injuries to ligaments and tendons are readily identified by MRI (see relevant sections below), and muscle trauma can be appreciated (Figs 9.11, 9.12). This has greatly expanded the role of the radiologist in evaluating the traumatized patient.

COMPLICATIONS OF FRACTURE

In open fractures, there is an increased potential for infection at the fracture site. Closed fractures are not as susceptible to this problem. Nevertheless there are potential problems in all fractures.

The tibia has long been recognized as a bone liable to delayed union or non-union. The reasons for this are obscure, but poor vascular supply and lack of immobilization have been cited. In practice it would appear that the reason for the high incidence of cases of delayed or non union may be due to the large number of 'high-energy' injuries seen in the tibia, particularly from auto-mobile fender injuries to pedestrians with a large amount of resulting necrosis of soft tissue and bone.

Delayed union   This may result from many causes (Table 9.2).

Non-union   This is the absence of bony union over a prolonged period (Table 9.3). The radiograph appearance is usually of a persistent fracture line, usually with sclerotic margins, and marked surrounding sclerosis (Fig. 9.13). MRI may have a role to play in the management of non-union with its ability to detect infective causes (Fig. 9.14).

Malunion is the term given to a fracture which heals in an un-satisfactory anatomic position, either with excessive overlap of fragments, or unsatisfactory angulation or displacement of the distal fragment (Fig. 9.15).

SPECIAL TYPES OF TRAUMA

Stress (Fatigue) Fractures

These fractures result from chronic repetitive forces which by themselves are insufficient to cause fracture, but over the course of time lead to the classic changes of a stress fracture. They occur in many bones and usually at characteristic sites, often as the

Table 9.2   Causes of Delayed Union

Mechanical	Poor apposition
	Inadequate stabilization
Pathological	Age—decreased osteoblastic activity
	Dietary—vitamin deficiency (C and D)
	Pathological fracture (underlying abnormality)
	Infection

Table 9.3   Causes of Non-union

1. Idiopathic (particularly tibia)
2. Poor stabilization
3. Infection
4. Pathological fracture
5. Massive initial trauma

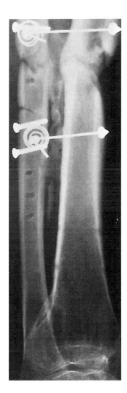

Fig. 9.13 Non-union of the tibia despite interosseous bone grafting and surgical wiring. There is sclerosis around the fracture line, without firm evidence of bone bridging, one year after the fracture.

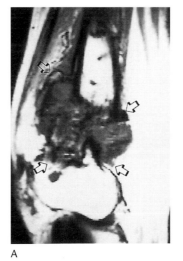 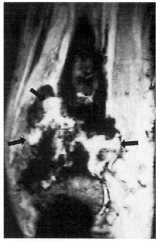

A   B

Fig. 9.14 **A.** MRI scan demonstrates tissue of mixed signal intensity in the fracture gap of non-union of the distal femur (arrows) on T$_1$ images. **B.** Areas of increased signal intensity are shown on T$_2$-weighted images (dark arrows), indicating foci of infection.

result of athletic activity: for example the 'march' fracture of the second and third metatarsal head, the stress fracture of the mid and distal tibia and fibula in long-distance runners and ballet dancers, and fractures of the proximal fibula in paratroopers.

The earliest diagnosis can be made by *radio-isotope scanning*, where activity will be seen before radiographic signs. When *radiographic signs* appear, they may take several forms, depend-

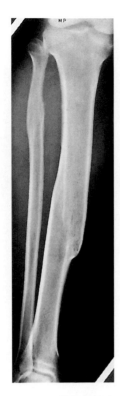

Fig. 9.15   Malunion of the tibial fracture, which has healed well but shows lateral angulation of the distal fragment.

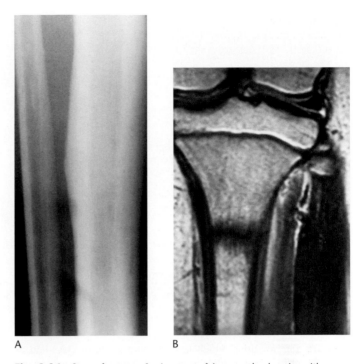

A   B

Fig. 9.16   Stress fracture. **A.** An area of increased sclerosis, with some dense periosteal new bone in the mid tibia. **B.** MRI may be helpful in early diagnosis before the plain radiographic signs become apparent.

ing upon the stage of healing or the chronicity of the stress factors. A hair-like lucency may be seen traversing the bone, although this may not be apparent without tomography. New bone formation around the fracture may be the only radiographic sign, or may accompany the cortical fracture (Fig. 9.16). MRI may be useful in making the diagnosis before any changes are seen radiographically (Fig. 9.16). If the patient continues the activity, a form of chronic fracture will occur with abundant sclerotic periosteal new bone and a persistent lucent fracture line with surrounding sclerosis (Fig. 9.17).

A type of stress fracture is said to account for the pars inter-articularis defects seen in *spondylolisthesis* (Fig. 9.18), whereby the continuance of the stress leads to a complete fracture, followed by non-union. Alternatively a congenital hypoplasia of the articular processes, or degenerative change within the posterior joints, may be the underlying cause. The defect in the pars is known as *spondylolysis*. When anterior displacement of the superior vertebral body on its neighbor is seen, spondylolisthesis is said to have occurred. Mild degrees of spondylolisthesis can occur when there is loss of articular cartilage at the posterior intervertebral joints as in degenerative disease. More severe spondylolisthesis results from pars interarticularis defects and is graded according to severity: Grade I—up to 25% displacement of the vertebral body; Grade II—up to 50%; Grade III—up to 75%; and Grade IV 100% displacement.

Avulsion Fractures

These occur from avulsion of bone fragments at the site of liga-mentous or tendinous attachments throughout the skeleton. Of

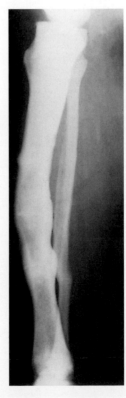

Fig. 9.17   Multiple stress fractures are seen, some with obvious horizontal lucencies running perpendicular to the bone cortex. The patient was a jogger who refused to give up jogging despite the pain!

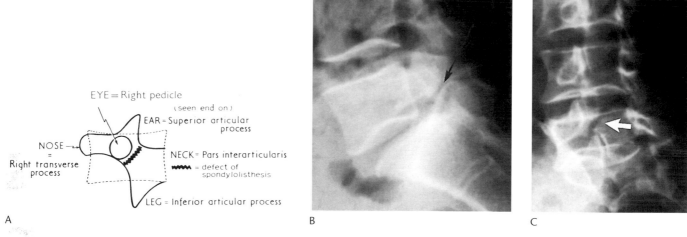

EYE = Right pedicle
(seen end on)

EAR = Superior articular process

NOSE =
Right transverse process

NECK = Pars interarticularis

= defect of spondylolisthesis

LEG = Inferior articular process

A   B   C

Fig. 9.18   A. Diagramatic representation of an oblique view of a lumbar vertebra, presenting the 'Scotty dog' appearance. The pars interarticularis defect corresponds to the dog's collar. **B** and **C.** Pars defect: oblique radiograph demonstrates the same appearances as in **A.** (Courtesy of Dr D.J. Stoker and Institute of Orthopaedics.)

note are abnormalities which have previously been classified as osteochondritis, but which represent avulsion fractures from chronic or repeated trauma. This includes *Osgood–Schlatter* disease and *Sinding-Larsen* disease, of the tibial tubercle and inferior patella respectively.

The diagnosis of Osgood–Schlatter disease is made clinically, although it can be suggested radiographically when there is clear elevation of fragments of the tibial tubercle separated from the underlying bone (Fig. 9.19). Fragmentation alone without dis-

placement does not constitute Osgood–Schlatter disease, and merely represents multiple ossification centers.

Common avulsion injuries at the origin of muscle tendon insertions are seen at the inferior border of the ischium (hamstrings) (Fig. 9.20), anterior inferior iliac crest (rectus femoris) (Fig. 9.21), and lesser trochanter (iliopsoas). See Table 9.4.

Pathological Fractures

Pathological fractures are fractures through bone that has been weakened by an underlying disease. This does not necessarily mean an underlying malignancy, although the term 'pathological fracture' tends to suggest it. Pathological fractures occur through bone that is weakened by such conditions as osteoporosis or osteomalacia, bone tumors (whether benign [Fig. 9.22] or malignant), or even tumor-like lesions of bone. In elderly patients, of course, underlying malignancy should be considered, especially if the fracture occurs in a site other than those usually seen in osteoporosis such as the femoral neck, or in cases in which the severity of the injury is inappropriate to the fracture created.

Post-traumatic Avascular Necrosis

This occurs from a traumatic severance of the blood supply to the bone or a fragment thereof. There are several bones in which this is likely to happen in areas where the blood supply is easily compromised. *Femoral neck* fractures may interrupt the vascular supply to the femoral head, as can posterior dislocation of the femoral head, with or without overt fractures of the head or acetabulum (Fig. 9.23). In fractures of the wrist involving the *scaphoid*, the proximal pole is at risk as the vascular supply enters the bone more distally (Fig. 9.24). Similarly, *talar waist* fractures threaten the proximal fragment. Post-traumatic avascular necrosis may occur in part of a bone as described above. It may also involve the growing epiphysis, as in the head of the second or third metatarsal (*Freiberg's disease*) or even the whole of a small bone, e.g. lunate (*Kienbock's disease*) (Fig. 9.25). Frequently there is no clear history of predisposing fracture. However there is evidence

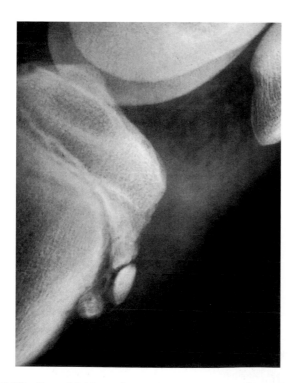

Fig. 9.19   Osgood–Schlatter disease. Fragmentation may be seen and a portion of the tibial tubercle ossification center is elevated.

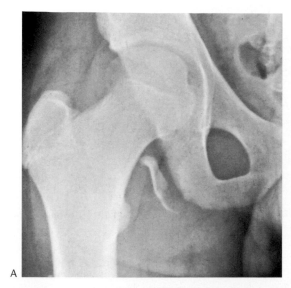

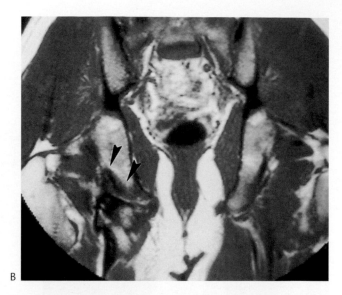

Fig. 9.20   A. Note an avulsion of the inferior border of the ischium at the site of insertion of the hamstrings. MRI of this injury (**B**) indicates the extent of injury to the underlying bone (arrowheads), not seen on the plain radiographs.

Table 9.4   Sites of Avulsion Fractures wiith Muscle Origin

Anterior superior iliac crest	Sartorius
Anterior inferior iliac crest	Rectus femoris
Ischial tuberosity	Hamstrings
Greater trochanter	Gluteals
Lesser trochanter	Iliopsoas
Posterior calcaneus	Achilles tendon
Olecranon process	Triceps
Superior patella	Quadriceps
Inferior patella (Sinding–Larsen)	Patella ligament
Tibial tuberosity (Osgood–Schlatter)	Patella ligament

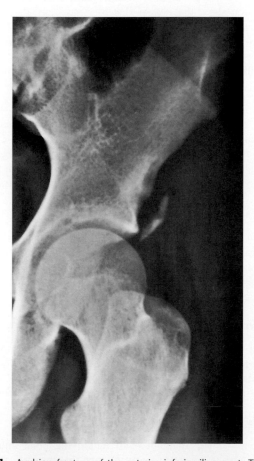

Fig. 9.21   Avulsion fracture of the anterior inferior iliac crest. This is the origin of the rectus femoris muscle.

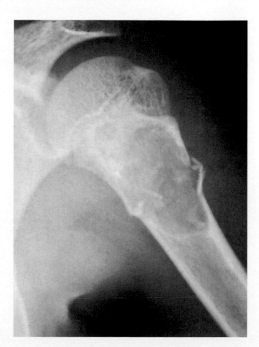

Fig. 9.22   Pathological fracture through a simple bone cyst of the proximal humerus.

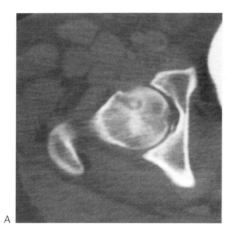

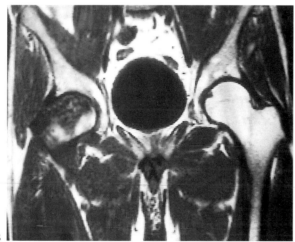

Fig. 9.23 A. CT shows a cortical fracture of the femoral head from previous posterior hip dislocation. A small intra-articular fragment is seen. **B.** MRI scan performed several weeks later indicates the typical findings of avascular necrosis.

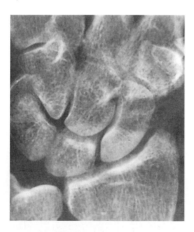

Fig. 9.24 Post-traumatic avascular necrosis of the proximal pole of the scaphoid. Although the fracture of the waist of the scaphoid has 'healed', avascular necrosis has occurred with resulting sclerosis.

that even conditions such as *Perthes disease* may result from a traumatic effusion, which is also responsible for the widening of the joint space that may be seen in the condition. This radio-

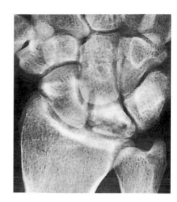

Fig. 9.25 Kienbock's disease: in fact, a form of traumatic avascular necrosis of the lunate.

graphic abnormality may be seen in the 'irritable hip syndrome' of children, which may progress to frank necrosis of the femoral head. This has been attributed to interruption of the vascular flow, possibly on the venous side, by the formation of granulation tissue. A similar scenario has been suggested for septic arthritis (pus within the joint), and hemophilia (blood within the joint).

In avascular necrosis, the necrotic bone usually becomes denser than the surrounding bone (Fig. 9.24) which in turn may become more osteopenic due to disuse. Studies on the femoral heads removed following fracture in the process of hip prosthesis implantation show that this is due to revascularization, when a thin layer of calcifying osteoid is laid down on the necrotic trabeculae. This feature may occur at any time from two months to two years following injury. Eventually collapse and fragmentation are likely to occur. MRI scan may be useful in the diagnosis.

Drillers' Disease (Vibration Syndrome)

Drillers' disease is seen in workers with vibrating machinery, usually after five or more years of use. Degenerative cysts are found in the bones of the wrist, and occasionally hand (Fig. 9.26). They are, however, indistinguishable from the cysts seen to result from heavy manual labor, and the exact etiology is uncertain.

Sudeck's Atrophy (Post-traumatic Reflex Dystrophy)

This is a rare condition in which, following injury to a limb, intense pain and swelling occurs, resulting in severe disuse osteoporosis. Interestingly, the initial injury may be relatively minor; the effects however are dramatic (Fig. 9.27). An associated neurovascular reaction may be present.

Transient Osteoporosis

This is a rare condition which usually affects the hip. Although this may represent a type of Sudeck's atrophy, a history of trauma is rare. Massive subarticular osteoporosis occurs, which is however self-limiting, with spontaneous resolution within 4–10 months.

Myositis Ossificans (Post-traumatic)

This usually occurs without overt underlying bone injury. The exact etiology is uncertain, but it may be due to ossification of a hematoma or reactive periosteal elements which have been

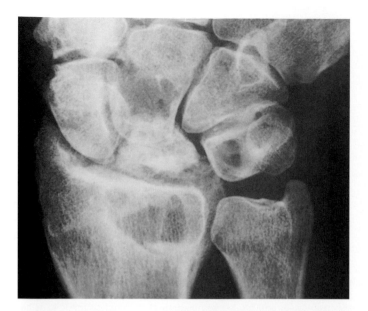

Fig. 9.26   Vibration syndrome. Fragmentation and flattening of the lunate due to avascular necrosis is typical of Kienbock's disease, accompanied by extensive cystic changes in the surrounding bones. These abnormalities occurred in a worker with compressed-air drills, who had been exposed to this repeated trauma for many years. (Courtesy of Dr D.J. Stoker and Institute of Orthopaedics.)

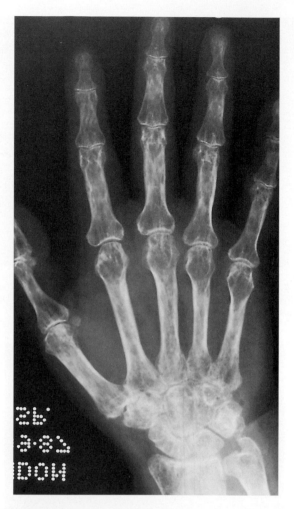

Fig. 9.27   Sudeck's atrophy: there was minor trauma to the forearm some weeks earlier. Note gross osteoporosis of the bones of the hand, wrist and forearm, most marked at the bone ends, but also causing cortical 'thinning' and resorption.

displaced into the soft tissues. The thigh is the commonest site. Hazy density in the soft tissues gives way to frank new bone formation, which may extend to the bone surface (Fig. 9.28). This may cause difficulty in distinguishing the lesion from parosteal osteosarcoma. Furthermore, unless adequate biopsy material is obtained, including the central and peripheral components of the lesion, histologic differentiation may also be difficult.

MRI has been shown to be a useful tool in the diagnosis of post-traumatic myositis ossificans, due to its ability to define the characteristic soft-tissue abnormality (see Fig. 9.12) which also may be seen before the changes are evident radiographically. A similar type of calcification or ossification may occur around joints following dislocation, and in cases of severe closed head injury (Fig. 9.29). Ligamentous avulsions or chronic ligamentous trauma may also result in calcification, such as calcification of the medial collateral ligament of the knee in cases of chronic sub-clinical trauma (Fig. 9.30) (*Pellegrini–Stieda lesion*).

Compartment Syndrome

Rarely, trauma to a limb will give rise to a potentially devastating situation whereby the tissue pressure within a closed 'compartment' causes progressive ischemia and ultimately necrosis. The compartments of the limbs consist of areas surrounded by rigid osseous and fascial planes. Tissue edema or hemorrhage may be the initiating factor and result from direct trauma and/or vascular interruption. The result of edema within a closed compartment is to raise the tissue pressure, thereby further decreasing vascular perfusion. Prompt fasciotomy is required. Volkmann's ischemia and contracture of the forearm, following fracture of the elbow, is probably a form of the compartment syndrome. Today the syndrome is most commonly seen in the leg as the result of road traffic accidents.

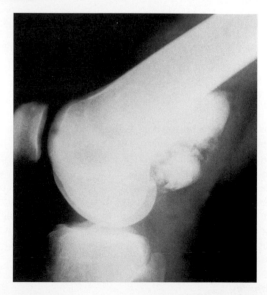

Fig. 9.28   Post-traumatic myositis ossificans. A well-defined bone density arises from the cortex of the distal femur and extends into the soft tissues. There was a history of blunt trauma, but even so, this lesion needs to be differentiated from parosteal osteosarcoma.

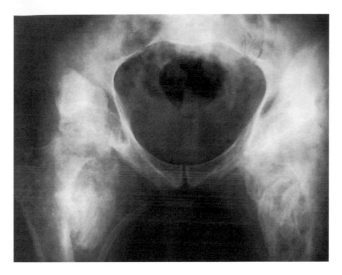

Fig. 9.29 Myositis ossificans associated with paraplegia. Very extensive soft-tissue ossification is visible round both hip joints. (Courtesy of Dr D.J. Stoker and Institute of Orthopaedics.)

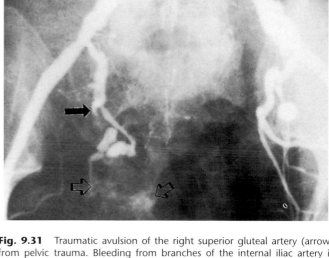

Fig. 9.31 Traumatic avulsion of the right superior gluteal artery (arrow) from pelvic trauma. Bleeding from branches of the internal iliac artery is also seen (open arrows). Marked diastasis of the right sacroiliac joint has occurred.

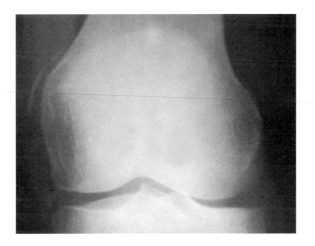

Fig. 9.30 Pellegrini–Stieda lesion. Post-traumatic calcification is shown in relation to the medial femoral condyle following a tear of the medial collateral ligament. (Courtesy of Dr D.J. Stoker and Institute of Orthopaedics.)

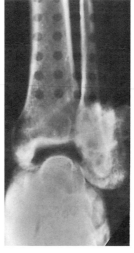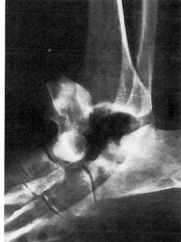

Fig. 9.32 Complete dislocation of the talus.

Arterial Injury

Vascular trauma generally occurs as the result of penetrating injury, and it may be caused by sharp bone fragments from a fracture, either at the time of injury or during manipulation. The popliteal artery is commonly injured from fractures or dislocations around the knee. Brachial artery injury may also result from supracondylar fractures of the humerus or elbow dislocations, particularly in children. Branches of the internal iliac artery—especially the superior gluteal, pudendal, and vesical—are at risk in pelvic ring fractures (see below), and are responsible for the massive blood loss and associated high mortality rates (Fig. 9.31).

Joint Injuries

Dislocations occur when there is a complete loss of normal articular contact between the bones comprising the joint (Fig. 9.32).

Subluxation refers to a partial loss of articular contact. *Diastasis* refers to separation of fibrous joints, e.g. symphysis pubis, sacroiliac joint (Fig. 9.33).

Joint injuries may be difficult to diagnose radiographically, as they frequently comprise ligamentous injury without obvious bone involvement. In addition, subtle avulsion fractures adjacent to joints may be the only indicator of gross ligamentous injuries. These are most commonly encountered around the *ankle*, where avulsions of the medial and lateral malleoli indicate collateral ligament disruption. Other important areas are the base of the *proximal phalanx of the thumb* (Fig. 9.34), and corner avulsions of the *tibial plateau*. Plain radiographic signs of injury such as effusion or hemarthrosis may be helpful. Stress views of the involved joint have been advocated, but this may require the patient to be sedated as they may be extremely painful to obtain.

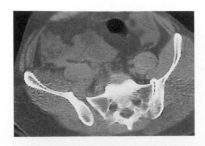

Fig. 9.33 CT image demonstrates complete diastasis of the right sacroiliac joint.

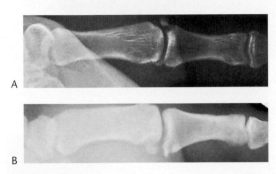

Fig. 9.34 Avulsion fractures of the proximal phalanx of the thumb. **A.** Fracture at the site of attachment of the radial collateral ligament. **B.** Fracture at the site of the attachment of the ulnar collateral ligament. In practice, the adductor of the thumb inserts in the same area, and may also be avulsed.

Assessment of Joints

Arthrography has traditionally been used to assess joint abnormalities (Fig. 9.35). *Ultrasound* has also been used, particularly to assess the shoulder joint for injuries to the rotator cuff (see below); CT is also useful in the shoulder, especially when combined with arthrography, when injuries of the glenoid labrum may be seen.

Magnetic resonance imaging (MRI) has made immense progress in recent years with its ability to define the soft tissues,

ligaments and tendons. Although originally finding favor for its ability to diagnose meniscal tears in the knee (Fig. 9.36), later work shows it can be useful for the shoulder (Fig. 9.35), ankle and wrist, where ligamentous and tendinous abnormalities may be demonstrated.

FRACTURES IN CHILDHOOD

Fractures in children differ from those in adults in several ways. They are often incomplete (torus or greenstick fractures) (Fig. 9.4), and 'plastic' fractures, without any cortical disruption, may occur. Children's bones have a greater capacity for remodeling than adults' bones, which allows for less exact corrective reduction, although rotational anomalies cannot be corrected by remodeling. Because of the hyperemia associated with fracture healing, there may be increased growth in the affected limb. This

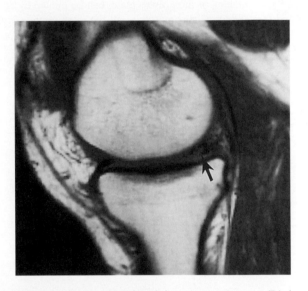

Fig. 9.36 Posterior horn tear of medial meniscus. MRI image (T_1) demonstrates a linear area of higher signal extending to the articular surface (arrow).

Fig. 9.35 Rotator cuff tear. **A.** Arthrography is performed by injecting contrast medium, with or without air, into the shoulder joint. Leakage of contrast into the subdeltoid bursa (arrows) indicates a rupture of the rotator cuff which normally separates the bursa from the joint. **B.** MRI demonstrates a large joint effusion, shown as high signal on this FLASH image. The effusion, which shows markedly increased signal intensity on this sequence, has tracked into the subdeltoid bursa (arrowheads), indicating rotator cuff rupture. In this case the subscapularis is seen to be retracted, with an irregular lateral margin (large arrows).

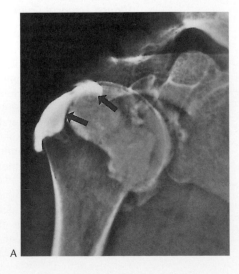

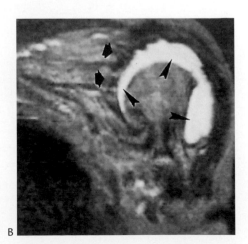

helps to restore length when overlap of the main fragments occurs, but on occasion also can cause unwanted increased length in a limb. Finally, because of the relatively weak epiphyseal plate, fractures through this region are common. Damage to the epiphyseal plate may result in partial or even complete growth arrest. The *Salter–Harris* classification of fractures of the epiphyseal plate is the one most commonly used (Figs 9.37, 9.38). Under this system, the potential for growth arrest increases with increasing type number, Types IV and V having the greatest potential for growth arrest (Fig. 9.39). However, it must be remembered that in a small child with uncalcified epiphyses, it may be difficult or impossible to accurately determine damage to the epiphyseal cartilage, and what may appear to be a simple Type I or II fracture may indeed represent a type IV or V injury, with the increased potential for growth arrest.

Growth arrest may take several forms, which have been classified by Bright. Type I and II growth arrests, which involve less than 25% of the area of the growth plate, can be treated by resection and implanting of inert material, but the more complex types may require radical resection and fusion with subsequent osteotomies or limb-lengthening procedures.

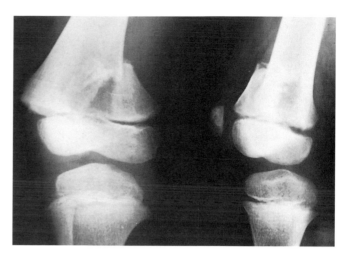

Fig. 9.38 Fracture-separation of the distal femoral epiphysis in an antero-medial direction, carrying with it a large fragment of the femoral metaphysis—the relatively common Salter–Harris Type II injury.

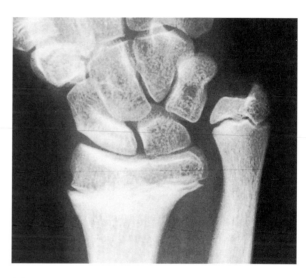

Fig. 9-39. Premature fusion of the distal radial epiphysis, following a fracture-separation seven years before, with relative overgrowth of the ulna.

Slipped Femoral Capital Epiphysis

This occurs in adolescent children and is probably related to trauma, which may be chronic. It represents a variety of Salter–Harris Type I fracture of the epiphyseal plate. It is commonly seen in boys approaching puberty, particularly those who are overweight and sexually immature. The incidence in girls however is rising, possibly as a result of an increase in sporting and physical activity. It may be bilateral (30–40%).

The epiphysis is displaced from the metaphysis, usually in a posterior and slightly inferior direction reflecting an anterior and superior slip of the femoral neck with respect to the epiphysis. 'Frog's-leg' views as well as anteroposterior views may be needed to make the diagnosis, and both hips should be examined because of the high incidence of bilateral involvement (Fig. 9.40).

Radiographic signs include blurring of the epiphyseal–metaphyseal junction due to superimposition; increased width of the epiphyseal plate; so-called elongation of the superior neck of

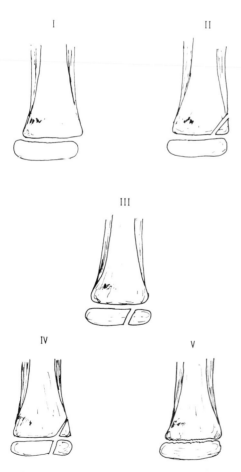

Fig. 9.37 Salter–Harris classification. I—injury through the epiphyseal plate only. II—Fracture through the epiphyseal plate and metaphysis. III—Fracture through the epiphyseal plate and epiphysis. IV—Fracture through the epiphyseal plate, metaphysis and epiphysis. V—Crush fracture of the epiphyseal plate.

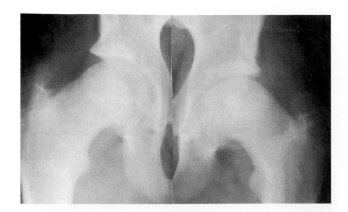

Fig. 9.40 Bilateral slipped capital femoral epiphyses. The diagnosis is more difficult when there is such symmetric abnormality. There is, however, obvious blurring of the epiphyseal line and elongation of the femoral neck. The femoral head does not project above the line of the femoral neck on either side.

the femur, whereby a line drawn along the superior neck fails to cut the epiphysis or cuts only a small portion (in normal patients this line usually cuts approximately one-fifth to one-fourth of the epiphysis); and loss of height of the epiphysis when compared to a normal contralateral hip. Careful follow-up of the contralateral hip is mandatory due to the high incidence of bilateral involvement.

A rare late complication of congenital slipped epiphysis is chondrolysis (*Waldenström's disease*), which ultimately causes joint space narrowing and early degenerative arthritis.

The Battered Child

In 1946 Caffey described a syndrome of subdural hematoma, associated with multiple fractures of the long bones, often in various stages of repair. This is the condition known today as the battered infant. In addition, clinical inspection of such cases may demonstrate bruises, burns, evidence of malnutrition and signs of neglect. Inconsistencies in the history given by the parents or guardian are usual.

Radiographic findings include fractures in different stages of healing, periosteal reactions (Fig. 9.41) particularly in the bones of the distal forearm or leg, multiple growth recovery lines, and injuries to the skull and ribs (Fig. 9.42). Epiphyseal separations and metaphyseal infractions are particularly common. Fractures in unusual sites (e.g. femoral shaft), and from apparently minor trauma, should also alert the physician to the possibility of non-

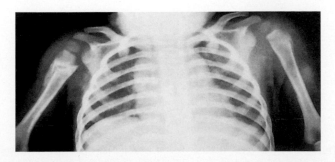

Fig. 9.41 Battered child. Healing fractures are seen in both proximal humeri.

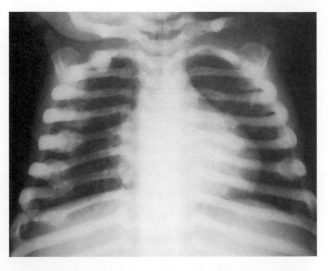

Fig. 9.42 Non-accidental injury. The radiograph shows multiple rib fractures at different stages of healing, probably the result of repeated compression injuries to the thorax. The child was admitted with a recent skull fracture. (Courtesy of Dr D.J. Stoker and Institute of Orthopaedics.)

accidental injury. Such findings warrant a complete skeletal survey and communication to the referring physician immediately, as many children subjected to battering die at a subsequent assault.

OTHER FORMS OF TRAUMA

Trauma may occur from a variety of other causes, including *ionizing radiation*, *frostbite* and rarely *electrical burns*, and *dysbaric osteonecrosis* (caisson disease).

Ionizing radiation may cause an area of osteonecrosis at the site of the insult whether from radiation therapy or other causes, e.g. the mouth in radium dial workers in the past. The affected bone generally exhibits a patchy sclerosis, and may fracture spontaneously. Secondary malignant degeneration may occur, usually to osteosarcoma after a latent period of more than five years.

Frostbite may give rise to acro-osteolysis (Fig. 9.43); in children there may be premature epiphyseal closure and growth arrest.

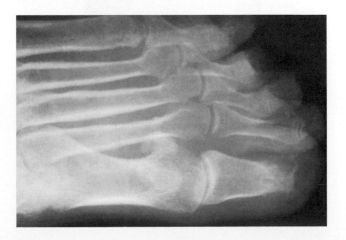

Fig. 9.43 Frostbite. Note acro-osteolysis of the toes, with almost complete resorption of the distal phalanges.

Caisson disease is found in deep-sea divers and tunnel workers, and is due to poor decompression giving rise to bubbles of nitrogen in the blood. These may block capillaries, causing avascular necrosis. Bone changes include areas of irregular bone density, usually in the long bones and due to medullary infarction, and subarticular infarctions, particularly in the humeral and femoral heads (Fig. 9.44). A similar pattern of subarticular bone infarction is seen in a variety of other conditions (Table 9.5). The changes of avascular necrosis are visible on radio-isotope bone scan and MRI long before they can be seen radiographically.

CHRONIC TRAUMA TO THE JOINTS *(Neuropathic Arthropathy)*

Brief mention will be made of this entity, although it is covered more fully in Chapter 10. Repeated trauma to the joints in the absence of normal pain and proprioceptive sensation will give rise to a severe destruction arthropathy, first described by Charcot (Figs 9.45–47). Although seen originally in cases of neurosyphilis, there is a variety of causes (Table 9.6).

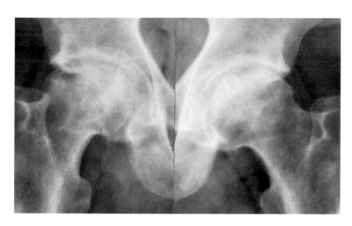

Fig. 9.44   Avascular necrosis of the hips. Note mixed sclerosis and lucency of the femoral heads, with collapse of the weight-bearing surface but maintenance of the joint spaces, indicating intact articular cartilage.

Table 9.5   Causes of Subarticular Bone Infarction—Avascular Necrosis

Caisson disease
Sickle-cell disease
Gaucher's disease
Pancreatitis
Chronic alcoholism (? pancreatitis)

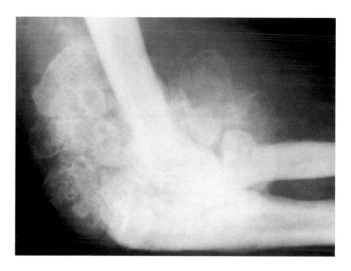

Fig. 9.46   Charcot joint: syringomyelia. The elbow joint shows marked irregularity, with abundant sclerosis, deformity and bone debris. On initial examination, the appearance resembles synovial osteochondromatosis. However, the generalized sclerosis and joint destruction indicate the diagnosis.

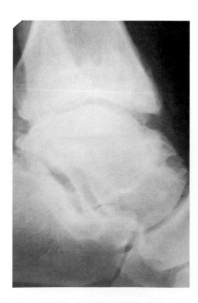

Fig. 9.45   Early Charcot joint, diabetic patient. Note irregularity of the talar dome, with increased density seen around the ankle joint.

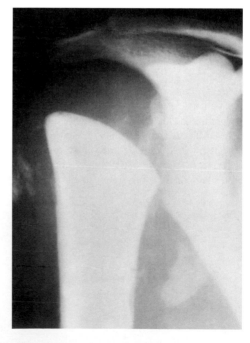

Fig. 9.47   Charcot joint: syringomyelia. Same patient as in Fig. 9-46. There is the appearance of a surgical 'amputation' of the head of the humerus. Glenoid destruction, joint debris, and increased radiodensity of the bones indicate the true nature of the abnormality.

Table 9.6 Causes of Charcot Joints

Diabetes (Fig. 9.45)
Neurosyphilis
Syringomyelia (Figs 9.46, 9.47)
Spina bifida
Leprosy
Congenital indifference to pain

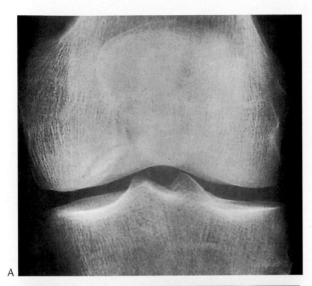

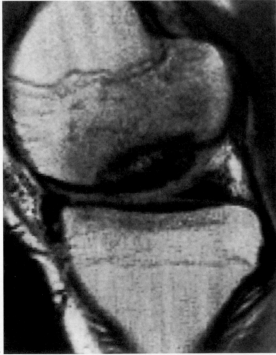

Fig. 9.48 Osteochondritis dissecans. **A.** Note defect in the femoral condyle, comprising a lucent ring with a more sclerotic center. **B.** MRI scan of avascular necrosis of the femoral condyle following subchondral fracture.

Most joints show evidence of disorganization, increased bone density, debris within the joint capsule, and bone destruction, giving rise to deformity—the so-called '5Ds' (Fig. 9.46). On occasion, however, a characteristic clear-cut destruction of the shaft of the bone is seen suggesting, at least superficially, a surgical procedure (Fig. 9.47).

OSTEOCHONDRITIS DISSECANS (Osteochondral Fractures)

Osteochondritis dissecans is really a misnomer, as the lesions clinically referred to as osteochondritis are usually the result of trauma, and indicate an osteochondral or chondral fracture occurring at an articular surface. After injury the detached portion of the bone may remain in situ, may be mildly displaced, or may become loose within the joint (Fig. 9.48; see Fig. 10.79).

The most common site of osteochondritis dissecans is the distal femur. The medial condyle is involved in 85% of cases, with the lesion classically on the lateral aspect of the medial femoral condyle (Fig. 9.48). Other forms of osteochondral fractures involve the weight-bearing surface of the joint, or the site of intra-articular ligamentous disruption (Fig. 9.49). Other sites of osteochondritis dissecans include the posterior patella and talar dome.

Other forms of osteochondral fractures occur with direct trauma to the articular surface, as seen in the Hill–Sachs deformity of the humeral head (see Ch. 10) from anterior dislocations, and the anterior femoral head defect following posterior dislocation of the hip (*Fig. 9.23*).

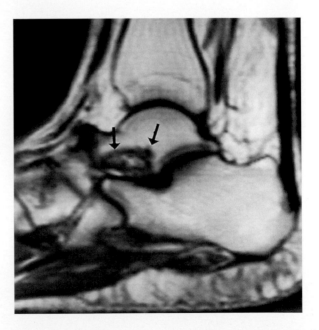

Fig. 9.49 Osteochondral fracture. Sagittal T_1 MRI of the ankle. There is a well-defined area of abnormal signal in the inferior border of the talus at the insertion of the interosseous ligament (arrows). The ligament itself cannot be seen, indicating disruption.

REFERENCES AND SUGGESTIONS FOR FURTHER READING

See end of Chapter 10.

10

SKELETAL TRAUMA: REGIONAL

Jeremy W.R. Young

THE SKULL

Head trauma, whether accidental or intentional, is a common event, with an incidence of almost 8 million cases each year in the United States. Approximately 500 000 are considered major injuries and half of these require emergency treatment. Overall, mortality rates are reported ranging from 5% to 50% and the majority of deaths in motor vehicle accidents are the result of head trauma.

The value of plain radiographic analysis of the skull continues to present a dilemma to physicians; despite the large number of publications refuting the clinical value of plain radiographs, they continue to be widely requested. The logical approach would be that if there has been sufficient injury to necessitate examination, computed tomography should be performed, since whether a fracture is present or not, intracranial hemorrhage may occur (Fig. 10.1).

Although not as sensitive as computed tomography, plain radiographs will demonstrate most skull fractures. The majority of these are linear and on occasion these may cause a diagnostic problem, simulating or being simulated by vascular grooves (see Ch. 54). In general, vascular grooves are less lucent and less sharply marginated, and are seen to branch and make curves rather than sharp angles.

Fractures which extend to the base of the skull may extend into the sphenoid sinus and an air–fluid level result. Otorrhea or rhinorrhea may occur in fractures of the skullbone. Fractures in the temporal bones are generally of two varieties: longitudinal (along the axis of the temporal bone), or transverse. Both may cause damage to the auditory or facial nerve, but longitudinal fractures are more likely to cause injury to the tympanic membrane and ossicles.

Depressed fractures of the skull may be readily apparent clinically but can be missed. In general, however, they have a typical radiographic appearance of a crescent of dense bone, due to overlapping fragments (Fig. 10.2). Tangential views provide the conclusive diagnosis in these cases. Intracranial hemorrhage may be suggested

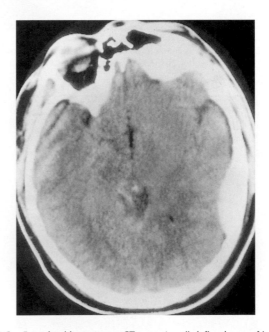

Fig. 10.1 Extradural hematoma: CT scan. A well-defined area of increased density is seen. The clear-cut convex inner margin is diagnostic of an extradural hematoma.

by shift of the calcified pineal gland on the frontal views of the skull.

CT is effective in detecting most skull fractures, particularly if 'bone windows' are used, although occasionally a fracture may be missed due to 'volume averaging'. These are usually clinically insignificant, however, unless there is concomitant intracerebral hemorrhage, which is usually readily recognized (Fig. 10.3).

Several studies suggest that MRI is not only more sensitive at detecting intracerebral trauma than CT, but may also demonstrate lesions earlier (Fig. 10.4). On the whole, however, MRI is less readily available than CT at this time.

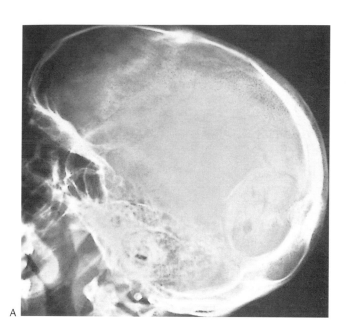

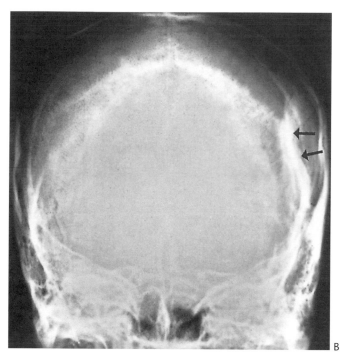

Fig. 10.2   Depressed skull fracture. **A.** A curvilinear density overlies the posterior parietal region on the lateral view. **B.** On the Townes view, the depressed nature of the defect can be appreciated (arrows).

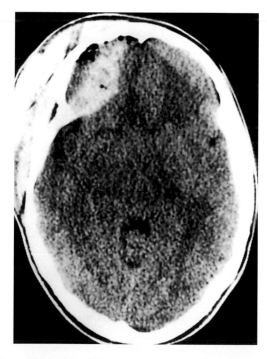

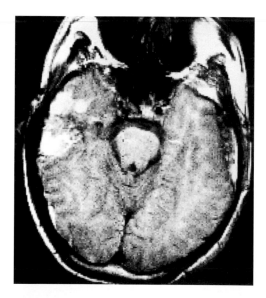

Fig. 10.4   MRI of right temporal lobe contusion (T_1-weighted). There is irregular high signal intensity within the temporal lobe, following trauma to the tempoparietal region of the skull.

Fig. 10.3   Skull fracture. CT scan demonstrates a large intra and cranial hematoma, with obvious high density blood in the right frontal lobe. Low density air 'bubbles' are also seen, indicative of fracture communicating to the outside environment, most likely via the frontal sinuses.

THE FACIAL BONES

Usually the result of automobile accidents or assaults, facial bone injury generally involves one of four areas: mandible, zygomatic arch and orbit, nasal bones, or complex fractures of the Le Fort varieties (see below).

Radiographic examination of the facial bones will include lateral, PA (occipito-frontal) and Waters (occipito-mental) views. These provide moderately good information, but overlying soft-tissue swelling can obscure detail considerably. Although additional views such as obliques may be helpful, CT has proved to be vastly superior to the plain film in the evaluation of facial trauma. Most recently, three-dimensional images have provided exquisite detail, not available by any other technique (Figs 10.5–7).

The *mandible* is most commonly fractured at its weak spot, adjacent to the canine tooth (Fig. 10.7). However, as it forms a 'ring' structure with the skull, there is a strong possibility of two fractures occurring, and this should always be excluded (Fig. 10.8).

The *nasal bones* are best identified on the lateral view, although the frontal views or occlusal film will determine displacement of the nasal septum.

On plain radiographs, the *zygomatic arch* and *orbital rim* are best seen on the occipito-mental (Waters) view, although the submento-vertical and Townes views are good for assessing the zygoma for depression. Fluid levels or opacification of the maxillary sinus are important hints of fractures extending into the sinus and may be the only sign of 'blow-out' fractures of the orbital floor. 'Blow-out' fractures may also involve the ethmoid sinus walls, and air may penetrate the periorbital space, giving rise to orbital emphysema (see Ch. 9).

Le Fort defined lines of weakness within the facial bones, leading to the classification system based on the type of fracture pattern (Figs 10.9, 10.10). In practice, pure symmetric Le Fort fractures of any one variety are rare, and a combination of the injuries usually occurs (Fig. 10.10).

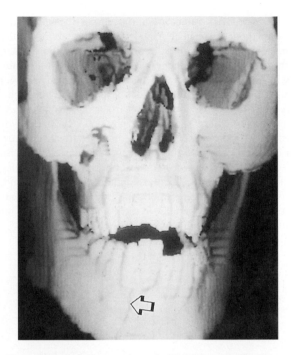

Fig. 10.7 Mandibular fracture (arrow): 3D CT. Exquisite detail is provided by the 3D reconstruction.

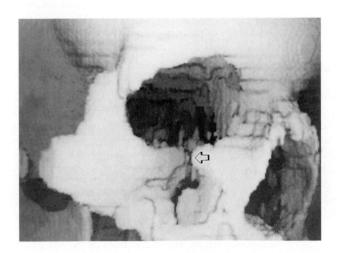

Fig. 10.5 Zygomatic fracture: 3D CT. The zygomatic arch is obviously depressed on the right, with a comminuted fracture involving the inferior orbital rim (arrow), and maxillozygomatic junction.

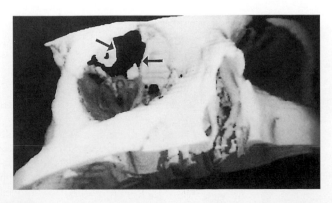

Fig. 10.6 Orbital 'blow-in' fracture: 3D CT. There is a large defect in the medial and posterior orbital walls (arrows).

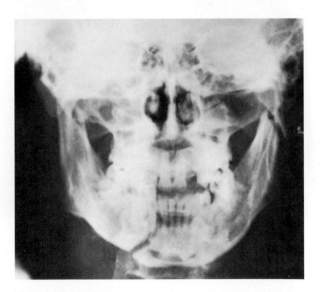

Fig. 10.8 Fractures of the mandible following direct injury. As with other bony rings, fractures in two places are common. Fractures involve the right canine region and the neck of the left condyle.

THE SPINE

Spinal trauma is a common cause of disability, with approximately 150 000 persons suffering from spinal injury in the United States each year. It is predominantly an affliction of the young, with 80% occurring below the age of 40. Spinal injuries are common in multitrauma patients, mainly from motor vehicle accidents and from falls. Cervical spine injury occurs in over 20% of such cases.

Examination of the patient in the acute setting may be difficult due to combative or uncooperative behavior, which may be the result either of head trauma or intoxication. Plain films are the primary method of evaluation and will detect abnormalities of alignment, as well as the majority of fractures. Additional methods of examination include tomography, CT and MRI. CT is able to clearly identify small bone fragments not seen on plain radiographs and has the advantage of better definition than tomography, as well as an ability to visualize the soft tissues. It also involves less radiation, may be quicker than tomography, and is only slightly more expensive. With the newer scanners, high-quality reconstruction in virtually any plane and three-dimensional images may also be obtained (Fig. 10.11). However, it must be remembered that despite the fact that CT is regarded by most authors as the 'gold standard' for examination of the spine, subtle undisplaced axially orientated fractures can be missed, at least in theory, and high-quality multi-directional tomography may prove superior in some cases.

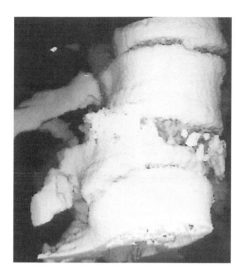

Fig. 10.11   3D CT of the spine. Note crush fracture of the body of L1, with anterior subluxation of T12 on L1.

MRI is becoming increasingly utilized in the spine, and has the advantage of detecting injury to the substance of the spinal cord, intervertebral disks, and supporting ligaments which cannot be evaluated by other techniques (Figs 10.12, 10.13). Also, it can easily define the later changes of post-traumatic syringomyelia.

Cervical Spine

Normal Radiographic Anatomy   An understanding of the anatomy of the normal cervical spine is obligatory for correct evaluation. The anatomic features are identified in Figure 10.14. Alignment should be assessed along several anatomic lines as shown. These are: the anterior and posterior spinal lines, joining the anterior and posterior aspects of the vertebral bodies along the line of the longitudinal ligaments; the spinolaminar line, which joins the anterior margins of the junction of the lamina and spinous processes; and the spinous process line, joining the tips of the spinous processes. In addition, a fifth line should be drawn between the posterior margins of the articular pillars. This line defines the posterior aspect of the articular pillars and allows assessment of the laminar space between the posterior pillar and spinolaminar line. Abrupt variation in this space has been shown to be an accurate method of

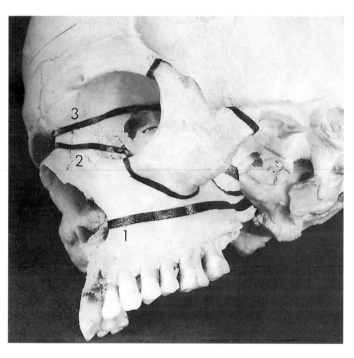

Fig. 10.9   Facial fractures lines. The lines of the common fractures are marked on the skull: 1. low transverse fracture; 2. pyramidal fracture; and 3. high transverse fracture. The numbers also relate to the Le Fort lines of weakness.

Fig. 10.10 CT of facial fracture. **A.** Fractures are identified through the anterior and lateral walls of the right maxillary sinus (arrows), and pterygoid plate (open arrow). There is complete opacification of the right antrum and nasal passage from hematoma, and a fluid level in the left antrum due to a maxillary fracture (not seen on this image). On another cut **B.** the zygomatic arch fracture is also seen (arrow), and there is obvious depression of the zygoma. The left maxillary fracture is also seen (open arrow).

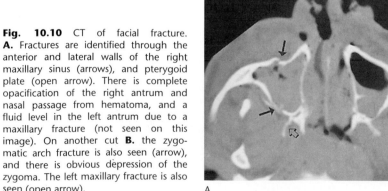

A

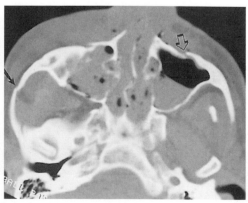

B

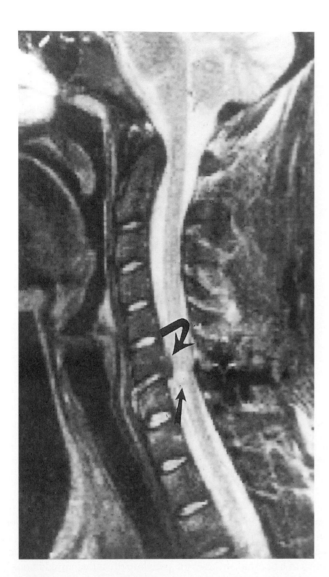

Fig. 10.12 MRI of the cervical spine: T$_2$-weighted image. There has been a fracture of C6, with mild posterior displacement of the dorsal fragment of the vertebral body (curved arrow). A focal area of high signal within the spinal cord at this level (straight arrow) indicates a focal cord injury.

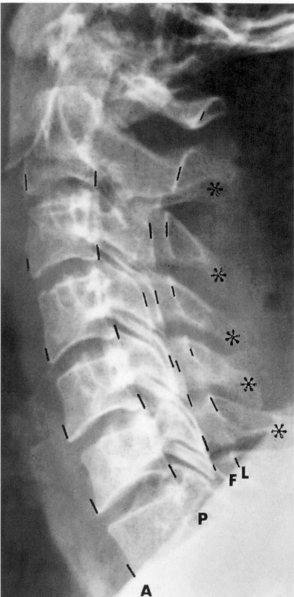

Fig. 10.14 Normal cervical spine. Five lines should be drawn in the mind. A and P are the anterior and posterior longitudinal lines respectively. These run along the margin of the anterior and posterior longitudinal ligament. L is the spinolaminar line, which runs between the anterior margin of the dorsal spines, outlining the posterior margin of the spinal canal. The asterisks represent the spinous line, along the posterior margin of the dorsal spines. F is the posterior pillar line, along the posterior margins of the articular pillars. N.B. Note divergence of the posterior pillar line in the upper and mid spine, due to mild positional rotation.

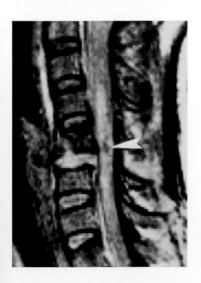

Fig. 10.13 MRI—spinal cord contusion. This gradient echo sequence shows a focal area of decreased signal in the cord posterior to the hyperflexion teardrop fracture of C5 (arrowhead), compatible with intracellular deoxyhemoglobin. There is surrounding high-signal edema.

determining rotational abnormality of a vertebral column, either with or without a fracture of the articular pillar (Figs 10.15, 10.16). Prevertebral soft-tissue measurements have traditionally been regarded as being a valuable indicator of injury or normality. Recently, however, Templeton et al (1987) have shown these to be of limited value, with the statistical likelihood of underlying injury occurring only at measurements above 7 mm at the C3 and C4 level, and a significant shift toward abnormality occurring only at measurements above 10 mm.

Radiographic Evaluation The condition of the patient will determine to a large extent the type and detail of the initial radiographic examination. The cross-table lateral view, with the patient supine, is the single most important radiographic examination and should be made as soon as the patient is stabilized. Evaluation of this film alone by an expert in the field will allow diagnosis of abnormality in the vast majority of cases. All seven vertebral bodies should be included on the radiographs. A normal cervical spine will demonstrate a gentle lordosis, but although lack of lordosis may be due to muscular spasm and indicate spinal injury, age, prior trauma, radiographic positioning, flexion of the spine, and the wearing of a hard collar (so commonly seen today) can all cause alteration in the natural lordosis.

In the lateral radiograph of the resting cervical spine, as well as a normal lordosis, there should be no disruption of the anterior spinal line. In flexion, the mid and upper segments of the spine move forward over the next inferior segment with concurrent sliding of each inferior articular facet over the superior facet of the level below, up to approximately 30% of the length of the articular surface. A unique phenomenon is seen in children up to the age of 8,

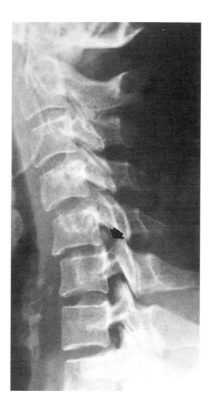

Fig. 10.16 Unilateral facet fracture-dislocation. There is a mild anterior subluxation of C5 on C6; also overlap of the posterior articular pillar lines at C6, but separation at C5, indicating rotation. The superior facet of C6 has been fractured and rotated forward with the anteriorly displaced inferior facet of C5 (arrow).

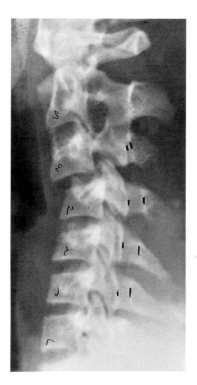

Fig. 10.15 Unilateral facet dislocation. There is an abrupt change in the laminar space (between the spinolaminar line and the posterior articular pillar line) at the C3/4 level, indicating rotation. There is also a mild anterior subluxation of C3 on C4.

approximately 25% of whom will demonstrate a 'pseudosubluxation' at the C2-3 level, attributed to laxity of the ligaments. This can be confirmed by examining the spinolaminar line, which will maintain a normal relationship in cases of pseudosubluxation. In addition, in approximately 20% of patients in this age group, over half of the anterior arch of the atlas lies above the tip of the dens. This should not be misinterpreted as atlanto-axial dislocation. Furthermore, the space between the posterior surface of the anterior arch of C1 and the anterior surface of the dens may widen in flexion up to 6 mm in children, although it remains constant in adults.

Kyphosis, or a localized flexion angulation, may be mild or severe, and can occur as a result of narrowing of the vertebral bodies anteriorly, as in a wedge compression fracture. Alternatively, widening of the interspinous distance and/or interfacet joints posteriorly indicates posterior ligamentous disruption, as seen in hyperflexion sprains (Fig. 10.17) (see below). Both of these appearances indicate a hyperflexion force as the cause of injury, and they may occur together. Asymmetry of the disk space is also a useful sign, and may indicate ligamentous damage to the longitudinal ligament at the site of widening.

Additional plain radiographic examination of the patient with a spine injury may include an anterior posterior (AP) view, and an open-mouth AP odontoid view. The incidence of injury to C7 in cervical injuries has been reported at 30%, although this figure would appear to be on the high side. Tomography or CT may be needed to visualize this region fully. Oblique views are reported to be useful for defining the neural foramina, and may clarify a

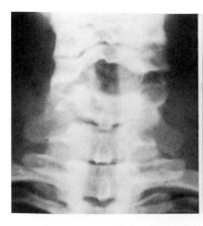
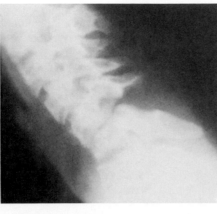

Fig. 10.17 Hyperflexion sprain/wedge compression fracture. There is a wedge compression fracture of C6 with marked widening of the interspinous distances of C5/6; also, widening of the facet joint at C5/6, with near 'perching' of the inferior facets of C5 on the superior facets of C6.

fracture of the articular pillars or a unilateral facet dislocation. 'Pillar views' of the cervical spine are also advocated by some authors. However, it can be argued that these additional views are superfluous; if an abnormality is not seen by routine plain film evaluation in a clinical setting suggestive of a fracture or dislocation, more definitive additional studies are mandatory in any case. These will include flexion/extension lateral radiographs, multidirectional tomography, CT, or MRI. These methods will provide additional information of abnormality, or confirm normality, and are indicated in the symptomatic patient whether the oblique and pillar views demonstrate abnormality or not.

Classification Most classification systems for cervical spine injury are based on the classic paper by Whitley and Forsythe (1960). These regard the forces acting on the spine as flexion, extension, rotation, compression, or a combination of the above. Each fracture force will be covered below.

Hyperflexion Injuries

These include hyperflexion sprain, flexion compression fractures, flexion teardrop fractures and, if rotation also occurs, unilateral facet lock.

Hyperflexion Sprain These injuries usually involve anterior subluxation of a vertebral body, with respect to the vertebra located inferiorly. Flexion extension views are invaluable in cases in which injury is expected but not immediately visible, or when minor abnormality such as asymmetry of a disk space or questionable 'fanning' of the spinous processes is seen. However, they should never be obtained when there is clear radiographic evidence of bone displacement or ligamentous injury. Also, in the acute setting, muscular spasm may prohibit movement of the spine, thus invalidating the findings.

Hyperflexion sprain is associated with posterior ligamentous injury of the spine. Depending upon the severity, the ligaments will be involved in the following order:

1. *Interspinous ligaments*, giving rise to widening of the interspinous distance.

2. The *ligamentum flavum* and *capsular ligaments*, which gives rise to more marked widening of the interspinous distance, and widening or subluxation of the facet joints (Figs 10.17, 10.18).

3. The *posterior longitudinal ligaments*, allowing widening of the posterior disk space. In such cases, ultimately total sub-

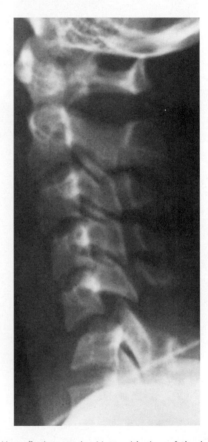

Fig. 10.18 Hyperflexion sprain. Note widening of the interspinous distance at C5/6, with additional widening of the facet joints, and superior subluxation of the facets of C4 on C5. The posterior intervertebral distance is also widened. This picture indicates severe ligamentous disruption.

luxation of the facets may occur, giving rise to bilateral locked facets (Fig. 10.19). This is usually associated with anterior subluxation of 50% or more of the vertebral body above the injury, and will cause stripping or rupture of the *anterior longitudinal ligament*.

Flexion Teardrop Fracture This occurs with flexion injuries when there is a compression fracture of the anterior aspect of the vertebral body inferior to the level of the injury (Fig. 10.20). This may also be associated with a posterior displacement of the

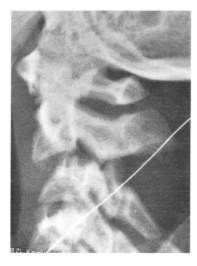

Fig. 10.19 Bilateral locked facet. C2 has leap-frogged over C3, and now lies with its inferior facets anterior to the superior articular facets of C3.

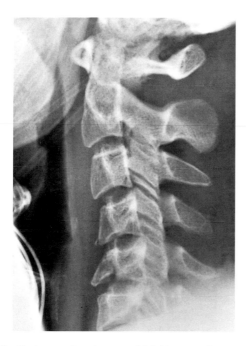

Fig. 10.20 Flexion teardrop fracture of C5. Note anterior compression of C5, with a fracture of the anterior inferior aspect. A very small avulsion is also seen at the anterior, inferior aspect of C4.

posterior portion of the affected vertebral body, causing spinal cord compression.

Unilateral Facet Dislocation When a rotational force is combined with hyperflexion, unilateral facet dislocation occurs. In such cases, the abnormal side rotates up and over the normal subjacent facet. The contralateral side acts as the fulcrum and is not involved in the injury. On the abnormal side, there is either 'locking' of the inferior articulation of the facet of the rotated vertebra anterior to the superior articulation of the facet of the normally positioned lower vertebral body, or—as occurs in approximately 30% of cases—there is a fracture through one of the articular facets, usually the superior facet of the lower vertebral body. In general

this fracture is horizontally orientated, indicating the rotational shearing nature of the force. Radiographically, the vertebral body of the rotated vertebra is displaced anteriorly, varying in degree up to approximately 20% of the vertebral body. Change in the laminar/facet interspace is an accurate assessment of rotational anomaly (Fig. 10.15). An apparent shift of the spinous process may be identified on the frontal view, due to its being 'rotated' away from the midline.

Wedge Fractures These occur when there is wedging of the anterior aspect of the vertebra, without ligamentous injury or posterior displacement of fragments. This usually means less than 30% compression of the anterior vertebra, and is associated predominantly with axial loading, as well as hyperflexion.

Hyperextension Injuries

In general, hyperextension injuries are associated with rupture of the anterior longitudinal ligament. This causes widening of the anterior disk space, and may cause prevertebral soft-tissue swelling. It must be remembered, however, that positioning of the head in the neutral position by a well-meaning passer-by, or the placement of a cervical collar at the scene of the accident, may largely restore any displacement, so that on initial inspection the radiograph can appear grossly normal. Hyperextension teardrop fractures may occur, usually at the anterior inferior aspect of the vertebral body involved, indicating the site of avulsion of the anterior longitudinal ligament. A further effect of hyperflexion, however, may be to cause an axial load on the posterior elements, giving rise to crush fractures of the articular pillars (Fig. 10.21) and narrowing of the interspinous distance. Fractures through the spinous process may also occur, due to axial compression. Facial injuries are often associated with these fractures.

Hangman's Fracture This injury, misnamed because of a superficial resemblance to fractures seen in victims of hanging, occurs with hyperextension of the head, and therefore a form of axial

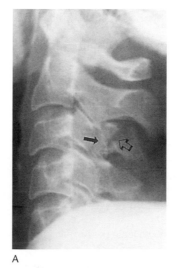
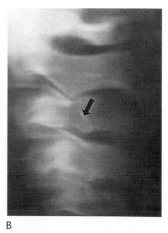

A   B

Fig. 10.21 Hyperextension fracture of the articular pillar of C3. **A.** There is obvious bone disruption of the posterior elements of C3, involving both the articular pillars (closed arrow) and lamina (open arrow). **B.** Tomography demonstrates the crush fracture of the articular pillar, with posterior displacement of the postero-inferior fragment (arrow).

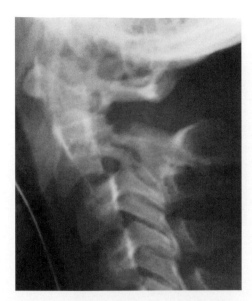

Fig. 10.22 Hangman's fracture. Classic oblique fractures through the pars interarticularis of C2 are associated with anterior subluxation of the body of C2.

loading on the posterior elements of the upper cervical spine caused by posterior rotation of the head in the sagittal plane (Fig. 10.22). The injurious force is in effect delivered by the occiput as it moves in an inferior and anterior direction, causing oblique fractures through the posterior arch of C2 which may extend into the body of C2. This fracture may be extremely unstable, although

the spinal cord is usually spared due to the large AP diameter of the spinal canal at this level. The fracture may also extend into the vertebral canal, risking injury to the vertebral artery. A similar fracture pattern may occasionally be seen at lower levels in the spine.

Axial Loading

Jefferson Fracture: Burst Fracture of C1 In these injuries, axial loading causes compression of the lateral masses of C1 between C2 and the occipital condyles. Because of the anatomy of the region, this gives rise to lateral displacement of the masses of C1 (Fig. 10.23), thus disrupting the ring. This can be appreciated on the AP odontoid view, but usually gives rise to anterior displacement of the atlas relative to the odontoid process. Prevertebral soft-tissue swelling is usual.

Burst Fracture This is caused by axial loading and the vertebra is shattered, often in all directions. The importance of this injury lies in the possibility of posterior displacement of fragments into the spinal canal.

Miscellaneous

Spinous Process Fracture This most commonly occurs at C7, and is often seen as an avulsion injury (clay shoveler's fracture). However, it may occur in direct trauma, or from compressive hyperextension (see above), or as the result of forced hyperflexion.

Odontoid Fractures Fractures of the odontoid have traditionally been divided into three types: Type I, in which the fracture is

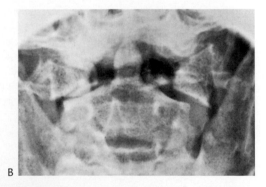

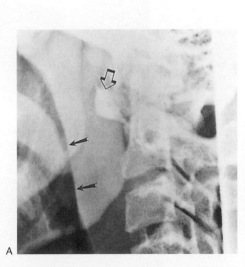

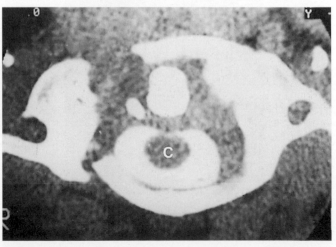

Fig. 10.23 Jefferson burst fracture of C1. **A.** The lateral view indicates anterior displacement of the anterior arch of C1 with respect to the odontoid process (open arrow). There is marked prevertebral soft-tissue swelling (closed arrows). **B.** The AP view demonstrates lateral displacement of the lateral masses of C2. **C.** Axial CT of Jefferson fracture of atlas. Contrast in subarachnoid space outlines cord.

through the upper aspect of the odontoid process; Type II, in which the fracture occurs through the base of the odontoid (Fig. 10.24), and Type III, where the fracture extends into the body of C2 (Fig. 10.25). More recently there has been a move toward classifying them as either high or low, the latter fractures extending into the body of C2 and hence representing the Type III fractures of the past. Non-united Type I fractures involving the superior aspect of the odontoid process are arguably the cause of the so-called os odontoideum, although a congenital non-union has also been suggested (Fig. 10.26). Odontoid fractures may be seen on the AP odontoid view, but should not be confused with artefacts from the posterior arch of the atlas (Mach effect) (Fig. 10.27), or overlying teeth. Type III (low) fractures extending into the body of C2 may cause disruption of the cortical 'ring' of the lateral aspect of the body of C2, seen on the lateral view (Fig. 10.25). There may also be an anterior tilt of the dens and hence anterior displacement of C1 with respect to the ring of C2.

Rotational Injuries Pure rotational injuries are rare, but may give rise to rotational (rotatory) subluxation. This is a condition of a rotational anomaly, usually of C1 on C2, which in children may give rise to torticollis. Although the condition may be self-limiting, occasionally it persists. It is best appreciated on open-mouth odontoid views, in the AP and both oblique projections, although tomography may be needed for full evaluation (Fig. 10.28).

Additional rotational injuries are those associated with axial loading or hyperextension, both of which can give rise to unilateral facet dislocation (see above).

Thoracolumbar Spine

Fractures in the thoracolumbar spine are generally the result of severe axial loading, as in falls from a height (crush fractures), or acute flexion injuries, commonly seen in seat-belt injuries in automobile accidents (see below). Rotational forces, however, may play a role, particularly in the upper lumbar region. As in the cervical spine, ligamentous injury can usually be appreciated by subluxation, either anterior or lateral. Widening of the interpedicular distance

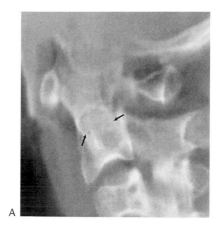

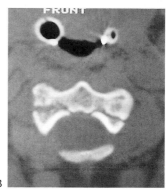

A

B

Fig. 10.25 Low (Type III) odontoid fracture. **A.** The lateral radiograph demonstrates interruption of the radiographic 'ring' of the body of C2 (arrows). **B.** CT demonstrates the nature of the fracture, through the body of C2.

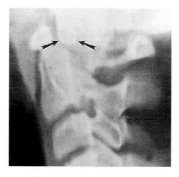

Fig. 10.26 Os odontoideum. The tip of the odontoid process is separated from the body, with smooth, well-corticated margins (arrows).

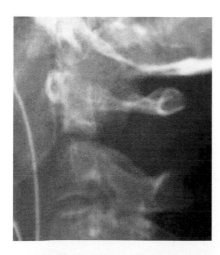

Fig. 10.24 Low (Type II) odontoid fracture. The fracture passes through the base of the odontoid process with slight separation, and anterior displacement of the odontoid process and ring of C1.

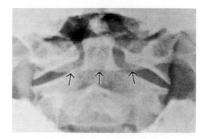

Fig. 10.27 Mach effect. An apparent fracture through the base of the odontoid process is due to the overlying posterior ring of C1 (arrows).

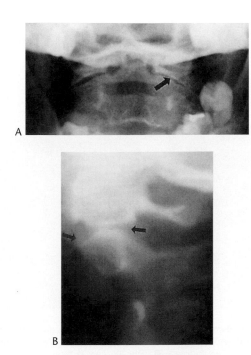

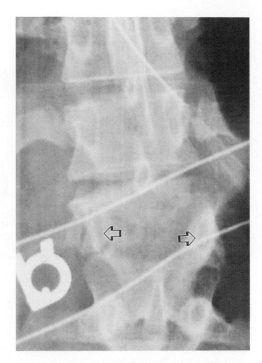

Fig. 10.28 Rotatory subluxation of C1 on C2. Despite a nearly perfect AP view **A.**, there is asymmetry of the C1/2 articulation with narrowing of the left (arrow), which cannot be attributed to patient positioning. This suggests a rotation of C1 on C2, confirmed **B.** by lateral tomograms, which indicate subluxation of the articular surfaces (arrowheads).

Fig. 10.29 Crush fracture L1. The interpedicular distance is widened, indicating lateral displacement of the pedicles, and hence 'bursting' of the ring formed by the vertebral body and posterior elements. Water-soluble contrast medium is present in the subarachnoid space.

or disk space, as well as paravertebral swelling in the thoracic region, are signs of injury which should be sought (Figs 10.29, 10.30).

Compression injuries cause 'burst fractures' or, when associated with flexion, wedge compression fractures, usually more marked at the anterior margin (Figs 10.31, 10.32). Lateral compression may also occur. Crush fractures are common in victims of falls, and are associated with fractures of the calcaneus, 'pilon' fractures of the tibial plafond, and vertical shear pelvic fractures (see below). These injuries therefore should warn of possible spinal trauma, particularly of the upper lumbar region. All forms of compression fracture require CT to evaluate for posterior displacement of fracture fragments and impingement upon the spinal cord.

Seat-belt Injuries These are caused by massive localized hyperflexion, typically the result of sudden deceleration, in an automobile accident, when the occupant is restrained by a lap seat belt. In general there is very little, or no, anterior wedging of the vertebral body, suggesting a distracting hyperflexion force. The fractures are subdivided into three groups. Type I, the 'Chance fracture', extends horizontally from the spinous process into the vertebral body, passing through the articular pillars and pedicles; Type II, the Smith fracture, is similar, but does not involve the spinous process (Fig. 10.33); Type III involves one side only, due to a rotational component of the force responsible.

THE PELVIS AND HIP

Much confusion has arisen over pelvic fractures, due to a lack of a logical and meaningful classification system. Traditionally, pelvic fractures were classified by reference to historical descriptions of

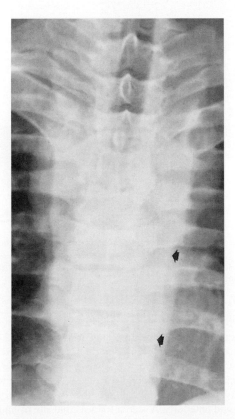

Fig. 10.30 Compression fracture: mild crush fracture of the body of T5, with a paraspinal soft-tissue 'mass' (arrows), due to hemorrhage.

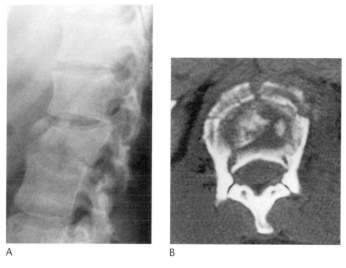

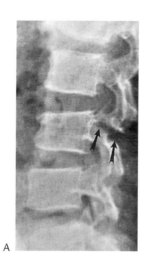

Fig. 10.31 Compression fracture of L2. **A.** Plain lateral radiograph indicates wedging of L2, with posterior bulging of the dorsal margin. **B.** CT scan demonstrates the extent of the impingement of the dorsal fragment upon the spinal canal.

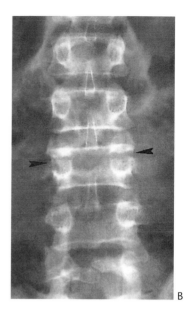

Fig. 10.33 Lap-belt injury: Smith fracture. **A.** There are horizontal fractures extending posteriorly from the dorsal surface of the vertebral body, through the pedicles (arrows). **B.** The AP view demonstrates the characteristic 'horizontal' defects in the pedicles (arrowheads).

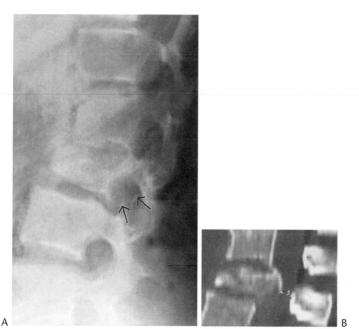

Fig. 10.32 Compression fracture L2. **A.** Again there is wedging and compression of L2, with evidence of body debris overlying the spinal canal (arrows). **B.** CT reconstruction indicates the position of the bone fragments and narrowing of the canal.

individual fractures, without any connection between them. These classifications included single fractures of the pelvis and thus were largely outdated by the work of Gertzbein and Chenoweth (1977) who demonstrated that there was always a second site of injury even in apparently single pelvic fractures. This is due to the fact that the pelvis is a bony ring, held together by ligamentous groups posteriorly and anteriorly. A search for a second site of injury should therefore always be made in fractures involving the pelvic ring.

The classification system of Young and Burgess (1987), developed from work by Pennal and Tile, which describes fractures relative to the force of injury, will be used in this text.

Lateral Compression Fractures   These are subdivided into three types, depending upon the severity of the injury and progressive involvement of the posterior pelvis (Fig. 10.34). Pubic rami fractures are invariably present, and generally run 'horizontally' or in the coronal plane. Alternatively they may present as 'buckle' fractures. A common association is a crush fracture of the sacrum (Fig. 10.35). Fracture of the medial wall of the acetabulum, with or without central dislocation of the femoral head, is also associated (Fig. 10.35). In Type I fractures, there is no ligamentous damage, and no posterior pelvic instability. However, with Type II injuries, there is medial displacement of the anterior pelvis on the side of injury, with either a fracture through the sacroiliac joint and iliac wing, or rupture of the posterior sacroiliac ligaments (Fig. 10.36). This allows some posterior instability. In Type III fractures, the lateral force on one side of the pelvis is transmitted through to the contralateral side, so that the force is directed outward (Figs 10.34C, 10.37). This causes 'opening' of the pelvis on the contralateral side, with associated posterior ligamentous disruption.

Anterior Posterior (AP) Compression Fracture   The damaging force in the AP (or PA) direction tends to cause 'opening' of the anterior pelvis (Fig. 10.35), with splaying of the symphysis pubis and/or fractures of the pubic rami, which, however, are in the vertical plane, in contrast to lateral compression fractures.

The more severe Types II and III fractures relate to increasing posterior ligamentous injury, and hence increasing instability (Figs 10.38–40). In Type II fractures, the anterior sacroiliac, sacrospinous and sacrotuberous ligaments are disrupted, allowing wide splaying of the anterior pelvis (Figs 10.38, 10.39). In Type III fractures, there is total disruption of the sacroiliac joint (Fig. 10.40). Fractures of the anterior and posterior acetabular pillars are common, and posterior hip dislocations are also associated, in contrast to lateral

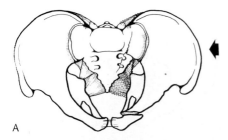
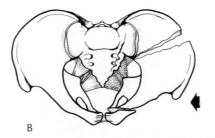
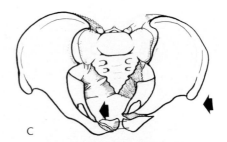

A   B   C

Fig. 10.34 Lateral compression pelvic fracture classification. **A.** Type I. Posteriorly positioned lateral force causes compression of the sacrum, and 'horizontal' or buckle fractures of the pubic rami. **B.** Type II. The force is delivered more anteriorly, causing inward rotation of the anterior pelvis around the anterior aspect of the sacroiliac joint. Either disruption of the posterior sacroiliac ligaments, or fracture of the iliac wing (shown here) results. **C.** Type III. The lateral force on one side is transmitted to the contralateral side, causing an externally directed force to 'open' the contralateral pelvis. Disruption of the major anterior ligamentous groups (anterior sacroiliac, sacrotuberous and sacrospinous) occurs. (Reproduced with permission of Urban-Schwartzenberg from Young and Burgess 1987.)

compression fractures when the medial wall of the acetabulum is at risk (see above).

Vertical Shear Fractures These commonly result from falls from a height. Fractures occur through the pubic rami and posterior pelvis, and are vertically oriented (Fig. 10.41). The large lateral hemipelvic fracture fragment containing the acetabulum is displaced superiorly.

Fractures of the posterior and superior acetabula are often associated with superior displacement of the femoral head. These injuries are associated with fractures of the lumbar vertebrae and calcaneus.

Mixed Fracture Pattern These arise from a combination vector of the forces causing injury, and give rise to a mixed pattern of

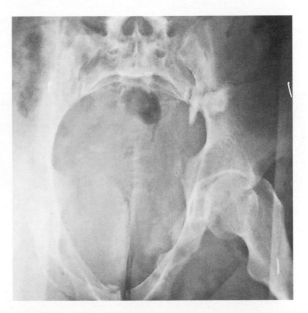

Fig. 10.36 Type II B lateral compression fracture. 'Horizontal' fracture of the right symphysis, and oblique fracture of the left iliac wing, arising from the sacroiliac joint. There is moderate medial displacement of the left anterior pelvis. (Reproduced with permission of Urban-Schwartzenberg from Young and Burgess 1987).

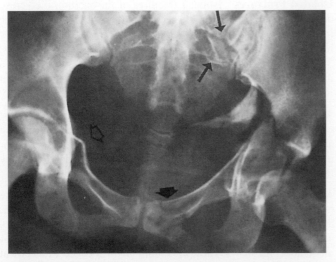

Fig. 10.35 Type I lateral compression fracture. A horizontal fracture of the left (closed arrow) and a buckle fracture of the right (open arrows) superior pubic ramus are seen. There is a crush fracture of the left sacrum (long arrows), and a fracture predominantly of the medial wall of the left acetabulum. (Reproduced with permission of Urban-Schwartzenberg from Young and Burgess 1987).

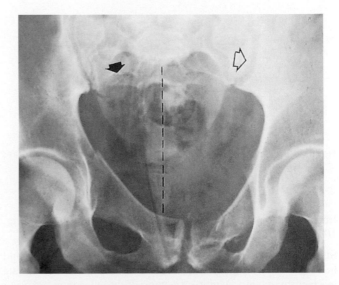

Fig. 10.37 Lateral compression Type III. There are crush fractures of the right sacrum (dark arrow) and left pubic rami. Note diastasis of the left sacroiliac joint (open arrow) and lateral displacement of the whole of the anterior pelvis to the left. Fractures of the right pubic rami are also seen.

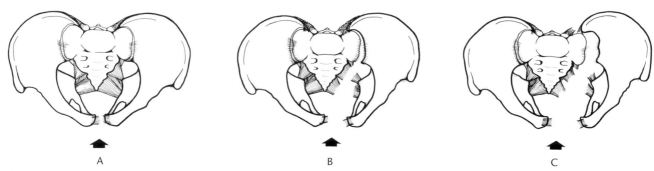

Fig. 10.38 Anteroposterior (AP) compression fracture classification. **A.** Type I. Diastasis of the symphysis pubis only. **B.** Type II. Diastasis of the symphysis pubis, disruption of the sacrospinous and sacrotuberous ligaments and anterior sacroiliac ligament. **C.** Type III. Total ligamentous disruption, including the posterior sacroiliac ligaments. (Reproduced with permission of Urban-Schwartzenberg from Young and Burgess 1987).

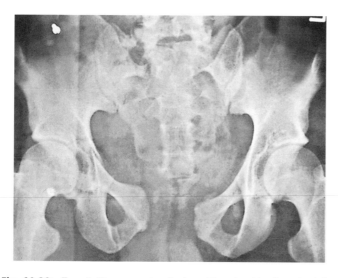

Fig. 10.39 Type II AP compression fracture. There is wide diastasis of the symphysis pubis and anterior left sacroiliac joint.

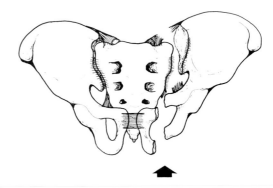

Fig. 10.41 Vertical shear fracture pattern. A superiorly directed force disrupts the left hemipelvis, with diastasis (or fracture) through the left sacroiliac region, and fractures of the pubic rami (or symphysis diastasis). The separated pelvic fragment containing the acetabulum is displaced superiorly. (Reproduced with permission of Urban-Schwartzenberg from Young and Burgess 1987).

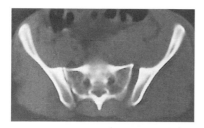

Fig. 10.40 Type III AP compression fracture. CT scan: complete diastasis of the left sacroiliac joint.

fracture, the commonest being a mixed anterolateral pattern (Fig. 10.42), with signs of both AP and lateral compression.

Straddle Fractures It is questionable whether this term should be used at all, as it gives no useful indication as to the underlying mechanism of injury. Multiple fractures of the pubic rami can occur from lateral, anterior–posterior compression or vertical shear fractures, and clues should be sought to the likely force vector, and to associated injuries (Fig. 10.43).

Isolated Fractures Isolated fractures of the sacrum, iliac crest, or inferior pubic ramus may occur, as these do not violate the integrity of the pelvic ring. Such sacral fractures are usually transverse and may be difficult to diagnose without a lateral view. Single fractures of a pubic ramus can be seen, resulting from a direct blow. However this is a rare occurrence, and additional injury to the pelvis should always be excluded.

Avulsion Injuries Avulsion injuries of the pelvis occur most commonly as the result of muscular exertion during sporting activities. The anterior superior iliac spine (sartorius), anterior inferior iliac spine (rectus femoris) and the ischial tuberosity (hamstrings) are the commonest sites.

Acetabular Fractures Acetabular fractures in general involve one or more of four regions: the posterior rim, the posterior pillar, the anterior pillar, or the quadrilateral plate. As expected, fractures of the posterior rim are usually caused by posterior dislocation of the femur (Fig. 10.44). These are commonly associated with cortical fractures of the anterior femoral head. Fractures of the posterior pillar may also be seen with posterior dislocations of the femur (Fig. 10.45), and, together with fractures of the anterior pillar, are common in AP compression fractures of the pelvis. By contrast, fractures involving the quadrilateral plate are usually associated

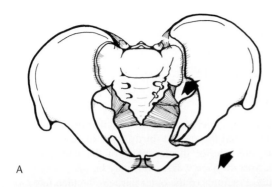

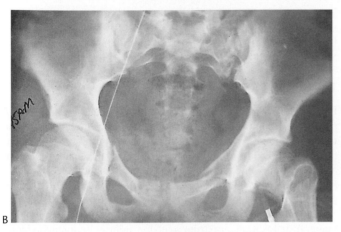

with lateral compression forces (Fig. 10.35). Undoubtedly CT provides the most detailed information about the fracture (Fig. 10.46), and there is a trend toward three-dimensional imaging of these fractures. The real advantage of conventional CT over plain radiography lies in its ability to detect small bone fragments within the joint space. Three-dimensional CT has been shown to miss small undisplaced fracture lines and intra-articular fragments, although it provides a dramatic representation of the overall fracture and orientation of fragments (Fig. 10.47).

MRI also has a role to play, particularly with its ability to detect avascular necrosis (see Ch. 9, Fig. 9.44), or injury to the internal structures, such as labral tears (Fig. 10.48).

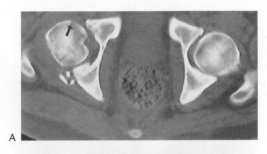

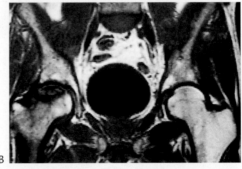

Fig. 10.42 Combined fracture pattern. **A.** AP and lateral compression. This type of injury gives fracture patterns of both AP and lateral compression, such as in **B**, where there are 'horizontal' fractures of the left pubic rami, indicating lateral compression, but disruption of the left sacroiliac joint, indicating AP compression.

Fig. 10.44 **A.** Posterior acetabular rim fracture shown on CT. There has been a posterior hip dislocation. A characteristic defect described by Richardson et al (1990), is seen in the anterior femoral head (arrow): it is similar to the Hill–Sachs deformity of the humeral head in anterior humeral dislocations. **B.** This type of dislocation may lead to post-traumatic avascular necrosis, as shown on this coronal MRI image.

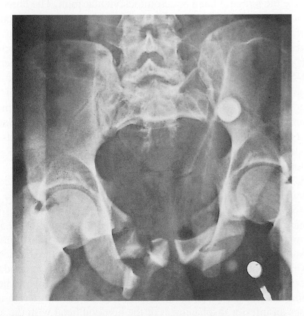

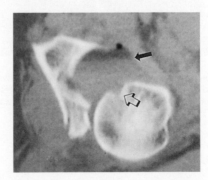

Fig. 10.43 The so-called 'straddle' fracture is not due to straddling, but, in this case, to AP compression. Diastasis of the left SIJ indicates a Type III AP compression fracture.

Fig. 10.45 Posterior acetabular pillar fracture. CT scan demonstrates an extensive fracture of the posterior acetabular pillar, again usually associated with posterior hip dislocation. A fat–fluid level is seen in the joint (arrow), with a small collection of air anteriorly, probably a 'vacuum' phenomenon. The cortical femoral head defect is again seen (open arrow).

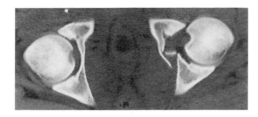

Fig. 10.46 Comminuted right acetabular fracture. CT indicates involvement of predominantly the quadrilateral plate, with disruption of the medial articular surface. A fracture through the anterior rim of the left acetabulum is also seen.

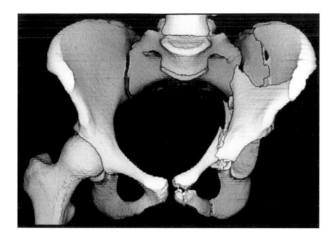

Fig. 10.47 3-D reformating of a fracture of the left pelvis and acetabulum, with computerized disarticulation. (Courtesy of Picker International.)

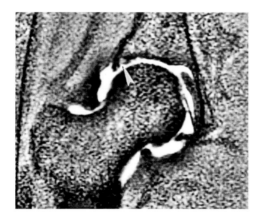

Fig. 10.48 Superior labral tear of right acetabulum. T$_1$-weighted image (fat suppression and intra-articular gadolinium) demonstrates irregularity of the superior labrum (arrowhead). (Courtesy of William Conway, M.D.)

RIB FRACTURES

The lower ribs are commonly fractured, often from relatively minor trauma. Pneumothorax and hemothorax may be associated and should be excluded.

In contrast, fractures of the first and second rib are usually from major trauma; serious associations including pneumothorax, hemopneumothorax, ruptured subclavian artery, pneumopericardium, and tracheobronchial fistula may be seen.

SHOULDER GIRDLE

The Clavicle

Fractures of the clavicle involve the middle third in 80%, the outer third in 15%, and the medial third in 5% of cases. Overriding of fragments and inferior displacement of the lateral fragment are common. Specific views, however, may be necessary to visualize the fracture. Fractures of the outer third are divided into two types: those in which disruption of the coracoclavicular ligaments does not occur (Type I), and those in which it does (Type II). Type II fractures are associated with greater displacement and a higher incidence of non-union.

The Scapula

Fractures of the scapula are relatively rare, comprising only 1% of all fractures. They usually occur from major direct blows, and thus are commonly associated with other injuries, frequently of the ribs and clavicle. They may occur in any of the anatomic regions of the scapula, but are most common in the body (50–70%). Fractures of the glenoid rim occur in approximately 20% of shoulder dislocations. Isolated fractures of the spinous process are rare. Fractures of the coracoid process may occur from anterior humeral dislocations, or from avulsion injuries (coracoclavicular ligament, coracobrachialis), and may also be seen from shotgun or rifle recoils.

Dislocations

Dislocations around the shoulder are relatively common and usually involve the humeral head or acromioclavicular joint. The humerus is most commonly dislocated *anteriorly* (95%) or, in practice, anteriorly, medially and inferiorly, coming to lie inferior to the coracoid process (Fig. 10.49). This may cause a cortical impaction both of the superior posterior aspect of the humerus (hatchet or Hill–Sachs deformity—(Fig. 10.50) and inferior aspect of the glenoid, or may give rise to injury of the anterior portion of the glenoid labrum (Bankart lesion—(Fig. 10.51). Although more common after multiple or recurrent dislocations, the Hill–Sachs defect can occur after a single episode, and merely represents an osteochondral fracture. Anterior dislocations present no diagnostic difficulty.

Posterior dislocations, however, may be difficult to appreciate, although they should not be missed. In general, they can be appreciated on the AP view by persistent internal rotation of the humerus and asymmetry of the glenohumeral joint (Fig. 10.52). An axillary view may be impossible to obtain, but a transthoracic or 'swimmers' view or oblique (Y) view will confirm the diagnosis.

An unusual *inferior dislocation* (*luxatio erecta*) is caused by severe hyperabduction of the arm, whereby the humeral head impinges upon the acromion, which in turn acts as a fulcrum and causes an inferior displacement of the humeral head with the arm 'locked' in abduction (Fig. 10.53).

Acromioclavicular separation is usually the result of a fall on the outstretched arm or point of the shoulder. The importance of acromioclavicular dislocation lies in the trauma to the coraco-

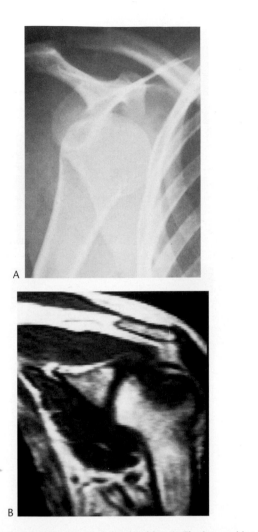

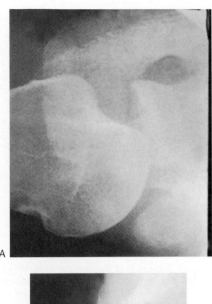

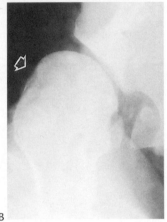

Fig. 10.49   Anterior dislocation of the shoulder. **A.** The humeral head lies medial and inferior to the glenoid in the subscapular fossa. **B.** MRI scan (T₁ weighting) following reduction of anterior dislocation demonstrates an area of decreased signal, indicating subarticular bone 'bruising', possibly leading to the later radiographic appearances of a Hill–Sachs deformity.

Fig. 10.50   Recurrent anterior dislocation of the shoulder. The characteristic defect is well shown in the axial projection **A.** A large defect of this nature can even be visualized clearly in the AP projection, but it is rarely possible to identify small defects on a simple frontal projection; a film in 60° internal rotation or a Stryker view **B.** is required.

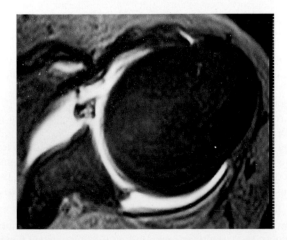

Fig. 10.51   Disruption of the anterior glenoid labrum seen by MR Arthrography. The disrupted anterior labrum is well shown by the high signal intensity gadolinium solution, within the joint capsule. Courtesy of William Conway, M.D.)

clavicular ligament. This injury has been classified as sprain (Grade I), subluxation (Grade II), and dislocation (Grade III) (Fig. 10.54). Grade III injuries are in general obvious on plain radiography, with both acromioclavicular and coracoclavicular separation. In Grade II injuries, stress views with weight-bearing may be needed. In Grade I injuries, mild widening of the acromioclavicular space, but not the coracoclavicular space, may be seen on stress views.

Rotator Cuff

This is the term applied to the conjoined tendons of the supraspinatus, infraspinatus, subscapularis and teres minor muscles. The rotator cuff passes between the humeral head and acromion before inserting into the greater tuberosity of the humerus. It separates the glenohumeral joint from the subdeltoid bursa. Ruptures, either partial or complete, may be diagnosed by arthrography, although ultrasound and MRI are gaining popularity as diagnostic tools (Fig. 10.55).

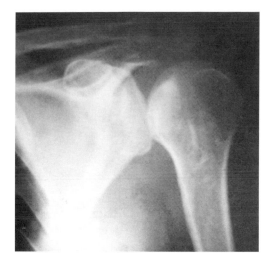

Fig. 10.52 Posterior dislocation of the shoulder. Note the circular appearance of the humeral head and the lack of parallelism between this and the glenoid fossa. The injury followed a severe electric shock causing muscle spasm, which had also precipitated compression fractures of the fifth and sixth thoracic vertebral bodies.

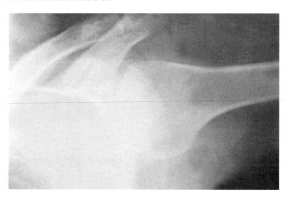

Fig. 10.53 Luxatio erecta. An unusual inferior dislocation of the humerus, which is 'locked' in abduction.

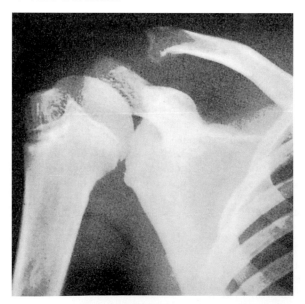

Fig. 10.54 Dislocation of the acromioclavicular joint following a fall on the point of the shoulder. The deformity is accentuated by examination in the erect position with weights being carried in both hands.

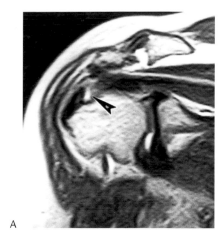

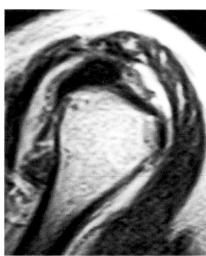

Fig. 10.55 MRI: rotator cuff injury. Paracoronal **A.** and parasagittal **B.** images demonstrate focal increased signal within the substance of the subscapularis tendon (arrowhead, **A**), indicative of a full thickness tear.

THE UPPER LIMB

Humerus

Most injuries result from falls on the outstretched arm, particularly in elderly (osteopenic) women. Fractures of the surgical neck or greater tuberosity are the commonest injuries. Spiral and oblique fractures are common, usually with displacement or angulation of the distal fragment (Fig. 10.56), often requiring open fixation. Radial nerve injury occurs in up to 30% of cases.

Intra-articular fractures may be mild, as in the Hill–Sachs lesion, or severe, leading to fragmentation and intra-articular bone fragments. A 'drooping' shoulder may be seen, possibly as a result of capsular, muscular and neurologic factors. Osteonecrosis has been reported in up to 50% of cases.

Supracondylar fractures are the commonest elbow injury in children (60%), resulting from a fall on the outstretched hand. No fracture line may be seen initially on the radiograph, but hemarthrosis with elevation of the anterior and/or posterior fat pads is highly suggestive. Volar displacement of the capitellum is also a helpful

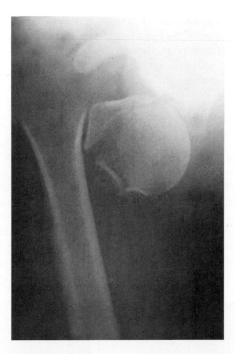

Fig. 10.56 Fracture of the surgical neck of the humerus: axial view. There is marked displacement of the distal humerus, with the comminuted fracture extending into the humeral head.

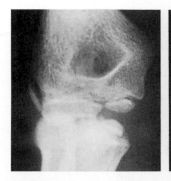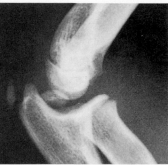

Fig. 10.58 Avulsion of medial epicondyle of the humerus. The center for the lateral epicondyle has ossified in this child, therefore the medial epicondyle should also have appeared. It is not in its normal location but lies within the medial compartment of the elbow joint.

sign (Fig. 10.57). These fractures, with associated vascular damage, may be of importance in the development of **Volkmann's ischemia** of the forearm. The second most common elbow fracture in children is that of the lateral epicondyle, although medial epicondylar fractures are also seen (Fig. 10.58).

Forearm Fractures

Fractures of the bones of the forearm are extremely common, particularly of the radial head, olecranon process, distal radius and ulna. The forearm effectively acts as a ring structure and apparent single fractures may be associated with additional injury, either ligamentous or bony. This 'closed ring' concept explains double forearm fractures (Fig. 10.59), i.e. Galeazzi fractures of the radius with distal ulnar dislocation (Fig. 10.60). and Monteggia fractures of the ulna with radial head dislocation (Fig. 10.61). It is therefore essential to examine the wrist and elbow carefully for additional injury in 'single bone' forearm fractures.

Fracture of the radial head is the commonest elbow injury in adults, usually occurring as a result of a fall on the outstretched arm. The fracture line may not be seen initially, but an elbow effusion is a good warning sign, warranting immobilization and repeat radiograph in 7–10 days.

Olecranon fractures result from falls onto the point of the elbow, or avulsions of the triceps insertions. They must be distinguished from the unfused ossification center in children and young adults.

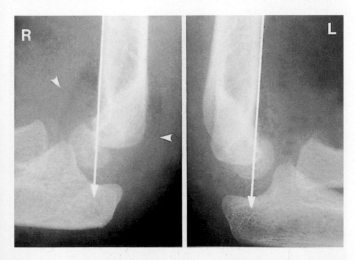

Fig. 10.57 Supracondylar fracture of humerus. The left humerus is normal; the line extending from the anterior cortex of the shaft passes through the middle third of the capitellum. A hemarthrosis of the right elbow joint displaces both fat pads and a similar line cuts the posterior third of the capitellum, indicating the anterior displacement of the fragment.

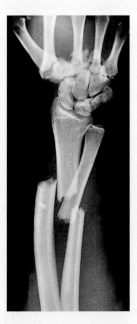

Fig. 10.59 Fractures through both forearm bones are seen. Apparent 'shortening' of the distal ulna, with marked angulation, suggests distal radio-ulnar joint injury.

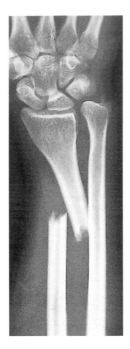

Fig. 10.60   Galeazzi fracture. Dislocation of the distal ulna accompanies the radial fracture.

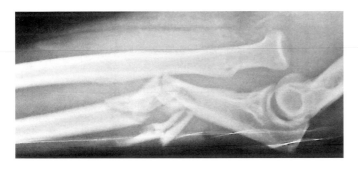

Fig. 10.61   Monteggia fracture-dislocation. There is a comminuted fracture of the ulna with dislocation of the radial head.

Injuries Around the Wrist

As mentioned above, injuries of the distal radio-ulnar joint are commonly associated with fractures of the radius and ulna, either alone or in combination. Injury to the wrist, and, in particular, disruption of the triangular fibrocartilage complex (TFCC), should be excluded in forearm fractures. TFCC disruptions may also be seen following a fall onto the outstretched hand. Arthrography is commonly used in evaluating TFCC disruptions, although MRI is gaining in popularity as a method of evaluating the wrist joint. The TFCC is, in general, well seen on MRI, although consistent visualization of the intercarpal ligaments has been less successful, and requires the highest quality of images.

The distal forearm is one of the commonest sites of fracture in the entire body, and most fractures are associated with eponyms.

In **Colles fracture**, the distal radius is fractured and angulated dorsally, giving rise clinically to the 'dinner-fork' deformity of the wrist (Fig. 10.62). The ulnar styloid is fractured in over 50% of cases, and there is almost invariably distal radio-ulnar dissociation.

Smith's fracture is the reverse of the Colles fracture, with volar angulation of the distal fragments of the radius (Fig. 10.59). In **Barton's fracture**, the fracture line extends through the dorsum of the distal radius to involve the articular surface. If the volar radial rim is involved, this is a *reverse Barton's fracture* (Fig. 10.63).

Fractures of the Carpus

The *scaphoid* bone is the most common carpal bone to be fractured. Once again, initial radiographic examination may be negative and a follow-up X-ray should be performed in 7–10 days after immobilization if there is a clinical suspicion (Fig. 10.64). Alternatively, a radionuclide bone scan may be helpful. Non-union and osteonecrosis of the proximal fragment are important complications, particularly in fractures of the proximal scaphoid, as the vascular supply enters in the middle of the bone. Dorsal avulsion fractures of the *triquetrum* are the second most common and may be appreciated

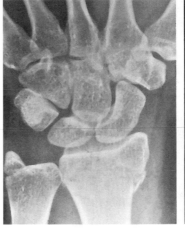
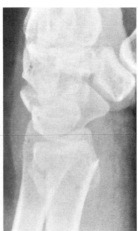

Fig. 10.62   Fracture of the distal radius with dorsal angulation of the distal fragment. Although frequently referred to as Colles fracture, the extension of the fracture to the articular surface, seen on the AP view, indicates that this is a Barton's fracture.

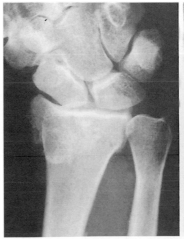
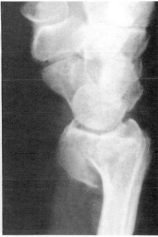

Fig. 10.63   Although commonly referred to as a Smith's fracture, the involvement of the articular surface indicates that this should more correctly be called a reverse Barton's fracture.

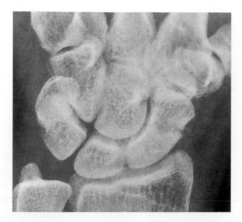

Fig. 10.64 Scaphoid fractures. There is a mild cortical irregularity of the radial side of the waist of the scaphoid. A faint fracture line extends through the waist.

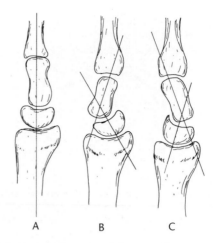

Fig. 10.66 A. Normal alignment of the wrist allows a continuous line to be drawn through the radius, lunate and capitate. **B.** Abnormal alignment: palmar flexion instability (volar intercalary segment carpal instability: VISI). The lunate is rotated toward the palmar surface of the wrist, with the capitate rotated toward the dorsal surface. **C.** Dorsiflexion instability (dorsal intercalary segment carpal instability: DISI)—the converse of **B.**

best on the lateral view. The other carpal bones are only rarely injured, except for the *hamate*, the hook of which may be detached acutely by blows on the proximal palm of the hand, or by chronic trauma, such as from holding a tennis racquet or golf club.

Dislocation of the Carpus

Dislocations of the carpus are complex, but are best appreciated by understanding two important concepts.

1. On the posteroanterior view, two major areas define the carpal relationship (Fig. 10.65): the proximal and distal carpal lines, following the proximal and distal margins of the scaphoid, lunate and triquetrum respectively. These lines should be roughly parallel, and the intercarpal joint spaces should be approximately equal.

2. On the lateral view of the normal wrist in its neutral position, a straight line can be drawn through the long axis of the radius, lunate and capitate (Fig. 10.66). This should intersect a line drawn along the long axis of the scaphoid at 30–60° (Fig. 10.67). A variation of the angle of any of these lines indicates carpal instability. Other patterns of instability are triquetrohamate instability (dissociation), and triquetrolunate dissociation, usually diagnosed by abnormal motion on fluoroscopy.

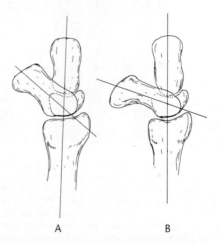

Fig. 10.67 A. In the normal wrist, the scaphoid long axis bisects the radial long axis at approximately 45° (30–60°). **B.** Rotatory subluxation: the long axis of the scaphoid is tilted in a volar direction.

Examination of carpal trauma has led to the concept of two 'injury arcs' in the wrist (Fig. 10.68), enabling a sequence of injuries to be predicted. The sequence usually begins on the radial side with rotatory subluxation of the scaphoid and scapholunate dissociation (see below). Stage II is the perilunate dislocation (see below), following failure of the radiocapitate ligament. In Stage III, injury to the radiotriquetral ligament and dorsal radiocarpal ligaments gives rise to triquetral malrotation and triquetrolunate dissociation; in Stage IV injury, there is disruption of the dorsal radiocarpal ligament, allowing complete dislocation of the lunate.

In *lunate dislocation*, the normal anatomy of the proximal carpal row is lost, and the lunate is usually seen to overlap the capitate, hamate and triquetrum on the PA view, also taking on a triangular, rather than a rectangular shape (Fig. 10.69). On the lateral projection, the lunate is seen overlying the volar aspect of the wrist, in an abnormal orientation.

In *perilunate (± trans-scaphoid fracture) dislocation*, the whole

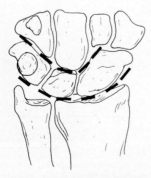

Fig. 10.65 Normal carpal relationship. The proximal and distal carpal lines define the normal carpal relationship on the PA projection.

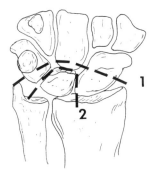

Fig. 10.68   Arcs of injury of the wrist. 1. The greater arc: pure injury of the greater arc gives rise to a trans-scaphoid, transcapitate, transhamate, and transtriquetral dislocation. 2. The lesser arc: injury here gives rise to lunate or perilunate dislocation.

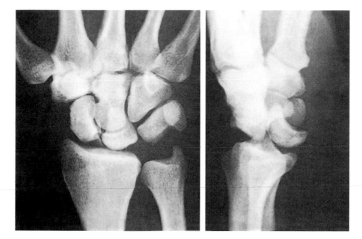

Fig. 10.69   Dislocation of the lunate. In the anteroposterior projection the lunate bone appears to be triangular instead of quadrilateral in shape, and the lateral projection shows clearly that it is displaced forward. The distal concavity no longer contains the base of the capitate. Because this appearance is perhaps intermediate between a lunate and a perilunate dislocation, it is better referred to as a dorsal midcarpal dislocation. A chip fracture of the proximal scaphoid is also present.

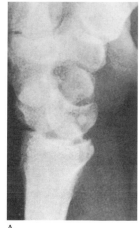
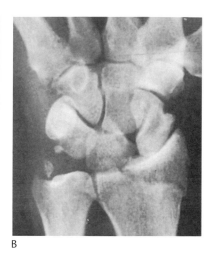

A   B

Fig. 10.70   **A,B** Perilunate dislocation of the carpus. With the exception of the lunate, the whole of the carpus has been dislocated dorsally in relation to the radius. Both the radial and ulnar styloid processes have been fractured. Note loss of articulation between lunate and adjacent carpal bones.

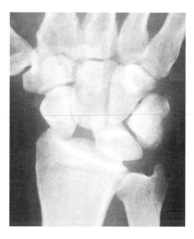

Fig. 10.71   Scapholunate dissociation: 'Terry-Thomas' or 'tooth gap' sign. There is wide separation of the scaphoid and lunate.

of the carpus (minus the proximal scaphoid pole in trans-scaphoid injuries), is dislocated posteriorly with respect to the lunate. This is usually evident on the PA view, but again is clear on the lateral projection (Fig. 10.70).

Scapholunate dissociation is identified by widening of the scapholunate joint, often exacerbated on clenching the fist (Terry-Thomas sign—(Fig. 10.71). This may be seen in rotational (rotatory) dislocation of the scaphoid.

Arthrography is currently the method of choice for examining the intercarpal ligaments. Some authors advocate injection of all three wrist compartments, although careful examination with video fluoroscopy after injection of the radiocarpal joint will define the vast majority of injuries (Fig. 10.72). Although MRI has been proposed as a diagnostic tool for intercarpal ligament disruptions, results to date have not been convincing.

The Hand

Hand injuries are common and usually present no diagnostic difficulty.

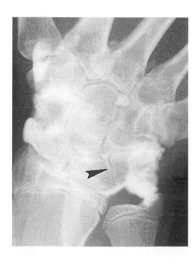

Fig. 10.72   Intercarpal ligament disruption: arthrogram. Injection of the radiocarpal joint has resulted in filling of the intercarpal joint as well. Contrast medium is seen passing between the lunate and triquetrum (arrowhead), indicating ligamentous disruption.

'*Bennett's fracture*' is a fracture-dislocation of the base of the first metacarpal with involvement of the articular surface, usually associated with 'dislocation' of the major fragment (Fig. 10.73).

Another important injury in the thumb is *avulsion* of the ulnar aspect *of the base of the proximal phalanx*, due to forced radial or posterior hyperextension. This injury is due to avulsion of either the ulnar collateral ligament or the adductor policis and creates instability and loss of forceful adduction if left untreated. Although named the 'mechanical bull' thumb, this injury is more common in skiing accidents, from falling into snow without releasing the ski pole. The '*boxer's' fracture* of the *fifth metacarpal* is a common injury presenting in accident and emergency departments (Fig. 10.74).

THE LOWER LIMB

The Femur

Fracture of the femoral neck and *intertrochanteric fractures* are common injuries following a fall, particularly in the elderly when osteoporosis is present (Fig. 10.75). Nevertheless, because of the age of many of the patients, underlying pathology such as metastasis should always be excluded. These fractures may be extremely difficult to define radiographically, and *radionuclide bone scan* may be necessary. A faint ill-defined linear density across the

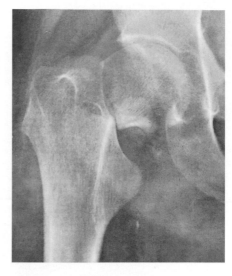

Fig. 10.75 A fracture of the femoral neck may be identified as a lucency interrupting the trabecular pattern, and the femur is externally rotated distal to the fracture.

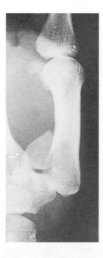

Fig. 10.73 Bennett's fracture-dislocation. The articular surface of the base of the first metacarpal is involved and the main portion of the bone is displaced proximally in relation to the trapezium.

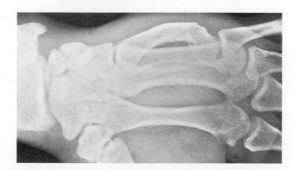

Fig. 10.74 Boxer's fracture: a fracture of the distal aspect of the fifth metacarpal, with volar angulation of the distal fragment.

femoral neck, interruption of trabecular lines, and subtle cortical disruptions may be the only radiological signs.

Fractures of the *femoral shaft* are almost always a sign of major trauma, often in multitrauma victims (see Fig. 9.3). In trivial trauma, underlying pathology should always be suspected.

Fractures of the *distal femur* are frequently intra-articular and give rise to angulation of the distal fragments and disruption of the knee joint.

The Knee and Lower Leg

Fractures around the knee include *femoral* fractures (see above), *patellar* fractures and *tibial plateau* fractures (Fig. 10.76). The only difficulty with patellar fractures may be in differentiating them from a bipartite patella when the fracture is single and involves the superior margins. This should be evident clinically and is usually clear radiographically although confusion may arise.

Fractures of the tibial plateau are obvious in general but on occasion may not be evident as a fracture line. A cross-table lateral radiograph may demonstrate a fat–fluid level of *lipohemarthrosis* in the suprapatellar bursa, indicating an intra-articular process (see Fig. 9.6). Tomograms may be needed in tibial plateau fractures to determine any depression of fragments. CT is also gaining popularity as a method of evaluating the extent of injury.

Injuries to the *menisci* traditionally have been examined by arthrography. However, in most centers MRI has superseded arthrography by virtue of its improved sensitivity and patient comfort. Not only can it define abnormality of the menisci (Fig. 10.77), but it can also identify abnormality of the supporting ligaments (Fig 10.78, 10.79), surrounding soft tissues (Fig. 10.80), and bony structures (Fig. 10.81).

Fractures of the *shaft of the tibia* are usually oblique or spiral, although transverse fractures also occur. There is invariably an associated fracture of the fibula, again indicating the association of double injuries with bony 'ring' structures. Complications of tibial fractures include a high incidence of open injuries and delayed union, usually the result of high-energy impact forces.

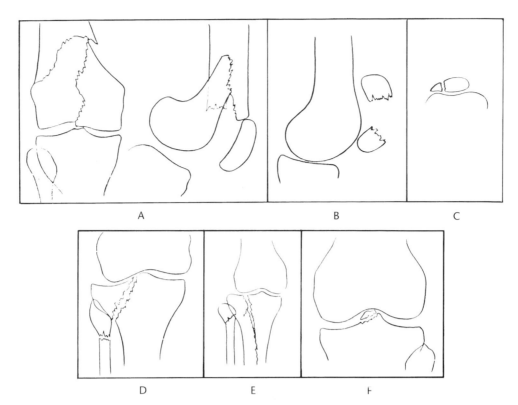

Fig. 10.76 Injuries of the knee and leg. **A.** Supracondylar fracture of the femur with extension to involve the articular surface. **B.** Transverse fracture of the patella with wide separation of fragments. **C.** Vertical fracture of the patella visible only in the axial projection. **D.** Fracture of the lateral condyle of the tibia and neck of fibula. This injury has resulted from forced abduction, with impact of the surface of the lateral femoral condyle upon the tibia. Involvement of the articular surface is minimal and this injury carries a good prognosis. **E.** A more severe fracture of the lateral tibial condyle with a crack running downward into the tibial shaft. This has been caused by complete rupture of the internal lateral ligament and the cruciate ligaments, so that the lateral margin of the femur has impacted upon the surface of the lateral tibial condyle to produce the injury. The articular surface is involved. The neck of the fibula is also fractured. **F.** Avulsion injury to extrasynovial intercondylar region of tibia.

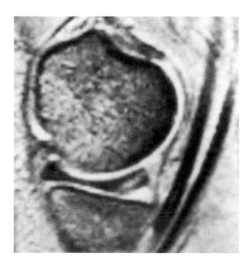

Fig. 10.77 MRI of meniscal injury, gradient echo sequence. There is irregularity of the posterior horn of the medial meniscus, with a linear area of increased signal extending through the meniscus to the inferior surface. These changes indicate a complete tear.

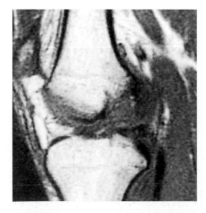

Fig. 10.78 MRI of anterior cruciate tear. There is loss of detail of the ligament, which is replaced by an amorphous collection of hematoma and debris.

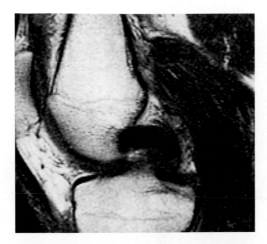

Fig. 10.79 Posterior cruciate tear. The ligament is disrupted in its mid and distal portions, with swelling, and loss of detail.

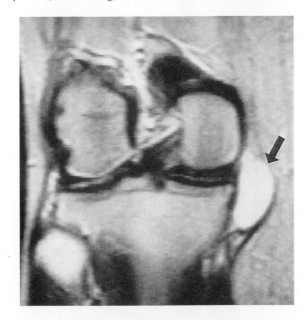

Fig. 10.80 Meniscal cyst: MRI (T₂). There is increased signal in a well-defined fluid collection (arrow) arising from the medial meniscus.

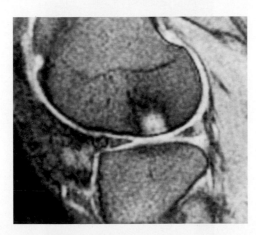

Fig. 10.81 Bone 'bruising' of the femoral condyle, following knee dislocation. MRI gradient echo image, showing the typical appearances of a focal area of increased signal.

Stress Fractures   These are found in those who inflict chronic stress on the leg (joggers, ballet dancers, etc). The proximal shaft is the commonest site, but they may occur at any site. Pain and increased uptake on radionuclide bone scan are the earliest signs. Periosteal reaction follows. Chronic stress fractures exhibit abundant surrounding sclerosis (see Fig. 9.17). Early diagnosis can be made by MRI, before radiographic changes become apparent (see Fig. 9.16).

The Ankle and Foot

The most detailed (and complex) classification of ankle fractures, that of Lauge-Hansen, is based on classifying the injury according to the nature of the causative force, much as in the pelvis and spine. However, as well as using the parameters of external rotation, abduction, adduction, and dorsiflexion, the classification is complicated by whether the foot is in pronation or supination at the time of injury. A similar system regards ankle injuries as being the result of forced supination or pronation, and forced adduction or abduction, with some variation being imparted by external (or rarely internal) rotation (Fig. 10.82) when injuries to the tibial plafond (usually posterior) may result. In practice, the injury patterns obtained using this less complicated system are the same as those described in the Lauge-Hansen classification.

Radiographically, symmetry of the ankle mortise should be sought, as asymmetry may be the only indication of significant ligamentous injury. In addition, the nature of the injury to the

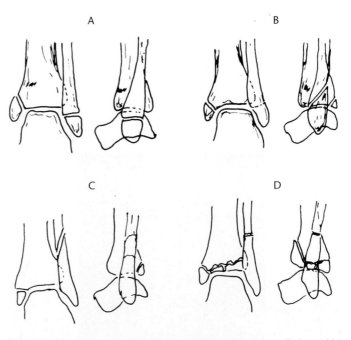

Fig. 10.82 Diagram of the major varieties of injuries of the ankle. **A.** Adduction/inversion injury of the ankle. The fracture on the tension side (lateral malleolus) is transverse. The medial malleolar fracture is oblique. **B.** Additional external rotation gives rise to an oblique or spiral fracture of the fibula ± fracture of the posterior aspect of the tibial plafond. **C.** Abduction (eversion) injury. The fracture on the tension side (medial malleolus) again is transverse; with external rotation, fracture of the posterior aspect of the tibial plafond may occur, as shown. **D.** Forced dorsiflexion. Comminution of the tibial plafond is expected, particularly involving the anterior aspect.

malleoli (i.e. whether horizontal or oblique) will indicate the side from which the force of injury was derived, the horizontal fracture occurring on the side of injury, and the oblique fracture on the opposite side. If no fracture is present, stress views may be indicated to evaluate for ligamentous damage. Again, however, MRI is gaining in popularity for evaluating the ankle, due to its ability to demonstrate ligamentous injury, particularly of the internal ligaments, and injuries to the surrounding tendons (Fig. 10.83).

Talar fractures are generally avulsions or fractures through the waist, usually as a result of forced dorsiflexion. These are often associated with dislocations of the ankle or subtalar joint (Fig. 10.84). Avascular necrosis of the proximal fragment is a common complication. Talar dislocation may also result from forced plantar flexion injuries.

Calcaneal fractures are a frequent finding in falls from a height, and may be associated with fractures of the thoracolumbar spine. They are generally predominantly shearing fractures, but with a certain crushing component, due to the anatomy of the region: the talus, and hence the tibia, is offset medially in relation to the body of the calcaneus. As such, the axial view of the talus may be helpful in the initial evaluation. Nevertheless, calcaneal fractures may be difficult to appreciate on plain radiographs. Flattening of Bohler's angle may be a helpful sign (Fig. 10.85). CT is particularly useful in the evaluation of calcaneal fractures (see Fig. 9.8D).

Other notable fractures of the foot include *avulsion of the base of the fifth metatarsal* which must be distinguished from an unfused epiphysis. In addition, the 'Jones' fracture of the proximal diaphysis of the fifth metatarsal may proceed to non-union, or delayed union. The *Lisfranc fracture-dislocation of the tarsometatarsal junction* is also an important injury, and although usually obvious (Fig. 10.86) is often overlooked when subtle. Malalignment of the second metatarsal and middle cuneiform on the frontal view is diagnostic in such cases. Failure to diagnose and treat this injury will give rise to significant long-term mid-foot problems.

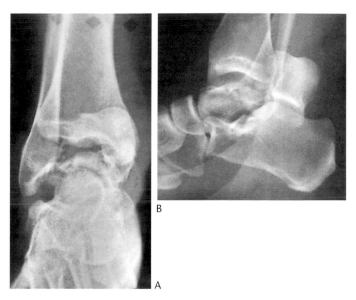

Fig. 10.84 **A,B** Fracture dislocation of the talus. There is a fracture through the waist of the talus, with complete dislocation of the posterior fragment.

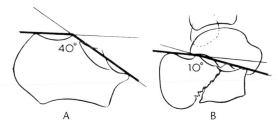

Fig. 10.85 Fracture of the calcaneus. The normal angle formed between the subtalar joint and the upper margin of the tuberosity of the calcaneus should be about 40°. Diminution of this angle should arouse suspicion of a fracture, but this may only be clearly shown in the axial projection. **A.** Normal Bohler's angle measurement. **B.** Increased angle with fracture of body of calcaneus.

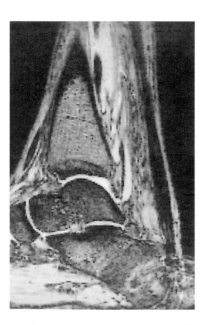

Fig. 10.83 MRI of the ankle: partial rupture of the Achilles tendon. There is widening of the tendon above its insertion, with areas of increased signal.

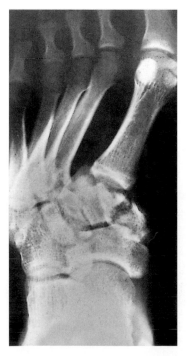

Fig. 10.86 Lisfranc fracture-dislocation. There are fractures through the medial cuneiform and bases of the second and third metatarsals, with lateral displacement of the first, second, third and fourth metatarsals.

REFERENCES AND SUGGESTIONS FOR FURTHER READING

Acheson, M. B., Livingston, R. R., Richardson, M. I. et al (1987) High-resolution CT scanning in the evaluation of cervical spine fracture: comparison with plain film examinations. *American Journal of Roentgenology*, **148**, 1179–1185.

Bloomberg, T. J., Nuttall, J., Stoker, D. J. (1978) Radiology in early slipped femoral capital epiphysis. *Clinical Radiology*, **29**, 657–667.

Bright, R. W. (1982) Partial growth arrest: identification, classification, and result of treatment. *Orthopedic Transactions*, **6**, 65–73.

Carrino J. A., McCauley T. R., Katz L. D., Smith R. C., Lange R. C., (1997) Rotator Cuff: Evaluation with fast spin-echo versus conventional spin echo MR imaging. *Radiology*. **202**: 533–539.

Crowe, J. E., Swischuk, L. E. (1977) Acute bowing fractures of the forearm in children: a frequently missed injury. *American Journal of Roentgenology*, **128**, 981–986.

Crues J. V. (1991). *MRI of the musculoskeletal system*. Raven Press, New York.

Daffner, R. H., Deeb, Z. L., Rothfus, W. E. (1986) Fingerprints of vertebral trauma—a unifying concept based on mechanisms. *Skeletal Radiology*, **15**, 518–525.

Daffner, R. H., Deeb, Z. L., Rothfus, W. E. (1987) Posterior vertebral body line: importance in the detection of burst fracture. *American Journal of Roentgenology*, **148**, 93–98.

Daffner R. H., Kennedy S. L. Fix T. J. (1996). The retropharyngeal prevertebral soft tissues revisited. *Emergency Radiology*. **3**: 247–252.

Daffner, R. H., Riemer, B. L., Lupetin, A. R., Dash, N. (1986) Magnetic resonance imaging in acute tendon ruptures. *Skeletal Radiology*, **15**, 619–625.

Dias, J. J., Stirling, A. J., Finlay, D. B. L., Gregg, P. J. (1987) Computerized axial tomography for tibial plateau fractures. *Journal of Bone and Joint Surgery*, **69B**, 84–89.

Eustace S., Brophy D., Denison W. (1997) Magnetic resonance imaging of acute orthopedic trauma to the lower extremity. *Emergency Radiology*, **4**: 30–37.

Fernbach, S. K., Wilkinson, R. H. (1984) Avulsion injuries of the pelvis and proximal femur. *American Journal of Roentgenology*, **137**, 581–586.

Foster, S. C., Foster, R. R. (1976) Lisfranc's tarsometatarsal fracture-dislocation. *Radiology*, **120**, 79–85.

Gertzbein, S. D., Chenoweth, D. R. (1977) Occult injuries of the pelvic ring. *Clinical Orthopaedics*, **128**, 201–207.

Goldberg, A. L., Rothfus, W. E., Deeb, Z. L. et al (1988) Impact of magnetic resonance on the diagnostic evaluation of acute cervicothoracic spinal trauma. *Skeletal Radiology*, **17**, 39–95.

Greaney, R. B., Gerber, F. H., Laughlin, R. I. et al (1983) Distribution and natural history of stress fractures in US marine recruits. *Radiology*, **146**, 339–346.

Harris, J. H. Jr., Harris, W. H. (1975) *The Radiology of Emergency Medicine*. Baltimore: Williams & Wilkins.

Hudson, T. M., Caragol, W. J., Kaye, J. J. (1976) Isolated rotatory subluxation of the carpal navicular. *American Journal of Roentgenology*, **126**, 601–605.

Judet, R., Judet, J., Letournel, E. (1964) Fracture of the acetabulum: classification and surgical approaches for open reduction. *Journal of Bone and Joint Surgery*, **46A**, 1615–1631.

Keen, J. S., Goletz, T. H., Lilleas, T. et al (1984) Diagnosis of vertebral fractures. A comparison of conventional radiography, conventional tomography, and computed axial tomography. *Journal of Bone and Joint Surgery*, **64A**, 586–594.

Lauge-Hansen, N. (1954) Fractures of the ankle: genetic roentgenologic diagnosis of fractures of the ankle. *American Journal of Roentgenology*, **71**, 456–462.

Lee R. R., (1997) MR imaging and cervical spine injury. *Radiology*. **1**: 617–618.

McArdle, C. B., Crofford, M. J., Mirfakhraee, M. et al (1986) Surface coil MR of spinal trauma. Preliminary experience. *American Journal of Neuroradiology*, **7**, 885–890.

Magid, D., Fishman, E. K. (1986) Computed tomography of acetabular fractures. *Seminars in Ultrasound, CT and MR*, **7**, 351–357.

Mirvis, S. E. (1989) Applications of MRI and 3-D CT in emergency medicine. *Annals of Emergency Medicine*, **18**, 1315–1321.

Mirvis, S. E., Geisler, F. H., Jelnick, J. J., Joslyn, J. N., Gellad, F. (1988) Acute cervical spine trauma: evaluation with 1.5 T MR imaging. *Radiology*, **166**, 807–816.

Mirvis, S. E., Young, J. W. R., Lim, C., Greenberg, J. (1986) Hangman's fracture: radiologic assessment in 27 cases. *Radiology*, **163**, 713–717.

Mirvis S. E., Young J. W. R. (1992). *Imaging in trauma and critical care*. Williams & Wilkins, Baltimore.

Orrison W. W., Benzel E. C., Willis B. K., Hart B. L., Epinosa M. C. (1995) Magnetic resonance imaging: evaluation of acute spine trauma. *Emergency Radiology*. **2**: 120–128.

Reckling, F. W. (1982) Unstable fracture-dislocations of the forearm (Monteggia and Galeazzi lesions). *Journal of Bone and Joint Surgery*, **64A**, 857–863.

Resnick, D. (ed) (1989) *Bone and Joint Imaging*. Philadelphia: W.B. Saunders.

Resnik, C. S., Gelberman, R. H., Resnick, D. (1983) Transcaphoid, transcapitate, perilunate fracture dislocation (scaphocapitate syndrome). *Skeletal Radiology*, **9**, 192–197.

Richardson, P., Young, J. W. R., Porter, D. (1990) CT detection of cortical fracture of the femoral head associated with posterior inferior dislocation. *American Journal of Roentgenology*, **155**, 93–94.

Rogers, L. R. (1982) *Radiology of Skeletal Trauma*. Edinburgh: Churchill Livingstone.

Rosen, R. A. (1970) Transitory demineralization of the femoral head. *Radiology*, **94**, 509–514.

Salter, R. B., Harris, W. R. (1963) Injuries involving the epiphyseal plate. *Journal of Bone and Joint Surgery*, **45A**, 587–622.

Scott, W. J. R., Fishman, E. K., Magid, D. (1987) Acetabular fractures: optimal imaging. *Radiology*, **165**, 537–539.

Templeton, P. A., Young, J. W. R., Mirvis, S. E., Buddemeyer, E. U. (1987) The value of retropharyngeal soft tissue measurement in trauma of the adult cervical spine. *Skeletal Radiology*, **16**, 98–104.

Thomason, M., Young, J. W. R. (1984) Os odontoideum. Case Report 261. *Skeletal Radiology*, **11**, 144–146.

Waddell, J. P., Johnston, D. W. C., Neidre, A. (1981) Fractures of the tibial plateau: a review of ninety-five patients and comparison of treatment methods. *Journal of Trauma*, **21**, 376–381.

Wang, S. C., Grattan-Smith, A. (1987) Thoracolumbar burst fractures: two 'new' plain film signs with CT correlation. *Australasian Radiology*, **31**, 404–409.

Whitley, J. E. N., Forsythe, H. F. (1960) Classification of cervical spine injuries. *American Journal of Roentgenology*, **83**, 633–641.

Yeager, B. A., Dalinka, M. K. (1985) Radiology of trauma to the wrist: dislocations, fracture dislocations, and instability patterns. *Skeletal Radiology*, **13**, 120.

Young, J. W. R., Burgess, A. R. (1987) *Radiologic Management of Pelvic Ring Fractures*. Baltimore: Urban-Schwartzenberg.

Young, J. W. R., Resnik, C. S., DeCandido, P., Mirvis, S. E. (1989) The laminar space in the diagnosis of rotational flexion injuries to the cervical spine. *American Journal of Radiology*, **152**, 103–107.

11

THE NORMAL CHEST: METHODS OF INVESTIGATION AND DIFFERENTIAL DIAGNOSIS

Janet Murfitt

With contributions from E. Rhys Davies, Richard W. Whitehouse, and Jeremy P. R. Jenkins

METHODS OF INVESTIGATION

1. Plain films:
   - PA, lateral
   - AP, decubitus, supine, oblique
   - Inspiratory–expiratory
   - Lordotic, apical, penetrated
   - Portable/mobile radiographs
2. Tomography
3. CT scanning
4. Radionuclide studies
5. Needle biopsy
6. Ultrasound
7. Fluoroscopy
8. Bronchography
9. Pulmonary angiography
10. Bronchial arteriography
11. MRI
12. Digital radiography and AMBER
13. Lymphangiography.

The *plain PA chest film* is the most frequently requested radiological examination. Visualization of the lung fields is excellent because of the inherent contrast of the tissues of the thorax. Lateral films should not be undertaken routinely. Comparison of the current film with old films is valuable and should always be undertaken if the old films are available. A current film is mandatory before proceeding to more complex investigations.

Simple linear tomography remains a useful investigation when CT is unavailable. It is helpful for confirming that an abnormality suspected on a plain film is genuine and that it is intrapulmonary, although the high kVp film has reduced the need for tomography in these circumstances. In addition it is still used in some centers to assess a peripheral lung mass, the lung apices and the abnormal hilum.

However, *conventional CT scanning* and *high-resolution thin-section CT scanning* are far superior for staging malignancy, detecting pulmonary metastases, and assessing chest wall and pleural lesions, the lung mass, the hilum and mediastinum. High-resolution scanning is of proven value in the diagnosis of diffuse lung disease, particularly in the early stages when the chest radiograph is normal, and for follow-up. In most centers high-resolution scanning is used for the detection of bronchiectasis, and surgery is undertaken without preoperative bronchography.

Radionuclide scanning is used as the first-line investigation of suspected pulmonary embolus in the majority of cases, with a normal scan excluding the presence of an embolus.

Pulmonary angiography remains the gold standard for the diagnosis of pulmonary embolism. It is usually undertaken in those patients with massive embolism when embolectomy or thrombolysis is contemplated. However, Spiral CT angiography is showing sensitivity and specificity rates approaching those of conventional angiography in the diagnosis of pulmonary embolism, and can demonstrate vessels of 2–3 mm size.

Ultrasound is of use for investigating chest wall and pleural lesions and lung lesions adjacent to the chest wall. It should be used for the localization of pleural fluid prior to a diagnostic tap or drainage to reduce the risk of a malpositioned catheter and pneumothorax. However, the acoustic mismatch between the chest wall and air-containing lung results in reflection of the ultrasound beam at the lung–pleura interface, so that normal lung cannot be demonstrated.

Biopsy of pulmonary lesions using a fine needle for aspiration has a high diagnostic yield for malignancy, excluding lymphoma, with a low incidence of complications. A cutting needle is associated with a higher complication rate but is more helpful in the diagnosis of lymphoma and benign lung conditions.

The value of *MRI* for diagnosing pulmonary disease is still in the assessment stage. No distinct advantage over high-resolution CT in the diagnosis of parenchymal disease has yet been shown but it is proven to be helpful in the diagnosis of hilar masses, lymphadenopathy and mediastinal lesions. With *digital radiography* the image is converted via an electronic image into a matrix of numbers. This allows easier storage and retrieval of images as well as transmission of images to other sites. At present the cost of such systems is high, however, and there is a lower spatial resolution than on conventional radiographs.

Using *Automatic Multiple Beam Equalization Radiography* (*AMBER*) the intensity of the X-ray beam is varied by using a horizontal beam to scan the chest caudally to cranially through detectors which modulate the beam intensity. The mediastinum and hidden areas of the lung are more clearly visualized at the cost of a higher radiation dose and edge artefacts.

Diagnostic pneumothorax is an obsolete procedure which was once used to differentiate a pleural-based from a pulmonary lesion. The *barium/contrast swallow* has been supplanted by CT for assessing the non-esophageal mediastinal mass but may be indicated in the investigation of conditions which may be associated with pulmonary changes such as scleroderma, hiatus hernia and achalasia. It is used for demonstrating broncho-esophageal fistulae, tracheal aspiration and vascular rings.

Chylous reflux with the formation of a chylothorax may be demonstrated by conventional *lymphangiography*.

THE PLAIN FILM

The PA View   By definition the patient faces the film chin up with the shoulders rotated forward to displace the scapulae from the lung fields. Exposure is made on full inspiration for optimal visualization of the lung bases, centering at T5. The breasts should be compressed against the film to prevent them obscuring the lung bases.

There is no general consensus regarding the kilovoltage used for chest radiography although the high kVp technique is becoming widely used. High kVp, low kVp or intermediate kVp techniques are used with various film-screen combinations, grids or air gap techniques.

Using a low kVp (60–80 kV) produces a high-contrast film (Fig. 11.1) with miliary shadowing and calcification being more clearly seen than on a high kV film. For large patients a grid reduces scatter. A FFD of 1.85 m (6 feet) reduces magnification and produces a sharper image. With high kilovoltages of 120–170 kVp the films are of lower contrast (Fig. 11.2A and B) with increased visualization of the hidden areas of the lung due to better penetration of overlying structures. The bones and pulmonary calcification are less well seen. The exposure time is

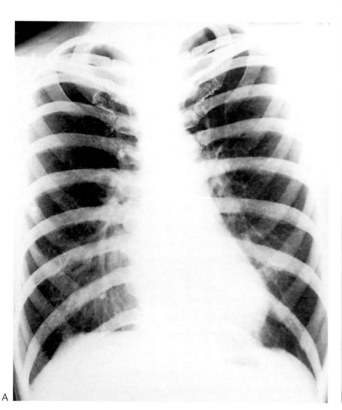

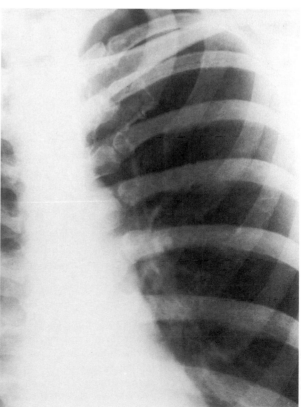

Fig. 11.1 A,B   Radiographs taken at 60 kVp.

shorter so that movement blur due to cardiac pulsation is minimized. A grid or air gap is necessary to reduce scatter and improve contrast. An air gap of 15–25 cm between patient and film necessitates an increased FFD of 2.44 m (8 feet) to reduce magnification.

An automatic exposure system and dedicated automatic chest unit are desirable in a busy department.

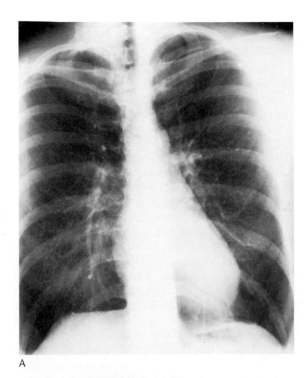

A

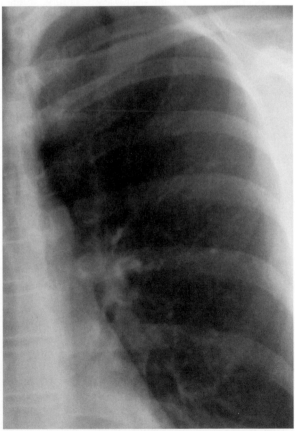

B

Fig. 11.2 A,B Radiographs of same patient as Fig. 11.1 taken at 170 kVp. Note the improved visualization of the main airways, vascular structures and the area behind the heart including the spine.

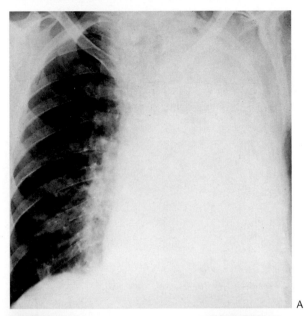

A

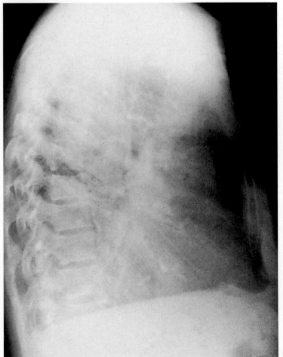

B

Fig. 11.3 A. Collapse and consolidation of the left lung. **B.** Lateral film. The appearances are less dramatic than on the PA film. Only the right hemidiaphragm is visible. The radiolucency of the lower vertebrae is decreased.

The Lateral View   A high kVp or normal kVp technique may be used with or without a grid. For sharpness the side of interest is nearest the film. With shoulders parallel to the film the arms are elevated, or displaced back if the anterior mediastinum is of interest.

Lesions obscured on the PA view are often clearly demonstrated on the lateral view. Examples of this are anterior mediastinal masses, encysted pleural fluid (Fig. 11.4) and posterior basal consolidation. In contrast, clear-cut lesions on the PA view may be difficult to identify on the lateral film because the two lungs are superimposed (Fig. 11.3). This is particularly so with a large pleural effusion.

Other Views   Although not frequently requested, additional plain films may assist with certain diagnostic problems before proceeding to the more complex and expensive techniques. The

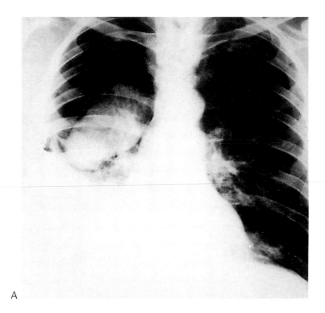

A

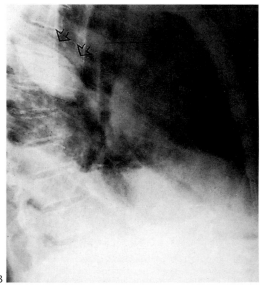

B

Fig. 11.4   Encysted pleural fluid. **A.** PA film. A large right pleural effusion and a large mass above. **B.** Lateral film. Loculated fluid is demonstrated high in the oblique fissure.

hidden areas of the PA film, rib destruction, cavitation, calcification, an air bronchogram and the main airways may all be more clearly seen on a *penetrated film*. *Oblique views* demonstrate the retrocardiac area, the posterior costophrenic angles and the chest wall, with pleural plaques being clearly demonstrated. In the AP position (as for patients unable to stand or portable radiographs) the ribs are projected over different areas of the lung from the PA view and the posterior chest is well shown. In contrast to the PA film the scapulae overlie the upper lungs and the clavicles are projected more cranially over the apices. The disk spaces of the lower cervical spine are more clearly seen whereas in the PA film the neural arches are visualized. When a portable radiograph is undertaken, the shorter FFD results in magnification of the heart and the longer exposure time in increased movement blur.

Good visualization of the apices requires projection of the clavicles upward, as in the *apical view* with the tube angled up 50–60°, or downward, as in the *lordotic view* with the patient in a lordotic PA position. In this view a middle lobe collapse shows clearly as a well-defined triangular shadow.

A subpulmonary effusion is frequently difficult to distinguish from an elevated diaphragm or consolidation. In the *supine* and *decubitus* positions (Fig. 11.5) free fluid becomes displaced. On the supine projection this results in the hemithorax becoming opaque with loss of the diaphragm outline, an apical cap, blunting of the costophrenic angle and decreased visibility of the pulmonary markings. On the PA view the apex of the effusion has a more lateral position than that of a normal diaphragm.

The decubitus films shows fluid levels particularly well. Small amounts of pleural fluid may be shown with the affected side dependent.

Paired *inspiratory* and *expiratory* films demonstrate air trapping and diaphragm movement. Small pneumothoraces and interstitial shadowing may be more apparent on the expiratory film.

Viewing the PA Film

Before a diagnosis can be made an abnormality, if present, must be identified. Knowledge of the normal appearance of a chest radiograph is essential. In addition the radiologist must develop a routine which ensures that all areas of the radiograph are scrutinized. Some prefer initially to view the film without studying the clinical information. Comparison of the current film with old films is important and often extremely helpful. A suggested scheme is as follows, examining each point in turn.

1.	Request form	Name, age, date, sex
		Clinical information
2.	Technical	Centering, patient position
		Markers
		Exposure
3	Trachea	Position, outline
4.	Heart and mediastinum	Size, shape, displacement
5.	Diaphragms	Outline, shape
		Relative position
6.	Pleura	Position of horizontal fissure
		Costophrenic, cardiophrenic angles
7.	Lung fields	Local, generalized abnormality
		Comparison of the translucency and vascular markings of the lungs

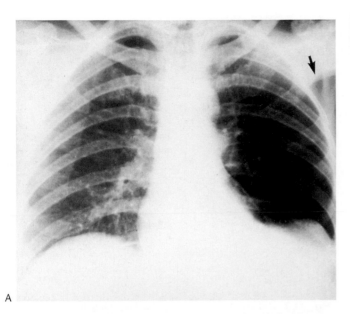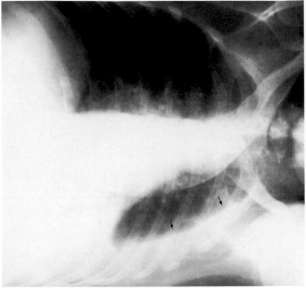

A   B

Fig. 11.5 Subpulmonary pleural fluid. **A.** Erect PA radiograph. There is apparent elevation of the left hemidiaphragm. Increased translucency of the left lung is due to a left mastectomy. Note the abnormal axillary fold (arrow). **B.** Left lateral decubitus film (with horizontal beam). Pleural fluid has moved to the most dependent part of the left lung (arrows).

8. Hidden areas	Apices, posterior sulcus
	Mediastinum, hila, bones
9. Hila	Density, position, shape
10. Below diaphragms	Gas shadows, calcification
11. Soft tissues	Mastectomy, gas, densities, etc.
12. Bones	Destructive lesions, etc.

Technical Aspects

Centering   If the film is well centered the medial ends of the clavicles are equidistant from the vertebral spinous processes at the T4/5 level. Small degrees of rotation distort the mediastinal borders, and the lung nearest the film appears less translucent. Thoracic deformities, especially a scoliosis, negate the value of conventional centering. The orientation of the aortic arch, gastric bubble and heart should be determined to confirm normal situs and that the side markers are correct.

Penetration   With a low kV film the vertebral bodies and disk spaces should be just visible through the cardiac shadow. Under-penetration increases the likelihood of missing an abnormality overlain by another structure. Overpenetration results in loss of visibility of low density lesions such as early tuberculous shadowing, although a bright light may reveal the abnormality.

Degree of Inspiration   On full inspiration the anterior ends of the sixth ribs or posterior ends of the tenth are above the diaphragms although the degree of inspiration achieved varies with patient build. Pulmonary diseases such as SLE and fibrosing alveolitis are associated with reduced pulmonary compliance, which may result in reduced inflation with elevation of the diaphragms. On expiration the heart shadow is larger and there is basal shadowing due to crowding of the normal vascular markings.

The Trachea

The trachea should be examined for narrowing, displacement and intraluminal lesions. It is midline in its upper part, then deviates slightly to the right around the aortic knuckle. On expiration deviation to the right becomes more marked. In addition there is shortening on expiration so that an endotracheal tube situated just above the carina on inspiration may occlude the main bronchus on expiration.

Its caliber should be even, with translucency of the tracheal air column decreasing causally. Normal maximum coronal diameter is 25 mm for males and 21 mm for females. The right tracheal margin, where the trachea is in contact with the lung, can be traced from the clavicles down to the right main bronchus. This border is the *right paratracheal stripe* and is seen in 60% of patients, normally measuring less than 5 mm. Widening of the stripe occurs with tracheal malignancy, mediastinal tumors, mediastinitis and pleural effusions. The left paratracheal line is rarely visualized.

The *azygos vein* lies in the angle between the right main bronchus and trachea. Enlargement occurs in the supine position but also with pregnancy, portal hypertension, IVC and SVC obstruction, right heart failure and constrictive pericarditis. On the erect film it should be less than 10 mm in diameter. Its size decreases with the Valsalva maneuver and on inspiration.

Widening of the carina occurs on inspiration. The normal angle is 60–75°. Pathological causes of widening include an enlarged left atrium (Fig. 11.6) and enlarged carinal nodes.

The Mediastinum and Heart

The central dense shadow seen on the PA chest film comprises the mediastinum, heart, spine and sternum. With good centering two-thirds of the cardiac shadow lies to the left of midline and one-

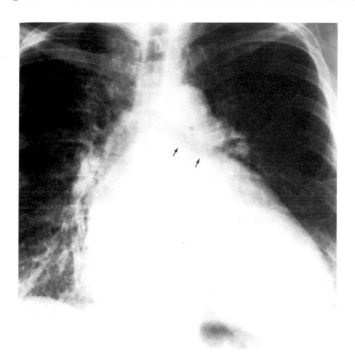

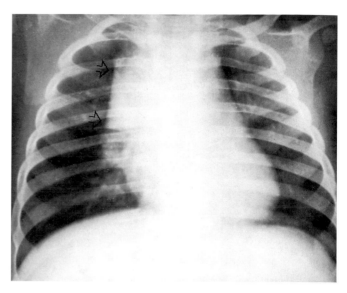

Fig. 11.7 Normal thymus in a child, projecting to the right of the mediastinum (arrows).

Fig. 11.6 Elevated left main bronchus (arrows) and widened carina. Patient with mitral valve disease and an enlarged left atrium.

third to the right, although this is quite variable in normal subjects. The *transverse cardiac diameter* and the *cardiothoracic ratio* are assessed. Measurement in isolation is of less value than when previous figures are available. An increase in excess of 1.5 cm in the transverse diameter on comparable serial films is significant. However the heart shadow is enlarged with a short FFD on expiration, in the supine and AP projections and when the diaphragms are elevated.

All borders of the heart and mediastinum are clearly defined except where the heart sits on the left hemidiaphragm. The right superior mediastinal shadow is formed by the SVC and innominate vessels; a dilated aorta may contribute to this border. On the left side the superior mediastinal border is less sharp. It is formed by the subclavian artery above the aortic knuckle.

Various junction lines may be visualized. These are formed by the pleura being outlined by the adjacent air-filled lung. The anterior junction line is formed by the lungs meeting anterior to the ascending aorta. It is only 1 mm thick and, overlying the tracheal translucency, runs downward from below the suprasternal notch, slightly curving from right to left. The posterior junction line, where the lungs meet posteriorly behind the esophagus, is a straight or curved line convex to the left some 2 mm wide and extending from the lung apices to the aortic knuckle or below. The curved pleuro-esophageal stripe, formed by the lung and right wall of the esophagus, extends from the lung apex to the azygos but is only visualized if the esophagus contains air. The left wall of the esophagus is not normally seen.

In young women the pulmonary trunk is frequently very prominent.

In babies and young children the normal *thymus* is a triangular sail-shaped structure with well-defined borders projecting from one or both sides of the mediastinum (Fig. 11.7). Both borders

may be wavy in outline, the 'wave sign of Mulvey', as a consequence of indentation by the costal cartilages. The right border is straighter than the left, which may be rounded. Thymic size decreases on inspiration and in response to stress and illness. The thymus is absent in DiGeorge syndrome. Enlargement may occur following recovery from an illness. A large thymus is more commonly seen in boys.

Adjacent to the vertebral bodies run the *paraspinal lines*, which are usually less than 10 mm wide. Enlargement occurs with osteophytes, a tortuous aorta, obesity, vertebral and adjacent soft-tissue masses, and a dilated azygos system.

A search should be made for abnormal densities, fluid levels, mediastinal emphysema and calcification. Spinal abnormalities may accompany mediastinal masses; for example, hemivertebrae are associated with neuroenteric cysts.

The Diaphragm

In most patients the right hemidiaphragm is higher than the left. This is due to the heart depressing the left side and not to the liver pushing up the right hemidiaphragm; in dextrocardia with normal abdominal situs the right hemidiaphragm is the lowest. The hemidiaphragms may lie at the same level, and in a small percentage of the population the left side is the higher; Felson (1923) reports an incidence of 3%. This is more likely to occur if the stomach or splenic flexure is distended with gas. A difference greater than 3 cm in height is considered significant.

On inspiration the domes of the diaphragms are at the level of the sixth rib anteriorly and at or below the tenth rib posteriorly. In the supine position the diaphragm is higher.

Both domes have gentle curves which steepen toward the posterior angles. The upper borders are clearly seen except on the left side where the heart is in contact with the diaphragm, and in the cardiophrenic angles when there are prominent fat pads. Otherwise loss of outline indicates that the adjacent tissue does not contain air, for example in consolidation or pleural disease.

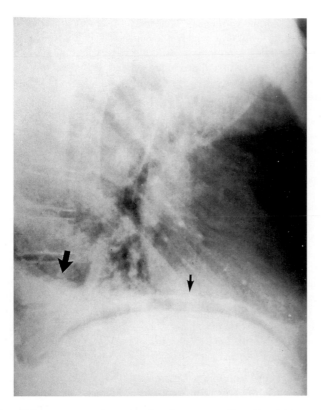

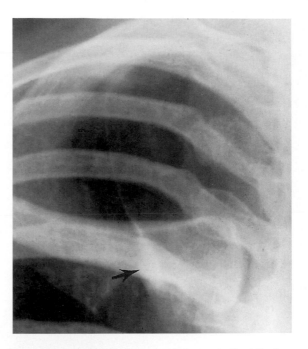

Fig. 11.9 Azygos fissure. The azygos vein is seen to lie at the lower end of the fissure (large arrow).

Fig. 11.8 Pneumoperitoneum after laparotomy. The thin right cupola (small arrow) is outlined by the adjacent aerated lung and the free abdominal gas. Posterior consolidation (large arrow) obscures the outline of the diaphragm posteriorly.

Free intraperitoneal gas outlines the undersurface of the diaphragm and shows it to be normally 2–3 mm thick (Fig. 11.8).

Congenital variations and other lesions of the diaphragm will be considered later.

The Fissures

The Main Fissures   The fissures separate the lobes of the lung but are usually incomplete allowing collateral air drift to occur between adjacent lobes. They are visualized when the X-ray beam is tangential. The horizontal fissure is seen, often incompletely, on the PA film, running from the hilum to the region of the sixth rib in the axillary line, and may be straight or have a slight downward curve. Occasionally it has a double appearance.

All fissures are clearly seen on the lateral film. The horizontal fissure runs anteriorly and often slightly downward. Both oblique fissures commence posteriorly at the level of T4 or T5, passing through the hilum. The left is steeper and finishes 5 cm behind the anterior costophrenic angle whereas the right ends just behind the angle.

Accessory Fissures   The *azygos* fissure is comma shaped with a triangular base peripherally and is nearly always right-sided (Fig. 11.9). It forms in the apex of the lung and consists of paired folds of parietal and visceral pleura plus the azygos vein which has failed to migrate normally. Enlargement occurs in the supine position. At postmortem the incidence is 1% but radiologically it is 0.4%. When left-sided, the fissure contains the hemiazygos vein.

The *superior accessory fissure* separates the apical from the basal segments of the lower lobes. It is commoner on the right side and has an incidence of 5%. On the PA film it resembles the horizontal fissure. The lateral film shows it running posteriorly from the hilum.

The *inferior accessory fissure* (Fig. 11.10) appears as an oblique line running cranially from the cardiophrenic angle toward the hilum and separating the medial basal from the other basal segments. It is commoner on the right side and has an incidence of 5%.

The *left-sided horizontal fissure* (Fig. 11.11) separates the lingula from the other upper lobe segments.

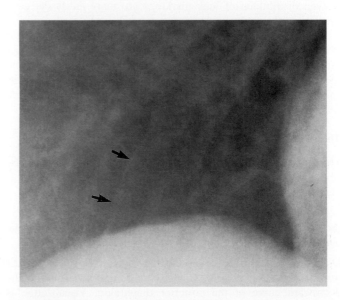

Fig. 11.10   Right inferior accessory fissure.

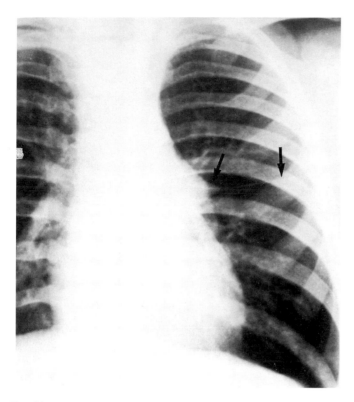

Fig. 11.11 Left-sided horizontal fissure.

The Costophrenic Angles

The normal costophrenic angles are acute and well defined but become obliterated when the diaphragms are flat. Frequently the cardiophrenic angles contain low density ill-defined shadows caused by fat pads.

The Lung Fields

By comparing the lung fields, areas of abnormal translucency or uneven distribution of lung markings are more easily detected. The size of the upper and lower zone vessels is assessed.

An abnormal shadow should be closely studied to ensure that it is not a composite shadow formed by superimposed normal structures such as vessels, bones or costal cartilage. The extent and location of the shadow is determined and specific features such as calcification or cavitation noted. A general survey is made to look for further lesions and displacement of the normal landmarks.

The Hidden Areas

The Apices   On the PA film the apices are partially obscured by ribs, costal cartilage, clavicles and soft tissues. Visualization is very limited on the lateral view.

Mediastinum and Hila   Central lesions may be obscured by these structures or appear as a superimposed density. The abnormality is usually detectable on the lateral film.

Diaphragms   The posterior and lateral basal segments of the lower lobes and the posterior sulcus are partially obscured by the downward curve of the posterior diaphragm. Visualization is further diminished if the film is not taken on full inspiration.

Bones   Costal cartilage or bone may obscure a lung lesion. In addition, determining whether a density is pulmonary or bony when overlying a rib may be difficult; AP, expiratory and oblique films may be helpful and preclude the need to proceed to CT.

The Hila

Normally the left hilum is 2.5 cm higher than the right. The hila should be of equal density and similar size with clearly defined concave lateral borders where the upper lobe vessels meet the pulmonary arteries. However there is a wide range of normal appearances. Any shadow which is not obviously vascular must be regarded with a high index of suspicion and investigated further. Old films for comparison are helpful in this situation.

Of all the structures in the hilum only the pulmonary arteries and upper lobe veins contribute significantly to the hilar shadows on the plain radiograph. Normal lymph nodes are not seen. Air can be identified within the proximal bronchi but normal bronchial walls are only seen end-on. The upper lobe bronchus may appear as a ring shadow adjacent to the upper outer hilum (Fig. 11.12), and is seen on the right side in 45% of cases and the left side in 50%. Normally there is less than 5 mm of soft tissue lateral to this bronchus. Thickening of the soft tissues suggests the presence of abnormal pathology such as malignancy.

The Inferior Pulmonary Ligament   This is a double layer of pleura extending caudally from the lower margin of the inferior pulmonary vein in the hilum as a sheet which may or may not be attached to the diaphragm and which attaches the lower lobe to the mediastinum. It is rarely identified on a simple radiograph but is frequently seen at CT.

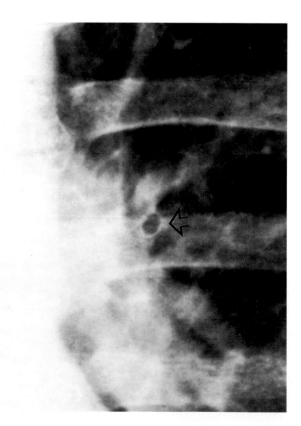

Fig. 11.12 Upper lobe bronchus seen end-on appears as a ring shadow.

The Pulmonary Vessels The left pulmonary artery lies above the left main bronchus before passing posteriorly, whereas on the right side the artery is anterior to the bronchus resulting in the right hilum being the lower. Hilar size is very variable. The maximum diameter of the normal descending branch of the right pulmonary artery is 10–16 mm for males (9–15 mm in females).

The upper lobe veins lie lateral to the arteries, which are separated from the mediastinum by approximately 1 cm of lung tissue. At the first intercostal space the normal vessels should not exceed 3 mm in diameter. The lower lobe vessels are larger than those of the upper lobes in the erect position, perfusion and aeration of the upper zones being reduced. In the supine position the vessels equalize. In the right paracardiac region the vessels are invariably prominent.

The peripheral lung markings are mainly vascular, veins and arteries having no distinguishing characteristics. There should be an even distribution throughout the lung fields.

Centrally the arteries and veins have different features. The arteries accompany the bronchi, lying posterosuperior, whereas veins do not follow the bronchi but drain via the interlobular septa eventually forming superior and basal veins which converge on the left atrium. This confluence of veins (Fig. 11.13) may be seen

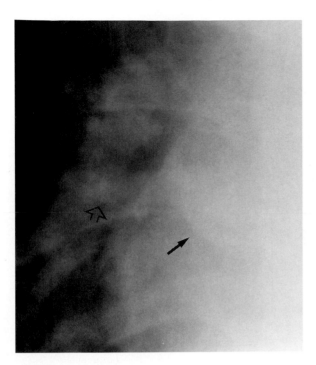

Fig. 11.13 Pulmonary vein (open arrow) draining into pulmonary confluence.

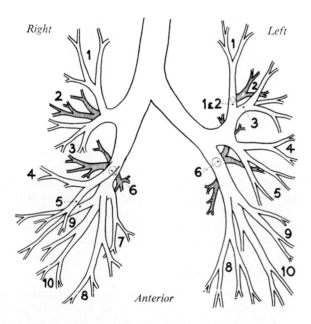

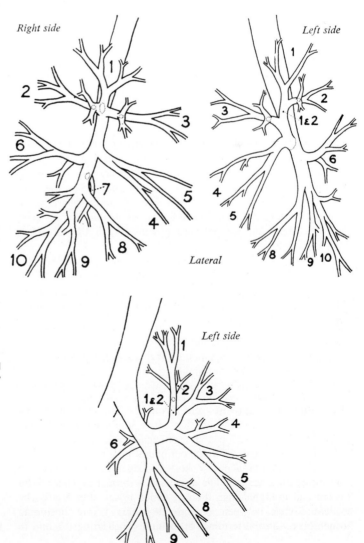

Fig. 11.14 Diagram illustrating the anatomy of the main bronchi and segmental divisions. Nomenclature approved by the Thoracic Society (reproduced by permission of the Editors of *Thorax*).

UPPER LOBE
1. Apical bronchus
2. Posterior bronchus
3. Anterior bronchus

Right   Left
MIDDLE LOBE   LINGULA
4. Lateral bronchus   4. Superior bronchus
5. Medial bronchus   5. Inferior bronchus

LOWER LOBE
6. Apical bronchus
7. Medial basal (cardiac)
8. Anterior basal bronchus   6. Apical bronchus
9. Lateral basal bronchus   8. Anterior basal bronchus
10. Posterior basal bronchus   9. Lateral basal bronchus
                                 10. Posterior basal bronchus

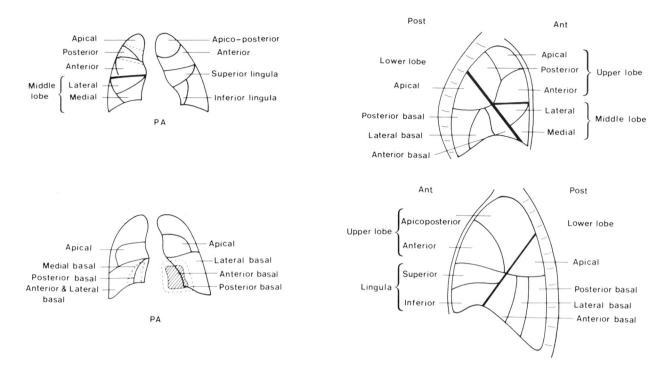

Fig. 11.15 Diagrams illustrating the approximate positions of the pulmonary segments as seen on the PA and lateral radiographs.

as a rounded structure to the right of midline superimposed on the heart, sometimes simulating an enlarged left atrium. It is visible in 5% of PA films according to Felson (1973). Pulmonary veins have fewer branches than arteries and are straighter, larger and less well defined.

The Bronchial Vessels These are normally not visualized on the plain chest film. They arise from the ventral surface of the descending aorta at the T5/6 level. Their anatomy is variable. Usually there are two branches on the left and one on the right which often shares a common origin with an intercostal artery. On entering the hila the bronchial arteries accompany the bronchi. The veins drain into the pulmonary veins and to a lesser extent the azygos system.

Enlarged bronchial arteries appear as multiple small nodules around the hilum and as short lines in the proximal lung fields. Enlargement may occur with cyanotic heart disease, and focal enlargement with a local pulmonary lesion. Occasionally enlarged arteries indent the esophagus.

Causes of Enlarged Bronchial Arteries
1. General—cyanotic congenital heart disease, e.g. pulmonary atresia, severe Fallot's tetralogy
2. Local—bronchiectasis, bronchial carcinoma.

The Pulmonary Segments and Bronchi The pulmonary segments (Figs 11.14, 11.15) are served by segmental bronchi and arteries but unlike the lobes are not separated by pleura. Normal bronchi are not visualized in the peripheral lung fields.

The right main bronchus is shorter, steeper and wider than the left, bifurcating earlier. The upper lobe bronchus arises after 2.5 cm and is higher than the left which arises after 5 cm. The bronchi divide between 6 and 20 times before becoming bronchioles with the terminal bronchioles measuring 0.2 mm in diameter. Each receives two or three respiratory bronchioles which connect with between 2 and 11 alveolar ducts. Each duct receives between 2 and 6 alveolar sacs which are connected to alveoli. The *acinus*, generally considered to be the functioning lung unit, is that portion of the lung arising from the terminal bronchiole (Fig. 11.16). When filled with fluid it is seen on a radiograph as a 5–6 mm shadow, and this comprises the basic unit seen in acinar (alveolar) shadowing.

The primary lobule arises from the last respiratory bronchiole. The secondary lobule is between 1.0 and 2.5 cm in size and is the smallest discrete unit of lung tissue surrounded by connective tissue septa. When thickened these septa become Kerley B lines (Fig. 11.17).

Other connections exist between the air spaces allowing collateral air drift. These are the pores of Kohn, 3–13 μm in size, which connect the alveoli, and the canals of Lambert (30 μm) which exist between bronchioles and alveoli.

The Lymphatic System The lymphatics remove interstitial fluid and foreign particles. They run in the interlobular septa, connecting with subpleural lymphatics and draining via the deep

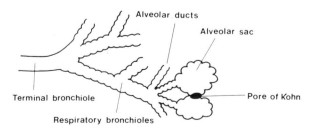

Fig. 11.16 A diagramatic representation of the acinus.

Table 11.2   Causes of Kerley Lines

Pulmonary edema
Mitral valve disease
Pneumoconiosis
Lymphangitis carcinomatosa
Sarcoidosis
Idiopathic (in the elderly)
Infections (viral, mycoplasma)
Interstitial pulmonary fibrosis
Alveolar-cell carcinoma
Lymphoma
Lymphangiectasia
Lymphatic obstruction
Lymphangiomyomatosis

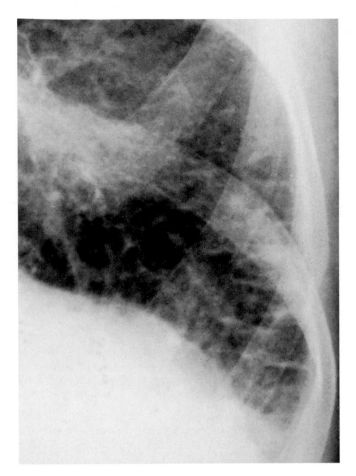

Fig. 11.17   Kerley B lines. Thickened interlobular septa in a patient with mitral valve disease.

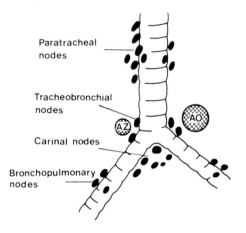

Fig. 11.18   The middle mediastinal nodes.

lymphatics to the hilum, with valves controlling the direction of flow. Normal lymphatics are not seen but thickening of the lymphatics and surrounding connective tissue produces Kerley lines, which may be transient or persistent. Thickened connective tissues are the main contributors to the substance of these lines (Tables 11.1, 11.2).

The Lymph Nodes   The intrapulmonary lymphatics drain directly to the bronchopulmonary nodes and this group is the first to be involved by spread from a peripheral tumor. A small number of intrapulmonary nodes are present and can occasionally be seen at CT but never on the plain film. The node groups and their drainage are well described (Fig. 11.18). Extensive inter-communications exist between the groups but the pattern of nodal involvement can sometimes indicate the site of the primary tumor.

Table 11.1   Kerley Lines

A Lines	Thin non-branching lines radiating from the hilum, 2–6 cm long. Thickened deep interlobular septa.
B Lines	Transverse non-branching thin lines at the lung bases perpendicular to the pleura, 1–3 cm long. Thickened interlobular septa.

Mediastinal nodes may be involved by tumors both above and below the diaphragm.

1. *The anterior mediastinal nodes* in the region of the aortic arch drain the thymus and right heart.
2. *The intrapulmonary nodes* lie along the main bronchi.
3. *The middle mediastinal nodes* drain the lungs, bronchi, left heart, the lower trachea and visceral pleura. There are four groups:
   a. Bronchopulmonary (hilar) nodes which drain into groups b and c. When enlarged they appear as lobulated hilar masses.
   b. Carinal nodes.
   c. Tracheobronchial nodes which lie adjacent to the azygos vein on the right side and near the recurrent laryngeal nerve on the left side.
   d. Paratracheal nodes are more numerous on the right side. There is significant cross drainage from left to right.
4. *The posterior mediastinal nodes* drain the posterior diaphragm and lower esophagus. They lie around the lower descending aorta and esophagus.
5. *The parietal nodes* consist of anterior and posterior groups situated behind the sternum and posteriorly in the intercostal region, draining the soft tissues and parietal pleura.

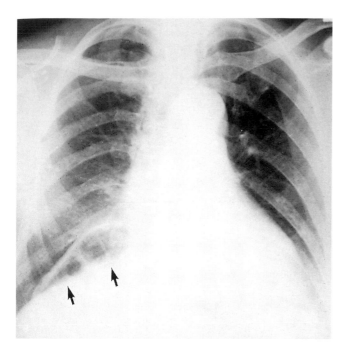

Fig. 11.19 Chilaiditi syndrome. Interposition of colon between liver and diaphragm. Note the colonic haustral pattern.

Below the Diaphragm

An erect chest film is preferred to an erect abdominal film for the diagnosis of a pneumoperitoneum. A search should be made for other abnormal gas shadows such as dilated bowel, abscesses, a displaced gastric bubble and intramural gas as well as calcified lesions. Interposition of colon between liver and diaphragm, *Chilaiditi syndrome* (Fig. 11.19), is a common and often transient finding particularly in the aged, the obvious haustral pattern distinguishing it from free gas. Subdiaphragmatic fat in the obese may be confused with free gas on a single film.

Soft Tissues

A general survey of the soft tissues includes the chest wall, shoulders and lower neck.

It is important to confirm the presence or absence of breast shadows. The breasts may partially obscure the lung bases. Nipple shadows are variable in position, often asymmetric, and frequently only one shadow is seen. Care is necessary to avoid misinterpretation as a neoplasm or vice versa. Nipple shadows are often well defined laterally and may have a lucent halo. Repeat films with nipple markers are necessary if there is any doubt.

Skin folds are often seen running vertically, particularly in the old and in babies. When overlying the lung fields they can be confused with a pneumothorax. However, a skin fold if followed usually extends outside the lung field.

The anterior axillary fold is a curvilinear shadow extending from the axilla onto the lung fields and frequently causing ill-defined shadowing which must be differentiated from consolidation.

At the apices the opacity of the sternocleidomastoid muscles curving down and slightly outward may simulate a cavity or bulla. The floor of the supraclavicular fossa often resembles a fluid level. A deep sternoclavicular fossa, commonly present in the elderly, appears as a translucency overlying the trachea and simulating a gas-filled diverticulum.

Subpleural thickening seen peripherally is often due to subpleural fat or prominent intercostal muscles rather than to pleural pathology.

Companion shadows are formed by the soft tissues adjacent to bony structures, are 2–3 mm thick, and are frequently seen running parallel to the upper borders of the clavicles and the inferior borders of the lower ribs.

Apical pleural thickening, 'the apical cap', has a reported incidence of 7% and occurs most commonly on the left side.

The Bones

All the bones should be surveyed. On occasions identification of an abnormality in association with pulmonary pathology may help to narrow the differential diagnosis. Sometimes a normal bony structure appears to be a lung lesion and further films such as oblique, lateral, inspiratory and expiratory or CT may be necessary.

The Sternum   The ossification centers are very variable in number, shape, position and growth rate. Usually there are single centers in the manubrium and xiphoid, with three or four centers in the body. Parasternal ossicles and, in infants, the ossification centers may be confused with lung masses.

The Clavicles   The rhomboid fossa is an irregular notch at the site of attachment of the costoclavicular ligament. It lies up to 3 cm from the medial end of the clavicle inferiorly and has a well-corticated margin. It is unilateral in 6% of cases and should not be mistaken for a destructive lesion. Superior companion shadows are a usual finding. The medial epiphyses fuse late and on occasions may appear as lung nodules.

The Scapulae   On the lateral film the inferior angle overlies the lungs and can simulate a lung mass. The spine of the scapula on the PA film casts a linear shadow which at first glance may seem to be pleural.

The Ribs   Companion shadows are common on the upper ribs. Pathological rib notching, as seen with aortic coarctation, should not be confused with the normal notch on the inferior surface just lateral to the tubercle. The contours of the ribs are evaluated for destruction. However the inferior borders of the middle and lower ribs are usually indistinct.

The first costal cartilage calcifies early and is often very dense, partly obscuring the upper zone. Costal cartilage calcification is rare before the age of 20. Central homogenous or spotty calcification occurs in females whereas there is curvilinear marginal calcification in males. On the lateral film the anterior end of the rib with its cartilage lying behind the sternum should not be confused with a mass.

The Spine   Routine evaluation is made for bone and disk destruction and spinal deformity. A scoliosis often results in apparent mediastinal widening, and oblique films may be necessary to fully visualize both lung fields. The ends of the transverse processes on the PA film may look like a lung nodule.

In the neonate the vertebral bodies have a sandwich appearance due to large venous sinuses. Residual grooves may persist in the adult.

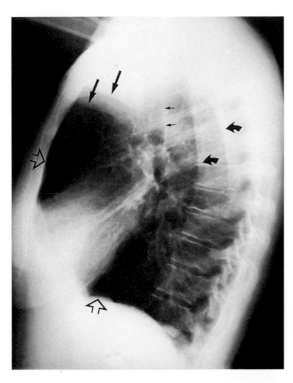

Fig. 11.20 Normal lateral film. Note the retrosternal and retrocardiac clear spaces (open arrows) and the increased translucency of the lower vertebrae. The axillary folds (large arrows) and scapulae (curved arrows) overlie the lung fields. The tracheal translucency is well seen (small arrows).

Viewing the Lateral Film

Routinely the left side is adjacent to the film to reduce cardiac magnification but if there is a specific lesion the side of interest is positioned adjacent to the film.

A routine similar to that used for the PA film should be employed. Important observations to make are (Fig. 11.20):

1. The Clear Spaces   There are two clear spaces; these correspond to the sites where the lungs meet behind the sternum and the heart. Loss of translucency of these areas indicates local pathology. Obliteration of the retrosternal space occurs with anterior mediastinal masses such as a thymoma (Fig. 11.21), aneurysms of the ascending aorta and nodal masses. Normally this space is less than 3 cm deep maximum; widening occurs with emphysema.

2. Vertebral Translucency   The vertebral bodies become progressively more translucent caudally. Loss of this translucency may be the only sign of posterior basal consolidation.

3. Diaphragm Outline   Both diaphragms are visible throughout their length, except the left anteriorly where it merges with the heart. A small segment of the right hemidiaphragm is effaced by the IVC. The posterior costophrenic angles are acute and small amounts of pleural fluid may be detected by blunting of these angles (Fig. 11.22).

The Fissures   The left greater fissure is steeper than the right and terminates 5 cm behind the anterior cardiophrenic angle. Loculated interlobar effusions are well shown and displacement or thickening of the fissures should be noted.

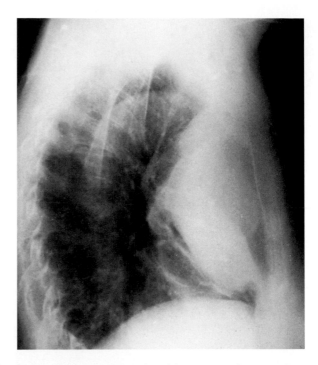

Fig. 11.21   Thymoma. Obliteration of the retrosternal space.

The Trachea   This passes down in a slightly posterior direction to the T6/7 level of the spine. It is partly overlapped by the scapulae and axillary folds. Anterior to the carina lies the right pulmonary artery. The left pulmonary artery is posterior and superior, and the veins are inferior. The venous confluence creates a bulge on the posterior cardiac border.

The normal posterior tracheal wall is invariably visible and measures less than 5 mm. This measurement includes both tracheal and esophageal walls plus the pleura. Widening may occur with disease of all these structures. A branch of the aorta seen end-on may appear as a nodule overlying the trachea and above the aortic arch. The right upper lobe bronchus is seen end-on as a circular structure overlying the lower trachea. Lying inferiorly is the left upper lobe bronchus seen end-on with its artery superiorly and vein inferiorly.

Shadowing seen in the region of the anterior cardiophrenic angle is thought to be due to *mediastinal fat* and the interface between the two lungs.

The *sternum* should be studied carefully in known cases of malignancy or when there is a history of trauma.

INTERPRETATION OF THE ABNORMAL FILM

Helpful Radiological Signs

The Silhouette Sign

Described by Felson (1950), the silhouette sign permits localization of a lesion on a film by studying the diaphragm and mediastinal outlines. These borders are seen because the adjacent alveoli are aerated. If this air is displaced the borders are obliterated and the lesion can be localized. Conversely if the border is retained and the abnormality is superimposed, the lesion must be lying either anterior or posterior. In 8–10% of people a short segment of

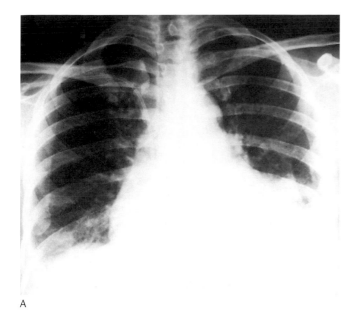

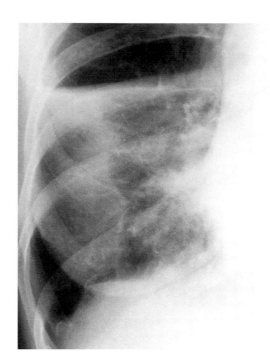

Fig. 11.23 Right middle lobe consolidation, demonstrating the silhouette sign with loss of outline of the right heart border.

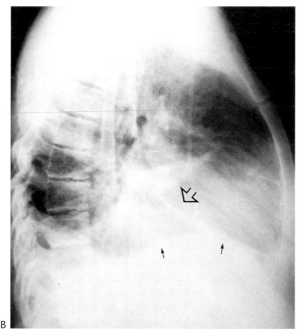

Fig. 11.22 A. PA film. A moderate sized left pleural effusion and a small right effusion. **B.** Lateral film. There is loss of translucency of the lower vertebrae, thickening of the oblique fissure (open arrow) and absence of the left hemidiaphragm, with loss of the right hemidiaphragm posteriorly.

the right heart border is obliterated by the fat pad or pulmonary vessels.

Obliteration of these borders may occur with pleural or mediastinal lesions as well as pulmonary pathology. The right middle lobe and lingula lie adjacent to the right and left cardiac borders, the apicoposterior segment of the left upper lobe lies adjacent to the aortic knuckle, the anterior segment of the right upper lobe and the middle lobe lie against the right aortic border. Pulmonary disease in these lobes and segments can obliterate the borders (Figs 11.23–25).

Using the same principle, a well-defined mass seen above the clavicles is always posterior whereas an anterior mass, being in contact with soft tissues rather than aerated lung, is ill defined. This is the *cervicothoracic sign*.

The *hilum overlay sign* helps distinguish a large heart from a mediastinal mass. With the latter the hilum is seen through the mass whereas with the former the hilum is displaced so that only its lateral border is visible.

The Air Bronchogram

Originally described by Fleischner (1941), and named by Felson (1973), the air bronchogram is an important sign showing that an opacity is intrapulmonary. The bronchus, if air-filled but not fluid-filled, becomes visible when air is displaced from the surrounding parenchyma. Frequently the air bronchogram is seen as scattered linear translucencies rather than continuous branching structures. It is most commonly seen within pneumonic consolidation and pulmonary edema. An air bronchogram is not seen within pleural fluid and rarely within a tumor, with the exception of alveolar-cell carcinoma and rarely lymphoma. It may be seen in consolidation distal to a malignancy if the bronchus remains patent (Fig. 11.26). An air bronchogram is usually a feature of alveolar shadowing but is described accompanying interstitial diseases such as sarcoidosis when there is extreme interstitial fibrosis. (See Table 11.3)

DIFFERENTIAL DIAGNOSIS

Alveolar (acinar/air space) Shadowing

The division of pulmonary shadowing into alveolar and interstitial is convenient but strictly incorrect; most disease processes involve both the interstitium and acinus on histologic examin-

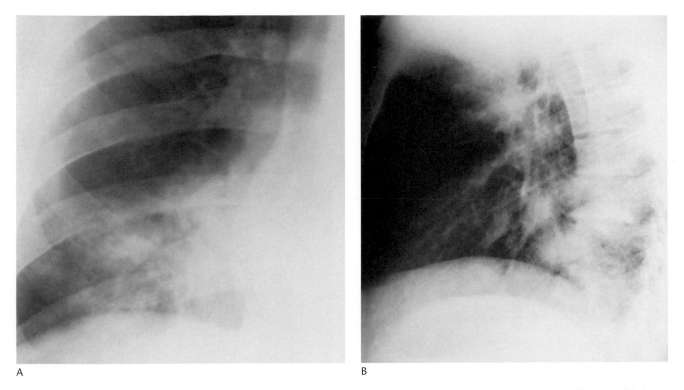

A   B

Fig. 11.24   Right lower lobe consolidation. **A.** Shadowing at the right base but the cardiac border remains visible. **B.** Lateral film. Consolidation in the posterior basal segment of the lower lobe with obliteration of the outline of the diaphragm posteriorly and loss of translucency of the lower vertebrae.

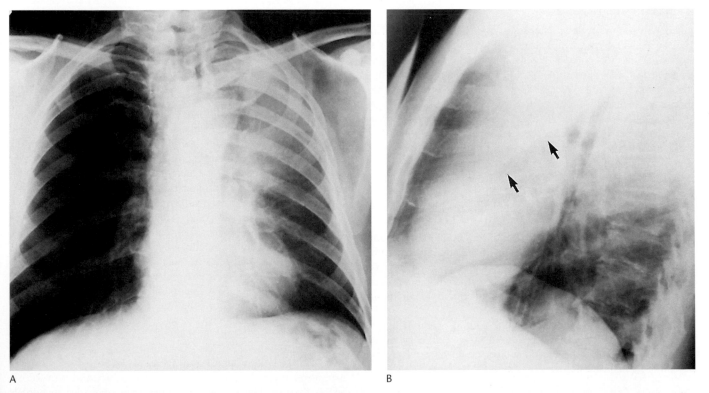

A   B

Fig. 11.25   Left upper lobe collapse. A carcinoma was present at the hilum. **A.** Shadowing in the upper zone with loss of outline of the upper cardiac border and aortic knuckle. There is tracheal deviation. **B.** Anterior displacement of the collapsed lobe and greater fissure.

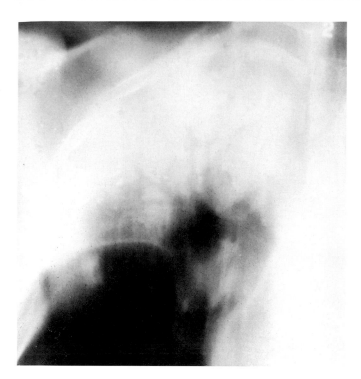

Fig. 11.26   Air bronchogram. An air bronchogram is clearly seen in the consolidated right upper lobe. A proximal carcinoma was present, although it is unusual for an air bronchogram to occur in the presence of a neoplasm.

Table 11.3   Causes of an Air Bronchogram

Common	Rare
Pneumonic consolidation	Lymphoma
Pulmonary edema	Sarcoidosis
Hyaline membrane disease	Alveolar proteinosis
(Fig. 11.27)	Alveolar-cell carcinoma
	Adult respiratory distress syndrome

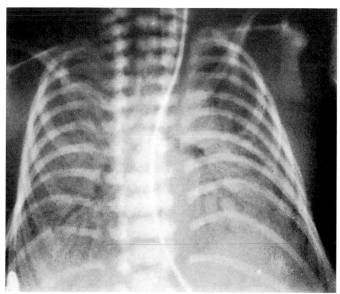

Fig. 11.27   Hyaline membrane disease. Extensive homogeneous consolidation with a prominent air bronchogram.

ation. When the distal airways and alveoli are filled with fluid, whether it is transudate, exudate or blood, the acinus forms a nodular 4–8 mm shadow. These shadows rapidly coalesce into fluffy ill-defined round or irregular cotton-wool shadows, non-segmental, homogenous or patchy, but frequently well defined adjacent to the fissures (Fig. 11.28). The acinar shadow is most evident on the edge of an area of consolidation. Vascular markings are usually obscured locally. The air bronchogram and silhouette sign are characteristic features. A ground-glass appearance or a generalized homogenous haze may be seen with a bat's wing or butterfly perihilar distribution (Fig. 11.29), sparing the peripheral lung fields which remain translucent. This pattern is commonly due to cardiac failure and clears quickly with treatment. Other causes include *Pneumocystis* infection, alveolar proteinosis and non-cardiac causes of pulmonary edema. Occasionally pulmonary edema is unilateral or peripheral.

Infective processes are usually localized, occasionally forming a round peripheral shadow which must be distinguished from a malignancy. If an infective process is bilateral and generalized it may well be due to an opportunistic infection. During resolution a mottled appearance can develop and this may give the impression that cavitation has occurred.

Consolidation in association with bulging pleural fissures may be seen with bacterial pneumonia, in particular due to *Pneumococcus* or Friedländer's bacillus, or in the presence of a central bronchial carcinoma.

The Diffuse Interstitial Pattern

'Diffuse interstitial pattern' is a radiological descriptive term and

does not imply that the disease process is confined to the interstitium. In many cases both the alveolar cavity and the interstitial tissues are abnormal.

Correlation between the plain film radiographic changes and the severity of the clinical respiratory symptoms is often poor, the plain film sometimes being normal in the presence of extensive interstitial disease. Earlier changes can be detected with high-resolution CT. A history of industrial dust exposure, bird fancying and disease processes such as rheumatoid arthritis is helpful.

The diffuse interstitial pattern (Fig. 11.30) is non-homogenous and includes various patterns including linear and septal lines, miliary shadows, reticulonodular and large nodular shadowing, honeycomb shadowing, peribronchial cuffing and the ground-glass pattern. Care is necessary to avoid mistaking normal vascular markings for early interstitial disease. Normal vessels are not seen in the periphery of the lung fields and unlike interstitial shadows vessels taper and branch. The presence of interstitial shadowing results in the normally visualized vessels becoming ill-defined and then lost. The zonal distribution of the shadowing is helpful in determining the differential diagnosis, for example asbestosis typically affects the lung bases whereas sarcoidosis spares the lung bases. Loss of volume may occur due to fibrosis but lobar collapse is not a feature. Other helpful features include lymphadenopathy and pleural effusions.

Table 11.4   Causes of Alveolar Shadowing

1. Pulmonary edema
   a. Cardiac
   b. Non-cardiac
      Fluid overload
      Hypoalbuminemia
      Uremia
      Shock lung (ARDS)
      Fat embolus
      Amniotic fluid embolus
      Drowning
      Hanging
      High altitude
      Blast injury
      Oxygen toxicity
      Aspiration (Mendelson syndrome)
      Malaria
      Inhalation of noxious gases
      Heroin overdose
      Drugs (e.g. nitrofurantoin)
      Raised intracranial pressure
2. nfections
   a. Localized
   b. Generalized, e.g. *Pneumocystis*, parasites, fungi
3. Neonatal
      Hyaline membrane disease
      Aspiration
4. Alveolar blood
      Pulmonary hemorrhage, haematoma
      Goodpasture's syndrome
      Pulmonary infarction
5. Tumors
      Alveolar-cell carcinoma
      Lymphoma, leukemia
6. Miscellaneous
      Alveolar proteinosis
      Alveolar microlithiasis
      Radiation pneumonitis
      Sarcoidosis
      Eosinophilic lung
      Polyarteritis nodosa
      Mineral oil aspiration and ingestion
      Drugs
      Amyloidosis

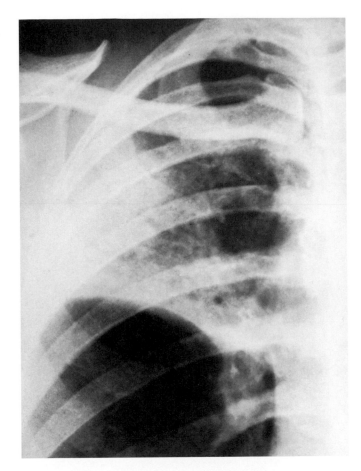

Fig. 11.28 Right upper lobe consolidation. Upper bowing of the horizontal fissure indicates some collapse. There is an acinar pattern with some confluence.

The miliary pattern has widespread small discrete opacities of similar size 2–4 mm in diameter. This pattern is most often seen with tuberculosis (Fig. 11.31). Dense opacities occur with calcification and metallic dust disease (Fig. 11.32).

Ground-glass shadowing is a fine granular pattern which obscures the normal anatomic detail such as the vessels and diaphragms, and which may be seen with an interstitial or with an alveolar pattern (see Tables 11.5–7).

Honeycomb Shadowing

The parenchymal destruction which may occur with end-stage interstitial pulmonary fibrosis can result in the formation of thin-walled cysts, the wall being 2–3 mm thick. When these cysts are 5–10 mm in size the term honeycomb shadowing is used. This condition is associated with an increased risk of pneumothorax, often of the tension type. Honeycomb shadowing is a particular feature of histiocytosis X. (See Table 11.8)

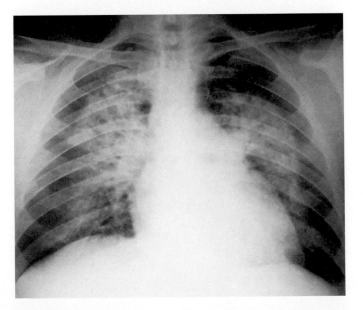

Fig. 11.29 Acute intra-alveolar pulmonary edema with a bat's wing distribution.

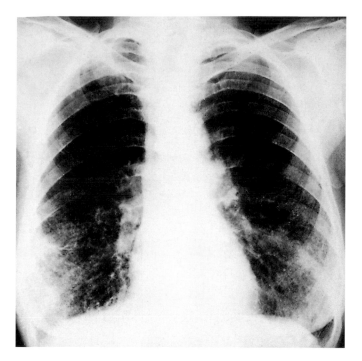

Fig. 11.30   Fibrosing alveolitis. Diffuse interstitial shadowing in the lower zones.

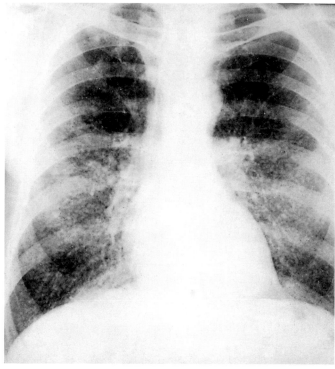

Fig. 11.32   Siderosis. Extensive dense miliary shadowing in an iron-foundry worker.

Table 11.5   **Causes of Miliary Shadowing**

Tuberculosis
Sarcoidosis
Coccidioidomycosis
Blastomycosis
Histoplasmosis
Chickenpox
Metastases
Alveolar microlithiasis
Secondary hyperparathyroidism
Dust inhalation:
    Tin
    Barium
    Beryllium
    Coal miner's pneumoconiosis
    Silicosis
Oil embolism (post-lymphangiography)
Hemosiderosis
Histiocytosis X
Bronchiolitis obliterans
Hyaline membrane disease

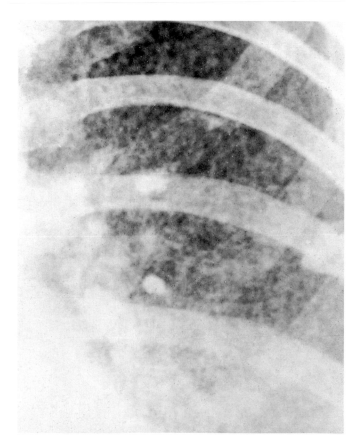

Fig. 11.31   Miliary tuberculosis. Widespread fine nodular shadowing without confluence.

The Single Pulmonary Nodule

Some 40% of solitary pulmonary nodules are malignant, with other common lesions being granulomas and benign tumors (See Table 11.9). A lateral film is often necessary to confirm that a lesion is intrapulmonary before investigating further. Typically an intrapulmonary mass forms an acute angle with the lung edge whereas extrapleural and mediastinal masses form obtuse angles (Fig. 11.33).

A nodule is assessed for its size, shape and outline and for the

Table 11.6 Causes of Large Nodular Shadows

Malignancy: metastases, alveolar-cell carcinoma, lymphoma, primary
Tuberculosis
Sarcoidosis
Hemosiderosis
Pulmonary infarcts, fat embolism
Pulmonary sequestration
Collagen disease: Wegener's granulomatosis, rheumatoid arthritis, etc.
Allergic lung disease: drugs, extrinsic allergic alveolitis
Alveolar shadowing: infections, pulmonary hemorrhage, pulmonary edema, hyaline membrane disease
Artefacts: skin nodules e.g. neurofibromatosis, clothing, hair
Pleural: tumors, loculated effusions

Table 11.7 Causes of Diffuse Interstitial Shadowing

Infections	Bacterial—tuberculosis, mycoplasma, etc.
	Viral
	Fungal
	Pneumocystis
	Parasites
Cardiac	Left heart failure
	Hemosiderosis
	Obstructed total anomalous pulmonary venous drainage
Neoplastic	Lymphangitis carcinomatosa
	Lymphoma
	Leukemia
Collagen diseases	SLE
	Polyarteritis nodosa
	Scleroderma
	Dermatomyositis
	Rheumatoid lung
Drugs	Busulfan
	Methotrexate
	Bleomycin
Dust disease	Coal miner's pneumoconiosis
	Asbestosis
	Silicosis
	Berylliosis
Honeycomb shadowing	
Miscellaneous	Idiopathic fibrosing alveolitis
	Sarcoidosis
	Amyloidosis
	Bronchiectasis
	Gaucher's disease
	Extrinsic allergic alveolitis
	Lipoid pneumonia
	Chronic interstitial pneumonia
	Gaucher's disease
	Histiocytosis X
	Tuberous sclerosis
	Neurofibromatosis
	Lymphangiomyomatosis

presence of calcification or cavitation. A search is made for associated abnormalities such as bone destruction (Fig. 11.34), effusions, lobar collapse, septal lines and lymphadenopathy. If previous films are available the doubling time can be assessed, that is the time taken for the volume of the mass to double. Usually malignant lesions have a doubling time of one to six months whereas benign lesions have a doubling time in excess of

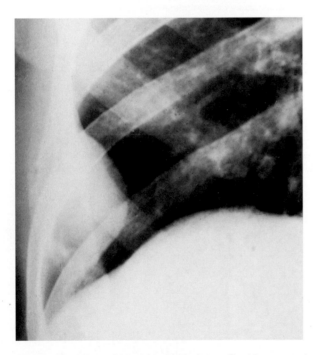

Fig. 11.33 Reticulum-cell sarcoma of right lower rib with an extrapleural mass.

18 months. Malignant lesions may grow spasmodically however. Masses larger than 4 cm are predominantly primary malignancies, metastases or pleural fibromas. Solitary metastases are rare, however. Tumors smaller than 10 mm cannot be seen clearly on a plain film and often appear as a 'smudge' shadow rather than a mass.

On occasions infective processes have a round appearance which is usually ill defined. Some change is seen at follow-up with simple consolidation after treatment.

Carcinomas are often upper zone with irregular, spiculated or notched margins. Calcification favors a benign lesion although a carcinoma may arise coincidentally at the site of an old calcified

Table 11.8 Causes of Honeycomb Shadowing

Common	Rare	Similar Appearances
Histiocytosis X	Tuberous sclerosis	Bronchiectasis
Scleroderma	Amyloidosis	Cystic fibrosis
Rheumatoid disease	Gaucher's disease	
Fibrosing alveolitis	Neurofibromatosis	
Pneumoconiosis	Chronic interstitial pneumonia	
Sarcoidosis	Lymphangiomyomatosis	

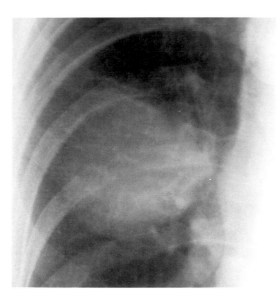

Fig. 11.34 Posteriorly positioned bronchial carcinoma with destruction of the adjacent rib.

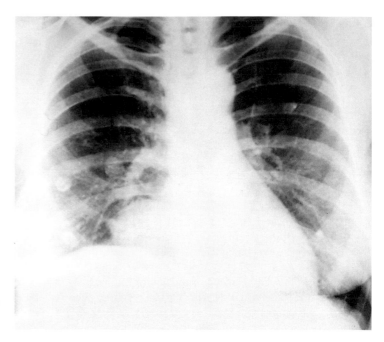

Fig. 11.36 Multiple calcified metastases from a chondrosarcoma of the right tenth rib.

focus. Popcorn calcification suggests a hamartoma (Fig. 11.35). Calcified metastases are rare, the primary tumor being usually an osteogenic or chondrosarcoma (Fig. 11.36).

Granulomas frequently calcify and are usually well defined and lobulated. Multiple lesions tend to be similar in size, whereas metastases are frequently of variable size but are well defined. *Arteriovenous malformations* characteristically have dilated feeding arteries and draining veins (Fig. 11.37); they are multiple in 30% of cases. *Rheumatoid nodules* are invariably subpleural. Most *bronchogenic cysts* are intrapulmonary, arising in the lower zones.

Multiple Pulmonary Nodules

Multiple small nodules 2–4 mm are called miliary shadows (see previously). In the majority of cases multiple nodules are metastases or tuberculous granulomata. Calcified nodules are generally benign except for metastases from bone or cartilaginous

tumors. The doubling time of metastases is highly variable, with a range of a few days to in excess of 2 years. It is well documented that thyroid metastases can persist unchanged for many years. (See Table 11.10)

Cavitating Lesions and Cysts

A cavity is a gas-filled space surrounded by a complete wall which is 3 mm or greater in thickness. Thinner-walled cavities are

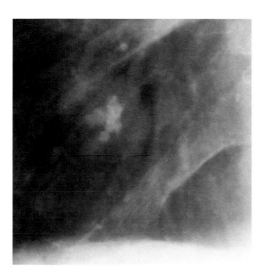

Fig. 11.35 Hamartoma with popcorn calcification.

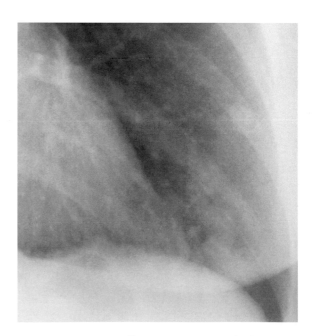

Fig. 11.37 Arteriovenous malformation with dilated feeding and draining vessels.

Table 11.9 Causes of a solitary pulmonary nodule

Malignant	Primary
	Secondary
	Lymphoma
	Plasmacytoma
	Alveolar-cell carcinoma
Benign	Hamartoma
	Adenoma
	Connective tissue tumors
Granuloma	Tuberculosis
	Histoplasmosis
	Paraffinoma
	Sarcoidosis
Infection	Round pneumonia,
	Abscess
	Hydatid
	Amebic
	Fungi
	Parasites
Pulmonary infarct	
Pulmonary hematoma	
Collagen diseases	Rheumatoid arthritis
	Wegener's granulomatosis
Congenital	Bronchogenic cyst
	Sequestrated segment
	Congenital bronchial atresia
	AVM
	Impacted mucus
Amyloidosis	
Intrapulmonary lymph node	
Pleural	Fibroma
	Tumor
	Loculated fluid
Non-pulmonary	Skin and chest wall lesions
	Artefacts

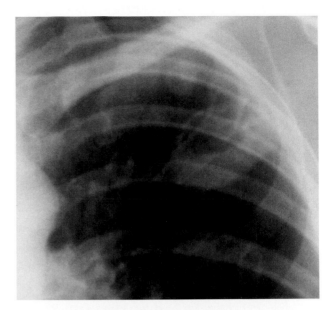

Fig. 11.38 Staphylococcal abscesses. Multiple cavitating abscesses in a young male heroin addict. Bilateral effusions also present.

called cysts or ring shadows. Cavitation occurs when an area of necrosis communicates with a patent airway. Particular features of importance are the location of the cavity, its outline, wall thickness, the presence of a fluid level, contents of the cavity, satellite lesions, the appearance of the surrounding lung and multiplicity of lesions. CT often provides additional helpful information. Fluid within a cavity can be demonstrated only when using a horizontal beam.

Common cavitating processes are tuberculosis, staphylococcal infections (Fig. 11.38) and carcinoma. The tumor mass itself or the distal lung may cavitate. (See Table 11.11)

Table 11.10 Causes of Multiple Pulmonary Nodules

Tumors	Benign—hamartoma, laryngeal papillomatosis
	Malignant—metastases, lymphoma
Infection	Granuloma —tuberculosis, histoplasmosis, fungi
	Round pneumonia
	Abscesses
	Hydatid cysts
Inflammatory	Caplan syndrome
	Wegener's granulomatosis
	Sarcoidosis
	Drugs
Vascular	Arteriovenous malformations
	Hematomas
	Infarcts
Miscellaneous	Mucus impaction
	Amyloidosis

The Site Tuberculous cavities are usually upper zone, in the posterior segments of the upper lobes or apical segments of the lower lobes. The site of lung abscesses following aspiration depends on patient position at the time but they are most often right-sided and lower zone. Traumatic lung cysts are often subpleural. Amebic abscesses are nearly always at the right base, the infection extending from the liver. Pulmonary infarcts are usually lower zone and sequestrated segments are left-sided.

The Wall of the Cavity Thick-walled cavitating lesions (Fig. 11.39) include acute abscesses, most neoplasms (usually squamous-cell), lymphoma, most metastases, Wegener's granulomas and rheumatoid nodules. Thin-walled lesions or ring shadows are usually benign and may be bullae (Fig. 11.40), pneumatoceles, cystic bronchiectasis, hydatid cysts, traumatic lung cysts, chronic inactive tuberculous cavities and neoplasms. Pneumatoceles often develop in children after a staphylococcal pneumonia, and a rapid change in size is a feature. In addition they frequently develop following pulmonary contusion and hydrocarbon ingestion.

Satellite lesions are a common feature of benign lesions, usually tuberculous. Multiple ring shadows, in the region of 6 mm in diameter, are seen with honeycomb shadowing.

Fluid Levels and the Meniscus Sign

Fluid levels are common in primary tumors, and irregular masses of blood clot or necrotic tumor may be present. Fluid levels are uncommon in cavitating metastases and tuberculous cavities. (See Table 11.12)

The meniscus sign is seen when an intracavitory body is surrounded by a crescent of air. It is commonly described with fungus balls such as an aspergilloma (Fig. 11.41). There is movement of the ball with change in the patient's position.

Ruptured hydatid cysts may have daughter cysts floating within the cavity, the *waterlily sign*. Other intracavitory lesions include inspissated pus, blood clot and cavernoliths. Blood clot may form within cavitating neoplasms, tuberculosis and pulmonary infarcts.

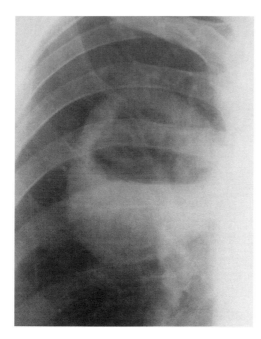

Fig. 11.39 Large irregular thick-walled cavitating neoplasm with air–fluid level.

Table 11.11 Cavitating Pulmonary Lesions

Infections	Staphylococcus
	Klebsiella
	Tuberculosis
	Histoplasmosis
	Amebic
	Hydatid
	Paragonimiasis
	Fungal
Malignant	Primary
	Secondary
	Lymphoma
Abscess	Blood-borne
	Aspiration
Pulmonary infarct	
Pulmonary hematoma	
Pneumoconiosis	PMF
	Caplan syndrome
Collagen diseases	Rheumatoid nodules
	Wegener's granulomatosis
Developmental	Sequestrated segment
	Bronchogenic cyst
	Congenital cystic adenomatoid malformation
Sarcoidosis	
Bullae, blebs	
Pneumatocele	Traumatic
	Infective
Traumatic lung cyst	

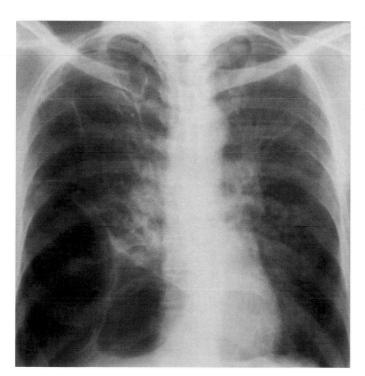

Fig. 11.40 Bullous emphysema with curvilinear shadows in the right lung and an associated paucity of vascular markings.

Calcification

Calcification is most easily recognized with low kVp films. In the elderly calcification of the tracheal and bronchial cartilage is common. Calcification of the bronchioles, *osteopathia racemosa*, is of no significance.

Tuberculosis is the commonest calcifying pulmonary process

with small scattered foci of various sizes, usually upper zone (Fig. 11.43). Chickenpox foci are smaller (1–3 mm), regular in size and widely distributed (Fig. 11.44). Characteristically the foci of *histoplasmosis* are surrounded by small halos.

Alveolar microlithiasis appears as tiny sand-like densities in the

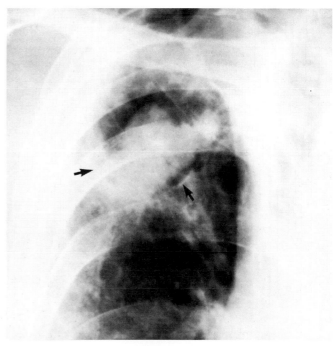

Fig. 11.41 Aspergillus mycetoma. A large mycetoma within an old tuberculous cavity in a fibrotic upper lobe. The mycetoma is surrounded by a halo of air.

Table 11.12   Fluid Levels on a Chest Radiograph

Intrapulmonary	
Hydropneumothorax	Trauma, surgery
	Bronchopleural fistula*
Esophageal	Pharyngeal pouch, diverticula
	Obstruction—tumor, achalasia
	Esophagectomy—bowel interposition
Mediastinal	Infections
	Esophageal perforation—endoscopy,
	trauma
Pneumopericardium	Diagnostic aspiration
	Surgery, trauma
Chest wall	Plombage with lucite balls (Fig. 11.42)
	Infections
Diaphragm	Hernias, eventration, rupture

*A bronchopleural fistula should be considered if a hydropneumothorax persists or enlarges after chest surgery.

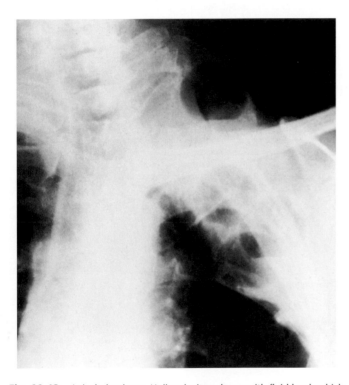

Fig. 11.42   Apical plombage. Hollow lucite spheres with fluid levels which have formed because of leakage of the walls of the spheres.

mid and lower zones, due to calcium phosphate deposits in the alveoli. Punctate calcification may develop within the pulmonary nodules of silicosis. Popcorn calcification is often present in hamartomas. Occasionally phleboliths are present in arteriovenous malformations. Very rarely a fine rim of calcification forms in the wall of a hydatid cyst.

Pleural plaques may contain irregular areas of calcification.

Lymph node calcification occurs in a number of conditions (Tables 11.13 and 11.4). An 'eggshell' pattern is characteristic of sarcoidosis and silicosis.

Calcification is not a feature of a primary lung malignancy. However a carcinoma may develop coincidentally adjacent to a calcified granuloma and therefore an area of eccentric calcification should not be presumed to exclude malignancy.

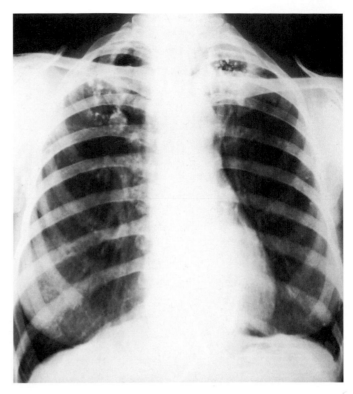

Fig. 11.43   Pulmonary tuberculosis. Numerous calcified foci in both upper zones with left upper lobe fibrosis.

Linear and Band Shadows

Normal structures such as the blood vessels and fissures form linear shadows within the lung fields. However, there are many disease processes which may result in linear shadows. Linear shadows are less than 5 mm wide, with band shadows defined as greater than 5 mm thick.

Pulmonary Infarcts   These are variable in appearance. Occasionally they form irregular thick wedge-shaped lines with the base adjacent to the pleura, but more usually they are nondescript areas of peripheral consolidation at the bases. Accompanying features are splinting of the diaphragm and a pleural reaction. Resolution tends to be slow, in contrast to infections which often resolve quickly except in the elderly.

Plate Atelectasis   Plate atelectasis, described by Fleischner 1941, is often seen postoperatively and is thought to be due to underventilation with obstruction of medium sized bronchi. These lines are several centimeters long, 1–3 mm thick and run parallel to the diaphragms extending to the pleural surface. Resolution is usually rapid.

Mucus-filled Bronchi   Also known as bronchoceles, these are bronchi distended with mucus or pus beyond an obstructing lesion but with aeration of the distal lung from collateral air flow. Causes to consider include bronchopulmonary aspergillosis, malignancy, benign tumors and bronchial atresia. Typically the bronchus has a gloved finger branching pattern with the fingers several millimeters wide (Fig. 11.45). They are more frequently found in the upper lobes.

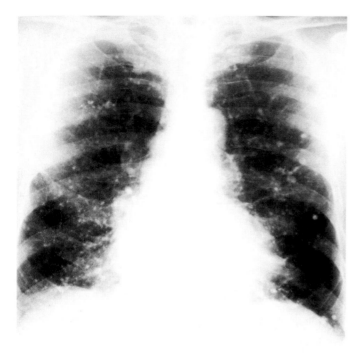

Fig. 11.44 Chickenpox. Widespread small calcified opacities following a previous chickenpox pneumonia.

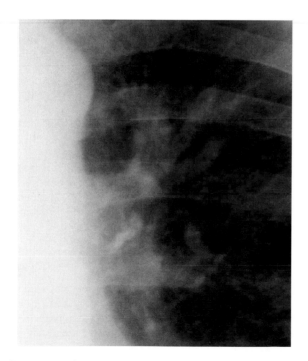

Fig. 11.45 Bronchocele with typical gloved finger branching pattern.

Sentinel Lines These are thought to be mucus-filled bronchi and appear as coarse lines lying peripherally in contact with the pleura and curving upward. They are often left-sided and associated with left lower lobe collapse. They may develop due to kinking of bronchi adjacent to the collapse.

Kerley B Lines These have been described previously. Unilateral

Table 11.13 Calcification on the Chest Radiograph

Intrapulmonary	Granuloma, infections:	tuberculosis, histoplasmosis, chickenpox, coccidioidomycosis, actinomycosis, hydatid cyst
	Chronic abscess	
	Tumors	
	Metastases: osteogenic sarcoma, chondrosarcoma	
	Cystadenocarcinoma	
	Arteriovenous malformation	
	Hamartoma, carcinoid	
	Hematoma	
	Infarct	
	Mitral valve disease	
	Broncholith—tuberculosis	
	Alveolar microlithiasis	
	Idiopathic	
	Rare	
	Metabolic—hypercalcemia	
	Silicosis, sarcoidosis	
	Rheumatoid arthritis	
	Amyloid	
	Osteopathia racemosa	
Lymph nodes	Tuberculosis	
	Histoplasmosis	
	Sarcoidosis	
	Silicosis	
	Lymphoma after irradiation	
Pleural	Tuberculosis	
	Asbestosis, talcosis	
	Old hemothorax, empyema	
Mediastinal	Cardiac	
	Valvular	
	Infarcted muscle	
	Tumors	
	Pericardial	
	Ventricular aneurysms	
	Vascular	
	Tumors	
Pulmonary artery	Pulmonary hypertension	
	Aneurysm	
	Thrombus	
Chest wall	Costal cartilage	
	Bone tumors, callus	
	Breast: tumors, fat necrosis	
	Soft tissue: parasites, tumors, etc.	

Table 11.14 Causes of Linear and Band Shadows

Pulmonary infarcts
Sentinel lines
Thickened fissures
Pulmonary, pleural scars
Bronchial wall thickening
Curvilinear shadows: bullae, pneumatoceles
Anomalous vessels
Artefacts
Plate atelectasis (Fleischner lines)
Kerley lines
Resolving infection
Mucus-filled bronchi (bronchocele)

Kerley lines usually indicate lymphangitis carcinomatosa but may be seen with early cardiac failure.

The normal and accessory *fissures* have been described.

Thickening of the Fissures This is often seen accompanying cardiac failure. Bulging fissures indicate lobar expansion which may occur with an acute abscess (Fig. 11.46), infections—most commonly *Klebsiella* but also *Pneumococcus*, *Staphylococcus* and *tuberculosis*—and in the presence of large tumors.

Old Pleural and Pulmonary Scars   Scars are unchanged in appearance on serial films. Pulmonary scarring is a common end result of infarction, appearing as a thin linear shadow often with pleural thickening and tenting of the diaphragm. Pleural scars extend to the pleural surface. Apical scarring is a common finding with healed tuberculosis, sarcoidosis and fungal disease (Fig. 11.47).

Curvilinear Shadows   These indicate the presence of bullae, pneumatoceles (Fig. 11.48) or cystic bronchiectasis.

Thickened Bronchial Walls   These cast thin parallel tramline shadows 1 mm thick which, when seen end-on, appear as ring shadows. They are a common finding in bronchiectasis, recurrent asthma, bronchopulmonary aspergillosis (Fig. 11.49), pulmonary edema and lymphangitis carcinomatosis. If the peribronchial interstitial space becomes thickened by fluid or tumor, the walls are less clearly defined.

Apical Shadowing

Apical pleural thickening, the 'pleural cap', has a reported incidence of 7% and is more commonly left-sided. It is crescent shaped, frequently irregular, and if bilateral is usually asymmetric. The significance is uncertain but it may represent old pleural thickening. If the thickening is irregular or markedly asymmetric or unduly prominent the underlying rib must be assessed for destruction as the possibility of a Pancoast (superior sulcus) tumor must be considered; this usually presents as a mass but in a quarter of cases it presents as a pleural cap (Fig. 11.50). (See Table 11.15)

The lung apex is a common site for tuberculosis and fungal diseases including *histoplasmosis*, *coccidioidomycosis*, *blastomycosis* and *aspergillosis*. Assessment of active disease is difficult in the presence of fibrotic changes. Previous films for comparison are invaluable.

Extrinsic shadows should be excluded (Fig. 11.51). Invariably in these cases the edge of the lesion is seen to extend beyond the limits of the lung and pleura into the soft tissues.

Signs of Loss of Volume

In the majority of cases loss of volume, or collapse, is caused by obstruction of a bronchus by tumor, mucus or foreign body, or extrinsic compression by nodes. More rarely it is due to bronchostenosis following trauma. With lobar or pulmonary collapse or fibrosis there is opacity of the affected lobe (s) with displacement or bowing of the pleural fissures (Fig. 11.52) and crowding of vascular markings within the collapse. Compensatory emphysema of the normal lung or lobes results in an increase in transradiancy with separation of the vascular markings. Mediastinal structures are displaced toward the affected side (Fig. 11.53), and the ipsilateral hemidiaphragm may become elevated. Crowding of the ribs on the affected side is common in children.

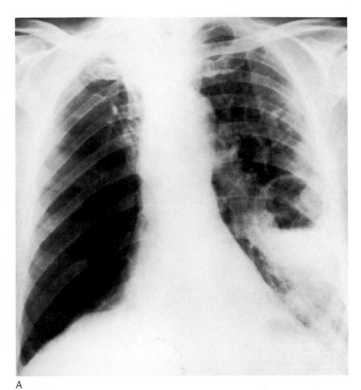

A

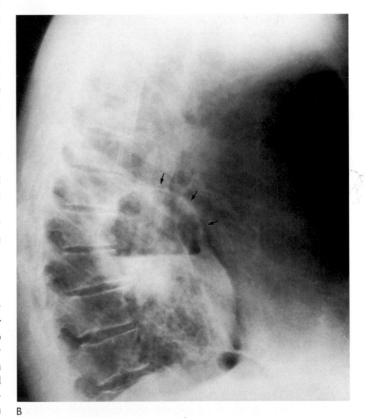

B

Fig. 11.46   **A.** A large lung abscess with a fluid level distal to a hilar carcinoma. There is an old right upper lobe collapse with compensatory emphysema. **B.** Note bulging of the oblique fissure adjacent to the abscess (arrows).

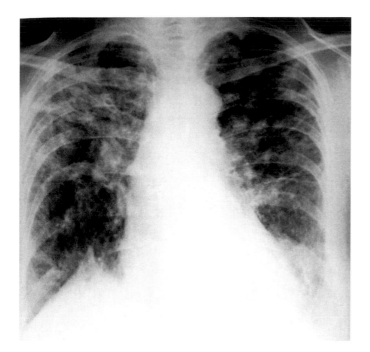

Fig. 11.47 Sarcoidosis. Fibrosis mainly affecting the upper zones with elevation of the hila and tenting of the right hemidiaphragm. A 55-year-old woman with a long history of sarcoidosis.

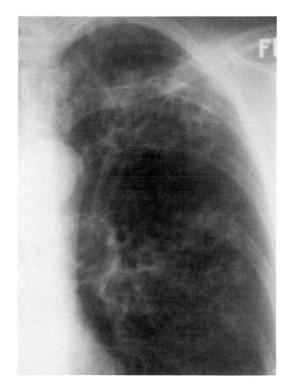

Fig. 11.49 Bronchiectasis due to bronchopulmonary aspergillosis.

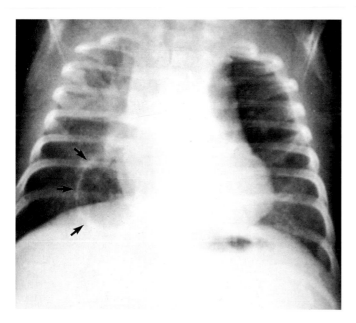

Fig. 11.48 Pneumatocele. Child with a staphylococcal pneumonia. Consolidation in the right upper lobe and a pneumatocele adjacent to the right heart border (arrows).

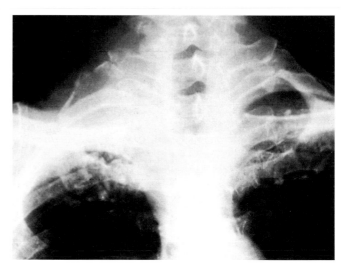

Fig. 11.50 Pancoast tumor. There is apical shadowing on the right side simulating pleural thickening. Note destruction of the first rib.

Lobar collapse displaces the hilum which changes shape. With major collapse there is herniation of the contralateral lung with displacement of the anterior mediastinal line. Obliteration of the bronchus at the site of the obstruction may be evident but this is more clearly seen at CT. The presence of a hilar mass with collapse can be identified by the 'Golden S sign' (Fig. 11.54). The central mass gives a convexity to the concave displaced fissure (as described by Golden) forming the shape of an S.

Hilar Enlargement

The normal pulmonary hilum has a very variable appearance. It is difficult to detect minor degrees of pathological enlargement and to distinguish a prominent pulmonary artery from a small mass lesion, although branch vessels can often be traced back to an enlarged artery. A hilum should be assessed for its position, size and density, with a comparison of the two hila. Any possible

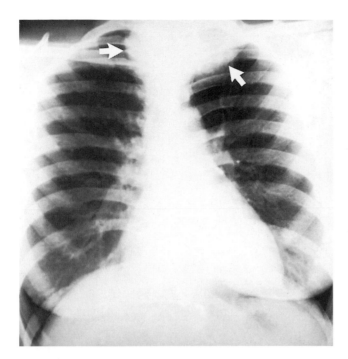

Fig. 11.51 A woman with her hair in a plait overlying the upper mediastinum and simulating mediastinal widening.

abnormality can be assessed further with contrast-enhanced CT or flexible bronchoscopy.

Bilateral hilar enlargement is commonly due to enlarged lymph nodes, which appear as lobulated masses, or to vascular enlargement. The adjacent bronchi may be slightly narrowed. Unilateral

Table 11.15   Common Causes of Apical Shadows

Pleural caps
Pleural fluid
Bullae
Pancoast tumor
Infections—tuberculosis
Pneumothorax
Soft tissue, e.g. companion shadows, hair, sternocleidomastoid muscles

enlargement is most commonly due to a neoplasm or vascular dilatation but is also seen with infections such as tuberculosis and whooping cough (see Table 11.16). Nodes affected by lymphoma are often asymmetrically involved (Fig. 11.55). Bilateral involvement occurs with sarcoidosis, silicosis and leukemia. Tuberculous lymphadenopathy without an identifiable peripheral pulmonary lesion is a common finding in the Asian population.

Small hila are usually the result of congenital cyanotic heart disease (see Table 11.17).

Unilateral Hypertranslucency

Comparison of the lung fields should reveal any focal or generalized abnormality of transradiancy. Increased transradiancy may be accompanied by signs of obstructive or compensatory emphysema such as splaying of the ribs, separation of the vascular markings, mediastinal displacement and depression of the hemidiaphragm.

Patient rotation and scoliosis are the commonest causes of increased transradiancy. (See Table 11.18) With rotation to the left, the left side becomes more radiolucent. Mastectomy is another important cause. An abnormal axillary fold is seen

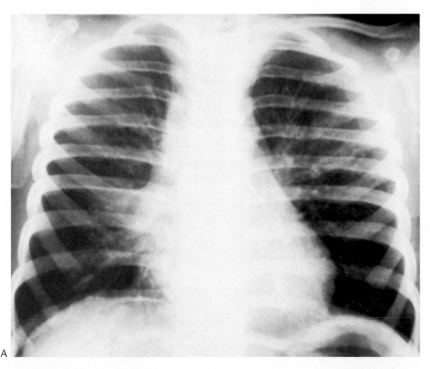

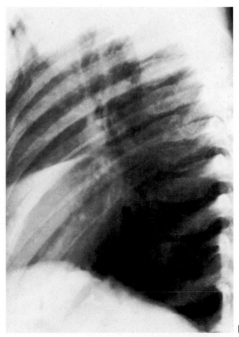

Fig. 11.52 Right middle lobe collapse. **A.** Loss of definition of the right heart border with adjacent shadowing. **B.** Lobar collapse with displacement of the fissures clearly shown.

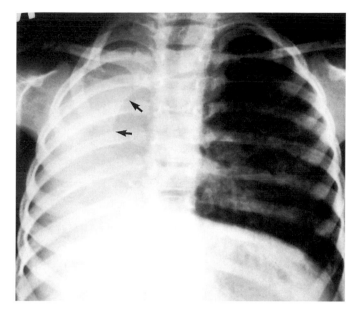

Fig. 11.53   Pulmonary agenesis. The right lung is absent. The heart and mediastinum are displaced to the right. Note herniation of the left lung across the midline (arrows). The rib spaces are narrowed on the right.

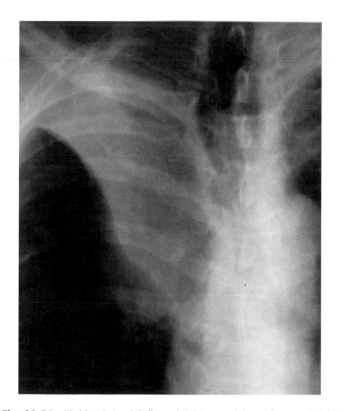

Fig. 11.54   'Golden S sign.' Collapsed right upper lobe with mass at right hilum.

following a radical mastectomy. However, the less extensive breast surgery favored currently is difficult to detect on the chest film.

With conditions such as *Macleod's* syndrome, congenital lobar emphysema and an inhaled foreign body an expiratory film will

Table 11.16   Causes of Hilar Enlargement

Unilateral	Apparent	Rotation
		Scoliosis
		Small contralateral hilum
	Lymph nodes	Tuberculosis
		Fungi
		Histoplasmosis
		Lymphoma
		Leukemia
		Carcinoma
	Tumors	Benign
		Malignant
	Pulmonary artery	Aneurysm
		Embolus
		Poststenotic dilatation
	Superimposed anterior/posterior mass	
	Pericardial defect	
	Normal	Especially left
Bilateral	Expiratory film	
	Lymph nodes	Lymphoma
		Carcinoma
		Leukemia
		Sarcoidosis
		Pneumoconiosis
		Glandular fever
		Whooping cough
		Tuberculosis
		Histoplasmosis
		Fungi
		Mycoplasma
	Pulmonary artery	Pulmonary hypertension
		Left heart failure
		Congenital heart disease
	Drugs	

demonstrate obstructive emphysema (Fig. 11.56). There is displacement of the mediastinum away from the affected side with depression of the ipsilateral diaphragm. Congenital lobar emphysema usually affects the right upper or middle lobes. A small pulmonary artery is a feature of *Macleod's* syndrome and congenital hypoplasia or absence of the artery.

The commonest causes of increased translucency of both lungs are asthma, emphysema and reduced pulmonary perfusion.

The Opaque Hemithorax

All the causes described of unilateral hypertranslucency may be responsible for an apparent contralateral increase in density. Penetrated, lateral and high kVp films are usually helpful. Signs of collapse, fluid levels, mediastinal displacement and rib abnormalities are important findings. Pulmonary agenesis is associated with hypoplastic ribs and is invariably left-sided.

Table 11.17   Causes of a Small Hilum

Unilateral	Apparent—rotation, scoliosis
	Normal—especially the left side
	Lobar collapse, lobectomy
	Hypoplastic pulmonary artery
	Macleod's syndrome
	Unilateral pulmonary embolus
Bilateral	Cyanotic congenital heart disease
	Central pulmonary embolus

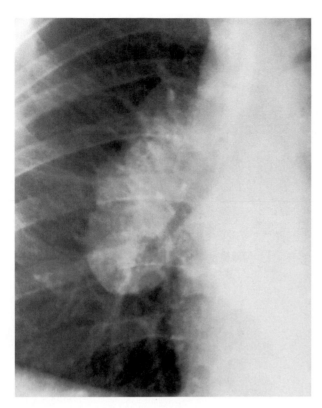

Fig. 11.55 A young man with Hodgkin's disease. An enlarged lobulated right hilum typical of glandular enlargement.

The Chest Film of the Elderly Person

With age the thorax changes shape and the AP diameter increases. A kyphosis develops so that the chin overlies the lung apex. Frequently only an AP film in the sitting position can be obtained, usually with a poor degree of inspiration so that the lung bases are poorly visualized.

Bone demineralization increases, with vertebral body compression and rib fractures being common. Bony margins become irregular. Costal cartilage and vascular calcification is prominent. Often there is calcification of the cartilaginous rings of the trachea and bronchi.

The major blood vessels become unfolded. On a lateral film the aorta is visualized throughout its length. Unfolding of the innominate and subclavian vessels results in widening of the upper mediastinum. Prominent hilar vessels accompany obstructive airways disease and the peripheral vessels become more obvious.

There may be changes due to old pathology with linear scars, pleural thickening, tenting of the diaphragm and calcified foci. Blunted costophrenic angles and flattened diaphragms are common findings in the elderly.

Limitations of the Plain Chest Film

Firstly the radiologist may fail to spot a lesion. Felson reported that 20–30% of significant information on a chest film may be overlooked by a trained radiologist.

Secondly a disease process may fail to appear as a visible abnormality on a plain film. Examples include miliary shadowing, metastases, early interstitial lung disease, bronchiectasis and

Table 11.18 Causes of Unilateral Hypertranslucency

Normal	Increased density contralateral lung, e.g. pleural effusion, thickening. Consolidation
Technical	Rotation, scoliosis
Soft tissue	Mastectomy
	Congenital absence pectoralis major
	Poliomyelitis
Emphysema	Compensatory: lobar collapse, lobectomy
	Obstructive: foreign body, tumor, Macleod's syndrome, congenital lobar emphysema
	Bullous
Vascular	Absent/hypoplastic pulmonary artery
	Obstructed pulmonary artery, e.g. by tumor, embolus
	Macleod's syndrome
Pneumothorax	

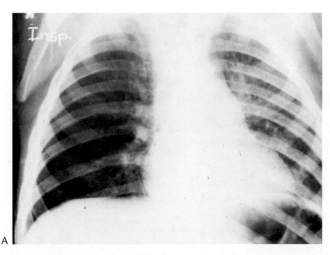
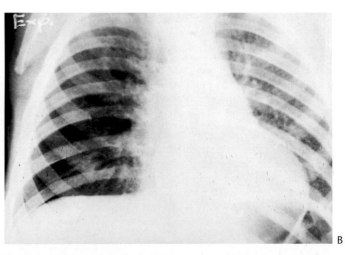

Fig. 11.56 Obstructive emphysema. This child inhaled a peanut. **A.** Inspiratory film shows a hypertransradiant right lung. **B.** Expiratory film. There is air trapping on the right side with further shift of the mediastinum to the left.

Table 11.19   Causes of an Opaque Hemithorax

Technical	Rotation, scoliosis
Pleural	Hydrothorax, large effusion
	Thickening, mesothelioma
Surgical	Pneumonectomy, thoracoplasty
Congenital	Pulmonary agenesis
Mediastinal	Gross cardiomegaly, tumors
Pulmonary	Collapse, consolidation, fibrosis
Diaphragmatic hernias	

small pleural effusions. Such lesions are demonstrated earlier using high-resolution CT. Inflamed bronchi are not easily seen and obstructive airways disease may be associated with a normal chest film. Small pulmonary emboli without infarction can rarely be diagnosed without a radionuclide study.

Finally, the shadow patterns themselves are rarely specific to a single disease process. For example, consolidation due to infection or following infarction may have identical appearances.

OTHER METHODS OF INVESTIGATION

Tomography

Tomography is performed:

1. To improve visualization of a lesion
2. To localize a lesion and to confirm it is intrapulmonary
3. To evaluate the hilum and proximal airways
4. To search for a suspected lesion, e.g. metastases
5. To evaluate the mediastinum and chest wall.

Technique   A recent chest film is mandatory. The examination should be closely supervised by the radiologist with particular attention to the radiographic technique, ensuring that the area of interest is included on the films taken. Linear tomography is usually adequate although more complex movements may be used. Cuts are routinely made at 1 cm intervals.

AP tomography, supplemented with lateral tomography, is satisfactory for peripheral lesions. The hilum is best visualized in the 55° posterior oblique position with the side of interest dependent (Fig. 11.57). On this view the bronchi are projected in profile. A penetrated view to show the carina is routinely obtained.

The Peripheral Mass   Features of diagnostic importance include calcification, cavitation, the outline of the mass, bronchial narrowing and the presence of an air bronchogram (Fig. 11.58). Spiculation is a strong indicator of malignancy.

The Hilum   Hilar tomograms are difficult to interpret. It is helpful to remember that normal sized nodes are not usually seen, and that enlarged nodes are well defined. The vessels, unlike a mass lesion, branch and taper. If a mass is identified the adjacent bronchi should be assessed for narrowing or occlusion.

Fluoroscopy

Fluoroscopy is of value for assessing chest wall and diaphragm motion, and for demonstrating mediastinal shift in cases of air

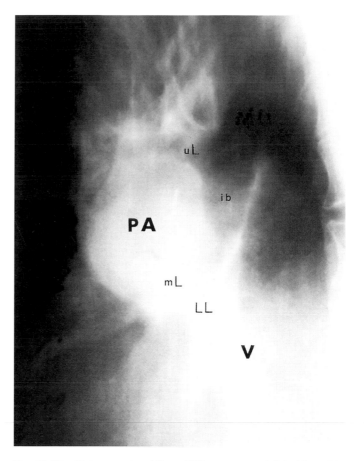

Fig. 11.57   Right posterior oblique (55°) tomogram of right hilum. PA = pulmonary artery; V = pulmonary vein; MB = main bronchus; uL = upper lobe bronchus; ib = intermediate bronchus; mL = middle lobe bronchus; LL = lower lobe bronchus.

trapping. It is helpful in uncooperative children when the radiograph is non-diagnostic due to movement and poor inspiration.

Screening may be used to differentiate pulmonary from pleural lesions by rotating the patient and noting movement of the lesion with respect to the sternum and spine. Pulsation is often a misleading sign; it may be transmitted to a mass lying adjacent to a vascular structure. Masses of vascular origin change size with the Valsalva maneuver and with patient position. Pulmonary lesions move with respiration whereas mediastinal lesions do not.

Radionuclide Scanning

E. Rhys Davies
Radionuclide scanning of the lungs is of most value in the diagnosis of pulmonary embolism, a normal scan excluding the diagnosis. However the major drawback of this technique is its lack of specificity, so that interpretation on occasions must be guarded. A report should be made in the light of a current chest film and a ventilation scan.

The main indications for this examination are:

1. Diagnosis of pulmonary embolism
2. Evaluation of emphysema

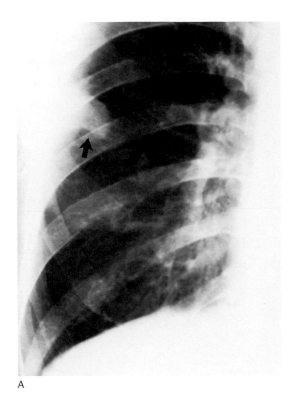

A

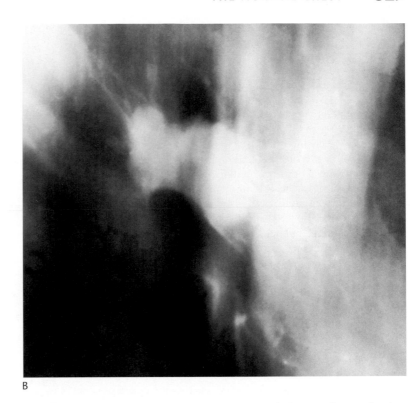

B

Fig. 11.58 Oat-cell carcinoma. **A.** Peripheral mass adjacent to the ribs. **B.** Oblique tomogram shows an irregular mass with thin strands extending into the surrounding lung.

3. To determine the extent of parenchymal disease, malignancy and infections associated with AIDS
4. Monitoring the effect of therapy.

The following techniques are essentially complementary to each other and to a chest radiograph taken within 24 hours of scanning.

1. Ventilation Studies

a. *Xenon-133*, with a principal photon energy of 80 keV and a half-life of 5.7 days, is still used. The gas is delivered to the mouthpiece of a rebreathing system and after a single deep inspiration a 10-second image is recorded. This record shows the distribution of inspired air, with areas of low activity representing poor ventilation. Next, the mixture of air and ^{133}Xe is rebreathed for some minutes to reach equilibrium, after which rebreathing is discontinued and serial images are recorded during the 'washout' phase. Persistent activity denotes air trapping, e.g. in an emphysematous bulla.

b. *Krypton-81m*, with a photon energy of 190 keV and a half-life of 13 seconds, is generated by the decay of cyclotron produced rubidium-81 (half-life 4.58 hours). Because of its short half-life, ^{81m}Kr is administered continuously during the investigation. Its distribution represents its rate of arrival and hence the ventilatory pattern. Naturally this pattern will be influenced by the posture of the patient as well as by disease. ^{133}Xe has the advantage of a relatively long shelf-life so that it is readily available at all times, but its photon energy peak is relatively close to that of ^{99m}Tc which is used for perfusion studies. The labeled microspheres for the perfusion studies are fixed in the pulmonary capillaries and

therefore the ventilation scan with krypton must precede the perfusion scan. This is an important disadvantage because it runs counter to the usual schemes of investigation. On the other hand, ^{81m}Kr can be separated satisfactorily from technetium and, despite the relative disadvantage of its cost and poor shelf-life, it is favored by most departments.

c. ^{99m}Tc-*labeled aerosols* have been developed in order to provide a relatively available ventilation technique. They have the disadvantage of disproportionate deposition of radioactivity in the larger air tubes.

It is essential to take anterior, posterior and posterior oblique views in all instances. Other tangential views may be helpful in individual cases.

2. Perfusion Studies

The principle of perfusion scanning is that particles greater than the size of the lung capillaries (80–100 μm) will be trapped during their first passage through the lungs.^{99m}Tc microspheres of uniform size, about 40 μm; are the most satisfactory agents. These are cleared from the lungs over the next 12 hours or so, and then they are gradually broken down and metabolized in the liver. The patient rests for 5–10 minutes to achieve circulatory equilibrium; 40–80 MBq are injected intravenously during several resting respiratory cycles, in the supine position. This achieves good mixing, so that lung activity is proportional to its perfusion. The more dependent parts of the lung are slightly better perfused than the remainder, so that the anterior basal segments are less well perfused than the posterior. It is important to remember this when interpreting the scan, but if the same position is used always, this normal variation will be taken into account more easily.

Anterior, posterior and both posterior oblique views are carried out and, in a normal scan, activity is found over the whole thorax except the mediastinum. The size of the mediastinal defect is determined mainly by the size of the heart. This normal pattern is altered whenever the perfusion of a region of lung is diminished. This occurs when there is mechanical obstruction of an artery (Fig. 11.59), or alveolar hypoxia due to air trapping, bronchial obstruction (Fig. 11.60), pneumonia or redistribution of blood flow as in mitral stenosis with pulmonary hypertension (Fig. 11.61). In normal lung, less than 1 in 1000 capillaries are occluded by microspheres and there is no hemodynamic upset. However, in severe pulmonary hypertension the capillary bed is already so reduced that a lung scan can be hazardous (especially if macro-aggregates are used, because they contain some particles up to 100 μm). Scanning is best avoided in these patients as it is unlikely to be useful.

3. Ventilation Perfusion Ratio (v/Q)

In normal scans the distribution of radioactivity is even and parallel in both ventilation and perfusion images. This pattern is disturbed in many diseases. Diminished ventilation leads reflexly to corresponding impaired perfusion, whereas the converse is not so, apart from exceptionally large or longstanding perfusion defects. Thus a bulla or collapsed segment will lead to impairment of activity in both scans, whereas embolus will lead to impaired perfusion and normal ventilation scans.

Pulmonary Embolism

The investigation of suspected pulmonary embolism is probably the most widespread indication for lung scintigraphy. Uncer-

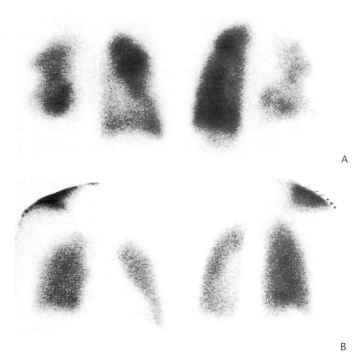

A

B

Fig. 11.59 **A.** Perfusion lung scan, ^{99m}Tc microspheres. There are several large defects in the right lung and a smaller defect in the left lung. **B.** Ventilation scan, ^{87m}Kr. There are no ventilation defects. These unmatched ventilation and perfusion scans are characteristic of pulmonary embolism.

tainties in clinical and plain radiographic diagnosis and the impossibility of using pulmonary angiography as the standard investigation have generated considerable demand for lung scintigraphy, with all its promise of being able to identify unperfused

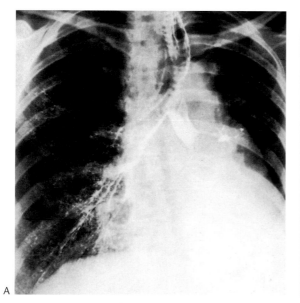
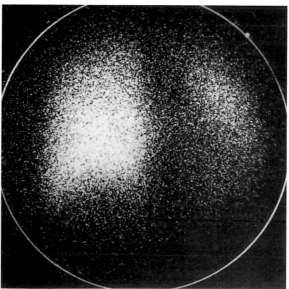

A

B

Fig. 11.60 Bronchial carcinoid. **A.** Bronchogram. There is a large filling defect in the left main bronchus and only a small amount of contrast medium has gone beyond it. The left lower lobe is collapsed. **B.** ^{99m}Tc-MAA scan, anterior projection. Right lung activity is even, and there is some activity in the left upper lobe, which is aerated, but none in the left lower lobe, which is not aerated or perfused.

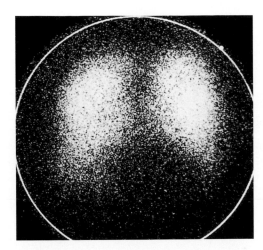

Fig. 11.61 Heart failure. ^{99m}Tc-MAA scan, anterior view. The cardiac defect is large; activity over the upper lobes is greater than over the lower lobes because of redistribution of blood flow due to heart failure.

segments of lung. Alas, it is rarely possible to verify the diagnosis pathologically, and in the face of justifiable clinical anxiety over the consequences of overlooking pulmonary embolus, it is important to indicate clearly the degree of probability that a scan is positive or negative.

The characteristic appearance of a pulmonary embolus is a perfusion defect corresponding to an identifiable segment or lobe without a matching ventilation defect. If there is no radiographic abnormality or if the perfusion defects are substantially larger than radiographic abnormalities, or are multiple, there is a high probability of pulmonary embolism. At the other extreme, normal perfusion excludes pulmonary embolus, and focal matched defects with no corresponding radiographic abnormality, or a perfusion defect smaller than a radiographic abnormality, have a low probability for pulmonary embolism (less than 10%). Matched V/Q defects, with or without radiographic abnormalities, make up the most difficult diagnostic group. Usually the patients are known to have pre-existing lung disease such as pulmonary tuberculosis, fibrotic sarcoidosis, asthma or chronic bronchitis, all of which will produce abnormal scans of this kind. Occasionally in this group it will be necessary to give some consideration to pulmonary angiography, particularly if anticoagulants are contraindicated.

With meticulous technique and careful consideration of the clinical and radiological features, a firm opinion can be given in the vast majority of instances. In a small minority, resolution of the problem will remain difficult. It is worth remembering that a subsegmental defect may be significant because of the intrinsic underestimation of the technique; and that an unmatched single segment defect has an intermediate probability of pulmonary embolus. It may be helpful to monitor the evolution of the signs by means of serial imaging and radiography if the clinical status in stable.

Scintigraphy may underestimate the extent of embolic disease in two important situations. First, minute peripheral embolization following fragmentation of clot may be overlooked if the emboli are distributed evenly. Second, partial occlusion of both main pulmonary arteries by a saddle embolus may produce a symmetric scan in the absence of total occlusion of the main pulmonary

artery, or a recognizable peripheral defect. Disparities between arteriogram and scintigram are more apparent than real once it is appreciated that the presence of a patent small artery on the angiogram does not necessarily mean there is good flow through its capillary bed. However an acute embolus can only be diagnosed on angiography if it is outlined clearly. The presence of arterial 'cut-off' is not adequate. A normal four-view scan at the time of a suspected embolus is virtually certain evidence against embolization.

Individual arteries cannot be identified without arteriography and it is generally accepted this should be done when embolectomy is being considered on clinical grounds.

Scintigraphy may be repeated without hazard and it has been suggested that a preoperative scan in high-risk patients (e.g. hip replacement) improves the ability to interpret postoperative scans. It is equally important sometimes to establish a baseline for future reference after an obvious embolus for the abnormalities resolve within weeks or months. Examinations that are normal or clearly positive can be judged objectively. Those that have an intermediate probability of embolus tend to be judged most subjectively and lead to difficult therapeutic decisions. Where the management protocol is aggressive, the tendency of the scan to underestimate will be an important consideration and full pedocaval phlebography will be done frequently. The call for pulmonary angiography also is most likely in such circumstances. Ventilation and perfusion studies are often useful both in the preoperative assessment of patients with large bullae and in their assessment after lobectomy.

Other lesions that can cause localized perfusion defects include lung tumors, pneumonia, exacerbation of chronic infection, tuberculosis, lung abscess, radiation pneumonitis, fibrosis, and underventilation associated with hypoplasia of pulmonary arteries. The value of scintigraphy in assessing these lesions is limited and their importance is that they should not be confused with pulmonary embolus. This can be achieved by meticulous examination of a chest radiography taken within 24 hours of the scans.

The investigation of pulmonary embolus is inseparable from the determination of its source. Ascending pedal phlebography is the traditional way of doing this and is still the best way of showing the precise location of the thrombus before operation. However, in any group of patients known to be at special risk, e.g. because of immobilization after operation, ^{131}I-fibrinogen given intravenously before operation will be incorporated into thrombi that are formed so that they can be detected by external counting. Usually the activity is measured at several points along both legs daily, and a rise of 30% between one of the counts and the adjacent counts is significant (Fig. 11.62). The method is much more reliable than clinical suspicion of deep vein thrombosis but loses its accuracy dramatically above the inguinal ligament.

The disadvantages of this technique are:

a. Radiopharmaceutical is administered preoperatively to all those at risk

b. The test cannot be applied to the ilio-femoral venous segment where the clinically significant thrombi are likely to be

c. Fibrinogen uptake in arthritic knees may complicate the interpretation.

Alternatively, the radiopharmaceutical being given for a lung scan can be divided into two equal amounts that are injected

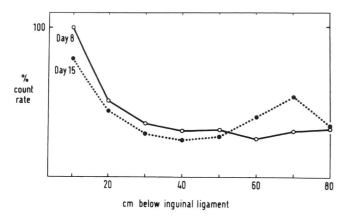

Fig. 11.62   Calf vein thrombosis. [131]I fibrinogen trace. On Day 8 the trace is normal, on Day 15 there is a significant rise of activity at 60 and 70 cm below the inguinal ligament, indicating thrombus formation in the calf.

synchronously into a dorsal pedal vein in each foot, with compression of superficial veins at the ankle. Rapid-sequence images of the limbs and abdomen can be taken to show the whole venous drainage including the inferior vena cava. Delayed transit, filling defects, adherence to intravenous thrombus and asymmetric pattern are indications of abnormality and the technique has many obvious advantages. The lung scan is then done in the usual way.

Gallium Scanning

[67]Ga citrate is well known for being taken up in areas of inflammation, granulocyte activity, and in some tumors (Fig. 11.63). It has a physical half-life of 78 hours and several photon peaks, the most useful being at 240 keV. After intravenous injection, it is bound in vivo to transferrin and lactoferrin, and is excreted in the bile and urine. Because it is concentrated in lactating breasts and excreted in maternal milk, breastfeeding should be discontinued temporarily if the investigation is unavoidable at this time. Images are usually taken at 6 hours but may be repeated up to 72 h if necessary.

The use of gallium citrate as an agent for detecting occult infection is usually directed extrathoracically, though unsuspected thoracic infections can sometimes be demonstrated. This is particularly so in the case of miliary tuberculosis presenting as pyrexia of unknown origin. The increased lung field activity is very subtle except when compared with the relative deficit over the heart. The detection of distant occult lesions, e.g. spine or renal tract, will help to confirm the diagnosis.

At one time, gallium-67 citrate scanning was advocated for staging carcinoma of the bronchus but it has now been superseded by high-resolution computed tomography.

The most practical use of ^{67}Ga scanning in lung disease is derived from the high affinity that granulomata have for the compound. For example, the granulomata of sarcoidosis can lead to a typical uptake pattern in the hila, right paratracheal lymph nodes, and the parotid and nasolacrimal glands. Further, in sarcoidosis the scan may be used to assess the extent of extrathoracic disease activity, and finally, to distinguish areas of active pulmonary disease from inactive fibrosis, a distinction that is not always possible from radiography (Goddard 1988, Cooke et al 1989) (Fig. 11.64).

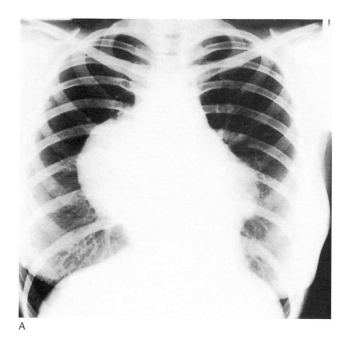

A

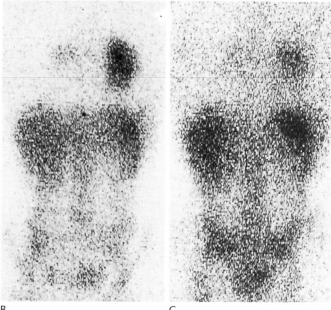

B   C

Fig. 11.63   Mediastinal lymphoma. **A.** PA chest radiograph. Anterior (**B**) and posterior (**C**) projections of ^{67}Ga citrate scan at 48 hours. There is high activity over the mediastinal abnormality. Note normal activity over lumbar spine, liver and spleen. The spleen is large but high activity is not in itself an indication that it is involved by lymphoma. Indeed the relatively low vascularity of splenic lymphoma may lead to lower activity than expected.

The role of ^{67}Ga citrate in detecting infection has been taken over to a large extent by ^{111}In leukocyte scanning. It is unusual to use the technique for pulmonary infections but it is important to recognize that abnormalities may be demonstrated in the lungs during leukocyte scanning. The labeling technique alters the properties of some of the white cells and makes them more liable to sequestration in the lungs, thereby giving an innocent slight but

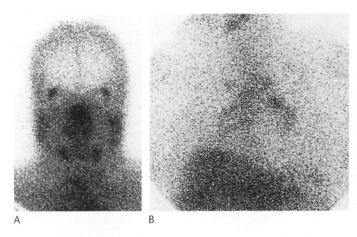

Fig. 11.64 Sarcoidosis. ^{67}Ga citrate scans of head (**A**) and chest (**B**), showing high activity in both hilar regions, the salivary glands, and more particularly the lacrimal glands.

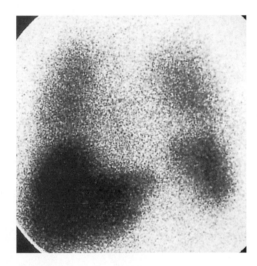

Fig. 11.65 ^{111}In leukocyte scan. There is normal activity in liver and spleen, and on each side of the heart there is pulmonary activity due to capillary trapping of damaged leukocytes.

diffuse activity on the scan. Careless injection technique may lead to overt clumping of cells. Finally, injection through central venous lines may lead to some disposition of white cells along the tube (Fig. 11.65).

CT of the Lungs

Richard W. Whitehouse

Technical Considerations Computed tomography of the thorax is a high radiation dose examination, capable of giving an effective dose 50–500 times higher than a conventional chest radiograph. The wide dose range is largely due to variations in technique between different operators.

Variation in breath holding between scans is a cause of misregistration of scan positioning in thoracic scanning. Some parts of the lung can be missed between adjacent sections with the possibility of small pulmonary parenchymal lesions being overlooked. The development of slip ring technology has allowed

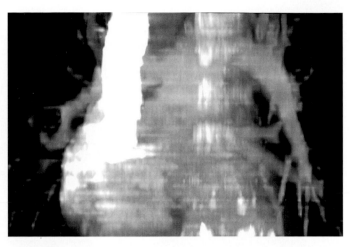

Fig. 11.66 Maximum intensity projection pulmonary angiogram (left anterior oblique view). The highest contrast density is in the superior vena cava. (Courtesy of Dr A. Horrocks.)

scanners to operate with continuous one direction rotation of the X-ray tube and detectors at one rotation per 1–2 seconds whilst the patient is motored smoothly through the scanner aperture. The resultant helical scan path may cover the entire thorax in a single breath hold and allows image reconstruction from any 360° data collection within the helix. Thus overlapping sections can be reconstructed through the entire thorax, overcoming this problem (*'spiral' scanning*). The same technique can be used during intravenous contrast infusion to demonstrate the pulmonary vessels. Postprocessing software can then produce a maximum intensity projection (MIP) pulmonary angiogram (Fig. 11.66).

The thorax contains tissues with CT numbers ranging from –1000 for air through lung parenchyma, fat and soft tissue, to cortical bone with a CT number of over 1500. Comprehensive evaluation of these tissues therefore requires interrogation of the grayscale image at a variety of window levels and widths. A wide

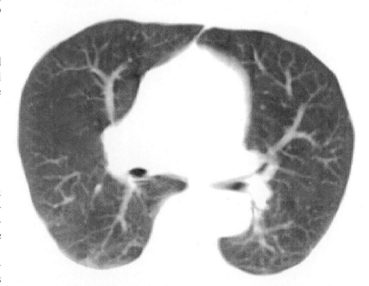

Fig. 11.67 Conventional 1 cm thick section through the mid chest, viewed on a lung window. Note the branching pulmonary vessels and the paucity of vessels at the sites of fissures.

window is necessary for bone and lung parenchyma, with a higher window level for bone, whilst a narrow window is necessary to demonstrate the smaller density differences that may be present between soft-tissue structures.

CT is a useful technique for guiding thoracic biopsy, both pulmonary fine needle aspiration and larger cutting needle biopsies of pulmonary, pleural and mediastinal masses.

Anatomic Considerations   Both the pulmonary arteries and the bronchi branch out from the hila to the lung periphery. Similarly the pulmonary veins radiate from the venous confluence and left atrium. CT through the upper or lower chest passes through these structures obliquely or in cross-section, resulting in a ring appearance for bronchi and filled circles or ovals for vessels. CT through the midpart of the thorax will demonstrate greater lengths of each individual structure as they arborize within the scan plane (Fig. 11.67). Careful reference to adjacent sections is therefore necessary to trace vessels and bronchi out from the hila to the apices and bases in order to demonstrate the continuity of these structures and to confirm whether small opacities in the pulmonary periphery are normal vessels or pulmonary nodules.

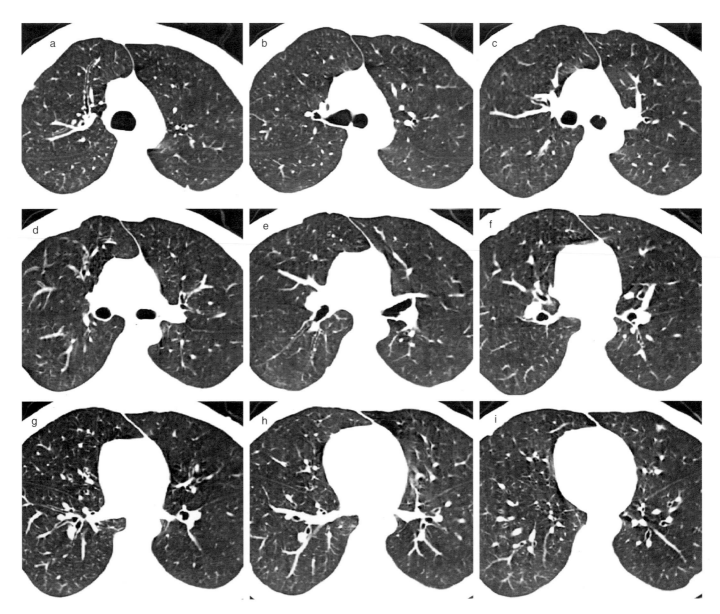

Fig. 11.68 High-resolution sections through the thorax demonstrate the segmental bronchi. **A.** Upper section; anterior division of the apical segmental bronchus of the right upper lobe is in the plane of section. **B.** Origin of right upper lobe bronchus is demonstrated at the level of the carina. **C.** Right anterior segmental upper lobe segmental bronchi are seen; on the left the apicoposterior upper lobe segmental bronchus is visible. **D.** The left upper lobe bronchus division into apicoposterior and anterior segmental bronchi is seen. **E.** The right lower lobe apical segmental bronchus origin is seen whilst on the left the main bronchus is dividing into upper and lower lobar bronchi. **F.** On each side the lower lobe bronchi are seen, with the lingular bronchus anteriorly on the left and the middle lobe bronchus anteriorly on the right. The left lower lobe apical segmental bronchus origin is evident. **G.** The right lower lobe bronchus has divided into medial, anterior, lateral and posterior segmental bronchi. **H.** The left lower lobe bronchus has divided into anterior, lateral and posterior basal segments. **I.** The basal segmental bronchi can be individually traced toward the lung bases.

The location of the pulmonary fissures on thick section (1 cm) CT scans can usually be inferred by a paucity of vessels in that region, whilst the fissures can usually be directly identified on thin-section high-resolution CT (compare Figs 11.67 and 11.68). The azygos fissure, when present, is clearly seen as it is perpendicular to the plane of section (Fig. 11.69). Careful interrogation of adjacent sections in both directions from the hila will usually allow identification of the segmental bronchi and often the subsegmental bronchi beyond this (Fig. 11.68).

Toward the lung bases, the apex of the right hemidiaphragm will usually appear centrally first, resulting in increased density in the middle of the lung image.

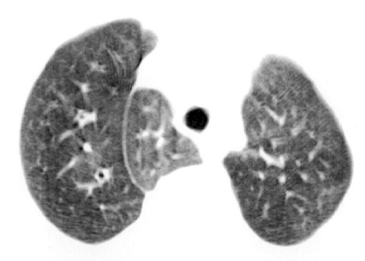

Fig. 11.69   The azygos fissure is clearly seen on CT.

Physiological Considerations   Respiratory phase: the density of the pulmonary parenchyma is strongly dependent upon the respiratory phase. In expiration there is a striking increase in density, particularly in the dependent part of the lung. This is likely to be due to reduced alveolar inflation with consequent crowding of the alveolar walls and pulmonary vasculature but may also have a contribution from altered perfusion. Lung parenchyma is best assessed by scanning in suspended full inspiration.

Posture: the influence of gravity on pulmonary vessel caliber is well demonstrated by CT. Dependent vessels are notably larger. Slightly increased parenchymal density, probably due to hypostatic parenchymal edema, may also be seen in the dependent part of the lungs on CT. This can be cleared by placing the patient prone and repeating the scan after a few minutes (Fig. 11.70). Scanning of the thorax with the patient in the decubitus position results in compression of the dependent lung, most noticeable during expiration, whilst the uppermost lung is in a state of relative inspiratory apnea and oligemia. Mediastinal structures may also move considerably under the influence of posture, particularly in patients with emphysema (Fig. 11.70).

Role of CT in Diseases of the Lung and Pleura

The chest radiograph usually reveals the anatomic distribution of lobar or segmental disease and can demonstrate generalized or diffuse pulmonary parenchymal abnormalities as an alteration in the pattern of pulmonary markings. High-resolution CT can confirm the location and extent of disease and can further characterize the location and pattern of disease (Fig. 11.71). Mediastinal or chest wall involvement by pulmonary pathology may also be demonstrated by CT (Fig. 11.72). Ascertaining the solitary nature of a pulmonary nodule or detection of other

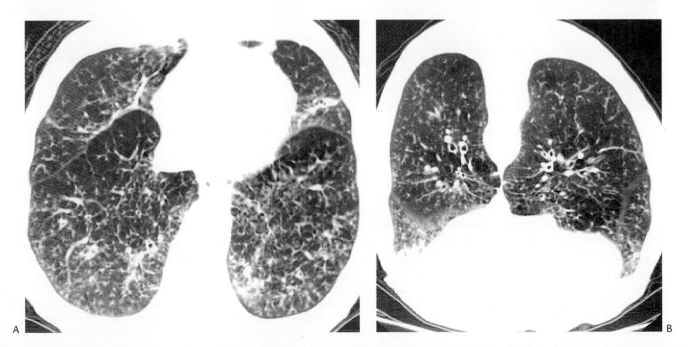

Fig. 11.70   A. Supine scan in chronic airways disease. The lungs are overinflated and postural increase in pulmonary density is evident posteriorly. **B.** Prone scan at the same level. The posterior increased density seen in **A** has cleared. Note the marked mobility of the mediastinum with the heart now flattened against the anterior chest wall.

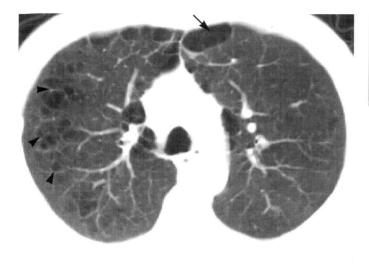

Fig. 11.71 Large areas of reduced pulmonary density (arrowheads) and bullae (arrow) in emphysema.

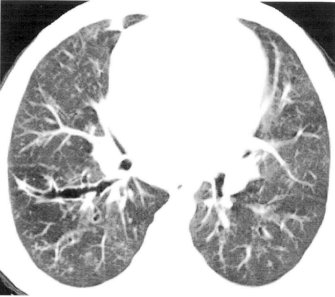

Fig. 11.73 Tubular bronchiectasis in a patient with cystic fibrosis.

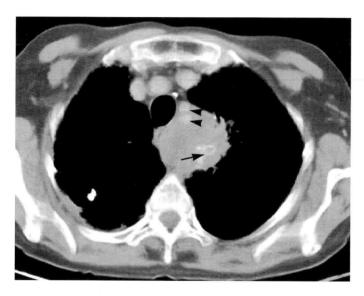

Fig. 11.72 Carcinoma of the lung incorporating calcification (arrow) from previous tuberculous granuloma. The tumor is extending into the mediastinum to encase the left common carotid and subclavian arteries (arrowheads).

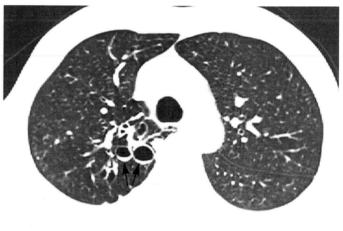

Fig. 11.74 Saccular bronchiectasis (arrows).

unsuspected nodules, determination of the probability of malignancy, contribution to staging prior to treatment and monitoring of response to treatment are all important roles for CT.

High-resolution CT (HRCT) The use of thin sections (1–3 mm) combined with a high spatial resolution reconstruction algorithm (e.g. the 'bone' algorithm) and targeting the scan to the lungs (i.e. using a field of view just large enough to encompass the region of interest) results in clear depiction of the distribution and higher definition of the appearance of pulmonary parenchymal disease. This has proved valuable in the demonstration and differential diagnosis of diverse interstitial pulmonary diseases. The severity and extent of bronchiectasis can be demonstrated

(Figs 11.73, 11.74). The technique can identify regions most suitable for biopsy at a time when the chest radiograph is normal.

Interstitial Diseases In *fibrosing alveolitis* and *systemic sclerosis*, CT demonstrates a typical peripheral distribution of disease involving the outer third of the lungs. This starts as a posterior basal subpleural crescent of increased attenuation, progressing to peripheral 'honeycombing'. The pleural and mediastinal interfaces may become irregular with a 'saw-tooth' margin (Fig. 11.75). In *asbestosis* HRCT may demonstrate subpleural curvilinear opacities, parenchymal bands, thickened inter- and intra-lobular lines, increased subpleural attenuation and honeycombing (Figs 11.76, 11.77). Pleural thickening and calcification will also be demonstrated in cases of asbestos-related pleural disease (Fig. 11.78). HRCT has a 100% positive predictive value in asbestosis with

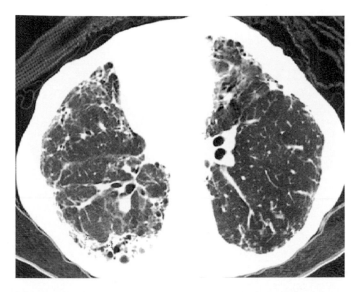

Fig. 11.75 HRCT 3 mm section. Fibrosing alveolitis. Note the predominantly peripheral involvement. (Courtesy of Dr P. M. Taylor.)

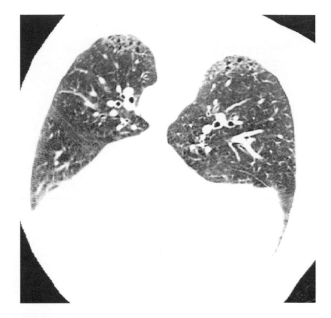

Fig. 11.77 HRCT asbestosis. Early subpleural increase in density on a prone scan. (Courtesy of Dr P. M. Taylor.)

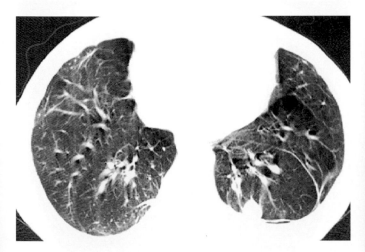

Fig. 11.76 HRCT asbestosis. Note the thickened septa and fibrous parenchymal and subpleural bands. (Courtesy of Dr P. M. Taylor.)

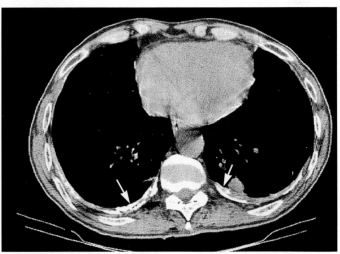

Fig. 11.78 HRCT soft-tissue window demonstrates asbestos-related pleural disease with posteromedial calcified pleural plaques (arrows).

pleural thickening. *Rounded atelectasis*, a fibrosing condition most commonly associated with asbestosis, is also clearly demonstrated on CT, the 'comet tail' of incurving vessels being characteristic (Fig. 11.79); other features include adjacent pleural thickening and an air bronchogram within the lesion. Recognition of these features may prevent unnecessary pulmonary resection for a supposed carcinoma but biopsy may be necessary as both *pulmonary carcinoma* and *pleural mesothelioma* are commoner in this group of patients. Irregular thickening of the interlobular septa, producing a reticular pattern, can be appreciated on HRCT in *lymphangitis carcinomatosa* before it is apparent on the chest radiograph (Fig. 11.80). In chronic *sarcoidosis* nodules at branchpoints of pulmonary vessels and bronchi may be seen, and beading of the bronchi is typical (Figs 11.81, 11.82). Air space opacification and thickening of the interlobular septa produces a characteristic 'crazy-paving' effect in *alveolar proteinosis*. *Lymphangioleiomyomatosis* is a condition only occurring in

women of reproductive age; the CT appearance is of multiple cystic spaces replacing the lung parenchyma. *Acute alveolar disease* is clearly demonstrated from whatever cause (Figs 11.83, 11.84), as is *miliary nodularity* (Fig. 11.85).

Pulmonary Nodules and Carcinoma   CT is the most sensitive imaging modality available for the identification of pulmonary nodules of 3 mm or greater in diameter, but is relatively insensitive to smaller nodules. The specificity for small nodules is also poor, with up to 60% of small nodules in patients with malignant disease being unrelated granulomata indistinguishable from metastases on CT. Most pulmonary metastases are found in the outer third of the lungs, more commonly toward the bases, and the majority of them are subpleural (Fig. 11.86). Spiral scanning has improved the detection rate for pulmonary nodules but has

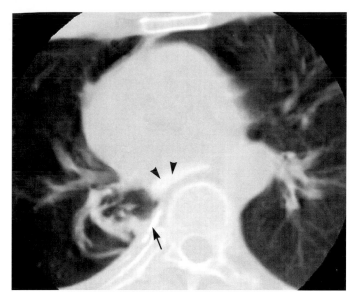

Fig. 11.79 Rounded atelectasis with 'comet tail' of vessels running into the mass which is adherent to the pleura. Adjacent calcified pleural plaque is evident (arrow). There is also oral contrast medium in the esophagus (arrowheads).

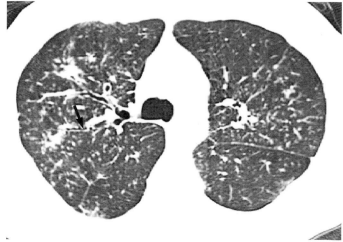

Fig. 11.81 HRCT sarcoidosis with beading of the segmental bronchial walls (arrow). (Courtesy of Dr P. M. Taylor.)

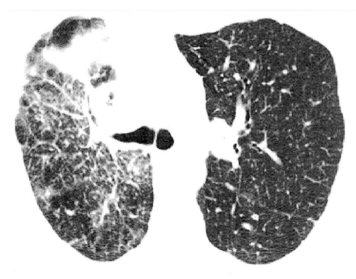

Fig. 11.80 HRCT lymphangitis carcinomatosa from carcinoma of the breast. Note the thickened interlobular septa. (Courtesy of Dr P. M. Taylor.)

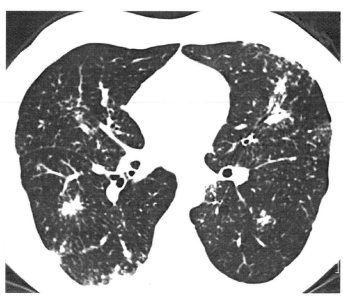

Fig. 11.82 HRCT sarcoidosis with patchy peribronchial shadowing.

not improved specificity. Assessment of the margins of pulmonary nodules is unreliable in differentiating benign from malignant disease. The presence of definite calcification in a pulmonary nodule suggests a granuloma and thus benign disease. However, scar carcinomas can arise in old tuberculous lesions (Fig. 11.72) and up to 14% of carcinomas demonstrate histologic calcification. Thus, to suggest benignity, the amount of calcification should represent over 10% of the nodule, the calcification should not be stippled and the lesion should not be greater than 3 cm in diameter. Unequivocal demonstration of fat density within a

pulmonary nodule is almost diagnostic of an *hamartoma*. Lack of growth of a nodule over a 2-year period is also indicative of benignity. Cavitation can be demonstrated early by CT but does not necessarily indicate malignancy (Fig. 11.87). In pulmonary malignancy CT can demonstrate spread to the hilum, mediastinum (Fig. 11.72), pleura, or chest wall and also allows assessment of mediastinal lymph nodes and the adrenal glands (common sites for metastatic spread).

HRCT should not be used for the detection of pulmonary nodules as non-contiguous sections are commonly performed in this technique.

Pleural Disease Differentiation of pulmonary from pleural disease is possible using CT. The distinction of a pleural effusion from subdiaphragmatic fluid is achieved by recognizing the relationship of the fluid to the diaphragm or its crura (Fig. 11.88).

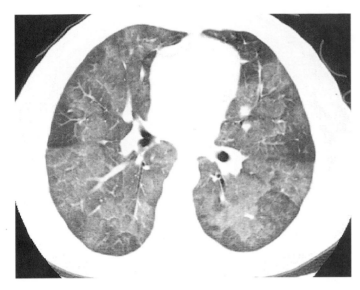

Fig. 11.83 HRCT diffuse alveolar disease in extrinsic allergic alveolitis. (Courtesy of Dr P. M. Taylor.)

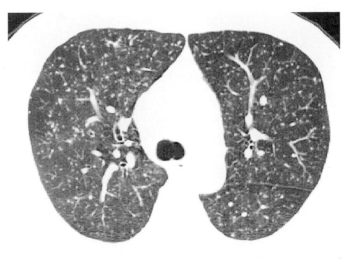

Fig. 11.85 HRCT miliary tuberculosis.

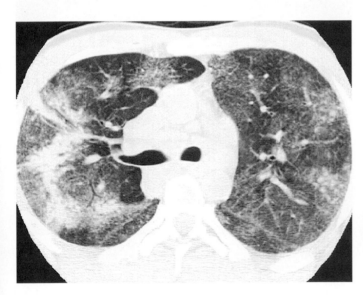

Fig. 11.84 HRCT acute sarcoidosis with widespread alveolar shadowing.

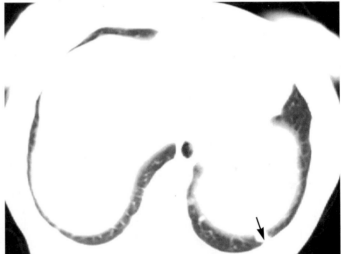

Fig. 11.86 Occult metastasis in the posterior costophrenic sulcus (arrow).

Pleural plaques in asbestos-related pleural disease are commonly discrete lesions arising over the diaphragmatic and posterolateral parietal pleura and may show characteristic calcification (Fig. 11.78). Pleural tumors (mesothelioma, metastatic adenocarcinoma, spread from thymic tumors) characteristically encase the lung, reducing its volume (Figs 11.89, 11.90).

MRI in Chest Diseases

Jeremy P. R. Jenkins

The role of MRI and its relation to other imaging techniques in chest diseases has yet to be defined and is still evolving. The main advantages of MRI include a multiplanar facility and a high intrinsic soft-tissue contrast discrimination, allowing vascular structures and lesions in the mediastinal and hilar regions to be defined separately from other tissues without the need for contrast-medium administration. Disadvantages of MRI include respiratory and cardiac motion artefacts and an inability to visualize small branching pulmonary vessels and bronchi, and lung parenchyma. These structures, however, are better depicted on CT. The introduction of faster MR scan times, enabling images to be obtained within a single breath hold, combined with a good signal-to-noise ratio (SNR), may alleviate some of these problems, as can the use of ECG- and respiratory-gated techniques. At present, MRI is unable to provide the same anatomic detail and spatial resolution in the lung as high-resolution CT. The ease of performance and wider availability of CT makes it the procedure of choice in the assessment of most lesions in the thorax, including lung metastases. MRI can be useful in certain situations, e.g. in the separation of mediastinal masses from normal or abnormal vessels, the illustration of the craniocaudal extent of large lesions and lesions at the lung apex, lung base and chest wall, and in the

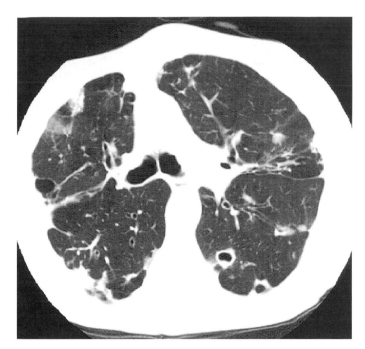

Fig. 11.87 HRCT rheumatoid lung with cavitating nodules, bronchiectasis and emphysema.

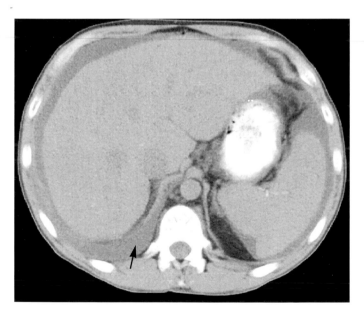

Fig. 11.88 Pleural effusion and ascites—note the relationship of the fluid to the right diaphragmatic crus with pleural fluid lying posterior to (and therefore above) the crus (arrow). Ascitic fluid is evident around the spleen and anterolateral to the liver.

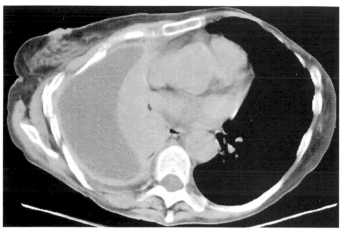

Fig. 11.89 Pleural metastatic tumor from carcinoma of the breast, encasing the lung with consequent volume loss, crowding of the ribs and a malignant effusion. Note the contralateral mastectomy.

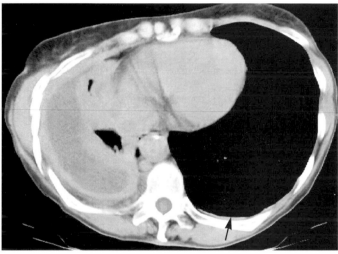

Fig. 11.90 Pleural mesothelioma. Similar characteristics to Fig. 11.89. Note the contralateral posterior pleural plaque indicating previous asbestos exposure (arrow).

assessment of pathology affecting major vessels and the brachial plexus (see Ch. 12).

Anatomic detail of *lung parenchyma* is limited on MRI due to respiratory and cardiac motion artefacts, an intrinsically low SNR from the lung air spaces, a poorer spatial resolution than conventional radiography and CT, and difficulty in precise localization of disease due to lack of normal anatomic landmarks. Normal lobar fissures and small peripheral pulmonary vessels and bronchi are not visualized, and alveolar and interstitial changes within the lung cannot be distinguished. Failure to visualize aerated lung is due to the magnetic susceptibility effects between air and soft tissue, creating magnetic field gradients at each alveolar wall interface. This effect is quite marked leading to shortening of the T_2 relaxation time of aerated lung to approximately 7 ms, compared with a T_2 of 80 ms for collapsed non-aerated lung. The use of minimum echo times (TE 7 ms) has been used with the T_1-weighted spin-echo sequence to compensate for this T_2 effect, and provides a 3.5 fold increase in the signal-to-ratio (SNR) from the lung compared with conventional TE values of 20 ms. MRI is unable to compete with thin-section high-resolution CT in the assessment or detection of small peripheral lung carcinomas, metastases, or calcifications. CT is the imaging method of choice in the detection and evaluation of lung nodules, including metastases. MRI can be useful, however, in differentiating lung nodules from vessels, particularly in the hilar region.

Cystic lesions of the lung (e.g. bronchogenic cysts and bronchial atresia with mucocele formation secondary to mucoid impaction) can be clearly demonstrated as areas of high signal on T_2-weighted images. Vascular lesions (e.g. scimitar syndrome and pulmonary A/V fistulae) may be missed on MRI due to lack of contrast from the low signal or signal void from flowing blood within the vessel and the surrounding air space. This problem can be overcome by the use of phase-sensitive flow sequences, which provide increased signal from coherently flowing blood.

There is considerable overlap in the MRI characteristics of parenchymal consolidation, which may be due to a variety of causes. In the experimental situation it has been possible to separate cardiogenic from non-cardiogenic pulmonary edema although the clinical utility is unclear. MRI may be of value in assessing activity of interstitial lung disease by the demonstration of excess water in active pathology. Granulation tissue and compressed lung enhance markedly following intravenous administration of gadolinium chelate. Chronic inactive disease and tumor enhance, but to a lesser degree.

Lung Biopsy

Techniques

1. *Open biopsy* is obtained at surgery and entails the risks of a thoracotomy and general anesthetic although an adequate specimen is obtained. With the increased use of percutaneous and endoscopic techniques, open biopsy is undertaken less often.

2. During **flexible bronchoscopy** biopsy can be made of central lesions. Brushings, washings and bacterial samples may be obtained. The success rate is high and the complication rate low.

3. **Catheter biopsy** is made with a French 7 or 8 catheter inserted via the cricothyroid membrane and screened into the relevant bronchus. Central masses can be biopsied.

4. **Percutaneous biopsy** has become a routine procedure in many centers. It may be performed with a fine needle (22–23 gauge) for aspiration or with a cutting needle using fluoroscopy, CT and, when appropriate, ultrasound.

The procedure is contraindicated in patients on anticoagulants or with a bleeding diathesis, or if the mass is thought to be vascular. It is inadvisable in patients with bullae, in those with pulmonary hypertension or with a central mass who have an increased risk of bleeding, and in patients who have had a pneumonectomy. Patient cooperation is essential and uncontrolled coughing a contraindication. Biopsy of a suspected hydatid cyst is inadvisable because of the theoretical risk of anaphylaxis.

Using aspiration fine needle biopsy the diagnostic yield is high for non-lymphomatous malignancy, in the region of 95% for a lesion exceeding 5 mm, but lower for benign lesions, around 75%. In addition there is a low complication rate. Large bore cutting needles may be used for pleural-based or very peripheral lung lesions having ascertained that the lesion is avascular at CT. There is a higher associated incidence of pneumothorax.

The site of the lesion must be determined. Biopsy is performed using biplanar screening or CT. Ultrasound can be used for pleural and chest wall lesions as well as peripheral lung masses. The shortest route is determined for passage of the needle avoiding vascular structures. The puncture site is marked and

anesthetized before inserting the needle on suspended respiration. Ideally the biopsy is taken from the periphery of a mass to avoid central necrotic tissue and to increase the likelihood of a positive biopsy. Some resistance is often experienced on entering the mass. Once its position is confirmed the biopsy is taken. With a fine needle suction is applied with a syringe and several passes are made with the needle. Ideally a cytologist should be at hand to prepare the slides.

Following the biopsy, films are taken to exclude a pneumothorax (Fig. 11.91). This has a reported incidence of some 15% although only one-third of these require drainage. The pneumothorax may not develop immediately and the patient should be observed for 4 hours, with a film taken at this time prior to discharge.

Complications reported include:

1. Pneumothorax
2. Hemoptysis—incidence 10%, usually transient
3. Intraparenchymal bleeding (5%)
4. Hemothorax
5. Empyema
6. Subcutaneous emphysema, pneumomediastinum
7. Seeding of malignant cells along the needle track
8. Air embolism (very rare)
9. Death (reported rate of 1:5–10 000).

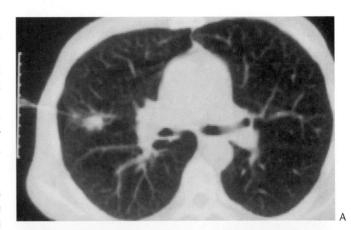

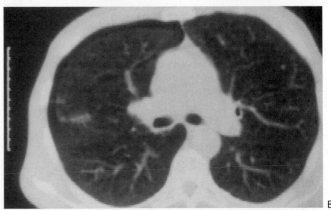

Fig. 11.91 **A.** CT percutaneous biopsy right lung mass (carcinoma). **B.** Small right pneumothorax.

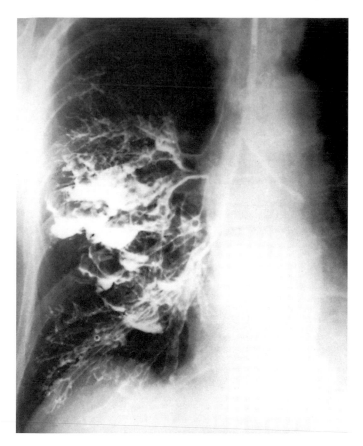

Fig. 11.92   Bronchogram. Patient with cystic bronchiectasis. The majority of the bronchi outlined with contrast medium are dilated.

Bronchography

Until recently bronchography was the definitive investigation for the diagnosis of bronchiectasis (Fig. 11.92) and for assessing the extent of the disease. High-resolution CT is now widely preferred (Fig. 11.93). Occasionally bronchography is used to investigate recurrent hemoptysis when all other investigations are negative and to demonstrate bronchopleural fistulae and congenital lesions such as sequestration and agenesis. Rarely it is used to elucidate the nature of a lesion by assessing bronchial distortion and displacement.

Severe or partial impairment of pulmonary function, massive hemoptysis, recent pneumonia, active tuberculosis and a history of allergy are recognized contraindications. A limited examination is performed if pulmonary function is reduced.

The technique is well described elsewhere. Approaches include cricothyroid puncture, nasal or transoral drip, and tracheal intubation under local or general anesthesia. Bronchography by contrast inhalation is not widely performed. Physiotherapy before and after the procedure, and atropine to reduce the secretions are essential. Films taken include AP, lateral, obliques and, if necessary, tomograms. Delayed films demonstrate distal filling. Cinebronchography has its exponents.

All the bronchi should be surveyed for evidence of narrowing, occlusion, intraluminal filling defects and dilated mucosal glands, as seen with bronchitis and bronchiectasis.

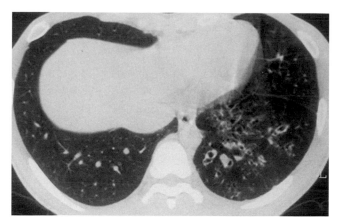

Fig. 11.93   High-resolution CT. Left lower lobe bronchiectasis.

Ultrasound

The acoustic mismatch between the chest wall and the adjacent aerated lung results in almost total reflection of the ultrasonic beam. Therefore ultrasound is useful only for assessing superficial pulmonary, pleural-based and chest wall lesions. It is helpful in the diagnosis and localization of pleural effusions and collections, and their drainage percutaneously, for subphrenic collections, in differentiating fluid from a mass lesion, and for studying diaphragm movement.

A 3.5 or 5.0 mHz transducer is preferred. Scanning can be performed with the patient sitting upright or supine. On supine scanning the right diaphragm and surrounding areas are clearly seen through the liver (Fig. 11.94). However, on the left side visualization is hampered by intervening bowel. Filling the stomach with water to use as an acoustic window and scanning obliquely improves visualization.

Pleural fluid appears as an echofree area outlining the pleural space (Fig. 11.95). Internal echoes may be due to blood or pus, with septa indicating loculation and a thick wall suggesting an empyema, within which gas may be occasionally identified.

If percutaneous drainage is undertaken a maximum of one litre should be aspirated at one sitting to prevent the development of 're-expansion' pulmonary edema. An 8–14 F catheter is left in situ, the size of the catheter chosen being matched to the viscosity of the aspirate.

Pleural-based masses are usually of low echogenicity and pleural thickening is easily identified. If consolidation is visualized fluid-filled or air-filled bronchi may be seen within it.

Pulmonary Angiography

The main indications are:

a. Diagnosis of pulmonary embolism
b. Evaluation of pulmonary hypertension
c. Diagnosis of vascular lesions, e.g. pulmonary hypoplasia, arteriovenous malformations, pulmonary artery aneurysms.

In the majority of cases embolism is excluded by a normal radionuclide perfusion scan. However for a definitive diagnosis,

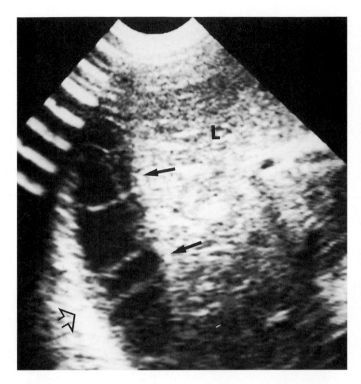

Fig. 11.94 Ultrasound scan of subphrenic abscess. There is a transonic area (arrows) between the liver (L) and diaphragm (open arrow). Strands crossing this area indicate loculation.

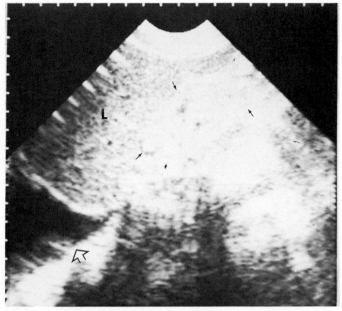

Fig. 11.95 Ultrasound scan of a pleural effusion. A patient in renal failure with acute glomerulonephritis. There is a moderate sized effusion (open arrow) seen as a transonic area in the posterior sulcus above the diaphragm. Note the highly echogenic kidney (small arrows).

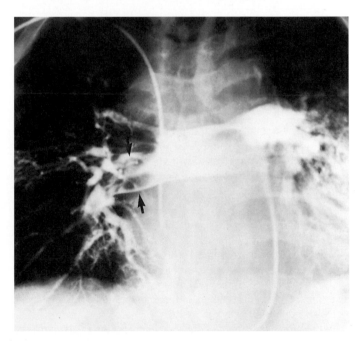

Fig. 11.96 Pulmonary angiogram. A 55-year-old man 4 days after a thoracotomy developed a DVT and pulmonary embolism. There are large thrombi (arrows) in the main arteries and peripheral perfusion is poor.

particularly if surgery is anticipated, angiography or contrast enhanced spiral CT is performed. In cases of pulmonary hypertension lower doses of contrast are used because of the increased risk of cardiogenic shock.

The right heart may be approached from the basilic vein after cutdown or via the femoral vein, provided femoral, iliac and IVC thrombus has been excluded by ascending phlebography or Doppler ultrasound examination in those cases of suspected embolism in order to prevent dislodging a large clot.

All procedures require ECG monitoring and pressure studies including right heart and pulmonary wedge pressures. A fairly rapid injection of a large bolus of contrast (50–60 ml at 20–25 ml/s) is necessary with a rapid film sequence (Fig. 11.96).

Improved arterial visualization is achieved with selective right and left artery injections, particularly if the peripheral vessels are of interest, but the main pulmonary artery only is injected if searching for a saddle embolus.

Magnification views help in the diagnosis of small peripheral emboli, as do occlusive balloons. DSA allows the use of smaller contrast volumes but disadvantages are the relatively poor resolution and artefacts due to chest motion affecting the quality of subtraction. DSA is not considered generally to be satisfactory for demonstrating small peripheral emboli.

Bronchial Arteriography

Angiography followed by embolization of bronchial and intercostal branches is a recognized treatment for life-threatening or recurrent severe hemoptysis, usually due to bronchiectasis or a mycetoma, when surgery is contraindicated. Its value is limited in the investigation of pulmonary abnormalities, malignant and benign lesions often having similar vascular patterns.

The anatomy of the bronchial arteries is very variable, the spinal branches often arising from the intercostal arteries or intercostal-bronchial trunks, in which case embolization should not be performed because of the risk of spinal cord infarction.

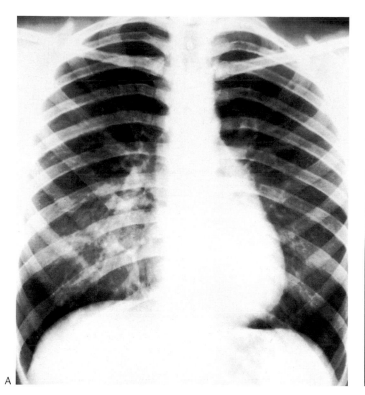

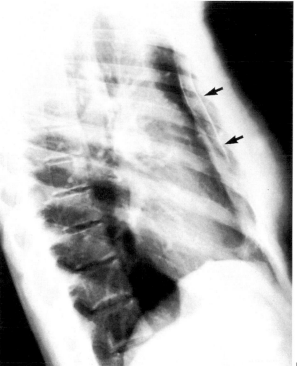

Fig. 11.97   Pectus excavatum (depressed sternum). **A.** Prominent shadowing adjacent to the right heart border. The heart is displaced to the left and has a straight left border. **B.** Note the posteriorly displaced sternum (arrows).

THE CHEST WALL

The Bones

The Clavicles   Old healed fractures are frequent findings. Erosion of the outer ends of the clavicles is associated with rheumatoid arthritis and hyperparathyroidism. Hypoplastic clavicles may be seen with the Holt–Oram syndrome and cleidocranial dysostosis.

Sternum   *Developmental abnormalities* such as perforation, fissures and agenesis are rare. Several sternal abnormalities are associated with congenital heart disease; examples include sternal agenesis, premature obliteration of the ossification centers and pigeon chest which are found with ventricular septal defects, and depressed sternum, associated with atrial septal defects and Marfan syndrome. Delayed epiphyseal fusion is a feature of cretinism, and double ossification centers in the manubrium commonly occur in Down syndrome.

In the presence of a *depressed sternum* (pectus excavatum) the anterior ribs are more vertical and the posterior ribs more horizontal than normal (Fig. 11.97); the heart is displaced to the left and posteriorly. It appears enlarged with a straight left border and indistinct right border with prominent lung markings and ill-defined shadowing in the right cardiophrenic angle. This should not be confused with consolidation. The lower thoracic spine is clearly seen through the heart.

Erosion of the sternum may occur with adjacent anterior mediastinal lymphadenopathy or tumors, aortic aneurysms and infective processes.

Primary *tumors* are rare and usually cartilaginous. The sternum may be the site of metastases, lymphoma and myeloma.

Sternal *fractures* occur with steering wheel injury, a thoracic spine injury being commonly associated.

The Ribs   *Rib notching* may affect the superior or inferior surface of the rib and be unilateral or bilateral.

Superior notching (Fig. 11.98) may be a normal finding in the elderly but has been reported in patients with rheumatoid arthritis, SLE, hyperparathyroidism, Marfan syndrome, neurofibromatosis and in paraplegics and polio victims.

Inferior notching (Fig. 11.99) develops as a result of hypertrophy of the intercostal vessels or with neurogenic tumors. Obstruction of the aorta results in reversed blood flow through the intercostal and

Table 11.20   Causes of Inferior Rib Notching

Unilateral	Blalock–Taussing operation	
	Subclavian artery occlusion	
	Aortic coarctation involving left subclavian artery or anomalous right subclavian artery	
Bilateral	Aorta	Coarctation, occlusion, aortitis
	Subclavian	Takayasu disease, atheroma
	Pulmonary oligemia	Fallot's tetralogy
		Pulmonary atresia, stenosis
		Truncus Type IV
	Venous	SVC, IVC obstruction
	Shunts	Intercostal-pulmonary fistula
		Pulmonary/intercostal arteriovenous fistula
	Others	Hyperparathyroidism
		Neurogenic
		Idiopathic

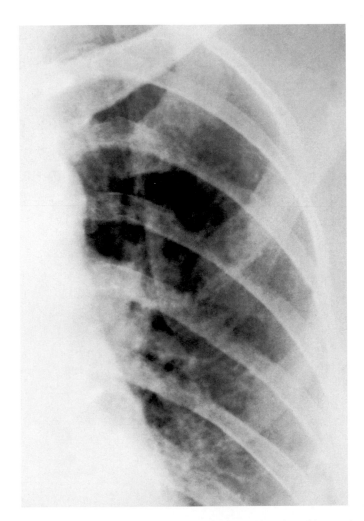

Fig. 11.98 Superior rib notching in a patient with a long history of paralysis following poliomyelitis.

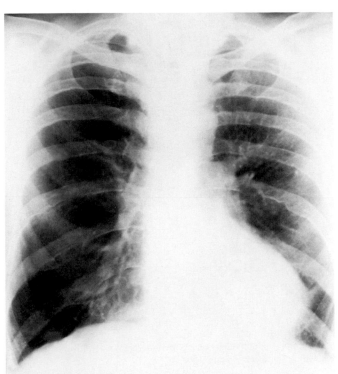

Fig. 11.99 Inferior rib notching. An elderly man who presented with hypertension. Coarctation of the aorta with rib notching most prominent in the fourth to eighth ribs.

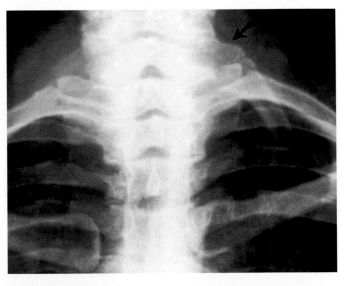

Fig. 11.100 Cervical ribs. Note the downward direction of the transverse process of C7 (arrow).

internal mammary arteries. With coarctation the first and second intercostal arteries and ribs are not affected, the arteries arising proximally from the costocervical trunk. The lower ribs are not affected unless the lower abdominal aorta is also involved. A preductal coarctation does not produce rib notching.

Congenital rib anomalies such as hypoplasia, bridging and bifid ribs are common. Hypoplastic first ribs, arising from T1, must be distinguished from cervical ribs (Fig. 11.100) which arise from C7, the transverse processes of which point caudally whereas the transverse processes of D1 are cranially inclined. Cervical ribs have an incidence of 1–2% and are usually bilateral but frequently asymmetric.

With Down's syndrome there are often only 11 pairs of ribs.

An *intrathoracic rib* is uncommon. It appears as a ribbon-like shadow near to the spine attached by one or both ends.

In *Tietze syndrome* the anterior ends of the ribs are usually normal but are occasionally enlarged or have a spotty appearance.

At *surgery* a rib may be removed (Fig. 11.101) or partially amputated. Periosteal stripping results in irregularity.

Soft-tissue masses such as a lipoma or neurofibroma may displace adjacent ribs and create a defect from pressure erosion.

Crowding of the ribs occurs with a scoliosis and major pulmonary collapse, in particular in children. It is an early sign of a

mesothelioma. Hyperinflation results in the ribs having a horizontal lie.

Fractures are often difficult to spot on the high kVp film. There may be an accompanying extrapleural hematoma, a pneumothorax or surgical emphysema. Callus may simulate a lung mass. The sixth to ninth ribs in the axillary line are the common sites for *cough fractures. Stress fractures* usually affect the first ribs.

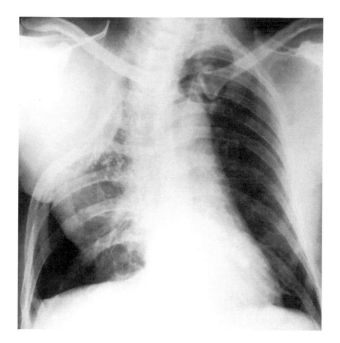

Fig. 11.101 Right thoracoplasty for tuberculosis. Removal of the upper ribs with collapse of the upper lobe.

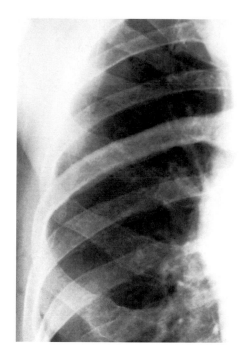

Fig. 11.102 Paget's disease. An enlarged sixth rib with a coarse trabecular pattern and of increased density.

Pathological fractures may be due to a local rib lesion or to a generalized reduction in bone mass as occurs with senile osteoporosis, myeloma, Cushing's disease and other endocrine disorders, steroid therapy and diffuse metastases. Cushing's disease is associated with abundant callus formation.

The *Looser's zones*, or pseudofractures, of osteomalacia represent areas of uncalcified osteoid and the resulting rib deformity creates a bell-shaped thorax.

Rib *sclerosis* occurs with generalized disorders such as osteopetrosis, myelofibrosis, fluorosis and metastases, or with localized lesions such as Paget's disease (Fig. 11.102), in which bony enlargement is characteristic. *Post-irradiation necrosis* results in un-united rib fractures, bony sclerosis or an abnormal trabecular pattern and soft-tissue calcification, and is often associated with a mastectomy.

Localized *rib expansion* occurs with fibrous dysplasia, myeloma, Gaucher's disease and benign tumors such as eosinophilic granuloma, hemangioma, chondroma, the brown tumors of hyperparathyroidism and aneurysmal bone cyst. In Hurler syndrome there is generalized expansion of the ribs, sparing the proximal ends, whereas in thalassemia expansion is most marked proximally and the trabecular pattern abnormal. Widening of the ribs is seen with rickets (Fig. 11.103) and scurvy. *Rib destruction* due to an infection or tumor of the soft tissues, lung or pleura is usually accompanied by an extrapleural mass. Characteristically actinomycosis infection is associated with a wavy periostitis of the ribs. Many malignant processes including metastases, lymphoma and myeloma commonly destroy the ribs.

The Thoracic Spine A survey is made to check for abnormal curvature or alignment, bone and disk destruction, sclerosis, paravertebral soft-tissue masses and congenital lesions such as butterfly vertebrae. Scoliosis and Klippel–Feil syndrome are associated with an increased incidence of congenital heart disease.

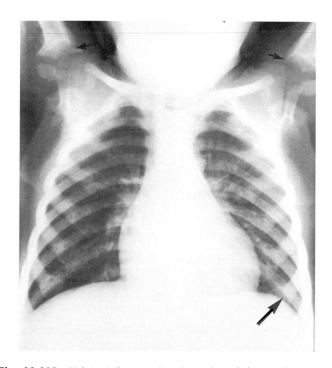

Fig. 11.103 Rickets. Enlargement and cupping of the anterior ends of the ribs. Note the metaphyseal changes in the humeri.

With a severe scoliosis, when the curve exceeds 60°, cardiorespiratory complications are common in adults.

With the *straight back syndrome* the normal kyphosis is reduced so that the sternum and spine are virtually parallel, resulting in compression of the mediastinum. Characteristically on the PA film the heart appears enlarged, is displaced to the left of midline and has a prominent left atrial appendage and aorta. On auscultation there is an ejection systolic murmur with accentuation on expiration.

Anterior erosion of the vertebral bodies sparing the disk spaces may occur with aneurysms of the descending aorta, vascular tumors, gross left atrial enlargement and neurofibromatosis, which may also cause posterior scalloping of the vertebral bodies and enlarged intervertebral foramina.

Destruction of a pedicle is typical of metastatic disease. A single dense vertebra, the ivory vertebra, is the classic appearance of lymphoma but is also seen with other conditions such as Paget's disease and metastases. Destruction of the disk with adjacent bony involvement is characteristic of an infective process.

Disk calcification may be idiopathic or post-traumatic and occurs in ochronosis and ankylosing spondylitis.

Soft Tissues

Artefacts   Hair plaits and fasteners, buttons, clothing and jewelry, etc., overlying the lungs may simulate a lung lesion. Tracing the edges of a lesion will show whether it extends beyond the lung margins, in which case the lesion is non-pulmonary. The suprasternal fossa, particularly in the elderly, may appear as a large translucency overlying the supraclavicular spine and should not be mistaken for a pharyngeal pouch.

Skin Lesions   Skin lesions including nevi and lipomas may simulate lung tumors. Multiple nodules occur with neurofibromatosis (Fig. 11.104). Pedunculated lesions have well-defined edges, being surrounded by air, and lung markings should be visible through the lesion. It is most helpful to examine the patient.

The Breast   Mastectomy is one of the commonest causes of a translucent hemithorax. With a simple mastectomy the axillary fold is normal, but following a radical mastectomy the normal downward curve of the axillary fold is replaced by a dense ascending line due to absence of pectoralis major (Fig. 11.105). In addition there may be a congenital absence of pectoralis major and minor, sometimes associated with syndactyly and rib abnormalities (*Poland syndrome*).

Surgical Emphysema   This often accompanies a pneumothorax (Fig. 11.106) and pneumomediastinum. After surgery an increase in the amount of emphysema on serial films suggests the development of a bronchopleural fistula.

Miscellaneous   Calcified nodes and parasites such as cysticercosis may overlie the lung fields. After lymphography contrast may be seen in the thoracic duct in the left upper zone where the duct drains into the innominate vein and there may be transient miliary shadowing in the lung fields due to oil emboli. Occasionally in patients who have undergone myelography with Myodil (Pantopaque) there is tracking of the residual Myodil along the intercostal nerves to give a bizarre appearance. This contrast medium is no longer in use.

The Diaphragm

The normal appearances of the diaphragm have already been described.

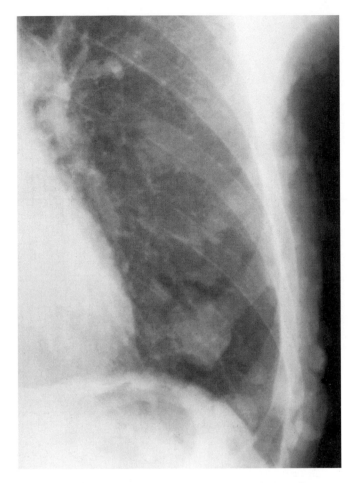

Fig. 11.104   Neurofibromatosis. Multiple soft-tissue lesions, those overlying the lung fields simulating intrapulmonary nodules.

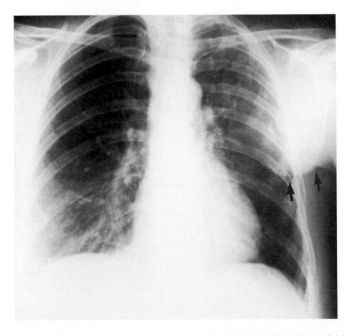

Fig. 11.105   Left mastectomy. Note the abnormal left axillary fold passing cranially (arrows). The left lung is hypertransradiant at its base. Note radiation necrosis of the upper ribs and soft-tissue calcification.

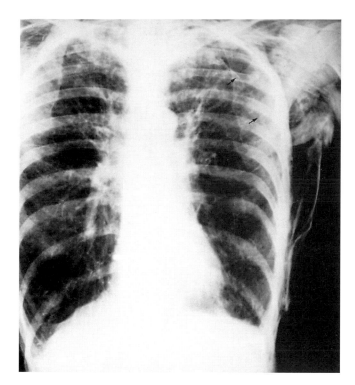

Fig. 11.106 Surgical emphysema following a small left pneumothorax (arrows) in a man with chronic obstructive airways disease.

Normal Variants

a. *Scalloping* (Fig. 11.107). Short curves of diaphragm, convex upward, are seen and this occurs predominantly on the right side.

b. *Muscle slips* (Fig. 11.107) are most commonly seen in tall, thin patients and in those with emphysema. They appear as small curved lines, concave upward, and are more common on the right side.

c. *Diaphragm humps* and *dromedary diaphragm* (Fig. 11.107). These variants are probably mild forms of eventration with incomplete muscularization of the hemidiaphragm but no muscle defect. They arise anteriorly and are usually right-sided, containing liver. There is no diaphragm defect. On the PA film the hump appears as a shadow in the right cardiophrenic angle and must be distinguished from a fat pad, lipoma, pericardial cyst and Morgagni hernia. On the lateral film the hump overlies the cardiac shadow and should not be confused with middle lobe consolidation. The dromedary diaphragm is a more severe form of diaphragm hump appearing as a double contour on the PA view.

d. *Eventration* (Fig. 11.108). This is nearly always left-sided, the hemidiaphragm being considerably elevated with characteristically marked mediastinal displacement to the right, a feature rarely seen with paralysis of the diaphragm. The muscle is thin and weak with movement reduced, paradoxical or absent on fluoroscopy. There may be an associated gastric volvulus with rotation along its long axis resulting in the greater curve being uppermost. Eventration must be distinguished from absence and rupture of the diaphragm as well as paralysis.

e. *Accessory diaphragm*. This rare condition is asymptomatic and usually right-sided. The hemithorax is partitioned by the accessory

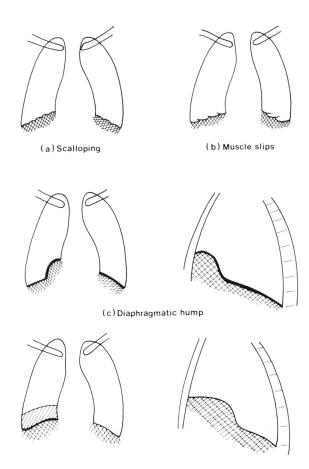

Fig. 11.107 Diagram to show the normal variants of the diaphragm.

diaphragm running parallel to the oblique fissure and resembling a thickened fissure. Its blood supply is often anomalous. Reported associations are other congenital lesions of the lungs such as anomalous venous drainage and lobar hypoplasia.

Diaphragm Movement

Respiratory excursion is easily assessed at fluoroscopy. Normally the left side moves slightly more than the right with an excursion of between 3 cm and 6 cm. Paradoxical movement occurs when the pressure exerted by the abdomen exceeds that of the weak diaphragm so that on inspiration or sniffing movement is upward. This occurs with diaphragm paralysis, eventration and sub-diaphragmatic infection. However paradoxical movement is also seen in a small number of normal subjects. Reduced excursion of the diaphragm frequently occurs with inflammatory processes either above or below the diaphragm; examples are subphrenic abscess and basal pneumonia.

The Elevated Diaphragm

The causes are listed in Table 11.21

Frequently no cause can be found to explain an elevated hemidiaphragm. The clinical history is important. It is essential to exclude an active lesion, particularly malignancy, by carefully assessing the lung fields, hila and mediastinum. Eventration is

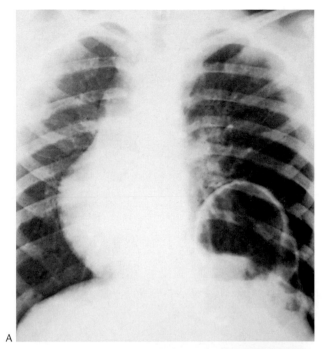

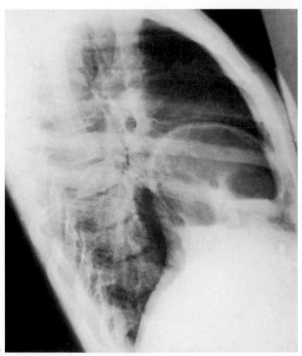

Fig. 11.108 Eventration. **A.** The left cupola is elevated and the heart displaced to the right. **B.** The lateral film shows the elevated left cupola with a distended stomach and a normal right cupola.

Table 11.21 Causes of Elevation of the Diaphragm

Bilateral	
1. Reduced pulmonary compliance	e.g. SLE, fibrosing alveolitis, lymphangitis carcinomatosa
2. Technical	Supine film, expiratory film
	Postoperative pain
3. Subdiaphragmatic	Ascites, obesity
	Bowel distension
	Abdominal mass, pregnancy
Unilateral	
1. Paralysis	Surgery and trauma
	Idiopathic
	Radiotherapy
	Neoplastic
	Diabetes mellitus
	Infections, TB glands, herpes zoster
2. Congenital	Eventration and humps
3. Pulmonary	Pulmonary and lobar collapse
	Pulmonary hypoplasia
	Pneumonectomy
	Pulmonary embolism
	Basal pneumonia
4. Pleural	Thickening
	Pleurisy
	Subpulmonary effusion
5. Bony	Scoliosis
	Rib fractures
6. Subdiaphragmatic	Gas-distended viscus
	Subphrenic abscess
	Pancreatitis
	Abdominal mass
	Hepatomegaly
	Splenomegaly

are very difficult to distinguish from a high diaphragm on plain films. Ultrasound is the definitive diagnostic investigation.

Splinting of the diaphragm occurs with upper abdominal inflammatory processes, basal pneumonia and embolism.

Determining whether diaphragm elevation is due to paralysis or an abdominal mass elevating the diaphragm may be difficult. The position of the liver edge should be noted. If the liver edge is low then there is probably a mass within or between the liver and diaphragm, whereas a normally positioned or high liver edge favors paralysis as a cause. On the left side the gastric bubble is assessed using the same principles.

A depressed diaphragm is seen with pulmonary hyperinflation and large pleural effusions.

Subphrenic Abscess

These are often associated with recent surgery or sepsis. A subphrenic abscess is more common on the right side, where it is more easily diagnosed than on the left side. Ultrasound and CT are the investigations of choice with percutaneous drainage if appropriate.

Plain film signs of a subphrenic abscess include:

1. Ipsilateral basal atelectasis and pleural effusion
2. Elevated hemidiaphragm with paradoxical or decreased movement

associated with marked cardiac displacement. Pleural thickening is often accompanied by tenting of the diaphragm, with loss of definition and obliteration or blunting of the costophrenic angles and thickened fissures. Subpulmonary fluid may be difficult to distinguish from an elevated diaphragm. Typically it has a straighter upper border and will change shape with patient position if it is not loculated. Loculated subpulmonary effusions

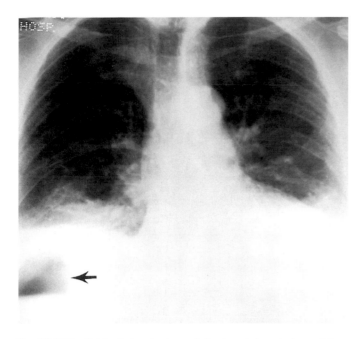

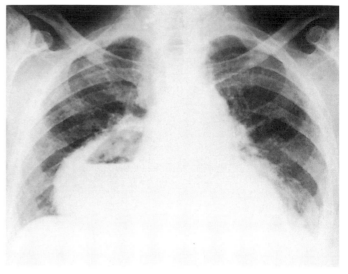

Fig. 11.110 Hiatus hernia. An elderly symptomatic patient. A large fluid level superimposed on the cardiac shadow: a typical appearance of a hiatus hernia.

Fig. 11.109 Right subphrenic abscess following cholecystectomy. A large gas shadow with an air–fluid level is seen below the right hemidiaphragm. There are bilateral effusions with patchy shadowing at the right base.

3. Abnormal gas shadow beneath the diaphragm due to infection with gas-forming organisms (Fig. 11.109); horizontal beam films improve visualization of the abscess cavity

4. Depression of the liver edge or gastric fundus.

The Thickness of the Diaphragm

The normal diaphragm is 2–3 mm thick. On the left side where the gastric bubble lies beneath the diaphragm, the stomach wall and diaphragm form a linear density 5–8 mm thick. However on the right side thickness cannot be assessed unless the inferior surface is outlined by free intraperitoneal gas. Thickening may be a normal variant but occurs with tumors of the diaphragm, stomach and pleura, subpulmonary fluid, diaphragm humps, and abdominal lesions including a subphrenic abscess, hepatomegaly and splenomegaly.

Tumors of the Diaphragm

Tumors of the diaphragm are rare. Benign lesions include lipomas, neurofibromas, fibromas and cysts. Pleural effusions are commonly present with sarcomas. Diaphragm tumors may appear as smooth or lobulated masses and need to be differentiated from lung and liver masses, hernias and diaphragm humps. CT is the most helpful investigation.

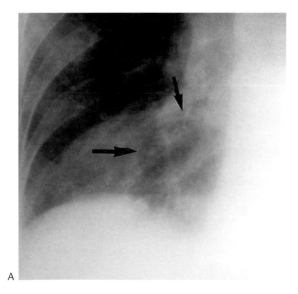

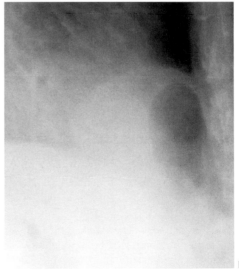

Fig. 11.111 Morgagni hernia. **A.** Soft-tissue mass in the right cardiophrenic angle with an associated gas shadow (arrowed). **B.** Hernia containing loop of bowel lying anteriorly in lateral view.

Hernias of the Diaphragm

The classic appearance of a *hiatus hernia*, with a fluid level superimposed on the cardiac shadow on the PA film, is well known (Fig. 11.110). A *Bochdalek hernia* arises posterolaterally through the pleuroperitoneal canal and is usually congenital, presenting at birth as respiratory distress. Ninety per cent are left-sided. The hernia may contain omentum, fat, spleen, kidney and bowel, in which case a gas shadow is seen within the mass. The ipsilateral lung is invariably hypoplastic with deviation of the mediastinum away from the side of the hernia. In the neonate this condition needs to be distinguished from cystic adenomatoid malformation of the lung.

The *Morgagni hernia* is usually asymptomatic, presenting in adults as an incidental finding on a chest film. They are right-sided and anterior, appearing as an homogenous shadow in the cardiophrenic angle. The hernia contains fat or occasionally bowel (Fig. 11.111).

Rupture of the Diaphragm

This is usually the result of trauma but may be idiopathic or related to previous surgery. Presentation is commonly acute but may be delayed in which case bowel strangulation may occur. Some 90% of cases are left-sided. Herniation of the stomach with gastric obstruction is common and must be distinguished from a pneumothorax and eventration. The gastric wall rarely abuts all the borders of the thoracic cage but if there is a diagnostic problem passage of a nasogastric tube or oral contrast should be helpful. Herniation of colon, spleen and kidney is less common. Appearances on the PA film may be normal if there is rupture without herniation, or the diaphragm may be elevated with an abnormal outline.

REFERENCES AND SUGGESTIONS FOR FURTHER READING

Alexander, G. (1966) Diaphragmatic movement and the diagnosis of diaphragmatic paralysis. *Clinical Radiology*, **17**, 79–83.

Armstrong, P., Wilson, A. G., Dee, P., Hansel, D. M. (1995) *Imaging of Diseases of the Chest*, 2nd edn. St. Louis: Mosby.

Bergin, C. J., Muller, N. L. (1985) CT in the diagnosis of interstitial lung disease. *American Journal of Roentgenology*, **145**, 505–510.

Boone, M. L., Swenson, B. E., Felson, B. (1964) Rib notching: its many causes. *American Journal of Roentgenology*, **91**, 1075–1088.

Campbell, J. A. (1963) The diaphragm in roentgenology of the chest. *Radiologic Clinics of North America*, **1**, 394–410.

Felson B, Felson H (1950) Localisation of intrathoracic lesions in the PA roentgenogram. Radiology 55: 363–374.

Felson, B. (1967) The roentgen diagnosis of disseminated pulmonary alveolar diseases. *Seminars in Radiology*, **2**, 3–21.

Felson, B. (1973) *Chest Roentgenology*. Philadelphia: W. B. Saunders.

Felson, B. (1979) A new look at pattern recognition of diffuse pulmonary disease. *American Journal of Roentgenology*, **133**, 183–189.

Fleischner, F. G. (1941) Linear shadows in the lung. *American Journal of Roentgenology*, **46**, 610–618.

Fraser, R. G., Pare, J. A. P., Fraser, R. S., Genereux, G. P. (1991) *Diagnosis of Diseases of the Chest*, 4th edn. Philadelphia: W.B. Saunders.

Freeman, L. M., Blaufox, M. D. (1980) Radionuclide studies of the lung. *Seminars in Nuclear Medicine*, **x**, 198–310.

Godwin, J. D., Tarver, R. D. (1985) Accessory fissures of the lung. *American Journal of Roentgenology*, **144**, 39–47.

Golden, R. (1925) The effect of bronchostenosis upon the roentgen-ray shadows in carcinoma of the bronchus. *American Journal of Roentgenology*, **13**, 21–30.

Goralnik, C. H., O'Connell, D. M., El Yousef, S. J., Haage, J. R. (1988) CT-guided cutting-needle biopsies of selected chest lesions. *American Journal of Roentgenology*, **151**, 903–907.

Greene, R., McCloud, T. C., Stark, P. (1977) Pneumothorax. *Seminars in Roentgenology*, **12**, 313–325.

Huston, J., Muhm, J. R. (1987). Solitary pulmonary opacities: plain tomography. *Radiology*, **163**, 481–485.

Jereb, M. (1980) The usefulness of needle biopsy in chest lesions of different sizes and locations. *Radiology*, **134**, 13–15.

Keats, T. E. (1979) *An Atlas of Normal Roentgen Variants that may Simulate Disease*, 2nd edn, pp. 427–500. Chicago: Year Book Medical Publishers.

Kerr, I. H. (1984) Interstitial lung disease: the role of the radiologist. *Clinical Radiology*, **35**, 1–7.

Khouri, N. F., Stitik, F. P., Erozan, Y. S. et al (1985) Transthoracic needle aspiration biopsy of benign and malignant lung lesions. *American Journal of Roentgenology*, **144**, 281–288.

Lavender, J. P. (1982) Radioisotope lung scanning and the chest radiograph in pulmonary disease. In: Steiner, R. E., Lodge, E. (eds). *Recent Advances in Radiology 6*. Edinburgh: Churchill Livingstone.

McCleod, R. A., Brown, L. R., Miller, W. E., DeRemee, R. A. (1976) Evaluation of the pulmonary hila by tomography. *Radiologic Clinics of North America*, **14**, 51–84.

Miller, W. E., Crowe, J. K., Muhm, J. R. (1976) The evaluation of pulmonary parenchymal abnormalities by tomography. *Radiologic Clinics of North America*, **14**, 85–104.

Milne, E. N. C. (1973) Correlation of physiologic findings with chest radiology. *Radiologic Clinics of North America*, **11**, 17–47.

Proto, A. V., Tocino, I. (1980) Radiographic manifestations of lobar collapse. *Seminars in Roentgenology*, **15**, 117–173.

Reed, J. C., Madewell, J. E. (1975) The air bronchogram in interstitial disease of the lungs. *Radiology*, **116**, 1–9.

Remy, J., Armand, A., Fardon, H. (1977) Treatment of haemoptysis by embolisation of bronchial arteries. *Radiology*, **122**, 33–37.

Ruskin, J. A., Gurney, J. W., Thorsen, M. K., Goodman, L. R. (1987) Detection of pleural effusions on supine chest radiographs. *American Journal of Roentgenology*, **148**, 681–683.

Sandler, M. S., Velchick, M. G., Alavi, A. (1988) Ventilation abnormalities associated with pulmonary embolism. *Clinics in Nuclear Medicine*, **13**, 450–458.

Savoca, C. J., Austin, J. H. M., Goldberg, H. I. (1977) The right paratracheal stripe. *Radiology*, **122**, 295–301.

Simon, G. (1975) The anterior view chest radiograph—criteria for normality derived from a basic analysis of the shadows. *Clinical Radiology*, **26**, 429–437.

Simon, G. (1978) *Principles of Chest X-ray Diagnosis*, 4th edn. London: Butterworths.

Simon, G., Bonnell, J., Kazantzis, G., Waller, R. E. (1969) Some radiological observations on the range of movement of the diaphragm. *Clinical Radiology*, **20**, 231–233.

Strickland, B. (1976) Sentinel lines—an unusual sign of lower lobe contraction. *Thorax*, **31**, 517–521.

Trapnell, D. (1973) The differential diagnosis of linear shadows in chest radiographs. *Radiologic Clinics of North America*, **11**, 77–92.

Vix, V. A., Klatte, E. C. (1970) The lateral chest radiograph in the diagnosis of hilar and mediastinal masses. *Radiology*, **96**, 307–316.

Radionuclide Scanning

Cooke, S. G., Davies, E. R., Goddard, P. R. (1989) Pulmonary uptake in gallium citrate scintigraphy – the 'negative heart' sign. *Postgraduate Medical Journal*, **65**, 885–891.

Goddard, P. R. (1988) Lung: pulmonary embolisms. In: Davies, E. R., Thomas, W. E. G. (Eds) *Nuclear Medicine: Applications to Surgery* Castle House Publications, Tunbridge Wells, pp. 199–202.

CT of the Lungs

Council, The Royal College of Radiologists (1994) *The Use of Computed Tomography in the Initial Investigation of Common Malignancies*, pp. 15–16. London: Royal College of Radiologists.

Muller, N. L. (ed.) (1991) Imaging of diffuse lung diseases. *Radiologic Clinics of North America*, **29**, 1043–1094.

Remy-Jardine, M., Remy, J., Farre, I., Marquette, C. H. (1992) Computed tomographic evaluation of silicosis and coal workers pneumoconiosis. *Radiological Clinics of North America*, **30**, 1155–1176.

Staples, C. A. (1992) Computed tomography in the evaluation of benign asbestos-related disorders. *Radiologic Clinics of North America*, **30**, 1191–1208.

Wegener, O. H. (1992) The lungs. In: *Whole Body Computed Tomography*, pp. 182–222. Massachusetts: Blackwell Scientific

Woodring, J. H. (ed.) (1990) Lung cancer. *Radiologic Clinics of North America*, **28**, 511–646.

MRI

Edelman, R. R., Hesselink, J. R., Zlatkin, M. B. (eds) (1996) *Clinical Magnetic Resonance Imaging*, 2nd edn. Philadelphia: WB Saunders.

Mayo, J. R. (1994) Magnetic resonance imaging of the chest: where we stand. *Radiologic Clinics of North America*, **32**, 795–809.

Naidich, D. P., Zerhouni, E. A., Siegelman, S. S. (eds) (1991) *Computed Tomography and Magnetic Resonance of the Thorax*, 2nd edn. New York: Raven Press.

12

THE MEDIASTINUM

Roger H. S. Gregson

With contributions from Richard W. Whitehouse and Jeremy P. R. Jenkins

Mediastinal disease is usually initially demonstrated on a chest radiograph and appears as a mediastinal soft-tissue mass, widening of the mediastinum or a pneumomediastinum. However the chest radiograph may appear normal in the presence of mediastinal disease, when computerized tomography (CT) subsequently reveals a small tumor or enlarged lymph nodes that have not deformed the outlines of the mediastinum on the plain film.

The commonest radiographic lesions in adults are undoubtedly lymph node masses, vascular abnormalities and a fixed hiatus hernia, and in infants and children it is the normal thymus gland. Mediastinal tumors and cysts and lymph node masses tend to predominate in surgically treated patients. The typical sites for the common and rare mediastinal masses are shown in Figure 12.1 and Table 12.1.

ANATOMY

The mediastinum is situated between the lungs in the centre of the thorax and extends from the thoracic inlet above to the central tendon of the diaphragm below, with the sternum anteriorly, the thoracic spine posteriorly and the parietal pleura laterally.

The differential diagnosis of a mediastinal mass is affected by its anatomic location and therefore from a radiological point of view it is useful to divide the mediastinum into three parts. The anterior division lies in front of the anterior pericardium and trachea, the middle division within the pericardial cavity but including the trachea, and the posterior division lies behind the posterior pericardium and trachea. Some normal structures such as the thoracic aorta and the mediastinal lymph nodes are present in all three divisions and some very large masses involve more than one division.

The anatomic structures that produce the outline of the mediastinum on a chest radiograph are discussed in Chapter 11, but the way that the various mediastinal lines as seen on a chest radiograph are formed becomes readily apparent on CT.

All the anatomic structures in the mediastinum are surrounded by fatty connective tissue and are well demonstrated by CT in the

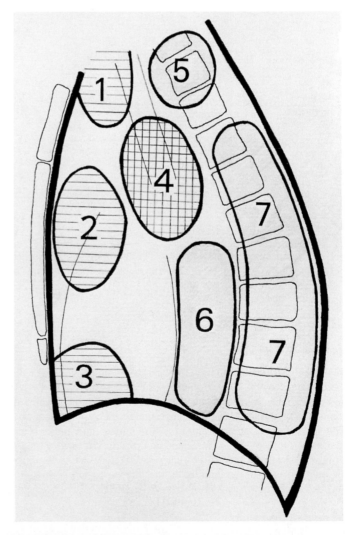

Fig. 12.1 Diagram illustrating the typical sites of the common and rare mediastinal masses listed in Table 12.1.

Table 12.1   The anatomic location of mediastinal masses

Position in mediastinum	Common lesions	Rare lesions
Anterior division	1. Tortuous innominate artery Lymph node enlargement Retrosternal goiter Fat deposition	Aneurysm of innominate artery Parathyroid adenoma Lymphangioma
	2. Lymph node enlargement Aneurysm of ascending aorta Thymoma Teratodermoid tumor	Sternal mass Lipoma Hemangioma
	3. Epicardial fat pad Diaphragmatic hump Pleuropericardial cyst	Morgagni hernia
Middle division	4. Lymph node enlargement Aneurysm of aortic arch Enlarged pulmonary artery Dilatation of superior vena cava Bronchogenic cyst	Tracheal lesion Cardiac tumor
Posterior division	5. Neurogenic tumor Pharyngo-esophageal pouch	
	6. Hiatus hernia Aneurysm of descending aorta Esophageal dilatation Dilatation of azygos vein	Neuroenteric cyst Pancreatic pseudocyst Sequestrated lung segment
	7. Neurogenic tumor Paravertebral mass	Bochdalek hernia Extramedullary hemopoiesis

normal adult, except the nerves. The anatomy is illustrated diagramatically at various levels through the mediastinum in Figure 12.2 and is discussed below.

CT OF THE MEDIASTINUM

Richard W. Whitehouse

Technical Considerations The greater proportion of the mediastinal volume is occupied by the heart and blood vessels and their contents. Adequate evaluation of the mediastinum therefore requires understanding and demonstration of the vascular anatomy. The use of intravenous contrast enhancement and rapid spiral scanning is ideal for CT demonstration of the mediastinum. Relatively low mA scans are usually satisfactory due to the large air and low soft-tissue content of the thorax; 5 mm collimation and extended spiral scans are therefore feasible.

Normal Appearances

If adequate mediastinal fat is present, the major vascular structures of the mediastinum, the trachea and the esophagus can be

accurately identified (Fig. 12.2) and abnormal masses distinguished. At the level of the sternoclavicular joints, an axial CT section will demonstrate the trachea as an air-filled round or horseshoe shaped structure lying centrally. Surrounding it in a clockwise direction from the right anterolateral position round to a posterior position lie the brachiocephalic trunk ('innominate artery'), the left common carotid artery, the left subclavian artery and the esophagus. Anterior to this ring of structures lie the right and left brachiocephalic veins. The right vein is rounded in cross-section, reflecting its vertical orientation, whilst the left vein is oval or tadpole shaped as it courses obliquely from left to right across the anterior mediastinum (Fig. 12.3A). On lower sections these veins join to form the superior vena cava, lying to the right of the ascending aorta (Fig. 12.3B, C). Dense intravenous contrast medium may cause significant artefacts from these veins; lower density contrast may be appropriate (200 mg I/ml) if dynamic contrast-enhanced scanning of the upper mediastinum or neck is performed.

A CT section at the level of the manubrio-sternal junction will demonstrate the arch of the aorta curving round to the left of the trachea with the superior vena cava and esophagus to the right of the anterior and posterior parts respectively (Fig. 12.3B). Sections below this will demonstrate the ascending and descending aortic limbs. The thymus lies anterior to the ascending aorta and may be seen as an arrowhead shaped structure in the anterior mediastinal fat. The azygos vein appears posterolaterally to the right of the esophagus and passes forward to join the superior vena cava over the top of the junction between the right main bronchus and right upper lobe bronchus (Fig. 12.3C), seen on the adjacent section (Fig. 12.3D). The division of the trachea into right and left main bronchi occurs at around the level of the fifth thoracic vertebra. The left pulmonary artery appears on this section as it passes over the top of the left main bronchus whilst the main pulmonary trunk and right pulmonary artery appear on lower sections (Fig. 12.3E), coursing from the left, adjacent to the ascending aorta, to the right, anterior to the bronchus intermedius, through the middle of the mediastinum. On sections below the carina, the left atrium appears anterior to the esophagus and descending aorta (Fig. 12.3F). The superior vena cava blends into the right atrium, becoming larger and less rounded in shape. The pulmonary trunk passes anterior to the aortic root to arise from the right ventricle (Fig. 12.3G). Posterior to the ascending aorta, the superior pericardial recess may cause a water density mass which should not be mistaken for a lymph node. At the level of the ventricles, the interventricular septum may be identified on contrast-enhanced scans as a soft-tissue density band between the denser contrast-laden blood in the ventricles (Fig. 12.3H). The diaphragmatic crura are clearly seen on lower sections, surrounding the aortic hiatus as curvilinear soft-tissue bands. The right crus is commonly longer and thicker than the left and can mimic a para-aortic mass on upper abdominal sections. The retrocrural space contains fat, the aorta, the azygos vein, thoracic duct and lymph nodes; the latter should not be greater than 6 mm in diameter.

The tissue planes contributing to the lines, edges and stripes identified on conventional chest radiographs can be directly identified and evaluated, thus the right paratracheal stripe is formed by the interface between the right upper lobe and the right lateral wall of the trachea. The *azygo-esophageal recess* is part of the right lower lobe, bounded by the posterior wall of the right main bronchus, the esophagus and the azygos vein. Carinal node enlargement expands into this space at an early stage. The *aorto-*

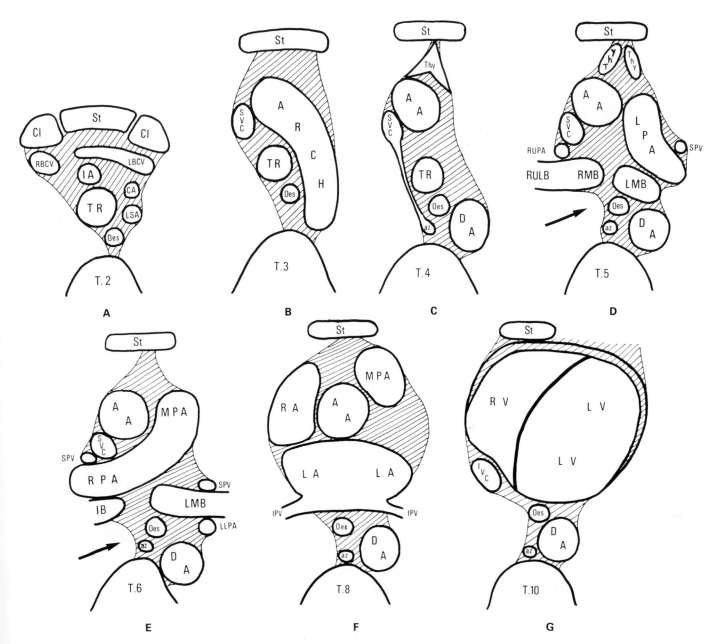

Fig. 12.2 Diagrams illustrating normal mediastinal anatomy at various levels through the thorax and features which can be identified by CT. **A.** Above the aortic arch through the sternoclavicular joints. **B.** Arch of aorta. **C.** Below the aortic arch through the aortopulmonary window. **D.** Left pulmonary artery. **E.** Main and right pulmonary arteries. **F.** Left and right atria. **G.** Left and right ventricles. Arch = arch of aorta; AA = ascending aorta; DA = descending aorta; IA = innominate artery; CA = left common carotid artery; LSA = left subclavian artery; MPA = main pulmonary artery; RPA = right pulmonary artery; LPA = left pulmonary artery; RUPA = right upper lobe pulmonary artery; LLPA = left lower lobe pulmonary artery; SPV = superior pulmonary vein; IPV = inferior pulmonary vein; SVC = superior vena cava; IVC = inferior vena cava; az. = azygos vein; RBCV and LBCV = right and left brachiocephalic or innominate veins; TR = trachea; RMB = right main bronchus; LMB = left main bronchus; IB = intermediate bronchus; RULB = right upper lobe bronchus; LV = left ventricle; RV = right ventricle; LA = left atrium; RA = right atrium; Es = esophagus; St = sternum; Cl = clavicle; Thy = thymus gland; → = azygo-esophageal recess.

pulmonary window is occupied by part of the left lower lobe, bounded by the descending aorta and the left pulmonary artery; nodal enlargement can again expand into this space, being detectable on both conventional chest radiography and on CT.

Clinical Applications

Mediastinal Masses   CT demonstrates the size, site, extent and contour of mediastinal masses. It will differentiate vascular from neoplastic masses and is particularly useful for evaluating regions poorly demonstrated on conventional radiographs, e.g. the retrocrural, retrosternal or subcarinal areas (Fig. 12.4). Characteristic fat or calcium densities may be demonstrated in dermoids or lipomas. Homogeneous water density and alteration in shape with posture may indicate a fluid-filled lesion and may also demonstrate a consistent relationship with a normal structure such

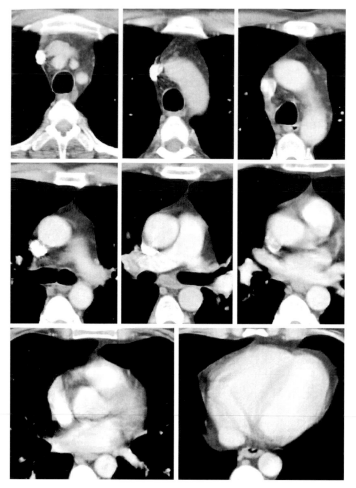

Fig. 12.3 Contrast-enhanced sections illustrating the vascular anatomy of the mediastinum.

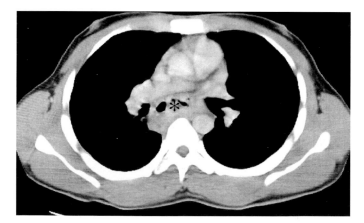

Fig. 12.4 Cavitating subcarinal mass (*), due to tuberculous adenopathy with esophageal erosion.

as the pericardium in the case of a pericardial cyst (Fig. 12.5). Thymic masses (Fig. 12.6) and diffuse thymic enlargement can be demonstrated. Diffuse mediastinal involvement by infiltrating malignant disease or fibrosis can also be demonstrated (Fig. 12.7).

Hilar Masses Hilar adenopathy can be distinguished from

prominent vessels, particularly if dynamic contrast enhancement is used. Subtle masses in the azygo-esophageal recess or aortopulmonary window can be demonstrated.

Paraspinal Masses Paraspinal masses are clearly demonstrated on CT. Appropriate section thickness and imaging on lung, bone and soft-tissue windows is imperative to assess the relationship of a lesion to the vertebrae, exit foramina, pleura, lung and associated tissues.

Vascular Abnormalities Dynamic contrast-enhanced spiral CT is an excellent method of demonstrating vascular pathology in the mediastinum. The entire length of the thoracic aorta can be imaged during peak contrast enhancement for the demonstration of aortic dissection or aneurysm (Figs 12.8–11). The central pulmonary artery and first to fourth order pulmonary artery branch thrombus can also be demonstrated by this technique in pulmonary thromboembolic disease but peripheral emboli may be missed. This technique may be of value where central emboli are

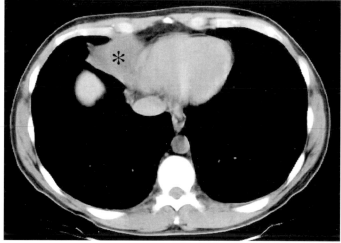

Fig. 12.5 Pericardial springwater cyst (*).

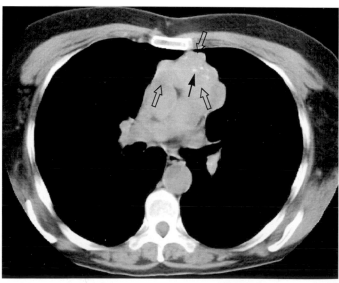

Fig. 12.6 Calcification (arrow) in a thymoma (open arrows).

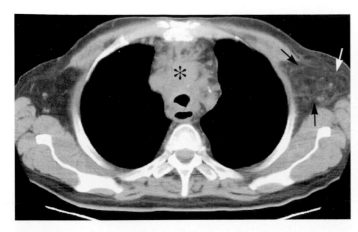

Fig. 12.7 Adenocarcinoma infiltrating the mediastinum (*) and obstructing the left brachiocephalic vein (note the edema in the left axilla (arrows).

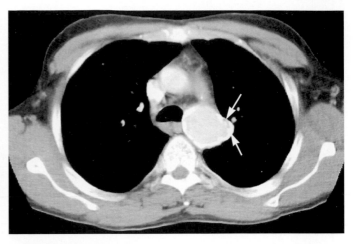

Fig. 12.9 Old, calcified post-traumatic aneurysm of the proximal descending aorta (arrows).

suspected or in patients unsuitable for conventional pulmonary angiography. Major vessel anomalies may be evident with or without intravenous contrast enhancement (Figs 12.12, 12.13).

Tracheo-bronchial Pathology CT allows the cross-sectional area and shape of the trachea and larger bronchi to be assessed. The use of spiral CT and subsequent image manipulation on a workstation can be used to produce 3D surface rendered, reformated or minimum-intensity projection images of the airways. This is valuable for the assessment of bronchial strictures or obstruction from tumors, after surgery, endotracheal tube removal or stenting procedures, and also in diseases such as relapsing polychondritis, tracheobronchomalacia (Fig 12.14) and the sleep apnea syndrome.

RADIOLOGICAL INVESTIGATION

Patients with mediastinal disease may be asymptomatic or present with symptoms and signs suggestive of intrathoracic pathology.

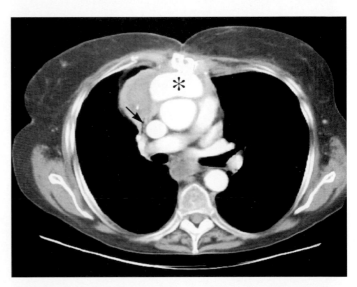

Fig. 12.10 False aneurysm of the ascending aorta (*), secondary to chronic osteomyelitis of the sternum from previous aortic valve replacement surgery. Note the bronchus entering the posterior aspect of the mass of thrombus (arrow) — the patient presented with hemoptysis.

The clinical presentation may be quite non-specific with symptoms such as chest pain, cough and weight loss, but more specific symptoms such as *dysphagia* or *stridor* are useful in localizing the mediastinal lesion to a particular anatomic site. A very specific clinical presentation such as myasthenia gravis raises the possibility of a thymoma, which occurs in about 10–15% of patients with this autoimmune neurological condition.

A variety of imaging modalities are available for investigating the mediastinum, but CT is undoubtedly the optimal radiological investigation for evaluating any mediastinal abnormality demonstrated on a high kV chest radiograph. The uses of CT include:

1. The investigation of an obvious mediastinal mass
2. The investigation of the wide mediastinum
3. The investigation of the abnormal hilum
4. The staging of malignant disease

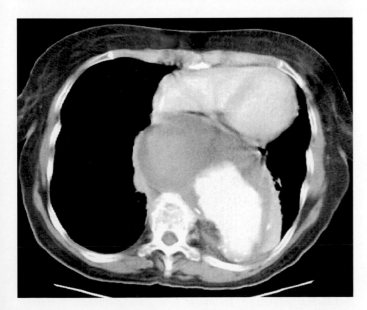

Fig. 12.8 Chronic, massive thoracic aortic aneurysm.

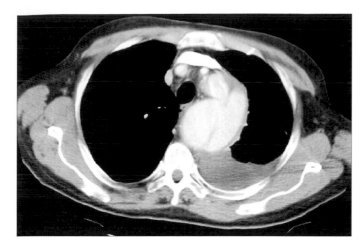

Fig. 12.11   Acute aortic dissection; note the hematoma over the left lung apex.

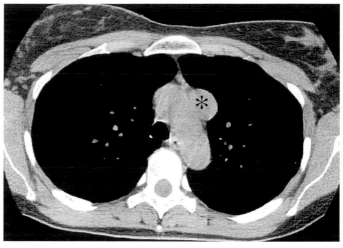

Fig. 12.13   Left-sided superior vena cava (*).

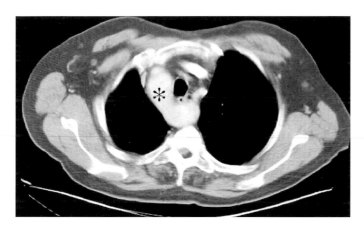

Fig. 12.12   Right-sided aortic arch (*).

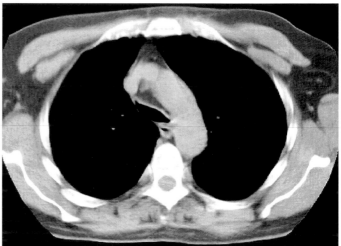

Fig. 12.14   Abnormal shape to the trachea due to distortion of the tracheal cartilage in tracheobronchomalacia.

5. The investigation of a suspected vascular abnormality
6. The detection of occult mediastinal disease.

The chest radiograph may be the only radiological investigation required to confirm the cause of a mediastinal abnormality such as a hiatus hernia, but CT is used to demonstrate the size and position of a mediastinal mass and to assess its attenuation value and relationship to the surrounding structures. Even with CT a histologic diagnosis cannot necessarily be made as many of the mediastinal lesions appear as masses with a similar soft-tissue attenuation value. Calcification is well demonstrated by CT, but it can occur in a number of mediastinal lesions as shown in Table 12.2 (p. 368). The presence of fat, however, is often diagnostic as it only occurs in a teratodermoid tumor, a mediastinal hernia and a lipoma or liposarcoma. The presence of fluid, which has an attenuation value of 0 to + 20 HU, indicates a mediastinal cyst, but if this contains either mucoid or hemorrhagic material the attenuation level is higher and the mass can be mistaken for a solid tumor. Necrosis and cystic degeneration within a solid tumor produce an attenuation level that is lower than that of soft tissue. CT can distinguish between lymphadenopathy, fat deposition and hemorrhage when there is mediastinal widening on a chest radiograph and can differentiate between a solid mass and a pulmonary vessel when there is an abnormal hilum. CT is used to demonstrate mediastinal lymphadenopathy as well as pulmonary and bone metastases in the staging of malignant disease and to detect occult mediastinal disease, such as a thymoma or enlarged lymph nodes in the mediastinum, when the chest radiograph appears normal. CT cannot distinguish between reactive hyperplasia and inflammatory or neoplastic causes of lymph node enlargement, because this is based on size criteria. A lymph node is regarded as normal if it has a short axis diameter of less than 10 mm; this results in a sensitivity and specificity for the diagnosis of mediastinal lymph node metastases of more than 80% in patients with bronchial carcinoma. A higher upper limit of normal increases the specificity at the expense of the sensitivity, which is decreased. CT can confirm the diagnosis of an aortic aneurysm or dissection, which can also be displayed as a 3D image by a surface shaded display technique or as an angiographic image by a maximum-intensity projection technique when a helical CT scanner is used.

Fine Needle Biopsy Fine needle biopsy of a mediastinal mass is useful and produces a pathological diagnosis in about 80% of patients. The procedure is done under local anesthetic using a 19–21 gauge needle with fluoroscopic or CT guidance to produce tissue samples for cytology and histology. This technique can be used instead of a diagnostic surgical procedure, but in about 20% of patients a specific diagnosis cannot be made because the small samples of tissue obtained limit the pathological interpretation, especially in the diagnosis of lymphoma. Aspiration of a mediastinal cyst can also be performed under ultrasound or CT guidance. The complications of these procedures include a minor pneumothorax in 15% of patients and a major pneumothorax in 3% of patients, as well as hemoptysis and a mediastinal hematoma.

Barium studies, angiography, radionuclide imaging and *ultrasound* are still used occasionally to confirm the diagnosis of a mediastinal lesion, and digital chest radiography certainly enhances the visualization of the mediastinum. *MRI* is being increasingly used to evaluate the mediastinum due to its ability to image in any plane and to demonstrate blood vessels without the need for contrast medium.

ANTERIOR MEDIASTINAL MASSES

Thyroid Tumor

Less than 5% of enlarged thyroid glands in the neck extend into the mediastinum to produce a retrosternal goiter. This can be due to non-toxic enlargement of the gland, thyrotoxicosis, carcinoma of the thyroid gland or Hashimoto's disease. An intrathoracic goiter also occasionally develops in a heterotopic thyroid gland in the anterior mediastinum.

A *retrosternal goiter* usually presents as a soft-tissue swelling that moves on swallowing in the root of the neck in a woman patient. The goiter is often asymptomatic, but can also produce dysphagia and stridor. Vocal cord paralysis or a superior vena caval compression syndrome indicate the development of malignancy.

A retrosternal goiter appears as an oval soft-tissue mass in the superior part of the anterior mediastinum, which extends down from the neck. The outline is well defined in the mediastinum but fades off into neck, due to its anterior location (a mass situated posteriorly in the thoracic inlet has a sharply defined upper and lower margin due to the posterior position of the lung apices). The soft-tissue mass more commonly projects to the right side of the mediastinum, with displacement and compression of the trachea to the left (Fig. 12.15). However, about 20% of thyroid goiters are retrotracheal, producing displacement of the esophagus posteriorly and the trachea anteriorly (Fig. 12.16). The soft-tissue mass may also contain central nodular, linear or crescent patterns of calcification. This is of course not a diagnostic radiological sign, because calcification also occurs in thymic tumors, teratodermoid tumors, aneurysms and enlarged lymph nodes, as shown in Table 12.2. Rapid increase in the size of the mass indicates internal hemorrhage into a cyst. The diagnosis is confirmed by either a *radionuclide scan*, using either ^{99m}Tc sodium pertechnetate or

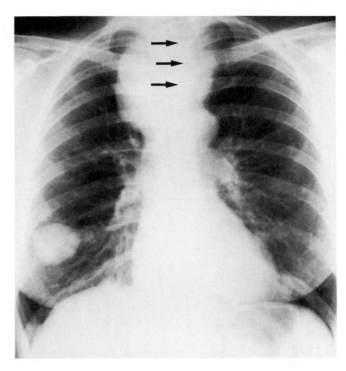

Fig. 12.15 Carcinoma of the thyroid. 53-year-old woman presenting with a painful goiter and dysphagia. PA film shows an oval mass in the superior part of the anterior mediastinum with displacement of the trachea (arrows) to the left and multiple pulmonary metastases.

^{123}I sodium iodide, which shows an area of increased activity extending below the sternal notch, or *CT*, which shows a mass of mixed attenuation containing soft tissue, cysts and calcification, extending from one of the lower poles of the thyroid gland (Fig. 12.16). This has a higher attenuation level than soft tissue on an unenhanced scan, due to its iodine content.

Thymic Tumor

The normal thymus gland is the commonest cause of mediastinal abnormality on a chest radiograph in infants. It produces a triangular soft-tissue mass which projects to one side of the mediastinum—often the right. The normal thymus gland becomes more prominent on an expiratory or slightly rotated film, but may disappeared radiologically in the presence of a severe neonatal infection, or after major surgery or the use of corticosteroids. The complete absence of the normal thymus gland occurs in immune deficiency disease involving the T lymphocytes, such as DiGeorge syndrome.

The commonest of the thymic tumors in the mediastinum are the benign and malignant *thymoma*. Enlargement of the thymus can also be due to *hyperplasia* of the gland, *thymic cysts, thymolipomas, lymphoma, germ cell tumors* and *carcinoid tumors*. About 30% of thymomas are malignant.

A thymoma usually presents as an anterior mediastinal mass on a chest radiograph in an adult patient. The thymoma is often asymptomatic, but can also present with myasthenia gravis. About 10–25% of patients with myasthenia have a thymoma and about 10–15% of patients with a thymoma have myasthenia gravis. It is

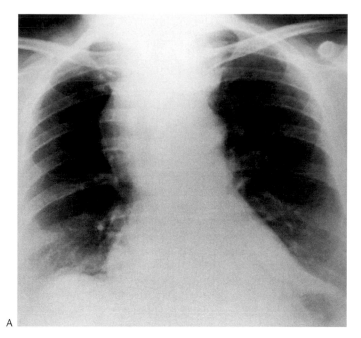

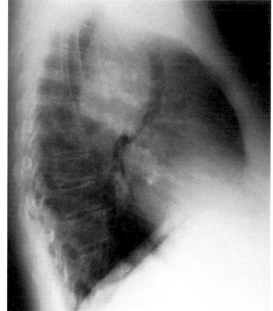

Fig. 12.16 Thyroid adenoma. 67-year-old woman presenting with a goiter. PA (**A**) and lateral (**B**) films show an oval mass in the superior part of the middle mediastinum with displacement of the trachea forward and to the right. CT scan with contrast enhancement (L + 50, W 500) (**C**) above the tracheal bifurcation shows a round mass of soft-tissue density (arrow), 8 cm in size, which contains calcification and cystic changes, in the middle mediastinum with compression of the trachea. Diagnosis confirmed by surgery.

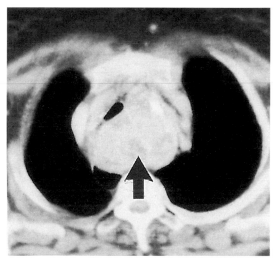

Table 12.2 The Causes of Calcification in a Mediastinal Mass

Anterior mediastinum
Aneurysm of ascending aorta
Retrosternal goiter
Thymoma
Tetratodermoid tumor
Lymphoma after radiotherapy
Hemangioma

Middle mediastinum

Lymph node enlargement	Tuberculosis
	Histoplasmosis
	Lymphoma after radiotherapy
	Sarcoidosis
	Silicosis
	Amyloidosis
	Mucin-secreting adenocarcinoma

Aneurysm of aortic arch
Bronchogenic cyst

Posterior mediastinum

Aneurysm of descending aorta	
Neurogenic tumor	Neuroblastoma
	Neurofibrosarcoma
	Ganglioneuroma

Neuroenteric cyst
Abscess
Hematoma
Leiomyoma of esophagus

most important to assess the mediastinum by CT in all patients with myasthenia, because surgical removal of a thymoma, or occasionally even the gland, may reduce or abolish the effects of this autoimmune neurological condition. A thymoma can also present with red-cell aplasia or hypogammaglobulinemia. *Thymic hyperplasia* occurs in association with thyrotoxicosis, Addison's disease, acromegaly, systemic lupus erythematosus, rheumatoid arthritis and after stress atrophy. It is important to realize that enlargement of the thymus gland following chemotherapy for Hodgkin's disease or testicular tumors can be due to rebound thymic hyperplasia and not recurrent disease in isolation. *Thymic carcinoids* can present with Cushing syndrome or hyperparathyroidism.

A thymoma appears as a round or oval soft-tissue mass which projects to one side of the anterior mediastinum when large, but may be undetectable on the chest radiograph if small, indicating the need for CT (Figs 12.6, 12.17). The soft-tissue mass may also contain a peripheral rim or central nodules of calcification. A very large soft-tissue mass with less radiographic density than ex-

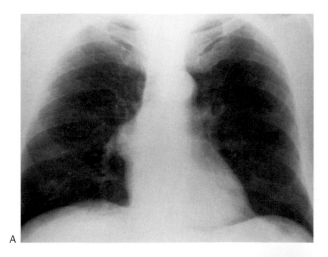

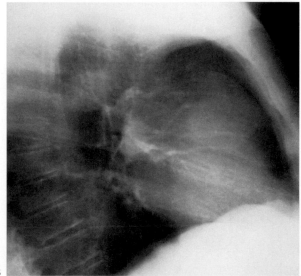

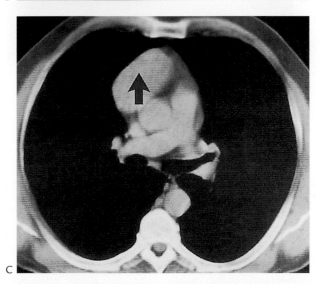

Fig. 12.17 Thymoma. 55-year-old man presenting with hypertension due to a pheochromocytoma. PA (**A**) and lateral (**B**) films show a round mass in the anterior mediastinum overlying the right hilum. CT scan with contrast enhancement (L + 50, W 500) (**C**) at the level of the tracheal bifurcation shows an oval mass of soft-tissue density (arrow), 7 cm in size, in the anterior mediastinum. Diagnosis confirmed by surgery.

pected for its size, and which alters in shape on respiration, is usually due to a *thymolipoma*. The presence of pleural metastases indicates a malignant thymoma, as these tumors tend to seed around the pleura (Fig. 12.18).

The diagnosis is confirmed by CT, which shows a mass of mixed attenuation containing soft tissue, calcification and cysts. Direct needle puncture of a thymoma with aspiration biopsy can be performed under CT or fluoroscopic guidance to confirm the diagnosis in patients with myasthenia gravis.

Teratodermoid Tumors

The commonest of the **germ-cell tumors** in the mediastinum are the *dermoid cyst* and the *benign* and *malignant teratoma*. This group of tumors also includes *choriocarcinomas, embryonal-cell carcinomas, endodermal sinus tumors* and *seminomas*. These tumors are all thought to arise from primitive germ-cell rests in the urogenital ridge. The dermoid cyst consists mainly of ectodermal tissues, whereas the solid teratoma usually contains tissues of ectodermal, mesodermal and endodermal origin. About 30% of teratodermoid tumors are malignant.

A teratodermoid tumor usually presents as an anterior mediastinal mass on a chest radiograph in a young adult patient. The tumor is often asymptomatic but can produce dyspnea, cough and chest pain, and may become infected to form an abscess, which can rupture into the mediastinum, the pleural cavity or the bronchial tree. The striking diagnostic symptom of trichoptysis is rare.

A benign dermoid cyst appears as a round or oval soft-tissue mass, which usually projects to only one side of the anterior mediastinum. The outline is well defined, but becomes irregular in very large tumors due to peripheral atelectasis in the surrounding compressed lung (Fig. 12.19). The soft-tissue mass may also contain a peripheral rim or central nodules of calcification, a fat–fluid level or a rudimentary tooth, which is of course a diagnostic radiological sign. Rapid increase in the size of the mass indicates either internal hemorrhage or the development of malignancy. An air–fluid level is present after rupture of an infected cyst into the bronchial tree. A malignant teratoma appears as a lobulated soft-tissue mass, which projects on both sides of the anterior mediastinum. The diagnosis is confirmed by CT, which shows a mass of mixed attenuation containing soft tissue, cyst fluid, fat, calcification or bone. Rarely, a teratodermoid tumor may occur in the posterior mediastinum.

Fat Deposition

The excessive deposition of fat in the mediastinum usually presents as an incidental finding, with widening of the superior part of the mediastinum and large epicardial fat pads on a chest radiograph in an obese adult patient. This can also occur in patients with Cushing syndrome, and in patients receiving long-term high-dose corticosteroid treatment. Steroids cause mobilization of body fat with its subsequent redistribution in the anterior mediastinum and cardiophrenic angles. This widening of the mediastinum can be difficult to differentiate from mediastinal hemorrhage, lymphadenopathy or a dissecting aortic aneurysm. The diagnosis is easily confirmed by CT, which shows an excessive amount of mediastinal fat (Fig. 12.20).

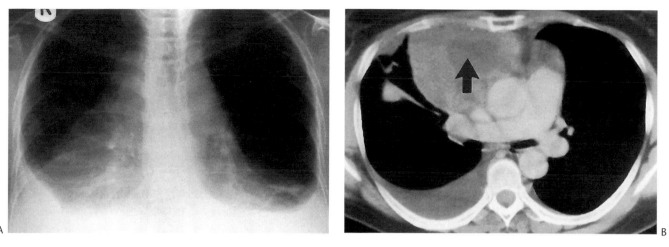

Fig. 12.18 Malignant thymoma. 43-year-old woman presenting with chest pain and dyspnea. PA film (**A**) shows widening of the mediastinum on the right with bilateral pleural effusions. CT scan with enhancement (L + 50, W 500) (**B**) at the level of the tracheal bifurcation shows an oval mass of mixed density (arrow), 9 cm in size, in the anterior mediastinum with a small pleural mass anteriorly on the right. Diagnosis confirmed by needle biopsy and surgery.

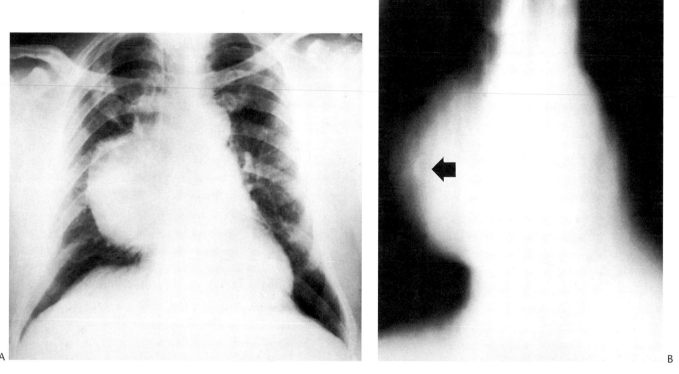

Fig. 12.19 Benign teratoma. 65-year-old man presenting with chest pain. PA film (**A**) and AP tomogram (**B**) show a large round mass which contains calcification (arrow) in the anterior mediastinum overlying the right hilum. Diagnosis confirmed by surgery.

Pleuropericardial Cyst

A pleuropericardial cyst usually presents as an anterior (or middle) mediastinal mass on a chest radiograph in an asymptomatic adult patient. About 75% of pleuropericardial cysts occur in the right anterior cardiophrenic angle (Fig. 12.21). The cysts have thin walls lined by mesothelial cells and contain clear fluid (hence their name of 'springwater' cysts). They appear as a round, oval or triangular soft-tissue mass in the anterior or middle mediastinum

and can alter in shape on respiration. The *differential diagnosis* of a soft-tissue lesion in the right anterior cardiophrenic angle includes an epicardial fat pad, a partial eventration of the right hemidiaphragm, right middle lobe or pleural pathology, a Morgagni hernia and a right atrial or pericardial tumor.

The diagnosis is confirmed by either ultrasound, which shows a transonic mass adjacent to the pericardium, or *CT*, which shows a thin-walled cyst containing fluid of low attenuation (0–20 HU) (Fig. 12.21). Direct needle puncture of a pleuropericardial cyst

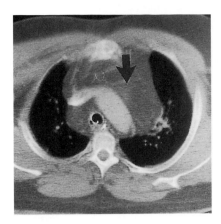

Fig. 12.20 Fat deposition. 40-year-old man presenting with chest pain after a road traffic accident and a widened mediastinum on a chest film. CT scan with contrast enhancement (L + 50, W 750) above the tracheal bifurcation shows excess deposition of fat throughout the mediastinum, particularly anteriorly (arrow).

with aspiration of its fluid contents can be performed under CT or ultrasonic guidance.

Morgagni Hernia

The foramen of Morgagni is a persistent developmental defect in the diaphragm anteriorly, between the septum transversum and the right and left costal origins of the diaphragm. A hernia through the foramen of Morgagni usually presents as an anterior mediastinal mass on a chest radiograph in an adult patient. The hernia is usually asymptomatic, but can produce retrosternal chest pain, epigastric discomfort and dyspnea. Strangulation of the contents of the hernial sac is rare.

More than 90% of Morgagni hernias are situated in the right anterior cardiophrenic angle (Fig. 12.22), due to the protective effect of the pericardium on the left. The smaller hernias contain omentum, which appears as a round or oval soft-tissue mass, but with a lower radiographic density than would be expected for its size. This can be difficult to differentiate from an epicardial fat pad, a pleuropericardial cyst or right middle lobe pathology, although occasionally the properitoneal fat line can be seen continuing upward from the anterior abdominal wall around the hernial sac on a lateral chest film. The larger hernias usually contain transverse colon, which appears as a soft-tissue mass containing either gas or an air–fluid level, but they can also contain liver, stomach or small intestine.

The diagnosis is confirmed by a barium meal and follow-through or a barium enema, which shows either upward tenting of the transverse colon toward the hernia or a loop of transverse colon above the diaphragm within the chest. The contents of the hernia are also easily confirmed by CT (Fig. 12.22).

Parathyroid Adenoma

An adenoma in an ectopic parathyroid gland in the chest usually presents with hypercalcemia in an adult patient with hyperparathyroidism. It is a rare tumor, occurring in the superior part of the anterior mediastinum, but due to its small size at presentation the mediastinum appears normal on a chest radiograph. It is also

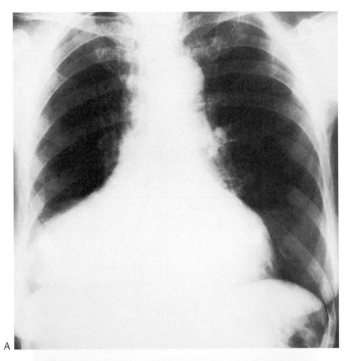

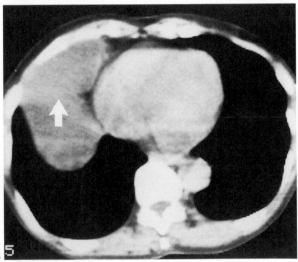

Fig. 12.21 Pleuropericardial cyst. 72-year-old woman presenting with dyspnea. PA film (**A**) shows a large oval mass in the right cardiophrenic angle and CT scan (L + 40, W 512) (**B**) below the tracheal bifurcation shows an oval mass (arrow), 10 cm in size, separate from the heart in the anterior and middle mediastinum. The density of the mass (average + 9 HU) is typical of cyst fluid.

difficult to identify at CT. The diagnosis is confirmed by a *radionuclide scan*, using ^{201}Tl chloride, with computerized subtraction of the thyroid image (using ^{99m}Tc sodium pertechnetate) to leave the parathyroid image, which shows an area of increased activity in the anterior mediastinum (Fig. 12.23).

Lymphangioma

A lymphangioma or cystic hygroma usually presents as a soft-tissue swelling that transilluminates in the root of the neck in

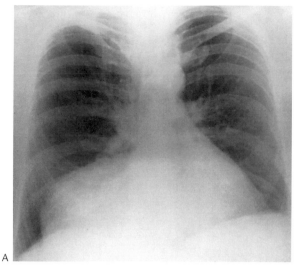

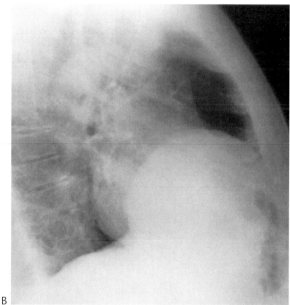

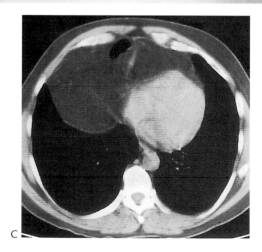

children. It is a rare mesenchymal tumor that occurs in the superior part of the anterior mediastinum and it appears as an oval soft-tissue mass which extends up into the neck and can alter in shape on respiration but does not displace the trachea. An associated chylothorax may also occur. The diagnosis is confirmed by ultrasound or CT.

Lipoma

A lipoma usually presents as an incidental mediastinal lesion on a chest radiograph in an asymptomatic adult patient. It is also a rare mesenchymal tumor, which occurs in the anterior (or posterior) mediastinum. It appears as a round or oval soft-tissue mass with a lower radiographic density than would be expected for its size, which can alter in shape on respiration (Fig. 12.24). Malignant degeneration into a liposarcoma may also occur. The diagnosis is confirmed by CT, which shows a solid mass of tissue of fatty attenuation (−50 to −100 HU) (Fig. 12.24).

Other Rare Anterior Mediastinal Masses

Apart from lymphangioma, lipoma and liposarcoma, other tumors of mesenchymal origin can also occur in the mediastinum; these include *fibroma, fibrosarcoma, hemangioma, hemangiopericytoma* and *hemangioendothelioma*. About 50% of mesenchymal tumors are malignant.

The small benign tumors are usually asymptomatic, whereas the large benign tumors and the malignant tumors tend to produce symptoms such as retrosternal chest pain, back pain or dysphagia, depending upon their anatomic location. They appear as a round

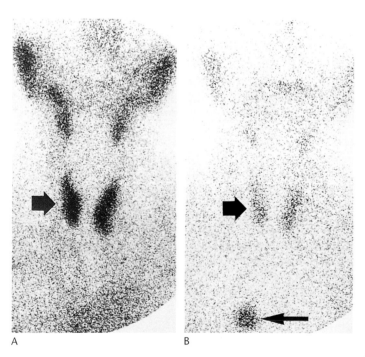

Fig. 12.22 Morgagni hernia. Asymptomatic 49-year-old man. PA (**A**) and lateral (**B**) films show a large round mass in the right cardiophrenic angle. CT scan (L + 50, W 500) (**C**) below the tracheal bifurcation shows an oval mass of fat density (arrow), 18 cm in size, which contains transverse colon in the anterior mediastinum.

Fig. 12.23 Parathyroid adenoma. 64-year-old woman presenting with hypercalcemia. Radionuclide scans with ^{99m}Tc (**A**) and ^{201}Tl (**B**) show activity in the salivary glands and thyroid gland (→) and in the parathyroid adenoma in the mediastinum (←). The latter is shown only on the thallium scan, even without computerized subtraction of scan A from scan B.

or oval soft-tissue mass in the anterior (or posterior) mediastinum or as widening of the mediastinum. The presence of phleboliths is of course diagnostic of a hemangioma.

A *plasmacytoma* of the sternum and an *osteochondroma* or a *chondrosarcoma* of a rib may also result in a tumor mass that involves the anterior mediastinum.

MIDDLE MEDIASTINAL MASSES

Lymph Node Enlargement

Lymph nodes occur in the anterior, middle and posterior mediastinum but are found predominantly in its middle division, where the paratracheal, tracheobronchial, bronchopulmonary (hilar) and subcarinal groups are situated (Fig. 11.18).

Enlargement of lymph node groups usually presents as a middle mediastinal mass on a chest radiograph in an adult patient. The enlarged lymph nodes are often asymptomatic, but can produce cough, dyspnea and weight loss or may be associated with generalized lymphadenopathy. There are many causes of enlargement of the mediastinal lymph node groups: these include metastatic disease, lymphoma, leukemia, sarcoidosis, tuberculosis, histoplasmosis, and other infections and granulomas.

Metastatic disease can produce enlargement of any of the lymph node groups within the mediastinum. The primary tumor is usually intrathoracic, such as a bronchial or esophageal carcinoma, but may occasionally be extrathoracic in origin—breast carcinoma, renal carcinoma, adrenal tumors, testicular tumors and tumors of the pharynx and larynx. Associated pulmonary metastases or lymphangitis carcinomatosa are also frequently present. A bronchial carcinoma situated either peripherally or centrally in the

lung metastasizes early to the mediastinal lymph nodes, producing either a unilateral hilar mass with an irregular outline (due to surrounding infiltration, atelectasis or consolidation), or widening of the superior part of the middle mediastinum due to superior vena caval compression syndrome. A bronchial carcinoma is the commonest primary tumor to metastasize to the mediastinal lymph nodes. A carcinoma of the breast may involve the lymph nodes of the internal mammary chain in the anterior mediastinum, and an esophageal carcinoma may involve the posterior mediastinal lymph nodes. A renal carcinoma or an adrenal neuroblastoma can metastasize to the hilar lymph nodes, usually on the right, whereas a testicular teratoma or seminoma usually metastasizes to the paratracheal lymph nodes.

Hodgkin's disease, the **non-Hodgkin's lymphomas** (including Castleman's disease) and the lymphatic leukemias usually involve the paratracheal and tracheobronchial lymph nodes, producing an asymmetric bilateral widening of the superior part of the middle mediastinum. Involvement of the subcarinal lymph nodes splays the carina, and unilateral or bilateral hilar masses can also occur. The lymphomas, particularly Hodgkin's disease, also frequently involve the anterior mediastinum, producing a lobulated soft-tissue mass due to indentation by the anterior ribs (Fig. 12.25).

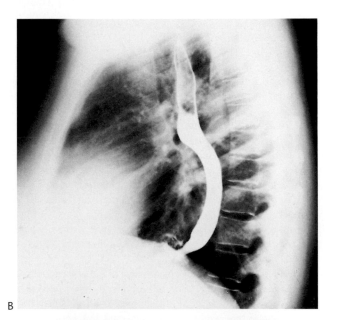

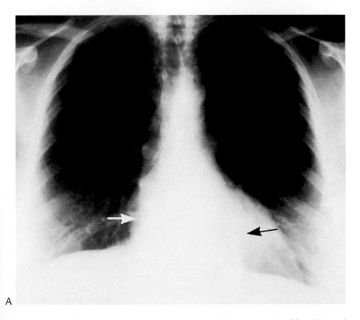

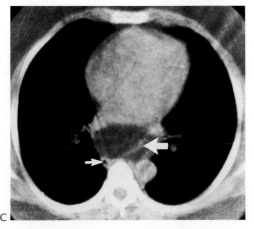

Fig. 12.24 Lipoma. Asymptomatic 42-year-old woman. PA film (**A**) and barium swallow (**B**) show an oval mass with less density than expected for its size, particularly in the lateral view, behind the heart. **C.** CT scan (L – 150, W 800) below the tracheal bifurcation shows an oval mass of fat density (←), 8 cm in size, in the posterior mediastinum, with displacement of the esophagus (→) to the right. (A and B courtesy of Dr P. Ho; C courtesy of Dr T.J. Bloomberg.)

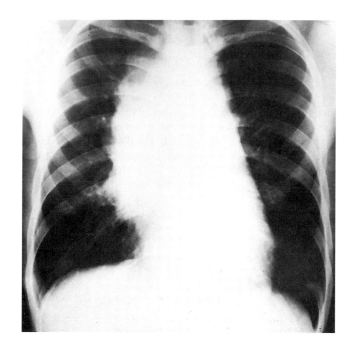

Fig. 12.25 Hodgkin's disease. 18-year-old man presenting with cervical lymphadenopathy. PA film shows asymmetric lobulated widening of the mediastinum, due to involvement of the middle and anterior mediastinal lymph nodes, particularly on the right.

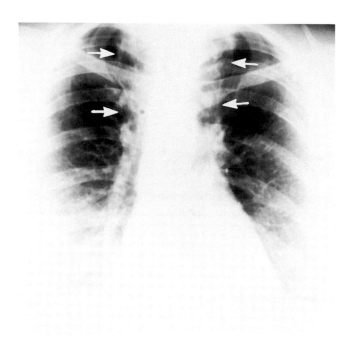

Fig. 12.26 Radiotherapy to the mediastinum. Asymptomatic 40-year-old woman with Hodgkin's disease in remission treated with mediastinal radiotherapy several years previously. PA film shows widening of the superior part of the mediastinum due to radiation fibrosis extending into the lungs (arrows).

Parenchymal lung disease may also occur, and lymph node calcification occasionally develops in Hodgkin's disease after irradiation.

Radiotherapy to the mediastinum produces a reduction in the size of lymph node masses in metastatic diseases which respond to radiation, such as lymphoma and seminoma during treatment, but may also produce a *chronic mediastinitis* with *fibrosis* extending into the lungs. This is quite characteristic and appears as a straight line, widening the mediastinum on both sides and corresponding to the treatment field (Fig. 12.26). This mediastinal fibrosis may also develop at lower therapeutic doses in patients who are also receiving cytotoxic chemotherapy, particularly cyclophosphamide.

Sarcoidosis typically causes enlargement of the bronchopulmonary lymph nodes, producing bilateral lobulated hilar masses with well-defined outlines. Sarcoid granulomas also frequently involve the tracheobronchial, right paratracheal and left aortopulmonary lymph nodes. Parenchymal lung disease commonly develops, and peripheral calcification occasionally occurs in the lymph nodes.

Primary tuberculous infection of the lung in children or young adult patients produces an area of consolidation in one of the lobes, with a unilateral hilar mass and an associated pleural effusion. Calcification may develop in both the primary Ghon focus and the mediastinal lymph nodes as healing occurs. Tuberculosis can also produce a unilateral paratracheal mass of lymph nodes without obvious pulmonary or pleural involvement (Fig. 12.27). This type of infection occurs in the adult immigrant population and in patients who are immunosuppressed.

In the USA, **fungal infection** such as *histoplasmosis, coccidioidomycosis* and *blastomycosis* may produce enlargement of the hilar or paratracheal lymph nodes. Calcification may also develop in the lymph nodes in healing histoplasmosis. The only fungus

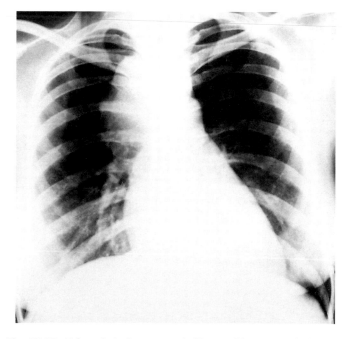

Fig. 12.27 Tuberculosis. Asymptomatic 29-year-old woman with chronic renal disease treated with immunosuppressive drugs. PA film shows a right paratracheal mass of enlarged lymph nodes in the middle mediastinum.

in the UK which causes unilateral hilar lymphadenopathy is *actinomycosis* and this can be difficult to differentiate from a bronchial carcinoma.

There are many other inflammatory causes of unilateral or bilateral lymphadenopathy: these include *infectious mononucleosis*

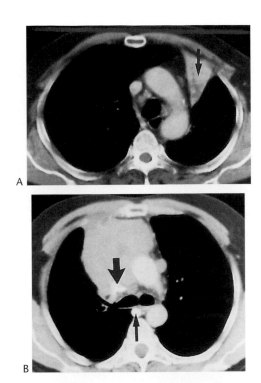

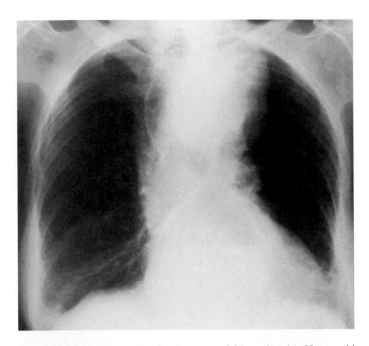

Fig. 12.28 A. Carcinoma of the bronchus. 67-year-old man presenting with hemoptysis and left upper lobe collapse seen on a chest film. CT scan with contrast enhancement (L + 50, W 500) above the tracheal bifurcation shows the left upper lobe collapse (↓) and two lymph nodes (both less than 10 mm in diameter) found to be involved with tumor at mediastinoscopy. **B.** Non-Hodgkin's lymphoma. 56-year-old man presenting with superior vena caval compression syndrome and a widened mediastinum on a chest film. CT scan with contrast enhancement (L + 50, W 500) at the level of the tracheal bifurcation shows a round mass of mixed soft-tissue density, 9 cm in size, in the anterior and middle mediastinum with compression of the superior vena cava (↓) and contrast medium filling the dilated azygos vein (↑). Diagnosis confirmed by surgical biopsy.

Fig. 12.29 Aneurysm of arch of aorta and hiatus hernia. 83-year-old woman presenting with dyspnea and hypertension. PA film shows a large round mass, which has some calcification in its wall, in the middle mediastinum, with displacement of the trachea to the right, and another large round mass containing an air–fluid level behind the heart in the posterior mediastinum.

or glandular fever, *measles, whooping cough*, mycoplasma infection, *adenoviruses* and a *pyogenic lung abscess*. Peripheral calcification may occur in the hilar nodes in patients with *silicosis*, and patients with *cystic fibrosis* may have enlarged hilar shadows due to enlarged lymph nodes or cor pulmonale.

The diagnosis of mediastinal lymph node enlargement is usually apparent on the chest radiographs, but can be confirmed by CT which shows the lymph node masses of soft-tissue attenuation distinct from the contrast-enhanced vascular structures (Fig. 12.28). Low-attenuation areas due to cyst formation or necrosis are occasionally seen in lymph nodes involved with Hodgkin's disease and metastatic testicular or squamous-cell tumors, particularly after treatment with radiotherapy or chemotherapy.

Aortic Aneurysm

The thoracic aorta passes through all the anatomic divisions of the mediastinum, and the great vessels arising from it lie in the superior part of the mediastinum. Abnormalities of the aorta and great vessels usually present as a mediastinal mass or widening of the mediastinum on a chest radiograph in an elderly patient. An unfolded aorta or a tortuous innominate artery is usually

asymptomatic but aortic aneurysms can produce chest pain, back pain, aortic incompetence, hoarseness and dysphagia. There are many causes of aneurysm of the thoracic aorta, including atherosclerosis, hypertension, blunt chest trauma, syphilitic aortitis, a mycotic origin and congenital anomalies such as coarctation of the aorta, Marfan syndrome and Ehlers–Danlos syndrome.

Aortic aneurysms produce either widening of the mediastinum or a round or oval soft-tissue mass in any part of the mediastinum with a well-defined outline and sometimes a peripheral rim of calcification (Figs 12.29, 12.30). Curvilinear calcification in an ascending aortic aneurysm can be due to either syphilitic aortitis or atherosclerosis. Displacement of the peripheral rim of calcification away from the wall of the aorta indicates a dissection. On fluoroscopy, aortic aneurysms appear as pulsatile masses, but this is not a diagnostic radiological sign because any mass lesion adjacent to the aorta transmits its pulsation. Aortic aneurysms may also involve adjacent bones, producing a pressure erosion defect of the sternum or anterior scalloping of one or two vertebral bodies.

The diagnosis can be confirmed by thoracic aortography or digital subtraction angiography but preferably by CT, which shows a dilated aorta containing a lumen of blood of high attenuation, due to contrast enhancement of the blood pool with water-soluble contrast medium (80–100 HU) and a layer of clot of lower attenuation on the wall of the aorta, which may contain calcification (Fig. 12.31), or by MRI (Fig. 12.40). The subintimal flap and false lumen of a *dissecting aortic aneurysm* can also be demonstrated by CT. Dissecting aortic aneurysms are now classified as Type A if they involve the ascending aorta (including the arch and descending aorta) and Type B if they involve only the descending aorta (see Ch. 25).

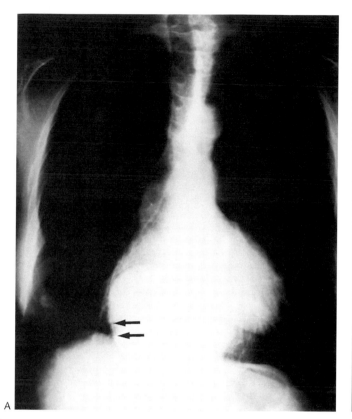

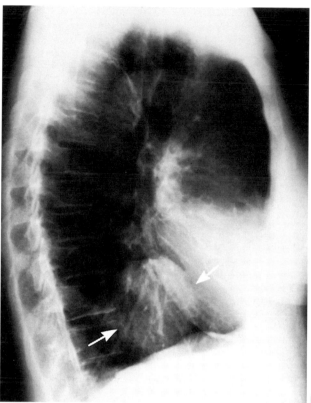

Fig. 12.30 Aneurysm of descending aorta. 59-year-old woman presenting with hematemesis from a benign gastric ulcer. PA (**A**) and lateral (**B**) films show a large round mass, which has some peripheral calcification in its wall (arrows) in the posterior mediastinum behind the heart. Diagnosis confirmed by ultrasound, using the liver as a window into the mediastinum.

A *tortuous innominate artery* occurs in about 20% of elderly patients with hypertension and produces widening of the superior part of the mediastinum on the right without displacement of the trachea to the left. However, a true aneurysm of the innominate or subclavian arteries is a rare cause of a mass in the superior part of the mediastinum.

The common *tortuous aneurysmal descending thoracic aorta* produces widening of the mediastinum on the left, often at the level of the left hilum. The hilar vessels can be seen through this apparent hilar mass, indicating that the descending thoracic aorta lies posterior to the hilum.

Dilatation of the main pulmonary artery can also produce an apparent left hilar mass, but in this case the main pulmonary artery lies anterior to the hilum. The causes of enlargement of the main pulmonary artery include primary or secondary pulmonary arterial hypertension, the poststenotic dilatation of pulmonary valve stenosis and a true pulmonary artery aneurysm.

Coarctation of the aorta, kinking of the aorta (pseudocoarctation) and *a right sided aortic arch* can also produce an abnormal mediastinal configuration. The diagnosis of these other vascular abnormalities is confirmed by CT in some cases or by MRI.

Dilatation of Mediastinal Veins

The superior vena cava lies in the middle mediastinum and the azygos vein lies in the posterior mediastinum. Dilatation of the veins in the mediastinum usually presents with cough, dyspnea and swelling of the ankles in an adult patient.

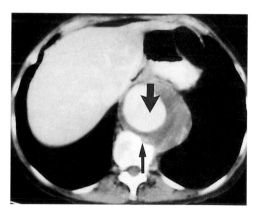

Fig. 12.31 Aneurysm of descending aorta. 45-year-old woman presenting with back pain. CT scan with contrast enhancement (L + 50, W 500) below the tracheal bifurcation shows an aneurysm of the descending aorta (↓), 8 cm in size, which contains thrombus, has calcification in its wall, and is eroding the adjacent lower thoracic vertebral body (↑).

Dilatation of the superior vena cava is produced by a raised central venous pressure, which occurs in congestive cardiac failure, tricuspid valve disease, constrictive pericarditis, a cardiomyopathy, a right atrial tumor, partial anomalous pulmonary venous drainage (to a right-sided superior vena cava) and a mediastinal tumor with a superior vena caval compression syndrome. A dilated superior vena cava produces widening of the superior part of the middle mediastinum on the right.

The causes of *dilatation of the azygos vein* include a raised central venous pressure, obstruction of the superior or inferior vena cava, portal hypertension, and congenital azygos continuation of the inferior vena cava. A dilated azygos vein produces an oval soft-tissue mass in the right tracheobronchial angle. This can be difficult to differentiate from an enlarged azygos lymph node, although the azygos vein alters in size with a change in posture or during the Valsalva maneuver.

Total anomalous pulmonary venous drainage (to a right- or left-sided superior vena cava) or an *isolated left-sided superior vena cava* produces an abnormally wide mediastinal configuration, whereas complete transposition of the great vessels produces an unusually narrow mediastinal configuration. A left superior inter-costal vein also produces an abnormal mediastinal configuration.

The diagnosis of these venous abnormalities is confirmed by phlebography but preferably by CT.

Bronchogenic Cyst

A bronchogenic cyst usually presents as a middle (or posterior) mediastinal mass on a chest radiograph in a child or young adult patient. The cyst is usually asymptomatic, but may produce stridor in children and cough, dyspnea and chest pain in adults. Infection with rupture into the bronchial tree is rare. The majority of bronchogenic cysts occur around the carina in the paratracheal, tracheobronchial or subcarinal regions. The cysts have thin walls lined by ciliated columnar epithelium of respiratory origin and contain mucoid material. They appear as a round or oval soft-tissue mass in the middle mediastinum, frequently on the right near the carina (Fig. 12.32), and can alter in shape on respiration. Rapid increase in the size of the mass indicates internal hemorrhage. An air–fluid level is present after rupture of an infected cyst into the bronchial tree.

The diagnosis is suggested by CT, which shows a mass containing fluid of either low attenuation (0–10 HU) or soft-tissue attenuation (10–50 HU) (Fig. 12.33), but is usually confirmed at surgery. A pericardial defect may occur in association with a bronchogenic cyst.

Rare Middle Mediastinal Lesions

Tracheal Tumors These include *carcinoma, cylindroma* and *plasmacytoma* and usually present with stridor in an adult patient. They are rare tumors, which occur in the middle mediastinum. They appear as narrowing of the tracheal lumen by a small soft-tissue mass. The diagnosis is confirmed by conventional tomography or CT.

Tracheobronchomegaly or the Mounier–Kuhn syndrome, and *tracheomalacia* may produce widening of the superior part of the mediastinum due to dilatation of the trachea.

POSTERIOR MEDIASTINAL MASSES

Neurogenic Tumors

The commonest of the neurogenic tumors in the mediastinum in adults are the *neurofibroma* and the *neurilemmoma* (or schwannoma), which develop from the peripheral intercostal nerves; the *ganglioneuroma* and the *neuroblastoma*, which arise

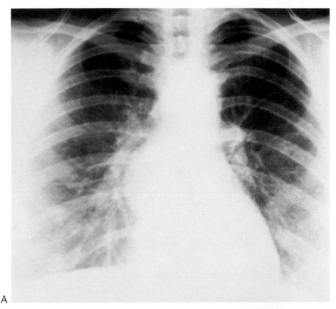

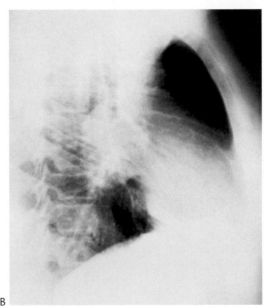

Fig. 12.32 Bronchogenic cyst. Asymptomatic 21-year-old woman. PA (**A**) and lateral (**B**) films show an oval mass in the middle mediastinum below the carina on the right. Diagnosis confirmed by surgery.

in the thoracic sympathetic ganglia, are the commonest of the neurogenic tumors in the mediastinum in children. This group of tumors also includes *neurofibrosarcomas, pheochromocytomas* and *chemodectomas*, which occur in paraganglionic nerve tissue. About 30% of neurogenic tumors are malignant.

A neurogenic tumor usually presents as a posterior mediastinal mass on a chest radiograph in a child or young adult patient. The tumor is often asymptomatic but can produce back pain and may extend through an intervertebral foramen into the spinal canal (hence their name of 'dumb-bell' tumors) to produce a spinal cord compression syndrome. A neurofibroma or neurofibrosarcoma in the mediastinum may be part of the generalized *neurofibromatosis* of von Recklinghausen's disease, but remember that a mediastinal

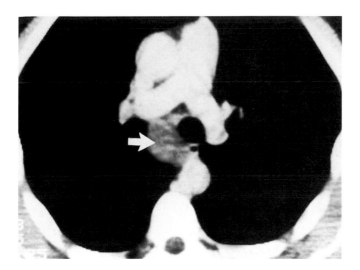

Fig. 12.33 Bronchogenic cyst. 25-year-old man presenting with cough. CT scan with contrast enhancement (L + 40, W 512) at the level of the tracheal bifurcation shows a round mass (→), 3 cm in size, in the middle mediastinum. The density of the mass (average + 45 HU) is typical of mucoid material.

the neurofibroma, due to its extensive mediastinal origin. A neuroblastoma may contain central spicules or a peripheral rim of calcification. This can also occur in neurofibrosarcomas and ganglioneuromas. However, calcification is generally not a feature of the benign neurogenic tumors and does not occur in the mediastinal lymph node metastases from an adrenal neuroblastoma.

Neurogenic tumors may also involve the posterior ribs or adjacent thoracic vertebrae. The benign tumors can produce splaying of several posterior ribs, a localized pressure erosion defect of one or two vertebral bodies, and of course rib notching. A bony destructive process indicates a malignant tumor. Enlargement of an intervertebral foramen is diagnostic of a dumb-bell neurogenic tumor, usually a neurofibroma. Rapid increase in the size of the mass or an associated pleural effusion indicates malignant degeneration.

The diagnosis is confirmed by CT, which shows a solid mass of soft-tissue attenuation which may contain calcification and involve the adjacent bones, or by MRI (Fig. 12.42, p. 385). Intraspinal extension is easily demonstrated by computer-assisted myelography or MRI. Rarely a neurogenic tumor may occur in the anterior or middle mediastinum.

Hiatus Hernia

A fixed or irreducible hiatus hernia is one of the commonest causes of a mediastinal mass and usually presents as a posterior mediastinal mass on a chest radiograph in an elderly patient. The hernia is often asymptomatic, but can produce dyspnea, retrosternal chest pain and epigastric discomfort. Incarceration of the stomach is rare.

mass in this neurocutaneous disease can also be caused by a *lateral thoracic meningocele.*

A neurogenic tumor appears as a round or oval soft-tissue mass with a well-defined outline in the paravertebral gutter, which usually projects to only one side of the posterior mediastinum (Fig. 12.34). A ganglioneuroma may appear as a rather elongated soft-tissue mass, in comparison to the more circular appearance of

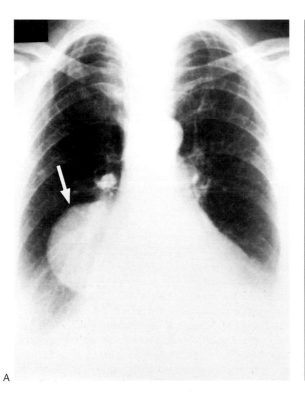

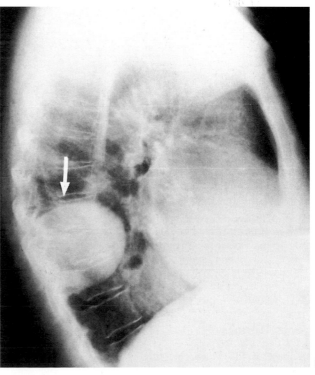

A

B

Fig. 12.34 Neurofibroma. Asymptomatic 57-year-old woman. PA (**A**) and lateral (**B**) films show a round mass in the posterior mediastinum behind the heart on the right. Lateral tomogram showed enlargement of the intervertebral foramen.

A hiatus hernia appears as a round soft-tissue mass containing an air–fluid level directly behind the heart, which lies to the left of the midline in the posterior mediastinum in about 70% of cases. The larger hernias can also contain liver, omentum and small intestine.

The diagnosis is easily confirmed by a penetrated PA film, a lateral film or a barium meal, which shows the stomach above the diaphragm within the chest (Fig. 11.110).

Esophageal Lesions

Lesions of the esophagus usually present with dysphagia in an adult patient, but can also produce an aspiration pneumonitis, due to spilling over of the esophageal contents into the trachea and main bronchi.

A *pharyngo-esophageal pouch* or Zenker's diverticulum is produced by herniation of the pharyngo-esophageal mucosa through Killihan's dehiscence, usually on the left, between the muscle fibres of the inferior constrictor muscle. The mediastinum appears normal on a chest radiograph when the pouch is small, but a large pouch appears as a round soft-tissue mass in the superior part of the posterior mediastinum, which contains an air–fluid level. The soft-tissue mass lies in the midline and displaces the trachea forward.

A *carcinoma* and even a *leiomyoma* of the esophagus may be large enough to produce a soft-tissue mass in the posterior mediastinum, and a large diverticulum of the lower esophagus occasionally produces a soft-tissue mass containing an air–fluid level behind the heart.

There are several causes of a dilated or *mega-esophagus*, and these include *achalasia* of the cardia, a *benign esophageal stricture*, a *carcinoma* of the esophagus, *presbyesophagus, systemic sclerosis* and South American *trypanosomiasis* or *Chagas disease*. The esophagus dilates proximal to the longstanding obstruction or due to the degeneration of Auerbach's plexus in its wall. A mega-esophagus produces widening of the posterior mediastinum behind the heart on the right, extending from the thoracic inlet to the diaphragm (Fig. 12.35). There is often an air–fluid level in the superior part of the posterior mediastinum, with the non-homogeneous mottled appearance of food particles mixed with air beneath it and no air in the fundus of the stomach. There may also be patchy pneumonic consolidation, bronchiectasis or even, occasionally, pulmonary fibrosis in both lower lobes, due to the recurrent aspiration pneumonitis.

The diagnosis of all esophageal lesions is confirmed by a barium swallow, which can also be useful in the investigation of other posterior mediastinal masses. The dilated esophagus is also easily confirmed by CT.

Esophageal lesions are discussed in more detail in Chapter 28.

Paravertebral Lesions

Paravertebral lesions of the dorsal spine usually present with back pain in an adult patient. Apart from *neurogenic tumors*, which have been discussed above, the differential diagnosis of a paravertebral mass includes a traumatic wedge *compression fracture* of a vertebral body with *hematoma* formation, a pyogenic or tuberculous *paraspinal abscess, multiple myeloma, disseminated lymphoma, metastatic carcinoma with paraspinal extension* and *extramedullary hemopoiesis*, which will be discussed below.

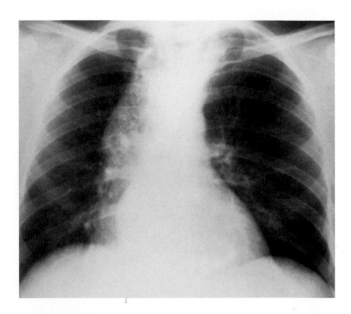

Fig. 12.35 Achalasia of the cardia. 31-year-old man presenting with dysphagia. PA film shows a dilated esophagus containing food behind the heart on the right, with absence of air in the gastric fundus. Diagnosis confirmed by barium swallow.

They appear as an elongated or lobulated soft-tissue mass with a well-defined outline, which usually projects on both sides of the posterior mediastinum (Fig. 12.36). Paravertebral masses also usually involve the adjacent thoracic vertebrae or intervertebral disk spaces. This allows the radiologist to differentiate between the inflammatory lesions, which usually produce narrowing of the intervertebral disk space as well as bone destruction, and the neoplastic lesions, which only produce bone destruction.

The diagnosis is confirmed by a penetrated PA film, or CT (Fig. 12.36). Direct needle puncture of a paravertebral mass with aspiration biopsy can be performed under CT or fluoroscopic guidance to establish the exact diagnosis.

Bochdalek Hernia

The foramen of Bochdalek is a persistent developmental defect in the diaphragm posteriorly, produced by a failure of the pleuroperitoneal canal membrane to fuse with the dorsal esophageal mesentery medially and the body wall laterally. A hernia through the foramen of Bochdalek usually presents either with acute respiratory distress in the neonatal period or as a posterior mediastinal mass in an adult patient. The hernia is usually asymptomatic in an adult patient, but can produce abdominal discomfort. Strangulation of the herniating bowel is rare.

About 90% of Bochdalek hernias occur in the left hemi-diaphragm, because of the protective effect of the liver on the right. The smaller hernias usually contain retroperitoneal fat, kidney or spleen, which appears as a soft-tissue mass in the posterior costophrenic angle. The smaller hernias can also contain the splenic flexure of the colon (Fig. 12.37).

The larger hernias contain jejunum, ileum and colon, which appears as multiple ring shadows in the hemithorax. The air-filled loops of bowel in the chest produce displacement of the heart and

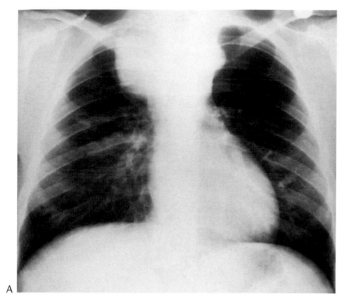

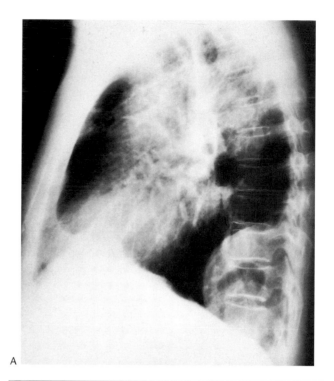

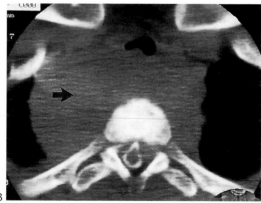

Fig. 12.36 Metastatic Ewing sarcoma paravertebral mass. 22-year-old man presenting with spastic paraparesis. **A.** PA film shows an asymmetric paravertebral mass in the posterior mediastinum. **B.** CT scan after myelography (L + 175, W 1400) shows an osteoblastic bone metastasis of the upper thoracic vertebral body of T2 with an associated paravertebral soft-tissue mass (arrow) which is compressing the trachea and the spinal canal.

mediastinum into the contralateral hemithorax and a compressed hypoplastic lung in the ipsilateral hemithorax. The larger hernias can also contain liver.

The diagnosis is confirmed by a barium meal and follow-through, which shows loops of small intestine and colon within the hemithorax (Fig. 12.37). A radionuclide scan, ultrasound or intravenous urography can confirm the diagnosis by showing liver, spleen or kidney above the diaphragm. The contents of the hernia are also easily confirmed by CT. Thirteen pairs of ribs may occur in association with a Bochdalek hernia.

Neuroenteric Cysts

The developmental anomalies produced by partial or complete persistence of the neuroenteric canal or its incomplete resorption include *gastrointestinal reduplications, enteric cysts, neuroenteric cysts, anterior meningoceles* and *cysts of the cord.*

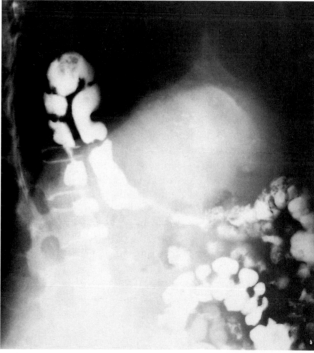

Fig. 12.37 Bochdalek hernia. Asymptomatic 65-year-old man. **A.** The lateral film shows an oval mass, which contains a loop of bowel, in the left posterior costophrenic angle. **B.** Barium meal and follow-through showed the splenic flexure of the colon within the hernia.

A neuroenteric cyst usually presents with respiratory distress or feeding difficulties in infants, whereas an anterior meningocele is usually asymptomatic. An enteric cyst may produce chest pain in children or young adult patients if peptic ulceration occurs within it. Infection with rupture into the esophagus is rare. These rare developmental cysts are closely related not only to the esophagus, to which there may be fibrous attachments, but also to the thoracic spine, in which there may be congenital bony abnormalities such as block vertebra, hemivertebra and butterfly vertebra (hence the split notochord syndrome). The cysts have thin walls lined by stratified squamous epithelium or ciliated columnar epithelium of both gastrointestinal and notochordal or neural origin and contain fluid material. They appear as a round or oval soft-tissue mass in the posterior mediastinum, frequently on the right. An air–fluid level is present after rupture of an infected cyst into the esophagus.

The diagnosis of a meningocele is confirmed by computer-assisted myelography, which shows the contrast medium entering the meningocele in the prone position. The diagnosis of an enteric cyst is occasionally confirmed by a barium swallow, if the barium sulfate actually enters the cyst. The diagnosis of neuroenteric cysts may be suggested by CT, which shows a mass of soft-tissue attenuation, but is usually confirmed by surgery.

Pancreatic Pseudocyst

A pseudocyst of the pancreas extending through the esophageal or aortic hiatus into the chest usually presents with dyspnea or dysphagia in an adult patient with acute pancreatitis. It is a rare abnormality which occurs in the posterior mediastinum and it appears as a round or oval soft-tissue mass behind the heart. A left basal pleural effusion or atelectasis in the lower lobes may also occur. The diagnosis is confirmed by CT, which shows a thin-walled cystic mass containing fluid of low attenuation (0–20 HU) extending from the abdomen into the chest through the aortic hiatus, behind the diaphragmatic crura.

Extramedullary Hemopoiesis

Extramedullary hemopoiesis in the chest usually presents as an incidental mediastinal lesion on a chest radiograph in children or young adult patients with a chronic hemolytic anemia, such as thalassemia major. It is a rare abnormality which occurs in the posterior mediastinum and it appears as a lobulated paravertebral soft-tissue mass behind the heart. The diagnosis is confirmed by a penetrated PA film or CT. Extramedullary hemopoiesis may also occur in myelofibrosis.

Other Rare Posterior Mediastinal Lesions

Apart from mesenchymal tumors, which have been discussed above, esophageal varices and a cyst of the thoracic duct may produce a soft-tissue mass in the posterior mediastinum. An osteochondroma or a chondrosarcoma of a vertebra or rib may also result in a tumor mass that involves the posterior mediastinum.

OTHER MEDIASTINAL LESIONS

Pneumomediastinum

Air in the mediastinum usually presents as an incidental finding on a radiograph in an asymptomatic child or adult patient, but it may produce chest pain, which is made worse by breathing or swallowing. The air usually tracks upward into the root of the neck to produce surgical emphysema. There are many causes of a *pneumomediastinum* and these include:

1. Perforation of the esophagus following endoscopy, dilatation of a stricture or insertion of an Atkinson or Celestin tube, or after prolonged vomiting as in the Mallory–Weiss syndrome
2. Rupture of the trachea or main bronchi following bronchoscopy or after blunt chest trauma
3. After sternotomy
4. Intermittent positive pressure ventilation, especially in neonates
5. Asthma
6. After prolonged coughing, as in whooping cough
7. During pregnancy, especially at the time of childbirth
8. Pneumoperitoneum due to any cause.

Air used to be deliberately introduced into the mediastinum during a diagnostic pneumomediastinum and it tracked into the mediastinum after diagnostic presacral pneumography, but today both these procedures are obsolete.

Air in the mediastinum appears as translucent streaks of gas outlining the blood vessels and other structures, with displacement of the parietal layer of the pleura laterally. A large volume of air tracks throughout the mediastinal tissue planes and up into the neck and so can easily be identified on a PA chest radiograph (Fig. 12.38), but a small volume of air behind the sternum or behind the heart can often only be seen on the lateral film.

The presence of chest pain and fever in a patient with a pneumomediastinum indicates *acute mediastinitis*; this is usually due to perforation of the pharynx, esophagus or trachea. In addition to the streaks of gas, the mediastinum may be widened by the edematous mediastinal tissues, which have a hazy outline, and there may be a small pleural effusion. An abscess occasionally develops from acute mediastinitis and appears as a round or oval soft-tissue mass (Fig. 12.39).

Chronic mediastinitis or *mediastinal fibrosis* usually presents with a superior vena caval compression syndrome. The commonest cause of chronic mediastinitis is radiotherapy (Fig. 12.26), but it may also be due to a chronic inflammatory condition such as tuberculosis or histoplasmosis. It can also occur in association with primary idiopathic retroperitoneal fibrosis, Riedel's thyroiditis, and drug treatment with methysergide or practolol. The mediastinum is usually widened and there may be narrowing of the trachea. The diagnosis is confirmed by superior vena cavography or digital subtraction angiography, which shows either complete occlusions or stenoses in the mediastinal veins with retrograde filling of dilated veins such as the jugular, azygos and internal mammary veins (Fig. 26.26).

Mediastinal Hemorrhage

Mediastinal hemorrhage usually presents with widening of the mediastinum on a chest radiograph in a patient who has sustained either blunt or penetrating chest trauma. Mediastinal hemorrhage can also be due to a leaking aortic aneurysm, and can occur in association with bleeding disorders and after anticoagulant or thrombolytic therapy. The diagnosis is confirmed by CT, which is particularly important following trauma as it may also show a

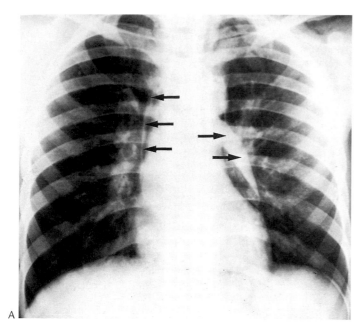

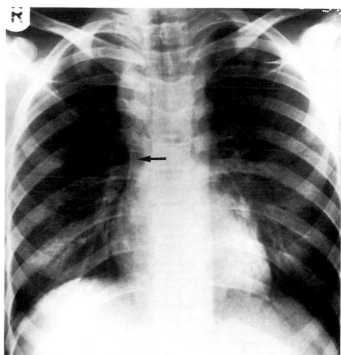

Fig. 12.39 Abscess. 15-year-old girl with a short history of pyrexia several days after a pharyngo-esophageal tear produced by an explosion of a well-known soda pop into her mouth as she opened the bottle with her teeth. PA film shows a right paratracheal mass in the middle mediastinum and traces of the resolving mediastinal gas (arrow).

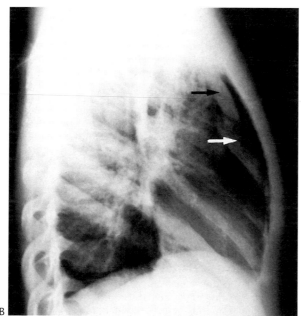

Fig. 12.38 Pneumomediastinum. 12-year-old boy with asthma. PA (**A**) and lateral (**B**) films show air in the mediastinum with displacement of the pleura (←) and demonstration of the thymus gland (→).

spinal fracture, pneumothorax, hemothorax or a false aneurysm. Arch aortography is, however, still essential in this situation.

MRI OF THE MEDIASTINUM

Jeremy P. R. Jenkins

MRI can stage certain mediastinal lesions more accurately than CT. The advantages of MRI include the differentiation of solid lesions from vessels, the direct visualization of the spinal canal and its neural contents, and the differentiation between chronic fibrosis (low signal) and recurrent lymphoma or tumor (inter-

mediate signal). In children MRI may be the preferred technique, obviating the need for intravenous contrast enhancement, but in adults CT is more often used in conjunction with MRI. MRI is particularly indicated when the administration of intravenous contrast medium is contraindicated or when vascular opacification is suboptimal. Surgical clips can produce significant streak artefacts on CT, whereas on MRI only a localized signal void is produced. In the postoperative patient, where residual or recurrent tumor is suspected, distortion of the hilar and mediastinal anatomy can be more easily assessed on MRI because of its multiplanar capability and greater intrinsic soft-tissue and vascular contrast discrimination.

Anterior Mediastinum

Mediastinal Thyroid   This is the commonest mass lesion in the thoracic inlet. Sagittal and transverse T_1-weighted scans demonstrate its extent and relationship to adjacent major vessels. The thyroid gland gives a signal intensity slightly greater than muscle on T_1-weighted images and a much more intense signal on T_2-weighted scans. Thyroid masses have longer relaxation times than normal thyroid and thus are of lower and higher signal on T_1- and T_2-weighted images respectively. Measurement of relaxation times is unhelpful in separating this lesion from other tumors. Hemorrhage within cysts can be shown but calcification is better demonstrated by CT. The internal architecture of this tumor, including cystic and necrotic changes, can be shown on T_2-weighted scans but better assessed using intravenous gadolinium-DTPA.

Thymus The *normal thymus* has a non-specific long T_1 and T_2 and appears of low signal, contrasting well with the high signal from surrounding fat on T_1-weighted scans but remaining isointense with fat on T_2-weighted images. The superior soft-tissue contrast resolution of MRI allowed the correct diagnosis to be made in a patient with an ectopic thymus in the posterior mediastinum because of its similarity in signal intensity characteristics to the normally positioned thymus. With increasing age, fat deposition within the normal thymus shortens its T_1 value, thereby reducing its contrast with adjacent fat.

The majority (90%) of *thymomas* are located in the anterior mediastinum and cannot be differentiated from other solid mediastinal tumors. Inhomogeneities in the tumor can occur due to cyst formation, necrosis or hemorrhage, and may be better delineated by the administration of gadolinium-chelate. A disadvantage of gadolinium-chelate enhancement in T_1-weighted images is the loss of contrast between fat and enhancing tumor, although this can be obviated by the use of frequency-offset fat suppression technique. *Malignant thymomas* cannot be differentiated from benign tumors on signal intensity appearances or on relaxation time measurements, but can be recognized by evidence of invasion of adjacent structures.

Cystic Mediastinal Masses MRI can demonstrate the cystic nature of lesions in the mediastinum when this is difficult to ascertain by other imaging techniques, including CT. *Simple cysts* typically have a very long T_1 and T_2, with a signal intensity similar to that of cerebrospinal fluid or urine. The actual signal intensity within the cyst does, however, depend upon its contents. It is important, therefore, to appreciate that the MRI appearance may be ambiguous and, in the presence of hemorrhage or an increase in the proteinaceous material within the cyst, may suggest a solid mass. The use of intravenous gadolinium chelate is helpful in confirming a solid mass lesion which demonstrates enhancement compared with a non-enhancing central cyst. A uniformly high signal intensity on T_1-weighted images, due to the presence of altered hemorrhage, is a typical feature of a benign cyst. In the assessment of *teratodermoids*, CT is superior to MRI because of its ability to detect calcification. Lipid is well shown by both techniques.

Middle Mediastinum

Nodal Disease There is debate as to the relative merits of ECG-gated or rapid-acquisition non-gated T_1-weighted images in the demonstration of mediastinal and hilar nodes. Both techniques provide equivalent morphological detail and reduce cardiac and respiratory motion artefacts, but the rapid-acquisition non-gated scans are more heavily T_1-weighted, providing greater soft-tissue contrast between lymph nodes and fat. It is generally agreed that MRI is slightly superior to CT in the detection of lymph node enlargement of the hilum but equivalent in the general assessment of enlarged nodes in the mediastinum. As hilar nodes are closely related to vessels, the superior contrast and multiplanar capability of MRI more than compensates for its slightly inferior spatial resolution. MRI can be of value in evaluating the *aortopulmonary window* and *subcarinal spaces*—areas that are difficult to delineate using the transverse plane of CT. MRI, however, has poorer spatial resolution and may not resolve small adjacent but separate nodes. *Calcification* within nodes, which may be useful as an estimate of benignity, is not easily detected. In patients with little mediastinal fat, small nodes can be difficult to define.

The diagnosis of nodal disease depends on the same *size* criteria as for CT. There is current debate as to the precise size criteria to be applied in different nodal areas, and also which dimension of the node (short or long axis) should be used for measurement. Generally, nodes greater than 10 mm are considered to be enlarged and involved by tumor. It should be recognized, however, that not all enlarged nodes are tumorous and that metastases can occur in normal-sized nodes. It is not possible from measured relaxation time values or other MRI criteria to distinguish between tumor-involved nodes and reactive hyperplastic nodes. An in vitro study of freshly removed lymph nodes from patients with lung cancer has shown significant ($p < 0.05$) differences in the mean T_1 values of tumorous (640 ms) and non-tumorous (566 ms) nodes. There was, however, too much overlap between the two groups for this to be of clinical relevance.

Although relaxation time values in themselves have limited value in the differentiation of pathology, the use of more sophisticated image analysis techniques, including texture analysis, may have great potential in detecting changes between tumor and non-tumor tissue which may not be demonstrable on visual inspection alone.

A new MRI lymphographic contrast agent, using an ultrasmall (<10 nm diameter) superparamagnetic iron oxide preparation, has been developed, with early experimental results indicating a clinical potential for imaging the lymphatic system. Following intravenous administration the ultrasmall iron oxide compound is able to bypass the mononuclear phagocytic system of the liver and spleen, cross capillary walls and achieve widespread tissue distribution, including lymph nodes and bone marrow. The particles accumulate in normal lymph nodes, reducing their signal intensity by a superparamagnetic effect. Malignant tissue is spared, and metastatic nodes, therefore, appear more intense than normal nodes. The use of such an agent could enable visualization of normal nodal anatomy and thus enhance the detection of nodal disease irrespective of size or anatomic distribution.

Lymphoma MRI is not able to characterize tissue reliably. Most malignancies have a non-specific long T_1 and T_2, and their enhancement characteristics using gadolinium-chelate are similar. Lymphoma usually has a homogeneous intermediate signal intensity on T_1-weighted images and appears isointense with fat on T_2-weighted scans. Nodular sclerosing Hodgkin's disease can appear heterogeneous, with low signal areas which are presumed to be due to a high fibrous content in this tumor type.

In the early post-treatment phase (8–12 weeks), responding lymphomas demonstrate heterogeneity in signal intensity, with a decrease in the T_2-weighted signal, associated with reduction in tumor size. Inactive residual masses assume a homogeneous low intensity signal pattern. Recurrent disease may be detected as an increase in signal intensity on the T_2-weighted images prior to evidence of a clinical relapse. Problems in interpretation, however, may result from intermixing of surrounding fat with an inactive mass. Postradiation or reactive inflammatory changes may also simulate active disease. A low signal from *fibrosis* is a more reliable indicator of tissue type than a high signal intensity which is not specific for tumor. MRI, nevertheless, has a role in the assessment of response to treatment and in the detection of recurrent mediastinal disease.

Great Vessels   Mediastinal disease can involve the mediastinal great vessels. Vascular abnormalities can be assessed with MRI without the need for the administration of intravenous contrast medium. The high intrinsic soft-tissue contrast, due to the low signal from flowing blood compared with the intermediate signal from the vessel wall and high signal from adjacent fat, gives MRI significant advantages over CT. Flow artefacts with signal within vessels during different phases of the cardiac cycle using conventional pulse sequences need to be recognized and correctly interpreted. MRI has been shown to be useful in the evaluation of central pulmonary embolism and pulmonary arterial hypertension. Peripheral emboli are poorly shown due to the intrinsic low signal from inflated lung.

Aorta   Both acquired and congenital lesions of the thoracic aorta can be shown to advantage with MRI, which has significant advantages over CT and angiography, particularly in the evaluation of *aortic aneurysms* and *coarctation* (see Ch. 25). The dimensions and extent of an aneurysm, the differentiation of a patent lumen from thrombus formation and the delineation of vessel wall from surrounding mediastinal fat can all be assessed. The use of multiplanar imaging allows the aortic valve and proximal origin of the great vessels to be demonstrated.

The origin and extent of *aortic dissection*, involvement of the arch and the dissecting flap can be well shown on MRI (Fig. 12.40). The distinction between slow-flowing blood and thrombus may be difficult on conventional pulse sequences and does require a more flow-sensitive sequence (phase-sensitive or gradient-echo even-echo rephasing). The ability to measure blood flow velocity in vivo using flow-sensitive sequences enables a clear separation between the true and false lumens to be made, together with an assessment of the re-entry site in aortic dissection (see Ch. 25). Three-dimensional gadolinium-enhanced MR angiography can provide a comprehensive mapping of the entire thoracic aorta and its major branches within a reasonably short time (approximately

4 min of data collection time). In this technique an intravenous infusion of gadolinium chelate is used to shorten the T_1 relaxation time of blood, making it possible to outline the aorta on a heavily T_1-weighted sequence without depending on the time-of-flight effect. This method uses a standard three-dimensional gradient-echo pulse sequence and the conventional body coil. A particular advantage of this technique is that the images are acquired without the need for ECG-gating or breath holding, useful in patients with arrhythmias or those who cannot breath hold. Also, the data set can be reformated in any imaging plane by post-processing. The main disadvantage is the requirement of a contrast injection, and most thoracic aorta pathologies can be diagnosed on conventional sequences without the use of gadolinium-chelate.

Mediastinal Veins   Superior vena caval infiltration or obstruction secondary to thoracic tumor can be well shown on transverse and coronal T_1-weighted images (Fig. 12.41). The same flow void phenomenon is observed in veins as in arteries, but signals within veins due to slow flow can be difficult to interpret. The distinction between slow flow and thrombus may require the use of phase-sensitive or gradient-rephasing sequences. Gadolinium-chelate can be useful in showing intraluminal tumor infiltration, which enhances compared with intraluminal thrombus (which shows no change in signal intensity). Gadolinium-chelate can also enhance slow-flowing venous blood, producing an increase in intraluminal signal, but this is usually more pronounced than that from tumor enhancement.

Tracheal Tumors   The reduced spatial resolution of MRI compared with CT accounts for the lower accuracy in the detection of 319 normal and 79 diseased bronchi confirmed bronchoscopically—40% normal and 70% diseased bronchi were visualized on MRI and 98% for both groups on CT. MRI and CT are considered equivalent in the visualization of larger airways,

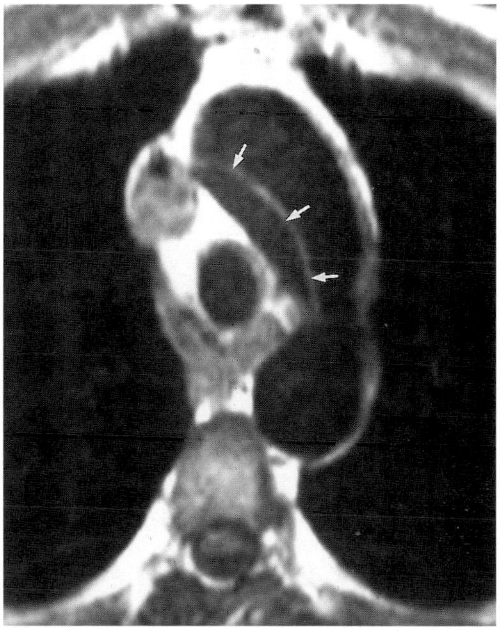

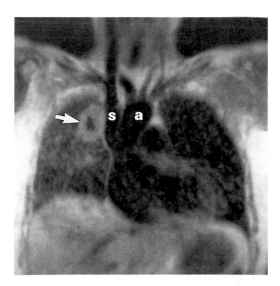

Fig. 12.40   Dissection flap (arrowed) in the aortic arch on an ECG-gated T_1-weighted spin-echo (700/20) image.

Fig. 12.41   Recurrent malignant fibrous histiocytoma of the right lung (arrowed) following previous lobectomy on coronal spin-echo (1100/26) image. The tumor is attached to and involves the lateral wall of the superior vena cava(s); a = aortic arch. (Reproduced with permission from Jenkins, J.P.R., Isherwood, I. 1987 Magnetic Resonance of the Heart: a Review. In: Rowlands, D. J. (ed) *Recent Advances in Cardiology 10*. Edinburgh: Churchill Livingstone.)

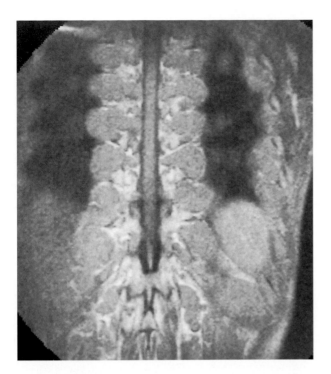

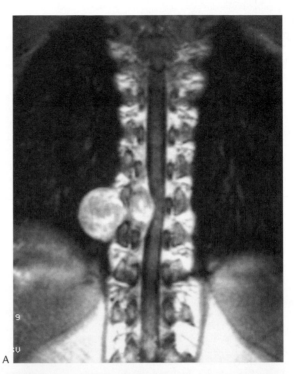

Fig. 12.42 Multiple paraspinal, intercostal and intra-abdominal neurofibromas in a patient with neurofibromatosis, on a coronal T$_1$-weighted (spin echo 700/40) image through the thorax.

but MRI has the possible advantage of imaging the whole trachea and major bronchi in a single oblique plane or by using a volume scanning technique. CT is superior, however, to MRI in the detection of endotracheal and endobronchial lesions.

Posterior Mediastinum

Neurogenic Tumors MRI is superior to CT in the detection and evaluation of neurogenic tumors within the posterior mediastinum (Figs 12.42, 12.43). This is due to the higher soft-tissue contrast discrimination, allowing direct visualization of the spine, spinal canal and cord (including nerve roots) without the need for intrathecal contrast medium, together with the multiplanar imaging facility. Calcification, which is common in neuroblastoma, is better shown by CT.

Esophageal Lesions Smooth muscle has similar values of relaxation time to skeletal muscle. There is therefore greater soft-tissue contrast between esophageal tumor (high signal) and muscle (low signal) on T$_2$-weighted images. Conventional T$_2$-weighted images of the mediastinum are, however, prone to significant motion artefacts and have a much lower SNR than T$_1$-weighted images. The advent of faster scanning techniques (by use of digital RF) has overcome some of these problems, improving image appearance. On T$_1$-weighted images there is reduced tumor-to-muscle contrast. The use of MRI affords no advantages over CT in the assessment of esophageal tumor, as MRI is unable to demonstrate small intraluminal and intramural tumors. Infiltration of the esophageal wall cannot be detected, and difficulty does occur in separating tumor from intraluminal contents in stenotic lesions. Tumor enhancement may be achieved by the use of gadolinium-chelate. Equivalent assessment of mediastinal infiltration can be demonstrated on both CT and MRI.

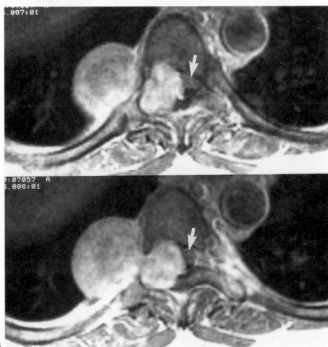

Fig. 12.43 Dumb-bell neurofibroma within a thoracic intervertebral foramen with intra and extraspinal extensions on coronal (**A**) and transverse (**B**) T$_1$-weighted gradient echo (300/14/90°) post gadolinium-chelate injection. Note the displacement of the adjacent thoracic cord (arrowed).

Extramedullary Hematopoiesis Extramedullary hematopoiesis has similar signal intensity characteristics to the spleen (long T$_1$/long T$_2$). The appearances are non-specific and indistinguishable from other mediastinal tumors. Similar morphological criteria to those applied to CT can be used with MRI.

Diaphragmatic Hernias Coronal and sagittal plane imaging are particularly useful in delineating the diaphragm, which has a low signal. The relationship of intrathoracic masses to the diaphragm can be well visualized, as can the contents of the hernial sac, which determine the signal intensity.

Fibrosing Mediastinitis CT is superior to MRI in the detection of calcification invisible on chest radiographs, a feature which is important in suggesting the diagnosis of fibrosing mediastinitis. A low signal on both T_1 and T_2-weighted images, due to the presence of fibrosis, is very often sufficiently different from that from tumor to suggest the correct diagnosis.

REFERENCES AND SUGGESTIONS FOR FURTHER READING

Adler, O. B., Rosenberger, A., Peleg, H. (1983) Fine needle aspiration biopsy of mediastinal masses. *American Journal of Roentgenology*, **140**, 893–896.

Baron, R. L., Lee, J. K. T., Sagel, S. S., Peterson, R. R. (1982) Computed tomography of the normal thymus. *American Journal of Roentgenology*, **142**, 121–125.

Baron, R. L., Levitt, R. G., Sagel, S. S., Stanley, R. J. (1981) Computed tomography in the evaluation of mediastinal widening. *Radiology*, **138**, 107–113.

Cohen, A. M., Creviston, S., Li Puma, J. P., Lieberman, J., Haaga, J. R., Alfidi, R. J. (1983) Nuclear magnetic resonance imaging of the mediastinum and hili. *American Journal of Roentgenology*, **141**, 1163–1169.

Crowe, J. K., Brown, L. R., Muhm, J. R. (1978) Computed tomography of the mediastinum. *Radiology*, **128**, 75–87.

Day, D. L., Gedgaudas, E. (1984) The thymus. *Radiologic Clinics of North America*, **22**, 519–538.

Egan, T. J., Neiman, H. L., Herman, R. J., Malave, S. R., Sanders, J. H. (1980) Computed tomography in the diagnosis of aortic aneurysm dissection or traumatic injury. *Radiology*, **136**, 141–146.

Fon, G. T., Bein, M. E., Mancuso, A. A., Keesey, J. C., Lupetin, A. R., Wong, W. S. (1982) Computed tomography of the anterior mediastinum in myasthenia gravis. *Radiology*, **142**, 135–141.

Gamsu, G., Webb, W. R., Sheldon, P. et al (1983) Nuclear magnetic resonance imaging of the thorax. *Radiology*, **147**, 473–480.

Glazer, H. S. (1989) Differential diagnosis of mediastinal pathology. *CT Review*, **1**, 41–51.

Heitzman, E. R., Goldwin, R. L., Proto, A. V. (1977) Radiological analysis of the mediastinum utilizing computed tomography. *Radiologic Clinics of North America*, **15**, 309–329.

Husband, J. E. S. (1989) Thymic masses and hyperplasia. *CT Review*, **1**, 53–63.

Kirks, D. R., Korobkin, M. (1981) Computed tomography of the chest in infants and children: techniques and mediastinal evaluation. *Radiologic Clinics of North America*, **19**, 409–419.

Lyons, H. A., Calvey, G. L., Sammons, B. P. (1959) The diagnosis and classification of mediastinal masses: a study of 782 cases. *Annals of Internal Medicine*, **51**, 897–932.

McLoud, T. C., Meyer, J. E. (1982) Mediastinal metastases. *Radiologic Clinics of North America*, **20**, 453–468.

Morrison, I. M. (1958) Tumours and cysts of the mediastinum. *Thorax*, **13**, 294–307.

Oudkerk, M., Overbosch, E., Dee, P. (1983) CT recognition of acute aortic dissection. *American Journal of Roentgenology*, **141**, 671–676.

Pugatch, R. D., Faling, L. J., Robbins, A. H., Spira, R. (1980) CT diagnosis of benign mediastinal abnormalities. *American Journal of Roentgenology*, **134**, 685–694.

Siegal, M. J., Sagel, S. S., Reed, K. (1982) The value of computed tomography in the diagnosis and management of pediatric mediastinal abnormalities. *Radiology*, **142**, 149–155.

Von Schulthess, G. K., McMurdo, K., Tscholakoff, D., De Geer, G., Gamsu, G., Higgins, C. B. (1986) Mediastinal masses: MR imaging. *Radiology*, **158**, 289–296.

Westcott, J. L. (1981) Percutaneous needle aspiration of hilar and mediastinal masses. *Radiology*, **141**, 323–329.

Wychulis, A. R., Payne, W. S., Clagett, O. T., Woolner, L. B. (1971) Surgical treatment of mediastinal tumours: a 40-year experience. *Journal of Thoracic and Cardiovascular Surgery*, **62**, 379–392.

CT of the Mediastinum

Costello, P. (1995) Thoracic imaging with spiral CT. In: Fishman, E. K., Jeffrey, R. B.: (eds) *Spiral CT: Principles, Techniques and Clinical Applications*, pp. 109–130. New York: Raven Press.

Wegener, O. H. (1992) The Mediastinum. In: *Whole Body Computed Tomography*, pp. 137–170. Massachusetts: Blackwell Scientific.

MRI of the Mediastinum

Herold, C. J., Zerhouni, E. A. (1992) The Mediastinum and Lungs. In: Higgins, C. B., Hricak, H., Helms, C. A. (eds) *Magnetic Resonance Imaging of the Body*, 2nd edn, ch. 22, pp. 461–523. New York: Raven Press.

Link, K. M. (1992) Great Vessels. In: Stark, D. D., Bradley, W. G. (eds) *Magnetic Resonance Imaging*, 2nd edn, ch. 46, pp. 1490–1530. St Louis: CV Mosby.

Matsumoto, A. H., Tegtmeyer, C. J. (1995) Contemporary diagnostic approaches to acute pulmonary emboli. *Radiologic Clinics of North America*, **33**, 167–183.

Prince, M. R., Narasimham, D. L. et al (1996) Three-dimensional gadolinium-enhanced MR angiography of the thoracic aorta. *American Journal of Roentgenology*, **166**, 1387–1397.

Scott, S (1995) Basic concepts of magnetic resonance angiography. *Radiologic Clinics of North America*, **33**, 91–113.

Weissleder, R., Elizondo, G., Wittenberg, L., Lee, A. S., Josephson, L., Brady, T. (1990) Ultrasmall superparamagnetic iron oxide; an intravenous contrast agent for assessing lymph nodes with MR imaging. *Radiology*, **175**, 494–498.

Zerhouni, E. A., Herold, C. J., Hahn, D. (1992) Mediastinum and Lung. In: Stark, D. D. Bradley, W. G. (eds) *Magnetic Resonance Imaging*, 2nd edn, ch. 45, pp. 1429–1489. St Louis: CV Mosby.

13

THE PLEURA

Michael B. Rubens and Simon P. G. Padley

Basic Anatomy The pleura is a serous membrane which covers the surface of the lung and lines the inner surface of the chest wall. The visceral pleura, over the lung, and the parietal pleura, over the chest wall, are continuous at the hilum, where a fold of pleura extends inferiorly to form the inferior pulmonary ligament. The two layers of pleura are closely applied to each other, being separated by a thin layer of lubricating pleural fluid. The parietal pleura, and the visceral pleura over the periphery of the lung are not normally visible radiographically. However, where the visceral pleura lines the interlobar fissures of the lung it is often visible, there being two layers of pleura outlined by aerated lung. The horizontal fissure of the right lung is often seen on a frontal chest film, and the oblique fissures will usually be seen on the lateral views. Some patients have one or more accessory fissures, the most common being the azygos fissure and the inferior accessory fissure of the right lower lobe. Occasionally anterior or posterior junction lines are seen in the frontal chest film, where the left and right lungs come into contact in the mediastinum.

Some Physiologic Considerations The normal anatomy of the lungs is maintained by a balance between different elastic forces of the chest wall and lungs. The lung has a natural tendency to collapse toward its hilum, and this is opposed by forces of similar magnitude in the chest wall tending to expand outward. The visceral and parietal layers of pleura are thus kept in close apposition. If increased fluid or air collects in the pleural space, the effect of the outward forces on the underlying lung is diminished, and the lung tends to retract toward its hilum. Therefore, in an erect patient a small pleural effusion which has gravitated to the base of the lung causes retraction of the lower part of the lung, but has comparatively little effect at the apex. Conversely, a small pneumothorax will collect at the apex and have little effect at the lung base. Obviously, large intrapleural collections will affect the entire lung. These basic patterns may be altered by the state of the underlying lung and the presence of pleural adhesions. Fibrotic, emphysematous or consolidated lung may not be able to retract and adhesions may prevent the usual distribution of air or fluid.

DISEASES OF THE PLEURA

Pleural Fluid

Fluid which accumulates in the pleural space may be transudate, exudate, pus, blood or chyle. Radiographically these produce similar shadows and are therefore indistinguishable. However, there may be clinical data to point to the etiology, or the chest film may show other abnormalities, such as evidence of heart failure or trauma, which indicate the cause. Sometimes the definitive diagnosis is only made after thoracentesis or pleural biopsy; not infrequently it remains obscure.

Transudates Transudates contain less than 3 g/dl of protein, and are usually clear or faintly yellow, watery fluids. A pleural transudate may be called a hydrothorax. They are often bilateral. The commonest cause is *cardiac failure*, when the effusion usually accumulates first on the right, before becoming bilateral. Other causes are *hypoproteinemia* (especially the nephrotic syndrome, hepatic cirrhosis and anemia), *constrictive pericarditis, Meigs' syndrome* and *myxedema*.

Exudates Exudates contain in excess of 3 g/dl of protein, and vary from amber, slightly cloudy fluid, which often clots on standing, to frank pus. A purulent pleural effusion is termed an empyema. The commonest causes of pleural exudate are *bacterial pneumonia, pulmonary tuberculosis, carcinoma of the lung, metastatic malignancy* and *pulmonary infarction*. Less common causes are *subphrenic infection, connective tissue disorders* (especially systemic lupus erythematosus and rheumatoid disease) and *non-bacterial* pneumonias. Unusual causes include *post-myocardial infarction syndrome, acute pancreatitis* and *primary neoplasia* of the pleura.

Hemothorax Bleeding into the pleural space is almost always secondary to open or closed trauma to the chest. Rarely, it is due to *hemophilia* or excessive *anticoagulation*. The effusions associated with pulmonary infarction and carcinoma of the lung are frequently blood-stained but rarely pure blood.

Chylothorax Chyle is a milky fluid high in neutral fat and fatty acids. Chylothorax may develop secondary to damage or obstruction of the thoracic lymphatic vessels. The commonest cause is chest *trauma*, usually surgical. Other causes include *carcinoma of the lung, lymphoma* and *filariasis. Lymphangiomyomatosis* is a rare cause.

Radiological Appearances of Pleural Fluid

Free Fluid Pleural fluid casts a shadow of the density of water or soft tissue on the chest radiograph. In the absence of pleural adhesions, the position and morphology of this shadow will depend upon the amount of fluid, the state of the underlying lung and the position of the patient. The most dependent recess of the pleura is the posterior costophrenic angle. A *small effusion* will, therefore, tend to collect posteriorly and in most patients 100–200 ml of fluid are required to fill this recess before fluid will be seen above the dome of the diaphragm on the frontal view (Fig. 13.1). Small effusions may thus be seen earlier on a lateral film than on a frontal film, but it is possible to identify effusions of only a few milliliters using decubitus views with a horizontal beam (Fig. 13.2), ultrasound or CT (Fig. 13.3). As more fluid accumulates, the costophrenic angle on the frontal view fills, and with increasing fluid a homogeneous opacity spreads upward, obscuring the lung base. Typically this opacity has a fairly well-defined, concave upper edge, is higher laterally than medially and obscures the diaphragmatic shadow (Fig. 13.4). Frequently fluid will track into the pleural fissures. If the film is sufficiently penetrated, pulmonary vessels in the lung masked by the effusion will be seen. A *massive effusion* may cause complete radiopacity of a hemithorax. The underlying lung will have retracted toward its hilum, and the space-occupying effect of the effusion will push the mediastinum toward the opposite side (Fig. 13.5). In the presence of a large effusion, lack of displacement of the mediastinum suggests that the underlying lung is completely

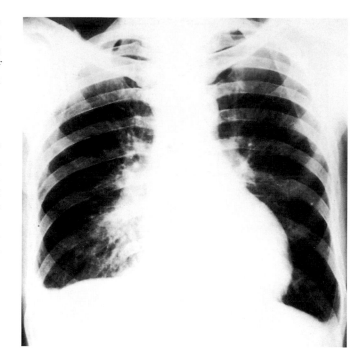

Fig. 13.1 Small bilateral pleural effusions. Man aged 58 with ischemic heart disease. The left costophrenic angle is blunted by a small effusion. The right pleural effusion is larger, and fluid is beginning to extend up the chest wall.

collapsed and when the effusion is of moderate size mediastinal shift toward the side of collapse may occur. This is likely to be due to carcinoma of the bronchus. In the presence of pleural disease the ipsilateral hemidiaphragm is usually elevated. However, the weight of a large effusion may cause inversion of the diaphragm, and this sign is probably best demonstrated by ultrasound.

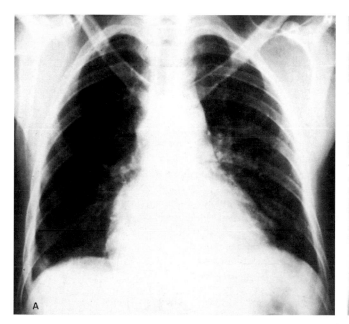

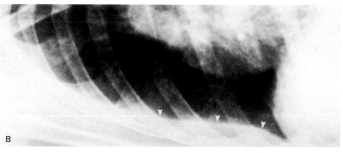

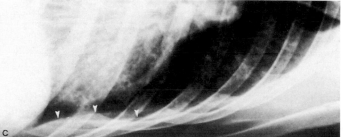

Fig. 13.2 Small bilateral pleural effusions. Man aged 34, renal transplant patient with cytomegalovirus pneumonia. The effusions probably relate to renal failure rather than the pneumonia. **A**. PA film shows subtle filling in of both costophrenic angles. **B** and **C**. Horizontal-beam right and left lateral decubitus films show obvious free pleural effusions collecting along the dependent lateral costal margins (arrowheads).

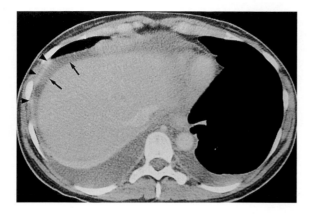

Fig. 13.3 CT scan through the dome of the right diaphragm. There are small pleural effusions in the posterior costophrenic recesses bilaterally. There is also a small volume of abdominal ascites (arrows) between the anterior surface of the liver and the undersurface of the diaphragm (arrowheads).

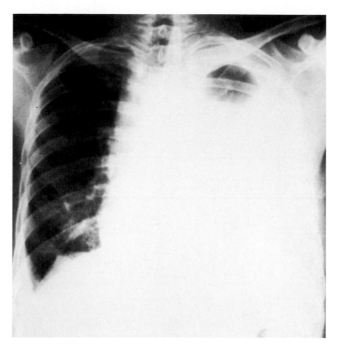

Fig. 13.5 Large pleural effusion. Man of 28 with well-differentiated lymphocytic lymphoma. PA film shows a large left pleural effusion extending over apex of lung and pushing the mediastinum to the right. A small right pleural effusion is also present, and right paratracheal shadowing represents lymphadenopathy.

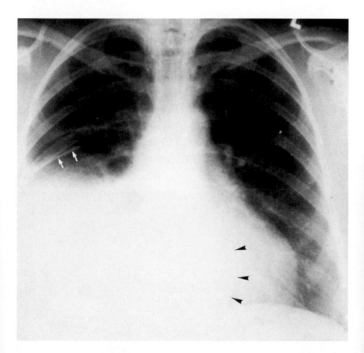

Fig. 13.4 Moderate-size pleural effusion in a woman of 56. Effusions of unknown etiology. PA film demonstrates typical pleural opacity with concave upper border, slightly higher laterally, and obscuring the diaphragm and underlying lung. Fluid is extending into the fissure (arrows) and also into the azygo-esophageal recess, producing a retrocardiac opacity (arrowheads).

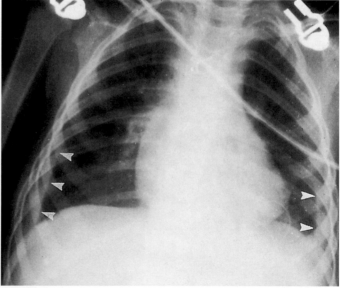

Fig. 13.6 Lamellar pleural effusions, post cardiac surgery. Erect AP film shows fluid filling both costophrenic angles and extending up the lateral chest wall (arrowheads).

Atypical distribution of pleural fluid is quite common. *Lamellar effusions* are shallow collections between the lung surface and the visceral pleura (Fig. 13.6), sometimes sparing the costophrenic angle. Strictly speaking, lamellar effusions represent interstitial pulmonary fluid. Occasionally quite large effusions accumulate between the diaphragm and undersurface of a lung, mimicking elevation of that hemidiaphragm. This is the so-called *subpulmonary pleural effusion*. The contour of the 'diaphragm' is altered, its apex being more lateral than usual, and there may be some blunting of the costophrenic angle or tracking of fluid into fissures (Fig.

13.7). On the left side increased distance between the gastric air bubble and lung base may be apparent. A subpulmonary effusion in a free pleural space will move with changes of posture, as can be demonstrated by horizontal-beam lateral decubitus or supine films. A large right pleural effusion may collect in the azygo-esophageal recess and mimic a retrocardiac mass (Figs 13.4 and

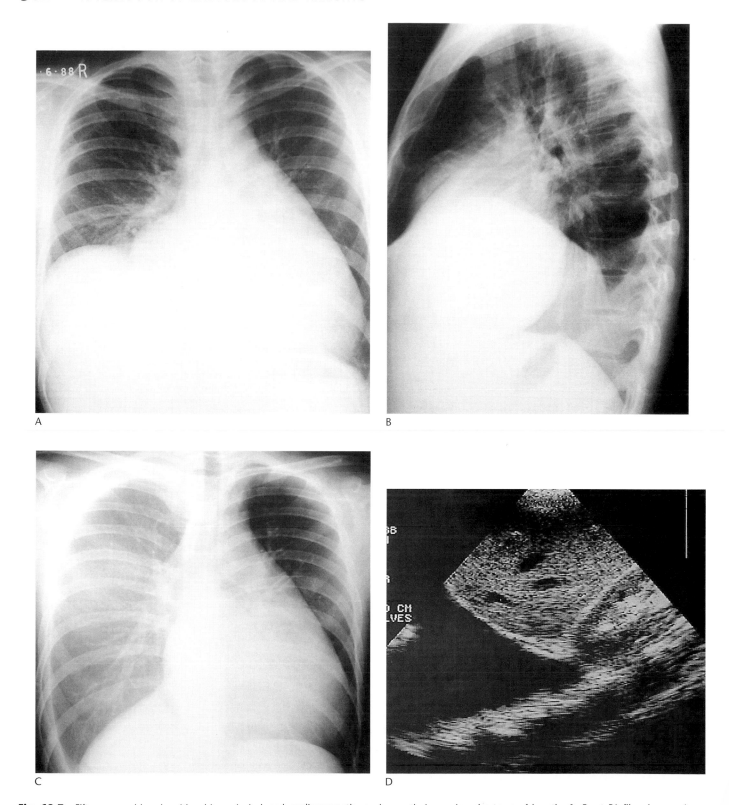

Fig. 13.7   Fifteen-year-old male with adriamycin induced cardiomyopathy and recently increasing shortness of breath. **A**. Erect PA film shows a large heart and apparent elevation of the right hemidiaphragm due to a large subpulmonic effusion. **B**. Lateral film shows fluid tracking up the posterior chest wall and blunting the posterior costophrenic recess. **C**. Supine chest radiograph obtained shortly afterward showing redistribution of pleural fluid. The appearances are now typical of a large supine pleural effusion with increased density of the right hemithorax. **D**. Ultrasound of the right lung base reveals a large anechoic space consistent with an uncomplicated pleural effusion.

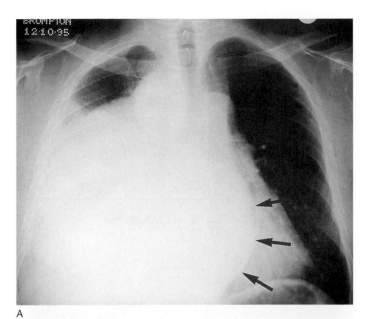

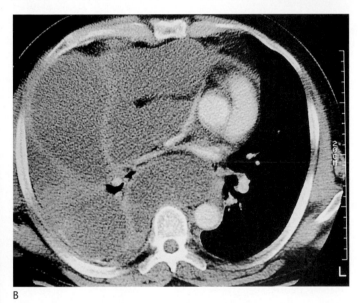

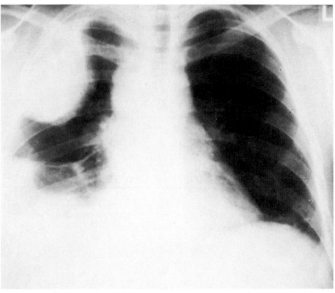

Fig. 13.9 Loculated pleural effusion in a man of 19 years with non-Hodgkin's lymphoma. Erect PA film shows well-circumscribed convex opacity adjacent to right upper costal margin and extending around apex of lung. Right paratracheal shadowing is partly due to lymph node enlargement, and partly due to loculated pleural fluid. Pleural fluid is also present at the right base extending into the horizontal fissure.

An encysted effusion is often associated with free pleural fluid or other pleural shadowing, and may extend into a fissure (Fig. 13.9). Loculated effusions tend to have comparatively little depth, but considerable width, rather like a biconvex lens. Their appearance, therefore, depends on whether they are viewed en face, in profile or obliquely. Fluoroscopy is often helpful in determining the best projection for radiographic demonstration. Extrapleural opacities tend to have a much sharper outline, with tapered, sometimes concave edges where they meet the chest wall. Peripheral pleurally based lung lesions may show an air bronchogram that will distinguish them from true pleural disease (Fig. 13.10). The differentiation between pleural thickening or mass

Fig. 13.8 Fifty-five-year-old male with adenocarcinoma of the pleura from an unknown primary site. **A**. PA chest radiograph reveals extensive opacification of the right hemithorax with a lobulated upper margin. There is shift of the azygo-esophageal line to the opposite side (arrows). **B**. Enhanced CT scan at the level of the main pulmonary artery showing mediastinal displacement due to the large loculated pleural fluid collection.

13.8). The reasons for atypical distribution of pleural fluid are often unclear, but it may be associated with abnormality of the underlying lung.

Loculated Fluid The pleural space may be partially obliterated by pleural disease, causing fusion of the parietal and visceral layers. Encapsulated and free pleural fluid can be distinguished by gravitational methods. Encapsulated fluid, however, may be difficult to differentiate from an extrapleural opacity, parenchymal lung disease or mediastinal mass, but there are some useful diagnostic points.

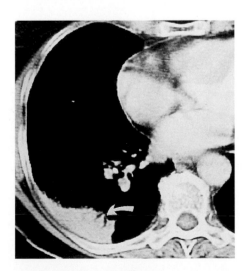

Fig. 13.10 Peripheral consolidation demonstrating the presence of an air bronchogram (arrow) in a patient with organizing pneumonia.

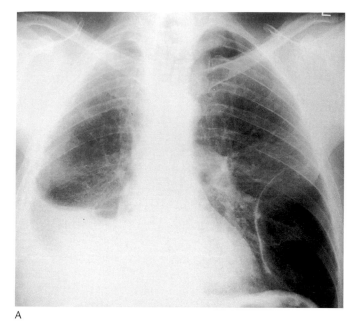
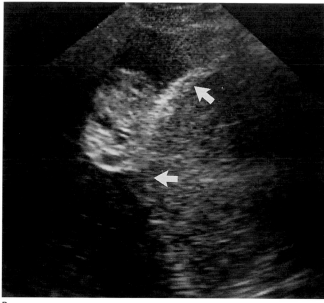

A   B

Fig. 13.11 A.   PA radiograph of a 55-year-old male patient with disseminated adenocarcinoma. The right hemidiaphragm is obscured by what appears to be a simple pleural effusion. (There is a large bulla at the left lung base.) **B**. Ultrasound of the right lung base reveals a tumor nodule on the dome of the diaphragm (arrows) surrounded by pleural fluid.

and loculated pleural fluid may be difficult on plain films, and CT and ultrasound are particularly useful in this context (Fig. 13.11).

Fluid may become loculated in one or more of the interlobar fissures. This is an uncommon occurrence and is most often seen in heart failure. The appearances depend upon which fissure is affected and the quantity of fluid. Fluid collecting in the horizontal fissure produces a lenticular, oval or round shadow, with well-demarcated edges. Fluid extending into the adjacent parts of the fissure may make it appear thickened. In both frontal and lateral projections the shadow appears rounded. Loculated fluid in an oblique fissure may be poorly defined on a frontal radiograph, but a lateral film is usually diagnostic since the fissure is seen tangentially, and the typical lenticular configuration of the effusion is demonstrated (Fig. 13.12).

Loculated interlobar effusions can appear rounded on two views. Following treatment they may disappear rapidly, and are hence known as 'pseudo-' or 'vanishing' tumors. They may recur in subsequent episodes of heart failure.

Empyema may be suspected on a plain film by the spontaneous appearance of a fluid level in a pleural effusion, but is best diagnosed by CT or ultrasound (Figs 13.13, 13.14). On CT an empyema usually has a lenticular shape and may compress the underlying lung. Fluid, with or without gas, may be present in the pleura and both layers of the pleura may be thickened. Since the likelihood of successful small bore catheter drainage decreases with time and the development of a pleural rind, rapid diagnosis and treatment should be the aim. If a complicated effusion be-comes chronic, *thickening* of the visceral or parietal pleura may occur. The former may prevent re-expansion of the lung, and

surgical decortication may be necessary if respiratory function is significantly impaired.

Multiple septations within an infected or reactive pleural collection may be broken down by the instillation of *fibrinolytic agents* such as *urokinase* (Fig. 13.15). Typically 100 000 IU of urokinase are instilled in 50 ml of normal saline. The drain is then clamped for 1 hour, after which free drainage or low pressure wall suction is reinstituted. This treatment, which may be repeated daily for up to 5 days, significantly increases the success rate of radiologically guided closed drainage and reduces the need for large bore drain insertion or surgical intervention. Regular (8-hourly) flushing of narrow bore catheters with 10 ml of normal saline will help to prevent the lumen becoming occluded with fibrinous debris.

Ultrasound Appearance of Pleural Fluid (Fig. 13.14)   Ultra-sound is an excellent method for locating loculated pleural fluid prior to diagnostic or therapeutic aspiration. The fluid may be anechoic or contain particulate material. It is possible to visualize septations in loculated collections and also to identify pleural thickening and masses. Transudates are almost always anechoic but exudates may or may not contain reflective material. The presence of pleural masses in association with an effusion is highly suggestive of malignant disease (Fig. 13.11B).

Pneumothorax

Pneumothorax is the presence of air in the pleural cavity. Air enters this cavity through a defect in either the parietal or the

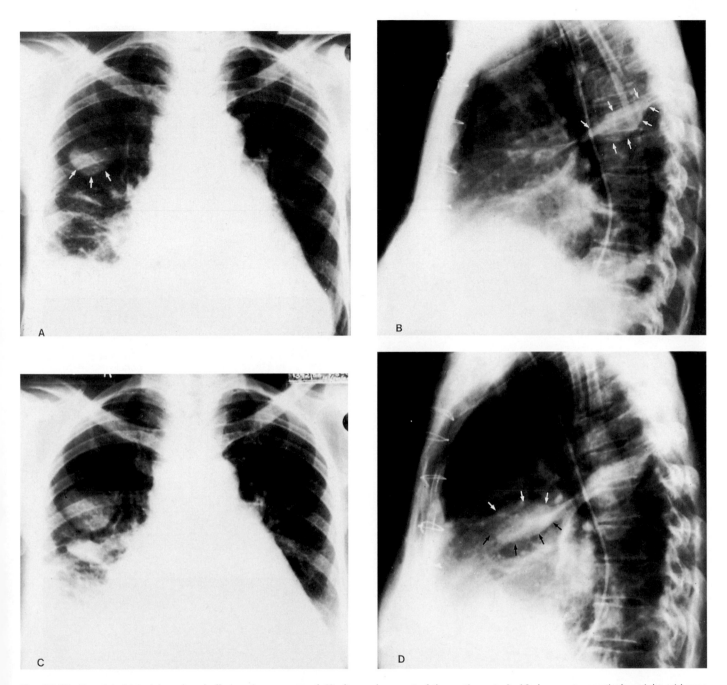

Fig. 13.12 Loculated interlobar pleural effusions in a woman of 60 after replacement of the aortic root. **A**. 19 days post-operatively a right mid-zone opacity appears (arrows), with a sharp lower margin and an indistinct upper margin. The right costophrenic angle has also filled in. **B**. Lateral projection demonstrates typical lenticular configuration of fluid loculated in the oblique fissure (arrows). **C**. Seven days later a second round opacity has appeared below the first. This opacity is well circumscribed. **D**. Lateral projection confirms that this is fluid loculated in the horizontal fissure (arrows).

visceral pleura. Such defects are the result of lung pathology, trauma or deliberate introduction of air, respectively giving rise to spontaneous, traumatic or artificial pneumothoraces. If pleural adhesions are present the pneumothorax may be localized, otherwise it is generalized. If air can move freely in and out of the pleural space during respiration it is an open pneumothorax, if no movement of air occurs it is closed, and if air enters the pleural space on inspiration, but does not leave on expiration, it is valvular. As intrapleural pressure increases in a valvular pneumothorax a tension pneumothorax develops.

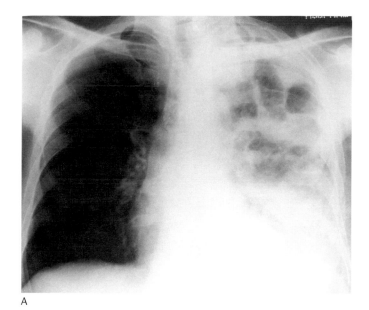

A

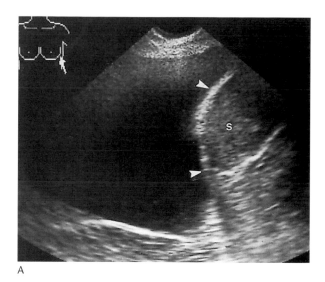

A

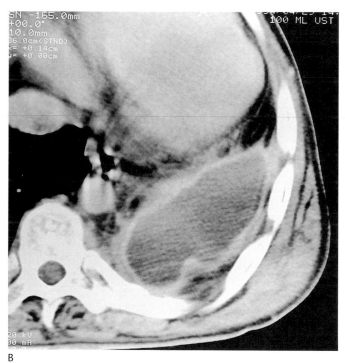

B

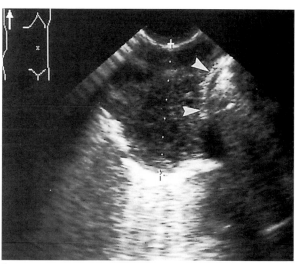

B

Fig. 13.13   Two patients with empyema. **A**. PA chest radiograph showing multiple fluid levels in a patient with a heavily loculated empyema complicating attempted pleurodesis. **B**. CT scan through the lower thorax in a patient with a right basal empyema collection. There is associated pleural thickening and compression of the adjacent lung parenchyma.

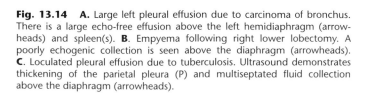

Fig. 13.14   **A**. Large left pleural effusion due to carcinoma of bronchus. There is a large echo-free effusion above the left hemidiaphragm (arrowheads) and spleen(s). **B**. Empyema following right lower lobectomy. A poorly echogenic collection is seen above the diaphragm (arrowheads). **C**. Loculated pleural effusion due to tuberculosis. Ultrasound demonstrates thickening of the parietal pleura (P) and multiseptated fluid collection above the diaphragm (arrowheads).

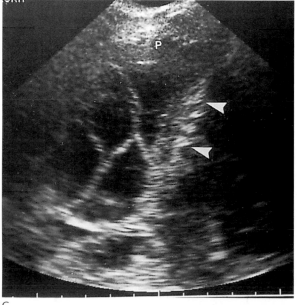

C

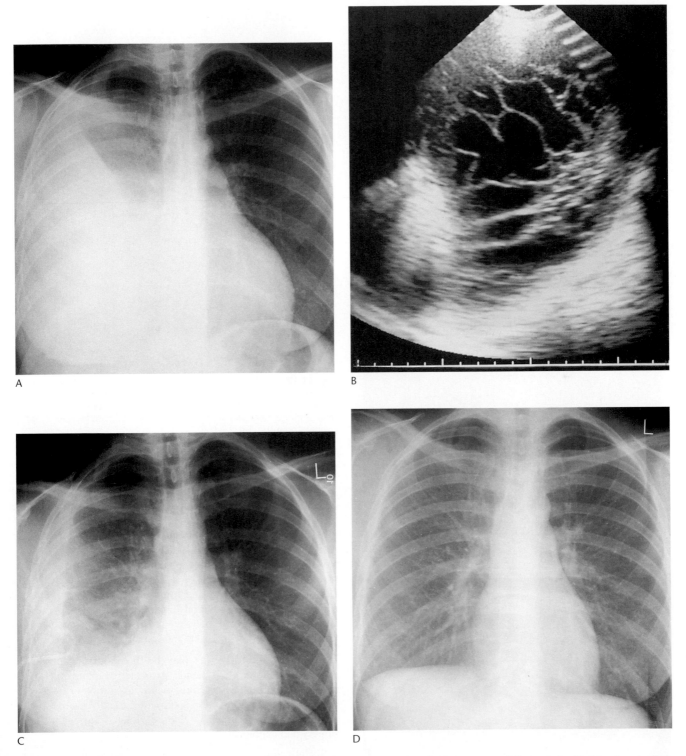

Fig. 13.15 Series of chest radiographs in a patient with a loculated parapneumonic pleural effusion successfully treated with intrapleural urokinase.
A. The initial chest radiograph demonstrates a large right pleural effusion which an ultrasound scan **B** shows to be heavily loculated.
C. PA radiograph 24 hours after fine bore catheter insertion and instillation of streptokinase. **D**. PA chest radiograph five months later.

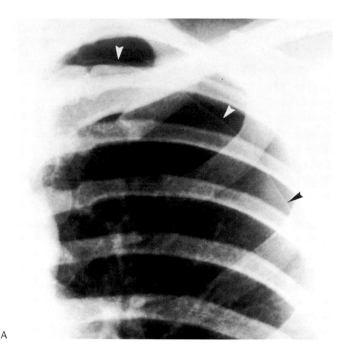

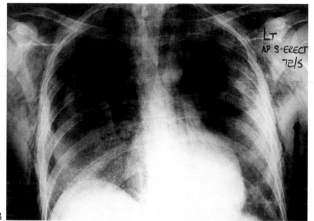

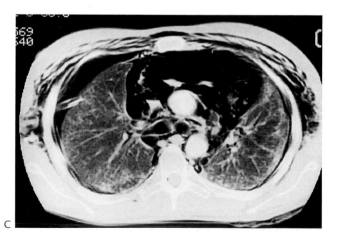

Fig. 13.16   A. Woman aged 22 with a spontaneous pneumothorax. PA film showing apical pneumothorax. The visceral pleural (arrowheads) separates aerated lung from the radiolucent pleural space. **B**. AP chest radiograph and **C** CT scan in a patient with *Pneumocystis carinii* pneumonia complicated by bilateral pneumothoraces and extensive mediastinal and surgical emphysema.

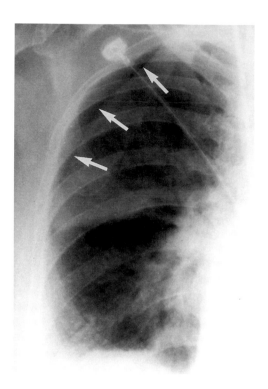

Fig. 13.17   Supine chest radiograph of an intubated patient. There is a skin fold projected over the right lung apex simulating a pneumothorax (arrows). Close inspection reveals lung markings extending beyond the skin fold, and no fine pleural line that should be visible with a genuine pneumothorax (cf. Fig. 13.16A).

Etiology

Spontaneous pneumothorax is the commonest type, and typically occurs in young men, due to rupture of a congenital pleural bleb. Such blebs are usually in the lung apex and may be bilateral.

In older patients chronic bronchitis and emphysema are common factors. Rarer causes include bronchial asthma, rupture of a tension cyst in staphylococcal pneumonia, rupture of a subpleural tuberculous focus, rupture of a subpleural tension cyst in carcinoma of the bronchus, and rupture of a cavitating subpleural metastasis. Other associations include many of the causes of interstitial pulmonary fibrosis (cystic fibrosis, histiocytosis, tuberous sclerosis, sarcoidosis and some of the pneumoconioses).

Traumatic pneumothorax may be the result of a penetrating chest wound, closed chest trauma (particularly rupture of a bronchus in a road accident), rib fracture, pleural aspiration or biopsy, lung biopsy, bronchoscopy, esophagoscopy, and positive-pressure ventilation. The pleura may also be violated during mediastinal surgery and nephrectomy.

Artificial pneumothorax as treatment for pulmonary tuberculosis is now of historical interest only, as is diagnostic pneumothorax.

Radiological Appearances   A small pneumothorax in a free pleural space in an erect patient collects at the apex. The lung apex retracts toward the hilum and on a frontal chest film the sharp white line of the visceral pleura will be visible, separated from the chest wall by the radiolucent pleural space, which is devoid of lung markings (Fig. 13.16). This should not be con-

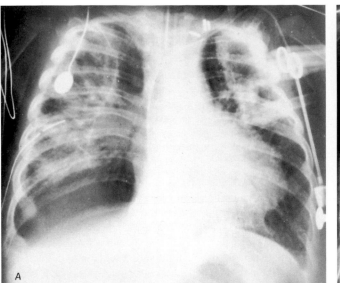
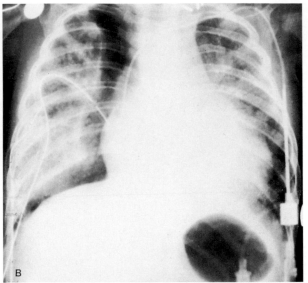

Fig. 13.18   Medial tension pneumothorax in a one-year-old-child on ventilator following closure of patent ductus arteriosus and resection of coarctation of aorta. **A**. Supine AP film demonstrates a right pneumothorax, the intrapleural air collecting anteriorly and medially, and the lung collapsing posteriorly and laterally. The pleural tube is situated laterally and is therefore not decompressing the pneumothorax. The right hemidiaphragm is depressed, and the mediastinum is displaced to the left, indicating a tension pneumothorax. **B**. Following insertion of another pleural tube more medially, the pneumothorax is smaller and the right hemidiaphragm and mediastinum have returned to their normal positions.

fused with the appearances of a skin fold, on which there is no discrete pleural line (Fig. 13.17). The affected lung usually remains aerated: however perfusion is reduced in proportion to ventilation and therefore the radiodensity of the partially collapsed lung remains normal. A small pneumothorax may easily go unseen and it may be necessary to examine the film with a bright light. An expiratory film will make a closed pneumothorax easier to see since on full expiration the lung volume is at its smallest, while the volume of pleural air is unchanged. Generally, expiratory radiographs are not routinely required. A lateral decubitus film with the affected side uppermost is occasionally helpful, as the pleural air can be seen along the lateral chest wall. This view is particularly useful in infants, since small pneumothoraces are difficult to see in supine AP films, as the air tends to collect anteriorly and medially (Fig. 13.18). Alternatively, a horizontal beam 'shoot through' lateral film may identify anterior pneumothoraces in the supine patient.

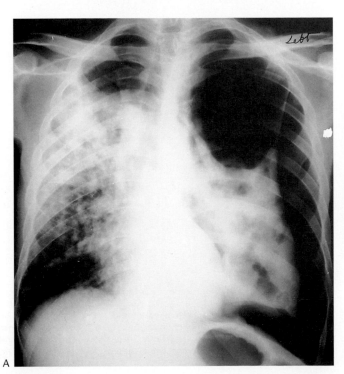

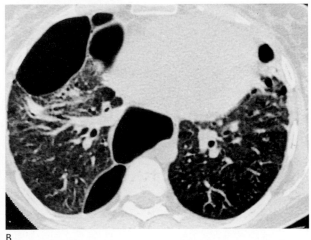

Fig. 13.19   A. Tension pneumothorax with a pleural adhesion. Elderly man with spontaneous pneumothorax secondary to extensive cavitating pulmonary tuberculosis. The left lung is prevented from collapsing completely by the extensive consolidation, and by tethering of an adhesion (arrowheads). The mediastinum is displaced to the right. **B.** Non-tension pneumothoraces in a 26-year-old female patient demonstrating multiple pleural adhesions causing loculation of air.

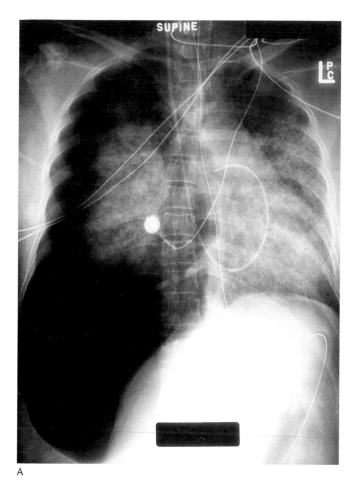

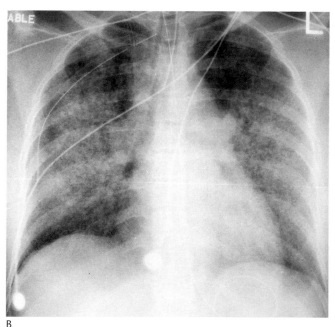

A large pneumothorax may lead to complete relaxation and retraction of the lung, with some mediastinal shift toward the normal side, which increases on expiration.

Tension pneumothorax   (Figs 13.18, 13.19A and 13.20) may lead to massive displacement of the mediastinum, kinking of the great veins and acute cardiac and respiratory embarrassment. Radiologically the ipsilateral lung may be squashed against the mediastinum, or herniate across the midline, and the ipsilateral hemidiaphragm may be depressed. On fluoroscopy the mediastinal shift to the contralateral side is greatest in inspiration, an observation that distinguishes a tension pneumothorax from a large pneumothorax not under strain.

Complications of Pneumothorax   Pleural adhesions may limit the distribution of a pneumothorax and result in a *loculated* or *encysted pneumothorax*. The usual appearance is an ovoid air collection adjacent to the chest wall, and it may be radiographically indistinguishable from a thin-walled subpleural pulmonary cavity, cyst or bulla. *Pleural adhesions* are occasionally seen as line

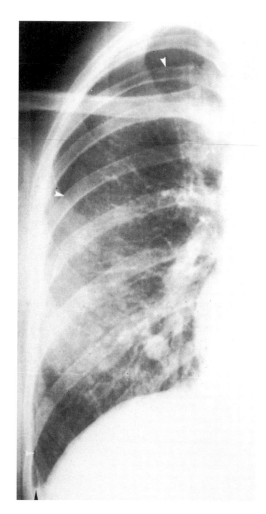

Fig. 13.20   A. Tension pneumothorax following a transbronchial lung biopsy. There is inversion of the right hemidiaphragm, and deviation of the mediastinum to the opposite side. **B**. Following insertion of a right-sided chest drain the diaphragm and mediastinum have returned to a normal position. The diffuse bilateral infiltrate is due to pre-existing pulmonary hemorrhage.

Fig. 13.21   Shallow hydropneumothorax in a man of 18 years. Spontaneous pneumothorax, probably due to rupture of subpleural cavitating metastatic osteogenic sarcoma. The primary tumor was in the right scapula, which has been removed, and pulmonary metastases are seen in the right lower zone. The visceral pleura is faintly seen (white arrowheads) and a short fluid level (black arrowhead) is present just above the right costophrenic angle.

shadows stretching between the two pleural layers, preventing relaxation of the underlying lung (Fig. 13.19). Rupture of an adhesion may produce a *hemopneumothorax*, or discharge of an underlying infected subpleural lesion, leading to a *pyopneumothorax*. Collapse or consolidation of a lobe or lung in association with a pneumothorax are important complications which may delay re-expansion of the lung.

Since the normal pleural space contains a small volume of fluid, blunting of the costophrenic angle by a short fluid level is commonly seen in a pneumothorax (Fig. 13.21). In a small pneumothorax this fluid level may be the most obvious radio-

logical sign. A larger fluid collection usually signifies a complication and represents exudate, pus or blood, depending on the etiology of the pneumothorax.

The usual radiological appearance of a *hydropneumothorax* is that of a pneumothorax containing a horizontal fluid level which separates opaque fluid below from lucent air above. This demonstration requires a horizontal beam film (Fig. 13.22), so that if the patient is not fit enough for an upright film a lateral decubitus film or 'shoot-through' lateral film may be indicated.

Bronchopleural Fistula

Bronchopleural fistula is a communication between the airway and the pleural space. It is most frequently a complication of complete or partial *pneumonectomy*, and is discussed under post-operative complications in Chapter 18. Other causes include *carcinoma of the bronchus* and *ruptured lung abscess*. The radiological appearance is that of a hydro- or pyo-pneumothorax.

Pleural Thickening

Blunting of a costophrenic angle is a frequent incidental finding on a chest X-ray. It is due to localized pleural thickening and usually results from a previous episode of pleuritis, although a previous history of chest disease is often lacking. In the asymptomatic patient and in the absence of other radiological abnormality it is of no other significance. It may mimic a small pleural effusion, and if a previous film is not available for comparison a lateral decubitus film or ultrasound scan will exclude free pleural fluid. Localized pleural thickening extending into the inferior end of an oblique fissure may produce so-called tenting of the diaphragm, and is of similar significance. This latter appearance may also result from basal intrapulmonary scarring, due to previous pulmonary infection or infarction.

Bilateral apical pleural thickening is also a fairly common finding. It is more frequent in elderly patients, and is not due to tuberculosis. Its etiology is uncertain, but ischemia is probably a factor. Such apical shadowing is usually symmetric (Fig. 13.23). Asymmetric or *unilateral apical pleural thickening*, however, may be of pathological significance, especially if associated with pain. If asymmetric, apical pleural shadowing may represent a *Pancoast tumor*, and it is important to visualize the adjacent ribs

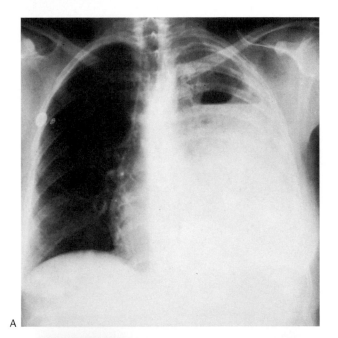

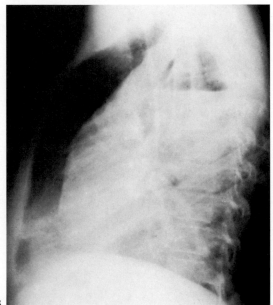

Fig. 13.22 Loculated pyo-pneumothorax in a woman of 45 following gunshot wound to chest. **A**. Erect PA film shows a fluid level in the left upper zone, and pleural thickening over the apex. **B**. Lateral film shows that the fluid level is situated posteriorly. The differential diagnosis lies between a pyopneumothorax and a lung abscess.

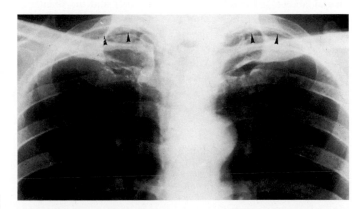

Fig. 13.23 Bilateral apical pleural thickening. An incidental finding in a 67-year-old man with ischemic heart disease. The apical pleural shadowing (arrowheads) is symmetric, although the edge is better seen on the left.

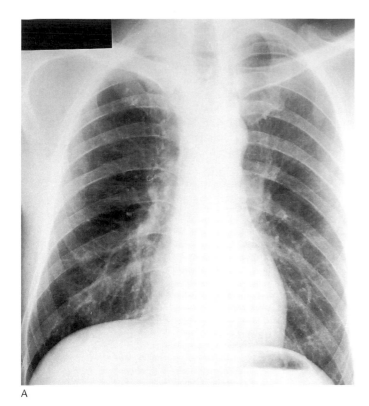

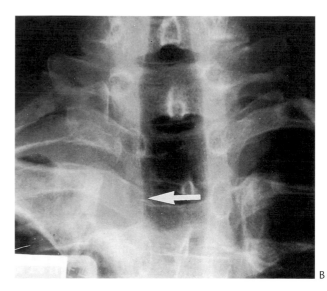

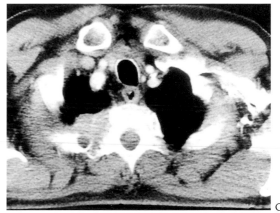

Fig. 13.24 Unilateral apical pleural thickening. Man aged 46 with pain in the right side of the neck and right arm. **A**. Dense pleural shadowing is present at the right apex. The left apex is clear. **B**. An AP view of the cervical spine demonstrates absence of the right pedicle of T3 (arrow). (Histology: anaplastic carcinoma.) **C**. CT demonstrates a right apical mass infiltrating the third thoracic vertebra.

and spine (Fig. 13.24). Penetrated films and tomography may be indicated, since evidence of bone involvement will almost certainly indicate a carcinoma.

More *extensive unilateral pleural thickening* is usually the result of a previous thoracotomy or pleural effusion. Empyema and hemothorax are especially likely to resolve with *pleural fibrosis*. Chronic pneumothorax is a rarer cause. These causes of pleural fibrosis all involve the visceral layer and the thickened pleura may calcify. If the entire lung is surrounded by fibrotic pleura, this is termed a *fibrothorax*. The pleural peel may be a few centimeters thick, and may cause reduced ventilation of the surrounded lung and subsequent decrease in volume of that hemithorax. If the chest X-ray shows that the vascularity of the affected lung is decreased relative to the other lung, then significant ventilatory restriction is likely and surgical decortication may be necessary.

Bilateral pleural plaques are a common manifestation of asbestos exposure, and occasionally more diffuse pleural thickening is seen.

Pleural Calcification

Pleural calcification has the same causes as pleural thickening. Unilateral pleural calcification is, therefore, likely to be the result of previous empyema, hemothorax or pleurisy, and bilateral

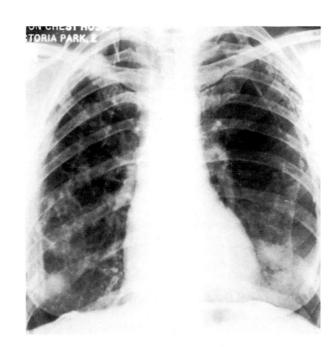

Fig. 13.25 Pleural calcification in a middle-aged woman with a history of recurrent episodes of pleurisy, presumed to be tuberculous. Extensive plaques of pleural calcification surround both lungs.

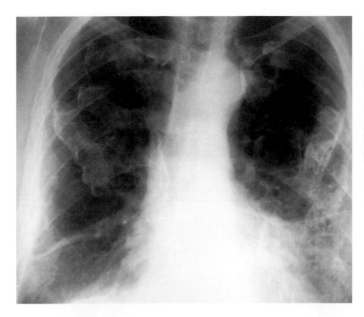

Fig. 13.26 Bilateral calcified pleural plaques seen en face over both lungs due to exposure to asbestos.

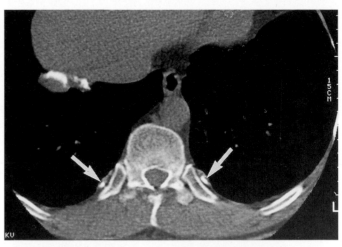

Fig. 13.28 CT demonstration of pleural abnormalities due to asbestos exposure in a middle-aged man. There are small calcified pleural plaques in the paraspinal gutters (arrows) and calcified pleural plaques over the right hemidiaphragm.

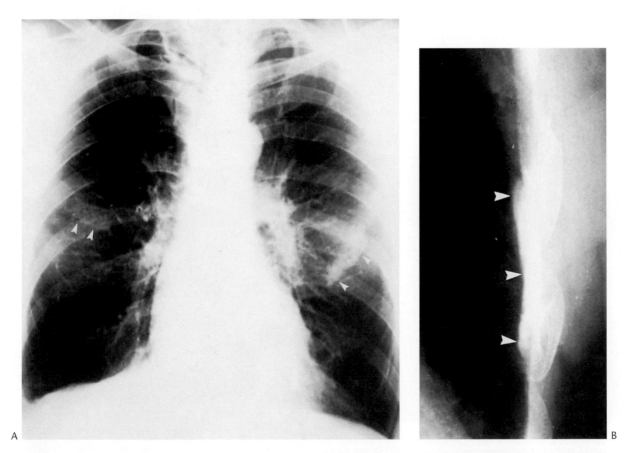

A

B

Fig. 13.27 Pleural calcification resulting from exposure to asbestos in a 51-year-old man with chronic obstructive airways disease. **A**. The lungs are hyperinflated. Calcified pleural plaques are present in both mid zones (arrowheads). **B**. An oblique film, aided by fluoroscopy, shows the left-sided plaque tangentially (arrowheads); it is situated in the parietal pleura, immediately deep to the ribs.

calcification occurs after asbestos exposure and in some other pneumoconioses, or occasionally after bilateral effusions. As with the incidental finding of pleural thickening, pleural calcification may be discovered in a patient who is not aware of previous or current chest disease.

The calcification associated with previous pleurisy, empyema or hemothorax occurs in the visceral pleura; associated pleural thickening is almost always present, and separates the calcium from the ribs. The calcium may be in a continuous sheet or in discrete plaques, usually producing dense, coarse, irregular shadows, often sharply demarcated laterally (Fig. 13.25). If a plaque is viewed en face it may cast a less well-defined shadow

and mimic a pulmonary infiltrate. However, a lateral view will often demonstrate the calcified plaque over the anterior or posterior pleura but it may be necessary to fluoroscope the patient to obtain the best tangential projection for demonstration of the plaque.

The calcification associated with asbestos exposure is usually more delicate and bilateral (Fig. 13.26). It is frequently visible over the diaphragm and adjacent to the axillae. Tangential views show it to be situated immediately deep to the ribs, and it is in fact located in the parietal pleura (Fig. 13.27). The most sensitive method for demonstrating a pleural plaque is HRCT (Fig. 13.28), and ultrasound can be helpful in differentiating a plaque from loculated fluid.

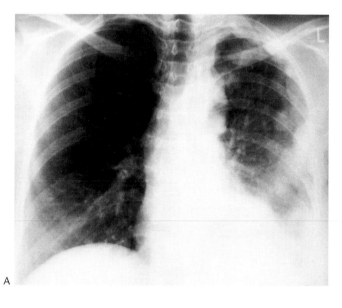

A

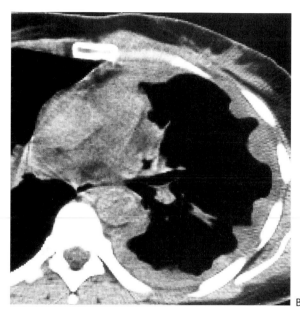

B

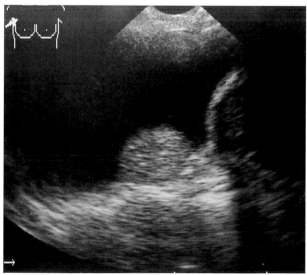

C

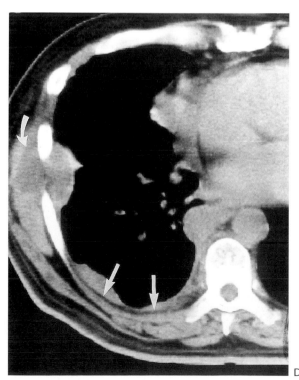

D

Fig. 13.29 A. Nodular pleural thickening due to metastatic carcinoma of the breast. Note the left mastectomy and surgical clips in the axilla. **B.** Same patient as **A**. CT demonstration of pleural deposits. The whole lung is encased by pleural tumor. **C.** Metastatic pleural tumor nodule in a patient with carcinoma of the ovary demonstrated by ultrasound. **D.** Pleural tumor deposits from adenocarcinoma of the esophagus. The largest nodule has crossed the pleural fat stripe, which is still visible elsewhere (arrows), and is invading the chest wall musculature (curved arrow).

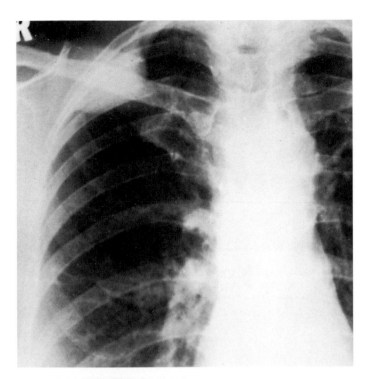

Fig. 13.30 Pleural fibroma or benign mesothelioma. Incidental finding in a 48-year-old woman with a past history of left apical tuberculosis. A sharply demarcated peripheral upper zone opacity is present, making an obtuse angle with the adjacent chest wall, and without other pleural abnormality. It was removed. Histology: benign fibrous mesothelioma.

Pleural Tumors

Primary neoplasms of the pleura are rare. Benign tumors of the pleura include local mesothelioma (or fibroma) and lipoma. The commonest malignant disease of the pleura is metastatic (Fig. 13.29), the most frequent primary tumors being of the bronchus and breast. Primary malignancy of the pleura (malignant mesothelioma) is usually associated with asbestos exposure.

Pleural fibromas usually present with finger clubbing and joint pains due to hypertrophic osteoarthropathy, but may be an incidental finding on a chest X-ray. The radiographic appearance is of a well-defined lobulated mass adjacent to the chest wall, mediastinum, diaphragm or a pleural fissure (Fig. 13.30). The mass may be small or occupy most of the hemithorax (Fig. 13.31). In the presence of osteoarthropathy, the diagnosis is almost certain, but if necessary, percutaneous needle biopsy is probably the investigation of choice.

Subpleural lipomas appear as well-defined rounded masses. They may change shape with respiration, being soft tumors, and if large enough may erode adjacent ribs. Since they comprise fat the CT appearance is diagnostic (Fig. 13.32).

Malignant Mesothelioma is usually due to prolonged exposure to asbestos dust, particularly crocidolite. The usual appearance is nodular pleural thickening around all or part of a lung (Fig. 13.33). A hemorrhagic pleural effusion may be present but the lung changes of asbestosis may be absent. The effusion may obscure the pleural masses. Often the mediastinum is central,

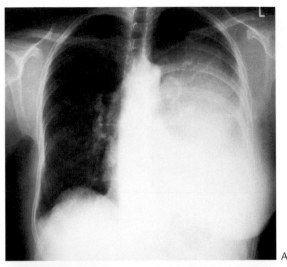

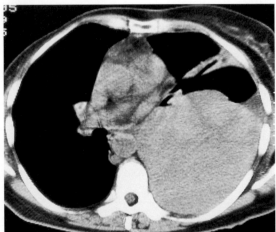

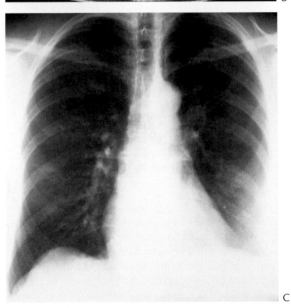

Fig. 13.31 A. Giant pleural fibroma in a patient with a distant history of a right mastectomy for carcinoma. **B**. CT scan in the same patient shows a large heterogeneous mass occupying most of the left hemithorax and associated with a small pleural effusion. There is no radiological evidence of chest wall invasion. **C**. Appearances immediately following surgery. The tumor was completely resected and there was no invasion of adjacent structures.

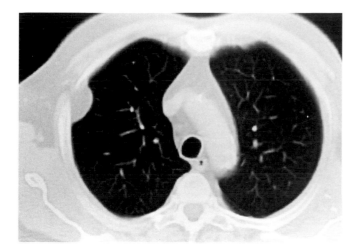

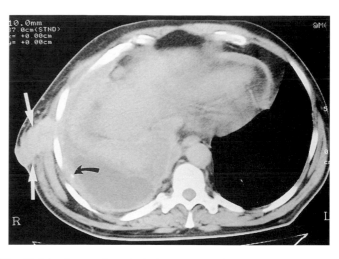

Fig. 13.32 **A.** Pleural lipoma. Incidental finding of a pleurally based opacity in the right mid zone (arrows). CT examination displayed on mediastinal window settings reveals a pleural mass of identical density to subcutaneous fat.

Fig. 13.34 CT scan through the lower thorax of a patient with malignant mesothelioma. There is metastatic tumor seeding along the biopsy tract (arrows). Note the fleck of pleural calcification (curved arrow).

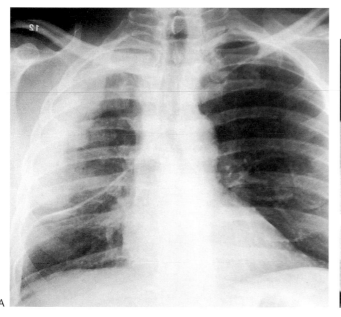

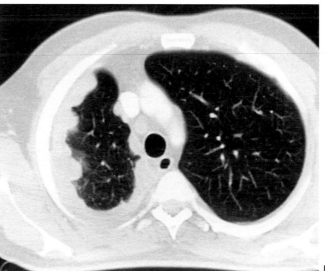

Fig. 13.33 Malignant mesothelioma. Abnormal chest radiograph (A) shows lobulated left pleural opacities. **B.** CT scan through the mid thorax demonstrates encasement of the right lung by nodular pleural tumor. Calcified pleural plaques were evident on other sections.

despite the presence of a large effusion, and this is thought to result from volume loss of the underlying lung secondary to either ventilatory restriction by the surrounding tumor, or bronchial stenosis by tumor compression at the hilum. Rib involvement may occur with malignant mesothelioma, but the presence of a pleural mass and adjacent rib destruction is more likely to be due to metastatic bone tumor, or possibly a primary bone tumor.

The extent of malignant mesothelioma is best assessed by CT.

CT may also help differentiate between malignant mesothelioma and benign pleural plaques. Nodular extension into fissures, pleural effusion and volume loss of the ipsilateral lung all suggest malignancy as does involvement of the mediastinal pleura and marked asymmetry of appearances. A tissue diagnosis may be obtained by *percutaneous needle biopsy*. Occasionally malignant mesothelioma is complicated by tumor seeding along biopsy or drainage tracts (Fig. 13.34).

REFERENCES AND SUGGESTIONS FOR FURTHER READING

Armstrong, P., Wilson, A. G., Dee, P., Hansell, D. M. (1995) *The Imaging of Diseases of the Chest*, 2nd edn. St Louis: Mosby-Year Book

Felson, B. (1973) *Chest Roentgenology*. Philadelphia: W.B. Saunders.

Fraser, R. G., Pare, J. A. P., Pare, P. D., Fraser, R. S., Genereux, G. P. (1989–91) *Diagnosis of Diseases of the Chest*, 3rd edn. Philadelphia: W. B. Saunders.

Simon, G. (1978) *Principles of Chest X-ray Diagnosis*, 4th edn. London: Butterworths.

The pleura

Albelda, S. M., Epstein, D. M., Gefter, W. B., Miller, W. T. (1982) Pleural thickening: its significance and relationship to asbestos dust exposure. *American Review of Respiratory Disease*, **126**, 621–624.

Henschke, C. I., Davis, S. D., Romano, P. M., Yankelvitz, D. F. (1989) The pathogenesis, radiological evaluation and therapy of pleural effusions. *Radiologic Clinics of North America*, **27**, 1241–1255.

Hillerdal, G. (1983) Malignant mesothelioma 1982: review of 4710 published cases. *British Journal of Diseases of the Chest*, **71**, 321–343.

Kawashima, A., Libshitz, H. I. (1990) Malignant pleural mesothelioma: CT manifestations in 50 cases. *American Journal of Roentgenology*, **155**, 965–969.

Leung, A. N., Müller, N. L., Miller, R. R. (1990) CT in differential diagnosis of diffuse pleural disease. *American Journal of Roentgenology*, **154**, 487–492.

McLeod, T. C., Flower, C. D. R. (1991) Imaging the pleura: sonography, CT and MR imaging. *American Journal of Roentgenology*, **156**, 1145–1153.

McLeod, T. C., Isler, R. J., Novelline, R. A., Putman, C. E., Simeone, J., Stark, P. (1981) The apical cap. *American Journal of Roentgenology*, **137**, 299–306.

Moskowitz, P.S., Griscom, N.T. (1976) The medial pneumothorax. *Radiology*, **120**, 143–147.

Müller, N. L. (1993) Imaging of the pleura. *Radiology*, **186**, 297–309.

Rasch, B. N., Carsky, E. W., Lane, E. T., Callaghan, J. P. O., Heitzman, E. R. (1982) Pleural effusion: explanation of some atypical appearances. *American Journal of Roentgenology*, **139**, 899–904.

Stark, D. D., Federle, M. P., Goodman, P. C., Padrasky, A. E., Webb, W. R. (1983) Differentiating lung abscess and empyema: radiography and computed tomography. *American Journal of Roentgenology*, **141**, 163–167.

Stuart, G., Silverman, M.D., Saini, S., Mueller, P.R. (1989) Pleural interventions. *Radiologic Clinics of North America*, **27**, 1257–1267.

Woodring, J. H. (1984) Recognition of pleural effusion on supine radiographs: how much fluid is required? *American Journal of Roentgenology*, **142**, 59–64.

Wright, F. W. (1976) Spontaneous pneumothorax and pulmonary malignant disease—a syndrome sometimes associated with cavitating tumours. *Clinical Radiology*, **27**, 211–222.

Yang, P-C., Luh, K-T., Chang, D-B., Wu, H-D., Yu, C-J., Kuo, S-H. (1992) Value of sonography in determining the nature of pleural effusion: analysis of 320 cases. *American Journal of Roentgenology*, **159**, 29–33.

14

TUMORS OF THE LUNG

Michael B. Rubens and Simon P. G. Padley

With a contribution from Jeremy P. R. Jenkins

A wide variety of neoplasms may arise in the lungs. While many lung tumors are overtly malignant and others are definitely benign, some fall both histologically and in their clinical behavior between these two extremes. Pulmonary tumors may be classified histologically or according to their presumed tissue of origin. However, it should be borne in mind that histopathologists do not always agree on the classification of an individual tumor. Carcinoma of the bronchus is by far the commonest and most important primary tumor of the lung.

CARCINOMA OF THE BRONCHUS

Carcinoma of the bronchus is the commonest fatal malignancy in adult males in the western world. It is commoner in men than in women, but the incidence in women is rising. Most cases occur between 40 and 70 years, and it is unusual below 30 years of age.

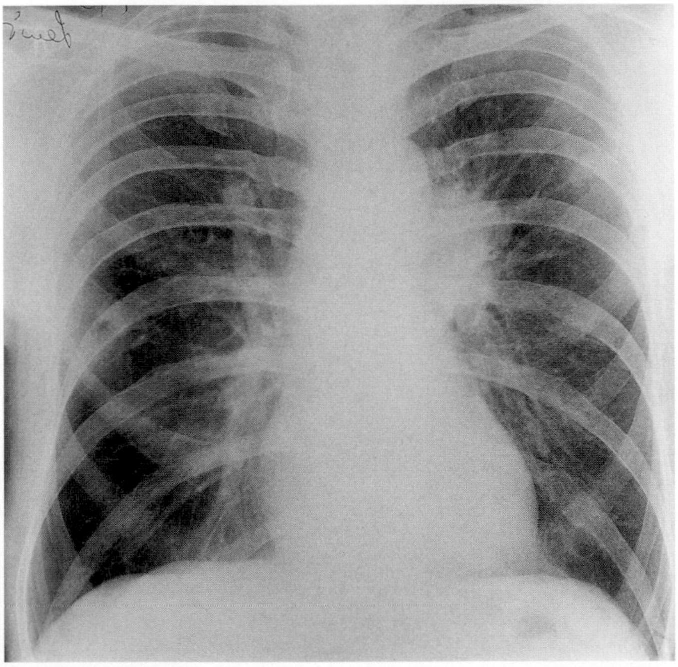

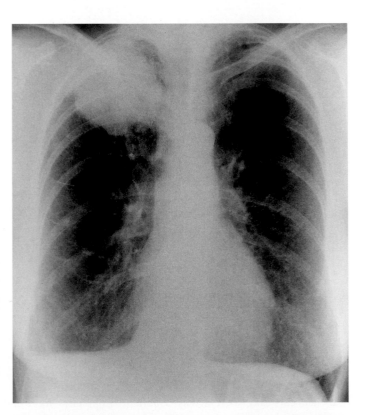

Fig. 14.1 Carcinoma of bronchus. The primary tumor is at the left hilum. Soft-tissue nodules in both lungs are metastases, and there is a lytic metastasis in the right eighth rib.

Fig. 14.2 Carcinoma of bronchus. A large, round soft-tissue mass is present at the right apex. Blunting of the right costophrenic angle is due to a small pleural effusion.

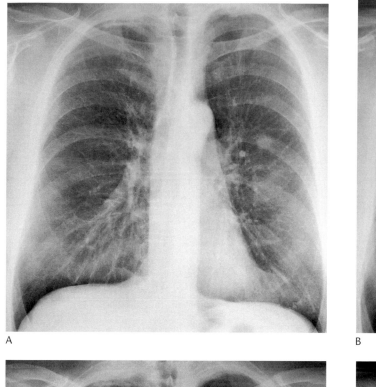

A

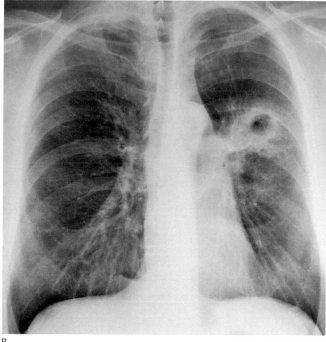

B

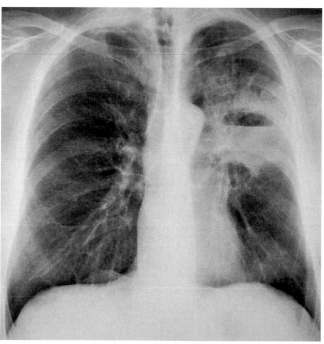

C

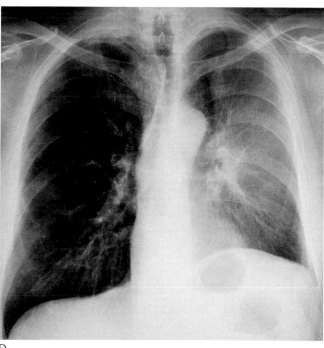

D

The most important single etiological factor is cigarette smoking. This is dose related, the risk being proportional to the number of cigarettes smoked. Other factors include atmospheric pollution and certain occupations. Smokers who are exposed to asbestos have an increased risk of lung cancer when compared to smokers without such exposure. Exposure to radioactivity and some industrial chemicals has caused increased mortality from lung cancer in some occupations. These include the mining of uranium, hematite and pitchblende, as well as working with gas retorts, chromates, nickel and arsenic.

Pathology

Most carcinomas of the lung fall into one of four types:

1. *Squamous-cell (or epidermoid) carcinoma*, which accounts for 30–50% of cases of primary lung cancer
2. *Adenocarcinoma* (including alveolar-cell carcinoma), accounting for 15–35% of cases
3. *Large-cell anaplastic carcinoma*, accounting for 10–15% of cases
4. *Small (oat) cell carcinoma*, accounting for 20–30% of cases.

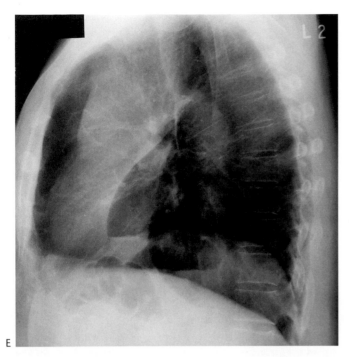

E

Fig. 14.3 Squamous-cell carcinoma of bronchus — natural history over 3 years in a patient who declined treatment. **A.** A small soft-tissue nodule is present in the left mid zone. **B.** 18 months later the tumor has enlarged and cavitated, and there is bulging of the aortopulmonary window, indicating lymph node enlargement. **C.** A further 6 months later, the tumor has further enlarged, and a fluid level is present in the cavity. Patchy consolidation is present in the left upper lobe. **D** and **E.** A further 3 months later there is now complete collapse of the left upper lobe, and the left hemidiaphragm is elevated due to phrenic nerve involvement.

Some lung cancers do not fall neatly into one of these categories, and may have components that resemble more than one type, e.g. *adenosquamous carcinomas*. Other rarer tumors are classified separately, e.g. *clear-cell carcinoma*, *basal-cell carcinoma* and *carcinosarcoma*.

Approximately 50% of lung cancers arise centrally, i.e. in or proximal to segmental bronchi (Fig. 14.1). The tumor arises in the bronchial mucosa and invades the bronchial wall. Tumor may grow around the bronchus and also into the bronchial lumen. Obstruction of the lumen leads to collapse, and often infection, in the lung distal to the tumor. Tumors that arise peripherally appear as soft-tissue nodules or irregular masses (Fig. 14.2), and invade the adjacent tissues. Signs of collapse or consolidation may occur, but are less obvious than with central tumors. Both central and peripheral tumors may be associated with hilar or mediastinal lymph node enlargement, and this is also a potential cause of central airway obstruction (Fig. 14.3). The tumor may also undergo central necrosis leading to cavitation. Peripheral tumors sometimes arise in pulmonary scars, and there is evidence that pulmonary fibrosis predisposes to neoplastic change. Although lung cancer usually presents as a single primary tumor, synchronous tumors are not rare (Fig. 14.4). Metastases from lung cancer may occur anywhere in the body, but hilar, mediastinal and supraclavicular lymph nodes are the commonest sites, followed by the liver, bones, brain, adrenal glands and skin. Lung cancer is a common cause of *lymphangitis carcinomatosa*.

The different cell types of lung cancer tend to show differences in behavior. *Squamous-cell cancers* tend to arise centrally, grow

relatively slowly and cavitate more often than other cell types. *Adenocarcinomas* usually arise peripherally, sometimes in fibrotic lung, and cavitate less often. *Small-cell tumors* have the fastest rate of growth and are usually disseminated at the time of presentation. They are usually central and are typically associated with mediastinal and hilar adenopathy, but rarely cavitate.

Clinical Presentation

Respiratory symptoms such as cough, wheeze, sputum production, breathlessness, chest discomfort and hemoptysis are the commonest presenting symptoms in patients with lung cancer. Other presentations include finger clubbing, superior vena caval obstruction, Horner's-syndrome, chest wall pain, dysphagia and signs of pericardial tamponade. An abnormal chest X-ray is a common presentation in patients who are symptom-free or who have non-specific symptoms. Patients may also present with symptoms of metastatic disease such as bone pain or signs of an intracranial tumor or general debility. Pneumonia, particularly if it does not respond to treatment, may be due to an underlying neoplasm. A small number of patients present with paraneoplastic syndromes such as hypertrophic osteoarthropathy, endocrine disturbance (e.g. inappropriate ADH secretion, Cushing's syndrome, hypercalcemia), peripheral neuropathy and recurrent peripheral venous thrombosis.

Radiological Features

The radiological features of lung cancer are a reflection of the pathology, and depend upon the size and site of the tumor and its histology.

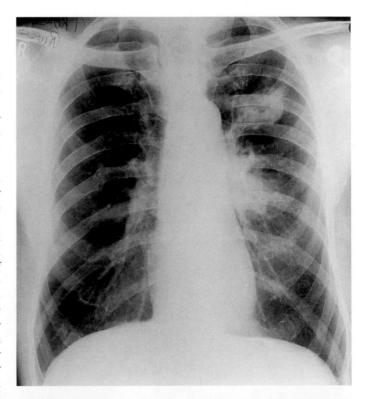

Fig. 14.4 Synchronous bronchial carcinomas. The soft-tissue mass overlying the left hilum was an adenocarcinoma in the apical segment of left lower lobe, and the mass in the left upper zone was an upper lobe squamous-cell carcinoma.

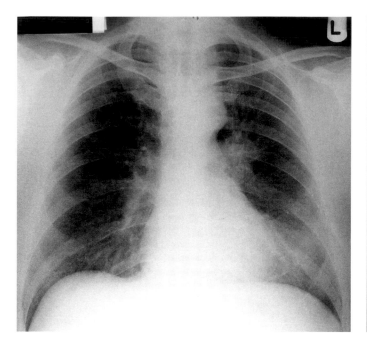

Fig. 14.5 Carcinoma of bronchus. The left hilum is enlarged by lymphadenopathy due to adenocarcinoma. The primary tumor is not visible.

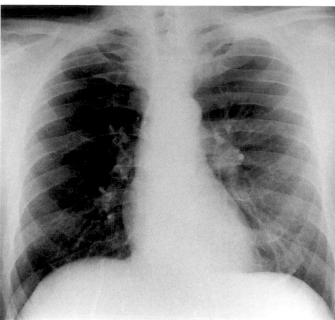

Fig. 14.6 Carcinoma of bronchus. Chest X-ray shows a dense left hilum, but no definite mass. Bronchoscopy showed a squamous carcinoma in the left main bronchus.

1. Hilar Enlargement This is a common radiographic manifestation of lung cancer. If the primary tumor is central this represents the tumor itself (Fig. 14.1). If the tumor is peripheral, it represents metastasis to bronchopulmonary lymph nodes (Fig. 14.5), and the primary tumor may or may not be visible. Occasionally, hilar involvement is subtle and presents as increased density of the hilum rather than as enlargement (Fig. 14.6). The true extent of nodal disease is best demonstrated by CT (Fig. 14.7) or MRI. Extensive hilar and mediastinal lymphadenopathy is frequently seen with small-cell tumors.

2. Airway Obstruction Bronchial narrowing due to tumor growth eventually causes collapse of the lung distal to the tumor. Depending on the location of the tumor, segmental or lobar collapse (Fig. 14.3) or, less often, collapse of an entire lung (Fig. 14.8) may be

Fig. 14.7 Carcinoma of bronchus. **A.** Chest X-ray shows a soft-tissue nodule in the left mid zone and prominence of the left hilum. **B.** Contrast-enhanced CT on lung window confirms left lower lobe mass, which proved to be an adenocarcinoma. **C** and **D.** CT on mediastinal windows shows left hilar lymphadenopathy, but more importantly there is very extensive mediastinal adenopathy surrounding the pulmonary arteries and extending into the subcarinal region and down into the azygo-esophageal recess.

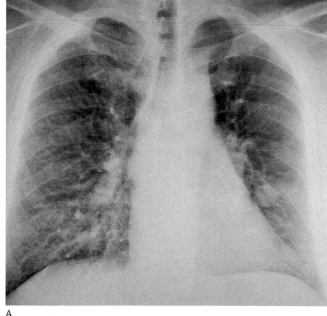

A

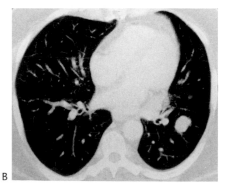

B

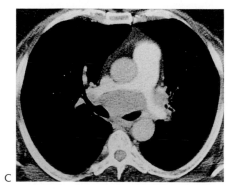

C

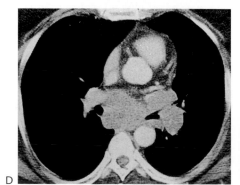

D

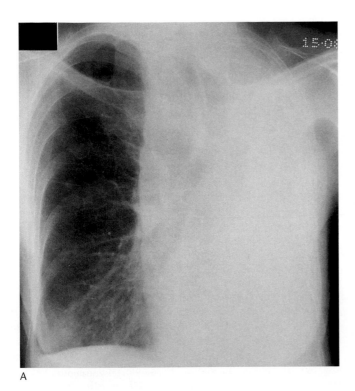

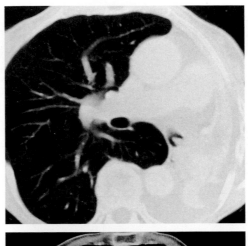

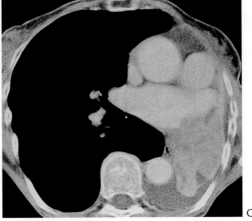

Fig. 14.8 Carcinoma of bronchus. **A.** Chest X-ray shows collapse of left lung. **B.** Contrast-enhanced CT on lung window confirms collapsed left lung, shows small pleural effusion and demonstrates tumor extending into the left main bronchus. **C.** CT on mediastinal window demonstrates tumor invading posterior wall of left atrium (confirmed at surgery).

seen. Prior to collapse of a lobe or segment, infection may develop distal to the bronchial obstruction. Consequently, segmental or lobar consolidation may be a manifestation of lung cancer, and since this is secondary to bronchial occlusion an air bronchogram is usually absent. As the primary tumor may be obscured by surrounding consolidation, the possibility of an underlying endobronchial lesion should always be considered in cases of segmental or lobar pneumonia which do not resolve despite appropriate treatment. Occasionally a tumor arising in a segmental or sub-

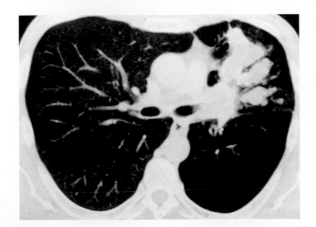

Fig. 14.9 Bronchocele due to carcinoma of bronchus. CT shows dilated, fluid-filled bronchi in lingula, secondary to carcinoma at left hilum.

segmental bronchus will lead to mucoid impaction and the development of a bronchocele or mucocele (Fig. 14.9).

3. Peripheral Mass A peripheral pulmonary mass on the chest X-ray is a common presentation of lung cancer (Figs 14.2, 14.3). If other features are present, such as hilar enlargement or bony metastases, then the malignant nature of the mass is easily appreciated (Fig. 14.1). Frequently, however, a mass is the only apparent abnormality and then the differential diagnosis is more difficult. There are no radiological features that can reliably differentiate between a benign and a malignant pulmonary nodule or mass. However, malignant tumors are usually larger than benign lesions at the time of presentation. Furthermore, peripheral lung cancers tend to have poorly defined, lobulated or umbilicated margins, or may appear spiculated (Fig. 14.10). *Satellite opacities* around the main lesion are more frequently seen with benign masses, but may be associated with carcinomas (Fig. 14.10). Diffuse or central *calcification* in a peripheral pulmonary mass is very suggestive of a benign lesion, but occasionally a calcified granuloma will have been engulfed by a malignant tumor. Bronchial carcinomas usually have a *doubling time* of between 1 and 18 months. Therefore, comparison with previous X-rays can be very helpful, and any mass or nodule that has not changed in appearance over a 2-year period is almost certainly benign.

Cavitation is visible in about 10–15% of peripheral lung cancers on plain X-rays (Figs. 14.3, 14.11) and is better demonstrated by CT (Fig. 14.12). It is due to either central necrosis of the tumor or abscess formation secondary to bronchial obstruction, and a fluid

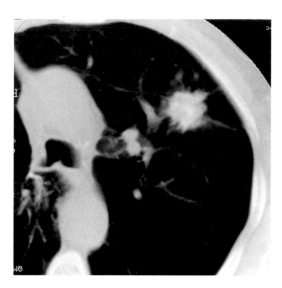

Fig. 14.10 Adenocarcinoma of bronchus. CT shows spiculated, soft-tissue mass with strands of tissue extending into the adjacent lung parenchyma.

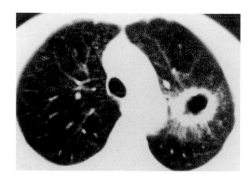

Fig. 14.12 Squamous-cell carcinoma of bronchus. CT shows a thick-walled cavitating mass with a spiculated outer surface and nodular inner surface.

level may be present within the cavity. Typically, malignant cavities are thick-walled with an irregular, nodular inner margin, but some may appear thin-walled. Since lung cancers tend to be associated with bronchial occlusion they virtually never show an air broncho-gram on the plain X-ray. However, it is not unusual to see an air bronchogram on the CT of an adenocarcinoma, and it is a common finding in alveolar-cell carcinoma.

Bronchial carcinomas arising at the lung apex were formerly regarded as an entity distinct from other lung cancers and were known as *Pancoast* or *superior sulcus tumors*. Histologically they are similar to other primary carcinomas of the lung. However, because of their location they have a tendency to invade ribs, the spine, the brachial plexus and the inferior cervical sympathetic ganglia. The plain film may show an obvious mass with associated bone destruction (Fig. 14.13), but frequently only asymmetric apical pleural thickening is visible, and the full extent of the tumor is best demonstrated by CT or MRI (Fig. 14.14). Bone involvement is often best shown by CT, but MRI can produce images in the coronal and sagittal planes which are ideal for

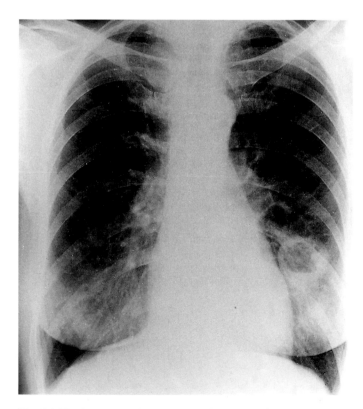

Fig. 14.11 Squamous-cell carcinoma of bronchus. Chest X-ray shows a cavitating mass with a fluid level in the left mid zone.

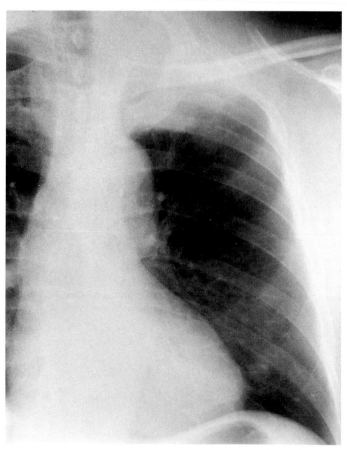

Fig. 14.13 Pancoast tumor. Chest X-ray shows a left apical mass with destruction of the second and third ribs posteriorly.

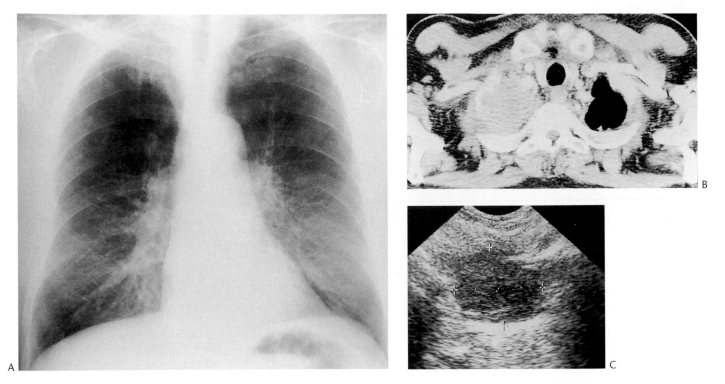

Fig. 14.14 Pancoast tumor. **A.** Chest X-ray shows asymmetric right apical pleural thickening. **B.** CT shows large right apical soft-tissue mass extending through chest wall into apex of right axilla. **C.** Ultrasound scan from right supraclavicular fossa shows apical pulmonary mass of relatively low echogenicity, and demonstrates the easiest route of access for percutaneous biopsy.

demonstrating the relationship of the tumor to the brachial plexus and subclavian vessels, and for showing involvement of the extrapleural fat over the lung apex (Fig. 14.15). However, for the purpose of percutaneous biopsy, these tumors are often most conveniently visualized by ultrasound scanning from the supraclavicular fossa (Fig. 14.14C).

4. Mediastinal Involvement Enlargement of mediastinal lymph nodes is a typical feature of small-cell tumors, but occurs with other bronchial carcinomas. The mediastinum appears widened and may have a lobulated outline (Fig. 14.16). In non-small-cell tumors lymph node involvement is less florid, and since its full extent may not be appreciated on the chest X-ray it is

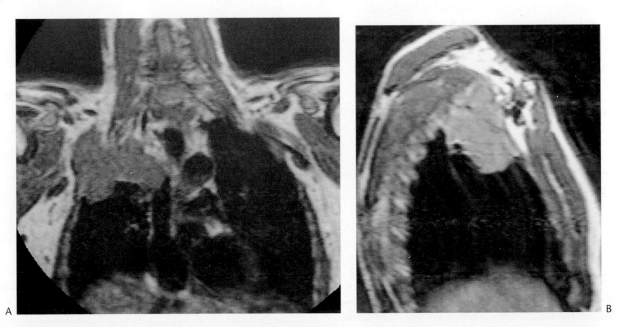

Fig. 14.15 Pancoast tumor. T_1-weighted coronal **A.** and sagittal **B.** MRI shows precise extent of right apical mass with obliteration of the extrapleural fat where the mass invades the chest wall and enters the root of the neck.

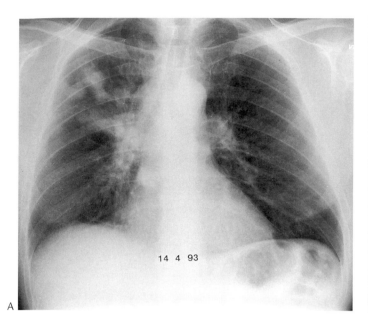

Fig. 14.16   Small-cell carcinoma of bronchus. **A.** Chest X-ray shows right upper lobe masses and extensive right paratracheal and right hilar lymphadenopathy. 5 months later, following chemotherapy the disease was in remission and the X-ray was normal. **B.** A further 2 months later the tumor has recurred with enlargement of the heart shadow due to pericardial effusion (confirmed by echocardiography).

best assessed non-invasively by CT or MRI (Figs 14.7A, 14.17B).

Enlarged mediastinal lymph nodes or central tumors may distort the *esophagus*. Barium swallow may, therefore, be used to assess the mediastinum, and is essential in patients with dysphagia (Fig. 14.18). In these patients esophageal compression or invasion may be demonstrated. Mediastinal invasion may involve the *phrenic nerve*, and in patients with lung cancer elevation of a hemidiaphragm suggests this complication or may be due to pulmonary collapse or subphrenic disease. Fluoroscopy or ultrasound scan of the diaphragm may be used to determine if an elevated dome moves paradoxically and is paralyzed.

Mediastinal spread of tumor may also cause *superior vena caval obstruction*, and this may be confirmed by superior vena cavography, dynamically enhanced CT or MRI. Invasion of the pericardium by metastatic lymph nodes or the primary tumor itself may result in pericarditis and pericardial effusion (Fig. 14.16).

5. Pleural Involvement   Pleural effusion may be due to direct spread of the tumor but may also be the result of lymphatic obstruction or be secondary to an obstructive pneumonitis. Pleural effusion also occurs as a sympathetic response to the tumor, in which case there is no cytologic or histologic evidence of pleural malignancy. Rarely, a cavitating subpleural tumor will cause a spontaneous pneumothorax.

6. Bone Involvement   Peripheral carcinomas may invade the ribs or spine directly (Figs 14.13–15). Hematogenous metastases from lung to bone are usually osteolytic (Fig. 14.1). They are often painful, and are identified earliest by isotope bone scan. Bone pain, particularly in the wrists, hands, ankles and feet, may also be due to hypertrophic osteoarthropathy. On plain films the affected bones show well-defined periosteal new bone formation. Isotope bone scan may be positive before radiographic changes are visible.

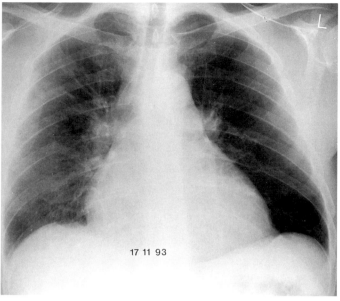

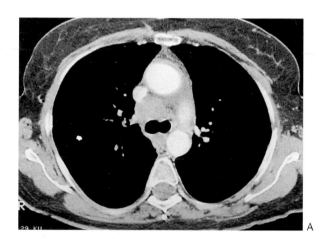

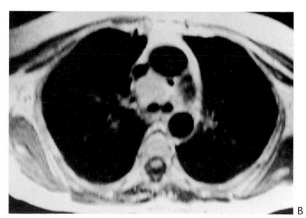

Fig. 14.17   Carcinoma of bronchus. Contrast-enhanced CT scan **A** and T₁-weighted MRI scan **B.** Axial scans at level of carina show similar anatomic detail, with retrocaval lymphadenopathy. In general, CT provides better spatial resolution, but MRI has better natural contrast.

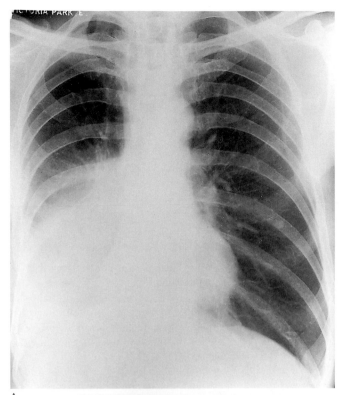

A

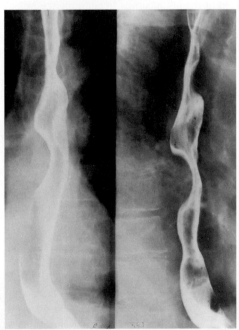

B

Fig. 14.18 Carcinoma of bronchus. **A.** Chest X-ray shows collapse and consolidation of right lower lobe. **B.** Barium swallow performed to investigate dysphagia shows extrinsic compression of mid esophagus by enlarged subcarinal lymph nodes.

Diagnostic Imaging and the Management of Carcinoma of the Bronchus

Imaging makes an important contribution to three aspects of the management of lung cancer. These are:

1. Making the diagnosis
2. Staging the tumor
3. Assessing treatment.

1. Making the Diagnosis The prognosis and treatment of lung cancer depends upon the general condition of the patient and on the histology of the tumor and its extent at the time of presentation. Small-cell tumors metastasize early and are usually disseminated at the time of presentation. Non-small-cell tumors metastasize later, the natural history of squamous-cell carcinoma being longer than that of adenocarcinoma and undifferentiated large-cell carcinoma. Moreover, small-cell tumors are more sensitive to chemotherapy than non-small-cell tumors. Therefore, when planning treatment it is important to know the histology of the tumor. Sputum cytology and bronchoscopic biopsies or washings usually provide the cell type of central tumors, but peripheral tumors may require percutaneous biopsy. This may be done with fluoroscopic, CT or ultrasound guidance (Fig. 14.19). Depending on the needle used the specimens may be suitable for cytologic or histologic evaluation, but in either case it is important to have available a pathologist skilled in examining small specimens.

2. Staging the Tumor Without treatment only about 1% of patients with lung cancer will survive 3 years from the time of diagnosis. Currently the main hopes for curative treatment lie with surgery for non-small-cell cancer, and chemotherapy for small-cell tumors. The main purposes of accurate staging of lung cancer are:

1. To identify those patients with non-small-cell tumors who will benefit from surgery
2. To avoid surgery in those who will not benefit, and
3. To provide accurate data for assessing and comparing different methods of treatment.

The TNM system (Table 14.1), where T describes the primary tumor, N the regional lymph nodes and M distant metastases, is widely used. The International Staging System (Table 14.2) based on the TNM system is designed to be used by thoracic surgeons

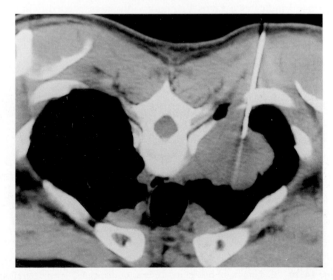

Fig. 14.19 Carcinoma of bronchus. CT of prone patient during percutaneous biopsy. The end of the biopsy needle is in the tumor.

Table 14.1   TNM Definitions for the International Staging System for Lung Cancer

Primary tumor (T)

TX	Tumor proved by the presence of malignant cells in bronchopulmonary secretions but not visualized roentgenographically or bronchoscopically, or any tumor that cannot be assessed as in a retreatment staging
TO	No evidence of primary tumor
T1S	Carcinoma in situ
T1	A tumor that is 3 cm or less in greatest dimension, surrounded by lung or visceral pleura, and without evidence of invasion proximal to a lobar bronchus at bronchoscopy
T2	A tumor more than 3 cm in greatest dimension, or a tumor of any size that either invades the visceral pleura or has associated atelectasis or obstructive pneumonitis extending to the hilar region. At bronchoscopy the proximal extent of demonstrable tumor must be within a lobar bronchus or at least 2 cm distal to the carina. Any associated atelectasis or obstructive pneumonitis must involve less than an entire lung
T3	A tumor of any size with direct extension into the chest wall (including superior sulcus tumors), diaphragm, or the mediastinal pleura or pericardium without involving the heart, great vessels, trachea, esophagus, or vertebral body; or a tumor in the main bronchus within 2 cm of the carina without involving the carina
T4	A tumor of any size with invasion of the mediastinum or involving the heart, great vessels, trachea, esophagus, vertebral body, or carina, or presence of malignant pleural effusion

Nodal involvement (N)

N0	No demonstrable metastasis to regional lymph nodes
N1	Metastasis to lymph nodes in the peribronchial or the ipsilateral hilar region, or both, including direct extension
N2	Metastasis to ipsilateral mediastinal lymph nodes and subcarinal lymph nodes
N3	Metastasis to contralateral mediastinal lymph nodes, contralateral hilar lymph nodes, ipsilateral or contralateral scalene, or supraclavicular lymph nodes

Distant metastasis (M)

M0	No (known) distant metastasis
M1	Distant metastasis present—specify sites

(From Mountain 1986.)

Table 14.2   Stages for International Staging System for Lung Cancer

Stage	Definition*
I	T1, N0, M0
	T2, N0, M0
II	T1, N1, M0
	T2, N1, M0
IIIA	T3, N0, M0
	T3, N1, M0
	T1–3, N2, M0
IIIB	Any T, N3, M0
	T4; any N, M0
IV	Any T; any N, M1

*See Table 14.1
(From Mountain 1986.)

considering tumor resection and by radiotherapists and oncologists treating more extensive disease.

Stage I indicates a T1 or T2 tumor without associated lymphadenopathy or distant metastases; such a tumor is likely to be amenable to surgical resection. Stage II tumors are similar primary tumors, but have associated ipsilateral hilar adenopathy; they are also potentially surgically curable, but the prognosis is less favorable. Stage IIIA tumors have extensive local intrathoracic disease which may be amenable to surgical resection; Stage IIIB tumors have local intrathoracic disease that is too extensive for resection, but may be treatable with radical radiotherapy. Stage IV tumors have distant metastases.

Thus, a tumor is likely to be inoperable if it extends directly into parietal pleura, chest wall, diaphragm or mediastinum, or is within 2.0 cm of the main carina. In addition, metastasis to contralateral hilar nodes, mediastinal nodes or more distantly precludes surgical cure. The plain chest film should be carefully scrutinized for evidence of spread of tumor. If the tumor appears localized and appears operable on bronchoscopy, *isotope bone scan* and *liver ultrasound* may be performed and, if the tumor still appears operable, the mediastinum should be assessed by CT or MRI (Fig. 14.20). Any node over 2 cm in diameter is likely to be involved, and nodes of 1 cm or less are usually regarded as normal. Nodes between 1 and 2 cm present a diagnostic problem, and the ability of CT to predict involvement by tumor is limited. However if the enlarged nodes are those that most directly drain the lung tumor, and other mediastinal lymph nodes are normal in size, the likelihood of malignant involvement is increased. In equivocal cases *mediastinoscopy* is indicated prior to subjecting the patient to thoracotomy. Positron-emission tomography using fluorodeoxy-

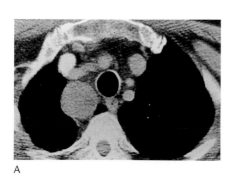

A

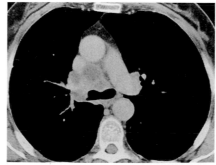

B

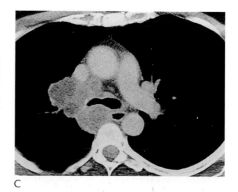

C

Fig. 14.20   Carcinoma of bronchus. Contrast-enhanced CT demonstration of mediastinal lymphadenopathy in 3 different patients. **A.** An enlarged right paratracheal node. **B.** Retrocaval and right hilar adenopathy. Ring enhancement of the glands indicates central necrosis. **C.** Retrocaval, subcarinal and right hilar adenopathy.

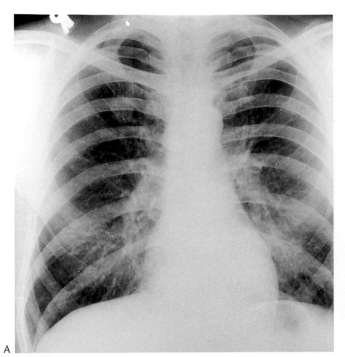
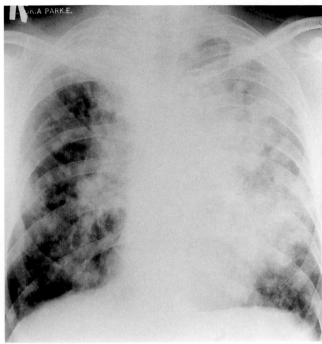

A
B

Fig. 14.21   Alveolar-cell carcinoma. **A.** Chest X-ray shows solitary right upper zone mass suggesting focal disease. **B.** 8 months later, despite right upper lobectomy (note excised sixth rib) the disease has rapidly progressed to the diffuse pattern with widespread nodules and consolidation.

glucose is a recently developed technique which may be useful in identifying lymph node involvement, and also more distant disease.

3. Assessing Treatment   Following chemotherapy for small-cell cancer, bulky mediastinal and hilar nodes and peripheral lesions may show complete regression (Fig. 14.16). Follow-up chest X-rays are required to detect local recurrence, although recurrent disease is often extrathoracic. These patients are also prone to opportunistic infections. Following radiotherapy radiation pneumonitis and pulmonary fibrosis may occur, and radiation esophagitis may be a consequence of mediastinal irradiation. Postoperative appearances are discussed in Chapter 18.

Alveolar-cell Carcinoma

Alveolar-cell carcinoma is also known as bronchiolar or bronchiolo-alveolar carcinoma, and is a subtype of adenocarcinoma with certain special features. It arises more peripherally than typical lung cancer, probably from type II pneumocytes. It accounts for 2–5% of all lung cancers, usually occurring between the ages of 50 and 70 years with an equal sex incidence. It is not associated with smoking but may be associated with diffuse pulmonary fibrosis and pulmonary scars.

These tumors arise within alveoli and produce areas of consolidation. It is uncertain whether they originate multi-centrically or focally; clinically two patterns are seen. The focal form arises as a solitary peripheral mass (Fig. 14.21) in which, unlike other forms of lung cancer, an air bronchogram is often visible. The diffuse form manifests itself as multiple acinar shadows throughout the lungs, often with areas of confluence, and the appearance may resemble pulmonary edema or bronchopneumonia. These features are elegantly demonstrated by CT which may

show any combination of ground-glass opacification, small nodular opacities, frank consolidation and thickened interlobular septa (Fig. 14.22). The focal form may spread via the airways and progress to the diffuse pattern (Fig. 14.21).

Metastatic Lung Disease

Metastases most commonly reach the lung hematogenously via the systemic veins and pulmonary arteries. They may originate at any site, but primary tumors of the breast, skeleton and urogenital system account for approximately 80% of pulmonary metastases. Lymphatic spread is less common and endobronchial spread is rare, usually being a manifestation of alveolar-cell carcinoma.

Approximately 3% of asymptomatic pulmonary nodules are metastases. The commonest primary tumors producing solitary pulmonary metastases are carcinomas of the *colon, kidney* and *breast*, *testicular tumors*, *bone sarcomas* and *malignant melanoma*. In about 75% of cases metastatic lung disease presents as multiple pulmonary nodules. Metastases to the lung are usually bilateral, affecting both lungs equally, with a basal predominance (Fig. 14.23). They are often peripheral and may be subpleural (Fig. 14.24).

Pulmonary metastases vary in size from a few millimeters in diameter (Fig. 14.25) to several centimeters. They tend to be spherical with a well-defined margin. An ill-defined margin may signify hemorrhage. *Cavitation* may occur in metastases from any primary site, but is more common in squamous carcinomas (Fig. 14.26) and sarcomas. Cavitation of a subpleural metastasis is a recognized cause of spontaneous pneumothorax. *Calcification* is unusual in pulmonary metastases, being seen most often in osteogenic sarcoma (Fig. 14.27), and rarely in chondrosarcoma and mucinous adenocarcinoma.

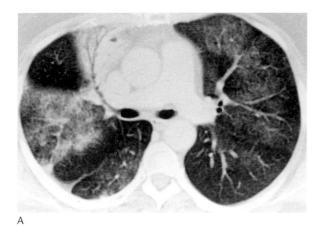

A

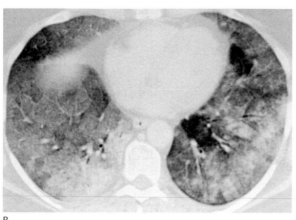

B

Fig. 14.22 Alveolar-cell carcinoma. **A, B** CT shows diffuse, small, nodular shadows, widespread ground-glass opacification and dense consolidation with an air bronchogram in the anterior segment of the right upper lobe.

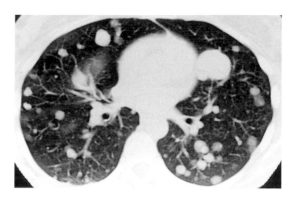

Fig. 14.24 Pulmonary metastases. Soft-tissue sarcoma. CT shows subpleural location of several of the metastases.

Endobronchial metastases are rare, the commonest primary tumors being carcinoma of kidney, breast and large bowel. They may occlude the airway and cause segmental or lobar collapse.

Lymphangitis Carcinomatosa This results from hematogenous metastases invading and occluding peripheral pulmonary lymphatics. The commonest primary sites are carcinoma of the lung, breast, stomach, pancreas, cervix and prostate. Lymphangitis carcinomatosa is usually bilateral, but lung and breast cancer may cause unilateral lymphangitis (Fig. 14.28). The chest X-ray shows coarse, linear, reticular and nodular basal shadowing, often with pleural effusions and hilar lymphadenopathy (Fig. 14.29). In the early stages of lung involvement the chest X-ray may suggest lymphangitis, but may not be diagnostic. In these cases a high-resolution CT scan may be undertaken to establish the diagnosis, when the typical appearance is nodular thickening of the inter-

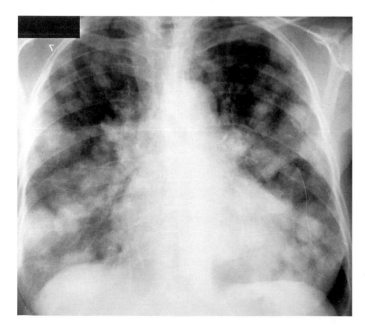

Fig. 14.23 Pulmonary metastases. Adenocarcinoma from unknown primary. Multiple, well-defined round opacities are present throughout both lungs.

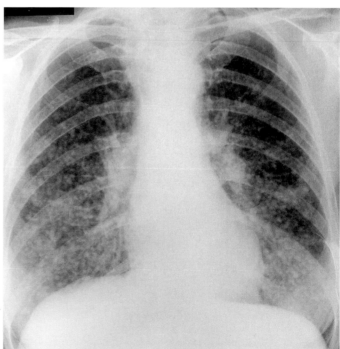

Fig. 14.25 Pulmonary metastases. Adenocarcinoma from unknown primary. Multiple small nodules are present throughout both lungs.

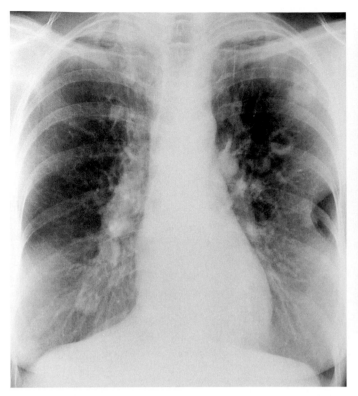

Fig. 14.26 Pulmonary metastases. Carcinoma of cervix. Multiple cavitating masses are present in both lungs.

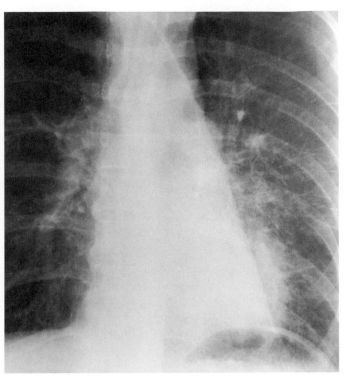

Fig. 14.28 Unilateral lymphangitis carcinomatosa. Carcinoma of the left lower lobe. There are several horizontal septal lines in the periphery of the left lung.

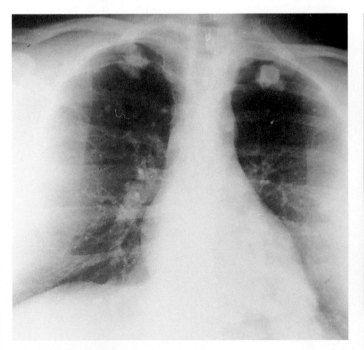

Fig. 14.27 Pulmonary metastases. Osteogenic sarcoma. Densely calcified masses are present in both lungs.

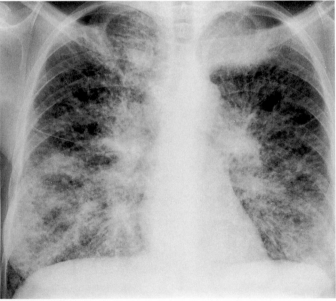

Fig. 14.29 Lymphangitis carcinomatosa. Carcinoma of cervix. Coarse reticular shadowing is present throughout both lungs, and there is bilateral hilar lymphadenopathy.

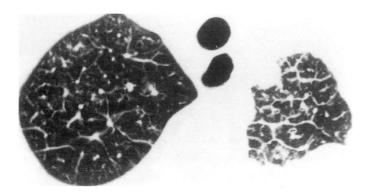

Fig. 14.30 Lymphangitis carcinomatosa. Breast cancer. HRCT shows marked nodular thickening of the interlobular septa and thickening of the centrilobular bronchovascular bundles in the left upper lobe, and early similar changes in the right upper lobe.

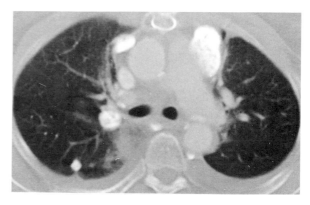

Fig. 14.32 Hodgkin's disease. CT shows extensive calcification in mediastinal lymph nodes in a patient previously treated for Hodgkin's disease.

lobular septa and thickening of the centrilobular bronchovascular bundles (Fig. 14.30).

INTRATHORACIC LYMPHOMA AND LEUKEMIA

Hodgkin's Disease

Hodgkin's disease is the commonest lymphoma. It is distinguished from other lymphomas by the presence of Reed–Sternberg cells. It is the commonest neoplasm of young adults with a peak incidence at 25–29 years of age, and a second, smaller peak at 70–74 years. The disease usually arises in lymph nodes, and hilar or mediastinal lymph node enlargement is seen

on the chest X-ray at the time of presentation in about 50% of cases. The lymphadenopathy is frequently bilateral but, unlike in sarcoidosis, it is often asymmetric and involves anterior mediastinal glands (Fig. 14.31). These retrosternal nodes may erode the sternum. CT may identify nodal disease not apparent on the chest X-ray, particularly in the retrosternal and paraspinal regions. Following treatment by radiotherapy or chemotherapy, lymph node calcification may occur (Fig. 14.32).

Involvement of lung parenchyma is seen in about 30% of cases. It is usually due to spread of disease from hilar lymph nodes along the peribronchial connective tissue space. The resulting pulmonary infiltrate may resemble lymphangitis carcinomatosa. Pulmonary involvement may also occur by direct extension from mediastinal lymph nodes across the pleura (Fig. 14.33). Lung

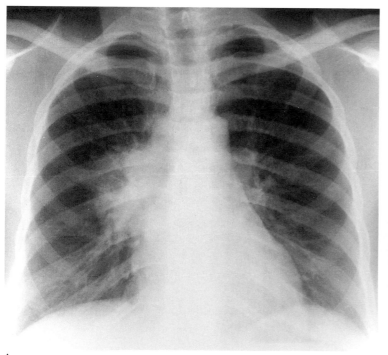

A

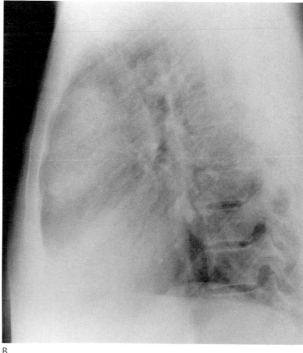

B

Fig. 14.31 Hodgkin's disease. **A.** Chest X-ray shows right hilar lymphadenopathy and the lateral film **B.** shows a large anterior mediastinal lymph node mass.

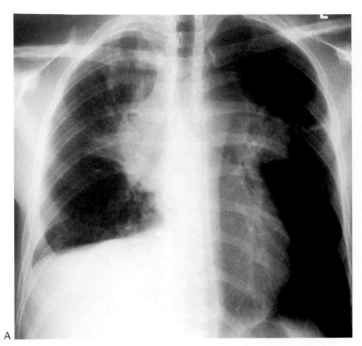

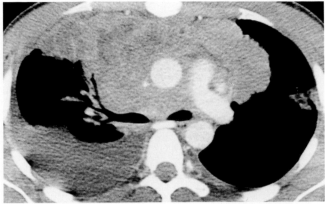

Fig. 14.33 Hodgkin's disease. **A.** Chest X-ray shows bilateral hilar adenopathy, mediastinal adenopathy, right upper lobe pulmonary shadowing and a right pleural effusion. **B.** Contrast-enhanced CT shows massive anterior mediastinal adenopathy, with direct infiltration of the right upper lobe and a large pleural effusion.

involvement in the absence of lymphadenopathy is rare if the patient has not already been treated. The pulmonary infiltrate may also appear as solitary areas of consolidation, larger confluent areas or miliary nodules. The pulmonary opacities may have an air bronchogram (Fig. 14.34) and may cavitate. Involvement of the bronchial wall may lead to areas of collapse and consolidation in the peripheral lung.

Pleural effusion occurs in approximately 30% of cases and is usually due to lymphatic obstruction. Pleural involvement by the disease itself is less common, but is a cause of pleural plaques and effusion.

Non-Hodgkin's Lymphoma

This group of diseases comprises nodular and diffuse lymphomas. The former were formerly known as giant follicular lymphoma and the latter included chronic lymphocytic leukemia, lymphosarcoma and reticulum-cell sarcoma or diffuse histiocytic lymphoma.

The radiographic manifestations of Hodgkin's and non-Hodgkin's lymphomas are similar (Fig. 14.35). However, the progression of

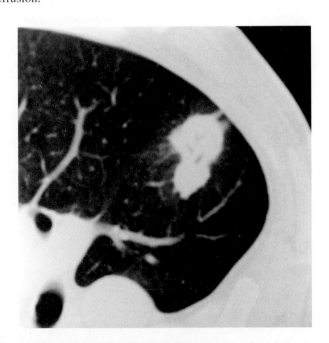

Fig. 14.34 Pulmonary lymphoma. CT shows an irregular soft-tissue mass with an air bronchogram.

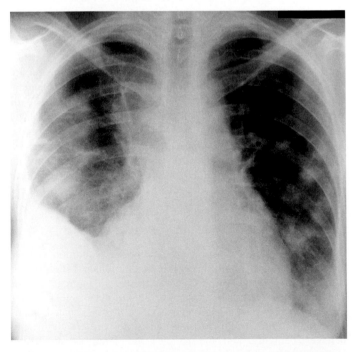

Fig. 14.35 Histiocytic lymphoma. Chest X-ray shows mediastinal adenopathy, multiple ill-defined pulmonary nodules and a right pleural effusion.

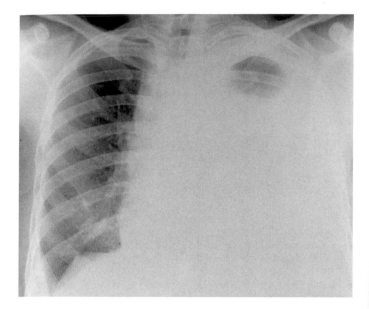

Fig. 14.36 Lymphocytic lymphoma. Chest X-ray shows a large left pleural effusion, a small right pleural effusion and right paratracheal adenopathy.

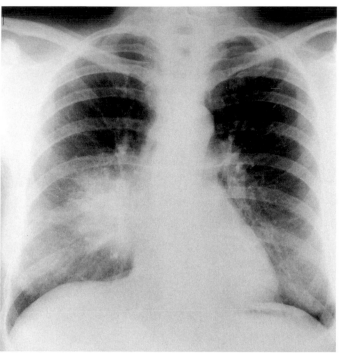

Fig. 14.37 Pseudolymphoma. Consolidation in the right middle lobe obscures the right hilum and heart border.

disease in the non-Hodgkin's group is less orderly with pulmonary and pleural involvement often preceding mediastinal disease. There is also a greater tendency for the pulmonary infiltrates to traverse fissures and involve the pleura (Fig. 14.36).

Leukemia

Radiographic abnormalities of the chest in leukemia are more commonly a manifestation of a complication of the disease rather than due to the disease itself. These complications include pneumonia, opportunistic infection, heart failure, pulmonary hemorrhage and reactions to therapy (drugs, transfusions and radiotherapy).

Mediastinal lymph node enlargement and pleural effusion are the commonest radiographic abnormalities due to leukemia. Mediastinal lymphadenopathy is unusual without evidence of lymphadenopathy elsewhere. It occurs most frequently in lymphatic and monocytic leukemias, but is rare in myeloid leukemia. Leukemic infiltrates in the lung are often a terminal event and are commoner in lymphatic leukemia than myeloid leukemia. The chest X-ray shows either bilateral streaky or reticular shadows similar to lymphangitis carcinomatosa or patchy consolidation.

Other Lymphoid Disorders

Pseudolymphoma This is a rare tumor-like condition characterized by solitary or multiple areas of pulmonary consolidation (Fig. 14.37), which are predominantly due to aggregations of mature lymphocytes and variable numbers of plasma cells. An air bronchogram is often visible and cavitation may occur. Lymphadenopathy and pleural effusion are rarely present. It usually behaves benignly, and the patients are often asymptomatic. However, there have been cases in which it appears to have undergone malignant transformation to pulmonary lymphoma.

Lymphocytic Interstitial Pneumonitis (LIP) This condition is microscopically similar to pseudolymphoma, but instead of being a focal abnormality it is characterized by a more diffuse interstitial infiltrate, and it may proceed to pulmonary fibrosis. It may develop as a solitary abnormality, or in association with a variety of autoimmune conditions such as Sjögren syndrome, but particularly in children there is an association with AIDS. Radiologically there is bilateral reticulonodular shadowing, sometimes with areas of consolidation, and there may be progression to honeycomb shadowing. Pleural effusions may occur, but lymphadenopathy is usually absent unless lymphomatous change occurs.

Lymphomatoid Granulomatosis This has been defined as 'an angiocentric, angiodestructive lymphoreticular, proliferative and granulomatous disease involving predominantly the lungs'. Hence, it was formerly thought of as a vasculitis. However, in approximately 50% of cases it progresses to a more typical lymphoma. Radiologically it usually appears as multiple ill-defined pulmonary nodules, often resembling metastases, although an air bronchogram is often seen. Cavitation occurs in about 10% of cases, but lymphadenopathy and pleural effusion are unusual.

PULMONARY SARCOMA

Although the lungs are a common site for metastatic sarcoma, primary sarcoma of the lung is rare. Prior to the AIDS epidemic ***Kaposi sarcoma*** occurred mostly as a tumor of skin; however, there are now increasing numbers of cases of pulmonary Kaposi sarcoma complicating AIDS. A localized form appears as segmental or lobar consolidation, but more commonly it is widespread with multiple nodular and linear opacities and areas of consolidation in both lungs. In addition, pleural effusions and hilar and mediastinal lymphadenopathy may be present.

Other primary pulmonary sarcomas may arise from any of the mesenchymal tissues in the lung. The most common are *fibrosarcoma*, *leiomyosarcoma* and *pulmonary artery angiosarcoma*; others include carcinosarcoma, pulmonary blastoma and malignant hemangiopericytoma. They most often present as a solitary pulmonary mass, radiographically indistinguishable from a carcinoma of the lung. Angiosarcoma of the pulmonary artery may present as a hilar mass and signs of pulmonary embolism and pulmonary arterial hypertension.

BRONCHIAL 'ADENOMA'

Bronchial 'adenoma' is a term that was formerly used to refer to a group of lesions that comprised two distinct pathological entities: carcinoid tumors and salivary gland type tumors. The salivary gland group is made up of adenoid cystic tumors (formerly known as cylindromas), mucoepidermoid tumors and mixed tumors. Carcinoids account for approximately 90% of bronchial 'adenomas' and adenoid cystic tumors for about 10%, the other salivary gland tumors being very rare. The term 'adenoma' implies a benign lesion, and since carcinoids and cylindromas may be locally invasive and may metastasize to local lymph nodes and beyond, the term has fallen into disuse.

Salivary Gland Type Tumors   These are mostly ***adenoid cystic carcinomas***, which usually arise in the trachea or major bronchi. They grow beneath the bronchial epithelium in a tubular fashion and extend outward into the bronchial wall. Local invasion is common. They present radiologically as a tumor mass with or without airway obstruction. ***Mucoepidermoid tumors*** are also locally invasive. ***Bronchial cystadenomas*** are small polypoidal tumors that project into the bronchial lumen and may, therefore, cause areas of atelectasis and infection, though they themselves are truly benign.

BRONCHIAL CARCINOID

Carcinoids are neuroendocrine tumors and are derived from bronchial APUD (amino precursor uptake decarboxylation) cells. These are the same cells which give rise to small-cell carcinoma. Bronchial carcinoids are described as either typical or atypical. Typical carcinoids tend to behave benignly, growing slowly and metastasizing infrequently. Atypical carcinoids have histologic and clinical features that lie between those of typical carcinoids and small-cell carcinoma, and approximately 50% will eventually metastasize.

Approximately 80% of carcinoids arise in lobar or main segmental bronchi (Fig. 14.38). Growth of tumor into the lumen may cause bronchial obstruction and collapse of the lung peripheral to the tumor. Lesser degrees of bronchial obstruction may result in recurrent segmental pneumonia, bronchiectasis or abscess formation, or air trapping in the lung distal to the tumor. If the tumor extends extrabronchially, lung infiltration may occur.

Peripheral carcinoids appear as well-circumscribed, round or ovoid solitary nodules (Fig. 14.39). On CT calcification may be seen within the tumor.

Carcinoids may produce a variety of hormones. These include serotonin, kallikrein, histamine, ACTH, insulin and substances

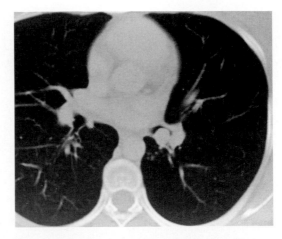

Fig. 14.38   Bronchial carcinoid. CT shows soft-tissue tumor in wall of left main bronchus, causing severe narrowing of the bronchial lumen.

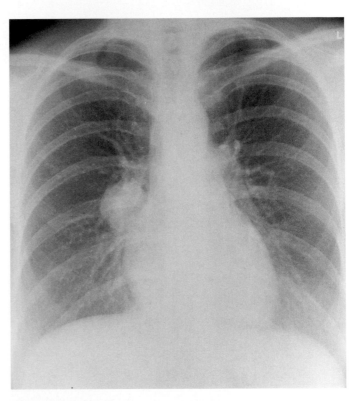

Fig. 14.39   Bronchial carcinoid. A well-defined, round, soft-tissue mass overlies the right hilum.

similar to antidiuretic hormone and gastrin. Rarely, production of these hormones may lead to clinical syndromes such as the carcinoid syndrome. Carcinoid syndrome due to a lung primary usually indicates hepatic metastases. Skeletal metastases from bronchial carcinoids may be osteoblastic.

PULMONARY HAMARTOMA

A hamartoma is a tumor which consists of an abnormal arrangement of the tissues normally found in the organ concerned. Most

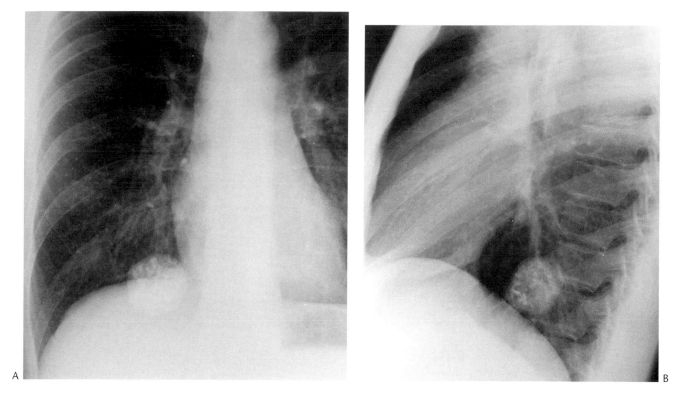

Fig. 14.40   Pulmonary hamartoma. **A, B** A well-defined, round soft-tissue mass with extensive, central 'popcorn' calcification is present in the right lower lobe.

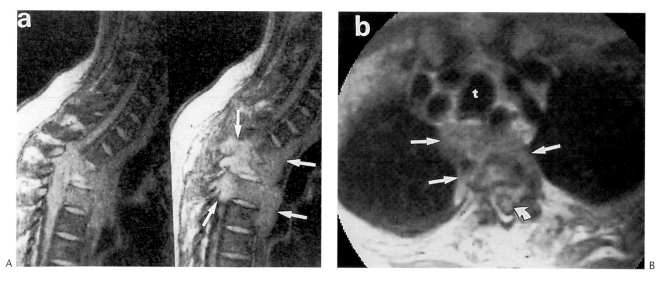

Fig 14.41   Posterior mediastinal carcinoma (straight arrows) infiltrating two adjacent thoracic vertebral bodies with partial collapse and extradural extension, on T_1-weighted (**A**) sagittal (spin echo 740/40) and (**B**) transverse (partial saturation recovery 500/18) scans. Note low signal from dural sac (curved arrow); t = trachea

pulmonary hamartomas have a large cartilaginous component, and there may also be an appreciable fatty component. They are rarely seen in childhood and most often present as a solitary pulmonary nodule in an asymptomatic adult. Unlike bronchial carcinoids, most pulmonary hamartomas are peripheral. They appear as well-circumscribed nodules varying in diameter from a few millimeters to several centimeters (Fig. 14.40). They do not

cavitate, and any low density within them represents fat. On the chest X-ray approximately 30% show calcification, often with a characteristic 'popcorn' appearance. On serial films they may be seen to grow slowly. CT may demonstrate or confirm the presence of fat or calcification within the nodule, allowing a precise diagnosis to be made. Rarely they arise endobronchially and may then present with signs of bronchial obstruction.

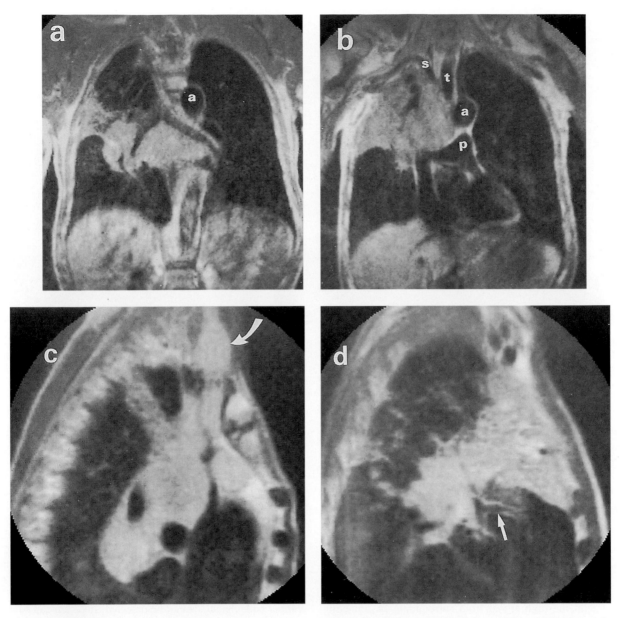

Fig 14.42 Carcinoma of the lung with lymphadenopathy and distal collapse/consolidation on (**A**, **B**) coronal T_1-weighted (spin echo 560/26) (**C,D**) parasagittal intermediate-weighted (spin echo 1200/60) images. The collapse/consolidation in the anterior and posterior segments of the right upper lobe shows heterogeneity and higher signal than the more uniform intensity of the central tumor, but clear separation is difficult. Nodal disease in the neck (curved arrow) is demonstrated in **C**. Straight arrow in **D** = middle lobe bronchus; a = aortic arch; p = left pulmonary artery; s = subclavian artery; t = trachea.

OTHER BENIGN PULMONARY TUMORS

This heading covers many rarities including *bronchial chondroma, pulmonary fibroma, pulmonary myxoma, plasma-cell granuloma (also known as histiocytoma, sclerosing granuloma, or inflammatory pseudotumor), bronchial lipoma, myoblastoma of the bronchus (or granular-cell tumor), bronchial papilloma* and *benign clear-cell tumor*. They are often asymptomatic, presenting as a solitary pulmonary nodule, although some may be multiple. Some may cause bronchial obstruction and therefore present with signs of lobar or segmental collapse or consolidation. In general, apart from lipomas, none of these tumors have features that allow a confident diagnosis based upon imaging alone.

MRI IN TUMORS OF THE LUNG

Jeremy P. R. Jenkins

CT is an established technique in the staging of lung carcinoma, with MRI currently used in a problem-solving role. Both CT and MRI are equally good at assessing tumor size. CT is more accurate in the demonstration of small nodules, except for those located close to hilar vessels, where MRI has the advantage. In tumors MRI has been shown to be more accurate than CT in evaluating mediastinal and vascular invasion. MR images of the lungs have a low signal-to-noise ratio (SNR). Contrast between tumor and lung is essentially independent of pulse sequence, due to the inherently low proton density and magnetic susceptibility between air and

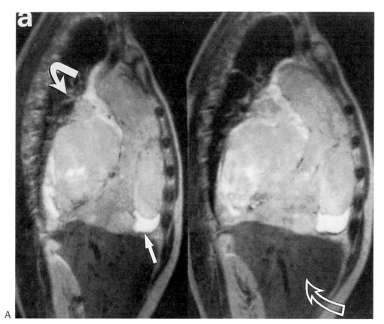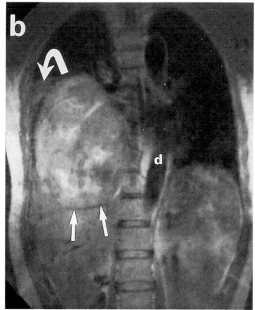

Fig 14.43 Large pleural fibrosarcoma compressing lung (curved closed arrow) and displacing liver (curved open arrow) on **A** two contiguous sagittal T$_2$-weighted (spin echo 1660/80) and **B** coronal T$_1$-weighted (spin echo 560/26) images. The liver is not directly infiltrated and neither is the anterior chest wall. The diaphragm can be seen as a low-intensity line (straight arrows), most clearly beneath a small anterior pleural effusion in **A**. d = descending aorta **C** (Reproduced with permission from: Jenkins, J.P.R. (1990) Magnetic resonance imaging in oncology. In: Johnson, R. J., Eddleston, B., Hunter, R. D. (eds) *Radiology in the Management of Cancer*. Edinburgh: Churchill Livingstone.)

soft tissue with aerated lung. Contrast and detail can be improved by enhancement of the mass with gadolinium-chelate. A major disadvantage of MRI compared with CT is that peripheral pulmonary vessels and lobar fissures are not visualized, making it difficult to demonstrate the position of a lung mass with respect to a lobe or segment.

Superior sulcus tumors can be better visualized by MRI than by CT, due to improved anatomic display on coronal and sagittal plane images (Fig 14.41). In a study of 31 patients with a superior sulcus tumor, the accuracy of MRI in the evaluation of tumor invasion of adjacent structures was 94%, compared with 63% by CT. T$_1$-weighted images showed the tumor as intermediate signal in contrast with the high signal from surrounding fat, enabling better delineation of chest wall invasion, adjacent vessels, brachial plexus, and spinal structures.

In a small series of patients with proximal lung carcinoma and distal lobar collapse, evaluated by dynamic contrast-enhanced CT and MRI, CT was more successful than MRI in differentiating tumor mass from collapsed lung (Fig 14.42). Dynamic contrast-enhanced CT was able to differentiate tumor from collapsed lung in 8 of 10 patients, whereas MRI demonstrated signal intensity differences in only half those patients. It should be noted that in 2 patients in whom differentiation between tumor and collapsed lung was not achieved by contrast-enhanced CT, MRI showed separation, suggesting a possible complementary role for the techniques. T$_2$-weighted sequences were most useful in demonstrating a higher signal (longer T$_2$) from the collapsed lung than from the tumor. It is likely that the use of gadolinium-chelate would improve the accuracy of MRI. MRI can identify any underlying mass lesions in a completely opacified hemithorax.

The *normal pleural space* cannot be resolved by MRI but adjacent *fat* is well shown. Early *chest wall invasion* by tumor is

better demonstrated on MRI than CT. T$_1$-weighted images provide good morphological detail and contrast discrimination between tumor (intermediate signal) and fat (high signal). The presence of a high signal within chest wall muscle on T$_2$-weighted images suggests more extensive invasion. The changes however are non-specific. Similar increased signal intensity can occur with inflammatory disease. *Rib destruction* is not well shown on MRI. Although cortical bone is better shown by CT, the extension of tumor into the marrow space is better identified on MRI. CT and MRI are unreliable in demonstrating mediastinal pleural infiltration, although the better contrast resolution of MRI has the greater potential. Microscopic invasion of the mediastinum by tumor without bulk change cannot be detected. Invasion can be assumed if interdigitation of tumor into the mediastinum or chest wall is present. The differentiation of pleural thickening can be further aided by the use of gadolinium-chelate injection. Interruption of the normal low signal intensity line of the pericardium, which is less than 2 mm thick and best delineated on coronal and transverse ECG-gated T$_1$-weighted images, suggests *pericardial invasion*. Similarly, interruption of the low intensity line of the diaphragm adjacent to a mass, on sagittal and coronal images, suggests infiltration (Fig 14.43). *Lymph node* assessment is discussed elsewhere (Ch. 12). Vascular invasion by tumor is more clearly demonstrated by MRI than by CT while CT is more sensitive in the detection of pleural effusions. On MRI, effusions are more clearly shown on T$_2$- or proton-density-weighted images as a high signal, compared with a low signal on T$_1$-weighted scans. MRI is helpful in differentiating pleural from parenchymal disease and has the potential to elucidate complex effusions. It is complementary to CT in the evaluation of pleural abnormalities, and can be used for the further assessment of focal non-calcified pleural lesions for which the level of confidence of CT in offering a diagnosis is low.

In these cases signal iso- or hypo-intensity (with respect to intercostal muscle) on T_2-weighted scans from the focal pleural lesion is a reliable predictor of benign (fibrotic) pleural disease. Lymphangitis carcinomatosa has the distinctive appearance of a hilar or mediastinal mass with peripherally dilated pulmonary lymphatics.

In the evaluation of distant metastases from carcinoma of the lung, MRI has the potential for characterizing some adrenal masses. On T_2-weighted images adrenal metastases have a high signal intensity (Fig. 36.15) whereas benign non-functioning adenomas give a low signal similar to surrounding liver. There is, however, some overlap, which limits its clinical value. MRI is a more sensitive technique than CT in the detection of liver and CNS metastases.

REFERENCES AND SUGGESTIONS FOR FURTHER READING

Adler, B., Padley, S., Miller, R. et al (1992) High-resolution CT of bronchoalveolar carcinoma. *American Journal of Roentgenology*, **159**, 275–277.

Altman, R. L., Miller, W. E., Carr, D. T. et al (1973) Radiographic appearances of bronchial carcinoid. *Thorax*, **28**, 433–434.

Armstrong, P (1995) Neoplasms of the Lungs, Airways and Pleura. In: Armstrong, P. et al (eds) *Imaging Diseases of the Chest*. Chicago: Year Book.

Arnold, A. M, Williams, C. J. (1979) Small cell lung cancer: a curable disease? *British Journal of Diseases of the Chest*, **73**, 327–348.

Aronchick, J. M., Wexler, J. A., Christen, B. et al (1986) Computed tomography of bronchial carcinoid. *Journal of Computer Assisted Tomography*, **10**, 71–74.

Balikian, J. P., Herman, P. G. (1979) Non-Hodgkin's lymphoma of the lungs. *Radiology*, **132**, 569–576.

Bateson, E. M. (1965) An analysis of 155 solitary lung lesions illustrating the differential diagnosis of mixed tumours of the lung. *Clinical Radiology*, **16**, 51–59.

Batra, P., Brown, K., Collins, J. D. et al (1988) Evaluation of intrathoracic extent of lung cancer by plain chest radiography, computed tomography and magnetic resonance imaging. *American Review of Respiratory Diseases*, **137**, 1456–1462.

Blank, N., Castellino, R. A. (1987) The mediastinum in Hodgkin's and non-Hodgkin's lymphomas. *Journal of Thoracic Imaging*, **2** (1), 66–71.

Bower, S. L., Choplin, R. H., Muss, H. B. (1983) Multiple primary carcinomas of the lung. *American Journal of Roentgenology*, **140**, 253–258.

Bragg, D. G. (1978) The clinical, pathological and radiographic spectrum of the intrathoracic lymphomas. *Investigative Radiology*, **13**, 2–11.

Bragg, D. G. (1987) Radiology of the lymphomas. *Current Problems in Diagnostic Radiology*, **16**, 183–206.

Bragg, D. G., Colby, T. V., Ward, J. H. (1986). New concepts in the non-Hodgkin lymphomas: radiologic implications. *Radiology*, **159**, 291–304.

Buy, J. N., Ghossain, M. A., Poirson, F. (1988) Computed tomography of mediastinal lymph nodes in non-small cell lung cancer: a new approach based on the lymphatic pathway of tumour spread. *Journal of Computer Assisted Tomography*, **12**, 545–552.

Cabanillas, F., Fuller, L. M. (1990) The radiological assessment of the lymphoma patient from the standpoint of the clinician. *Radiologic Clinics of North America*, **28**, 683–695.

Castellino, R. A. (1986) Hodgkin disease: practical concepts for the diagnostic radiologist. *Radiology*, **159**, 305–310.

Castellino, R. A. (1991) The non-Hodgkin's lymphomas: practical concepts for the diagnostic radiologist. *Radiology*, **178**, 315–321.

Chiles, C., Ravin, C. E. (1985) Intrathoracic metastases from an extrathoracic malignancy; radiographic approach to patient evaluation. *Radiologic Clinics of North America*, **23**, 427–438.

Cho, S. R., Henry, D. A., Beachley, M. C., Brooks, J. W. (1981) Round (helical) atelectasis. *British Journal of Radiology*, **54**, 643–650.

Choplin, R. H., Rawamoto, E. H., Dyer, R. B. et al (1986) Atypical carcinoid of the lung: radiographic features. *American Journal of Roentgenology*, **146**, 665–668.

Coppage, L., Shaw, C., Curtis, A. M. (1987) Metastatic disease to the chest in patients with extrathoracic malignancy. *Journal of Thoracic Imaging*, **2**(4): 24–37.

Corrin, B., Liebow, A. A., Friedman, P. J. (1975) Pulmonary lymphangiomyomatosis. *American Journal of Pathology*, **79**, 348–383.

Daly, B. D. T., Faling, L. J., Gunars Bite, P. A. C. (1987) Mediastinal lymph node evaluation by computed tomography in lung cancer: an analysis of 345 patients grouped by TNM staging, tumor size and tumor location. *Journal of Thoracic and Cardiovascular Surgery*, **94**, 644–672.

Davis, S. D., Zirn, J. R., Govoni, A. F. (1990) Peripheral carcinoid tumor of the lung: CT diagnosis. *American Journal of Roentgenology*, **155**, 1185–1187.

Dee, P. M., Arora, N. S., Innes, D. I. (1982) The pulmonary manifestations of lymphomatoid granulomatosis. *Radiology*, **143**, 613–618.

Epstein, D. M. (1990) Bronchioloalveolar carcinoma. *Seminars in Roentgenology*, **25**, 105–111.

Falaschi, F., Battolla, L., Mascalchi, M., et al (1996) Usefulness of MR signal intensity in distinguishing benign from malignant pleural disease. *American Journal of Roentgenology*, **166**, 963–968.

Feigin, D. S., Siegelman, S. S., Theros, E. G. et al (1977) Non-malignant lymphoid disorders of the chest. *American Journal of Roentgenology*, **129**, 221–228.

Forster, B. B., Müller, N. L., Miller, R. R. et al (1989) Neuroendocrine carcinomas of the lung: clinical, radiologic and pathologic correlation. *Radiology*, **170**, 441–445.

Gefter, W. B. (1990) Magnetic resonance imaging in the evaluation of lung cancer. *Seminars in Roentgenology*, **25**, 73–84.

Heath, D., Reid, R. (1985) Invasive pulmonary haemangiomatosis. *British Journal of Diseases of the Chest*, **79**, 284–294.

Heelan, R. T., Demas, B. E., Caravelli, J. F. et al (1989) Superior sulcus tumors: CT and MR imaging. *Radiology*, **170**, 637–641.

Heitzman, E. R., Markarian, B., DeLise, C. T. (1975) Lymphoproliferative disorders of the thorax. *Seminars in Roentgenology*, **10**, 73–81.

Henschke, C. I., Davis, S. D., Romano, P. M., Yankelevitz, D. F. (1989) The pathogenesis, radiologic evaluation, and therapy of pleural effusions. *Radiologic Clinics of North America*, **27**, 1241–1255.

Herbert, A., Wright, D. H., Isaacson, P. G., Smith, J. L. (1984) Primary malignant lymphoma of the lung: histopathologic and immunologic evaluation of nine cases. *Human Pathology*, **15**, 415–422.

Lahde, S., Paivansalo, M., Rainio, P. (1991) CT for predicting the resectability of lung cancer: a prospective study. *Acta Radiologica*, **32**, 449–454.

Lewis, E. R., Caskey, C. I., Fishman, E. K. (1991) Lymphoma of the lung: CT findings in 31 patients. *American Journal of Roentgenology*, **156**, 711–714.

Libshitz, H. I. (1989) Imaging and staging of lung cancer. *Current Opinion in Radiology*, **1**, 21–24.

Libshitz, H. I. (1990) Computed tomography in bronchogenic carcinoma. *Seminars in Roentgenology*, **25**, 64–72.

Lillington, G. A., Stevens, G. M. (1976) The solitary nodule. The other side of the coin. *Chest*, **70**, 322–323.

Madewell, J. E., Feigin, D. S. (1977) Benign tumors of the lung. *Seminars in Roentgenology*, **12**, 175–186.

Maile, C. W., Moore, A. V., Ulreich, S. et al (1983) Chest radiographic-pathologic correlation in adult leukemia patients. *Investigative Radiology*, **18**, 495–499.

Mayo, J. R. (1994) Magnetic resonance imaging of the chest: where we stand. *Radiologic Clinics of North America*, **32**, 795–809.

McLoud, T. C., Bourgouin, P. M., Greenberg, R. W. et al (1992) Bronchogenic carcinoma: analysis of staging in the mediastinum with CT by correlative lymph node mapping and sampling. *Radiology*, **182**, 319–323.

Mountain, C. F. (1986) A new international staging system for lung cancer. *Chest*, **89** (suppl), 225S–233S.

Müller, N. L., Miller, R. R. (1990) Neuroendocrine carcinomas of the lung. *Seminars in Roentgenology*, **25**, 96–104.

Munk, P. L., Müller, N. L., Miller, R. R. et al (1988) Pulmonary lymphangitic carcinomatosis: CT and pathologic findings. *Radiology*, **166**, 705–709.

Naidich, D. P. (1990) CT/MR correlation in the evaluation of tracheobronchial neoplasia. *Radiologic Clinics of North America*, **28**, 555–571.

Nessi, R., Ricci, P. B., Ricci, S. B. et al (1991) Bronchial carcinoid tumors: radiologic observations in 49 cases. *Journal of Thoracic Imaging*, **6**(2), 47–53.

North, L. B., Libshitz, H. I., Lorigan, J. G. (1990) Thoracic lymphoma. *Radiologic Clinics of North America*, **28**, 745–762.

Padovani, B., Mouroux, J., Seksik, L. et al (1993) Chest wall invasion by bronchogenic carcinoma: evaluation with MR imaging. *Radiology*, **187**, 33–38.

Pancoast, H. K. (1932) Superior sulcus tumor: tumor characterized by pain, Horner's syndrome, destruction of bone and atrophy of hand muscles. *Journal of the American Medical Association*, **99**, 1391–1396.

Ray, J. F., Lawton, B. R., Magnin, G. E. et al (1976) The coin lesion story: update 1976. *Chest*, **70**, 332–336.

Rigler, L. G. (1955) The roentgen signs of carcinoma of the lung. *American Journal of Roentgenology*, **74**, 415–428.

Romney, B. M., Austin, J. H. M. (1990) Plain film evaluation of carcinoma of the lung. *Seminars in Roentgenology*, **25**, 45–63.

Siegelman, S. S., Khouri, N. F., Scott, W. W. et al (1986) Pulmonary hamartoma: CT findings. *Radiology*, **160**, 313–317.

Templeton, P. A., Zerhouni, E. A. (1990) MR imaging in the management of thoracic malignancies. *Radiologic Clinics of North America*, **27**, 1099–1111.

Templeton, P. A., Caskey, C. I., Zerhouni, E. A. (1990) Current uses of CT and MR imaging in the staging of lung cancer. *Radiological Clinics of N. American* 28: 631–646.

Various authors (1977) Pulmonary neoplasms. *Seminars in Roentgenology*, **12**, 161–246.

Webb, W. R., Gatsonis, C., Zerhouni, E. A. et al (1991) CT and MR imaging in staging non-small cell bronchogenic carcinoma: report of the Radiologic Diagnostic Oncologic Group. *Radiology*, **178**, 705–713.

Woodring, J. H. (1990) Unusual radiographic manifestations of lung cancer. *Radiologic Clinics of North America*, **28**, 599–618.

15

PULMONARY INFECTIONS

Simon P. G. Padley and Michael B. Rubens

Inflammatory disease of the lung may be referred to as either pneumonia or pneumonitis. Although these terms are interchangeable, *pneumonia* usually implies an infection by pathogenic organisms resulting in consolidation of lung, whereas *pneumonitis* tends to refer to those inflammatory processes that primarily involve the alveolar wall, e.g. fibrosing alveolitis in the UK or usually interstitial pneumonia in the USA. Pneumonias may be classified on the basis of morphology or etiology.

ACUTE PNEUMONIA

A causative organism is only likely to be found in 50% of cases, usually because of prior treatment with antibiotics or an inability to provide a satisfactory sputum specimen. Of these organisms there will be approximately a third each of bacterial, non-bacterial and viral. Of the bacterial causes the *pneumococcus (Streptococcus pneumoniae)* is most common, with much smaller numbers of *Staphylococcus aureus, Haemophilus influenzae, Klebsiella pneumoniae* and *Legionella pneumophila*.

Of the non-bacterial causes *Mycoplasma pneumoniae* is most common. In fact, it is the most common proven cause of primary pneumonia in the UK at the present time. Other non-bacterial causes found in small numbers are *Chlamydia psittaci* (psittacosis) and *Coxiella burnetii* (Q fever). The viruses are almost all *influenza* and *cold viruses*. Mixed infections are found in approximately 10% of cases.

Lobar pneumonia commences as a localized infection of terminal air spaces. Inflammatory edema spreads to adjacent lung via the terminal airways and pores of Kohn, and causes uniform consolidation of all or part of a lobe.

In lobar pneumonia the usual homogeneous lung opacification is limited by fissures and affected lobes retain normal volume and often show air bronchograms. The onset may be so acute that opacification is often at its maximum on the initial radiograph. However, consolidation may not be obvious on the initial radiograph. *Streptococcus pneumoniae* classically causes lobar pneumonia. The classic appearance of lobar pneumonia is increasingly

uncommon, partly because early antibiotic treatment aborts the progression of disease. Consolidation may not spread uniformly throughout the lobe. From the initial focus of infection inflammatory edema spreads via the air passages and the pores of Kohn, and as a result consolidation may conform to segmental boundaries. Occasionally rounded lesions with ill-defined margins appear, especially in children, producing a so-called 'round pneumonia'. Kerley B lines may appear in the affected area from a temporary overloading of lymphatics and edema of interlobular septa. The distribution of the inflammatory exudate can be influenced to some degree by the effect of gravity, best seen in the immobile patient. Resolution is accompanied by diminution of the density of the opacity as air returns to the lobe, and it is usually complete, with the lung architecture being restored to normal.

Bronchopneumonia is a multifocal process which commences in the terminal and respiratory bronchioles and tends to spread segmentally. It may also be called lobular pneumonia, and produces patchy consolidation. The commonest causes are *Staphylococcus aureus* and Gram-negative organisms.

In clinical practice the most useful classification is according to the causative organism, since this is what influences the management and outcome of the infection. Unfortunately, it is not possible to diagnose the organism from radiology alone. However, radiology is important in confirming the presence and location of pneumonia, as well as following its course. Moreover, the chest radiograph may indicate complications of a pneumonia such as pleural effusion, empyema, pneumothorax, atelectasis, abscess formation and scarring.

Bacterial Pneumonias

Streptococcus pneumoniae This is a common cause of pneumonia in all age groups, and particularly in young adults. Typically it produces lobar consolidation (Fig. 15.1), which is often basal but may occur anywhere in the lung. The volume of the consolidated lung is normal, and an air bronchogram may be visible. Occasionally edema of the interlobular septa causes septal lines.

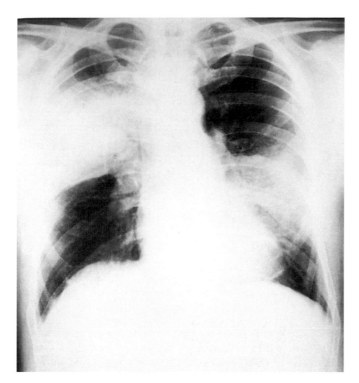

Fig. 15.1 Pneumococcal pneumonia. Lingular and right upper lobe consolidation with sparing of the apex.

Pleural effusion, empyema and cavitation are unusual if the infection is treated promptly, but may be seen in debilitated patients. Resolution is usually complete.

Staphylococcus aureus This is a common cause of pneumonia in debilitated patients. It may also cause superinfection in influenza (Fig. 15.2). Hematogenous infection of the lungs may occur in

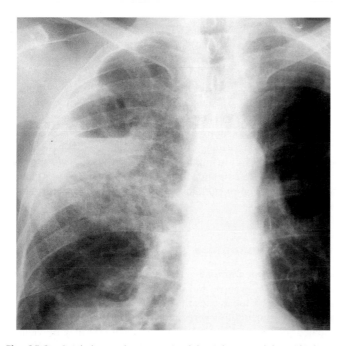

Fig. 15.2 Staphylococcal pneumonia of the right upper lobe with abscess formation.

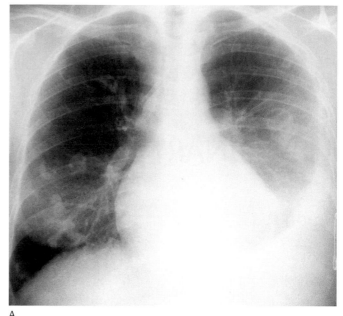

A

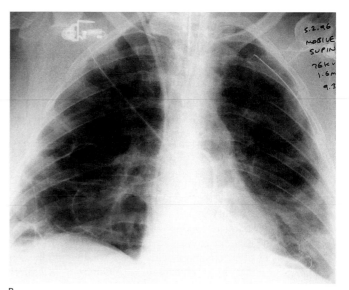

B

Fig. 15.3 A. Hematogenous staphylococcal abscess formation in an intravenous drug abuser. There are multiple thin-walled cavities and an associated left pleural effusion. **B.** Multiple large thin-walled pneumatoceles in a different intravenous drug abuser with staphylococcal tricuspid endocarditis.

septicemia, and is a common complication of intravenous drug abuse; when dissemination is hematogenous the typical appearance is of multiple poorly defined rounded nodules that develop rapidly over a few days (Fig. 15.3). Usually cavitation is evident, especially on later examinations. When pneumonia occurs as a complication of intravenous drug abuse echocardiography should be undertaken since in most of these patients the source of septic emboli is an infective endocarditis on the tricuspid valve.

Infection may also be the result of inhalation, typically causing a bronchopneumonia with multiple, patchy areas of consolidation (Fig. 15.4). Confluence of these areas may develop. Again cavitation is common, and in children pneumatoceles frequently develop.

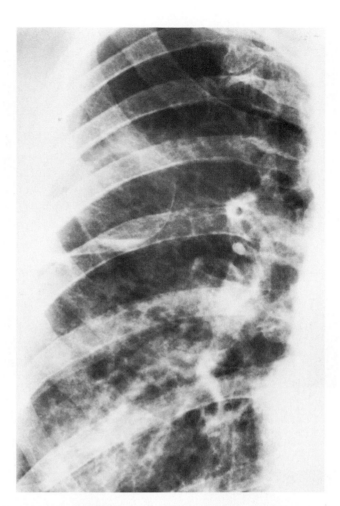

Fig. 15.4 Staphylococcal bronchopneumonia. A pneumatocele has developed in the right upper lobe. The radiograph eventually returned to normal.

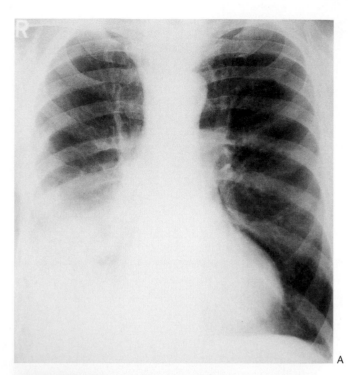

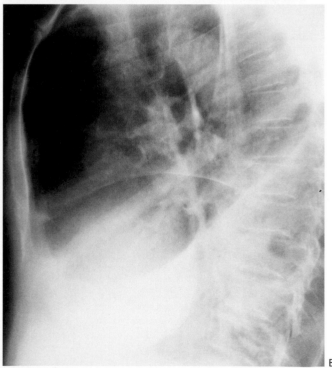

Fig. 15.5 A, B. *Klebsiella* pneumonia. There is consolidation in the right lower lobe with associated loss of volume evident on the lateral view.

Pleural effusion, empyema and areas of atelectasis are common complications.

***Klebsiella* Pneumonia**   This is due to *Friedländer's bacillus* and typically occurs in elderly debilitated men. There is usually lobar consolidation (Fig. 15.5), more often right-sided, and frequently upper lobe. The volume of the affected lung is maintained, or may be increased causing bulging of the fissures. Cavitation is common (Fig. 15.6) and if there is healing with fibrosis then cavities may become permanent and mimic TB. A bronchopneumonic pattern may also occur (Fig. 15.7).

Legionnaire's Disease   In 1976 an explosive epidemic of severe respiratory illness occurred at an American Legionnaires' convention in Philadelphia. It was a rapidly extending pneumonia complicated by shock, mental confusion, respiratory and renal failure, unresponsive to the usual antibiotics, with a case fatality of 16%. A previously unknown Gram-negative bacillus was eventually isolated and given the name *Legionella pneumophila*. The organism is ubiquitous in water, multiplying in water coolers, air conditioners and showers, and infection takes place from inhalation of an aerosol mist. It is prone to attack smokers and the debilitated. Radiographically there is spreading consolidation, and although it may be confined to one lobe initially it soon extends to others and to the opposite lung (Fig. 15.8). Another characteristic feature is

the slow resolution over several weeks, but this is usually complete. Small *pleural effusions* are common; abscess and pneumatocele formation are rare.

Haemophilus influenzae   This is a commensal of the upper respiratory tract, but since it is sometimes found in large numbers in the sputum in association with chronic lung diseases and treatment

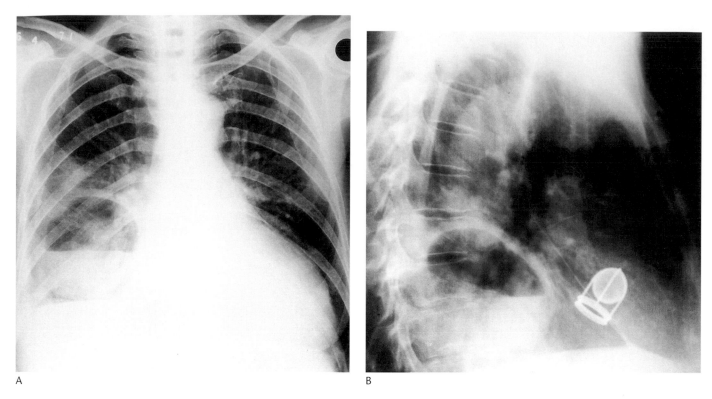

A   B

Fig. 15.6 A, B. *Klebsiella* pneumonia. There is a large cavity in the right lower lobe following cavitation of pneumonic consolidation. An aortic valve replacement is present.

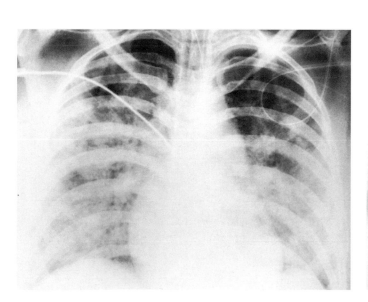

Fig. 15.7 *Klebsiella* septicemia. There is diffuse patchy alveolar shadowing with air bronchograms.

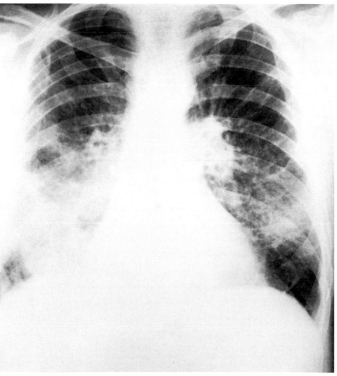

Fig. 15.8 Legionnaire's disease. There is bilateral consolidation, more marked on the right.

aimed at its eradication is often followed by clinical improvement, it is accorded a potentially pathogenic role. It is a secondary invader found in chronic bronchitis, cystic fibrosis and debilitated states. It is also found in influenza and other virus infections. Any pulmonary opacities found in *Haemophilus* infection are disseminate and bronchopneumonic; there are no characteristic radiographic appearances (Fig. 15.9).

Other Gram-negative Pneumonias

Pseudomonas aeruginosa* and *Escherichia coli These are two of the many Gram-negative organisms which normally inhabit the upper respiratory tract and gastrointestinal tract and may cause pneumonia or other infections in debilitated patients. They are likely to be pathogenic in patients with chronic lung disease such as cystic fibrosis, as well as in patients who are immunosuppressed or have diabetes. Infections also tend to occur following major surgery and in patients who have received long-term broad-spectrum antibiotics. Thus they are particularly prone to colonize patients on long-term mechanical ventilation. Pneumonia normally results from inhalation, but may also be hematogenous in origin. The radiographic appearances are of a bronchopneumonia which is often basal.

Melioidosis Melioidosis, a disease of tropical countries of the East, is caused by *Pseudomonas pseudomallei*. It may manifest years after the patient has left an endemic area. There are two pulmonary forms: a septicemic disseminate infection with necrotizing lesions, and a chronic apical pneumonia which breaks down to form a thin-walled cavity.

Tularemia. Discovered in Tulare, California, infection with *Francisella tularensis* is endemic amongst small mammals and is spread by ticks. Humans acquire the infection either by inoculation or inhalation. Remarkably few organisms are required to cause illness. In the bacteremic form there are small oval pulmonary lesions and hilar adenopathy (Fig. 15.10). Inhalation infection causes one or more areas of consolidation, also with hilar adenopathy. Untreated the consolidated lung cavitates and fibroses and may then mimic tuberculosis.

Mycoplasma Pneumonia

Mycoplasma pneumoniae This is the only member of the mycoplasma group that is commonly pathogenic in man. Although classed as bacteria these organisms are unlike other common bacterial species, being smaller and lacking rigid cell walls containing peptidoglycan. As a result they are not susceptible to antibiotics that affect cell wall synthesis such as the penicillins. Due to these morphological and structural differences mycoplasma pneumonia is often referred to as an **atypical** or **non-bacterial pneumonia**. This term was originally given to an illness where the systemic symptoms overshadowed those due to pneumonia, and where the course of disease was less dramatic but more prolonged than typical pneumonia. Atypical pneumonia is now known to have a number of causes in addition to mycoplasma, which is the commonest, and these include adenovirus, psittacosis and Q fever. Mycoplasma is most frequently encountered in young adults and is the commonest isolate from primary pneumonias in the UK, accounting for 10–20% of cases, but only in a small proportion does it cause a major respiratory illness.

The earliest radiographic signs are fine reticular or nodular shadows followed by the appearance of consolidation, which may

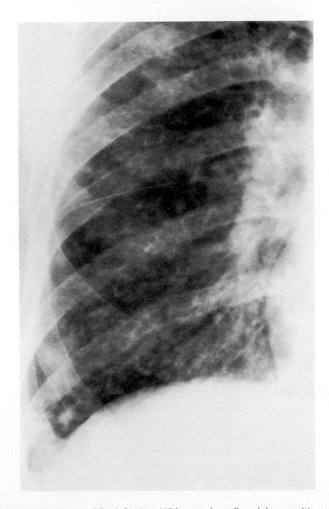

Fig. 15.9 *Haemophilus* infection. Widespread small nodular opacities are evident.

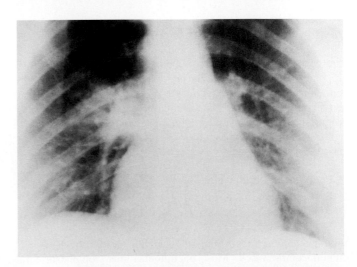

Fig. 15.10 Tularemia. There is right hilar nodal involvement and perihilar consolidation.

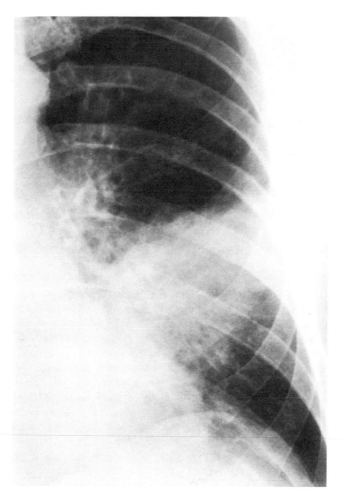

Fig. 15.11 Mycoplasma pneumonia. There is a patch of left mid zone consolidation obscuring the left heart border.

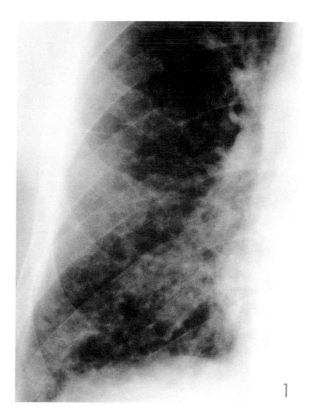

Fig. 15.12 Adenovirus chest infection. There is reticulonodular infiltrate, most marked in a bronchovascular distribution at the right base.

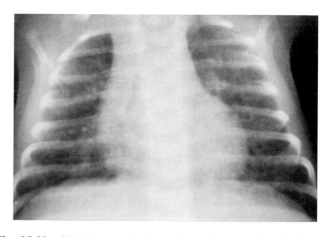

Fig. 15.13 CMV pneumonia. Two and a half month old child. There is reticular nodular shadowing throughout both lungs.

be segmental or lobar, and is usually unilateral (Fig. 15.11). Lymph node enlargement and pleural effusion are uncommon and cavitation is rare.

Viral Pneumonias

Viral pneumonia usually commences in distal bronchi and bronchioles as an interstitial process with destruction of the epithelium, edema and lymphocytic infiltration. There may also be focal inflammation of the terminal bronchioles and alveoli and progression to hemorrhagic pulmonary edema.

The radiological appearances of a viral pneumonia are very varied, but often include:

1. Peribronchial shadowing (Fig. 15.12)
2. Reticulonodular shadowing (Fig. 15.13)
3. Patchy or extensive consolidation (Fig. 15.14).

Viral pneumonia is uncommon in adults, unless the patient is immunocompromised. Most pneumonias that complicate viral infections in adults are due to bacterial superinfection. However, viral pneumonias are not rare in infants and children.

Influenza Virus Pneumonia as a complication of influenza is normally due to secondary bacterial infection, often *Staphylococcus aureus, Streptococcus pneumoniae* or *Haemophilus*. However, the very young, the elderly and debilitated patients may develop a primary viral pneumonia with patchy consolidation. Occasionally, especially during influenza epidemics, a fulminating hemorrhagic pneumonia may be seen with widespread consolidation indistinguishable from non-cardiogenic pulmonary edema or adult respiratory distress syndrome (Fig. 15.14). If the patient survives, extensive pulmonary fibrosis may develop.

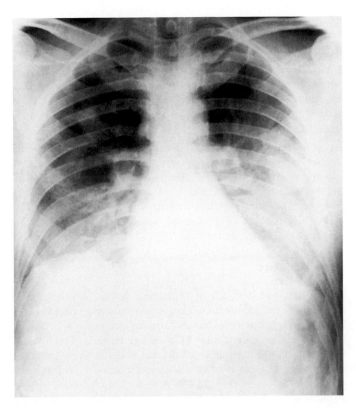

Fig. 15.14 Influenza A. Hemorrhagic consolidation was present at postmortem.

Herpes Varicella Zoster Varicella pneumonia occurs more often in adults than in children. In the acute phase of infection the chest radiograph may show widespread nodular shadows up to 1 cm in diameter, and clinically the pneumonia will be concurrent with the typical skin rash (Fig. 15.15). Following recovery a small proportion of these nodules calcify and, if multiple, may produce

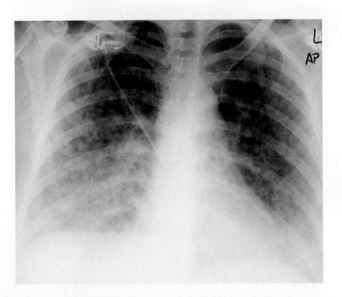

Fig. 15.15 Chickenpox pneumonia occurring during pregnancy. There is widespread, predominantly nodular shadowing throughout both lungs. The patient made a complete recovery.

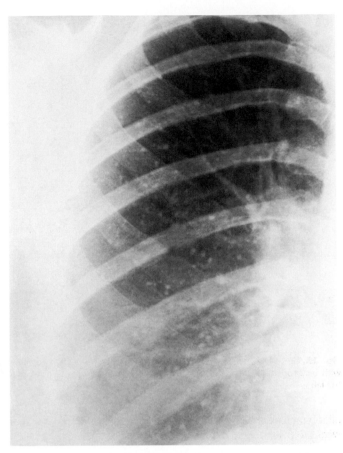

Fig. 15.16 Multiple calcified varicella scars.

a characteristic radiographic appearance (Fig. 15.16). These patients are usually able to give a history of severe chickenpox as an adult.

Measles Giant-cell Pneumonia In addition to the common secondary respiratory infections associated with measles, there is a specific pulmonary viral infection characterized by multinucleate giant cells with cytoplasmic inclusions in the respiratory epithelium. Although a disease of childhood, it has been recorded in adults. The mediastinal and hilar nodes are commonly enlarged but other radiographic abnormalities are variable and include streaky basal linear shadows, widespread reticular shadows and diffuse ill-defined nodular opacities (Fig. 15.17). Remarkably swift resolution can take place, over the course of a few days.

Infectious Mononucleosis Less than 10% of cases have intrathoracic manifestations during the disease. The commonest abnormality on the chest X-ray is lymph node enlargement, and the lungs may show an isolated opacity or reticulonodular shadows.

Chlamydial and Rickettsial Pneumonias

Psittacosis and Ornithosis Usually acquired by contact with sick parrots or domestic fowl, this infection is due to *Chlamydia psittaci*. The pneumonia usually presents as patchy or lobar consolidation, although nodular shadows may be seen. There is often

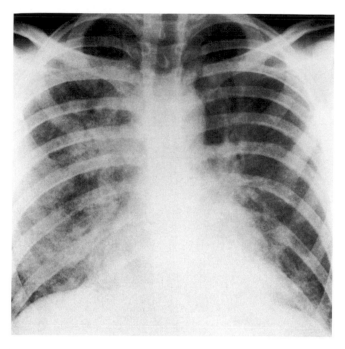

Fig. 15.17   Measles giant-cell pneumonia. Extensive ill-defined opacities with air bronchograms. The changes are more marked on the right than the left.

hilar lymphadenopathy. The radiographic changes may take several weeks to resolve.

Q Fever   This is usually acquired by contact with cattle or sheep and is due to *Coxiella burnetii*. The pneumonia typically presents as rounded areas of consolidation, up to 10 cm in diameter, in both lungs, lobar consolidation, or linear densities due to atelectasis. Lymph node enlargement is unusual. The radiographic changes may take a month or more to resolve, during which time the ill-defined opacities become more sharply defined, smaller and denser. Rarely Q fever produces an endocarditis, meningoencephalitis or hepatitis.

Rocky Mountain Spotted Fever   This tick-borne disease is endemic to the southern USA as well as the Rocky Mountains. It may cause patchy consolidation, pleural effusions, and be complicated by secondary bacterial pneumonia. Overall there is a 5% mortality.

Scrub Typhus   This rickettsial disease is endemic in the countries of the Pacific basin, and causes pulmonary abnormalities in approximately 10% of cases. The radiographic pattern is diverse and takes the form of interstitial, lobar or widespread pulmonary opacities. The latter presentation resembles adult respiratory distress syndrome both clinically and radiographically, but it clears rapidly with appropriate treatment.

Lung Abscess

Suppuration and necrosis of pulmonary tissue may be due to tuberculosis, fungal infection, malignant tumor and infected cysts. However, the term lung abscess usually refers to a cavitating lesion secondary to infection by pyogenic bacteria. This is most frequently due to aspiration of infected material from the upper respiratory tract, and is often associated with poor dentition and periodontal infection (Fig. 15.18). A variety of organisms may be responsible, and anaerobic bacteria are frequently found in the sputum. Occasionally there is a history of loss of consciousness and presumed aspiration. Other causes of lung abscess include staphylococcal (Fig. 15.19) and *Klebsiella* pneumonia, septic pulmonary emboli (Fig. 15.3) and trauma.

Radiographically an abscess may or may not be surrounded by consolidation. Appearance of an air–fluid level indicates that a communication with the airways has developed. The wall of the abscess may be thick at first, but with further necrosis and coughing up of infected material it becomes thinner (Fig. 15.18).

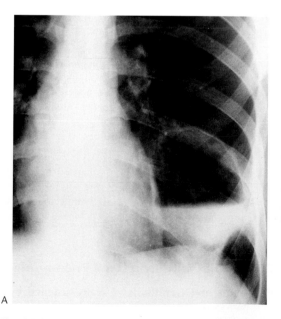
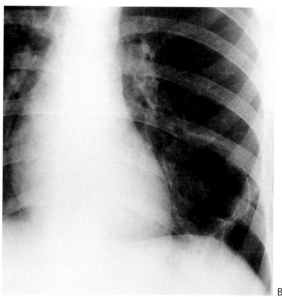

A   B

Fig. 15.18   **A.** Lung abscess. There was poor dental hygiene. Mixed anaerobic growth. **B.** Several weeks later a thin-walled pneumatocele remains.

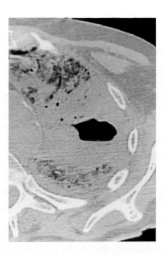

Fig. 15.19 Staphylococcal abscess in a patient with adult respiratory distress syndrome. A cavity with a fluid level is present within a dense area of consolidation.

Aspiration and Inhalation

The effects of aspiration of particulate or liquid foreign material into the lungs are twofold: those due to mechanical bronchial obstruction and those due to the irritant properties of the aspirate. When the cough reflex is suppressed by stupor, alcohol or drugs, aspiration of food from the stomach during vomiting is likely to occur. The inflammatory response excited by vegetable matter is intense and commonly followed by secondary infection with commensals and anaerobic organisms. Aspiration of infected material from nasal and oral sepsis is a common cause of lung abscess. The radiological patterns are therefore those of atelectasis or suppurative bronchitis and pneumonia. Metallic or inorganic particles may excite little response, the mechanical effects of uncomplicated atelectasis or obstructive emphysema predominating, and they may remain undetected for long periods.

Aspiration of mineral oils results in **lipoid pneumonia** (Fig. 15.20). The prolonged use of liquid paraffin for constipation is the usual cause and a precipitating factor is chronic esophageal obstruction. The oil floats to the top of any residue in the esophagus, the optimal position for aspiration. The oil is almost inert and the reaction is indolent, granulomatous and fibrotic; any lung damage is permanent. Radiographically there are dense well-defined tumor-like masses or an extensive bilateral opacity spreading outward from the hilar regions. Vegetable oils and animal fats such as milk induce a greater inflammatory response and the opacities are ill defined and bronchopneumonic. Influenced by gravity, the lesions of aspiration and inhalation are found predominantly in the posterior parts of the lungs. Small aspirates are common in the aged from incompetence of the closing mechanism of the larynx. These recurrent aspirations produce coarse peribronchial thickening, small patches of pneumonia and eventually fibrosis and bronchiectasis.

Mendelson's Syndrome This is a chemical pneumonia caused by aspiration of acid gastric contents during anesthesia. An intense bronchospasm is rapidly followed by a flood of edema throughout the lungs, resulting in hypoxia and requiring high ventilation pressures. The radiographic appearance of massive pulmonary edema taken together with the clinical presentation is pathognomonic (Fig. 15.21).

In cases of *near drowning* the lungs show widespread, ill-defined alveolar opacities due to pulmonary edema. The effects of

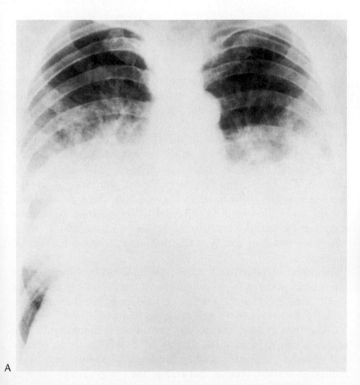

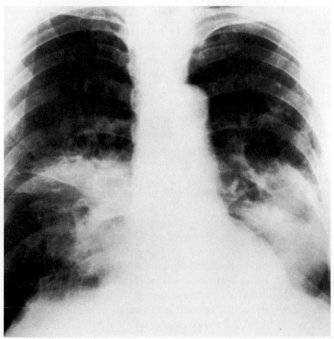

A   B

Fig. 15.20 **A.** Lipoid pneumonia. Aspiration of liquid paraffin. **B.** Eight years later there has been significant clearing but severe residual fibrosis is now present.

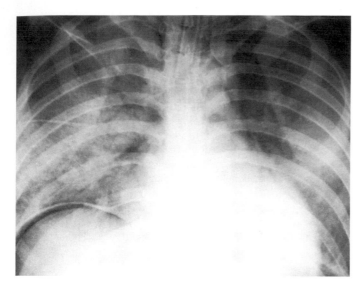

Fig. 15.21 Mendelson's syndrome. Postoperative aspiration of gastric contents.

salt water are less severe and of shorter duration than those due to hypotonic fresh water.

Inhalation of Irritant Gases Inhalation of gases such as ammonia, chlorine and nitrogen dioxide produces an acute focal or diffuse pulmonary edema followed by functional derangements indicative of bronchiolar and alveolar damage. It is a cause of *bronchiolitis obliterans*. Widespread tubular bronchiectasis and severe emphysema have been reported as sequels to accidental smoke inhalation.

PULMONARY TUBERCULOSIS

Mycobacterium tuberculosis is responsible for most cases of tuberculosis; fewer than 5% of cases are caused by atypical mycobacteria. Infection from milk is now rare where pasteurized milk is available. Infection is usually by inhalation of organisms from open cases of the disease. Transmission is by droplet inhalation, and the dose of viable organisms received is critical. Children, the immunocompromised, especially HIV-positive patients, and some immigrant groups are particularly susceptible. All these factors are reflected in the recommendations current in the UK concerning isolation of patients, treatment of contacts and general control measures. A chest radiograph is part of these control measures, and follow-up of contacts for two years may be judged necessary.

The occupational risk of hospital personnel is, in general, minimal and only a pre-employment chest radiograph is needed. Annual chest radiographs are not required. Those judged to be at higher risk should be offered an annual chest radiographic examination. Staff in any institution who will be in regular contact with children should have a chest radiograph as part of a pre-employment check, but routine periodic radiography is not necessary.

There are racial differences in the incidence of tuberculosis; in Britain it is 30 times more common in immigrants from the Indian subcontinent than in the indigenous population. Other factors that predispose to infection are old age, poor nutrition, alcoholism, silicosis, diabetes, pregnancy, malignant disease and immuno-suppression, especially by HIV infection.

Previous infection or BCG vaccination render most patients hypersensitive to tuberculoprotein. Possession of such hyper-sensitivity influences the course of the disease, and it is traditional to classify tuberculosis as *primary*, if the patient is not sensitized, and *post-primary* if the patient is. Most cases of post-primary infection are due to reactivation of previous infected foci, often many years after first infection. Occasionally, a primary infection progresses to the post-primary phase without an intervening latent period.

Primary Pulmonary Tuberculosis Most cases of primary pulmonary tuberculosis are subclinical, although there may be fever, respiratory symptoms or erythema nodosum. Organisms settle and multiply in an alveolus anywhere in the lungs, but most commonly in a subpleural site in the well-ventilated lower lobes. There is an area of peripheral consolidation (the Ghon focus), and spread from this along the draining lymphatics may lead to enlargement of regional lymph nodes. This combination is referred to as a primary complex. Subpleural infection may cause a serous effusion. Activation of the immune system usually leads to resolution, healing and fibrosis at this stage. Usually a fibrous capsule walls off the lesion and dystrophic calcification may occur. If the response to infection is weak the disease may progress and there is little difference between lesions of primary and post-primary evolution. This may manifest as further consolidation, possibly with cavitation, and bronchogenic spread of infection. Rupture of a cavity into the pleura may cause *pneumothorax, pleural effusion* or *empyema*, and erosion into a pulmonary vessel may lead to hematogenous spread and *miliary infection*.

Lymphadenopathy is a common feature of primary infection, but is rare in post-primary tuberculosis except in the HIV-positive population. Enlarged lymph nodes may press on adjacent airways and cause pulmonary collapse or air trapping with hyperinflation. Caseating nodes may also erode into airways, causing broncho-pneumonia, and into vessels causing miliary infection.

Post-primary Pulmonary Tuberculosis This follows the primary infection after a latent interval, however short or long, and is due to either reactivation or reinfection. It is now generally accepted that almost all post-primary tuberculosis is due to reinfection.

The lesions usually start in the subapical parts of the upper lobes or in the apical segment of the lower lobes as small areas of exudative inflammation. These extend, coalesce, caseate and cavitate. Typically there is a large cavity with several smaller satellite cavities, often bilateral but more advanced on one side. Cavity walls are lined by tuberculous granulation tissue and traversed by fibrotic remnants of bronchi and vessels. A vessel which has not been totally obliterated may dilate—a Rasmussen aneurysm.

Dispersal of infection from the cavities to other parts of the lungs takes place as in the primary form, and results in numerous small areas of caseous pneumonia, often in the lower lobes. Massive dispersal may lead to caseation of a whole lobe.

Adhesions usually limit pleural spread but sometimes the lung becomes encased in a thick coating of caseous material, fibrosis and hyaline connective tissue. Small cavities that heal leave radiating fibrotic strands puckering the lung. Large cavities become lined by columnar or squamous epithelium and are prone to secondary infection or fungal colonization.

Radiology of Tuberculosis

Pulmonary Changes

Consolidation in Primary Infection   This may involve any part of the lung, and the appearance is non-specific unless there is coincidental lymphadenopathy. The area involved may be small or affect an entire lobe, and an air bronchogram may be visible (Figs 15.22, 15.23). Occasionally consolidation appears as a well-defined nodule or nodules. Healing is often complete without any

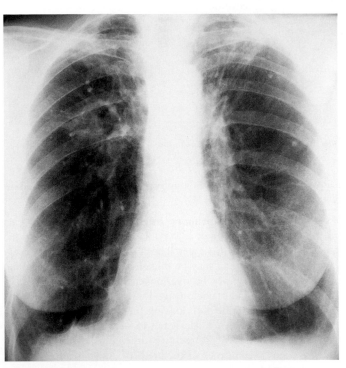

Fig. 15.24   Healed tuberculosis. There is bilateral upper lobe fibrosis with elevation of both hila. Basal emphysema has developed. There are multiple calcified granulomas in the mid and upper zones.

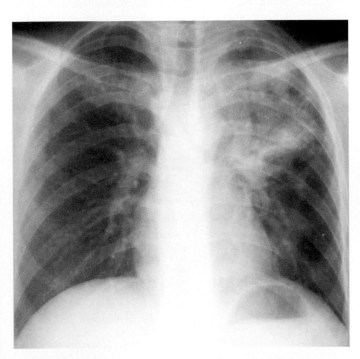

Fig. 15.22   Tuberculous pneumonia. Air bronchograms are present in the left upper lobe consolidation. Less marked right upper lobe consolidation is also present.

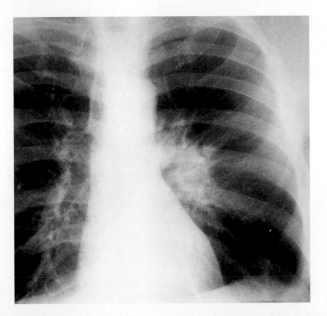

Fig. 15.23   Tuberculosis. There is left hilar enlargement and perihilar consolidation.

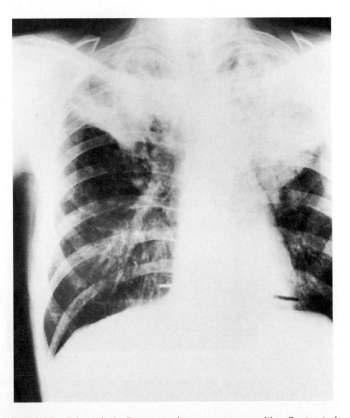

Fig. 15.25   Tuberculosis. Dense non-homogeneous opacities. Contracted right upper lobe.

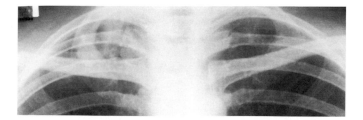

Fig. 15.26 Tuberculosis. Minimal right apical lesion.

sequelae on the chest radiograph although fibrosis and calcification may occur (Fig. 15.24).

Consolidation in Post-primary Infection This usually appears in the apex of an upper or lower lobe, and almost never in the anterior segments of the upper lobes. The consolidation is often patchy and nodular and may be bilateral (Fig. 15.25). A minimal apical lesion can easily be overlooked because of overlapping shadows of ribs and clavicle (Fig. 15.26). Comparison with the opposite side is then helpful, looking for asymmetries of density. The apical projection was designed to overcome this difficulty, but is rarely useful. Progressive infection is indicated by extension and coalescence of the areas of consolidation, and the development of cavities (Fig. 15.27).

Simultaneously there may be fibrosis and volume loss indicating healing (Fig. 15.24). Cavities may be single or multiple, large or small and thin- or thick-walled. Fluid levels are sometimes visible within cavities. With fibrosis there is often obliteration of cavities. However, larger cavities may persist and areas of bronchiectasis and emphysema may develop. Healed lesions often calcify. Since the upper lobes are predominantly involved, the effects of fibrotic contraction are seen as the trachea being pulled away from the midline, elevation of the hila and distortion of the lung parenchyma (Fig. 15.28). Chronic cavities are often colonized by *Aspergillus* and other fungi, and mycetomas may develop (Fig. 15.29). Disease activity is monitored by periodic radiographs, the appearance of new lesions or the extension of old ones indicating continued activity whereas contraction indicates that the balance has been tilted in favor of healing. Once the radiographic signs have stabilized, any subsequent change in size or density must be regarded as suspicious of reactivation, fungal colonization or complication by neoplasm.

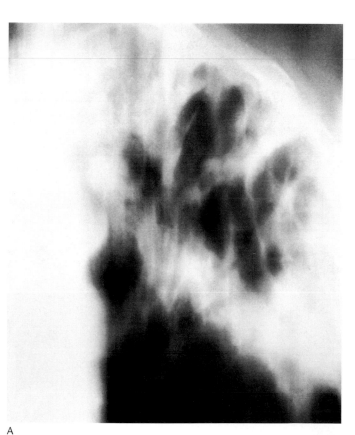

A

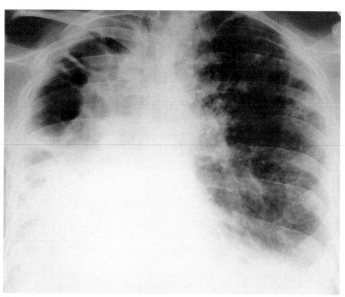

B

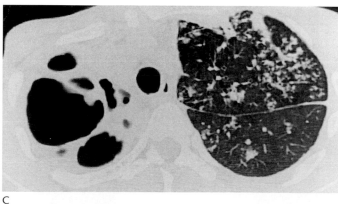

C

Fig. 15.27 Tuberculosis. **A.** Linear tomogram shows multiloculated destruction of the left upper lobe. **B** and **C.** Chest radiograph and CT scan demonstrating almost complete destruction of the right lung due to pulmonary tuberculosis. The CT reveals bronchopneumonic spread to the opposite lung.

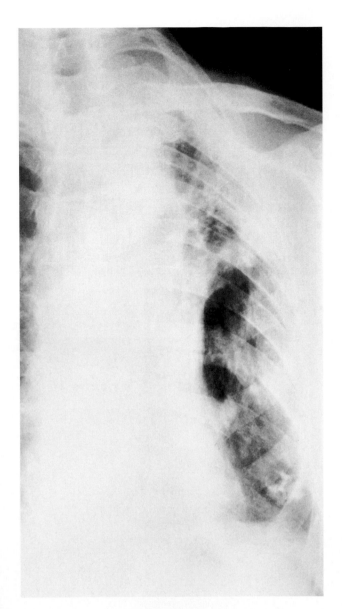

Fig. 15.28 Tuberculosis. There is fibrotic shrinkage of the left upper lobe with mediastinal and hilar displacement and apical pleural thickening.

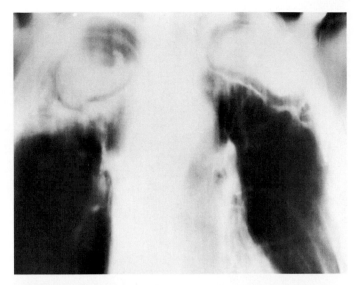

Fig. 15.29 Bilateral aspergillomas. Tomogram through the apices demonstrates presence of air around fungal masses.

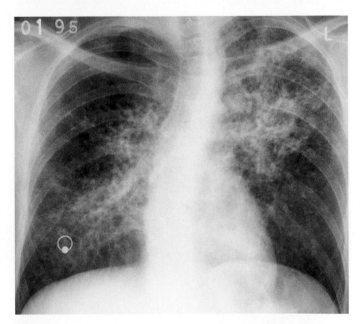

Fig. 15.30 Extensive bronchopneumonic spread of tuberculosis in an HIV-positive patient.

Tuberculous Bronchopneumonia This may occur in both primary and post-primary infection, causing patchy, often nodular, areas of consolidation (Figs 15.27C, 15.30).

Miliary Tuberculosis This is due to hematogenous spread of infection and may be seen in both primary and post-primary disease. In the former the patient is often a child, and in the latter case the patients are often elderly, debilitated or immunocompromised. At first the chest radiograph may be normal, but then small, discrete nodules, 1–2 mm in diameter, become apparent, evenly distributed throughout both lungs (Fig. 15.31). These nodules may enlarge and coalesce, but with adequate treatment they slowly resolve. Occasionally, some may calcify.

Tuberculoma This is a localized granuloma due to either primary or post-primary infection. It usually presents as a solitary well-defined nodule, up to 5 cm in diameter. Calcification is common but cavitation is unusual (Fig. 15.32).

Lymphadenopathy Hilar and mediastinal lymphadenopathy is a common feature of primary infection and may be seen in the presence or absence of peripheral consolidation. Following healing, involved nodes may calcify. Lymphadenopathy is usually unilateral but may be bilateral, in which case the differential diagnosis includes lymphoma and sarcoidosis. It is often more pronounced in children (Fig. 15.33).

Pleural Changes

Pleural effusion complicating primary infection is usually unilateral and due to subpleural infection. Pulmonary consolidation

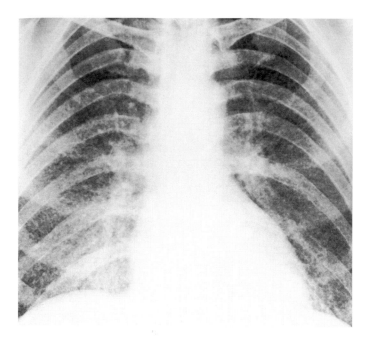

Fig. 15.31 Miliary tuberculosis. There are innumerable well-defined nodules present.

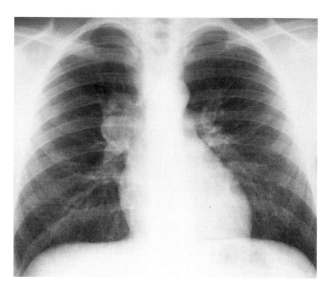

Fig. 15.33 Tuberculosis. There is right hilar lymph node enlargement.

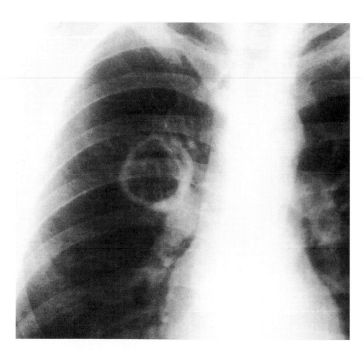

Fig. 15.32 Tuberculoma. A well-defined cavity is projected adjacent to the right hilum.

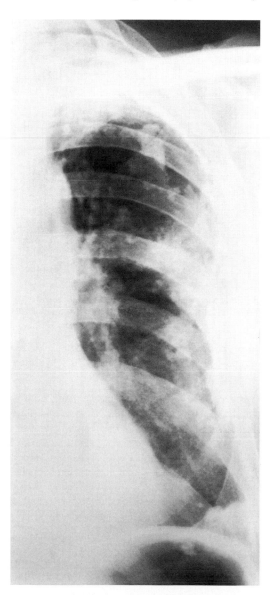

Fig. 15.34 Tuberculosis. There is generalized pleural thickening with extensive pleural calcification.

and/or lymphadenopathy may or may not be apparent. At presentation the effusion may be large and relatively asymptomatic. These effusions usually resolve without complication. Pleural effusion in post-primary infection, however, often progresses to empyema. Healing is then complicated by pleural thickening and often calcification (Fig. 15.34). Uncommon complications of tuberculous empyema are bronchopleural fistula, osteitis of a rib, pleurocutaneous fistula and secondary infection. Previous thoracoplasty may also complicate the appearances.

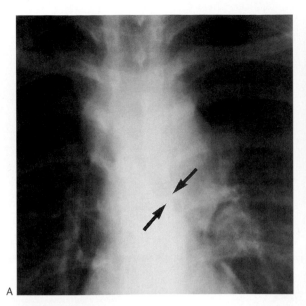
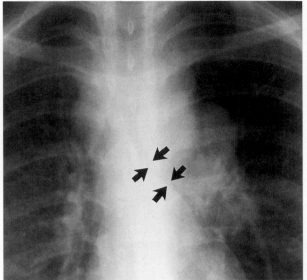

Fig. 15.35 Tuberculous lymphadenopathy. **A.** There is mediastinal and left hilar lymph node enlargement causing some narrowing of the left main bronchus. **B.** One month later appearances have significantly progressed with enlargement of the hilar and mediastinal nodes and increased left main bronchial narrowing.

Pleural thickening over the apex of the lung often accompanies the fibrosis of healing apical tuberculosis.

Pneumothorax may complicate subpleural cavitatory disease.

Airway Involvement

This may be secondary to lymphadenopathy or endobronchial infection and may therefore complicate both primary and post-primary disease. Compression of central airways by enlarged nodes may cause pulmonary collapse or air trapping (Fig. 15.35). Healing of endobronchial infection with fibrosis may also result in bronchostenosis. The lung distal to bronchial narrowing may develop bronchiectasis.

OTHER MYCOBACTERIAL PULMONARY INFECTIONS

There are a number of related bacilli with morphology and staining properties very similar to those of the tubercle bacillus. Of these atypical mycobacteria, those most frequently the cause of human disease are *M. xenopi*, *M. kansasii* and *M. battei*. Their infectivity is low but their sensitivities to drugs differ from that of *M. tuberculosis*. In general they cause less fibrosis and are less prone to spread but more prone to cavitate than *M. tuberculosis* infections. A common pattern is of a cluster of small opacities grouped around a central lucency. The cavities are thin-walled. Pleural disease, miliary disease and node enlargement are rare. These differences are not however sufficient, in an individual case, to differentiate them from *M. tuberculosis* infections.

BRANCHING BACTERIA

Actinomycosis *Actinomyces israelii* is a commensal of the oropharynx and may rarely cause pulmonary infection by aspiration or direct extension from esophagus or mediastinum. Classically it causes abscess formation, pleural invasion, osteomyelitis of ribs,

and sinuses to the chest wall. Apical disease may mimic tuberculosis, and occasionally a patchy pneumonia may develop. Presentation nowadays is most often as a mass-like area of consolidation which may resemble lung cancer (Fig. 15.36).

Nocardiosis *Nocardia asteroides* is a saprophyte found world-wide in soil. Infection usually occurs as a result of inhalation by debilitated individuals. Most commonly there is non-segmental, cavitating pneumonia, often with pleural effusion or empyema. It may also present as a solitary pulmonary nodule, with or without cavitation, and occasionally with hilar lymphadenopathy (Figs 15.37, 15.38).

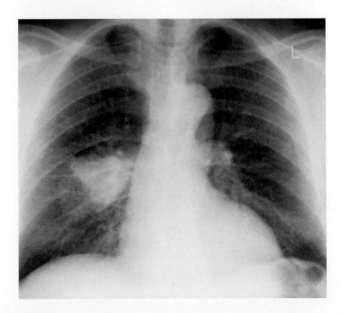

Fig. 15.36. Actinomycosis. There is a dense mass-like area of consolidation in the right mid zone.

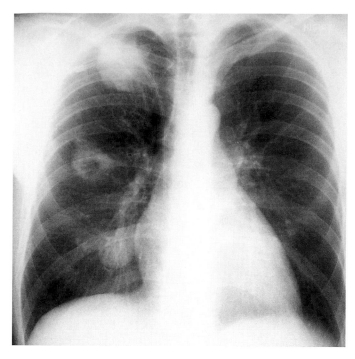

Fig. 15.37 *Nocardia asteroides* pneumonia. There are multiple cavities within the right lung, one of which has cavitated.

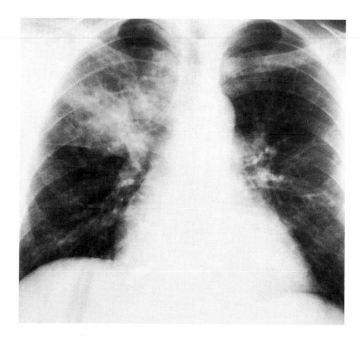

Fig. 15.38 Nocardiosis. There is non-homogeneous consolidation in the right upper lobe.

FUNGAL INFECTIONS

Histoplasmosis Infection with *Histoplasma capsulatum* is usually due to inhalation of soil or dust contaminated by bat or bird excreta. Although widespread it rarely causes chest infection, except in the eastern USA. Infection is usually subclinical and

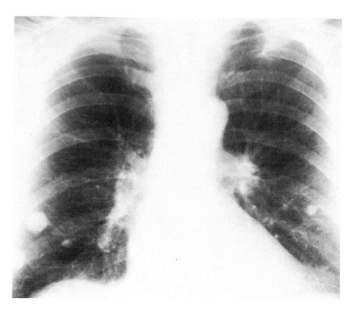

Fig. 15.39 Histoplasmosis. Calcified nodules of varying size are present in both lungs. Calcified right hilar nodes are also present.

heals spontaneously, sometimes leaving small, calcified pulmonary nodules (Fig. 15.39) or calcified hilar or mediastinal nodes. When many nodules are scattered throughout the lungs they closely resemble the scars of miliary tuberculosis or varicella pneumonia except that they tend to be rather more variable in size (Fig. 15.40). Rarely a calcified node may erode and obstruct a bronchus.

Progression of one or more of these foci leads to larger nodules. Hilar node enlargement is common and may be the only visible manifestation. Locally progressive disease may also take the form of consolidation, acute or chronic, the latter associated with fibrosis and cavitation (Fig. 15.41). The presence of

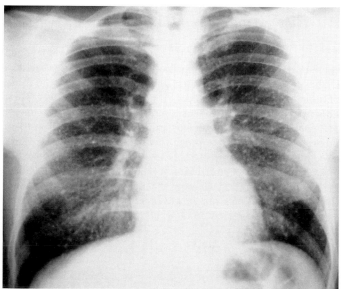

Fig. 15.40 Histoplasmosis. Incidental finding of multiple calcified pulmonary nodules.

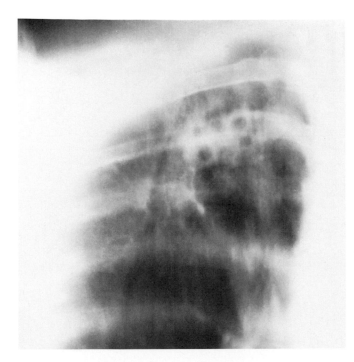

Fig. 15.41 Histoplasmosis. Chronic disease at the right apex. Tomogram shows multiple small cavities. Diagnosis confirmed at lobectomy.

cavitation within an area of lung distorted by fibrosis produces an appearance similar to tuberculosis.

When massive inhalation of organisms occurs the presentation may be one of wheezing, dyspnea, a dry cough and fever. The chest radiograph shows diffuse small nodular shadows (Fig. 15.42)

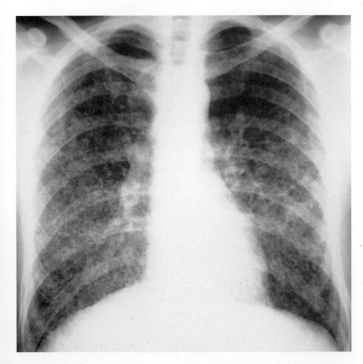

Fig. 15.42 Acute histoplasmosis following massive exposure whilst visiting a bat-infested cave. There are widespread bilateral well-defined 3–5 mm nodules.

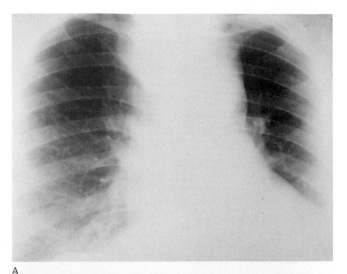

A

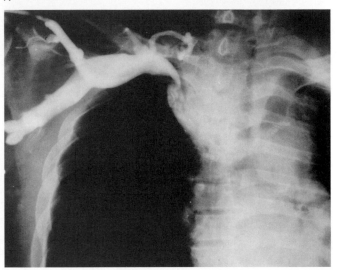

B

Fig. 15.43 Fibrosing mediastinitis following histoplasmosis. **A.** Chest X-ray shows widening of the upper mediastinum. **B.** Right arm phlebogram demonstrating compression of the right innominate vein. There is also a degree of tracheal narrowing.

which, following resolution, may calcify (Fig. 15.40). A histoplasmoma may resemble a tuberculoma, being round, usually well circumscribed and often calcified. Pleural disease and hematogenous spread are rare.

An uncommon late manifestation of histoplasmosis is a *fibrosing mediastinitis* which can cause stenosis of the venae cavae, esophagus, trachea, bronchi or central pulmonary vessels (Fig. 15.43). The chest radiograph will then show a widened mediastinum. Large hilar shadows with opacities extending into the lungs and Kerley B lines may appear.

Coccidioidomycosis *Coccidioides immitis* causes endemic disease in parts of the south west USA. Some 60% of infections are asymptomatic and the commonest radiographic finding is a nodule which calcifies as it heals. However *C. immitis* may cause a pneumonic illness, and the chest radiograph may show patchy consolidation which may cavitate and be associated with pleural effusion or hilar or mediastinal adenopathy. Alternatively single

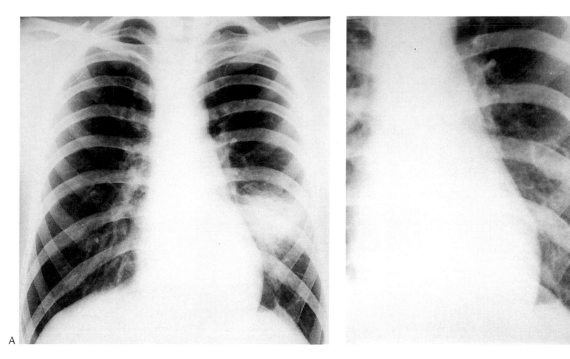

A   B

Fig. 15.44   Coccidioidomycosis. **A.** A non-specific patch of consolidation is present in the left lower lobe. **B.** One year later a thin-walled cavity is evident.

or multiple pulmonary nodules may develop, up to 3 cm in diameter, and these have a tendency to form thin-walled cavities (Fig. 15.44). The fungus may also cause isolated mediastinal or hilar adenopathy and so raise the possibility of lymphoma or sarcoidosis in the differential diagnosis. Rarer manifestations are progressive upper lobe consolidation with fibrosis and cavitation, similar to tuberculosis, and miliary disease.

Blastomycosis   *Blastomyces dermatitidis* is found in parts of the south east USA, and may cause infection similar to other fungi. Hence presentations include an asymptomatic solitary nodule, a pneumonic illness with chronic consolidation, lymphadenopathy, fibronodular disease or miliary disease. Cavitation is occasionally seen, but calcification is rare. Unlike histoplasmosis and coccidioidomycosis fibrosis is uncommon, and once lesions have healed, scars are frequently inconspicuous.

Cryptococcosis (torulosis)   *Cryptococcus neoformans* is a yeast form of fungus found worldwide. Infection is mostly subclinical, but may be important in debilitated patients. It may present with a pleural-based mass (torulosis), possibly cavitating, that may be indistinguishable radiographically from lung cancer (Fig. 15.45). Nodal enlargement and cavitation are unusual. However other presentations include segmental or lobar consolidation and miliary nodules. As with most fungal infections almost any radiographic pattern may occur.

Candidiasis   *Candida albicans* is a normal mouth commensal which, when conditions are favorable, causes moniliasis (thrush), a superficial surface infection. It is rarely invasive unless the patient is immunocompromised. Lung infection, when it occurs, is probably from hematogenous spread. The pulmonary lesion is a chronic pneumonia which breaks down with the formation of an abscess. A mycetoma may develop in the abscess, which is then indistinguishable from aspergilloma.

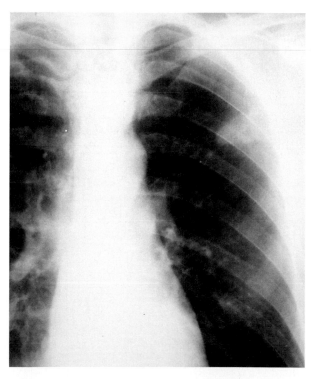

Fig. 15.45   Cryptococcus. A pleurally based mass-like area of consolidation in the left upper lobe is present in a patient who also had cryptococcal meningitis.

Mucormycosis   The *Mucorales* group of fungi are best known as causes of a spreading destructive infection of the face and sinuses in diabetics or the immunosuppressed. Lung infection is a rapidly progressive, dense, cavitating bronchopneumonia.

Aspergillosis *Aspergillus fumigatus* is widespread in the atmosphere and it is inevitable that man inhales the spores from time to time. It is capable of multiplying in air passages when the conditions are favorable. The pulmonary manifestations are grouped into three categories:

1. *Aspergilloma* Any chronic pulmonary cavity may be colonized by fungus. Such cavities are mostly secondary to tuberculosis, histoplasmosis or sarcoidosis, and are, therefore, usually in the upper lobes. The fungal hyphae form a ball or mycetoma which lies free in the cavity.

The *chest radiograph* may show a density surrounded by air within a cavity, but this is best shown by tomography (Fig. 15.29) or CT. By altering the position of the patient the ball is seen to be mobile. There is almost always pleural thickening related to the mycetoma. The differential diagnosis of a mycetoma in a cavity includes *blood clot, cavitating tumor, lung abscess* and *hydatid cyst*.

Mycetomas are associated with development of vascular granulation tissue in the cavity wall, which may bleed. Life-threatening hemoptysis may be difficult to treat surgically, and may be better managed by *bronchial* or *intercostal artery embolization*.

2. *Invasive Aspergillosis* In immunocompromised individuals *Aspergillus* may cause primary infection of the lung. This may be a bronchopneumonia, lobar consolidation or multiple nodules (Fig. 15.46). On high-resolution CT scanning a halo of increased attenuation in the surrounding lung may be seen (Fig. 15.47). Histologically this corresponds to surrounding hemorrhagic inflammation, and although this finding on CT scanning is not completely diagnostic, it is highly suggestive. Cavitation is common, and following bone marrow transplantation often occurs

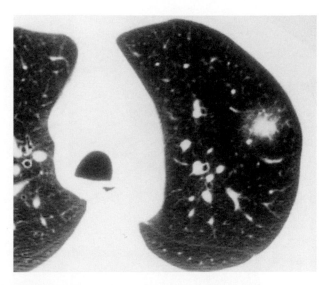

Fig. 15.47 Invasive aspergillosis. High-resolution CT through a left upper lobe nodule demonstrating a halo of increased attenuation. Pathologically this correlates with a surrounding zone of hemorrhagic necrosis.

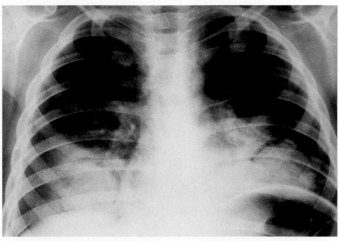

Fig. 15.48 Invasive aspergillosis in a patient with acute lymphoblastic leukemia. A necrotizing pneumonia in both lower zones has cavitated, mimicking the formation of fungus balls.

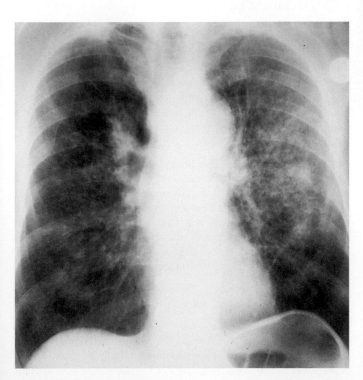

Fig. 15.46 Invasive aspergillosis. There is widespread bronchopneumonic change in a patient receiving chemotherapy for oat-cell carcinoma.

when the white-cell count recovers. The appearances may then mimic an intracavitatory mycetoma (Fig. 15.48) although in contrast to aspergilloma formation in the immunocompetent patient, in the immunosuppressed patient this will occur in an area of previously normal lung.

3. *Allergic Bronchopulmonary Aspergillosis* *Aspergillus* is the commonest cause of pulmonary eosinophilia in the UK; the patient is usually an asthmatic in whom the fungus has colonized the lobar and segmental bronchi, where it produces a Type III reaction. Patients present with a cough and wheeze and often expectorate mucus plugs which contain fungi.

In the acute phase the chest radiograph shows patchy consolidation, often in the upper zones. Mucus plugging may cause lobar collapse (Fig. 15.49), and dilated mucus-filled bronchi may be visible as finger-like, tubular shadows (Fig. 15.50). Appearances may return completely to normal with appropriate treatment.

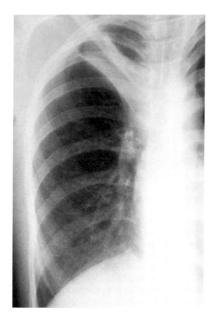

Fig. 15.49 Asthmatic with allergic bronchopulmonary aspergillosis. Mucus plugging has resulted in collapse of the right upper lobe. Complete resolution followed treatment.

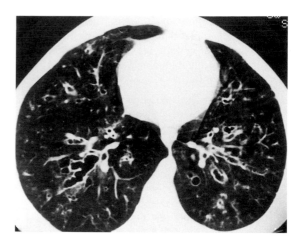

Fig. 15.51 Allergic bronchopulmonary aspergillosis. High-resolution CT demonstrating widespread bronchiectasis of the medium and large airways.

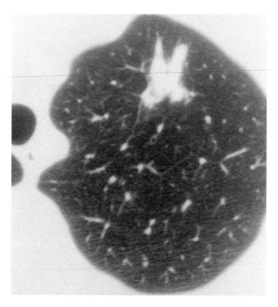

Fig. 15.50 Allergic bronchopulmonary aspergillosis. High-resolution CT scan demonstrating finger-like opacities due to dilated mucus-filled bronchi.

However, with repeated attacks there may be pulmonary fibrosis and bronchiectasis. Fibrotic changes tend to occur in the upper zones. Bronchiectasis may produce ring shadows and tramline shadows. Unlike other causes of bronchiectasis, allergic bronchopulmonary aspergillosis may produce changes that are more severe in the central airways than peripherally (Fig. 15.51).

The condition pursues an intermittent course over many years and the frequency of chronic changes increases with the number of acute episodes. Within areas previously the site of transient opacities, the bronchi dilate and contain plugs of tough, stringy mucus mixed with small numbers of the aspergillus. Mucoid impaction is a dilated bronchus packed tightly with this material. Because of their thickened walls, bronchi may be visible as tubes, rings or cavities or, if impacted, as bulbous 'gloved finger' or branching opacities. Air may return to impacted bronchi if the material is coughed up. Plugging of central bronchi can lead to collapse of lobes or whole lungs. Continued damage and repair by fibrosis will lead to focal emphysema, permanent shrinkage and eventually end-stage upper lobe fibrosis. Thus, although pulmonary opacities are transient, in only a minority of cases does the chest radiograph become completely normal between acute episodes. A mycetoma may form, not always in the upper lobes.

PROTOZOAL INFECTIONS

Pneumocystis This is discussed under 'Acquired immune deficiency syndrome' (see p. 452).

Toxoplasmosis This is a protozoal disease widespread in mammals and birds; human acquisition is from cats or uncooked meat.

Although *toxoplasmosis* rarely involves the lungs, it may on occasion be responsible for an interstitial pneumonia, in which case the chest radiograph may show patchy consolidation and mediastinal lymphadenopathy.

Entamoeba histolytica This protozoon is also found worldwide although amebiasis tends to occur in the tropics and subtropics. Involvement of the chest is usually secondary to hepatic infection and is therefore usually right-sided. A hepatic amebic abscess may erode the diaphragm and cause diaphragmatic elevation, pleural effusion, basal consolidation and lower lobe cavitation. *Ultrasound* scan may reveal liver abscesses, and allows assessment of the diaphragm and pleural spaces.

METAZOAN INFECTIONS

Loeffler's Syndrome This may be caused by many parasitic worms, including *Ascaris*, *Taenia*, *Ankylostoma* and *Strongyloides*, all of which may lodge in or migrate through the lungs at some stage of their life cycles. The term *Loeffler's syndrome* is now applied to almost any transient pulmonary opacities of a predominantly eosinophilic histology associated with a blood eosinophilia. The heavier the infestation the more profuse are the pulmonary lesions. *Strongyloides stercoralis* in particular is capable of causing widespread opacities and a serious pulmonary illness. Such *hyper-infection* can be activated by immunosuppression.

Schistosomiasis   Schistosomiasis may cause pulmonary eosinophilia. If the eggs lodge in pulmonary arteries of less than 100 μm, the lesions they cause are small granulomas like miliary tuberculosis or sarcoidosis, but if they lodge in arteries of larger size the irritation causes vascular necrosis and fibrotic occlusion. The latter results in pulmonary hypertension if sufficient vessels are occluded. A third type of reaction results in diffuse interstitial fibrosis.

Paragonimiasis   Infestation is usually acquired in the tropics from eating infected shellfish. The commonest reactions in the lung are formation of multiple 1–2 cm diameter cysts and bronchopneumonic shadowing, which may resemble tuberculosis. The dead flukes may calcify.

Armillifer armillatus   This is usually acquired by eating infected snakes. The larvae may migrate to the lungs where they encyst, die and calcify. The typical radiographic appearance is of multiple thin-walled cysts in a subpleural distribution. Dead larvae may calcify and be visible within the cysts as coils, targets or signet ring shapes.

Hydatid Disease   This is caused by *Echinococcus granulosus*. Dogs are the principal reservoir of the adult worm, and most mammals serve as intermediate host for the larvae (echinococci). The hydatid is a parasitic echinococcal cyst consisting of three layers: an adventitia formed of compressed host tissue, a middle layer of friable ectocyst and an inner germinal layer from which is produced large numbers of scolices which are the heads of developing worms. Daughter cysts are formed if the viability is threatened but in the lung the cyst is unilocular (Fig. 15.52). Cysts mainly occur in the lungs and liver. Approximately 20% of the pulmonary cysts are bilateral, and about 10% are associated with hepatic cysts. Uncomplicated pulmonary hydatid cysts appear as well-circumscribed, round or oval, homogenous masses, which may be up to 10 cm in diameter. Calcification is rare. Cysts may rupture into the pleura or bronchi. Following rupture into a bronchus an air–fluid level may appear or the ectocyst may separate from the adventitia so that a double-walled cyst may be seen. The choice of treatment of pulmonary hydatid disease lies between medical therapy (albendazole) or surgery, when the cyst must be removed intact.

CONGENITAL ABNORMALITIES THAT PREDISPOSE TO PULMONARY INFECTION

Cystic Fibrosis   This is an autosomal recessive condition that occurs in 1 in 2000 live births and produces a generalized disease of exocrine glands and mucous glands. The latter produce abnormally viscous mucus which impairs mucociliary function and in the chest predisposes to frequent chest infections and development of bronchiectasis. It is now relatively common for patients to survive into adulthood, but overall the prognosis remains poor, with most deaths being a direct result of respiratory complications. *Pseudomonas aeruginosa, Staph. aureus, Haemophilus influenzae* and *Klebsiella* species are frequent causes. The early radiographic changes may be limited to hyperexpansion, but eventually after repeated episodes of infection, a combination of bronchial wall thickening and dilatation and scarring produces a characteristic pattern. Clusters of ring shadows, some containing air–fluid levels, may be visible, together with evidence of air trapping, lobar or segmental collapse or consolidation. The latter usually indicates superadded infection. As respiratory failure progresses cor pulmonale may develop, as may repeated episodes of hemoptysis which may be life threatening. Repeated pneumothoraces, often resistant to tube drainage, are a further potentially fatal complication (see Ch. 16).

Hypogammaglobulinemia   This predisposes to bacterial infections with resultant bronchiectasis in long-term survivors.

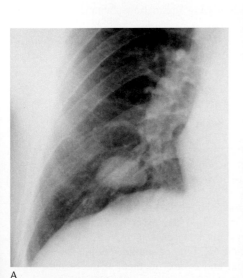

A

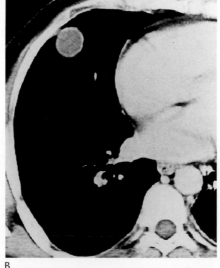

B

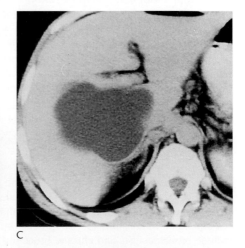

C

Fig. 15.52   Pulmonary hydatid disease. **A.** Well-defined right basal pulmonary mass. **B.** The CT scan reveals the well-defined wall and cystic contents. **C.** This patient also had a large hepatic hydatid cyst.

Chronic Granulomatous Disease Only in rare instances do patients with this condition survive to adult life. Phagocytosis is normal but the polymorphs are incapable of destroying the ingested bacteria at a normal rate. Children suffer from recurrent pneumonias, but with increasing age these become less frequent. The lungs usually show bilateral interstitial fibrosis. Other thoracic complications are bronchiectasis and granulomatous mediastinitis.

Impaired Neutrophil Chemotaxis Phagocytic cells are attracted to sites of bacterial infection by chemotactic substances released by the organisms or locally produced by the host. Activated complement is one such host substance. Instances have been found of impaired neutrophil chemotactic responses which have an adverse effect on the frequency and severity of infections. Abscesses and skin sepsis are the common manifestations and recurrent staphylococcal pneumonias are not infrequent.

Congenital Dyskinetic Ciliary Syndromes The 'immotile cilia syndrome' was the term originally applied to this group of conditions, but this is too restrictive since it is now known that there can be abnormalities of synchrony as well as total immotility. This collective term encompasses a heterogeneous mixture of structural and functional abnormalities of cilia. It is now postulated that the beating of embryonic cilia determines organ situs; if the beat is abnormal the situs will be randomly allocated and 50% will have situs inversus. Sperm tails are also cilia, and males with the condition will be infertile, hence explaining the combination of bronchiectasis, situs inversus and male infertility in *Kartagener's syndrome*.

Impairment of mucociliary clearance renders the lungs more susceptible to bronchopulmonary infections, but this is only a serious problem if the infections are repeated and severe. The radiographic signs are those of bronchiectasis, atelectasis and chronic obstructive airways disease.

Young's Syndrome This is a combination of obstructive azoospermia, sinusitis and chronic pulmonary infections. The latter begin in childhood and eventually most patients develop bronchiectasis. There is no structural abnormality of cilia but mucociliary transport is impaired. Spermatogenesis is normal, but the infertility of these men is due to a progressive obstruction of the epididymis by inspissated secretions.

Congenital Pulmonary Sequestration This is an abnormality in which some lung tissue develops separated from the normal airways and pulmonary vessels. The blood supply is derived from the descending aorta. Sequestrated segments are situated basally in contact with the diaphragm, and appear solid when uncomplicated. They may become infected and develop a communication with the bronchial tree, following which they may cavitate and show a fluid level (Fig. 15.53).

ACQUIRED CONDITIONS THAT PREDISPOSE TO PULMONARY INFECTION

Systemic conditions that are associated with decreased immunity include old age, poor nutrition, diabetes, alcoholism, connective tissue disorders, many malignant diseases and AIDS.

Pulmonary abnormalities that predispose to chest infections include bronchiectasis and chronic bronchitis. In addition general anesthesia, especially if prolonged, may be associated with pneumonia.

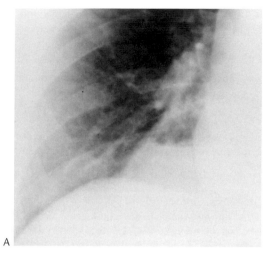
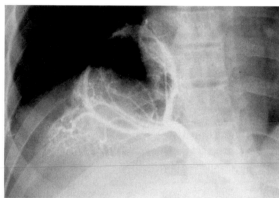

Fig. 15.53 Pulmonary sequestration. **A.** The chest radiograph demonstrates a cavitating mass-like lesion in the right lower lobe. Note the preservation of the heart border and diaphragm. **B.** Angiogram demonstrating the typical blood supply from a side branch of the subdiaphragmatic aorta.

Iatrogenic causes include cancer chemotherapy, steroids, immunosuppression following organ transplantation, and radiotherapy.

Chronic infection of the paranasal sinuses and *esophageal obstruction* may cause pneumonia or lung abscesses due to aspiration.

PULMONARY INFECTIONS IN IMMUNOCOMPROMISED PATIENTS—NON-AIDS

Pulmonary opportunistic infections are a common complication in immunocompromised patients. The radiographic appearances are often non-specific, and despite the high morbidity and mortality associated with chest infection in these patients a definitive diagnosis may be difficult to reach. In order for the radiologist to have a meaningful input into the assessment of the immunocompromised patient with acute chest symptoms the underlying cause of immunodeficiency, type of immunosuppressive therapy, white blood cell count and overall medical status of the patient must be known. Whilst the role of the radiologist in these patients has primarily been one of detection and monitoring of pulmonary abnormalities, the introduction of HRCT now makes it possible to offer earlier and more specific diagnostic information. Furthermore HRCT allows prediction of the relative chances of obtaining a positive diagnosis from transbronchial versus percutaneous biopsy, particularly when other techniques have proved non-diagnostic.

Immunodeficiency may occur as a result of impaired cell-mediated immunity (T-cells), for example in patients with lymphoma, patients who have undergone bone marrow transplantation or who are immunosuppressed following solid organ transplantation. Reduced humoral immunity (B-cells) is most commonly seen in patients with myeloma, non-Hodgkin's lymphoma and lymphoblastic leukemia. Reduced granulocyte number and/or function is encountered in patients with leukemia and in those undergoing immunosuppressive therapy following transplantation.

Bacterial Pneumonias   These are the most frequent pulmonary infections in the immunocompromised patient and rapid progression may occur. In addition to the common pathogens, debilitated patients—including diabetics and patients on steroid therapy—are also prone to the legionella group of bacteria. When tuberculosis occurs in this patient group it is usually due to reactivation. *Nocardia asteroides* has a predilection for immuno-suppressed patients.

Invasive Aspergillosis   This may occur in patients following solid organ or bone marrow transplantation. Diagnosis may be difficult, and CT should be considered early in the investigation of the immunocompromised patient with clinical evidence of chest infection but a normal chest radiograph. The radiographic pattern is discussed elsewhere.

***Candida albicans* Pneumonia**   This may occur in severely immunosuppressed patients with leukemia or lymphoma, and lung disease usually develops as part of hematogenous dissemination, often as a preterminal event (Fig. 15.54). As a result there is frequently evidence of oral, cutaneous or hepatic disease.

The radiographic changes are non-specific, with widespread interstitial or alveolar disease or lobar segmental consolidation. Occasionally, multiple nodules occur. Other fungi may cause disease in immunocompromised patients, as discussed above (Figs 15.55, 15.56).

ACQUIRED IMMUNE DEFICIENCY SYNDROME (AIDS)

AIDS is due to infection by the human immunodeficiency virus (HIV), and classically exposes the patient to infections normally resisted by cell-mediated immunity. The syndrome comprises

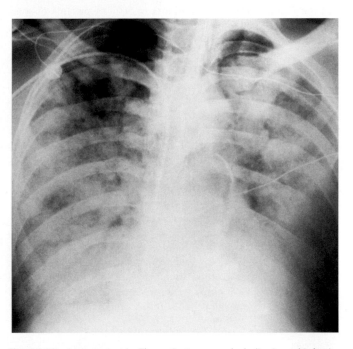

Fig. 15.55   Mucormycosis. The patient was an alcoholic. Fungal infection followed Rocky Mountain spotted fever. Mixed infection with Gram-negative organisms. Postmortem confirmation.

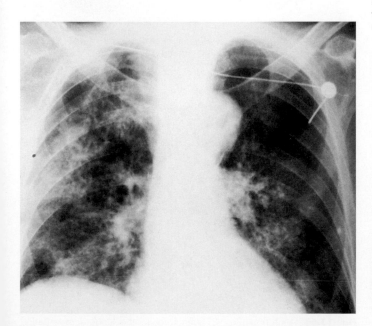

Fig. 15.54   *Candida albicans* bronchopneumonia. Mixed infection with Gram-negative organisms. Chronic alcoholic. Postmortem confirmation.

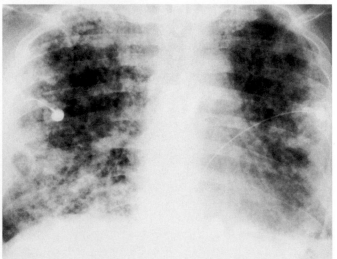

Fig. 15.56   Disseminated cryptococcosis. Mixed infection with Gram-negative organisms. Patient on steroids for systemic lupus.

opportunistic infections and certain rare malignancies, and in the UK is most often seen in homosexual males, drug addicts and hemophiliacs. Although a wide variety of infectious and non-infectious pulmonary diseases occur in AIDS, the commonest remains opportunistic infection.

***Pneumocystis carinii* Pneumonia (PCP)**   This protozoal infection occurs in all groups of immunocompromised patients with reduced cell-mediated immunity. It is particularly common in the AIDS population; approximately 60–80% of all patients with AIDS will suffer at least one episode of PCP during the course of their illness. Approximately 40% of patients will have recurrent episodes of PCP despite the use of prophylaxis. Furthermore PCP was the initial AIDS-defining illness in 50% of patients in some earlier series. Symptomatically, patients present with dry cough and shortness of breath, frequently accompanied by a pyrexia. Whilst the radiographic appearances may be normal early in the disease in up to 10% of patients and the degree of dyspnea may be in advance of the radiographic changes, most patients will develop perihilar and mid and lower zone bilateral interstitial or ground-glass infiltrate (Fig. 15.57). This may rapidly progress to involve the entire lung (Fig. 15.58). On HRCT scanning the characteristic appearances are of a ground-glass infiltrate extending from the hilar regions into the surrounding lung, occasionally demonstrating a geographic pattern. Cavities, usually thin-walled, but occasionally with a wall up to several millimeters in thickness, may develop (Fig. 15.59). Although appearances may return entirely to normal some residual scarring and cyst formation is not uncommon. Pneumothorax is a well recognized complication of *Pneumocystis carinii* pneumonia, usually in association with cystic change (Fig. 15.60). When pneumothorax occurs later in the course of disease, tube drainage may be ineffective and pleurodesis may be required. Extensive mediastinal and surgical emphysema may develop, and this combination of clinical

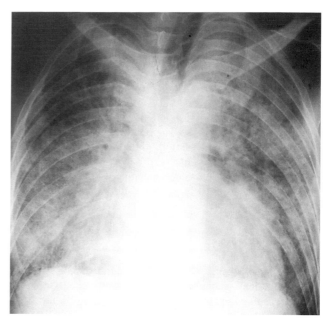

Fig. 15.58 *Pneumocystis carinii* pneumonia. Extensive bilateral consolidation.

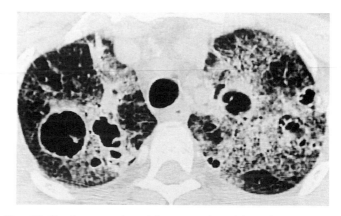

Fig. 15.59 *Pneumocystis carinii* pneumonia. High-resolution CT scan through the apices demonstrating ground-glass infiltrate associated with multiple thin-walled cavities.

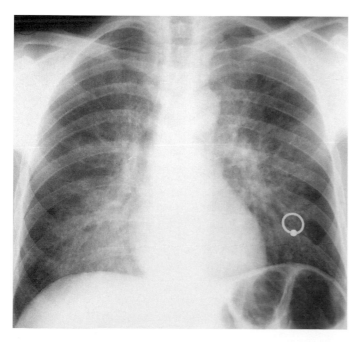

Fig. 15.57 *Pneumocystis carinii* pneumonia. There is widespread bilateral mid and lower zone ground-glass infiltrate.

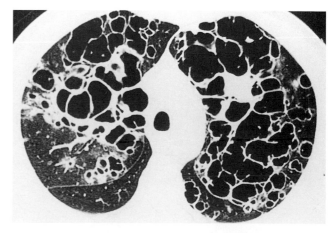

Fig. 15.60 High-resolution CT scan through the lungs demonstrating multiple areas of cystic destruction following repeated *Pneumocystis* infection. (Courtesy of C. D. R. Flower, Addenbrooke's Hospital, Cambridge.)

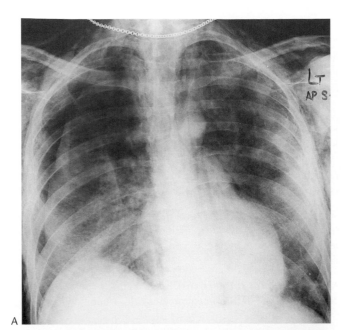

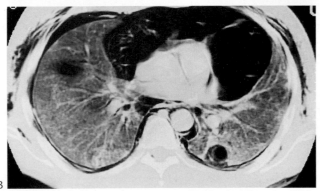

Fig. 15.61 *Pneumocystis carinii* pneumonia. Chest radiograph (**A**) and CT scan (**B**) demonstrating extensive mediastinal and surgical emphysema with bilateral pneumothoraces.

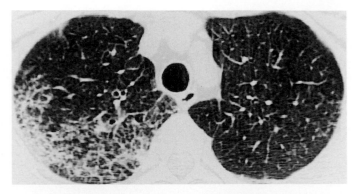

Fig. 15.62 *Pneumocystis carinii* pneumonia. Asymmetric interstitial infiltrate in the right apex, barely visible on the chest radiograph, in a patient on aerosolized pentamidine.

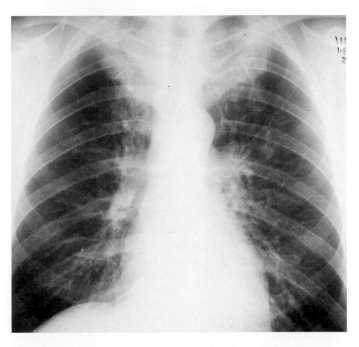

Fig. 15.63 *Pneumocystis carinii* pneumonia. Chest radiograph demonstrating bilateral apical infiltrates in a patient on aerosolized pentamidine prophylaxis.

features has a poor outlook (Fig. 15.61). Many less common manifestations of PCP are well recognized and include miliary disease, discrete pulmonary nodules, pleural effusions and mediastinal lymphadenopathy. Mediastinal lymph nodes may become calcified, particularly well seen on CT scanning. Many AIDS patients in the West will undergo prophylactic treatment with aerosolized pentamidine, and these patients are more likely to develop atypical patterns of disease including an apical distribution of involvement (Figs 15.62, 15.63), calcified hilar and abdominal nodes and viscera, and pulmonary cystic disease. PCP may present with unilateral disease and occasionally may mimic a bacterial pneumonia, with focal or lobar consolidation. Miliary disease is occasionally encountered (Fig. 15.64).

Whilst the radiographic changes may be highly suggestive of PCP the diagnosis is usually made on examination of induced sputum, which has a yield of approximately 80–90%. When induced sputum examination is negative in patients with clinical and radiological features of PCP, including desaturation on exercise, a trial of therapy may be commenced. It is usual to reserve bronchoscopy for patients who subsequently fail to respond to a trial of therapy.

Bacterial Pneumonia AIDS patients are prone to community acquired pneumonia such as *Streptococcus pneumoniae, Staphylococcus aureus* and *Pseudomonas aeruginosa*. Whilst disease progression may be unusually rapid and severe in this patient group, with cavitation and pleural effusions being more frequent than in non-immunocompromised patients, most commonly the pattern of disease is the same as in the normal population. Bacterial infections may occur relatively early in the course of AIDS whilst the CD4+ count remains high, and repeated bacterial chest infections are now included in the CDC list of AIDS-defining illnesses.

Mycobacterial Infection Mycobacterial infection is also common in the AIDS population; equally, AIDS is commonly detected underlying a new case of TB. Indeed the HIV-positive rate in patients with active TB in the United States is between 4 and 40%, depending on the population center.

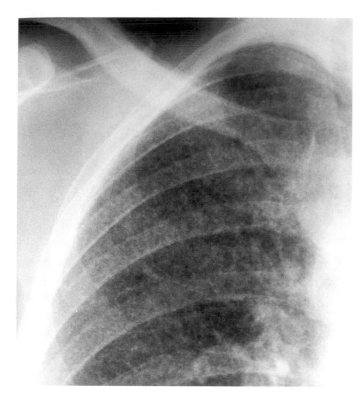

Fig. 15.64 *Pneumocystis carinii* pneumonia causing miliary shadowing. Appearances resolved on appropriate treatment.

Mycobacterium tuberculosis (MTB)   Radiological manifestations of MTB depend on the degree of immunosuppression. In the early stages of HIV infection appearances are similar to those of reactivation TB in the normal population. When the CD4+ count falls in the later stages of HIV disease, appearances become more in keeping with primary TB. Cavitation becomes less common and mediastinal nodal enlargement typically shows marked central low density change with a rim of enhancing tissue (Fig. 15.65). Lung changes include non-specific areas of pulmonary consoli-

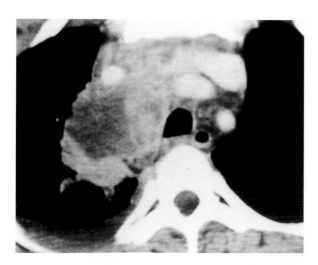

Fig. 15.65 Tuberculous lymph node enlargement in a patient with AIDS. There is a central low density area surrounded by a rim of enhancing nodal material.

dation and the presence of round or branching pulmonary nodules. Occasionally a miliary pattern is seen.

Mycobacterium Avium Intracellulare (MAI)   MAI is frequently isolated in the AIDS population and is a common postmortem finding. Despite this there is frequently no clinical evidence of infection prior to death. Although in the immunocompetent population MAI is usually confined to the chest, in the HIV-positive group the infection is almost always disseminated and may be identified from a bone marrow aspirate or blood culture. Within the chest appearances are similar to MTB, although pleural effusions are more common with MAI and miliary disease is particularly uncommon.

Atypical mycobacterial infections   These occur with a similar frequency in the AIDS population as in the general population. However miliary disease is considerably more common in the AIDS population.

Multiple drug resistant TB (MDRTB)   This is considerably more common in the AIDS population and is becoming an increasingly major problem.

Cytomegalovirus (CMV)   Although CMV inclusion bodies are a frequent finding in lung material from AIDS patients, CMV rarely causes clinical infection; when identified in patients with acute pulmonary disease it is often in association with other pathogenic organisms (Fig. 15.66).

Toxoplasmosis   There is a high prevalence of previous exposure in the HIV-positive adult population. However genuine pulmonary involvement is distinctly unusual, despite the frequent occurrence of CNS toxoplasmosis. The chest radiographic appearances are non-specific.

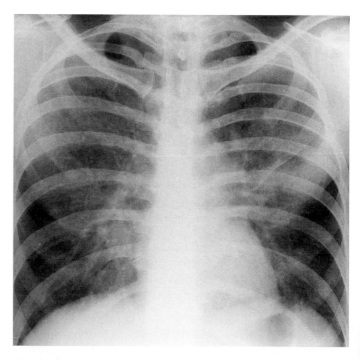

Fig. 15.66 Cytomegalovirus in AIDS. Although CMV is rarely a cause of pneumonia in isolation, on occasion other organisms are not identified.

Fungal Infection

Fungal infections are relatively rare in the AIDS population, and when there is pulmonary involvement there is often disseminated disease.

Histoplasma Capsulatum infection occurs in patients who have visited or reside in areas where the organism is endemic, such as the central USA and Central and South America. The disease is usually widely disseminated, and when pulmonary abnormalities are evident they normally take the form of a diffuse non-specific interstitial infiltrate or bilateral discrete non-calcified nodules. Lymphadenopathy occurs more frequently than in *Pneumocystis carinii* pneumonia. The diagnosis is usually made from bone marrow aspirate and culture.

Coccidioides immitis is also widespread in the central USA and occasionally causes Coccidioidomycosis in exposed AIDS patients. The radiographic features are non-specific with a bilateral nodular or reticulonodular infiltrate, usually without mediastinal and hilar lymph node enlargement. Occasionally, solitary pulmonary nodules occur with this infection.

Cryptococcus Neoformans   When *Cryptococcus* causes clinical disease in the HIV population it is usually due to infection of the brain or meninges, and when pulmonary disease occurs it is usually in association with CNS disease. Radiographic changes are non-specific and include single or multiple nodules, consolidation with or without cavitation, interstitial infiltrates and enlargement of mediastinal lymph nodes.

Aspergillus Fumigatus   Aspergillus is an infrequent fungal infection in the HIV population, occasionally causing pneumonic disease or discrete pulmonary nodules (Fig. 15.67).

Non-infectious Pulmonary Disease in AIDS

Kaposi's Sarcoma   occurs in approximately 10% of patients with AIDS. Usually there is evidence of cutaneous or visceral disease when there is lung involvement. Kaposi sarcoma usually appears as ill-defined nodules (Fig. 15.68), sometimes associated with pleural effusions and lymphadenopathy. Occasionally Kaposi sarcoma may present with a diffuse pulmonary infiltrate. When there is pulmonary involvement, disease is usually evident

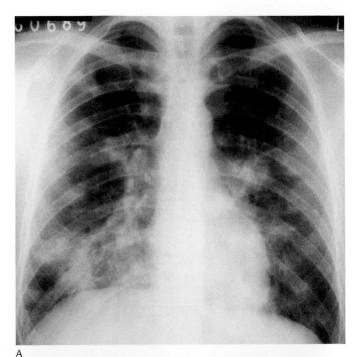

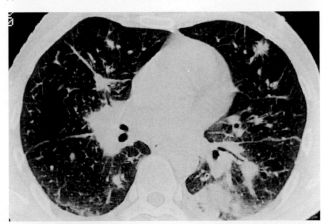

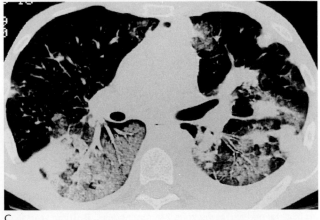

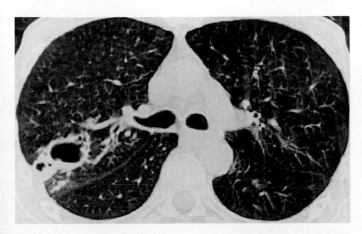

Fig. 15.67   Right upper lobe cavity colonized by aspergillus in an AIDS patient.

Fig. 15.68   Kaposi sarcoma. **A.** Multiple poorly defined pulmonary nodules are present bilaterally in a patient with bronchial and cutaneous Kaposi sarcoma. **B** and **C.** CT scans of two different patients demonstrating multiple poorly defined pulmonary nodules with a mid and lower zone and peribronchovascular predominance.

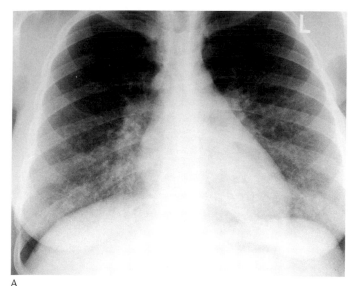

A

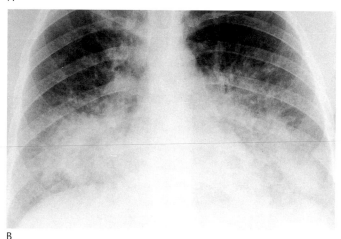

B

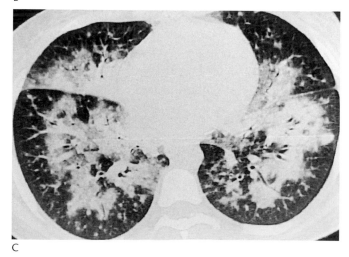

C

bronchoscopically as distinctive raised erythematous plaques within the airways. If these plaques become sufficiently enlarged they may occlude segmental bronchi resulting in atelectasis.

A variety of lymphoproliferative disorders are associated with AIDS including lymphocytic interstitial pneumonitis, seen most frequently in the non-AIDS population in association with Sjögren's syndrome and SLE. When occurring in the AIDS population it is most frequent in children although adult cases are regularly encountered. The radiological appearances are most commonly a mid and lower zone reticular or reticulonodular infiltrate. Although it is radiographically indistinguishable from opportunistic infection, slow progression of radiological change is suggestive of the diagnosis (Fig. 15.69). Neither pleural nor lymph node enlargement is associated with LIP, and if present should prompt a search for an alternative diagnosis. Bronchiectasis may occasionally occur. Features of LIP may regress as the degree of immunocompromise progresses.

Non-specific Pneumonitis is a relatively poorly defined condition that occurs in the immunosuppressed patient with or without AIDS. It has been attributed to a variety of causes including unidentified viral infection, drug therapy and irradiation. Symptoms in patients with histologic confirmation of the diagnosis are variable although reduction of the diffusing capacity of the lungs appears to be a more constant feature. The chest radiographic appearances are non-specific. Appearances may be normal or there may be alveolar or interstitial infiltrate; differentiation from other opportunistic infection is therefore not possible. Bronchiectasis has been observed to develop in a number of cases (Fig. 15.70). Failure to respond to treatment for infective causes and a relatively indolent course should raise the possibility of this diagnosis in a susceptible patient.

Lymphoma, rarely confined to the thorax, is well described in AIDS patients. When the presentation is with thoracic disease, there may be atypical mediastinal nodal enlargement, pleural or

Fig. 15.69 Lymphocytic interstitial pneumonitis. **A.** Chest X-ray demonstrating bilateral mid and lower zone 2–5 mm nodules. **B.** Three years later there is an extensive mid and lower zone pulmonary infiltrate. **C.** High-resolution CT scan demonstrating the bronchovascular distribution of confluent infiltrate with more peripheral discrete nodules. Transbronchial biopsy confirmed the diagnosis of lymphocytic interstitial pneumonitis.

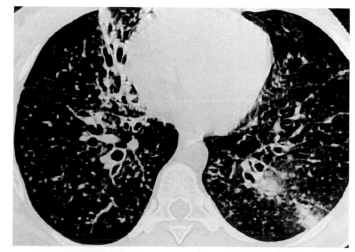

Fig. 15.70 Non-specific interstitial pneumonitis. A nodular infiltrate with patches of confluence is present in addition to widespread bronchiectasis, most marked in the middle lobe. The appearances have been slowly evolving over three years.

pericardial effusions, areas of pulmonary infiltrate or single or multiple pulmonary masses (Figs 15.71, 15.72).

Occasionally patients with AIDS develop **primary lung tumors**, with an increased incidence relative to the general population.

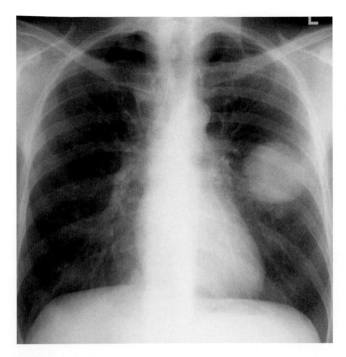

Fig. 15.71 AIDS-related lymphoma. There is a well-defined mass in the left mid zone. Percutaneous needle biopsy was undertaken to confirm the diagnosis.

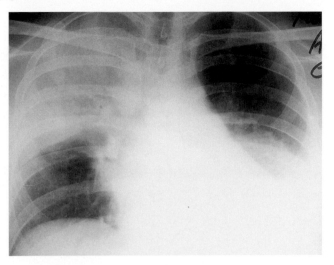

Fig. 15.72 AIDS-related lymphoma causing extensive consolidation in the right upper lobe. Infiltration of the left lower lobe in association with a pleural effusion is also evident.

SUGGESTIONS FOR FURTHER READING

Armstrong, P., Wilson, A. G., Dee, P., Hansell, D. M. (1995) Infections of the Lung and Pleura. In: *Imaging of Diseases of the Chest*, 2nd edn. St Louis: Mosby–Year Book.

Armstrong, P., Wilson, A. G., Dee, P., Hansell, D. M. (1995) AIDS and Other Forms of Immunocompromise. In: *Imaging of Diseases of the Chest*, 2nd edn. St Louis: Mosby–Year Book.

Berkmen Y. M. (1980) Uncommon acute bacterial pneumonias. *Seminars in Roentgenology*, **15**, 17–24.

Berkmen, Y. M. (1980) Aspiration and inhalation pneumonias. *Seminars in Roentgenology*, **15**, 73–84.

Fanta, C. H., Pennington, J. E. (1981) Fever and new lung infiltrations in the immunocompromised host. *Clinics in Chest Medicine*, **2**, 19–37.

Genereux, G. P., Stilwell, G. A. (1980) The acute bacterial pneumonias. *Seminars in Roentgenology*, **15**, 9–6.

Janower, M. L., Weiss, E. B. (1980) Mycoplasmal, viral and rickettsial pneumonias. *Seminars in Roentgenology*, **15**, 25–34.

Miller, W. T. (ed) (1996) Fungus diseases of the chest. *Seminars in Roentgenology*, **31**, 1.

Moore, E. H. (1991) Diffuse lung disease in the current spectrum of immuno-compromised hosts (non-AIDS). *Radiological Clinics of North America*, **29:5**, 983–998.

Naidich, D. P., McGuiness, G. (1991) Pulmonary manifestations of AIDS: CT and radiographic correlations. *Radiological Clinics of North America*, **29:5**, 999–1018.

Palmer, P. E. S. (1979) Pulmonary tuberculosis—usual and unusual radio-graphic presentations. *Seminars in Roentgenology*, 141(3): 204–243.

Reeder, M. M., Palmer, P. E. S. (1980) Acute tropical pneumonias. *Seminars in Roentgenology*, **15**, 35–49.

Schwartz, J., Baum, G. L. (1970) Fungal diseases of the lungs. *Seminars in Roentgenology*, **5**, 13–54.

16

DISEASES OF THE AIRWAYS; COLLAPSE AND CONSOLIDATION

Michael B. Rubens and Simon P. G. Padley

TRACHEA AND BRONCHI

The Trachea

Congenital Abnormalities *Tracheo-esophageal fistula* may occur as an isolated anomaly. On the plain film, air may be visible in the esophagus (Fig. 16.1), but the diagnosis is usually made by a contrast study of the esophagus. Barium or low osmolarity

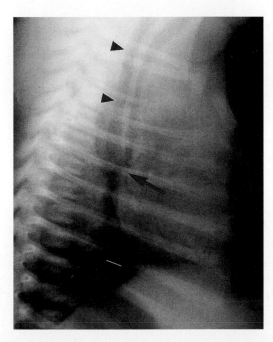

Fig. 16.1 Tracheo-esophageal fistula. A lateral chest radiograph shows the fistula between the trachea and the esophagus (arrow). The esophagus is air-filled (arrowheads).

contrast medium must be used. If a simple swallow does not show the fistula, contrast medium should be injected into a nasogastric tube with the patient prone. As the tube is withdrawn the fistula is usually seen. Tracheo-esophageal fistula may also be associated with esophageal atresia. Other causes of tracheal narrowing are hypoplasia of the tracheal cartilage, and compression by a distended esophageal pouch.

Tracheal Narrowing Tracheal narrowing may be due to an extrinsic mass or mediastinal fibrosis or an intrinsic abnormality of the tracheal wall. *Laryngotracheobronchitis* or *croup* is the commonest cause of tracheal narrowing. It is usually viral and affects the upper trachea, most often in young children. Pyogenic bacteria and tuberculosis may cause a more generalized acute tracheitis. Tuberculosis may cause fibrosis and chronic tracheal stenosis.

Fibrosing mediastinitis, which may be due to tuberculosis or histoplasmosis, can cause both tracheal and bronchial stenosis. Rarer chronic inflammatory causes of tracheal narrowing include *sarcoidosis, chronic relapsing polychondritis* (Fig. 16.2), *Wegener's granulomatosis, rhinoscleroma* and *tracheopathia osteoplastica*.

Sabersheath trachea is a condition which usually occurs in elderly men and is almost invariably seen in association with chronic obstructive airways disease. The tracheal wall is normal and the abnormal configuration of the lumen is probably a reflection of abnormal intrathoracic pressures. The return of the trachea to a normal caliber in its extrathoracic portion supports this theory.

Primary *tumors* of the trachea are rare. Benign tumors present as small, well-defined intraluminal nodules. They are mostly papillomas, fibromas, chondromas or hemangiomas, Malignant tumors of the trachea tend to occur close to the carina. They are mostly squamous, adenoid cystic or adeno-carcinomas (Fig. 16.3). They may cause a localized mass or a long stricture. Their extraluminal extent is best assessed by CT (Fig. 16.4).

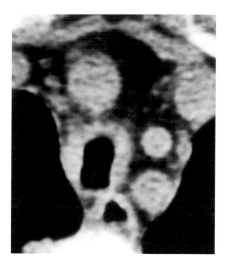

Fig. 16.2 CT scan through the trachea at the level of the great vessels demonstrating diffuse tracheal wall thickening. Compare with the normal tracheal wall thickness demonstrated in Fig. 16.4B. Biopsy was consistent with relapsing polychondritis.

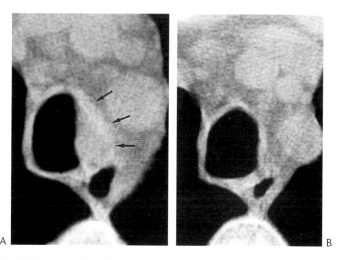

Fig. 16.4 Adenoid cystic carcinoma of the trachea. **A.** CT demonstrates a mass within the left lateral tracheal wall causing only slight distortion of the lumen. The extraluminal component extends into the adjacent mediastinal fat (arrows). **B.** CT image 2 cm cranial to the lesion demonstrates normal tracheal wall thickness.

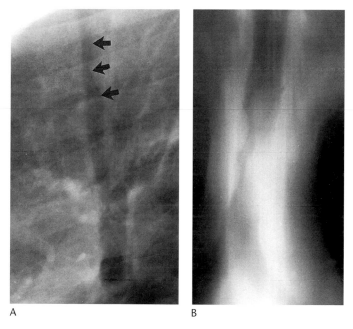

Fig. 16.3 Squamous carcinoma of the trachea. **A.** Close up of the lateral chest X-ray demonstrates narrowing of the trachea with irregularity of the posterior wall (arrows). **B.** AP tomogram demonstrating lobulated filling defects within the tracheal air column.

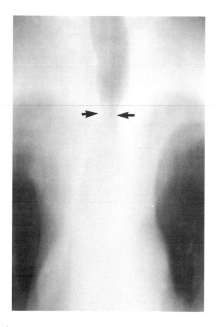

Fig. 16.5 There is a stricture (arrows) of the trachea following tracheostomy 10 years earlier.

Tracheal stenosis may be the result of previous injury. This includes incomplete laceration of the trachea as well as iatrogenic causes such as previous tracheostomy or prolonged tracheal intubation (Fig. 16.5). Stricture development following prolonged intubation is thought to be secondary to ischemia of the tracheal mucosa due to overinflation of the cuff of the endotracheal tube. Low pressure cuffs have now become widespread to prevent this complication. Other rare causes of tracheal wall thickening and stenosis are *amyloidosis, tracheopathia osteoplastica* and *tracheomalacia*.

Tumors of the thyroid, esophagus or lung may displace or compress the trachea, and if malignant may invade the trachea. Rarely the trachea is the site of metastases from a distant primary tumor such as melanoma.

Tracheal Widening   The normal dimensions of the trachea have been assessed using a variety of techniques, most recently computed tomography. The trachea becomes slightly larger with increasing age. On CT scanning the maximum coronal diameter of the trachea is 23 mm in a male and 20 mm in a female. Dilatation of the trachea is rare, and it may result from a defect of connective tissue. This may be an isolated abnormality as in *tracheobronchomegaly* (Mounier–Kuhn syndrome—Fig. 16.6) or associated with Ehlers–Danlos syndrome or cutis laxa. In

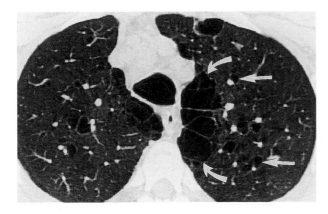

Fig. 16.6 Mounier–Kuhn syndrome. There is dilatation of the trachea in association with bronchiectasis (arrows). There are also multiple paraseptal bullae (curved arrow).

Mounier–Kuhn syndrome the trachea may be as wide as the vertebral bodies and of uneven contour, with bulging of the mucosa between the cartilage rings. The dilatation may proceed no further than the main bronchi, or it may be associated with a generalized bronchiectasis. The hypothesis that it results from a defect of connective tissue receives some support from its occasional association with Ehlers–Danlos syndrome, a generalized connective tissue disorder.

The Bronchi

Bronchiectasis *Bronchiectasis* is the irreversible dilatation of one or more bronchi, and is usually the result of severe, recurrent or chronic infection. Childhood pneumonias, especially *pertussis* and *measles*, and *tuberculosis* are important causes. Other predisposing factors include *chronic sinusitis, bronchial obstruction and abnormalities of the cilia, mucus and immune system* (e.g. *Kartagener syndrome*—Fig. 16.7), *cystic fibrosis and agamma-globulinemia*). Non-infective causes include bronchopulmonary aspergillosis and inhalation of noxious fluids or gases. In addition bronchiectasis is seen in association with intrinsic connective tissue abnormalities such as Ehlers–Danlos syndrome, Marfan syndrome and tracheobronchomegaly, and rarely in association with more common conditions such as rheumatoid disease and Sjögren syndrome.

Bronchiectasis may be localized or generalized. It is frequently basal but, in tuberculosis and cystic fibrosis, it usually involves the upper zones. Dilated bronchi may produce tramline shadows (Fig. 16.8) or ring shadows (Fig. 16.9), and dilated, fluid-filled bronchi may cause 'gloved finger' shadows. Accumulation of pus or secretions in ectatic bronchi may produce fluid levels (Figs 16.7, 16.9). Chest infections frequently complicate bronchiectasis so that areas of consolidation may obscure the above signs. *Bronchography* was until relatively recently the definitive method of diagnosing bronchiectasis but has now been completely superseded by HRCT. Traditionally bronchiectasis has been described as cylindrical, varicose or saccular.

Cylindrical (or tubular) bronchiectasis (Fig. 16.10) produces a dilated bronchus with parallel walls, in *varicose bronchiectasis* the walls are irregular, and in *saccular (or cystic) bronchiectasis* (Fig. 16.11) the airways terminate as round cysts. In an individual

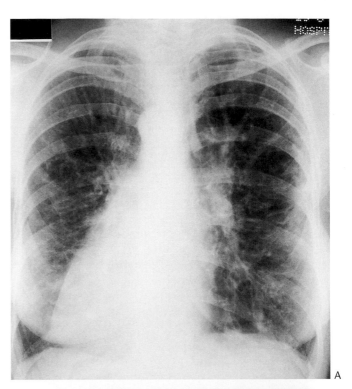

A

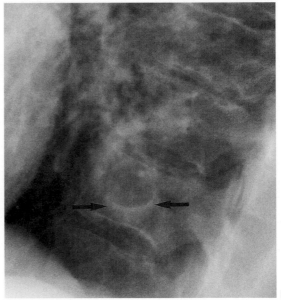

B

Fig. 16.7 Kartagener syndrome. **A.** There is dextrocardia and widespread bronchiectasis, most obvious at the left base. **B.** A lateral view demonstrates an air–fluid level (arrows) within a dilated bronchus.

patient it is common to see more than one pattern. Bronchiectasis usually involves the peripheral bronchi more severely than the central bronchi. Although it has long been held that in bronchopulmonary aspergillosis this pattern may be reversed, overall the distribution and morphology of bronchiectatic change demonstrated by CT gives no more than a clue to the underlying etiology.

The CT signs of bronchiectasis are those due to thickened, dilated bronchi, which may or may not contain fluid (Fig. 16.12).

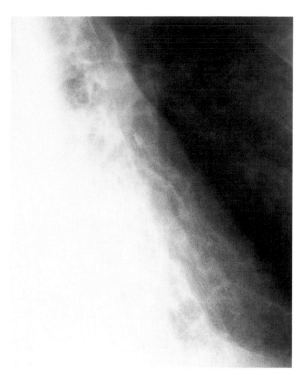

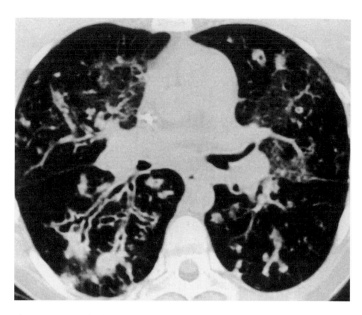

Fig. 16.10 Cylindrical or tubular bronchiectasis. CT image at the level of the hila demonstrates widespread bronchiectasis, particularly well seen in the apical segment of the right lower lobe. The bronchi fail to taper and have irregular thickened walls.

Fig. 16.8 Bronchiectasis. Tramline shadows are visible through the heart shadow.

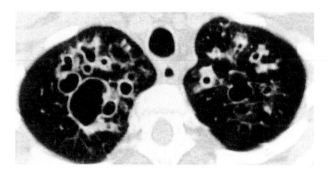

Fig. 16.11 Cystic bronchiectasis. A CT image through the upper lobes demonstrates multiple ring shadows. More caudal images reveal these to be due to irregularly dilated bronchi.

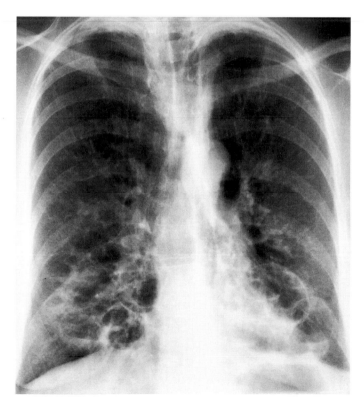

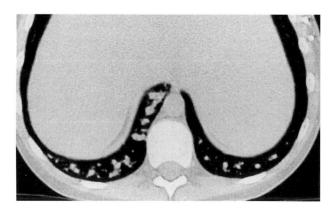

Fig. 16.9 Bronchiectasis. Multiple ring shadows, many containing air–fluid levels, are present throughout the lower zones of this patient with cystic bronchiectasis.

Fig. 16.12 Bronchiectasis with mucus plugging. A CT scan through the posterior costophrenic recesses showing multiple fluid-filled dilated bronchi causing a string of rounded opacities in the posterior costophrenic angle. (Same patient as illustrated in Fig. 16.13.)

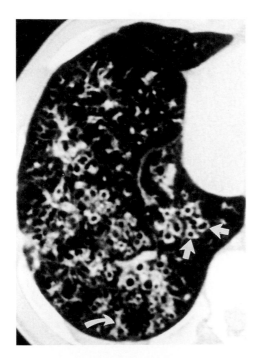

Fig. 16.13 Bronchiectasis. CT image through the right lower lobe reveals dilated subsegmental bronchi. Note how the bronchi are larger than the accompanying vessels. Several bronchi demonstrate the signet ring sign (arrows). Plugging of peripheral smaller bronchi is evident (curved arrow).

The common appearances of bronchiectasis on CT include nontapering bronchi, extending into the peripheral third of the lung. This is best appreciated when the bronchus lies in the plane of the CT section (Fig. 16.10). Normally the bronchus is the same size as or fractionally larger than the adjacent artery, although attention to the arterial bifurcation should be made to avoid overdiagnosis. When the bronchus is more markedly dilated and passes through the axis of the scan a typical signet ring appearance may be seen (Fig. 16.13). The wall of the bronchus may or may not be thickened. On expiratory scans there is frequently evidence of air trapping (Fig. 16.14). Peripheral airways may become plugged producing small subpleural branching opacities (Fig. 16.13).

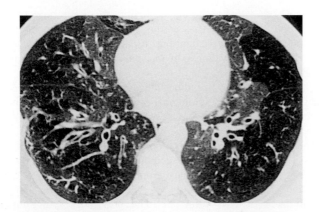

Fig. 16.14 Bronchiectasis with air trapping. CT image at end expiration demonstrates areas of relatively higher and lower attenuation. The lower attenuation areas indicate air trapping.

Bronchial arteriography is sometimes useful in the management of hemoptysis secondary to bronchiectasis. Severe hemoptysis may be secondary to bronchial artery hypertrophy. If the site of bleeding can be identified, it may be treated by therapeutic embolization.

Cystic Fibrosis

Cystic fibrosis was formerly a condition seen only in children. However, with improved management many patients now reach adulthood (see Ch. 19).

The increased viscosity of the bronchial secretions in cystic fibrosis causes bronchial obstruction. This leads to air trapping and also predisposes to bronchiectasis. The *chest radiograph* may, therefore, show signs of air trapping with flattening of the diaphragm, bowing of the sternum and increased dorsal kyphosis, and also signs of bronchiectasis (Fig. 16.15). Peribronchial thickening, peripheral nodular opacities and ring shadows may be visible. Areas of emphysema may develop. Chest infections are common, *staphylococci* and *Pseudomonas* being important pathogens, so that areas of consolidation may be seen (Fig. 16.15). In response to chronic pulmonary infection the hilar lymph nodes may enlarge. The central pulmonary arteries may also enlarge due to pulmonary arterial hypertension. In later stages of the disease spontaneous pneumothorax may occur (Fig. 16.16).

OBSTRUCTIVE AIRWAYS DISEASE

Chronic obstruction to bronchial airflow is an abnormality that unites the group of conditions termed *chronic obstructive pulmonary disease* (COPD) or *chronic obstructive airways disease (COAD)*. This group is the most common form of chronic lung disease and includes chronic bronchitis, pulmonary emphysema and asthma, which are discussed in this section.

Definitions

Chronic bronchitis This is defined in clinical terms as 'a chronic cough without demonstrable cause, with expectoration on most days during at least three consecutive months for more than two consecutive years'.

Asthma Asthma is a clinical term referring to 'widespread narrowing of the bronchi, which is paroxysmal and reversible'.

Emphysema This is defined in morphologic terms as 'an increase beyond the normal in the size of the air spaces distal to the terminal bronchioles, with dilatation and destruction of their walls'.

Clinically and radiologically a patient may have manifestations of more than one kind of chronic obstructive airways disease.

Asthma

The clinical syndrome of asthma results from hyper-reactivity of the larger airways to a variety of stimuli, causing narrowing of the bronchi, wheezing and often dyspnea.

Extrinsic or atopic asthma is usually associated with a history of allergy and raised plasma IgE. An important cause of extrinsic

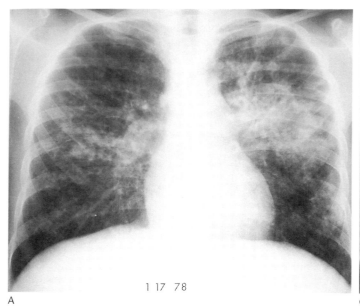

A   1 17 78

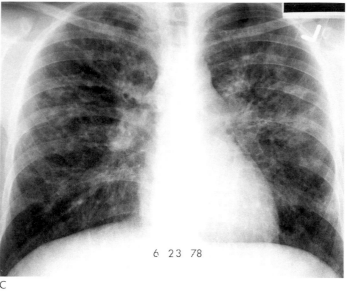

C   6 23 78

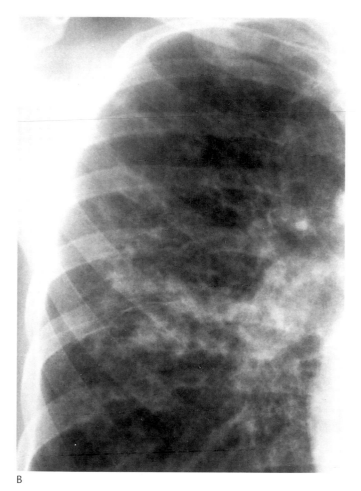

B

Fig. 16.15 Cystic fibrosis. **A.** Chest X-ray during an acute chest infection showing left perihilar and right mid zone consolidation. **B.** Close-up of the right mid zone demonstrating multiple ring shadows and tramlines due to extensive bronchiectasis. **C.** Six months later the acute changes have resolved leaving a background of bronchiectasis.

asthma is aspergillosis; this is discussed in detail in Chapter 15. *Intrinsic* or non-atopic asthma may be precipitated by a variety of factors such as exercise, emotion and infection. In acute exacerbation of chronic bronchitis due to a chest infection, wheezing is a common feature.

The role of radiology in asthma is limited. Most asthmatics show a normal chest X-ray during remissions. During an asthmatic attack the chest X-ray may show signs of hyperinflation (Fig. 16.17), with depression of the diaphragm and expansion of the retrosternal air space. Mediastinal emphysema may occur secondary to a rupture at terminal bronchiolar level or beyond, and occasionally this may lead to a pneumothorax. The peripheral pulmonary vessels appear normal, but if the central pulmonary arteries are enlarged, irreversible pulmonary arterial hypertension is probably present. The importance of radiology is to exclude complications such as a pulmonary infection, atelectasis due to mucus plugging or pneumothorax.

Chronic Bronchitis

The most consistent pathological finding in chronic bronchitis is hypertrophy of the mucus-secreting glands of the bronchi. Their secretions are more viscous than usual, leading to interference with the mucociliary transport mechanisms and plugging of the small airways.

Chronic bronchitics are almost always smokers, and are usually male. Other important etiological factors are urban atmospheric pollution, a dusty work environment and low socio-economic group.

The role of radiology in chronic bronchitis is to detect and assess complications of the condition and also to detect coincidental diseases. Pulmonary emphysema is a common complication which can be assessed radiographically, as can the development of cor pulmonale. The presenting symptoms of pulmonary tuberculosis and lung cancer can be masked by chronic bronchitis, and again the chest X-ray may help.

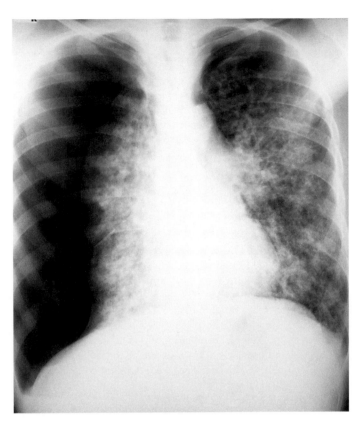

Fig. 16.16 Cystic fibrosis. There are widespread bronchiectatic changes and a large right pneumothorax. A small left apical pneumothorax is also present.

Radiological Appearances Approximately 50% of patients with chronic bronchitis have a normal chest X-ray. In patients with a plain film abnormality, the signs are due to emphysema, superimposed infection or possibly bronchiectasis.

An appearance which suggests chronic bronchitis is the so-called '*dirty chest*' (Fig. 16.18). There is generalized accentuation

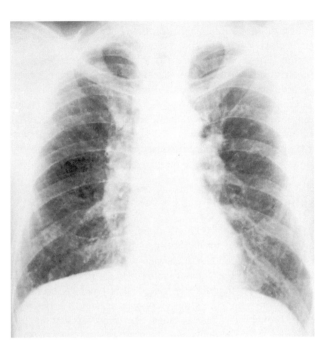

Fig. 16.18 Chronic bronchitis in a man of 62. Small poorly defined opacities are present throughout both lungs, producing the 'dirty chest'. This contrasts with the clear lungs in Fig. 16.17B.

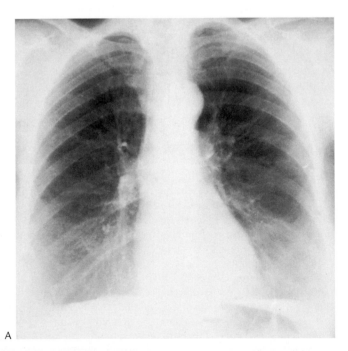

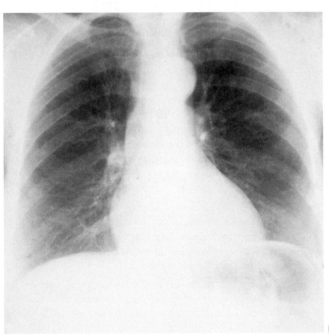

A   B

Fig. 16.17 Asthma in a woman of 64. **A.** During an asthmatic attack the lungs are hyperinflated, the diaphragms being depressed and flattened. **B.** During remission the chest radiograph is normal.

of the bronchovascular markings. Small, poorly defined opacities may be seen anywhere in the lungs, but their perception can be extremely subjective. There is some correlation between the 'dirty chest' and the presence of perivascular and peribronchial edema, chronic inflammation and fibrosis. If this pattern is particularly obvious, with fine linear shadows and hazy nodular opacities, the appearance may resemble interstitial fibrosis, lymphangitis carcinomatosis or bronchiectasis.

Thin tramline or tubular shadows may also be seen, suggesting bronchiectasis, but the precise nature of these shadows is uncertain. These opacities are usually related to the hila, and may be clearly demonstrated by tomography, but again are only suggestive and not diagnostic of chronic bronchitis.

If emphysema with air trapping is present the lung volumes increase, the diaphragm becomes flattened and the retrosternal air space increases. The number and size of the peripheral vessels decrease, and the central pulmonary arteries may enlarge. If cor pulmonale supervenes the heart enlarges.

Emphysema

As stated above, emphysema is defined in morphologic terms as enlargement of the airways beyond the terminal bronchi, with dilatation and destruction of their walls. Classification of emphysema is also based, in part, on morphology, and a basic knowledge of lung structure is therefore pertinent. The trachea, bronchi and terminal bronchioles are strictly conducting airways. Beyond the terminal bronchioles, gas exchange takes place, so that respiratory bronchioles, alveolar ducts and alveolar sacs are both conducting and respiratory structures. The alveoli are purely respiratory in function. The secondary pulmonary lobule is a unit of lung structure supplied by between three and five terminal bronchioles; lung distal to a terminal bronchiole is called an acinus, and a secondary pulmonary lobule, therefore, comprises 3–5 acini.

Types of Emphysema and Associated Conditions

Involvement of the secondary pulmonary lobule by emphysema may be non-selective or selective.

1. *Panacinar emphysema* is a non-selective process characterized by destruction of all of the lung distal to the terminal bronchiole. It is sometimes termed panlobular emphysema. The lung may be involved locally or generally, but distribution throughout the lung is rarely uniform. It may be associated with centriacinar emphysema, especially in chronic bronchitis, and is also seen in α_1-antitrypsin deficiency.

2. *Centriacinar emphysema* is a selective process characterized by destruction and dilatation of the respiratory bronchioles. The alveolar ducts, sacs and alveoli are spared until a late stage. It is sometimes called centrilobular emphysema and is frequently found in association with chronic bronchitis.

3. *Paraseptal emphysema* involves the periphery of the secondary lobules, usually in the lung periphery, sometimes combined with pan- or centri-acinar emphysema, and occasionally causes bulla formation.

4. *Paracicatricial emphysema* refers to distension and destruction of terminal air spaces adjacent to fibrotic lesions, and is most frequently seen as a result of tuberculosis.

5. *Obstructive emphysema* is strictly a misnomer, and the condition is better termed 'obstructive hyperinflation', since the distal airways are dilated but not necessarily destroyed. It is discussed here for the sake of completeness. It occurs when a larger bronchus is obstructed in such a way that air enters the lung on inspiration but is trapped on expiration. Such one-way valve obstruction may be due to an inhaled foreign body (e.g. peanuts or teeth) or due to an endobronchial or peribronchial tumor. The lung beyond the obstruction becomes hyperinflated.

6. *Compensatory emphysema* is another process that is better regarded as hyperinflation. If part or all of a lung collapses, shrinks or is removed, the resulting space is occupied by displacement of the mediastinum or diaphragm, or usually, more significantly, by hyperinflation of the unaffected or remaining lung. This is discussed in the section on lobar collapse later in this chapter.

7. A *bulla* is an emphysematous space with a diameter of more than 1 cm in the distended state, and its walls are made up of compressed surrounding lung or pleura, depending on its location.

Emphysema may be classified according to the presence or absence of air trapping at respiratory bronchiolar level. Panacinar, obstructive and congenital lobar emphysema are associated with air trapping and usually cause symptoms. Centriacinar, paraseptal and compensatory emphysema are not associated with air trapping and are usually asymptomatic.

Radiological Appearances

1. Panacinar Emphysema The radiographic features of panacinar emphysema are the results of destruction of lung tissue altering the vascular pattern, interference of ventilation decreasing lung perfusion, and air trapping. The effects of panacinar emphysema are almost always apparent clinically by the time the radiographic manifestations occur, but a normal chest X-ray virtually excludes severe generalized emphysema.

The main radiographic signs are (Fig. 16.19):

a. Reduction of pulmonary vascularity peripherally

b. Hyperinflation of the lungs

c. Alteration of the cardiac shadow and central pulmonary arteries.

The vascular pattern in affected areas of lung is attenuated. Involvement of the lung may be localized or generalized, but if generalized is usually patchy. Involved areas have fewer vessels than normal, and those vessels that remain are small. Mild degrees of vascular attenuation are difficult to perceive, so it is worth comparing the size of vessels in different zones. If vessels are diminished in caliber and number in a particular zone, compared to another, that zone is likely to be emphysematous.

Peripheral vascular attenuation is due to a number of factors. Perfusion of emphysematous lung is less than normal, and pulmonary blood flow is diverted to less affected areas of lung. Pulmonary vessels are displaced around emphysematous areas and bullae. Small arteries are obliterated by the primary emphysematous process, but these vessels are too small to be visualized radiographically, and this process, therefore, probably does not contribute to the oligemic appearances, but may be a factor in increased radiolucency of affected areas.

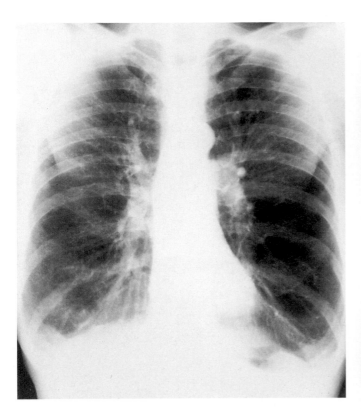

Fig. 16.19 Emphysema in a man of 54. The lungs are hyperinflated, the diaphragm being low and flat. The peripheral vascular pattern is attenuated in the right mid and left mid and lower zones. The central pulmonary arteries are enlarged, indicating pulmonary arterial hypertension. The heart is elongated.

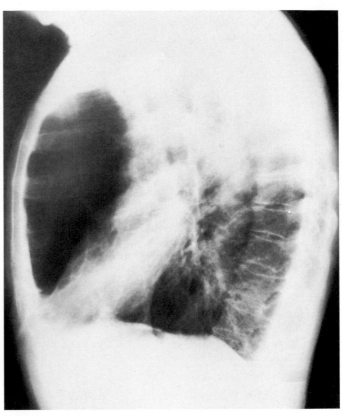

Fig. 16.20 Emphysema in a man of 52. Lateral film shows increased lung volume, which is producing a barrel chest. The retrosternal space is deeper than normal and extends more inferiorly than normal.

Panacinar emphysema has a tendency to affect the lung bases and may cause diversion of blood flow to the upper zones, which should not be mistaken for pulmonary venous hypertension. In α_1-antitrypsin deficiency the changes of emphysema tend to be basal. Air trapping causes hyperinflation of the lungs, and may lead to flattening of the diaphragm and increased anteroposterior diameter of the thorax. Flattening of the diaphragm is often best seen on the lateral projection, the level of the diaphragm often being as low as the eleventh rib posteriorly. Some normal individuals can push their diaphragm as low on full inspiration, but on expiration the diaphragm will rise 5–10 cm, whereas in emphysema excursion of the diaphragm is usually less than 3 cm. In severe emphysema the diaphragm may actually be inverted.

The 'barrel chest' is caused by bowing of the sternum and increased thoracic kyphosis. The retrosternal air space may increase in depth, and extend inferiorly between the anterior surface of the heart and the sternum (Fig. 16.20).

The heart often appears long and narrow. This is probably due primarily to the low position of the diaphragm altering the projection of the heart. Enlargement of the central pulmonary arteries usually signifies pulmonary arterial hypertension (Fig. 16.19). If cor pulmonale develops, the heart may enlarge due to right ventricular dilatation. In patients with emphysema who develop left heart failure, the signs of hyperinflation may decrease, and the level of the diaphragm will rise. This is due to pulmonary edema decreasing the compliance of the lung and thus reducing the lung volume. In these patients the distribution of edema fluid within emphysematous lung may be bizarre.

CT is more sensitive than the plain chest X-ray in detecting the presence and distribution of emphysema (Fig. 16.21). Vascular attenuation may be detected earlier, and bullae may be identified by CT when not visible on the chest X-ray. In addition expiratory scans may identify areas of air trapping.

2. Bullous Disease of the Lungs Bullae are usually present in the lung in association with some form of emphysema, but occasionally bullae occur locally in otherwise normal lung (Fig. 16.22). They commonly occur in paraseptal emphysema, and in emphysema associated with scarring, but clinically the most important bullae are those due to panacinar emphysema, with or without chronic bronchitis.

Bullae appear as round or oval translucencies varying in size from 1 cm in diameter to occupation of almost an entire hemithorax (Fig. 16.23). They may be single or multiple, and are usually peripheral. In asymptomatic patients and in those with pulmonary scarring, bullae tend to be apical, but in chronic obstructive airways disease bullae are found throughout the lungs (Fig. 16.21). Their walls may be visible as a smooth, curved, hairline shadow. If the walls are not visible, displacement of vessels around a radiolucent area may indicate a bullous area.

Bullae are usually air-filled but may become infected and filled with fluid. Associated inflammatory change may be present in the surrounding lung. A bulla will show a fluid level if it is partially fluid-filled, or will appear solid if completely fluid-filled (Fig. 16.24).

A giant bulla may be difficult to differentiate from a loculated

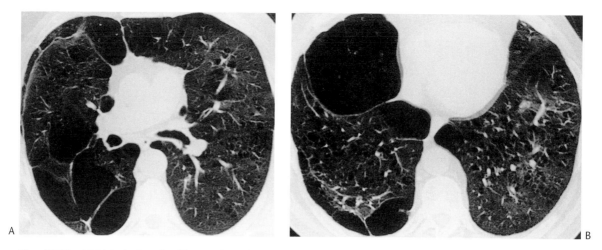

Fig. 16.21 Multiple bullae. **A.** CT scan through the level of the right main pulmonary artery reveals multiple bullae predominantly in the right lung. **B.** CT scan further toward the lung bases revealing several further bullae. Some of these have well-defined walls.

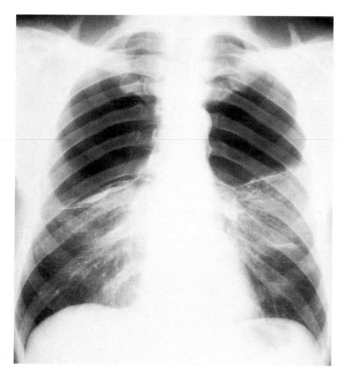

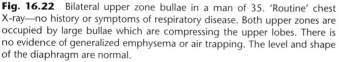

Fig. 16.22 Bilateral upper zone bullae in a man of 35. 'Routine' chest X-ray—no history or symptoms of respiratory disease. Both upper zones are occupied by large bullae which are compressing the upper lobes. There is no evidence of generalized emphysema or air trapping. The level and shape of the diaphragm are normal.

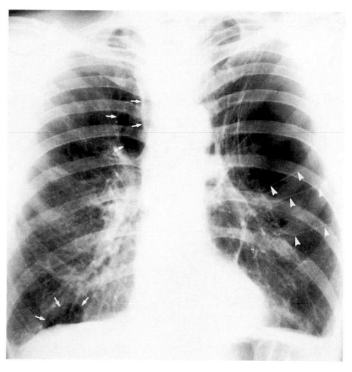

Fig. 16.23 Emphysema with bullae in a man of 61. The lungs are hyperinflated. A giant bulla occupies most of the left hemithorax, compressing the left lung. Strands of lung tissue (arrowheads) are seen crossing this bulla. Small bullae (arrows) are also present in the right lung.

pneumothorax, and CT may be necessary to demonstrate the wall of the bulla or thin strands of lung tissue crossing it.

3. Emphysema with Chronic Bronchitis Many patients with chronic obstructive airways disease have emphysema *and* chronic bronchitis. The chest X-ray may then show a combination of changes of hyperinflation, pulmonary arterial hypertension and increased bronchovascular markings of the so-called '*dirty chest*'.

At one end of the clinical spectrum is the '*pink puffer*' who, by major effort, ventilates sufficient alveoli to maintain normal blood gases; since there is no hypoxemia, normal pulmonary artery pressure is preserved. Pink puffers tend to have predominantly panacinar emphysema, and the chest X-ray shows peripheral vascular attenuation and hyperinflation. This appearance may be termed the 'arterial deficiency' pattern.

At the other end of the clinical spectrum is the '*blue bloater*', who chronically retains carbon dioxide due to poor alveolar ventilation. The respiratory center becomes insensitive to the persistently raised concentration of arterial carbon dioxide, and chronic cyanosis occurs. Chronic hypoxemia causes pulmonary

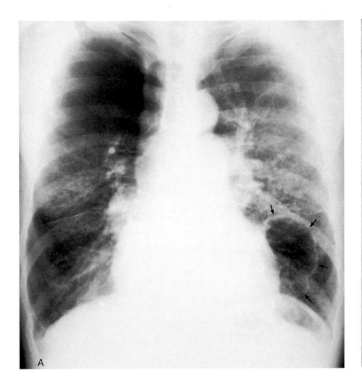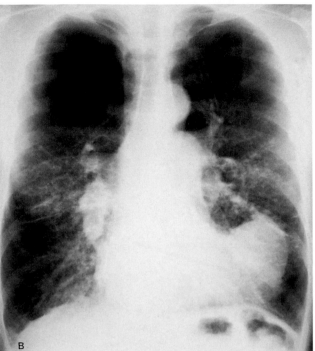

Fig. 16.24 Emphysema with infected bulla in a man of 48. **A.** The lungs are hyperinflated. The right upper zone is occupied by a large bulla, and another bulla is seen adjacent to the left heart border (arrows). The central pulmonary arteries are enlarged. **B.** Following a chest infection the left-sided bulla has filled with fluid and appears completely opaque.

arteriolar constriction, and in due course pulmonary arterial hypertension and cor pulmonale occur. Blue bloaters tend to have centriacinar emphysema and less extensive panacinar emphysema. The chest X-ray shows increased bronchovascular markings, enlarged central pulmonary arteries and possibly cardiac enlargement. This appearance may be termed the 'increased markings' pattern of emphysema, and signs of hyperinflation are rarely severe. Most patients with chronic bronchitis and emphysema exhibit features between these extremes.

4. Unilateral or Lobar Emphysema (Macleod or Swyer–James Syndrome) Classically the syndrome is based on the chest X-ray appearance of a hypertransradiant hemithorax. It is probably the result of a childhood viral infection causing bronchiolitis and obliteration of the small airways; the involved distal airways are ventilated by collateral air drift, and air trapping leads to panacinar emphysema. However, CT of patients shows that although one lung tends to be more affected than the other, there are usually bilateral abnormalities characterized by bronchiectasis and areas of hypertransradiancy.

The affected lung is hypertransradiant, due to decreased perfusion, and may be smaller than normal. The ipsilateral pulmonary artery is visible, but small, and the peripheral vascular pattern is attenuated. Air trapping occurs in the affected lung, which tends to maintain its volume on expiration, resulting in displacement of the mediastinum to the more normal side, and restriction of the ipsilateral hemidiaphragm (Fig. 16.25).

The syndrome may also be illustrated by radionuclide scanning, when a perfusion scan will show reduced flow to the affected lung, and a ventilation scan, using xenon, will demonstrate air trapping.

The differential diagnosis of the chest X-ray appearance includes proximal interruption of the pulmonary artery, the hypogenetic

lung syndrome and pulmonary artery obstruction due to embolism. However, none of these entities exhibits air trapping.

5. Centriacinar Emphysema This occurs principally in chronic bronchitis and uncomplicated coal miner's pneumoconiosis. The radiological appearance is that of the primary condition. In later stages panacinar and bullous emphysema may become apparent.

6. Obstructive 'Emphysema' Obstructive hyperinflation may affect an entire lung, a lobe or a segment. The cause—such as an inhaled foreign body or tooth, or a central tumor—may be apparent on the chest X-ray. The vascular pattern of the affected part of the lung is attenuated, and this area may appear hypertransradiant. Fluoroscopy or an expiratory film will demonstrate air trapping in the affected area with deviation of the mediastinum to the normal side, and restriction of the ipsilateral hemidiaphragm on expiration.

7. Compensatory 'Emphysema' The radiological signs resulting from collapse or removal of all or part of a lung are discussed in the section on lobar collapse (Ch. 13).

8. Congenital Lobar Emphysema This is discussed in Chapter 19.

Bronchiolitis

The term bronchiolitis encompasses a range of conditions.

1. Acute Bronchiolitis This occurs in children, usually in the first year of life, and is most commonly the result of respiratory syncytial virus infection. The condition is usually self limiting; nevertheless, in the UK, it is the main cause of pediatric hospital admission during the winter months. When it is due to adenovirus

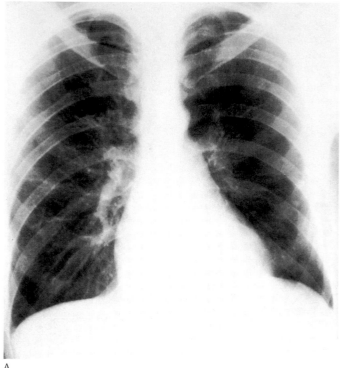

A

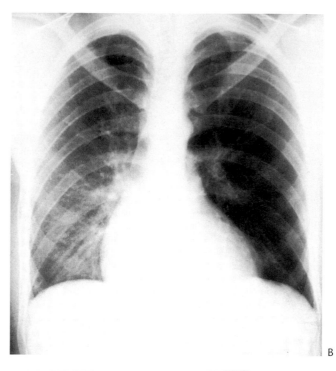

B

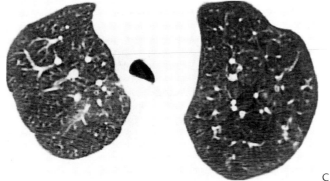

C

Fig. 16.25 Unilateral emphysema in a man of 30 with a history of repeated chest infections as a child, but no current respiratory symptoms. **A.** Inspiratory film shows normal right lung and hypertransradiant left lung with small left pulmonary artery. **B.** Expiratory film demonstrates displacement of mediastinum to the right and restricted movement of the left hemidiaphragm, indicating air trapping in the left lung. **C.** CT scan through the upper lobes of a different patient with unilateral emphysema. At end expiration there is air trapping within the left lung where the vessels are relatively attenuated.

infection there is a markedly increased risk of subsequent development of bronchiolitis obliterans (see below). Radiologically the appearances are most frequently hyperinflation of the lungs and perihilar prominence and indistinctness.

2. **Obliterative Bronchiolitis**   Bronchiolar occlusion may result from a viral bronchiolitis (often in childhood), from inhalation of toxic fumes, drug therapy (classically penicillamine), rheumatoid disease or may be cryptogenic. Obliterative bronchiolitis resulting from childhood viral infection may present in adult life as unilateral or lobar emphysema (see above). In addition there is a cryptogenic variety. The chest radiograph may show evidence of pulmonary hyperinflation, and decreased vascularity in the mid and lower zones. Changes on HRCT include bronchial dilatation with or without patchy areas of hypertransradiancy, probably due to air trapping (Fig. 16.26). In some patients small branching opacities, corresponding pathologically to small airways plugged with granulation tissue, can be seen in the lung periphery (Fig. 16.27).

3. **Panbronchiolitis**   Diffuse panbronchiolitis, often referred to as Japanese panbronchiolitis because of its relative frequency in Japan and the Far East, is a disorder characterized by bronchial

inflammation and chronic sinus infection. Eventually pulmonary function tests become obstructive, and bronchiectasis and respiratory failure may develop. Although the chest radiograph may demonstrate mid and lower zone nodules, becoming more profuse and widespread as the disease progresses, the bronchiolitis is best demonstrated by HRCT. This demonstrates small branching opacities which pathologically correspond to respiratory bronchioles surrounded by and containing an inflammatory infiltrate. Treatment involves low-dose long-term erythromycin and supportive measures.

Cryptogenic Organizing Pneumonitis and Bronchiolitis Obliterans Organizing Pneumonia (COP and BOOP)

COP and *BOOP*, two recently recognized entities, are effectively the same condition, described independently in the UK and the USA at approximately the same time. To avoid confusion with the largely separate condition of obliterative bronchiolitis, COP is suggested as the preferred term. They are likely to represent one possible response of the lung to an inflammatory stimulus.

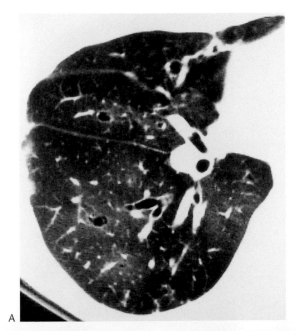

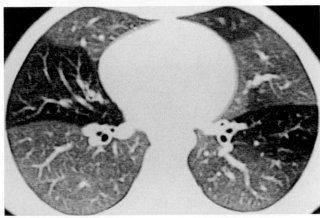

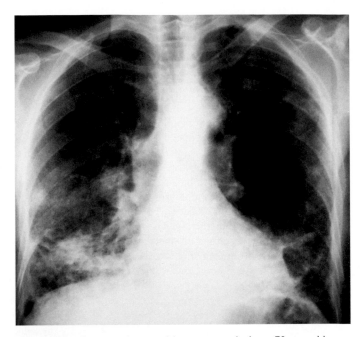

Fig. 16.28 Cryptogenic organizing pneumonia in a 70-year-old man with chronic consolidation. The appearances had been unchanged for several weeks despite multiple courses of antibiotics.

Patients are typically middle aged, and there is no preponderance of either sex. Frequently the patient has had a systemic illness lasting a few weeks or months with a non-productive cough, dyspnea, malaise and a low-grade fever. Often antibiotics have been administered without response, and no organism has been identified. The chest radiograph usually demonstrates consolidation which is patchy and chronic (Fig. 16.28). On HRCT there is air space consolidation, usually in the lower half of the lungs: in 50% of cases with a predominantly subpleural distribution, and in 30–50% of cases in a peribronchovascular distribution (Fig. 16.29). Lung biopsy, which

Fig. 16.26 Obliterative bronchiolitis due to graft versus host disease. **A.** Close-up view of the right lower-zone reveals patchy areas of higher and lower attenuation and thin-walled dilated bronchi. **B.** Obliterative bronchiolitis in a different patient. A CT scan obtained at end expiration shows marked variation in the CT attenuation within the lungs. The relatively hypodense areas have failed to deflate due to small airways disease.

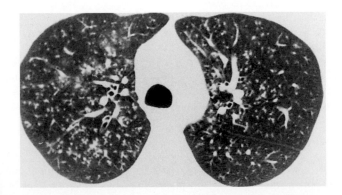

Fig. 16.27 Obliterative bronchiolitis. There are multiple branching opacities representing occluded small airways, in this case secondary to inhaled amyl nitrate. Open lung biopsy confirmed the presence of bronchioles plugged with granulation tissue.

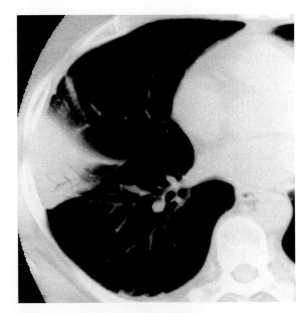

Fig. 16.29 Cryptogenic organizing pneumonia. There is a wedge-shaped pleurally based patch of consolidation containing an air bronchogram. The diagnosis was confirmed following a percutaneous needle biopsy.

characteristically demonstrates small airways and adjacent air spaces plugged with granulation tissue, may be required to make the diagnosis, and there is usually a dramatic clinical and radiological response to corticosteroid therapy.

Bronchocele and Mucoid Impaction

Obstruction of a segmental bronchus may lead to accumulation of secretions and pus in the lung distally. If collateral air drift allows the affected lung to remain aerated a bronchocele or bronchial mucocele may develop. The obstruction may be congenital or due to endobronchial tumor or inhaled foreign body, or to inflammatory stricture or extrinsic compression. Mucoid impaction in asthma, allergic bronchopulmonary aspergillosis and cystic fibrosis may produce a similar obstruction. The typical appearance on the chest radiograph is a group of oval or cigar-shaped shadows, which may appear to branch (Fig. 16.30): they lie along the axis of the bronchial tree and point toward the hilum.

Bronchial Atresia

Bronchial atresia is an uncommon condition that usually presents as an incidental well-defined pulmonary opacity, most frequently in the left upper lobe. The surrounding lung is emphysematous, a feature best demonstrated on CT (Fig. 16.31). Pathologically there is mucus impaction and dilatation distal to a short atresia in a segmental bronchus. Although the diagnosis can be suggested confidently from the typical HRCT appearances, resection of the affected segment is often undertaken due to the remote possibility of a small occluding neoplasm. The majority of cases occur in the left upper lobe, with the right upper lobe and lower lobes being involved with reducing frequency.

THE LUNGS—COLLAPSE AND CONSOLIDATION

Collapse

Partial or complete loss of volume of a lung is referred to as collapse or atelectasis. Current usage has made these terms synonymous, and they imply a diminished volume of air in the lung with associated reduction of lung volume. This contrasts with consolidation, in which a diminished volume of air in the lung is associated with normal lung volume. There are several different mechanisms which may cause pulmonary collapse.

Mechanisms of Collapse

1. Relaxation or Passive Collapse   This is the mechanism whereby the lung tends to retract toward its hilum when air or increased fluid collects in the pleural space. It is discussed above under diseases of the pleura.

2. Cicatrization Collapse   As discussed in the section on the pleura, normal lung expansion depends upon a balance between outward forces in the chest wall and opposite elastic forces in the lung. When the lung is abnormally stiff, this balance is disturbed, lung compliance is decreased and the volume of the affected lung is reduced. This occurs with pulmonary fibrosis.

3. Adhesive Collapse   The surface tension of the alveoli is decreased by surfactant. If this mechanism is disturbed, as in the

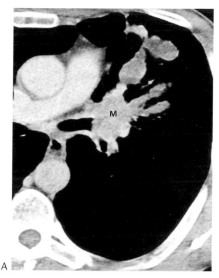

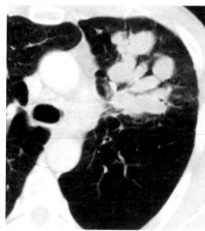

Fig. 16.30 Bronchocele secondary to a left hilar tumor. **A.** On mediastinal windows there are fluid density opacities radiating out from the left hilar mass (M). **B.** A scan at a slightly more cranial level on lung window settings shows multiple rounded opacities in the left upper lobe due to mucoid impaction within obstructed bronchi.

respiratory distress syndrome, collapse of alveoli occurs, although the central airways remain patent.

4. Resorption Collapse   In acute bronchial obstruction the gases in the alveoli are steadily taken up by the blood in the pulmonary capillaries and are not replenished, causing alveolar collapse. The degree of collapse may be modified by collateral air drift if the obstruction is distal to the main bronchus, and also by infection and accumulation of secretions. If the obstruction becomes chronic, subsequent resorption of intra-alveolar secretions and exudate may result in complete collapse. This is the usual mechanism of collapse seen in carcinoma of the bronchus.

Radiological Signs of Collapse   The radiographic appearance in pulmonary collapse depends upon the mechanism of collapse, the degree of collapse, the presence or absence of consolidation, and the pre-existing state of the pleura. Signs of collapse may be considered as direct or indirect. Indirect signs are the results of compensatory changes which occur in response to the volume loss.

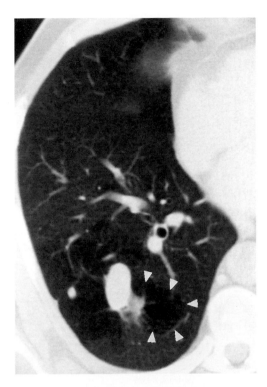

Fig. 16.31 Bronchial atresia. There is a well-defined opacity in the right lower lobe surrounded by a patch of emphysematous lung (arrowheads).

Direct Signs of Collapse

1. Displacement of Interlobar Fissures This is the most reliable sign, and the degree of displacement will depend on the extent of the collapse.

2. Loss of Aeration Increased density of a collapsed area of lung may not become apparent until collapse is almost complete. However, if the collapsed lung is adjacent to the mediastinum or diaphragm, obscuration of the adjacent structures may indicate loss of aeration.

3. Vascular and Bronchial Signs If a lobe is partially collapsed, crowding of its vessels may be visible; if an air bronchogram is visible, the bronchi may appear crowded.

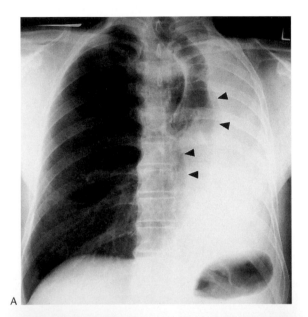

A

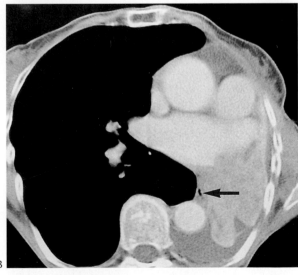

B

Fig. 16.33 Complete collapse of the left lung due to a left hilar tumor. **A.** The chest radiograph demonstrates deviation of the trachea and shift of the mediastinum to the left. Air–soft tissue interfaces are seen due to herniation of the right lung across the midline (arrowheads). **B.** CT scan demonstrates herniation of both the retrosternal lung and the azygo-esophageal reflection. The esophagus contains a small amount of air (arrow).

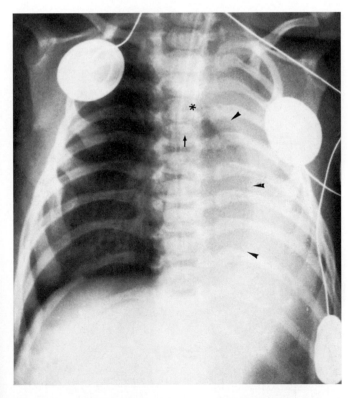

Fig. 16.32 Complete collapse of the left lung. A newborn child with complex cyanotic heart disease. The tip of the endotracheal tube (arrow) is beyond the carina (asterisk) and down the right bronchus, causing collapse of the left lung and compensatory hyperinflation of the right lung which has herniated across the midline (arrowheads).

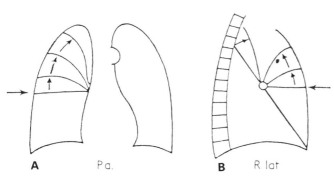

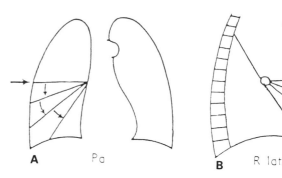

Fig. 16.34 Right upper lobe collapse. **A.** PA projection. Note how lesser fissure is drawn upward, and often curved, toward the apex and mediastinum. **B.** Right lateral view. Lesser fissure also displaced upward. Note some forward displacement of greater fissure above the hilum.

Fig. 16.36 Right middle lobe collapse. In both projections the lesser fissure is drawn downward. In the PA view the fissure finally merges with the mediastinum and disappears. Note in the lateral view that the lower part of the greater fissure may be displaced forward.

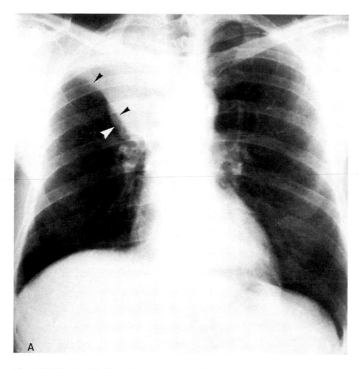

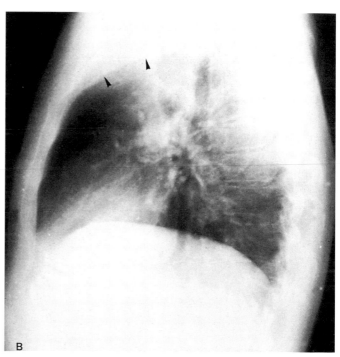

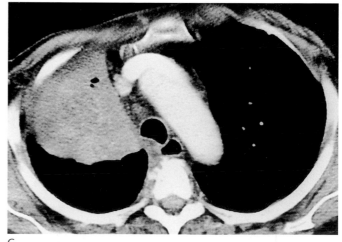

Fig. 16.35 **A.** PA film shows a mass (white arrowhead) above the right hilum, and elevation of the horizontal fissure (black arrowheads). There is compensatory hyperinflation of the right lower lobe. **B.** Lateral film shows anterior displacement of part of oblique fissure (arrowheads). **C.** CT scan of right upper lobe collapse in a different patient images on mediastinal window settings.

Indirect Signs of Collapse

1. Elevation of the Hemidiaphragm   This sign may be seen in lower lobe collapse, but is rare in collapse of the other lobes.

2. Mediastinal Displacement   In upper lobe collapse the trachea is often displaced toward the affected side, and in lower lobe collapse the heart may be displaced.

3. Hilar Displacement   The hilum may be elevated in upper lobe collapse, and depressed in lower lobe collapse.

4. Compensatory Hyperinflation   The normal part of the lung may become hyperinflated, and it may appear hypertransradiant, with its vessels more widely spaced than in the corresponding area of the contralateral lung. If there is considerable collapse of a lung, compensatory hyperinflation of the contralateral lung may occur, with herniation across the midline.

Patterns of Collapse   An air bronchogram is almost never seen in resorption collapse, but is usual in passive and adhesive collapse, and may be seen in cicatrization collapse if fibrosis is particularly dense.

Pre-existing lung disease such as fibrosis and pleural adhesions may alter the expected displacement of anatomic landmarks in lung collapse. There also tends to be a reciprocal relationship between the compensatory signs: e.g. in lower lobe collapse, if diaphragmatic elevation is marked, hilar depression will be diminished.

Complete Collapse of a Lung

Complete collapse of a lung, in the absence of pneumothorax or large pleural effusion or extensive consolidation, causes opacification of the hemithorax, displacement of the mediastinum to the affected side and elevation of the diaphragm. Compensatory hyperinflation of the contralateral lung occurs, often with herniation across the midline (Fig. 16.32). Herniation most often occurs in the retrosternal space, anterior to the ascending aorta,

but may occur posterior to the heart or under the aortic arch (Fig. 16.33).

Lobar Collapse

The following descriptions apply to collapse of individual lobes, uncomplicated by pre-existing pulmonary or pleural disease. The line drawings (Figs 16.34, 16.36, 16.38, 16.40, 16.43) represent the alteration in position of the fissures, as seen in the frontal and lateral projections, resulting from increasing degrees of collapse. Only the fissures are represented. The indirect signs of collapse are not indicated.

Right Upper Lobe Collapse   (Figs 16.34, 16.35) The normal horizontal fissure is usually at the level of the right fourth rib anteriorly. As the right upper lobe collapses, the horizontal fissure pivots about the hilum, its lateral end moving upward and medially toward the superior mediastinum, and its anterior end moving upward toward the apex. The upper half of the oblique fissure moves anteriorly. The two fissures become concave superiorly. In severe collapse the lobe may be flattened against the superior mediastinum, and may obscure the upper pole of the hilum. The hilum is elevated, and its lower pole may be prominent. Deviation of the trachea to the right is usual, and compensatory hyperinflation of the right middle and lower lobes may be apparent.

Right Middle Lobe Collapse   (Figs 16.36, 16.37). In right middle lobe collapse the horizontal fissure and lower half of the oblique fissure move toward one another. This can best be seen in the lateral projection. The horizontal fissure tends to be more mobile, and therefore usually shows greater displacement. Signs of right middle lobe collapse are often subtle on the frontal

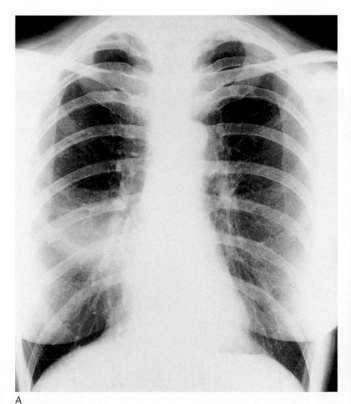

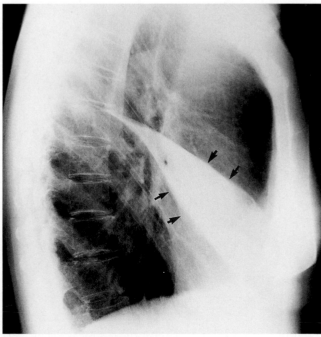

A   B

Fig. 16.37   Right middle lobe collapse. **A.** PA film shows loss of definition of the right heart border indicating loss of aeration of the middle lobe. **B.** A lateral film shows partial collapse of the middle lobe evident as a wedge-shaped opacity (arrows).

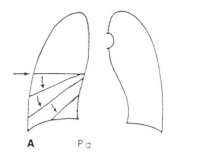
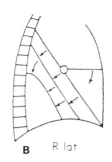

Fig. 16.38 Right lower lobe collapse. In the PA projection the greater fissure is not visible until the collapse is fairly complete. The lesser fissure is displaced downward as in collapse of the middle lobe. The degree of displacement seen may be greater in collapse of the lower lobe than of the middle lobe, as the middle lobe tends to retract toward the hilum and the fissure may disappear. In the lateral view, the oblique fissure moves backward, tending to retain its obliquity. The upper part of the oblique fissure may curve backward and downward, so becoming visible in the PA projection.

posteriorly to the diaphragm, close to the sternum, anteriorly. The position of these fissures on the lateral projection is the best index of lower lobe volumes. When a lower lobe collapses its oblique fissure moves posteriorly but maintains its normal slope. In addition to posterior movement, the collapsing lower lobe causes medial displacement of the oblique fissure, which may then become visible in places on the frontal projection.

Right lower lobe collapse causes depression of the horizontal fissure, which may be apparent on the frontal projection. Increased opacity of a collapsed lower lobe is usually visible on the frontal projection. A completely collapsed lower lobe may be so small that it flattens and merges with the mediastinum, producing a thin, wedge-shaped shadow. On the left this shadow may be obscured by the heart, and a penetrated view with a grid may be required for its visualization. If complete *left lower lobe collapse* is still in doubt, a right oblique film may demonstrate the

projection, since the horizontal fissure may not be visible, and increased opacity does not become apparent until collapse is almost complete. However, obscuration of the right heart border is often present, and may be the only clue in this projection. The *lordotic AP projection* brings the displaced fissure into the line of the X-ray beam, and may elegantly demonstrate right middle lobe collapse. Since the volume of this lobe is relatively small, indirect signs of volume loss are rarely present.

Lower Lobe Collapse (Figs 16.38–41) The normal oblique fissures extend from the level of the fourth thoracic vertebra

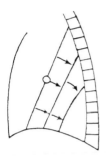

Fig. 16.40 Left lower lobe collapse. No fissure is visible in the PA projection. The lateral view shows that the greater fissure is displaced posteriorly as in collapse of the right lower lobe. The upper part of the fissure may also be drawn downward as well as backward.

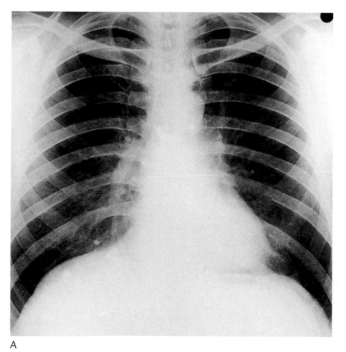

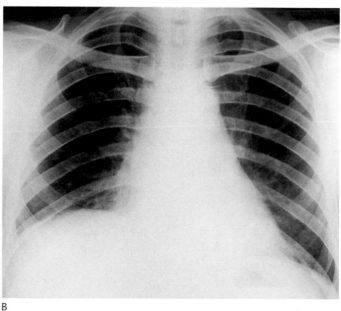

Fig. 16.39 Right lower lobe collapse. **A.** Normal preoperative film. **B.** Following coronary artery bypass surgery there is right lower lobe collapse with depression and medial rotation of the hilum, elevation of the right hemidiaphragm and hyperinflation of the right upper lobe.

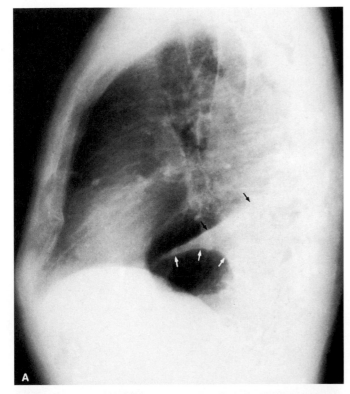

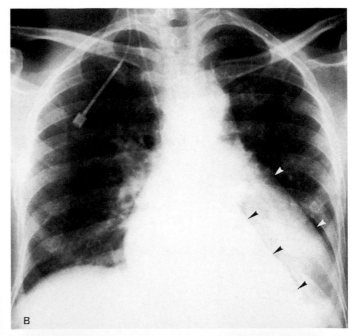

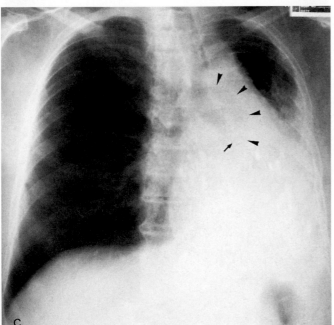

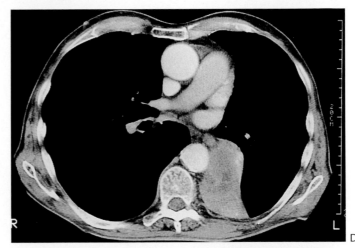

Fig. 16.41   A. 66-year-old man with squamous-cell carcinoma of the left lower lobe. The oblique fissure is displaced posteriorly (black arrows). The left hemidiaphragm is obscured by the collapsed lobe, but the position of the stomach bubble (white arrows) indicates that the left hemidiaphragm is elevated. **B.** Postoperative film of patient with aortic valve replacement. The shadow of the collapsed left lower lobe (black arrowheads) is seen through the shadow of the heart (white arrowheads). **C.** 57-year-old man with oat-cell carcinoma occluding the left bronchus (arrow). The left lower lobe is collapsed, obscuring the left hemidiaphragm. The mediastinum is shifted to the left, and part of the hyperinflated right lung has herniated across the midline (arrowheads). **D.** Left lower lobe collapse demonstrated on CT. There is mixed density within the collapsed lung, probably due to fluid-filled bronchi.

wedge of tissue between spine and diaphragm. Mediastinal structures and parts of the diaphragm adjacent to the non-aerated lobe are obscured.

The hilum is usually depressed and rotated medially, and upper lobe hyperinflation is evident, but diaphragmatic elevation is not usual.

Lingula Collapse   (Fig. 16.42) The lingula is often involved in collapse of the left upper lobe, but it may collapse individually, when the radiological features are similar to right middle lobe collapse. However, the absence of a horizontal fissure on the left makes anterior displacement of the lower half of the oblique fissure and increased opacity anterior to it important signs. On the frontal projection the left heart border becomes obscured.

Left Upper Lobe Collapse (Figs 16.42–44) The pattern of upper lobe collapse is different in the two lungs. Left upper lobe collapse is apparent on the lateral projection as anterior displacement of the entire oblique fissure, which becomes oriented almost parallel to the anterior chest wall. With increasing collapse

the upper lobe retracts posteriorly and loses contact with the anterior chest wall. The space between the collapsed lobe and the sternum becomes occupied by either hyperinflated left lower lobe

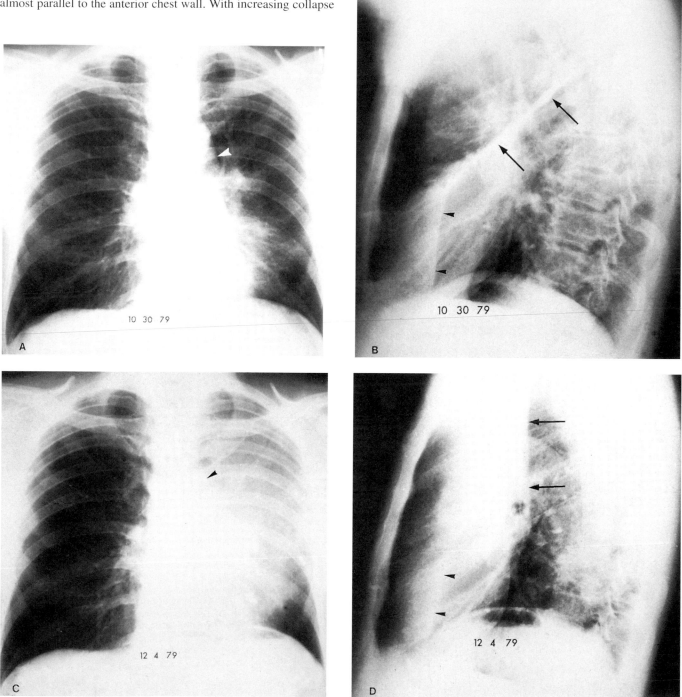

Fig. 16.42 Lingula and left upper lobe collapse in a man with carcinoma at the left hilum. **A.** PA film shows hazy left heart border, indicating loss of aeration of the lingula. A mass is present in the aortopulmonary window (arrowhead). **B.** Lateral film shows collapse-consolidation of the lingula, with anterior displacement of the lower part of the oblique fissure (arrowheads). The upper part of the oblique fissure (arrows) is thickened, but in normal position. **C.** Five weeks later the left upper lobe has collapsed. A hazy opacity covers most of the left hemithorax. Vessels in the hyperinflated left lower lobe can just be seen through the haze, and the aortic knuckle is obscured (arrowhead). **D.** Lateral film shows that the oblique fissure is now displaced anteriorly (arrows).

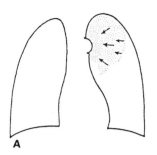
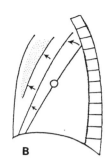

Fig. 16.43 Left upper lobe collapse. **A.** The greater fissure does not become visible in the PA projection. When the degree of collapse is fairly complete the lobe shows a uniform loss of translucency (this may be due to accompanying consolidation), which increases in density as the degree of collapse increases. Vessel markings seen through this opacity are those in the overexpanded lower lobe. **B.** In the lateral view, initially the fissure moves bodily forward, the lingula remaining in contact with the diaphragm. With increasing collapse the lingula retracts upward, and the bulk of the upper lobe moves posteriorly, and becomes separated from the sternum by aerated lung. This is usually overexpanded lower lobe, though occasionally a portion of the right lung may herniate across the midline.

or herniated right upper lobe. With complete collapse, the left upper lobe may lose contact with the chest wall and diaphragm and retract medially against the mediastinum. On a lateral film, therefore, left upper lobe collapse appears as an elongated opacity extending from the apex and reaching, or almost reaching, the diaphragm; it is anterior to the hilum and is bounded by displaced oblique fissure posteriorly, and by hyperinflated lower lobe anteriorly.

A collapsed left upper lobe does not produce a sharp outline on the frontal view. An ill-defined hazy opacity is present in the upper, mid and sometimes lower zones, the opacity being densest near the hilum. Pulmonary vessels in the hyperinflated lower lobe are usually visible through the haze. The aortic knuckle is usually obscured, unless the upper lobe has collapsed anterior to it,

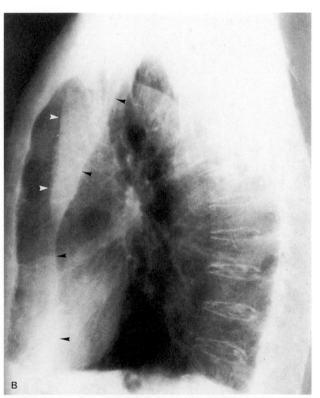

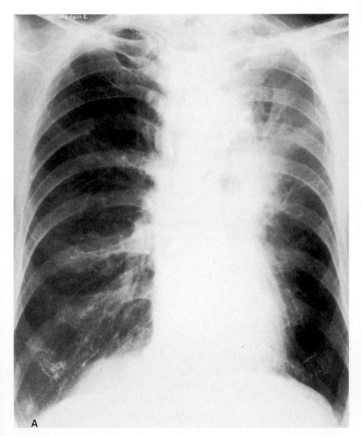

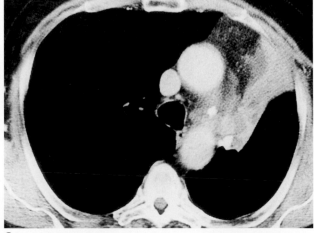

Fig. 16.44 Left upper lobe collapse due to squamous-cell carcinoma. **A.** PA film shows typical upper zone haze, through which is seen the elevated and enlarged left hilum, and vessels of the hyperinflated lower lobe. The contour of the aortic knuckle is indistinct, but the descending aorta is sharply outlined. **B.** Lateral film shows the collapsed left upper lobe between the anteriorly displaced oblique fissure (black arrows) and part of the hyperinflated lower lobe. **C.** CT demonstration of left upper lobe collapse. Calcified lymph nodes due to previous tuberculosis are visible.

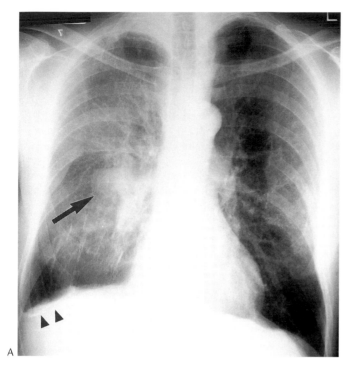

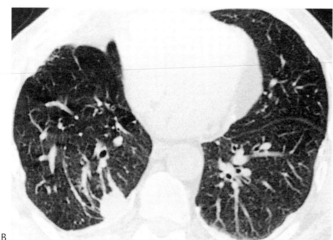

Fig. 16.45 Rounded atelectasis in a patient with a history of asbestos exposure. **A.** Chest radiograph shows en face pleural plaque on the right with calcified pleural plaques over the dome of the right diaphragm (arrowheads). There is the suggestion of a right infrahilar mass. **B.** High-resolution CT demonstrates indrawing of the bronchovascular structures into a pleurally based mass. The appearances are typical of rounded atelectasis. There is widespread calcified pleural plaque.

allowing it to be outlined by lower lobe. If the lingula is involved, the left heart border is obscured. The hilum is often elevated, and the trachea is often deviated to the left.

Rounded Atelectasis (Fig. 16.45) This is an unusual form of pulmonary collapse which may be misdiagnosed as a pulmonary mass. It appears on the plain film as a homogenous mass, up to 5 cm in diameter, with ill-defined edges. It is always pleural-based and associated with pleural thickening. Vascular shadows may be seen to radiate from part of the opacity, resembling a comet's tail. The appearance is caused by peripheral lung tissue

folding in on itself. It is often related to asbestos exposure, but may occur secondary to any exudative pleural effusion. It is not of any other pathological significance. The CT appearance is usually diagnostic, and enables differentiation from other pulmonary masses.

Consolidation

Functionally the pulmonary airways can be divided into two groups. The proximal airways function purely as a conducting network; the airways distal to the terminal bronchioles are also conducting structures, but, more importantly, are the site of gaseous exchange. These terminal airways are termed acini, an acinus comprising respiratory bronchioles, alveolar ducts, alveolar sacs and alveoli arising from a terminal bronchiole. Consolidation implies replacement of air in one or more acini by fluid or solid material, but does not imply a particular pathology or etiology. The smallest unit of consolidated lung is a single acinus, which casts a shadow approximately 7 mm in diameter. Communications between the terminal airways allow fluid to spread between adjacent acini, so that larger confluent areas of consolidation are generally visible and are frequently not confined to a single segment.

The commonest cause of consolidation is acute inflammatory exudate associated with pneumonia. Other causes include *cardiogenic pulmonary edema, non-cardiogenic pulmonary edema, hemorrhage* and *aspiration. Neoplasms* such as alveolar-cell carcinoma and lymphoma can produce consolidation, and *alveolar proteinosis* is a rare cause. In an individual patient, consolidation may be due to more than one basic etiology. For example, a patient with major head trauma may be particularly susceptible to infection, aspiration and non-cardiogenic pulmonary edema.

When consolidation is associated with a patent conducting airway an *air bronchogram* (Fig. 16.46) is often visible. This sign is produced by the radiographic contrast between the column of air in the airway and the surrounding opaque acini. If consolidation is secondary to bronchial obstruction, however, the air in the conducting airway is resorbed and replaced by fluid, and the affected area is of uniform density.

The volume of purely consolidated lung is similar to that of the normal lung since air is replaced by a similar volume of fluid or solid. However, collapse and consolidation are often associated with one another. When consolidation is due to fluid, its distribution is influenced by gravity, so that in acute pneumonitis consolidation is often denser and more clearly demarcated inferiorly by a pleural surface, and is less dense and more indistinct superiorly.

Ultrasound may demonstrate consolidation in adjacent lung (Fig. 16.47). When air bronchograms are evident on the chest radiograph these may be manifest as echogenic linear structures. When the bronchi become fluid-filled they are more clearly demonstrated as echo-free branching structures.

Lobar Consolidation

Consolidation of a complete lobe produces a homogenous opacity, possibly containing an air bronchogram, delineated by the chest wall, mediastinum or diaphragm and the appropriate interlobar fissure or fissures. Parts of the diaphragm and mediastinum adjacent to the non-aerated lung are obscured.

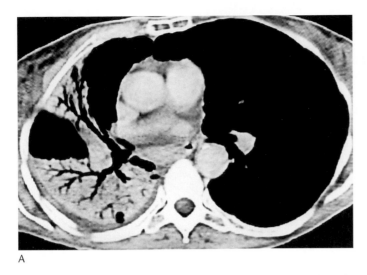

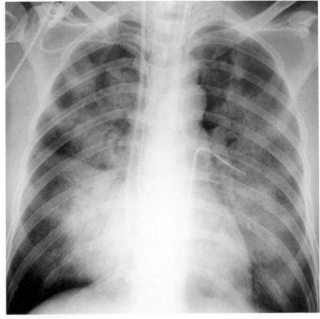

Fig. 16.46 Air bronchogram. **A.** CT shows patent air-filled bronchi surrounded by widespread pulmonary consolidation due to an acute bacterial chest infection. **B.** Chest radiograph of a different patient following aspiration of gastric contents demonstrating widespread air space shadowing containing air bronchograms.

Right Upper Lobe Consolidation (Fig. 16.48) This is confined by the horizontal fissure inferiorly and the upper half of the oblique fissure posteriorly, and may obscure the right upper mediastinum.

Right Middle Lobe Consolidation (Fig. 16.49) This is limited by the horizontal fissure above, and the lower half of the oblique fissure posteriorly, and may obscure the right heart border.

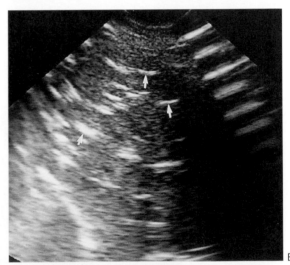

Fig. 16.47 **A.** Right lower lobe consolidation associated with volume loss demonstrated on CT. Note the air-filled bronchi. **B.** Ultrasound scan. The air bronchograms are evident as echogenic linear structures (arrows). **C.** Fluid bronchograms in a different patient (arrows); arrowheads indicate the position of the diaphragm.

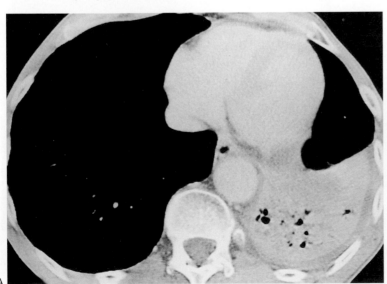

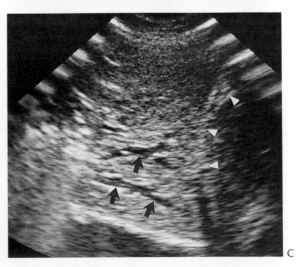

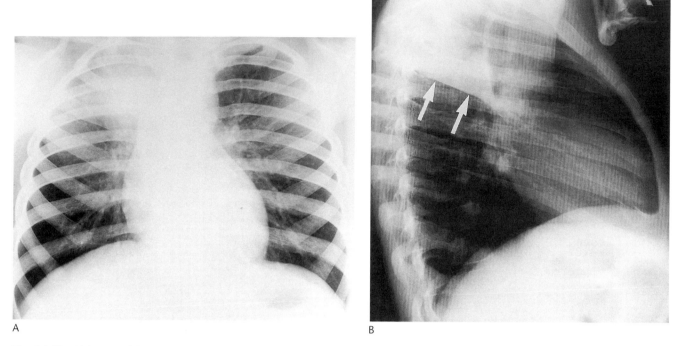

Fig. 16.48   Right upper lobe consolidation in a 6-year-old boy with aortic valve disease. **A.** Opacity in the right upper zone obscures the upper mediastinum. **B.** The lateral film shows consolidation anterior to the upper part of the oblique fissure (arrows), mostly in the posterior segment of the right upper lobe.

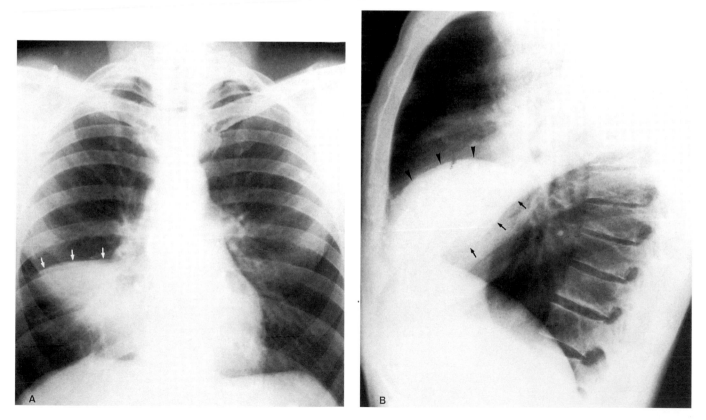

Fig. 16.49   Right middle lobe consolidation. 37-year-old man with squamous-cell carcinoma of the right middle lobe. **A.** PA film shows homogeneous opacity limited by horizontal fissure (arrows) and obscuring the right heart border. **B.** Lateral film shows consolidation bounded by horizontal fissure (arrowheads) and lower half of oblique fissure (arrows).

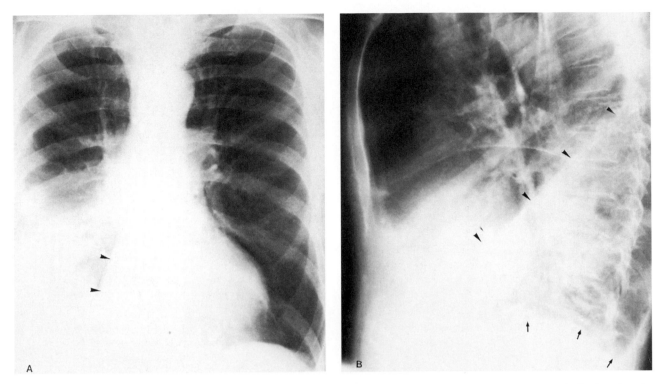

Fig. 16.50   Right lower lobe consolidation. Pneumonia complicating chronic bronchitis. **A.** PA film shows right lower zone shadowing obscuring the diaphragm but not the right heart border (arrowheads). **B.** Lateral film shows shadowing with air bronchogram, limited by oblique fissure anteriorly (arrowheads). The left hemidiaphragm is visible (arrows) but the right is obscured.

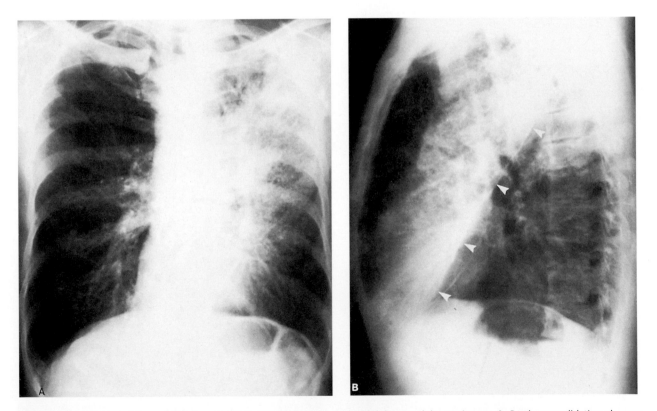

Fig. 16.51   Left upper lobe and lingula consolidation. A 70-year-old man with left upper lobe carcinoma. **A.** Patchy consolidation obscures the left heart border and aortic knuckle. **B.** The consolidation is bounded posteriorly by the oblique fissure (arrowheads).

Lower Lobe Consolidation   (Fig 16.50) This is limited by the oblique fissure anteriorly, and may obscure the diaphragm.

Left Upper Lobe and Lingula Consolidation   (Fig. 16.51)

These are limited by the oblique fissure posteriorly. Lingula consolidation may obscure the left heart border, and consolidation of the upper lobe may obscure the aortic knuckle.

REFERENCES AND SUGGESTIONS FOR FURTHER READING

Atelectasis Part I (1996) *Journal of Thoracic Imaging*, **11**, 91–149.

Bergin, C. J., Müller, N. L., Miller, R. R. (1986) C T in the qualitative assessment of emphysema. *Journal of Thoracic Imaging*, **1**, 94–103.

Breatnach, E., Kerr, I. H. (1982) The radiology of cryptogenic obliterative bronchiolitis. *Clinical Radiology*, **33**, 657–661.

Carr, D. H., Pride, N. B. (1984) Computed tomography in preoperative assessment of bullous emphysema. *Clinical Radiology*, **35**, 43–45.

Fletcher, C. M., Pride, N. B. (1984) Editorial. Definitions of emphysema, chronic bronchitis, asthma and air flow obstruction: 25 years on from the CIBA Symposium. *Thorax*, **39**, 81–85.

Macleod, W. M. (1954) Abnormal transradiancy of one lung. *Thorax*, **9**, 147–153.

Padley, S. P. G., Adler, B. D., Hansell, D. M. et al (1993) Bronchiolitis obliterans: high resolution CT findings and correlation with pulmonary function tests. *Clinical Radiology*, **47**, 236–240.

Patheram, I. S., Kerr, T. H., Collins, J. V. (1981) Value of chest radiographs in severe acute asthma. *Clinical Radiology*, **32**, 281–282.

Proto, A. V., Tocino, I. (1980) Radiographic manifestations of lobar collapse. *Seminars in Roentgenology*, **15**, 117–173.

Robbins, L. L., Hale, C. H. (1945) The roentgen appearance of lobar and segmental collapse of the lung; preliminary report. *Radiology*, **44**, 107–114.

Schneider, H. J., Felson, B., Gonzalez, L. L. (1980) Rounded atelectasis. *American Journal of Roentgenology*, **134**, 225–232.

Simon, G. (1964) Radiology and emphysema. *Clinical Radiology*, **15**, 293–306.

Swyer, P. R., James, G. C. W. (1953) A case of unilateral emphysema. *Thorax*, **8**, 133–136.

Thurlbeck, W. M., Churg, A. M. (eds) (1995) *Pathology of the Lung*, 2nd edn, pp 739–826. New York: Thieme Medical.

Thurlbeck, W. M., Simon, G. (1978) Radiographic appearance of the chest in emphysema. *American Journal of Roentgenology*, **130**, 429–440.

Tomashefski, J. F. (1977) Definition, differentiation and classification of COPD. *Postgraduate Medicine*, **62**, 88–97.

Vock, P., Spiegel, T., Fram, E. K. et al (1984) CT assessment of the adult intrathoracic cross section of the trachea. *Journal of Computer Assisted Tomography*, **8**, 1076–1082.

Webb, W. R., Müller, N. L., Naidich, D. P. (1996) *High Resolution CT of the Lung*, pp 227–270. Philadelphia: Lippincott–Raven.

17

DIFFUSE LUNG DISEASE

Simon P. G. Padley and Michael B. Rubens

There are many causes of diffuse lung disease in addition to infection, neoplasia or a primary abnormality of the airways. The chest radiograph remains the basic radiological tool in the investigation of these patients. However plain radiography is a relatively insensitive test, and is normal in 10–20% of patients with histologically proven interstitial lung disease.

Computed Tomography

There is no doubt that computed tomography (CT) and, particularly, high-resolution CT (HRCT) can play a major role in the assessment of patients with chronic diffuse lung disease (CDLD) (Table 17.1). HRCT has been shown to have a high sensitivity and specificity, and as a result there has been much recent interest in the role of this imaging technique in the diagnosis and management of many diffuse lung diseases. Because there is no superimposition of structures HRCT allows better assessment of parenchymal abnormalities compared with plain radiography. Conventional CT uses contiguous 10 mm-thick sections and is ideal for many clinical situations, but due to volume averaging there is some loss of fine detail. To avoid volume averaging HRCT uses thin-section CT images 1–2 mm thick and 10–15 mm

Table 17.1 Indications for the Use of HRCT in Diffuse Lung Disease

1. Confirmation of abnormality in patients with symptoms suggestive of diffuse lung disease with a normal or near normal chest radiograph.
2. Further assessment in patients with an abnormal but non-diagnostic chest radiograph.
3. As a guide to the site and method of biopsy.
4. As a guide to the assessment of disease activity, especially in fibrosing alveolitis.
5. To diagnose superimposed complications such as infection or tumor when they are clinically suspected but not visible on the chest radiograph.
6. To determine the relative importance of each condition in patients with more than one chronic diffuse lung disease.

apart. Resolution is further improved by using a high-spatial-frequency algorithm. This combination produces images with striking anatomic detail. Almost all recently installed CT scanners have the ability to generate HRCT images of high quality.

HRCT is particularly useful in patients with suspected CDLD but with normal radiographs or with questionable abnormalities on the chest radiograph. In many cases HRCT allows the radiologist to make a confident diagnosis, and in some cases biopsy can be avoided. In others the site and type of biopsy (open lung biopsy, biopsy at video assisted thoracoscopic surgery—(VATS or transbronchial biopsy) most likely to provide the diagnosis can be suggested.

HRCT has been shown to be particularly accurate in the diagnosis of many common causes of CDLD including fibrosing alveolitis, sarcoidosis, lymphangitis carcinomatosa, silicosis and asbestosis. HRCT is also remarkably accurate in the diagnosis of some of the rarer causes of CDLD such as lymphangioleiomyomatosis and pulmonary histiocytosis X. HRCT has a further role in the assessment of disease activity in some types of CDLD, particularly in fibrosing alveolitis and sarcoidosis.

SARCOIDOSIS

Sarcoidosis is a multisystem disease of unknown etiology. Pathologically it is characterized by the development of non-caseating granulomas which either resolve or become fibrotic. It may occur at any age but usually presents in young adults. Although worldwide in distribution there are racial differences in incidence, natural history and radiographic patterns. There is evidence of a genetic predisposition from clustering of familial cases and a higher frequency in monozygotic than dizygotic twins. Blacks are 12 times more likely to develop sarcoidosis than whites, and black females are twice as susceptible as black males. Patients most commonly present with one or more of erythema nodosum, arthralgia, an abnormal chest radiograph and respiratory symptoms. The diagnosis is usually made by the combination of symptoms, clinical signs and histology. When the chest radiograph is abnormal transbronchial biopsy is usually diagnostic and demonstrates non-caseating epithelioid granulomas. Within the lungs these are distributed along the bronchovascular bundles and adjacent to pleural surfaces and interlobular septa. Healing frequently involves fibrosis which may progress whilst the disease remains active. The final radiographic appearances range from normal to severe fibrosis. A Kveim test is occasionally performed to confirm the diagnosis. A Kveim test requires an intradermal inoculation of an extract of sarcoid tissue. The resulting skin reaction is biopsied and is deemed positive if it displays typical sarcoid histology.

Radiological Appearances Sarcoidosis commonly causes *thoracic lymphadenopathy* and *parenchymal lung opacities*. Adenopathy almost always precedes pulmonary shadowing, but they are often present simultaneously. The chest radiograph is abnormal at some time in 90% of patients with sarcoidosis.

Typically there is bilateral, symmetric hilar enlargement involving both tracheobronchial and bronchopulmonary nodes (Fig. 17.1). Bilateral hilar lymph node enlargement, in the correct clinical setting, is often regarded as sufficient evidence of sarcoidosis to negate the need for biopsy. Right paratracheal lymphadenopathy is also common, and left paratracheal adenopathy is occasionally seen. Enlargement of other mediastinal nodes is rarely appreciated on the chest radiograph but may be seen on CT (Fig. 17.2). If the hilar adenopathy is very asymmetric or anterior mediastinal adenopathy is a feature, other diagnoses should be considered. Rarely the involved lymph nodes may calcify, sometimes peripherally, causing 'egg-shell' calcification (Fig. 17.3).

Nodal enlargement usually resolves, and recurrence following resolution is unusual. In some patients nodal enlargement may persist for many years and despite a long period of non-progression the development of parenchymal disease may still occur. Overall approximately 50% of cases will progress from radiographically evident bilateral hilar lymph node enlargement to nodal and pulmonary disease. Virtually all patients with intra-

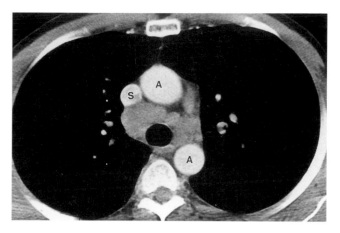

Fig. 17.2 Sarcoidosis. There are multiple mediastinal lymph nodes. S = superior vena cava; A = aorta.

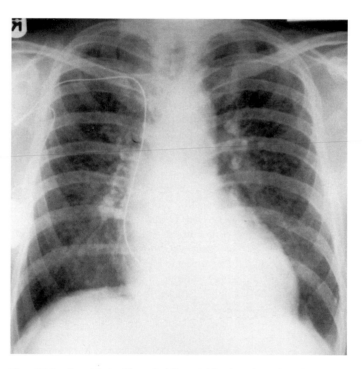

Fig. 17.3 Sarcoidosis. There is bilateral hilar lymph node calcification. Some of the nodes are calcified peripherally ('egg-shell' calcification). A pacing electrode is present. Heart block is an occasional complication of sarcoidosis.

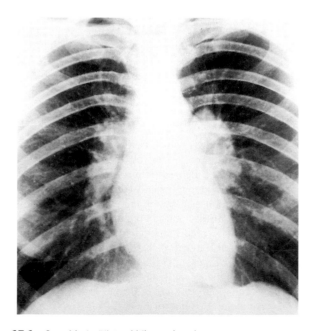

Fig. 17.1 Sarcoidosis. Bilateral hilar node enlargement.

thoracic adenopathy due to sarcoid develop pulmonary granulomas histologically. It is therefore not surprising that the incidence of parenchymal abnormality is significantly higher on HRCT scanning than on chest radiography. Typically HRCT reveals multiple small irregular nodular opacities which, although widespread, tend to have a predominantly peribronchovascular and subpleural distribution (Fig. 17.4). The mid zones are most profusely involved and nodules may be so numerous as to create fine ground-glass opacification or appear as miliary shadows (Fig. 17.5). Larger nodules of the order of 1 cm in diameter may be present. They may be well or poorly marginated and may coalesce to form larger opacities (Fig. 17.6). Air bronchograms

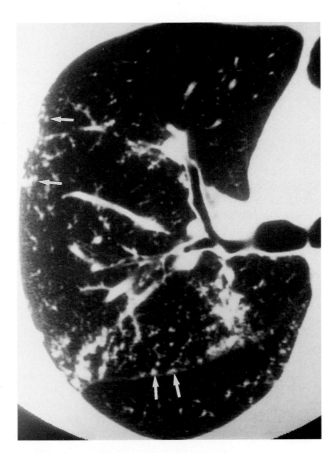

Fig. 17.4 Sarcoidosis. HRCT scan through the right lung shows nodularity of the bronchovascular bundles due to multiple sarcoid granulomas. Nodules are also evident in the subpleural regions adjacent to the chest wall and major fissure (arrows).

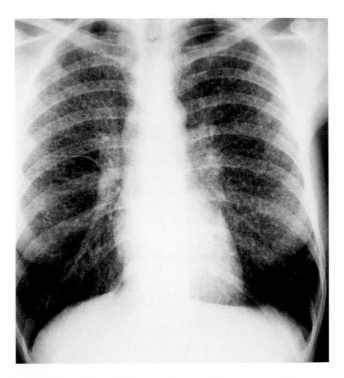

Fig. 17.5 Sarcoidosis. Miliary, nodular opacities are present throughout both lungs. One year later the appearances were entirely normal.

are occasionally visible, and rarely nodules may cavitate. Parenchymal nodules evident on chest radiography often appear most profuse in the lung bases where the anteroposterior dimension of the lungs is maximized. A reticular pattern may be evident, usually radiating from the hila. Septal lines are uncommon. When present they do not indicate lymphatic obstruc-

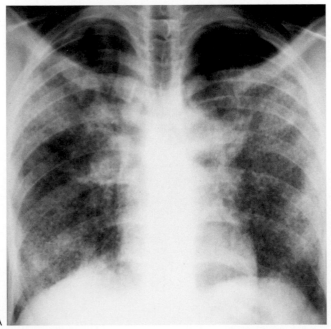

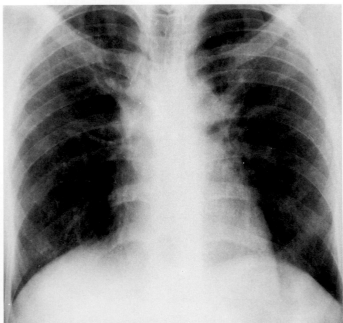

Fig. 17.6 Sarcoidosis. **A.** Miliary nodules with areas of coalescence peripherally. **B.** After resolution of the nodular shadowing there is mild mid and upper zone linear scarring.

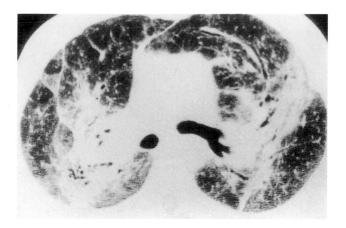

Fig. 17.7 HRCT scan at the level of the hila showing conglomerate fibrotic masses with radiation into the surrounding lung.

tion from nodal disease but rather reflect micronodular disease related to intralobular septa.

Nodules up to 2–3 cm in size are rarely seen in the UK but are recognized in the USA, most commonly in Afro-Caribbean patients.

Most cases of parenchymal involvement resolve completely, but approximately one-third develop *pulmonary fibrosis*. This tends to involve the mid and upper zones more than the bases (Fig. 17.6). The commonest pattern is of a few inconspicuous linear mid zone scars. Coarse linear shadows, ring shadows and bullae may be seen in more severe cases. Occasionally, confluent fibrotic areas develop and on HRCT a typical perihilar and posterior mid zone pattern is evident (Fig. 17.7).

Unusual manifestations of sarcoidosis include basal septal lines, pleural effusions, spontaneous pneumothorax and broncho-stenosis. Rarely endobronchial disease may result in fibrotic strictures causing segmental or even lobar collapse. Evidence of air trapping is well recognized on expiratory HRCT scanning (Fig. 17.8).

Gallium-67 This isotope is taken up by involved lymph nodes and lung, and has been used to assess the activity and extent of the disease.

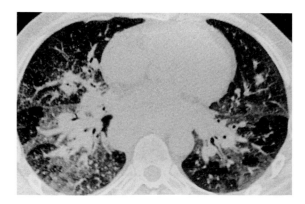

Fig. 17.8 Sarcoidosis. Expiratory HRCT scan through the lower zones. There is air trapping as evidenced by areas of parenchyma that remain of lower attenuation on expiration. Some of these correspond to individual secondary pulmonary nodules.

THE PNEUMOCONIOSES

The pneumoconioses are diseases caused by inhalation of *inorganic dusts*. The diagnosis depends on a history of exposure to the dust, and an abnormal chest radiograph and respiratory function tests. Only occasionally is a lung biopsy required to confirm the diagnosis. The history of exposure may include living near a mine or a factory or living with an exposed worker, as well as working directly with dust. Dusts may be termed active or inactive. Active dusts are fibrogenic in the lung, and inactive dusts are relatively inert. Inhaled dusts—such as coal dust—are often a combination of active and inactive materials. The important active dusts are asbestos and silica. The reaction of an individual to dust exposure depends on several factors in addition to the nature of the dust, including the duration of exposure, concentration of particles and individual susceptibility.

Dust particles larger than 5 μm in diameter are usually deposited onto the bronchial and bronchiolar walls and are coughed up. Smaller particles may reach the alveoli. Asbestos fibers are the exception, fibers longer than 30 μm sometimes penetrating the lung parenchyma.

Silicosis

Exposure to silica may occur in granite, slate and sandstone quarrying, gold mining, sandblasting and in foundry, ceramic and pottery works. Exposure of several years may lead to pulmonary fibrosis. Fibrosis may continue after exposure has ceased.

Radiology *Simple silicosis* causes multiple, nodular shadows, 2–5 mm in diameter (Fig. 17.9). These initially appear in the mid and upper zones, eventually involving all lung zones but relatively sparing the bases. HRCT confirms that they are most profuse in the mid and upper zones but also demonstrates a

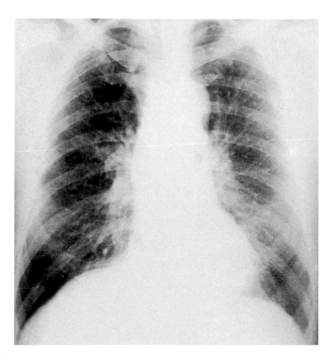

Fig. 17.9 Simple silicosis. Multiple, small nodules are present throughout both lungs.

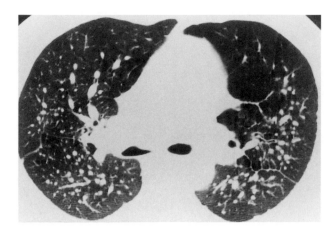

Fig. 17.10 Simple silicosis. CT scan demonstrates multiple well-defined pulmonary nodules, most numerous in the posterior lung parenchyma.

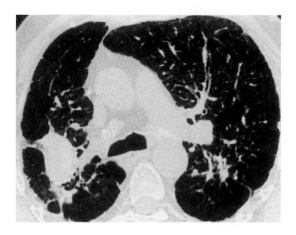

Fig. 17.12 Early complicated silicosis. CT scan demonstrates coalescence of nodules into pulmonary masses.

predilection for the posterior aspect of the lungs not evident on the chest radiograph (Fig. 17.10). The nodules are well defined, uniform in density and size (2–5 mm) and rarely calcify. Linear shadows and septal lines may also appear. In *complicated silicosis* the nodules become confluent and form homogenous, non-segmental areas of shadowing. This tends to occur in the upper lobes, and the areas of fibrosis may migrate toward the hila, creating areas of emphysema in the lung periphery. These changes may be seen on plain radiography (Fig. 17.11), but are detected at an earlier stage by conventional or HRCT (Fig. 17.12).

When complicated silicosis develops the possibility of tuberculosis should be considered although cavitation of 'massive shadows' may also be due to ischemic necrosis (Fig. 17.11). HRCT also has a role in patients with silicosis in whom the pulmonary function tests and radiological appearances do not correlate. The impairment in pulmonary function correlates with the severity of emphysematous changes, often best assessed with HRCT, rather than the profusion of pulmonary nodules.

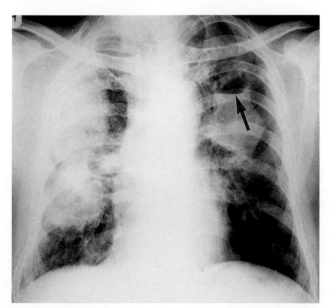

Fig. 17.11 Progressive massive fibrosis (PMF). Large confluent masses have formed. Cavitation is evident on the left (arrow).

Extensive fibrosis may be complicated by pulmonary arterial hypertension and cor pulmonale. Hilar lymphadenopathy is common in silicosis, and the nodes may calcify diffusely or with a peripheral 'egg-shell' pattern (Fig. 17.13). Patients with silicosis and rheumatoid disease may develop *Caplan's syndrome*, but like massive fibrosis this is commoner in coal worker's pneumoconiosis.

Coal Worker's Pneumoconiosis

Coal dust is mostly carbon, but it may contain silica. Coal workers are prone to coal worker's pneumoconiosis, silicosis, chronic bronchitis and emphysema. Coal dust is not fibrogenic and deposits in the lung are surrounded by emphysema. The corresponding radiographic appearance is simple pneumoconiosis. As in silicosis, simple pneumoconiosis may progress to a complicated variety with the development of *progressive massive fibrosis (PMF)* (Fig. 17.14). This is usually associated with prolonged exposure and sometimes a complicating factor such as infection or an autoimmune process.

In *simple pneumoconiosis*, small, faint, indistinct nodules, 1–5 mm in diameter, appear in the mid zones. Eventually nodules may be seen throughout the lungs, but remain most numerous in the mid zones. The development of PMF is marked by coalescence of the small nodules or the appearance of larger opacities of 1 cm diameter or more. As in silicosis, areas of massive fibrosis associated with coal worker's pneumoconiosis are usually mid or upper zone and bilateral; they are round or oval and tend to migrate toward the hila creating peripheral areas of emphysema and bullae. The fibrotic masses may calcify or cavitate (Fig. 17.14). Simple coal worker's pneumoconiosis does not usually develop further if exposure ceases, but PMF often does progress.

Patients with rheumatoid disease and coal worker's pneumoconiosis may develop *Caplan's syndrome*. Multiple, round, well-defined opacities, 1–5 cm in diameter, may appear in the lungs (Fig 17.15). These usually appear in crops, and are often accompanied by cutaneous rheumatoid nodules. These represent necrobiotic nodules, but if the underlying pneumoconiosis is not appreciated they may be misdiagnosed as metastases. Nodules may regress, remain static, calcify or cavitate (Fig. 17.16).

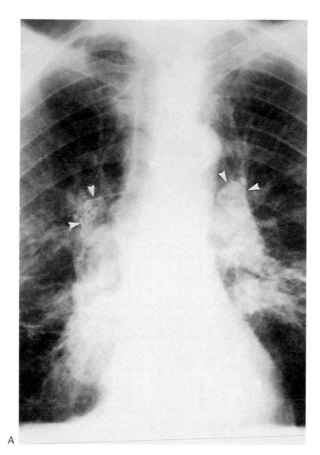

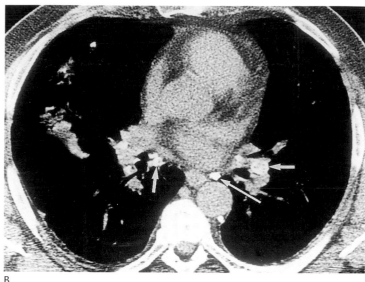

Fig. 17.13 Silicosis. **A.** There is bilateral hilar lymphadenopathy. Many of the nodes are calcified, some of them peripherally. **B.** Similar changes on CT.

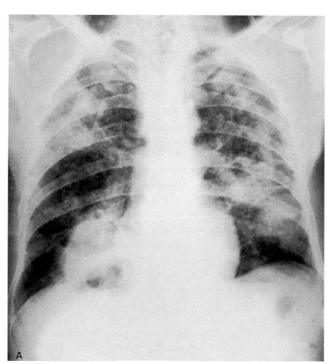

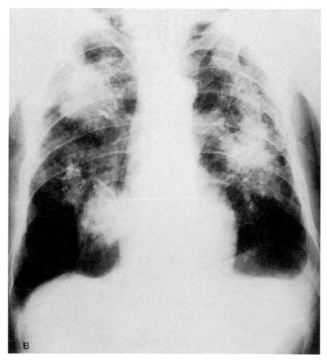

Fig. 17.14 Progressive massive fibrosis in a coal miner of 52. **A.** Nodular opacities are present throughout both lungs, and several areas of more confluent shadowing are present. **B.** Four years later, lower zone masses have migrated centrally, leaving peripheral areas of emphysema. The upper lobe opacities have enlarged.

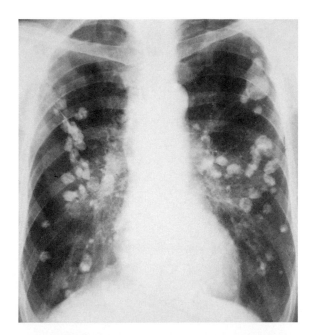

Fig. 17.15 Male aged 54 with Caplan's syndrome. Coal worker with rheumatoid arthritis. Multiple rounded opacities are present (some partly calcified).

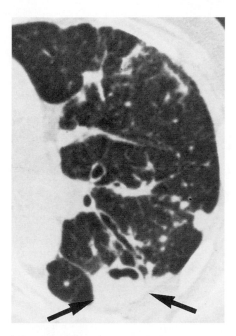

Fig. 17.16 Caplan's syndrome. There is a left-sided cavitating pulmonary nodule (arrows) on a background of pneumoconiosis.

Asbestosis

Asbestos exposure may occur in asbestos mining and processing, in construction and demolition work, in ship building and in the manufacture of some textiles. Living near such workplaces, or with exposed workers, also carries some risk of exposure. Manifestations of exposure may not become apparent for many years.

The four types of asbestos that commonly cause disease are chrysolite, crocidolite, amosite and anthophyllite. *Chrysolite* (or white asbestos) is the commonest, and *crocidolite* (or blue asbestos) is the most pathogenic. The fibrosis is probably the result of physical and chemical irritation in addition to an autoimmune mechanism. Inhaled fibers, sometimes longer than 30 µm, may reach the alveoli and penetrate the pleura and occasionally the diaphragm. The fibers gravitate to the lower lobes, so that changes are more severe in the lower zones than in the mid and upper zones.

Symptoms of asbestosis are often not apparent until 20 or 30 years after exposure. Malignant disease is an important complication. Lung cancer is relatively common, especially when asbestos exposure is combined with cigarette smoking. Compared to the non-smoker without exposure to asbestos, asbestos alone increases the likelihood of lung cancer by a factor of 5, cigarette smoking alone by a factor of 10, and the combination of asbestos and cigarettes by a factor of 50. The combination of asbestos and cigarettes also predisposes to carcinomas of the esophagus, larynx and oropharynx. Mesothelioma of the pleura is the other malignancy closely associated with asbestos exposure, and may develop after a latent period of 20 years. Other neoplasms associated with asbestos exposure are carcinomas of the large bowel and renal tract and peritoneal mesothelioma.

Radiological Appearance Asbestos exposure may produce changes in the lung parenchyma and in the pleura. Pleural changes, which include plaques, calcification, diffuse thickening and effusion, are seen on the chest X-ray more often than parenchymal changes.

Pleural Plaques These develop bilaterally. They tend to occur in the mid zones and over the diaphragm (Fig. 13.26) and are the most frequent manifestation of previous exposure. Small plaques may be difficult to see on the standard chest radiograph, but may be demonstrated with oblique views, preferably aided by *fluoroscopy*, or by *ultrasound* or *HRCT* (Fig. 13.28). The plaques often calcify and may produce bizarre opacities, sometimes resembling holly leaves (Fig. 13.26). Small pleural effusions may occasionally occur, unrelated to malignancy, but large effusions suggest an underlying carcinoma or mesothelioma.

Pulmonary Fibrosis This may be seen with or without pleural changes. While the chest radiograph remains the first investigation in patients with suspected asbestosis, HRCT is indicated in those patients with clinical or functional abnormalities compatible with asbestosis in whom the chest radiograph is normal or shows questionable abnormalities. Between 5 and 25% of asbestos-exposed patients with a normal chest radiograph have HRCT abnormalities suggestive of asbestosis. On plain radiography the earliest signs are a fine reticular or nodular pattern in the lower zones (Fig. 17.17). With progression this becomes coarser and causes loss of clarity of the diaphragm and cardiac shadow—the so-called *'shaggy heart'* (Fig. 17.18). Eventually the whole lung may become involved, but the basal preponderance persists and areas of emphysema may develop. HRCT demonstrates fibrosis initially in the periphery of the lung (Fig. 17.18). Parenchymal bands that extend inward from the pleural surface may develop with resultant distortion in the lung

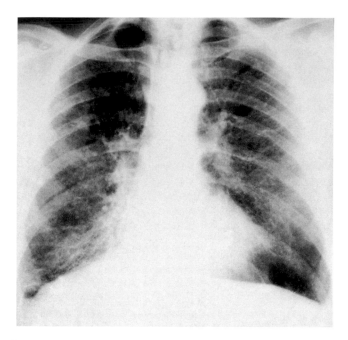

Fig. 17.17 Asbestos exposure of 25 years. Fine reticulonodular shadowing in the mid and lower zones is best seen on the right. Bullous disease is present at the left base.

architecture. Subpleural linear opacities may also be present (Fig. 17.19). A pattern of interstitial fibrosis indistinguishable from idiopathic pulmonary fibrosis may develop, and the presence of asbestos-related pleural disease can be helpful in differentiating between the two conditions.

Berylliosis

Acute berylliosis causes a chemical pneumonitis which radiographically has the appearance of non-cardiogenic pulmonary edema. *Chronic berylliosis* is a systemic disease characterized by widespread non-cavitating granulomas. The thoracic radiological manifestations are identical to sarcoidosis (Fig. 17.20).

Other Pneumoconioses due to Inactive Dusts

Inactive dusts do not cause fibrosis in the lungs, but may produce changes on the chest X-ray simply by accumulating in the lungs. Symptoms are usually absent.

Siderosis This is due to prolonged exposure to iron oxide dust. Widespread reticulonodular shadowing occurs. When exposure ceases the shadowing may regress. In *silicosiderosis* fibrosis may occur, with a picture resembling that of silicosis.

Stannosis This condition is caused by inhalation of tin oxide. Multiple, very small, very dense, discrete opacities of 0.5–1 mm diameter are distributed throughout the lungs. Particles may collect in the interlobular lymphatics and produce dense septal lines. The opacities are denser than calcium because of the high atomic number of tin.

Barytosis This results from inhalation of particulate barium sulphate, causing very dense nodulation throughout the lungs. Following cessation of exposure the shadows regress.

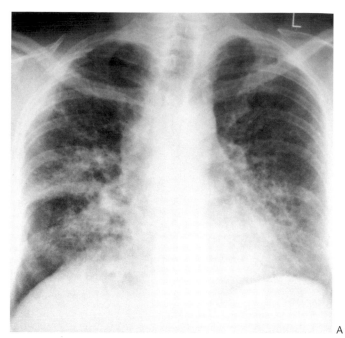

A

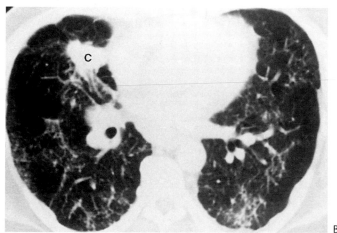

B

Fig. 17.18 Asbestosis. **A.** Chest radiograph demonstrating loss of clarity of the cardiac silhouette (shaggy heart). **B.** HRCT reveals linear opacities and also a carcinoma (C) adjacent to the right heart border.

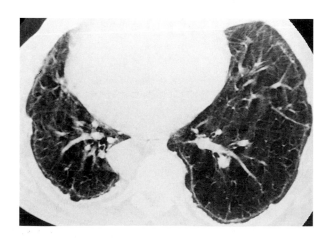

Fig. 17.19 HRCT demonstrating an extensive subpleural linear stripe due to asbestosis.

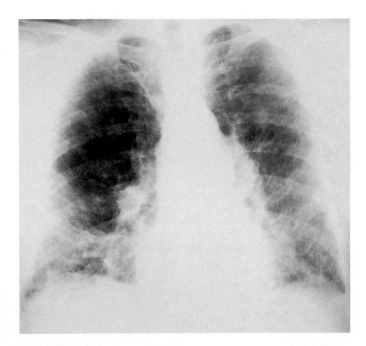

Fig. 17.20 Berylliosis. The patient had spent 35 years in the glass-blowing industry making neon lights. The chest radiograph shows diffuse reticular shadowing. The appearance is indistinguishable from end-stage sarcoidosis.

ASPIRATION AND INHALATION

Aspiration of liquid or solid material into the airways may cause mechanical obstruction, and depending on the nature of the aspirate, a variable amount of inflammation.

Mendelson's Syndrome This is due to aspiration of acid gastric contents by the anesthetized patient. Intense bronchospasm is followed by a chemical pneumonitis. The chest radiograph shows widespread pulmonary edema. Similar changes are seen in patients after near-drowning.

Lipoid Pneumonia This results from aspiration of mineral oil, which is usually being taken for chronic constipation. Aspirated oil tends to collect in the dependent parts of the lungs where it causes a chronic inflammatory response. The chest radiograph usually shows large, dense, tumor-like opacities.

Petrol or Paraffin Aspiration This may cause a pneumonitis, which is usually basal. It may be followed by the development of pneumatoceles.

Inhalation of Irritant Gases Chlorine, ammonia and oxides of nitrogen may produce pulmonary edema followed by obliterative bronchiolitis and emphysema.

Oxygen Toxicity This may occur following prolonged administration of oxygen in concentrations above 50%. Damage to the alveolar epithelium causes pulmonary edema followed by interstitial fibrosis.

EXTRINSIC ALLERGIC ALVEOLITIS

Extrinsic allergic alveolitis, also known as *hypersensitivity pneumonitis*, is an allergic inflammatory granulomatous reaction of the lungs caused by the inhalation of dusts containing certain organisms or proteins. Inhaled particles less than 10 μm in diameter are capable of reaching the alveoli, where their potential for causing damage to the gas-exchanging parts of the lungs is considerable. If the particles are antigenic and the lung previously sensitized, a hypersensitivity reaction ensues. Antibodies are meant to neutralize potentially harmful foreign material, but sometimes the combination of antigen and antibody is itself damaging and constitutes a disease process. In *farmer's lung* the offending organism is usually *Micropolyspora faeni* from damp moldy hay. *Pigeon breeders* inhale dust from feathers or desiccated droppings containing bird serum protein. *Mushroom growers* are affected by fungal spores from the compost used. *Sugar cane workers* exposed to moldy sugar cane residue may develop bagassosis. *Air-conditioning systems* may circulate fungal spores and amebae. A similar reaction in the lungs may be induced by drugs, in this case blood borne, the most common examples being *nitrofurantoin* and *salazopyrine*.

Precipitating antibodies directed specifically against the antigen are found in the serum of patients but their presence only implies exposure, not necessarily disease. Some 40% of pigeon breeders have precipitins but few suffer from the disease. However the presence of precipitins to extracts of budgerigar excreta in those exposed is stronger evidence in favor of disease. The immunological reactions are predominantly Type III, that is, free-circulating antigen and antibody combine in the presence of complement to form complexes which are deposited in the alveolar walls. Activation of complement sets in train a sequence of reactions liberating a variety of damaging substances. The timescale of the reaction is intermediate, which corresponds well with the clinical presentation. Type IV reactions also play a part, and here the antibody is produced and transported by lymphocytes which then aggregate at the site where the reaction takes place. The granuloma, a characteristic feature of Type IV reactions, is the fundamental histologic lesion of extrinsic allergic alveolitis.

Typically the patient develops headache, fever, chills, a cough and dyspnea 5 or 6 hours after exposure. Smaller and more frequent exposure to the antigen may result in progressive dyspnea, and is typical of disease due to budgerigars. On auscultation there are usually inspiratory crepitations. Lung function tests show restricted ventilation and impaired gas transfer but little airways obstruction. The best test is a bronchial challenge by the inhalation of the allergen to reproduce the symptoms and functional abnormalities. It is now rarely used, but it was instrumental initially in establishing the pathogenesis of the disease.

Treatment is by removal from exposure or, if that is not possible, reduction of contact to a minimum. Steroids are of doubtful value. In only 50–60% of patients does the lung function return to normal and some continue to deteriorate after elimination of exposure.

Radiological Appearances The radiographic appearances are dependent on the length of allergen exposure and the balance between continuing inflammatory change and the development of fibrosis. A mixture of inflammatory and fibrotic changes is the most common pattern. In the early stages the chest radiograph may be normal, but may show diffuse fine nodular opacities or a generalized, 'ground-glass' haze (Fig. 17.21). HRCT frequently reveals a combination of small (1–3 mm) pulmonary nodules and areas of ground-glass change even in those patients with a normal

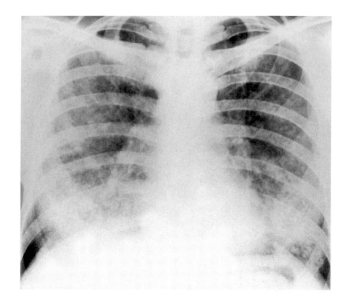

Fig. 17.21 Farmer's lung. Patchy alveolar opacification superimposed on a miliary nodulation. The costophrenic angles are clear.

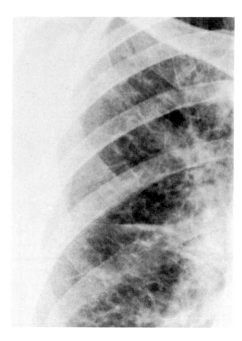

Fig. 17.23 Allergic alveolitis due to monoamine oxidase inhibitor drug. The interstitial shadowing was generalized throughout both lungs. Complete resolution within 7 days.

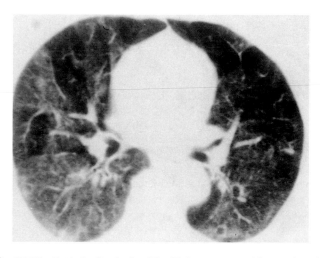

Fig. 17.22 Extrinsic allergic alveolitis. CT demonstrates widespread patchy areas of increased attenuation (ground-glass shadowing) representative of areas of inflammatory change.

chest radiograph (Fig. 17.22). Patchy consolidation and septal lines, similar to pulmonary edema, may also be seen in acute attacks (Fig. 17.23). With the development of fibrosis reticulo-nodular shadows may progress to coarse linear opacities, typically in the mid and upper zones. Finally, severe contraction of the upper and mid zones with 'honeycombing', cyst formation and bronchiectasis may occur.

Lung fibrosis, often with an upper lobe predominance, is a common end-stage of a number of disparate diseases, including extrinsic allergic alveolitis, cryptogenic fibrosing alveolitis, tuberculosis, bronchopulmonary aspergillosis, ankylosing spondylitis and many others. At this stage it is often impossible to differentiate between them on the basis of the chest radiograph although HRCT frequently still allows the underlying etiology to be identified.

CONNECTIVE TISSUE DISEASES

This group of conditions, also known as the collagen vascular diseases, comprises a number of chronic inflammatory, auto-immune disorders. They may involve any tissue in any part of the body; joints, serous membranes and blood vessels are frequently involved, and all connective tissue diseases involve the lungs and pleura to some extent. The acute inflammatory episodes characteristically lead to fibrosis and collagen production. While many patients show clinical or radiological features that allow the diagnosis of a specific connective tissue disorder, some patients exhibit signs of more than one of the conditions. Consequently it is not always possible to make a precise diagnosis.

Conventionally, the connective tissue diseases comprise rheumatoid arthritis, systemic lupus erythematosus (SLE), systemic sclerosis (SS), mixed connective tissue disease, polyarteritis nodosa (PAN) and dermatomyositis/polymyositis (PMS). CREST syndrome is a subset of SS characterized by cutaneous calcinosis, Raynaud's phenomenon, esophageal abnormalities, sclerodactyly and telangiectasis. Mixed connective tissue disease consists of combined features of SLE, SS and PMS. The term 'overlap syndrome' has been extended to include almost any combination so that it now lacks a precise definition.

Systemic Lupus Erythematosus (SLE)

SLE is typically a disease of young women (F:M=9:1), and blacks are affected more frequently than whites. Features usually include some or all of a butterfly facial rash, arthralgias, Raynaud's phenomenon, renal involvement and CNS disease. The lungs or pleura are involved in approximately 50% of cases. Interstitial fibrosis is relatively rare, occurring in less than 5% of cases.

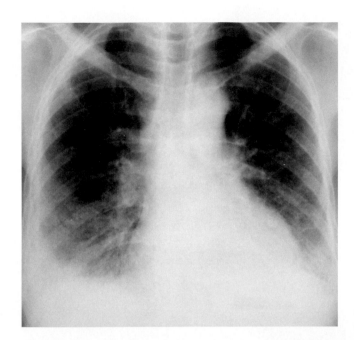

Fig. 17.24 Systemic lupus erythematosus. Bilateral pleural effusions are present.

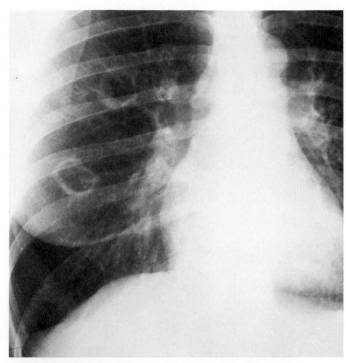

Fig. 17.25 Rheumatoid disease. Two cavitating necrobiotic nodules are visible in the right lung.

Pleuritic pain with a small *pleural effusion* is a common manifestation, and may occur bilaterally (Fig. 17.24). Movement of the diaphragm is decreased secondary to the pleurisy and may cause areas of *atelectasis* in the lower lobes. This may produce bilateral, horizontal basal band shadows and elevation of the diaphragm on the chest radiograph. The reduction in lung volume is not usually accompanied by pleural or parenchymal disease, even on HRCT. It is probably a reflection of SLE-related chest wall or diaphragmatic myopathy.

Patchy Consolidation This may be seen, sometimes with cavitation, and is most often due to infection, pulmonary edema or pulmonary infarction. Lupus pneumonitis and diffuse pulmonary hemorrhage occasionally occur. Vascular thrombosis, either in the lungs or elsewhere, is related to the lupus anti-coagulant which paradoxically increases coagulability in vivo.

Enlargement of the Cardiac Shadow This may be due to pericardial effusion, myocarditis or endocarditis, and should be investigated by cardiac ultrasound in the first instance.

Rheumatoid Disease

Rheumatoid disease may cause pleural effusions, pulmonary nodules, fibrosing alveolitis and bronchiolitis obliterans. These occur more often in males than females, occasionally being apparent before joint disease. Overall, only a few per cent of patients with rheumatoid arthritis develop fibrosing alveolitis although conversely rheumatoid arthritis is a relatively common etiology in a mixed population of patients with fibrosing alveolitis.

Pleural Effusion Effusions are the commonest thoracic manifestation. These may be unilateral or bilateral, are usually larger than in SLE and are often asymptomatic. Rheumatoid pleural effusions often become chronic but may resolve with pleural

fibrosis. Rarely a cholesterol effusion may develop and remain unchanged over several years.

Rheumatoid Pulmonary Nodules These are uncommon but are characteristic of this condition (Fig. 17.25). The necrobiotic nodules are usually associated with subcutaneous nodules, and are similar histologically. They produce well-defined, round opacities up to 7 cm in diameter and may be single or multiple. In Caplan's syndrome rheumatoid nodules develop against a background of simple pneumoconiosis. The two diseases modify each other in a distinctive fashion and numerous round opacities up to 5 cm in diameter, resembling metastases, may appear (Fig. 17.15). The solid fibrotic lesions eventually become hyalinized and may calcify. The syndrome was first described in coal miners but it is also found in asbestosis, silicosis and other industrial pneumoconioses.

Fibrosing Alveolitis This is apparent on the chest radiograph in approximately 5% of patients. However evidence of interstitial fibrosis is more common on HRCT, pulmonary function testing and histologic examination. It usually produces basal reticulo-nodular shadowing, but may progress to honeycombing and severe volume loss (Fig. 17.26).

Obliterative bronchiolitis is a potential cause of respiratory failure and the chest radiograph may be normal, although evidence of small airways disease may be evident on HRCT.

Progressive upper lobe fibrosis with bullous cystic changes indistinguishable from those found in ankylosing spondylitis has also been reported.

Systemic Sclerosis

Systemic sclerosis has the highest incidence of pulmonary fibrosis

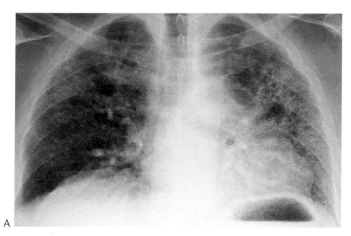
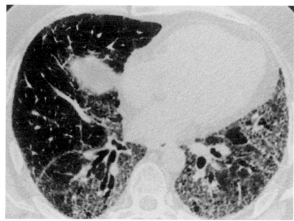

Fig. 17.26 Rheumatoid disease. Chest radiograph (**A**) and HRCT (**B**) demonstrating typical subpleural honeycomb changes of pulmonary fibrosis. There is considerable volume loss.

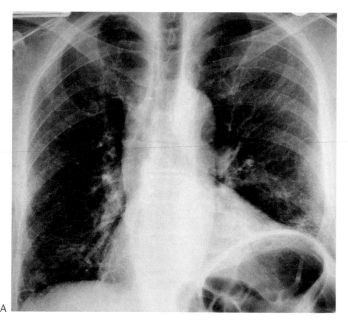

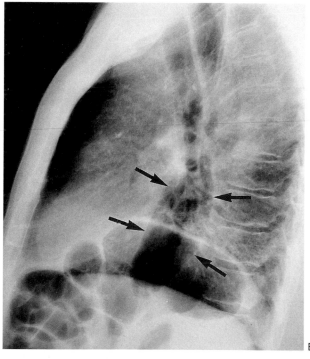

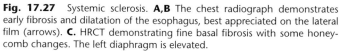

Fig. 17.27 Systemic sclerosis. **A,B** The chest radiograph demonstrates early fibrosis and dilatation of the esophagus, best appreciated on the lateral film (arrows). **C.** HRCT demonstrating fine basal fibrosis with some honeycomb changes. The left diaphragm is elevated.

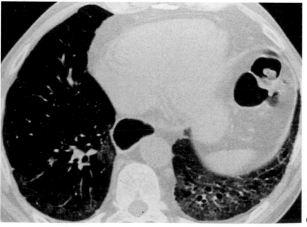

amongst the connective tissue diseases, with almost all patients eventually developing lung disease that is indistinguishable from idiopathic pulmonary fibrosis. However progression is slower and outlook slightly better than in the idiopathic form. Esophageal involvement resulting in abnormal motility may cause reflux and aspiration. Occasionally a dilated esophagus, sometimes demonstrating an air–fluid level, is visible on the chest radiograph (Fig. 17.27). Pulmonary artery hypertension may be seen with or without pulmonary fibrosis. As in other conditions with fibrosing alveolitis, the usual appearance on the chest radiograph is of basal reticulonodular shadowing, with progressive pulmonary volume loss (Fig. 17.27). Eventually honeycomb change may develop. Egg-shell lymph node calcification is a recognized feature.

Associated pleural disease is rare. There is a predisposition to *lung cancer*.

Other Connective Tissue Disorders

Dermatomyositis and Polymyositis Primary lung involvement is unusual. A basal fibrosing alveolitis may occur and involvement of the pharyngeal muscles may predispose to aspiration pneumonitis (Fig. 17.28).

Ankylosing Spondylitis In 1–2% of cases of longstanding ankylosing spondylitis, upper lobe fibrosis develops. It is usually bilateral and associated with apical pleural thickening. The

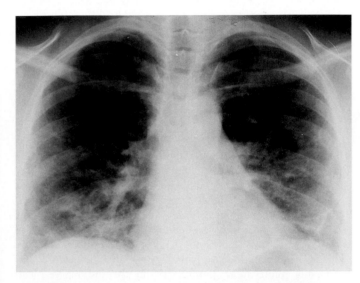

Fig. 17.28 Polymyositis. There is volume loss due to basal fibrosis.

radiological appearances are indistinguishable from other causes of upper lobe fibrosis. With severe fibrosis bullae develop and may become colonized by *Aspergillus* (Fig. 17.29).

Sjögren's Syndrome Sjögren's syndrome comprises dry eyes, dry mouth and one of the other connective tissue disorders. If the latter is missing it is called the sicca syndrome or primary Sjögren's syndrome. Women are more often affected than men. The salivary, lacrimal and mucous glands of the mouth, nose, eyelids, pharynx, bronchial tree and stomach may all be the site of the pathological changes which consist of a massive lymphoid infiltration with eventual atrophy of the gland acini. There are minor salivary glands in the lip and this is the easiest site for diagnostic biopsy. Although sarcoidosis may involve the salivary glands, with the same functional effects, it is by convention excluded from the definition of Sjögren's and sicca syndromes. In addition to the features of an associated connective tissue disease there may also be pleural effusion, fibrosing alveolitis, recurrent chest infections and lymphocytic interstitial pneumonitis. As a result there is no characteristic pattern.

Systemic Vasculitides

This section also includes diseases that have traditionally been classified together as *pulmonary angiitis* and *granulomatosis*. This subgroup comprises Wegener's granulomatosis, allergic angiitis and granulomatosis (Churg–Strauss syndrome), necrotizing sarcoid granulomatosis, lymphoid granulomatosis and bronchocentric granulomatosis.

Wegener's Granulomatosis Classic Wegener's granulomatosis is a necrotizing vasculitis which involves the upper respiratory tract, the lungs and the kidneys. There is a limited variant which is more or less confined to the thorax.

Symptoms referable to the upper air passages are almost always present at some time in the course of the disease: nasal obstruction, purulent discharge, sinusitis, chronic ulceration—even, in some cases, necrosis of nasal cartilage and bone. Cough, hemoptysis and pleurisy are usually accompanied by constitutional symptoms of malaise, weakness and fever. Rheumatoid

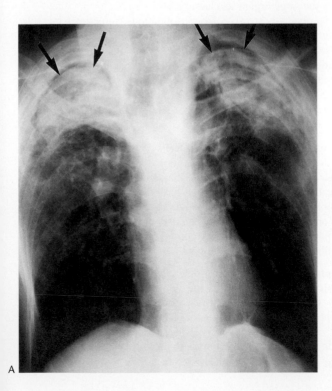

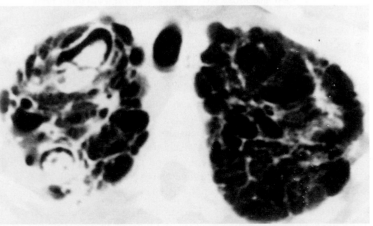

Fig. 17.29 Ankylosing spondylitis. **A.** Chest radiograph demonstrating bilateral apical mycetoma (arrows). **B.** Ankylosing spondylitis in a different patient with mycetoma formation confirmed on CT.

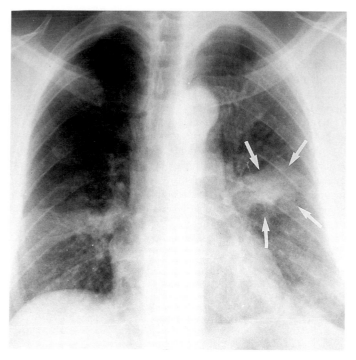

Fig. 17.30 Wegener's granulomatosis. There are several poorly defined pulmonary masses, the largest in the left mid zone (arrows).

and antinuclear factors are commonly found in the blood. Untreated, the disease has a poor prognosis with an average survival of five months, but steroids and cyclophosphamide have transformed the outlook.

Lesions occur in any part of the respiratory tract and take the form of inflammatory necrosis in the walls of small arteries and veins leading to occlusion of the lumen. Granulation tissue containing lymphocytes, polymorphs and giant cells represents a reparative process, but this also undergoes necrosis. The necrotic granulation tissue forms rubbery pulmonary masses which may be single or multiple. Granulomatous masses up to several centimeters in diameter may be apparent on the chest radiograph (Fig. 17.30). These are fairly well defined and often cavitate; they may resolve spontaneously, while new masses appear. Cavitating lesions may have thick or thin walls, depending on how much of the necrotic material is expectorated. Multiple cavities can closely mimic tuberculosis.

A diffuse pattern of disease, where the area of involved lung is still aerated but contains vaguely reticular or irregular nodular opacities, is also recognized. Relapse may occur in previously affected areas.

Other frequent radiographic signs are small pleural effusions and paranasal sinus opacification. Occasional complications are pneumothorax and subglottic stenosis, and granulomas may also develop in the trachea or bronchi and cause pulmonary collapse. Reactive hilar or mediastinal lymphadenopathy may be seen.

Polyarteritis Nodosa (PAN) Classic PAN is a vasculitis of medium sized arteries which involves the kidneys and liver more often than the lungs. There is inflammation in and around the vessel, followed by necrosis of the wall, which is thereby weakened and gives way, forming small aneurysms, the 'nodosa'

of the title. Vessels are also occluded by the process. It is predominantly a male disease, in the ratio 3:1. The protean symptomatology reflects the widespread distribution of the lesions, affecting gut, skin, kidney, heart, central nervous system, joints and muscle. Visceral angiography shows aneurysms or other arterial abnormalities in over 60% of cases.

PAN may be associated with eosinophilia, and may present as asthma with transient pulmonary opacities. Pulmonary edema may occur secondary to cardiac or renal failure, and areas of consolidation may be due to pulmonary hemorrhage.

Radiological Appearances Abnormalities in the lungs are unusual but nodules, segmental opacities, atelectasis, small pleural effusions and diffuse interstitial fibrosis may be found. Opacities are usually transient, except for those caused by diffuse fibrosis.

The rare disease of **relapsing polychondritis** has similarities to polyarteritis nodosa and the two conditions are sometimes found together. There is inflammation, necrosis and fibrosis of cartilage and other tissues with a high glycosaminoglycan content. The destruction of the cartilage of the bronchial tree produces collapsible airways and ultimately fibrotic strictures. The lungs are exposed to the risk of infection because of defective clearance of secretions.

Allergic Granulomatosis and Angiitis (*Churg–Strauss Disease*) This lies at one end of a scale with classic polyarteritis nodosa at the other (see below), the middle ground being occupied by the overlap syndrome with features common to both. Like classic PAN, allergic granulomatosis and angiitis is a generalized necrotizing vasculitis but with certain differences. The lungs are always involved; it occurs in patients with asthma; there is a blood eosinophilia; the pathology is granulomatous; and eosinophils figure more prominently in the infiltrations. The differences are therefore mostly of degree rather than of kind. It is to be suspected in asthmatics with a multisystem disorder and affects the same organs as classic PAN.

Lung opacities are alveolar consolidations, sometimes massive, or a diffuse coarse reticulation, and typically they wax and wane. Infarcts following pulmonary arteritis account for some of the opacities. Sometimes the presentation is acute, suggesting a precipitating insult, and this hypersensitivity vasculitis can be induced by drugs, serum sickness or infection. Henoch–Schönlein purpura is a vasculitis of this type. These transient lung opacities are nodular, diffuse or patchy.

Necrotizing Sarcoid Granulomatosis Unlike other angiocentric granulomatous diseases this condition spares the upper airways, glomeruli and systemic circulation, and shares histologic and clinical features of sarcoidosis. It has been suggested that a more appropriate name would be nodular sarcoidosis. Within the lungs there are sarcoid-like granulomata and a granulomatous vasculitis. Multiple or solitary pulmonary nodules, with or without infiltrates, and hilar lymph node enlargement are the radiological features.

Lymphomatoid Granulomatosis This is similar to Wegener's granulomatosis but involves the lymphoreticular tissues. Indeed many of the features of this condition also occur in various lymphomas and it is probable that it may be a form of lymphoma itself. Indeed approximately 10% of cases will develop more classic features of lymphoma. Radiology is non-specific and biopsy is required for diagnosis.

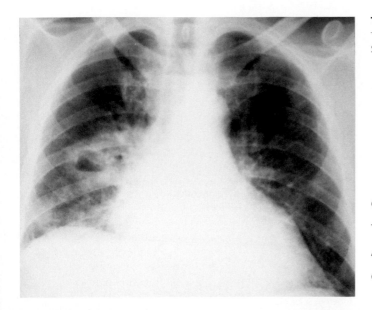

Fig. 17.31 Bronchocentric granulomatosis. There is a cavitating pulmonary mass. Diagnosis was made following resection.

Table 17.2   Pulmonary Eosinophilia: Types and Causes

Simple pulmonary eosinophilia
    Parasites
        Ascaris lumbricoides
        Ankylostoma
        Strongyloides
        Taenia
        Toxocara
    Drugs
        PAS
        Aspirin
        Penicillin
        Nitrofurantoin
        Sulfonamides
Chronic pulmonary eosinophilia
    Etiology uncertain
Tropical pulmonary eosinophilia
    Filariasis
Asthmatic pulmonary eosinophilia
    Aspergillus fumigatus
Connective tissue disorders
    Wegener's granulomatosis
    Other systemic vasculitides

Bronchocentric Granulomatosis This condition resembles allergic bronchopulmonary aspergillosis. Vasculitis is probably only a secondary phenomenon to airways disease and only occurs adjacent to necrotizing granulomatous lesions. The disease may occur in asthmatics, in which case there may be pulmonary and peripheral eosinophilia and precipitins to aspergillus. When the disease encountered in non-asthmatics, the patients are older and have milder symptoms. Radiologically the appearances are non-specific. There may be a single or multiple opacities, consolidation, atelectasis, cavitation or a reticulonodular infiltrate (Fig. 17.31). Changes are usually unilateral. Diagnosis requires biopsy.

PULMONARY EOSINOPHILIA

A number of conditions cause transient opacities on the chest radiograph in association with an excess of eosinophils in the blood. The pulmonary opacities are due to an eosinophilic exudate. These conditions may be referred to as the PIE syndrome (pulmonary infiltrates with eosinophilia).

Simple Pulmonary Eosinophilia (*Löffler's syndrome*) This is usually a mild, transient condition. A large number of allergens have been found to be responsible, but often the cause is not identified. Table 17.2 lists some of the causes. The chest radiograph shows areas of ill-defined, non-segmental consolidation which may change position over a few days, but usually resolve within a month.

Chronic Pulmonary Eosinophilia This rare condition is associated with fever, malaise, cough and prolonged eosinophilia. One-third of patients give a history of asthma or atopy. Pathological examination demonstrates alveolar exudate containing eosinophilia and macrophages and mild alveolar wall infiltration. A few patients will have eosinophilic infiltration in other organs, including the myocardium. The radiological features are similar to Löffler's syndrome, but persist for a month or more, and the areas of consolidation tend to be peripheral in distribution

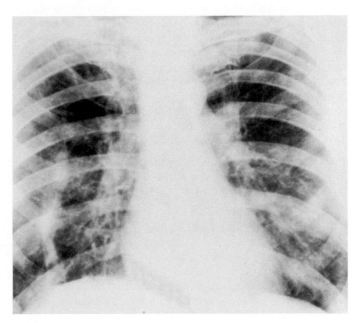

Fig. 17.32 Chronic eosinophilic pneumonia. Alveolar opacities distributed peripherally. The vertical band in the right lung is characteristic.

(Fig. 17.32). A particularly distinctive pattern that is virtually diagnostic in the appropriate clinical setting is a vertical band of consolidation paralleling the chest wall but separated from it, not being restricted by interlobular fissures. This distribution is even more apparent on CT (Fig. 17.33). The differential diagnosis of this radiological appearance should include cryptogenic organizing pneumonia, particularly when the changes are peripheral and basal. Treatment with steroids usually produces a dramatic radiological and symptomatic improvement although initial doses need to be high and therapy at a reduced dose may need to be prolonged.

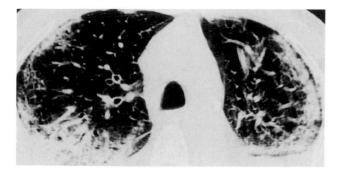

Fig. 17.33 Chronic eosinophilic pneumonia in a retired farmer. There is consolidation paralleling the chest wall bilaterally. Small pleural effusions are present due to concurrent heart failure.

Tropical Pulmonary Eosinophilia This is caused by *filariasis* and presents with a cough, wheeze and sometimes fever. The chest radiograph shows fine, bilateral, diffuse nodular shadowing, with occasional confluent areas.

Asthmatic Pulmonary Eosinophilia This is most commonly caused by *Aspergillus fumigatus* but often no allergen is identified. In uncomplicated asthma the chest radiograph is usually normal between attacks or may show hyperinflation during an episode of wheezing. In chronic severe asthma hyperinflation may persist. Lobar or segmental collapse due to bronchial mucosal swelling and mucus plugging may occur and often resolves completely and rapidly. When asthmatic pulmonary eosinophilia develops bronchial casts may be coughed up during attacks, and there may be fever. The chest radiograph may then show transient shadows, but after repeated attacks there may also be signs of fibrosis and bronchiectasis.

Pulmonary Eosinophilia Associated with the Systemic Vasculitides The radiographic features are those of the underlying connective tissue disorder.

DIFFUSE PULMONARY FIBROSIS

Pulmonary fibrosis may be a localized or generalized occurrence. Localized pulmonary fibrosis is commonly the result of pneumonia or radiotherapy. Diffuse pulmonary fibrosis is usually the result of a systemic condition or is due to inhalation of dusts or fumes (see Table 17.3).

Fibrosing Alveolitis

Fibrosing alveolitis describes a number of conditions in which there is pulmonary fibrosis associated with a chronic inflammatory reaction in the alveolar walls. It includes such conditions as diffuse idiopathic pulmonary fibrosis, diffuse interstitial fibrosis and Hamman–Rich disease. The etiology is frequently uncertain, but many cases are associated with a known cause (see Table 17.3).

Cryptogenic Fibrosing Alveolitis

This condition is also known as *usual interstitial pneumonitis* (UIP) and may be regarded as an interstitial pneumonitis. Histologically most cases show fibrosis and cellular infiltrate

Table 17.3 Diffuse Pulmonary Fibrosis: Causes

Cryptogenic fibrosing alveolitis
Radiation
Drugs and poisons
Connective tissue diseases
    Systemic sclerosis
    SLE
    Rheumatoid disease
Organic and inorganic dusts
    Pneumoconioses
    Silicosis
    Extrinsic allergic alveolitis
Noxious gases
Chronic pulmonary venous hypertension
Adult respiratory distress syndrome
Infection
    Tuberculosis
    Fungi
    Viral
Sarcoidosis
Histiocytosis
Neurofibromatosis
Tuberous sclerosis
Lymphangiomyomatosis

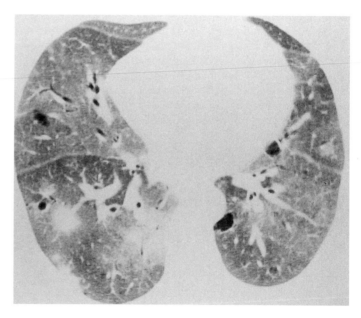

Fig. 17.34 Desquamative interstitial pneumonitis (DIP). There is diffuse ground-glass change throughout the lungs due to inflammatory infiltrate. Note the relatively low density of the larger bronchi and small bullae compared with the remainder of the lungs.

confined to the alveolar walls. Some cases show mononuclear cells in the alveoli and may be termed *desquamative interstitial pneumonitis* (DIP) (Fig. 17.34). Rarer variants are associated with bronchiolitis obliterans and diffuse alveolar damage, lymphocytic interstitial pneumonitis or a giant-cell interstitial pneumonitis.

Patients present with increasing dyspnea, a dry cough, finger clubbing, widespread basal crackles, and impaired ventilation and gas exchange. The disease may be rapidly progressive with death from respiratory or cardiac failure within a few weeks, or it may continue for many years. Desquamative histology has a better

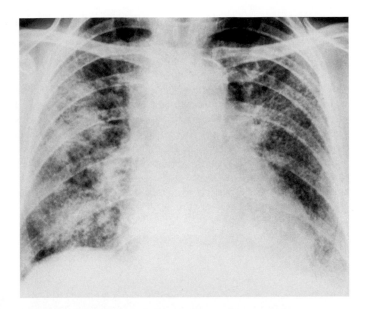

Fig. 17.35 Cryptogenic fibrosing alveolitis. Miliary opacities and a little reticulation. The apices are spared.

prognosis, but it can hardly be called benign, with a reported mortality of 27% and a mean survival time of 12 years. Carcinoma of the lung of all histologic types, including bronchioloalveolar cell, complicates the disease process in about 10% of cases.

The earliest **radiographic change** is bilateral, basal, groundglass shadowing. This is followed by a fine nodular pattern, and then coarser, linear shadows develop, predominantly basally but spreading throughout the lungs (Fig. 17.35). There is progressive pulmonary volume loss. Ring shadows appear and may produce a honeycomb pattern (Fig. 17.36), and basal septal lines may be visible. Pleural effusion is rare.

HRCT is of particular value in idiopathic pulmonary fibrosis, in which the appearances may be sufficiently diagnostic to avoid the necessity of an open lung biopsy (Fig. 17.37). In addition HRCT allows some assessment of the relative degrees of inflammation and fibrosis, and so is able to predict the likelihood of success of steroid therapy (Fig. 17.38). Hilar and mediastinal lymph node enlargement is well recognized, but only usually apparent on CT. Pleural effusions are rare. Cor pulmonale, pulmonary embolism and infection are all complications that may further contribute to radiographic changes.

Histiocytosis X (Langerhans Cell Histiocytosis)

The three variants of this disease—Letterer–Siwe disease, Hand–Schüller–Christian disease and eosinophilic granuloma—involve the lung in approximately 20% of cases. Eosinophilic granuloma usually involves the skeleton, but may be confined to the lungs, when there is a male:female preponderance of 5:1.

Eosinophilic granuloma of the lung may present without symptoms, or with a dry cough, dyspnea or spontaneous pneumothorax. Histologically there is infiltration of alveolar walls by histiocytes and eosinophils, followed by fibrosis. The presence of Langerhans cells is regarded as specific. There is no association with atopy or allergy and there is no blood eosinophilia.

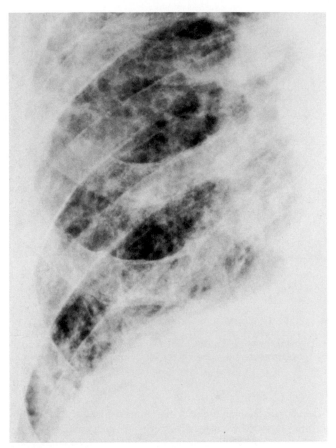

Fig. 17.36 Cryptogenic fibrosing alveolitis. Ring shadows are well seen in the right lower zone due to coarse fibrosis and honeycomb formation.

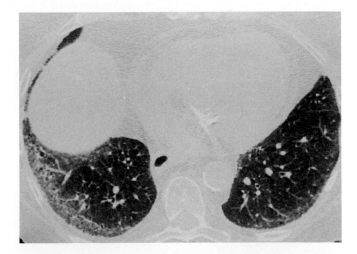

Fig. 17.37 Cryptogenic fibrosing alveolitis. HRCT through the lung bases shows subpleural fibrosis. Lung biopsy is likely to reveal established fibrosis.

Radiology The earliest reported manifestation is ill-defined transient patchy consolidation, but this is rarely seen. A fine reticulonodular pattern throughout both lungs, but predominantly in the mid and upper zones is more usual (Fig. 17.39). The diagnosis usually requires confirmation with lung biopsy, although the HRCT changes are characteristic and show a mixture

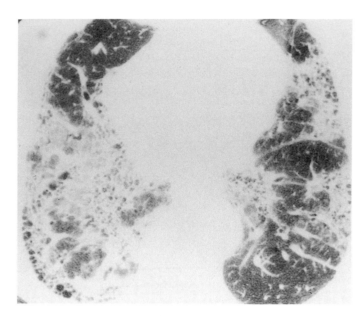

Fig. 17.38 Cryptogenic fibrosing alveolitis. HRCT shows a mixture of fibrosis and areas of ground-glass change. Histologic assessment of lung biopsy is likely to reveal a mixture of inflammation and fibrosis. This patient may benefit from steroids although the established fibrous component may remain.

of discrete nodules and cystic spaces, sometimes with sparing of the lung bases. The range of severity of lung involvement and associated pulmonary impairment is wide. As fibrosis progresses, a coarser linear pattern appears, with development of ring shadows, honeycombing and bullae. The lung volumes are usually normal. There is a 20% incidence of spontaneous pneumothorax. In severe cases transplantation has been under-

taken, although even then the disease may recur in the donor lungs (Fig. 17.40).

Tuberous Sclerosis

This is an autosomal dominant neurocutaneous disorder that classically consists of the triad of mental retardation, epilepsy and adenoma sebaceum. Only about 1% of patients with tuberous sclerosis will develop lung involvement. The majority of patients developing lung involvement are older and with a lower incidence of mental retardation than the population of tuberous sclerosis patients as a whole. If pulmonary disease does develop it is often the most important clinical consequence of the disease. Recurrent pneumothoraces are frequent (Fig. 17.41), and respiratory failure

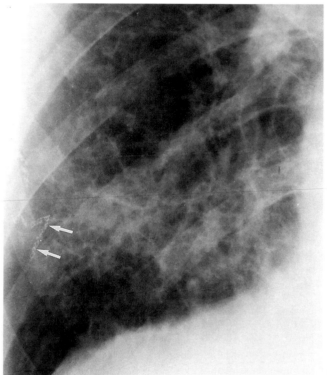

B

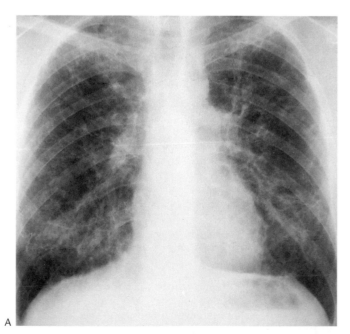

A

C

Fig. 17.39 Histiocytosis. **A,B** Fine reticulonodular shadowing is present throughout both lungs, producing a honeycomb pattern. Note the line of biopsy staples (arrows). **C.** CT demonstrates cystic spaces and discrete nodules characteristic of histiocytosis.

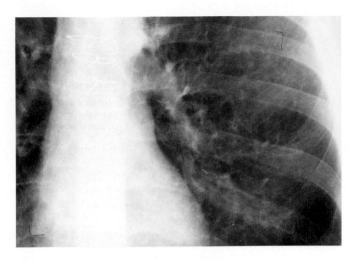

Fig. 17.40 Histiocytosis recurring following transplantation. Note the sternotomy suture wires.

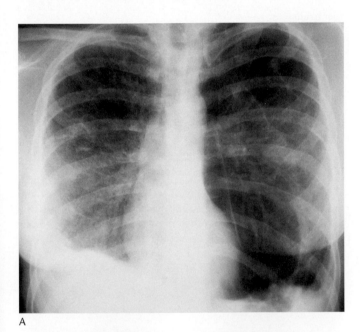

A

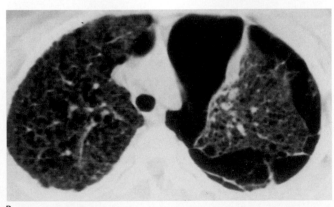

B

Fig. 17.41 Tuberous sclerosis. **A.** There is a fine reticular infiltrate. The right costophrenic angle is blunted following pleurodesis. There is a loculated left pneumothorax. **B.** HRCT demonstrates multiple thin-walled cystic spaces, and loculated pneumothorax.

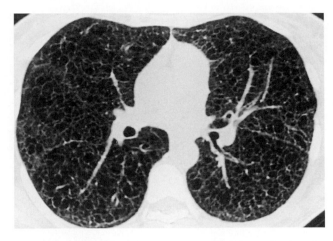

Fig. 17.42 Tuberous sclerosis. The lungs are almost completely replaced by multiple thin-walled cysts.

or cor pulmonale is often progressive and fatal. Diffuse hyperplasia of smooth muscle in the small airways, alveolar walls and peripheral vessels produces reticulonodular shadowing and eventually *honeycombing* on the chest radiograph.

As with histiocytosis X the diagnosis can be suggested with HRCT, which demonstrates multiple thin-walled cysts, with normal areas of intervening lung, usually affecting all lung zones equally (Fig. 17.42), although apical sparing has been suggested in some series. Chylous pleural effusions are rare but may be large, bilateral and persistent.

Lymphangioleiomyomatosis (LAM)

The condition is radiologically and pathologically very similar to tuberous sclerosis. There is proliferation of smooth muscle and lymphatics in the alveolar walls, interlobular septa and pleura. However in LAM the distribution of muscle proliferation is initially perilymphatic, and the disease may also involve the mediastinal and retroperitoneal lymph nodes. Hence chylothorax and chyloperitoneum are commoner than in tuberous sclerosis. LAM is confined to females, and almost all are premenopausal. Clinical features of pneumothorax, dyspnea and hemoptysis are the same as those encountered in tuberous sclerosis. Anti-estrogen therapy has resulted in some improvement in prognosis.

The chest radiographic and HRCT features (Fig. 17.43) are identical to tuberous sclerosis apart from occasional associated changes in the ribs.

Neurofibromatosis

Pulmonary fibrosis occurs in approximately 10% of patients with neurofibromatosis Type I. Disease progression is slow, in contrast to tuberous sclerosis. Radiographically neurofibromatosis may produce reticular shadowing and honeycombing on the chest radiograph. Bullae may develop in the mid and upper zones (Fig. 17.44).

Adult Respiratory Distress Syndrome (ARDS)

ARDS may be due to a large number of causes (Table 17.4). It presents as acute respiratory failure in patients without previous lung disease and usually follows major trauma or shock.

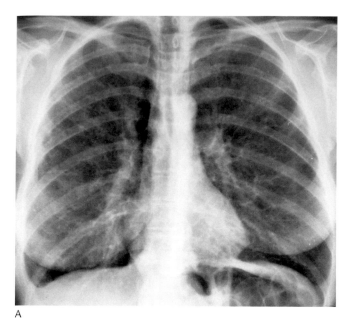

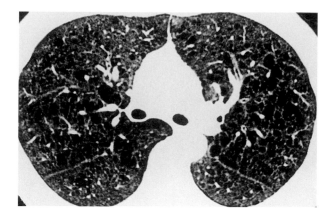

Fig. 17.44 Neurofibromatosis. There are multiple thin-walled cysts replacing the normal lung parenchyma.

Table 17.4   Causes of ARDS

Major trauma
Septicemia
Hypovolemic shock
Fat embolism
Near-drowing
Mendelson syndrome
Burns
Viral pneumonia
Pancreatitis
Oxygen toxicity
Disseminated intravascular coagulopathy

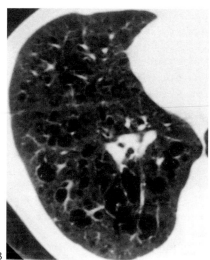

Fig. 17.43 Lymphangioleiomyomatosis. **A.** Amber chest radiograph demonstrating normal lung volumes and multiple thin-walled cysts. **B.** HRCT shows normal lung between the discrete cystic spaces.

Clinically the patient becomes hypoxemic 12–24 hours after the precipitating event. There is then progressive respiratory failure over several days, usually requiring ventilatory support. During this time there may be superimposed infection, or various complications of positive pressure ventilation may develop. In excess of 50% of cases are fatal, and survivors may be left with chronic lung disease.

The corresponding pathological processes are a hemorrhagic pulmonary edema in the acute phase, followed by resolution or, more often, fibrosis.

Radiographically, bilateral, patchy alveolar shadows appear in the first 24 hours (Fig. 17.45). These become more extensive over the next few days (Fig. 17.46). Pleural effusions are unusual, and the heart does not enlarge. At this stage Gram-negative pneumonia frequently develops, and cavitation and pleural effusions may be seen.

Pneumomediastinum, pneumothorax and subcutaneous emphysema, in addition to interstitial barotrauma, may result from the need for aggressive ventilatory support (Fig. 17.47). If the patient survives, there is gradual clearing of the alveolar

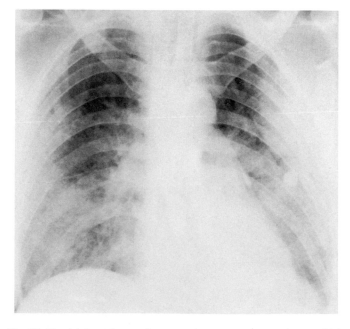

Fig. 17.45 Adult respiratory distress syndrome. Fat embolism from multiple skeletal trauma. Diffuse alveolar opacities.

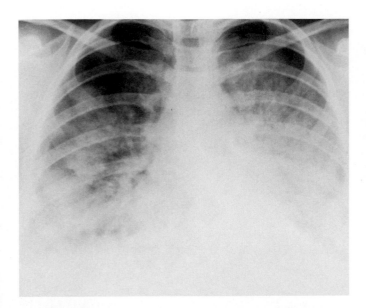

Fig. 17.46 Staphylococcal toxic shock. Extensive alveolar opacification. *Staphylococcus aureus* was isolated from a vaginal tampon.

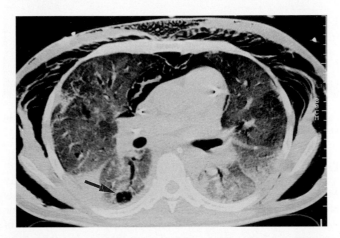

Fig. 17.47 ARDS. CT demonstrates extensive mediastinal and subcutaneous emphysema as well as a parenchymal bulla (arrow) possibly related to high-pressure ventilation. Note the typical anterior–posterior density gradient in lung attenuation due to the effects of gravity.

shadowing, which is replaced by evidence of pulmonary fibrosis. The lung volumes may be decreased and reticular shadowing may develop. A minority of patients fully recover.

PULMONARY HEMORRHAGE AND HEMOSIDEROSIS

Hemorrhage into the lungs and airways may complicate lung cancer, pneumonia, bronchiectasis, pulmonary venous hypertension, blood dyscrasias, anticoagulant therapy, disseminated intravascular coagulation and trauma. Multifocal bleeding into the alveoli not associated with any of these conditions may be referred to as pulmonary hemosiderosis.

Pulmonary Hemosiderosis

This may be either idiopathic or associated with renal disease. In *Goodpasture syndrome* pulmonary hemosiderosis occurs with a

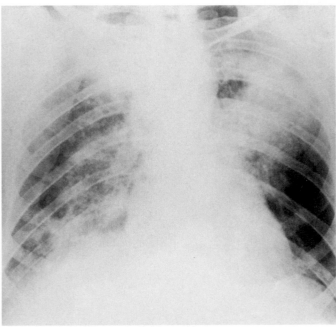

Fig. 17.48 Pulmonary hemorrhage. Goodpasture syndrome. Large alveolar opacities.

glomerulonephritis associated with circulating antiglomerular basement membrane antibodies. Immunofluorescence microscopy shows a linear deposit of the immunoglobulin on the glomerular capillaries, sometimes with similar deposits on the alveolar capillaries. In other cases the nephritis may be due to Wegener's granulomatosis, systemic lupus erythematosus, polyarteritis nodosa or penicillamine hypersensitivity.

Infection, fluid overload, smoking and inhalation of toxic fumes are factors which are known to precipitate episodes of bleeding. Pulmonary function tests often indicate airways obstruction and there may be an increased uptake of inhaled radioactive CO by the leaked blood. The latter test is useful in differentiating hemorrhage from edema and infection. Treatment regimes include steroids, immunosuppression and plasmapheresis, and these are more effective in Goodpasture syndrome than in the other types.

Hemoptysis is a common symptom but its severity does not match the large volumes of blood lost into the lungs, since most of it is beyond the mucociliary clearing processes. Bleeding is severe enough to cause anemia, even at times requiring blood transfusion. Macrophages with engulfed red cells and hemosiderin fill the alveolar spaces and infiltrate the walls. These macrophages in the sputum or bronchoalveolar lavage fluid are a diagnostic feature. After repeated attacks of bleeding, interstitial fibrosis is initiated but this is not sufficiently extensive to cause gross scarring or destruction of lung architecture.

Radiology During an acute episode of pulmonary hemorrhage patchy, ill-defined areas of consolidation appear on the chest radiograph (Fig. 17.48). They may become confluent and demonstrate an air bronchogram. The appearance may be indistinguishable from pulmonary edema. HRCT is more sensitive than the chest radiograph in detecting abnormalities in patients with suspected pulmonary hemorrhage (Fig. 17.49). When bleeding stops, the opacities resolve within a few days. Following repeated

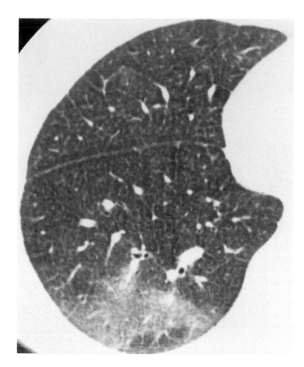

Fig. 17.49 Acute pulmonary hemorrhage. There is ground-glass change in the posterior aspect of the right lung, due to alveolar hemorrhage. Note the generalized nodularity due to the effects of recent hemorrhage.

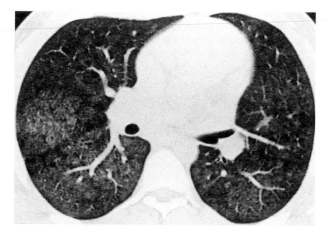

Fig. 17.50 Pulmonary hemosiderosis, chronic phase. There is diffuse ill-defined nodular change, mainly in the posterior aspect of the lungs.

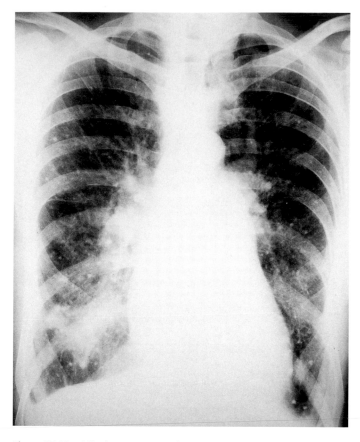

Fig. 17.51 Mitral stenosis with pulmonary ossification due to hemosiderosis.

episodes of bleeding, pulmonary fibrosis may develop and produce a diffuse hazy nodular or reticular pattern (Fig. 17.50).

Patients with nephritis are prone to pulmonary edema and pneumonia, and the differentiation from pulmonary hemorrhage may be difficult. Pneumonic consolidation tends to resolve more slowly than edema or hemorrhage. Cardiomegaly, septal lines and pleural effusion suggest cardiogenic pulmonary edema.

Pulmonary hemosiderosis is also well recognized in some patients with heart disease which chronically elevates left atrial pressure, such as occurs secondary to mitral stenosis. The radiographic features in the lungs are distinctive, consisting of a permanent miliary stippling due to the focal nature of the bleeding (Fig. 17.51).

DRUG-INDUCED PULMONARY DISEASE

Many drugs in common use are toxic to the lungs and may produce diffuse pulmonary abnormalities. Although in some patients there is a clear temporal relationship between the onset of symptoms and the introduction of drug therapy, in others there may be a lag time of several years before lung disease becomes clinically apparent. As a result the development of toxicity may go undetected.

When interpreting a chest radiograph with diffuse shadowing it is important to be aware of what therapy the patient has received or is undergoing. Some drugs are intrinsically toxic to the lungs (e.g. many cancer chemotherapeutic agents) and their effect on the lung may be dose-related or cumulative. Other drugs seem to cause pulmonary abnormalities in a minority of recipients who show a hypersensitivity or idiosyncratic response. There are a variety of lung responses to drug toxicity. HRCT has been shown to be more sensitive than chest radiography in the detection of parenchymal changes in those patients suspected of having drug-induced lung disease.

Pulmonary Fibrosis Many cytotoxic drugs (e.g. azathioprine, bleomycin, busulfan, cyclophosphamide, chlorambucil) and non-cytotoxic drugs (amiodarone, nitrofurantoin) cause alveolitis which may progress to pulmonary fibrosis. The fibrogenic effect of cytotoxic drugs is enhanced by radiotherapy and high levels of inspired oxygen. The chest radiograph may show reticulonodular shadowing, often with a basal predominance (Fig. 17.52).

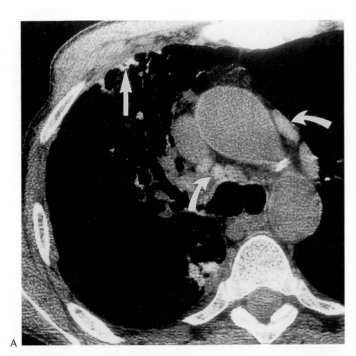

A

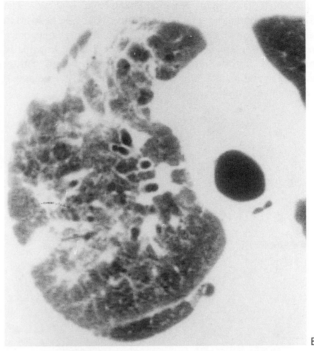

B

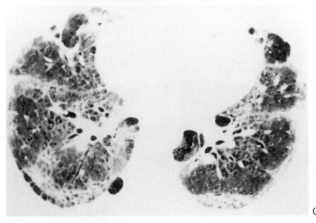

C

Fig. 17.52 A. Amiodarone toxicity. There are enlarged mediastinal lymph nodes (curved arrows). Note the area of dense peripheral consolidation due to amiodarone deposition (arrow). **B.** Same patient on lung windows demonstrating coarse fibrosis. **C.** Lung fibrosis in a different patient on long-term pizotifen therapy.

Pulmonary Eosinophilia Para-aminosalicylic acid (PAS), aspirin, penicillin, nitrofurantoin, sulfonamides and methotrexate are some of the substances that may produce an eosinophilia and pulmonary infiltrates. This hypersensitivity may, after prolonged drug administration, lead to pulmonary fibrosis.

ARDS This may result from the administration of a variety of agents, particularly cytotoxic agents such as cyclophosphamide, bleomycin and busulfan (Fig. 17.53).

Bronchiolitis Obliterans This condition may be drug induced, most commonly as a result of penicillamine therapy.

SLE Reaction Some drugs—such as penicillin, procainamide, isoniazid and methyldopa—may cause pleural effusions, pneumonitis and pulmonary fibrosis.

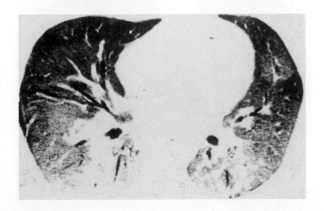

Fig. 17.53 ARDS reaction to methotrexate administration. Compare with Fig. 17.47.

Pulmonary Edema Pulmonary edema may be a complication of narcotic overdose. It may also be caused by overinfusion of intravenous fluids and by hypersensitivity to transfused blood or blood products.

Pulmonary Thromboembolism This may arise from the use of oral contraceptives.

Opportunistic Infection Drugs that suppress the immune system (e.g. cancer chemotherapeutic agents and steroids) predispose to infection. Pneumonias that are likely to be seen in this context may be due to tuberculosis, Gram-negative bacteria, viruses, *Pneumocystis* and *Aspergillus*.

Mediastinal Adenopathy Phenytoin and amiodarone may cause lymph node enlargement (Fig. 17.52).

Pulmonary Talcosis Chronic intravenous drug abuse may lead to pulmonary talcosis as a result of chronic deposition of magnesium silicate (talc) within the lungs. The most common source of intravenous talc is as a binding agent used in most tablets, which may then be ground up and injected. The pulmonary inflammatory reaction produced by talc deposition may initially appear as a fine nodular or ground-glass appearance on the chest radiograph and HRCT scan (Fig. 17.54). Eventually the pulmonary fibrosis results in severe emphysema, with a radiological pattern that may resemble progressive massive fibrosis or end-stage sarcoidosis (Fig. 17.55).

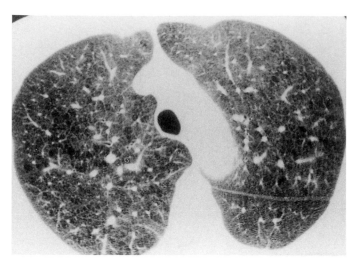

Fig. 17.54 Pulmonary talcosis due to repeated injection of ground-up tablets. There is diffuse increase in attenuation of the lung compared with the trachea.

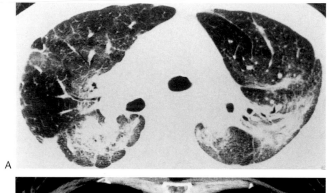

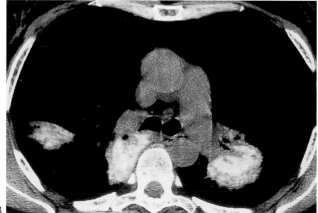

Fig. 17.55 Pulmonary talcosis. **A.** There are perihilar masses with radiating strands of fibrosis distorting the surrounding pulmonary architecture. Compare with Fig. 17.7. **B.** CT scan on mediastinal window setting in a different patient demonstrating high attenuation in the perihilar masses.

AMYLOIDOSIS

Amyloid is a proteinaceous substance with specific chemical and staining properties. Amyloidosis is a group of conditions in which amyloid in unusually large amounts is deposited in connective tissue, around parenchymal tissue cells and in the walls of blood vessels. The conditions are grouped into primary and secondary categories according to whether there is a prior precipitating cause. Secondary amyloidosis may arise as a complication of chronic infection such as tuberculosis, osteomyelitis, bronchiectasis or leprosy, but in Western countries infection now assumes less importance and the most common causes are rheumatoid disease and neoplasia.

Both primary and secondary amyloidosis can occur in localized and generalized forms. Once generalized amyloidosis is established, it tends to be progressive and has a poor prognosis when vital organs become involved. In 75% of cases of the generalized disease there are amyloid deposits in the mucosa of rectal biopsy specimens. Secondary amyloid does not invoke an inflammatory response in the lungs, whereas primary amyloid does. For this reason secondary amyloidosis in the lungs seldom causes symptoms, and the chest radiograph is normal unless the initiating cause is intrapulmonary.

Primary amyloidosis may produce a variety of abnormalities in the airways and lungs. There may be multiple nodular angular opacities which can cavitate or calcify (Fig. 17.56). These nodules may be up to several centimeters in size and grow slowly. Calcification is usually in the form of fine stippling. Alternatively there may be diffuse reticulonodular shadowing or honeycombing due to diffuse deposition of amyloid within alveolar walls, lobular septa and pulmonary arterioles. Occasionally amyloid deposition is confined to hilar and mediastinal lymph nodes. Alternatively lymph node involvement may accompany tracheobronchial or parenchymal amyloid. Enlarged lymph nodes may contain calcification, and nodal size is occasionally massive.

Tracheobronchial amyloid may take the form of a solitary endobronchial tumor mass or polyp, or it may grow down the trachea and into the bronchi in the form of nodular submucosal plaques. Radiologically, the effects are those of obstruction,

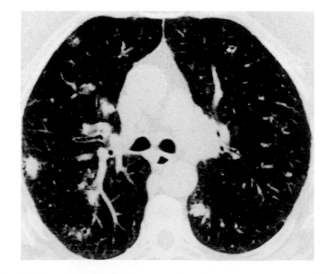

Fig. 17.56 Amyloidosis. CT scan reveals multiple small pulmonary nodules scattered through the lungs. In this patient these were non-calcified.

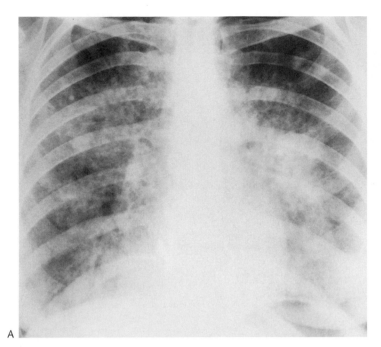
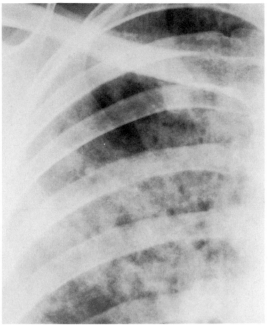

Fig. 17.57 **A.** Pulmonary alveolar proteinosis. Central alveolar patchy densities and vague nodulation. **B.** Close-up. Ill-defined alveolar opacities; air bronchogram visible.

namely atelectasis, distal bronchiectasis and infection. There is a nodularity of the wall of the air passages and multiple strictures. Surgical resection may be required. Amyloid material is sometimes found in relation to bronchial neoplasms, and caution is required in the interpretation of biopsy appearances since they may not be typical of the whole lesion.

Tracheopathia osteoplastica is a condition of cartilaginous masses lining most of the trachea and major bronchi. The masses contain amyloid deposits, calcific bodies and ossifications. It is thought to be an end-stage of tracheobronchial amyloidosis.

PULMONARY ALVEOLAR PROTEINOSIS

This is a rare disease of unknown etiology in which Type II pneumocytes overproduce a proteinaceous lipid-rich material to a degree that overwhelms the capacity of the lung to remove it. This is probably the result of a response by the lungs to an irritant. Histologically there is a striking lack of reaction within the alveolar walls. The disease is three times more common in men than in women and can occur at any age.

The radiographic appearance resembles pulmonary edema, with small, acinar, perihilar opacities present in both lungs (Fig. 17.57). These opacities may become confluent. There may be thickening of the interlobular septa in addition to ground-glass shadowing and consolidation on HRCT, producing the 'crazy paving' appearance that is typical of this condition (Fig. 17.58). The disease predisposes to pulmonary infection from both common respiratory pathogens and opportunistic organisms. It may also be associated with lymphoma, leukemia and immuno-globulin deficiency. Diagnosis is made by lung biopsy or bronchoalveolar lavage. Approximately 25% of cases are fatal within 5 years.

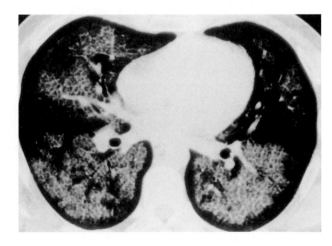

Fig. 17.58 Alveolar proteinosis. Typical crazy paving appearances with alveolar filling and septal wall thickening.

PULMONARY ALVEOLAR MICROLITHIASIS

This is a disease of unknown etiology which may be familial. It is characterized by the presence of multiple, fine sand-like calculi in the alveoli. The calculi are calcified and produce widespread, minute, but very dense opacities on the chest radiograph (Fig. 17.59). The strikingly abnormal radiograph contrasts with a relative lack of symptoms, although later in the disease there may be pulmonary fibrosis.

IDIOPATHIC PULMONARY OSSIFICATION

This rare condition has also been described under a variety of

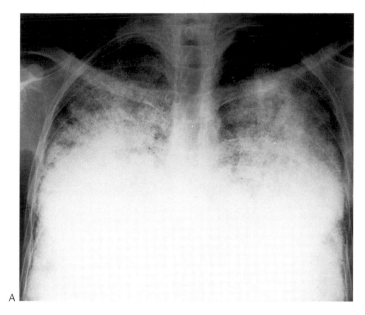
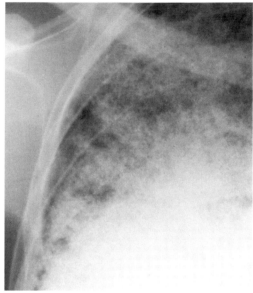

Fig. 17.59   A. Pulmonary alveolar microlithiasis. Multiple, fine, dense opacities are visible throughout the lungs. **B.** Magnified view of the right lung.

other names, including ossifying pneumonitis, bony metaplasia of lung and arboriform pulmonary ossification. In its usual form the delicate branching or lace-like pattern of dystrophic bone formation in the lower parts of the lungs is sufficiently distinctive to suggest the diagnosis. The cause is unknown and there are no symptoms attributable to the condition.

REFERENCES AND SUGGESTIONS FOR FURTHER READING

Aberle, D. R., Gamsu, G., Ray, C. S., et al (1988) Asbestos-related pleural and parenchymal fibrosis: detection with high-resolution CT. *Radiology*, **166**, 729–734.

Adler, B. D., Padley, S. P. G., Müller, N. L., et al (1992) Chronic hypersensitivity pneumonitis: high-resolution CT and radiographic features in 16 patients. *Radiology*, **185**, 91–95.

Akira, M., Yokoyama, K., Yamamoto, S., et al (1991) Early asbestosis: evaluation with high-resolution CT. *Radiology*, **178**, 409–416.

Begin, R., Ostiguy, G., Fillion, R., et al (1991) Computed tomography scan in the early detection of silicosis. *American Review of Respiratory Disease*, **144**, 697–705.

Bergin, C. J., Muller, N. L., Vedal, S., et al (1986) CT in silicosis: correlation with plain films and pulmonary function tests. *American Journal of Roentgenology*, **146**, 477–483.

Blesovsky, A. (1966) The folded lung. *British Journal of Diseases of the Chest*, **60**, 19–22.

Breatnach, E., Kerr, I. H. (1982) The radiology of cryptogenic obliterative bronchiolitis. *Clinical Radiology*, **33**, 657–661

Brennan, S. R., Daly, J. J. (1979) Large pleural effusions in rheumatoid arthritis. *British Journal of Diseases of the Chest*, **73**, 133–140.

Buschman, D. L., Waldron, J. A., King, T. E. (1990) Churg-Strauss pulmonary vasculitis: high-resolution computed tomography scanning and pathologic findings. *American Review of Respiratory Disease*, **142**, 458–461.

Caplan, A. (1953) Certain unusual radiological appearances in the chest of coal-miners suffering from rheumatoid arthritis. *Thorax*, **8**, 29–37.

Caplan, A. (1962) Correlation of radiological category with lung pathology in coal-workers' pneumoconiosis. *British Journal of Industrial Medicine*, **19**, 171–179.

Cotes, E., Gibson, J. C., McKerrow, C. B., et al (1983) A long term follow-up of workers exposed to beryllium. *British Journal of Industrial Medicine*, **40**, 13–21.

Demling, R. H. (1987) Smoke inhalation injury. *Postgraduate Medicine*, **82**, 63–68.

Doig, A. T. (1976) Barytosis: a benign pneumoconiosis. *Thorax*, **31**, 30–39.

Epler, G. R., McLoud, T. C., Gaensler, E. A., et al (1978) Normal chest roentgenograms in chronic diffuse infiltrative lung disease. *North American Journal of Medicine*, **298**, 934–939.

Epler, G. R., McLoud, T. C., Gaensler, E. A. (1982) Prevalence and incidence of benign asbestos pleural effusion in a working population. *Journal of the American Medical Association*, **247**, 617.

Farrelly, C. A. (1982) Wegener's granulomatosis: a radiological review of the pulmonary manifestations at initial presentation and during relapse. *Clinical Radiology*, **33**, 545–551.

Feigin, D. S. (1986) Talc: understanding its manifestations in the chest. *American Journal of Roentgenology*, **146**, 295–301.

Frazier, A. R., Miller, R. D. (1974) Interstitial pneumonitis in association with polymyositis and dermatomyositis. *Chest*, **65**, 403–407.

Gaensler, E. A., Carrington, C. B. (1977) Peripheral opacities in chronic eosinophilic pneumonia: the photographic negative of pulmonary edema. *American Journal of Roentgenology*, **128**, 1–13.

Gaensler, E. A., Carrington, C. B. (1980) Open biopsy for chronic diffuse infiltrative lung disease: clinical, roentgenographic and physiological correlation in 502 patients. *Annals of Thoracic Surgery*, **30**, 411–426.

Gaensler, E. A., Carrington, C. B., Coutre, R. E., et al (1972) Pathological, physiological and radiological correlations in the pneumoconioses. *Annals of the New York Academy of Sciences*, **200**, 574–607.

Hansell, D. M., Moskovic, E. (1991) High-resolution computed tomography in extrinsic allergic alveolitis. *Clinical Radiology*, **43**, 8–12.

Hartman, T. E., Primack, S. L., Swensen, S. J., et al (1993) Desquamative interstitial pneumonia: thin section CT findings in 22 patients. *Radiology*, **187**, 787–790.

Hunninghake, G. W., Fauci, A. S. (1979) Pulmonary involvement in the collagen vascular diseases. *American Review of Respiratory Disease*, **119**, 471–503.

Julsrud, P. R., Brown, I. R., Li, C-Y., Rosenow, E. C., Crowe, J. K. (1978) Pulmonary processes of mature-appearing lymphocytes: pseudolymphoma, well-differentiated lymphocytic lymphoma and lymphocytic interstitial pneumonitis. *Radiology*, **127**, 289–296.

Kuhlman, J. E. (1991) The role of chest computed tomography in the diagnosis of drug-related reactions. *Journal of Thoracic Imaging*, **6**, 52–61.

Kuhlman, J. E., Hruban, R. H., Fishman, E. K. (1991) Wegener's granulomatosis:

CT features of parenchymal lung disease. *Journal of Computer Assisted Tomography*, **15**, 948–952.

Landay, M. J., Christensen, E. E., Bynum, L. J. (1978) Pulmonary manifestations of acute aspiration of gastric contents. *American Journal of Roentgenology*, **131**, 587–592.

Levin, D. C. (1971) Proper interpretation of pulmonary roentgen changes in systemic lupus erythematosus. *American Journal of Roentgenology*, **111**, 510–517.

Locke, G. B. (1963) Rheumatoid lung. *Clinical Radiology*, **14**, 43–53.

Lynch, D. A., Rose, C. S., Way, D., et al (1992) Hypersensitivity pneumonitis: sensitivity of high-resolution CT in a population-based study. *American Journal of Roentgenology*, **159**, 469–472.

McDonald, T. J., Neel, H. B., DeRemee, R.A. (1982) Wegener's granulomatosis of the subglottis and the upper portion of the trachea. *Annals of Otology, Rhinology and Lanyngology*, **91**, 588–592.

MacFarlane, J. D., Diepe, P.A., Rigden, B. G., Clark, T. J. H. (1978) Pulmonary and pleural lesions in rheumatoid disease. *British Journal of Diseases of the Chest*, **72**, 288–300.

McLoud, T. C., Epler, G. R., Colby, T. V., Gaensler, E. A., Carrington, C. B. (1986) Bronchiolitis obliterans. *Radiology*, **159**, 1–8.

Mayo, J.R., Müller, N.L., Road, J., et al (1989) Chronic eosinophilic pneumonia: CT findings in six cases. *American Journal of Roentgenology*, **153**, 727–730.

Mendelson, C. L. (1946) The aspiration of stomach contents into the lungs during obstetric anesthesia. *American Journal of Obstetrics and Gynecology*, **52**, 191–205.

Müller, N. L., Miller, R. R., Webb, W. R., et al (1986) Fibrosing alveolitis: CT–pathologic correlation. *Radiology*, **160**, 585–588.

Müller, N. L., Staples, C. A., Miller, R. R., et al (1987) Disease activity in idiopathic pulmonary fibrosis: CT and pathologic correlation. *Radiology*, **165**, 731–734.

Neeld, E. M., Limacher, M. C. (1978) Chemical pneumonitis after the intravenous injection of hydrocarbon. *Radiology*, 129(1):36.

Padley, S. P. G., Hansell, D. M., Flower, C. D. R., et al (1991) Comparative accuracy of high resolution, computed tomography in the diagnosis of chronic diffuse infiltrative lung disease. *Clinical Radiology*, **44**, 222–226.

Padley, S. P. G., Adler, B., Hansell, D. M., et al (1992) High-resolution computed tomography of drug-induced lung disease. *Clinical Radiology*, **46**, 232–236.

Primack, S. L., Hartman, T. E., Hansell, D. M., et al (1993) End-stage lung disease: CT findings in 61 patients. *Radiology*, **189**, 681–686.

Remy-Jardin, M., Degreef, J. M., Beuscart, R., et al (1990) Coal workers pneumoconiosis: CT assessment in exposed workers and correlation with radiographic findings. *Radiology*, **177**, 363–371.

Remy-Jardin, M., Remy, J., Deffontaines, C., et al (1991) Assessment of diffuse infiltrative lung disease: comparison of conventional CT and high-resolution CT. *Radiology*, **181**, 157–162.

Remy-Jardin, M., Remy, J., Wallaert, B., et al (1993) Pulmonary involvement in progressive systemic sclerosis: sequential evaluation with CT, pulmonary function tests, and bronchoalveolar lavage. *Radiology*, **188**, 499–506.

Sargent, E. N., Gordonson, J. S., Jacobson, G. (1977) Pleural plaques: a signpost of asbestos dust inhalation. *Seminars in Roentgenology*, **12**, 287–297.

Schurawitzki, H., Stiglbauer, R., Graninger, W., et al (1990) Interstitial lung disease in progressive systemic sclerosis: high-resolution CT versus radiography. *Radiology*, **176**, 755–759.

Staples, C. A., Gamsu, G., Ray, C. S., et al (1989) High resolution computed tomography and lung function in asbestos-exposed workers with normal chest radiographs. *American Review of Respiratory Diseases*, **139**, 1502–1508.

Talner, L. B., Gmelich, J. T., Liebow, A. A., Greenspan, R. H. (1970) The syndrome of bronchial mucocele and regional hyperinflation of the lung. *American Journal of Roentgenology*, **110**, 675–686.

Turner-Warwick, M. (1974) A perspective view on widespread pulmonary fibrosis. *British Medical Journal*, **ii**, 371–376.

Turner-Warwick, M., Dewar, A. (1982) Pulmonary haemorrhage and pulmonary haemosiderosis. *Clinical Radiology*, **33**, 361–370.

Wells, A. U., Hansell, D. M., Corrin, B., et al (1992) High resolution computed tomography as a predictor of lung histology in systemic sclerosis. *Thorax*, **47**, 738–742.

Yoshimura, H., Hatakeyama, M., Otsuji, H., et al (1986) Pulmonary asbestosis: CT study of subpleural curvilinear shadow. *Radiology*, **158**, 653–658.

18

CHEST TRAUMA; THE POSTOPERATIVE CHEST; INTENSIVE CARE; RADIATION

Simon P. G. Padley and Michael B. Rubens

TRAUMA

The thorax may be affected by direct trauma, or by effects of trauma elsewhere in the body. Direct trauma may be the result of penetrating or non-penetrating injury. The usual causes of penetrating injury are shooting, stabbing and shrapnel wounds.

Thoracic surgery is a special category of penetrating trauma. Non-penetrating injuries may be caused by falls, blows or blasts. Automobile accidents resulting in deceleration injuries are increasing in frequency. Trauma to other areas of the body may have thoracic complications. For example, bone fractures may cause fat emboli, and pulmonary complications following abdominal surgery are common.

Radiological Techniques The severely injured patient, the post-operative patient and the patient in the intensive care ward are true tests of the radiographer's skill. In no areas of radiography are good-quality films more necessary, and in no other group of patients are good-quality films more difficult to produce.

The injured patient is usually brought to the X-ray department, where, if possible, an erect PA film should be taken. A high-kV technique is desirable in order to see mediastinal detail, but if this is not possible a penetrated grid radiograph should be taken. A lateral film may be useful. If the patient is severely injured it is necessary to make do with supine films. In the acute stage, multiple views for rib fractures are not indicated, since it is complications of the fractures that really matter, whether or not fractures are seen.

The use of *computed radiography* is becoming more common-place in the intensive care setting. Whilst the X-ray source is a standard portable generator, the image is captured on a phosphor plate detector which is then laser scanned to produce a digital chest radiograph. This technique has advantages over conventional radiography since the latitude of the detector system is wide, reducing the need for repeat examinations for technical reasons, and maintaining a consistent quality of image between examinations. Although the radiograph can be laser printed onto film, in common with all digital information, the radiograph may be sent to a remote location for reporting or viewing, and the current radiograph can be compared with previous films retrieved from a digital archive.

Ultrasound is an excellent method for examining the pleura, diaphragm and subphrenic areas. *Aortography*, *CT* and *trans-esophageal ultrasound* may be indicated when vascular injuries are suspected.

The postoperative patient and the patient in the intensive care

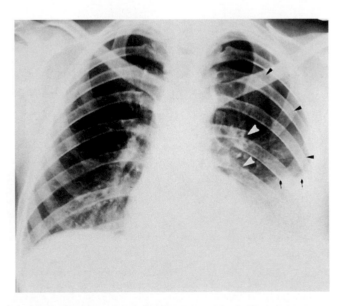

Fig. 18.1 Rib fractures and hemopneumothorax in a woman injured in an automobile accident. The left seventh and eighth ribs are fractured (white arrowheads). A pneumothorax (black arrowheads) is present, and a fluid level (arrows) is seen in the pleural space.

ward will usually be examined with mobile X-ray equipment. An erect PA film, with the patient sitting up, is preferable, but a supine film at end inspiration is better than a film taken with the patient slouched and at end expiration. The highest kV and mA possible and high-speed screens will minimize motion blurring. Horizontal-beam lateral decubitus films are often useful to assess pleural fluid, pneumothoraces and fluid levels.

The films of intensive care ward patients need to be examined with full clinical information, since many of the pathological processes to which these patients are susceptible produce similar radiographic manifestations. Serial films need to be evaluated for general trends, as day-to-day changes may not be apparent, and special attention needs to be given to monitoring and life-support devices.

Injuries to the Thoracic Cage

Rib fractures are common, and may be single, multiple, unilateral or bilateral. Healed rib fractures are a fairly frequent incidental finding on the chest X-ray. Acute rib fractures are often difficult to see if there is no displacement, and their presence may only be inferred by surrounding hematoma producing an extrapleural opacity. In cases of chest trauma, the chest X-ray is more important in detecting a complication of rib fracture than the fracture itself. However, fracture of the first three ribs is often associated with major intrathoracic injury, and fracture of the lower three ribs may be associated with important hepatic, splenic or renal injury.

Complications of rib fracture include a flail segment, pneumothorax, hemothorax and subcutaneous emphysema. A *flail segment*

is usually apparent clinically, the affected part of the chest wall being sucked in during inspiration, possibly compromising the underlying lung. The chest X-ray will show several adjacent ribs to be fractured in two places, or bilateral rib fractures.

The fractured ends of ribs may penetrate underlying pleura and lung and cause a *pneumothorax, hemothorax, hemopneumothorax* (Fig. 18.1) or *intrapulmonary hemorrhage*. Air may also escape into the chest wall and cause *subcutaneous emphysema* (Fig. 18.2).

Stress fractures of the first and second ribs are sometimes an incidental finding on the chest X-ray. *Cough fractures* usually affect the sixth to ninth ribs in the posterior axillary line, but may not be visible until callus has formed.

Fractures of the *sternum* usually require a lateral film or CT for visualization.

Fractures of the *thoracic spine* may be associated with a paraspinal shadow which represents hematoma.

Fractures of the *clavicle* may be associated with injury to the subclavian vessels or brachial plexus, and posterior dislocation of the clavicle at the sternoclavicular joint may cause injury to the trachea, esophagus, great vessels or nerves of the superior mediastinum.

Herniation of lung tissue is usually associated with obvious rib fractures, but may only be apparent on tangential views in full inspiration.

Injuries to the Diaphragm

Laceration of the diaphragm may result from penetrating or non-penetrating trauma to the chest or abdomen. Ruptures of the left

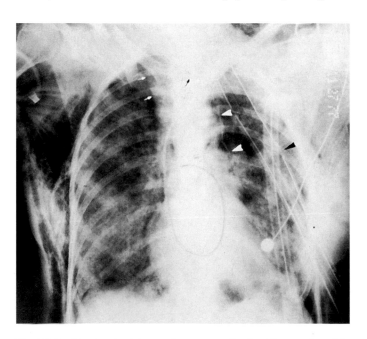

Fig. 18.2 Massive chest trauma in a woman involved in an automobile accident. Gross subcutaneous emphysema extends over the chest wall, outlining muscle planes. The right clavicle is fractured. Several ribs were fractured, but this is not seen on this film. Mediastinal emphysema separates pleura from the descending aorta (white arrowheads). A mediastinal hematoma is present (white arrows). Widespread lung contusion is obscured by the subcutaneous emphysema. Note tracheostomy tube (black arrow), left pleural tubes, with side hole indicated (black arrowhead), Swan–Ganz catheter and ECG lead.

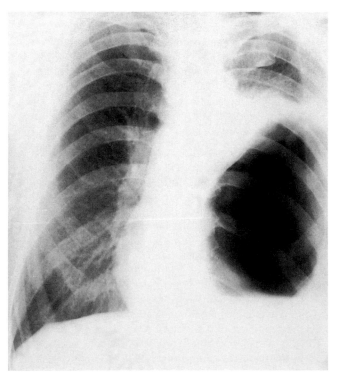

Fig. 18.3 Rupture of diaphragm in a man of 58 who fell from a building 13 years before, breaking ankles and injuring chest, and now presented with persistent vomiting. The chest radiograph demonstrates distended stomach in the left hemithorax, confirmed by barium swallow. Thoracotomy revealed stomach herniating into left pleural cavity through a 5 cm rent in the left hemidiaphragm.

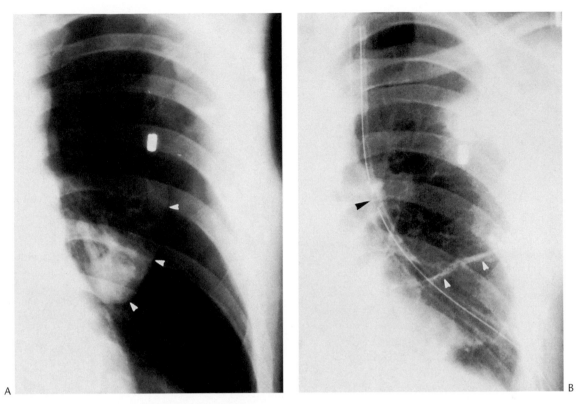

Fig. 18.4 Penetrating chest injury—man with bullet wound. **A.** Large pneumothorax (arrowheads), and bullet in chest wall. **B.** Following insertion of pleural tube (black arrowhead), the lung re-expands, revealing hematoma in bullet track. Band shadow in lower zone (white arrowheads) represents subsegmental atelectasis.

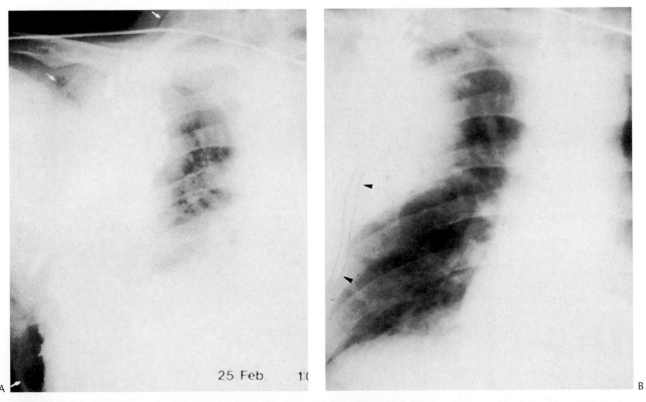

Fig. 18.5 Pulmonary contusion and hemothorax in a man with a gunshot injury. **A.** Subcutaneous emphysema is present over the chest wall (arrows), and dense shadowing extends over most of the hemithorax. **B.** Following the insertion of a pleural drain (arrowheads) the lower half of the shadowing, due to blood in the pleural space, has gone. The remaining opacity is pulmonary contusion. A few bullet fragments are visible above the contusion.

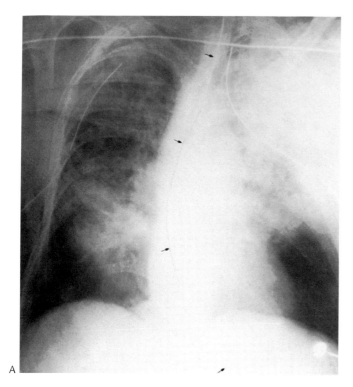

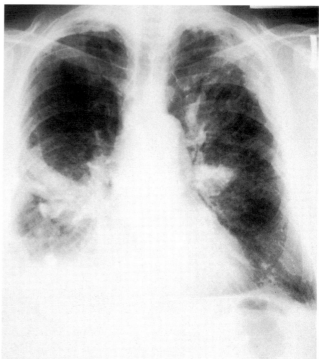

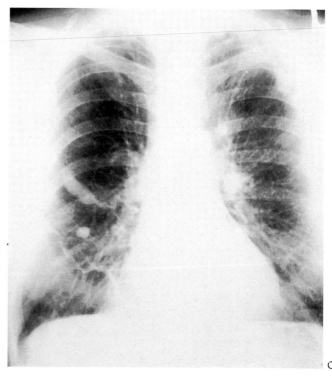

Fig. 18.6 Pulmonary contusion and hematoma in a youth of 18 trampled on by a bull. **A.** Extensive consolidation is present throughout both lungs, particularly in the left upper zone. Subcutaneous emphysema is seen over the right hemithorax. Bilateral pleural tubes and a nasogastric tube (arrows) are present. **B.** Six days later the contusion has resolved and multiple pulmonary hematomas and some extrapleural hematomas have become visible. **C.** One month later the hematomas are smaller.

hemidiaphragm are encountered more frequently in clinical practice than ruptures on the right. The typical plain film appearance is of obscuration of the affected hemidiaphragm and increased shadowing in the ipsilateral hemithorax due to herniation of stomach, omentum, bowel or solid viscera (Fig. 18.3), although such herniation may be delayed. Ultrasound may demonstrate diaphragmatic laceration and free fluid in both the pleura and peritoneum. Barium studies may be useful to confirm herniation of stomach or bowel into the chest.

Injuries to the Pleura

Pneumothorax, as mentioned above, may be a complication of rib fracture, and is then usually associated with a hemothorax (Fig. 18.1). If no ribs are fractured, pneumothorax is secondary to a pneumomediastinum, pulmonary laceration or penetrating chest injury (Fig. 18.4). Pneumothorax due to a penetrating injury is liable to develop increased pressure, resulting in a tension pneumothorax which may require emergency decompression.

Hemothorax may also occur with or without rib fractures (Fig. 18.5), and is due to laceration of intercostal or pleural vessels. If a pneumothorax is also present a fluid level will be seen on a horizontal-beam film (Fig. 18.1).

Pleural effusion may also result from trauma. Open injuries to the pleura are prone to infection and development of an empyema.

Injuries to the Lung

Pulmonary contusion is due to hemorrhagic exudation into the alveoli and interstitial spaces and appears as patchy, non-segmental consolidation (Figs 18.5, 18.6). Shadowing appears within the first few hours of penetrating or non-penetrating trauma, usually shows improvement within 2 days, and clears within 3–4 days (Fig. 18.7). When contusion due to a bullet

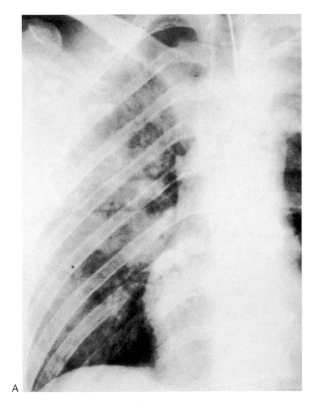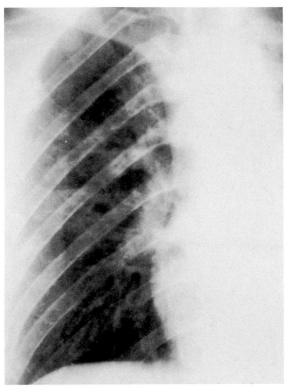

A   B

Fig. 18.7 Pulmonary contusion in a man following an automobile accident. **A.** Extensive consolidation throughout right lung. Left lung was clear. No rib fractures. **B.** Four days later the shadowing has resolved.

wound clears, a longitudinal hematoma in the bullet track may become visible (Fig. 18.4).

Pulmonary lacerations as a result of non-penetrating trauma may appear as round thin-walled cystic spaces. When the injury is acute, the laceration may be obscured by pulmonary contusion, but as the surrounding consolidation resolves, laceration will become evident. If the laceration is filled with blood it appears as a homogenous round opacity, and if partly filled with blood it may show a fluid level (Fig. 18.8). Such pulmonary hematomas or blood cysts gradually decrease in size, but may take a few months to resolve completely (Fig. 18.9). Pulmonary hematomas are often multiple (Fig. 18.6).

Torsion of a lung is a rare result of severe thoracic trauma, usually to a child. The lung twists about the hilum through 180°. If unrelieved the lung may become gangrenous and appear opaque on the chest X-ray.

Atelectasis and compensatory *hyperinflation* after a chest injury may be due to aspiration of blood or mucus into the bronchi. Atelectasis may also occur secondary to decreased respiratory movement.

Pulmonary edema as a manifestation of the adult respiratory distress syndrome may occur after major trauma.

Fat embolism is a rare complication of multiple fractures, due to fat globules from the bone marrow entering the systemic veins and embolizing to the lungs. Poorly defined nodular opacities appear throughout both lungs. The opacities resolve within a few days. The diagnosis is confirmed if fat globules are present in the sputum or urine.

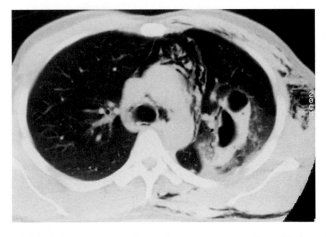

Fig. 18.8 Pulmonary contusion and pulmonary laceration. CT through the chest demonstrates mediastinal and chest wall emphysema following trauma. There is also a thin-walled loculated air/fluid collection within the lung due to a pulmonary laceration surrounded by ground-glass change indicative of contusion.

Injuries to the Trachea and Bronchi

Laceration or rupture of a major airway is an uncommon result of severe chest trauma, usually in an automobile accident. Fracture of the first three ribs is often present, and mediastinal emphysema and pneumothorax are common (Fig. 18.10). The injury is usually

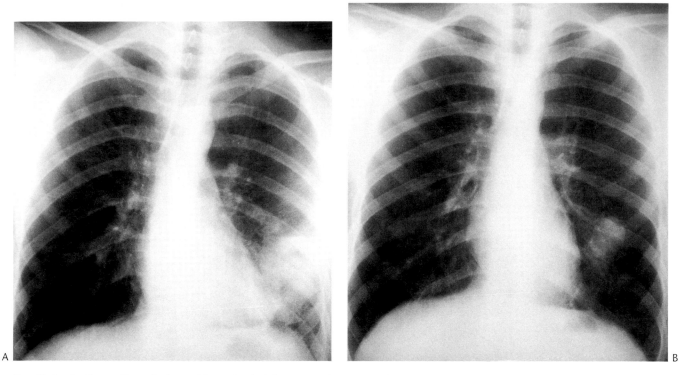

Fig. 18.9 **A.** Chest radiograph obtained immediately following a stab wound to the chest. There is a pulmonary hematoma evident on the left. **B.** Radiograph three months later demonstrates only partial resolution.

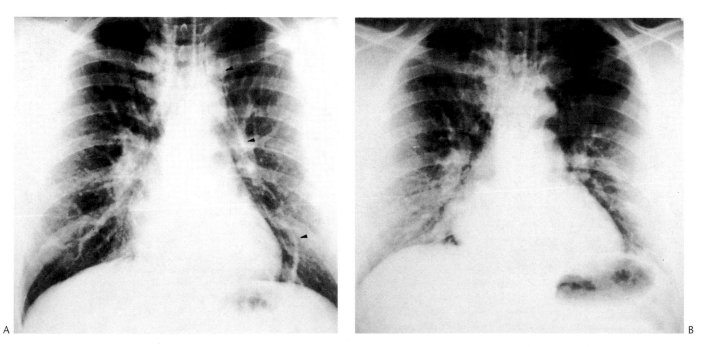

Fig. 18.10 Ruptured trachea with dyspnea and chest pain in a man suffering a deceleration injury. **A.** Pneumomediastinum with linear lucencies in the mediastinum and displacement of mediastinal pleura (arrowheads). **B.** One hour later, following a bout of coughing, a left pneumothorax has developed. Bronchoscopy revealed a ruptured trachea.

in the *trachea* just above the carina, or in a *main bronchus* just distal to the carina. If the bronchial sheath is preserved there may be no immediate signs or symptoms, but tracheostenosis or bronchiectasis may occur later. Tomography may be helpful in diagnosis, but bronchoscopy is the best diagnostic method in the acute stage.

Injuries to the Mediastinum

Pneumomediastinum and *mediastinal emphysema* describe the presence of air between the tissue planes of the mediastinum. Air may reach here as a result of interstitial pulmonary emphysema, perforation of the esophagus, trachea or a bronchus, or from a penetrating chest injury. Interstitial pulmonary emphysema is a result of alveolar wall rupture due to high intra-alveolar pressure, and may occur during violent coughing, asthmatic attacks or severe crush injuries, or be due to positive pressure ventilation. Air dissects centrally along the perivascular sheath to reach the mediastinum. Rarely, air may dissect into the mediastinum from a pneumoperitoneum. A pneumomediastinum may extend beyond the thoracic inlet into the neck, and over the chest wall. Pneumothorax is a common complication of pneumomediastinum, but the converse never occurs.

Pneumomediastinum usually produces vertical translucent streaks in the mediastinum. This represents gas separating and outlining the soft-tissue planes and structures of the mediastinum. Gas shadows may extend up into the neck (Fig. 18.11), or dissect extrapleurally over the diaphragm, or extend into the soft-tissue planes of the chest wall, causing subcutaneous emphysema (Figs 18.11, 18.12). The mediastinal pleura may be displaced laterally,

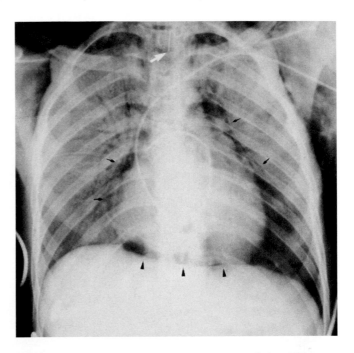

Fig. 18.12 Complications of positive pressure ventilation. Diffuse consolidation in a boy aged 15 following presumed viral pneumonia. Note endotracheal tube (white arrow) and Swan–Ganz catheter, both well positioned. Pneumomediastinum is indicated by linear lucencies in the mediastinum, lateral displacement of the mediastinal pleura (black arrows) and infrapericardial air, producing the 'continuous diaphragm' sign (arrowheads). There is extensive bilateral subcutaneous emphysema.

and become visible as a linear soft-tissue shadow parallel to the mediastinum (Figs 18.2, 18.10–12). If mediastinal air collects beneath the pericardium the central part of the diaphragm may be visible, producing the 'continuous diaphragm' sign (Fig. 18.12).

Sometimes it may be difficult to differentiate between *pneumopericardium* and pneumomediastinum. In pneumopericardium gas does not extend beyond the aortic root or much beyond the main pulmonary artery (Fig. 18.21). In pneumomediastinum, gas often outlines the aortic knuckle and extends into the neck. In pneumopericardium a fluid level is often seen on horizontal-beam films, and the distribution of air may alter with changes in the patient's position. The patient's position has little or no effect on a pneumomediastinum. Pneumomediastinum is relatively more common in neonates and infants, and may displace the thymus or resemble a lung cyst.

Mediastinal hemorrhage may result from penetrating or nonpenetrating trauma, and be due to venous or arterial bleeding. Many cases are probably unrecognized, as clinical and radiographic signs are absent. Important causes include automobile accidents, aortic rupture and dissection, and introduction of central venous catheters. There is usually bilateral mediastinal widening (Fig. 18.13), but a localized hematoma may occur (Figs 18.2, 18.30).

Aortic rupture is usually the result of an automobile accident. Most non-fatal aortic tears occur at the aortic isthmus, the site of the ligamentum arteriosum. Only 10–20% of patients survive the acute episode, but a small number may develop a chronic aneurysm at the site of the tear. The commonest acute radiographic signs are widening of the superior mediastinum, and

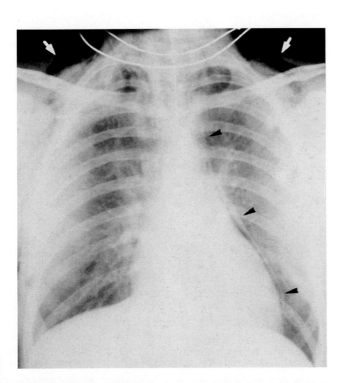

Fig. 18.11 Pneumomediastinum in a man after an automobile accident. Note linear lucencies in the mediastinum extending into the neck, and subcutaneous emphysema over the supraclavicular fossae (arrows). The mediastinal pleura is outlined by air and displaced laterally (arrowheads).

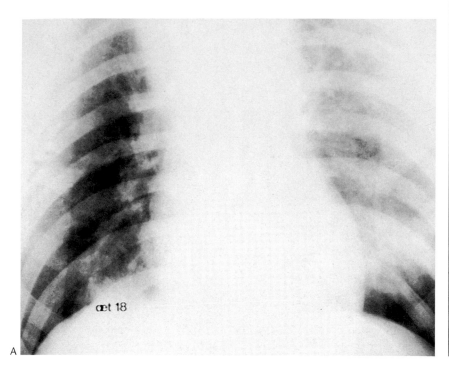

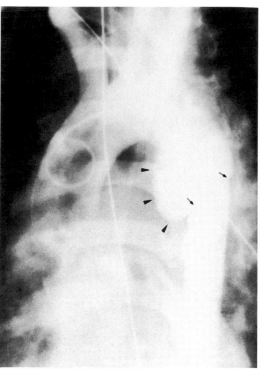

Fig. 18.13 Mediastinal hemorrhage in a youth of 18 after an automobile accident. **A.** Chest radiograph shows bilateral widening of the superior mediastinum. The aorta is obscured. **B.** Arch aortogram demonstrates an aneurysm of the aortic isthmus (arrowheads) with intimal tear (arrows).

obscuration of the aortic knuckle (Fig. 18.13). Other radiographic signs include deviation of the left main bronchus anteriorly, inferiorly and to the right, and rightward displacement of the trachea, a nasogastric tube or the right parasternal line. A left apical extrapleural cap or a left hemothorax may be visible. Whilst aortography is the definitive investigation, CT, trans-esophageal echocardiography or MRI may be diagnostic. In everyday practice many departments will have emergency access to a CT scanner but will not be centers of cardiothoracic surgery. A properly conducted CT scan demonstrating a normal media-stinum has a very high negative predictive value for the presence of aortic rupture. However, if CT is equivocal or shows a media-stinal hematoma then generally angiography will be required prior to surgery (Fig. 18.14).

Cardiac injury may result from penetrating or blunt trauma. Penetrating injuries are usually rapidly fatal but may cause tamponade, ventricular aneurysm or septal defects. Blunt trauma may cause myocardial contusion and infarction and may be associated with transient or more permanent rhythm disturbance.

Esophageal rupture is usually the result of instrumentation or surgery (Fig. 18.15), but occasionally occurs in penetrating trauma, and is rarely spontaneous due to sudden increase of intra-esophageal pressure (Boerhaave syndrome). Clinically there is acute mediastinitis; radiographically there are signs of pneumo-mediastinum, with or without a pneumothorax or hydropneumo-thorax, which is usually left-sided. The diagnosis should be confirmed by a swallow using water-soluble contrast medium or barium. The former is safer; the latter is radiographically superior

but carries a theoretical risk of granuloma formation in the mediastinum.

Chylothorax due to damage to the thoracic duct may become apparent hours or days after trauma. Thoracic surgery is the commonest cause.

THE POSTOPERATIVE CHEST

Intrathoracic surgery is performed most frequently for resection of all or part of a lung, or for cardiac disease. This section will discuss the usual acute and long-term changes apparent radio-graphically following such surgery, followed by a description of complications of thoracic and of non-thoracic surgery.

THORACOTOMY

Lung resections are usually performed posterolaterally through the fourth or fifth intercostal space. Part of a rib may be resected, the periosteum may be stripped or the ribs may simply be spread apart following a muscle incision (Fig. 18.16). Rib fractures sometimes occur, but often the surgical route is not obvious on the chest X-ray, or is marked only by some narrowing of the intercostal space, or some overlying soft-tissue swelling and subcutaneous emphysema.

Following *pneumonectomy* it is important for the remaining lung to be fully ventilated, and for the mediastinum to remain

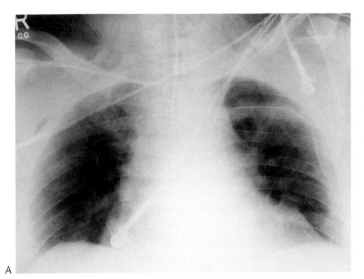

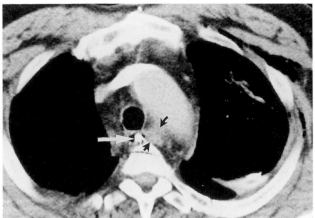

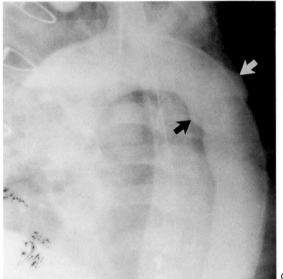

Fig. 18.14 Aortic rupture. 56-year-old male patient with a severe deceleration injury and a remote history of sternotomy for coronary artery bypass grafting. **A.** Supine chest radiograph demonstrates questionable mediastinal widening, surgical emphysema and a left chest tube. **B.** Contrast-enhanced CT scan at the level of the aortic arch reveals a small mediastinal hematoma (black arrows) adjacent to the esophagus, which contains a nasogastric tube. The mediastinum is of normal width. **C.** Arch aortogram demonstrating an intimal tear at the usual site (arrows).

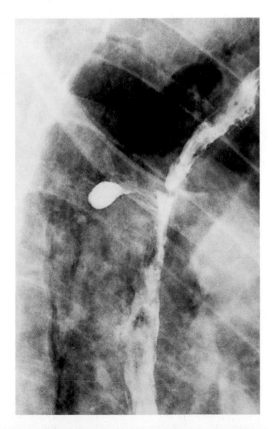

Fig. 18.15 Esophageal rupture following difficult endoscopy. Following the procedure a check radiograph demonstrated pneumomediastinum (not shown) and a localized perforation was detected on contrast swallow.

close to the midline. Excessive mediastinal shift may compromise respiration and venous return to the heart. On the initial postoperative film the trachea should be close to the midline, the remaining lung should appear normal or slightly plethoric, and the pneumonectomy space usually contains a small amount of fluid. A drainage tube may or may not be present in the space. Over the next several days the pneumonectomy space begins to obliterate by gradual shift of the mediastinum to that side, and accumulation of fluid. The space is usually half-filled within about a week, and completely opacifies over the next 2–3 months (Fig. 18.17). If the mediastinum moves toward the remaining lung, this may indicate too rapid accumulation of fluid in the pneumonectomy space, or atelectasis in the remaining lung. A sudden shift may indicate a bronchopleural fistula (Fig. 18.18).

Following *lobectomy* the remaining lung should expand to fill the space of the resected lobe. Immediately postoperatively, pleural drains are present, preventing accumulation of pleural fluid, and the mediastinum may be shifted to the side of the operation. With hyperinflation of the remaining lung the mediastinum returns to its normal position. When the drains are removed a small pleural effusion commonly occurs but usually resolves within a few days, perhaps leaving residual pleural thickening.

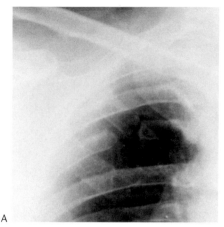

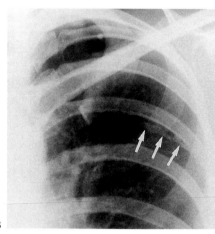

Fig. 18.16 A. Typical sharply truncated rib defect following right thoracotomy (right upper lobectomy for carcinoma). **B.** Late post-surgical changes following periosteal stripping at time of left fifth interspace thoracotomy for mitral valvotomy. There is a wavy line of calcification below the affected rib (arrows).

With *segmental* or *subsegmental lung resections* a cut surface of the lung is oversewn, and air leaks are fairly common, sometimes causing persistent pneumothorax which may require prolonged drainage. Wire sutures or staples may be visible at the site of a bronchial stump or lesser lung resection.

Complications of Thoracotomy

Postoperative Spaces   These may persist following lobectomy and segmental or subsegmental resections. They are air spaces that correspond to the excised lung. Fluid may collect in them, but they usually resolve after a few weeks or months. If they persist and are associated with constitutional symptoms, increasing fluid and pleural thickening, an empyema or bronchopleural fistula should be suspected.

Empyema   Empyema complicating pneumonectomy, or rarely lobectomy, usually occurs a few weeks after surgery, although it may occur months or years later. Rapid accumulation of fluid may push the mediastinum to the normal side. If a fistula develops between the pneumonectomy space and a bronchus or the skin, the air–fluid level in the space will suddenly drop (Fig. 18.18). Increasing gas in the pneumonectomy space may also indicate infection by a gas-forming organism.

Bronchopleural Fistula   This is a communication between the bronchial tree (or lung tissue) and the pleural space. The commonest cause is a complication of *lung surgery*, but it may be the result of rupture of a *lung abscess*, erosion by a *lung cancer* or *penetrating trauma*. Bronchopleural fistula complicating complete or partial lung resection may occur early, when it is due to faulty closure of the bronchus, but it more commonly occurs late due to infection or recurrent tumor of the bronchial stump. The usual radiographic appearance is the sudden appearance of, or increase in the amount of, air in the pleural space, with a corresponding decrease in the amount of fluid in the space. A fluid level is almost always present (Fig. 18.18). If fluid enters the airways and is aspirated into the remaining lung, widespread consolidation may be seen on the chest X-ray. Sinography of the pleural space or bronchography may demonstrate the fistula.

Pleural Fluid   This is usually seen on the chest X-ray following thoracic surgery. If the amount is excessive it may be due to bleeding or chylothorax.

Diaphragmatic Elevation   Elevation may indicate phrenic nerve damage and is best assessed by fluoroscopy or ultrasound.

Other pulmonary complications of thoracic surgery include *atelectasis*, *aspiration pneumonia*, *pulmonary embolism* and *pulmonary edema*, both cardiogenic and non-cardiogenic. These may also complicate non-thoracic surgery and are discussed below.

CARDIAC SURGERY

Most cardiac operations are performed through a *sternotomy* incision, and wire sternal sutures are often seen on the postoperative films (Figs 18.35, 18.36). Mitral valvotomy is now rarely performed via a *thoracotomy* incision (Fig. 18.16), but this route is still used for surgery of coarctation of the aorta, patent ductus arteriosus, Blalock–Taussig shunts and pulmonary artery banding.

Following cardiac surgery, some widening of the cardiovascular silhouette is usual, and represents bleeding and edema. Marked widening of the mediastinum suggests significant *hemorrhage*, but the necessity for re-exploration is based upon the overall clinical situation (Figs 18.19, 18.20). Some air commonly remains in the pericardium following cardiac surgery, so that the signs of *pneumopericardium* may be present (Fig. 18.21).

Pulmonary opacities are very common following open heart surgery, and left basal shadowing is almost invariable, representing *atelectasis*. This shadowing usually resolves over a week or two. Small *pleural effusions* are also common in the immediate postoperative period.

Pneumoperitoneum is sometimes seen, due to involvement of the peritoneum by the sternotomy incision. It is of no pathological significance.

Violation of left or right pleural space may lead to a *pneumothorax*. Damage to a major lymphatic vessel may lead to a *chylothorax* or a more localized collection—a *chyloma*. *Phrenic nerve damage* may cause paresis or paralysis of a hemidiaphragm.

Surgical clips or other metallic markers have sometimes been used to mark the ends of coronary artery bypass grafts. *Prosthetic heart valves* are usually visible radiographically, but they may be difficult to see on an underpenetrated film. Their assessment—fluoroscopically, angiographically or ultrasonographically—is outside the scope of this chapter.

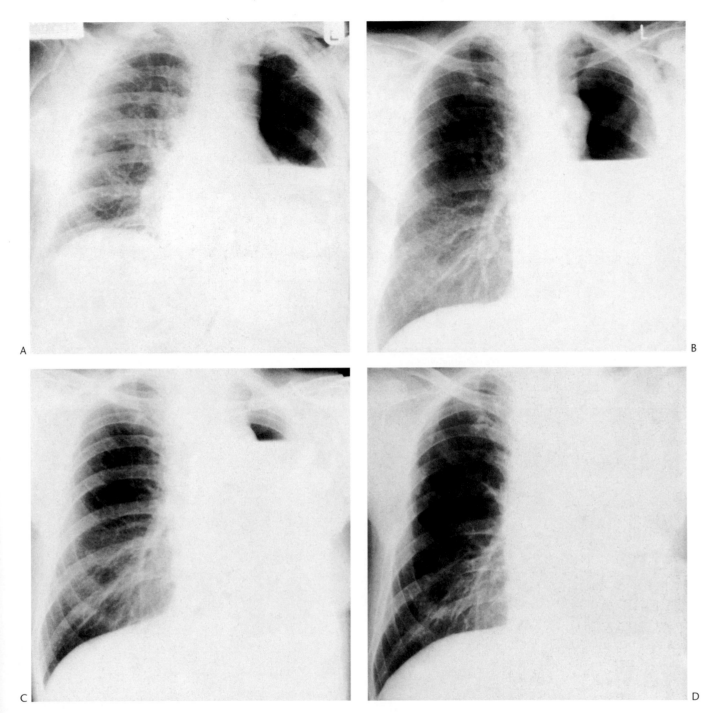

Fig. 18.17 Normal post-pneumonectomy appearance. 1 day **A**, 6 days **B**, 5 weeks **C** and 8 weeks **D** postoperatively. The pneumonectomy space is gradually obliterated by the rising fluid level and mediastinal shift.

Sternal dehiscence may be apparent radiographically by a linear lucency appearing in the sternum and alteration in position of the sternal sutures on consecutive films. The diagnosis is usually made clinically and may be associated with osteomyelitis. A first or second rib may be fractured when the sternum is spread apart. The importance of this observation is that it may explain chest pain in the postoperative period.

Acute mediastinitis may complicate mediastinal surgery

although it is more commonly associated with esophageal perforation or surgery. Radiographically there may be mediastinal widening or pneumomediastinum, and these features are best assessed by CT scan (Figs 18.22, 18.23).

Chronic mediastinal infection including sternal osteomyelitis may follow median sternotomy, and may be difficult to differentiate from postsurgical granulation tissue and hematoma. Mediastinal gas may persist for some weeks or months after

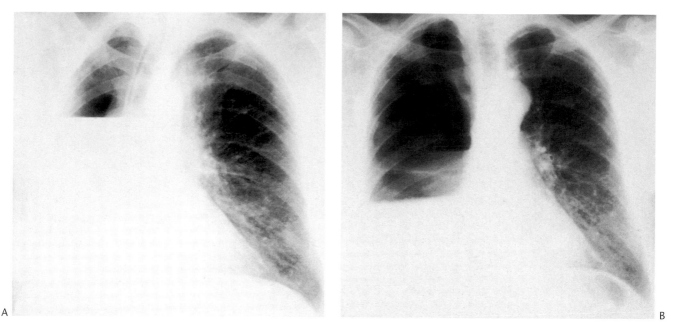

Fig. 18.18 Bronchopleural fistula. **A.** 13 days after right pneumonectomy the space is filling with fluid and the mediastinum is deviated to the right. **B.** Two days later, after the patient coughed up a large amount of fluid, the fluid level has dropped and the mediastinum has returned to the midline. Bronchoscopy confirmed a right bronchopleural fistula.

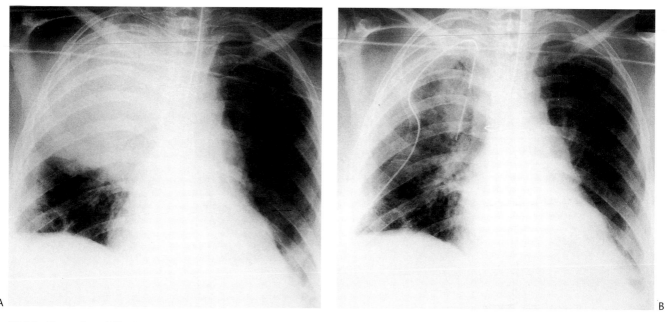

Fig. 18.19 Hemorrhage following cardiac transplantation. **A.** Four hours following return from surgery the chest radiograph reveals opacification of the right upper zone. Ultrasound at the patient's bedside confirmed a large fluid collection. **B.** After insertion of a chest drain there has been partial resolution of the appearances.

surgery, and only increasing amounts of gas on subsequent examination is a reliable indication of the presence of a gas-forming organism.

The *postpericardotomy syndrome* is probably an autoimmune phenomenon, usually occurring in the month after surgery. It presents with fever, pleurisy and pericarditis. Pleural effusions may be visible and the cardiac silhouette may enlarge. Ultrasound

will demonstrate pericardial fluid. Patchy consolidation may occur in the lung bases.

LATE APPEARANCES AFTER CHEST SURGERY

Following thoracotomy, the appearance of the chest X-ray may return to normal, or evidence of surgery may persist. Resected

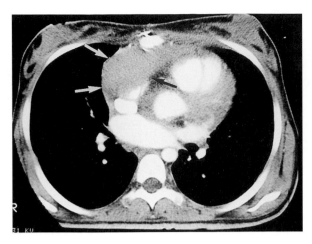

Fig. 18.20 Mediastinal hematoma. Enhanced CT scan demonstrates a soft-tissue density non-enhancing mass in the anterior mediastinum three days following cardiac surgery (arrows).

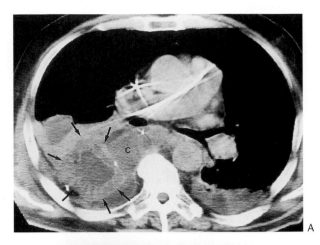

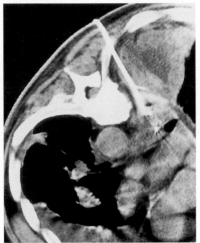

Fig. 18.22 Infected mediastinal collection following esophagectomy. **A.** The gastric conduit (arrowheads) is discernible separately from the collection (C) and small bilateral effusions. **B.** Drainage accomplished by CT-guided pigtail catheter insertion with the patient in a semi-prone position.

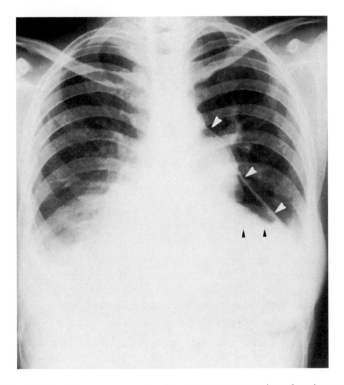

Fig. 18.21 Hemopneumopericardium in a woman two days after closure of atrial septal defect. The pericardium is outlined by air (white arrowheads) which does not extend as high as the aortic arch. A fluid level (black arrowheads) is present in the pericardium, and there are bilateral pleural effusions.

ribs or healed rib fractures are usually obvious (Figs 18.13, 18.24). There may be irregular regeneration of a rib related to disturbed periosteum. A rib space may be narrowed where a thoracotomy wound has been closed (Fig. 18.24). Rib notching may result from a Blalock–Taussig shunt between subclavian and pulmonary arteries. Pleural thickening often remains after a thoracotomy.

Rearrangement of the remaining lung occurs after lobectomy, so that the anatomy of the fissures may be altered. Following esophageal surgery, stomach or loops of bowel may produce unusual soft-tissue opacities or fluid levels if they have been brought up into the chest (Fig. 18.25). A contrast swallow frequently clarifies the appearances.

Surgery is now rarely performed for pulmonary tuberculosis, but many patients who have had such surgery are still alive. The object of surgery was to reduce aeration of the infected lung, usually an upper lobe. *Thoracoplasty* involved removal of the posterior parts of usually three or more ribs so that the underlying lung collapsed (Fig. 18.26). Occasionally, thoracoplasty was combined with pneumonectomy for the treatment of chronic tuberculous empyema. An alternative approach was *plombage*, which was the extrapleural insertion of some inert material to collapse the underlying lung. Solid or hollow *lucite balls* (Fig. 18.27) were commonly used. Other substances included crumpled *cellophane packs* and *kerosene (paraffin)* (Fig. 18.28).

THORACIC COMPLICATIONS OF GENERAL SURGERY

Atelectasis   This is the commonest pulmonary complication of thoracic or abdominal surgery (Fig. 18.25B). Predisposing factors are a long anesthetic, obesity, chronic lung disease and smoking.

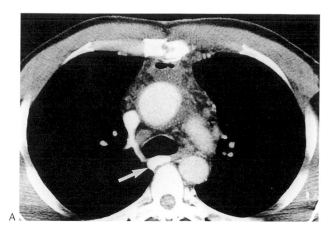

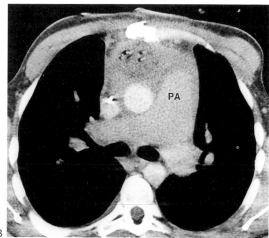

Fig. 18.23 Post-surgical mediastinitis. Two cases. **A.** CT 3 weeks following aortic valve replacement in a patient with signs of infection. There is a small retrosternal air and fluid collection, subsequently drained. Note the enlarged azygos vein (arrow) due to previous SVC thrombosis. **B.** Infected mediastinal collection in a different patient several weeks following ASD closure. Note the large pulmonary trunk (PA).

It is a result of retained secretions and poor ventilation. Postoperatively it is painful to breathe deeply or cough. The chest X-ray usually shows elevation of the diaphragm, due to a poor inspiration. Linear, sometimes curved, opacities are frequently present in the lower zones, and probably represent a combination of subsegmental volume loss and consolidation (Fig. 18.4B). These shadows usually appear about 24 hours postoperatively and resolve within two or three days.

Pleural Effusions These are common immediately following abdominal surgery and usually resolve within two weeks. They may be associated with pulmonary infarction. Effusions due to subphrenic infection usually occur later.

Pneumothorax When it complicates extrathoracic surgery pneumothorax is usually a complication of positive pressure ventilation or central venous line insertion. It may complicate nephrectomy.

Aspiration Pneumonitis This is common during anesthesia but fortunately is usually insignificant. When significant, patchy consolidation appears within a few hours, usually basally or around

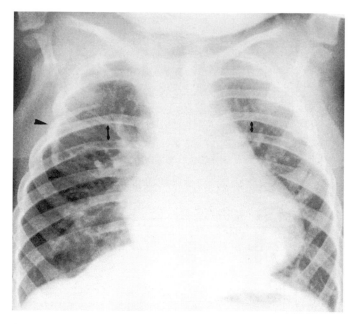

Fig. 18.24 Post-thoracotomy ribs. Right thoracotomy with partially excised regenerating right fourth rib (arrowhead) after repair of tracheo-esophageal fistula. Left thoracotomy, indicated by narrowed fifth intercostal space, for pulmonary artery banding for multiple ventricular septal defects.

the hila (Fig. 18.29). Clearing occurs within a few days, unless there is superinfection.

Pulmonary Edema In the postoperative period edema may be cardiogenic or non-cardiogenic. The latter includes fluid overload and the adult respiratory distress syndrome.

Pneumonia Postoperative atelectasis and aspiration pneumonitis may be complicated by pneumonia. Postoperative pneumonias, therefore, tend to be associated with bilateral basal shadowing.

Subphrenic Abscess This usually produces elevation of the hemidiaphragm, pleural effusion and basal atelectasis. Loculated gas may be seen below the diaphragm, and fluoroscopy may show splinting of the diaphragm. Subphrenic abscess can be demonstrated by CT or ultrasound.

Pulmonary Embolism This may produce pulmonary shadowing, pleural effusion or elevation of the diaphragm. However, a normal chest X-ray does not exclude pulmonary embolism, and the initial investigation of choice is a perfusion lung scan. There is also an emerging role for spiral CT scanning in the investigation of acute pulmonary embolism.

THE PATIENT IN INTENSIVE CARE

Patients are admitted to an intensive care ward postoperatively, following major trauma or following circulatory or respiratory failure. A number of monitoring and life-support devices may be used in their care. Radiology plays an important part in the management of these devices.

Central Venous Pressure (CVP) Catheters These are used to monitor right atrial pressure. The end of a CVP line needs to be intrathoracic, and is ideally in the superior vena cava (Fig.

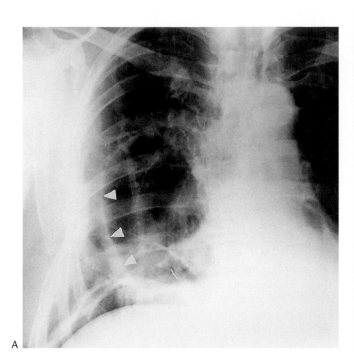

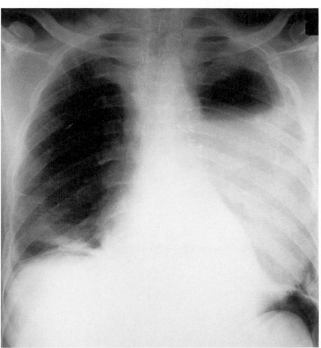

Fig. 18.25 **A.** Ivor Lewis esophagectomy. There is a rib defect, air under the diaphragm and a gas-filled gastric conduit in the right chest. This is outlined by a rim of pleural fluid (arrowheads). **B.** Dilated gastric pull-up in a different patient. An air–fluid level is seen in the distended conduit due to outflow obstruction at the site of the mobilized pylorus. Right basal atelectasis is present.

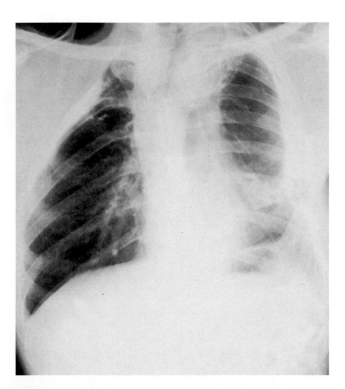

Fig. 18.26 Thoracoplasty. The first five right ribs have been removed. Left upper lobe fibrosis, bilateral apical calcification and extensive left pleural calcification are due to tuberculosis.

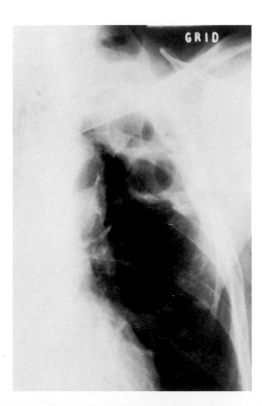

Fig. 18.27 Plombage. Several hollow balls have been inserted extra-pleurally at the left apex. The balls are slightly permeable, and the shallow fluid levels do not indicate a complication.

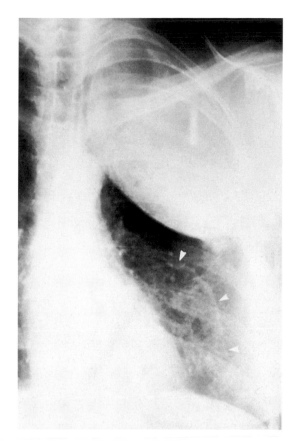

Fig. 18.28 Oleothorax. Plombage has been performed by instilling kerosene (paraffin) extrapleurally through a thoracotomy with excision of the fifth rib. A thin rim of calcification has developed in the extrapleural collection. Some keresone has tracked inferiorly behind the lung and produced a calcified pleural plaque which is seen en face (arrowheads).

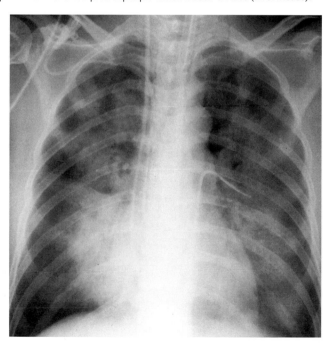

Fig. 18.29 Admission chest radiograph of a patient with acute viral encephalitis was clear. Six hours later a film following emergency intubation reveals extensive bilateral basal and perihilar air space shadowing due to massive aspiration of gastric contents.

18.33B). CVP lines may be introduced via an antecubital, subclavian or jugular vein. Subclavian venous puncture carries a risk of pneumothorax and mediastinal hematoma (Fig. 18.30). Rarely, perforation of the subclavian vein leads to fluid collecting in the mediastinum or pleura (Fig. 18.31). All catheters have a potential risk of coiling and knotting, or fracture leading to embolism.

Swan–Ganz Catheters These are used to measure pulmonary artery and pulmonary wedge pressures. The latter is an index of left atrial pressure. Swan–Ganz catheters are usually introduced via an antecubital or jugular vein. An inflatable balloon at the catheter tip guides it through the right heart. Ideally the end of the catheter should be maintained 5–8 cm (2–3 in) beyond the bifurcation of the main pulmonary artery in either the right or left pulmonary artery (Figs 18.12, 18.34). When the pulmonary wedge pressure is measured the balloon is inflated, and the flow of blood carries the catheter tip peripherally, to a wedged position. After the measurement has been made the balloon is deflated and the catheter returns to a central position, otherwise there is a risk of pulmonary infarction. The inflation balloon is radiolucent. The balloon should normally be kept deflated to minimize the risk of thrombus formation.

Nasogastric Tubes These may not reach the stomach or may coil in the esophagus (Fig. 18.32) or occasionally are inserted into the trachea and into the right bronchus (Fig. 18.33).

Endotracheal Tubes These are used for access to the airways for ventilation and management of secretions, and also to protect the airway. The chest X-ray is important in assessing the position

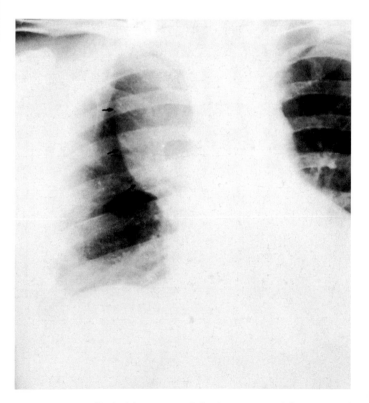

Fig. 18.30 Mediastinal hematoma. Following unsuccessfully attempted placement of a central venous line via the right subclavian vein, a large extrapleural hematoma (arrows) is present.

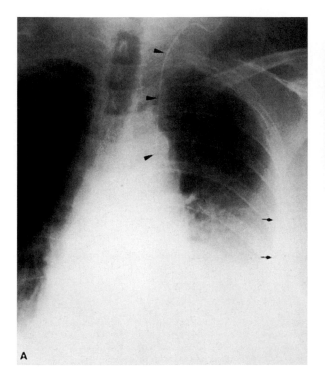

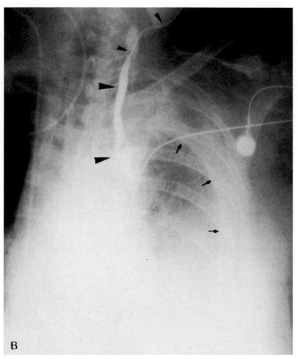

Fig. 18.31 Perforation of innominate vein. **A.** A central venous catheter (arrowheads) has been introduced via the left jugular vein. Its tip points inferiorly, rather than to the right along the axis of the innominate vein. A pleural effusion (arrows) is present. **B.** Next day the effusion is larger. Injection of contrast medium into the catheter (larger arrowheads) demonstrates extravasation and communication with the pleural effusion.

of the tip of the endotracheal tube relative to the carina. Extension and flexion of the neck may make the tip of an endotracheal tube move by as much as 5 cm. With the neck in neutral position the tip of the tube should ideally be about 5–6 cm above the carina. A tube that is inserted too far usually passes into the right bronchus (Fig. 18.34), with the risk of collapse of the left lung. If the inflated cuff of the tube dilates the trachea, there is a risk of ischemic damage to the tracheal mucosa. A late complication of an overinflated cuff is tracheostenosis.

Tracheostomy Tubes   These are usually inserted for long-term ventilatory support, either percutaneously using a Seldinger type technique, or by formal surgical tracheostomy. The tube tip should be situated centrally in the airway at the level of T3 (Fig. 18.2). Acute complications of tracheostomy include pneumothorax, pneumomediastinum and subcutaneous emphysema. Long-term complications include tracheal ulceration, stenosis and perforation.

Positive Pressure Ventilation   Complications may include interstitial emphysema, pneumomediastinum, pneumothorax and subcutaneous emphysema (Fig. 18.12).

Pleural Tubes   These are used to treat pleural effusions and pneumothoraces. If the patient is being nursed supine, the tip of the tube should be placed anteriorly and superiorly for a pneumothorax, and posteriorly and inferiorly for an effusion. A radiopaque line usually runs along pleural tubes, and is interrupted where there are side holes. It is important to check that all the side holes are within the thorax (Figs 18.2, 18.4). Tracks may remain on the chest X-ray following removal of chest tubes, causing tubular or ring shadows. When doubt remains about tube position then CT scanning should be considered (Fig. 18.35).

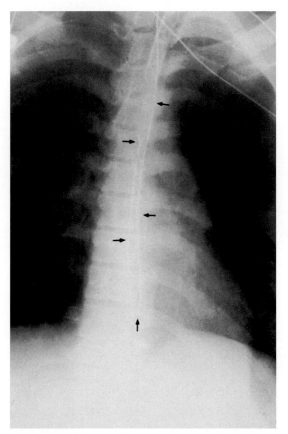

Fig. 18.32 Nasogastric tube coiled in esophagus. The tube does not reach the stomach, but has folded back on itself (arrows).

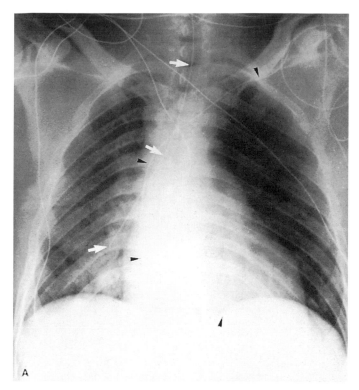

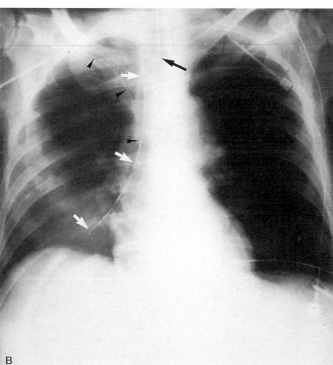

Fig. 18.33 Nasogastric tubes in right bronchus. **A.** The nasogastric tube (arrows) passes down the trachea and into the right bronchus. The patient had been 'fed' via the tube, causing patchy consolidation in the right lung. A temporary pacing electrode (arrowheads) is present. **B.** This patient, with chronic renal failure, developed peritonitis following peritoneal dialysis. Drains are present in the abdomen. A nasogastric tube (white arrows) has been passed beyond an endotracheal tube (black arrow) and into the right bronchus! Two venous lines are present; the right-sided catheter (arrowheads) is well placed for central venous pressure measurements.

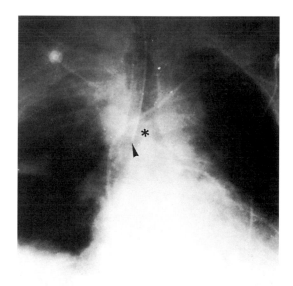

Fig. 18.34 Endotracheal tube too low. The tip of the endotracheal tube (arrowhead) is beyond the carina (asterisk) and in the right bronchus. A well-positioned Swan–Ganz catheter is present.

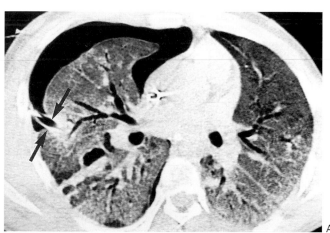

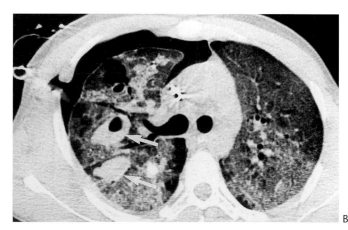

Fig. 18.35 **A,B** Multiple injuries following automobile accident. CT obtained due to a persistent pneumothorax despite apparently satisfactory tube position. The chest tube can be seen entering the lung parenchyma (black arrows). Note also the extensive parenchymal changes due to ARDS, and the right-sided pulmonary hematomas (white arrows).

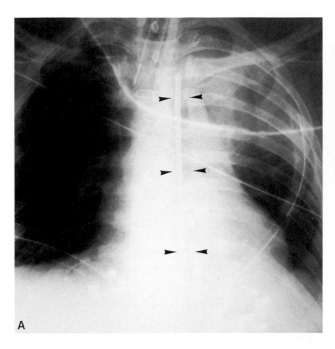

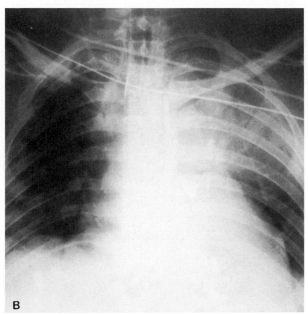

Fig. 18.36 Intra-aortic balloon pump. Post-coronary artery bypass surgery. **A.** Bilateral pleural and mediastinal drains and endotracheal tube are present. The pump is well sited, and its balloon is seen to be inflated (arrowheads). **B.** The drains have been removed. When this radiograph was exposed the balloon was deflated.

Mediastinal Drains These are usually present following sternotomy. Apart from their position, they look like pleural tubes.

Intra-aortic Balloon Pumps These are used in patients with cardiogenic shock, often following cardiac surgery. The pump comprises a catheter, the end of which is surrounded by an elongated, inflatable balloon. It is inserted via a femoral artery and is positioned in the descending thoracic aorta. The pattern of inflation and deflation of the balloon is designed to increase coronary perfusion during diastole, and to reduce the left ventricular afterload. The ideal position of the catheter tip is just distal to the origin of the left subclavian artery (Fig. 18.36). If the catheter tip is advanced too far it may occlude the left subclavian artery, and if it is too distal the balloon may occlude branches of the abdominal aorta.

Pacemakers These may be permanent or temporary. Temporary epicardial wires are sometimes inserted during cardiac surgery, and may be seen as thin, almost hair-like metallic opacities overlying the heart. Temporary pacing electrodes are usually inserted transvenously via a subclavian or jugular vein (Fig. 18.33A). If a patient is not pacing properly, a chest X-ray may reveal that the position of the electrode tip is unstable, or a fracture in the wire may be seen (Fig. 18.37). A full discussion of the radiology of pacemakers is outside the scope of this chapter.

RADIATION INJURY OF THE LUNG

Radiation injury of the lung usually results from treatment of a pulmonary or mediastinal neoplasm by radiotherapy. It may also be a complication of the treatment of breast cancer. The changes

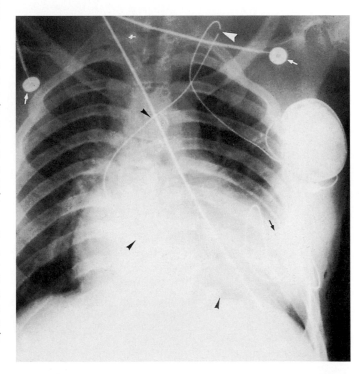

Fig. 18.37 Fractured pacing wire. Patient with surgically repaired complete atrioventricular canal. A permanent transvenous pacing system is present; the power unit is in the left axilla; the electrode (arrowheads) reaches the right ventricle by traversing the innominate vein, superior vena cava and right atrium. The electrode is fractured (white arrowhead). Note disconnected epicardial electrodes (black arrow) and ECG electrodes (white arrows).

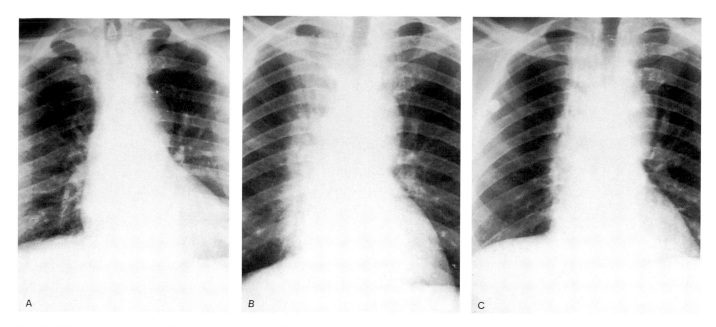

Fig. 18.38 Radiation pneumonitis in a man of 45 with diffuse histiocytic lymphoma who developed upper thoracic spinal cord compression. **A.** After surgical decompression the lungs are clear and the patient commenced radiotherapy to the spine. **B.** Ten weeks later there is paraspinal consolidation with air bronchograms. **C.** 14 weeks after treatment paraspinal pulmonary fibrosis has developed. The changes correspond to the shape of the treatment portal.

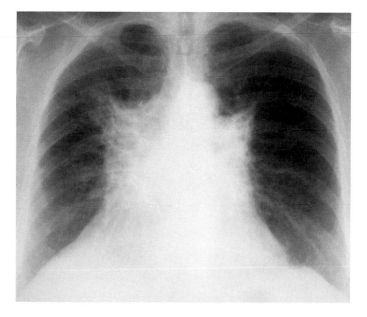

Fig. 18.39 Mediastinal fibrosis following radiotherapy several years previously. The sharp margins of the fibrosis correspond to the edges of the radiation field.

seen on the chest X-ray are often remarkably geometric, and correspond to the shape of the treatment portal.

The earliest pathological changes in the lung are alveolar and bronchiolar desquamation and accumulation of exudate in the alveoli. This is followed by organization and fibrosis.

The effect of radiation on the lung depends upon several factors. Healthy lung tissue is more resistant to damage than diseased lung. Previous radiotherapy and associated chemotherapy increase the likelihood of fibrosis. The total dose, the time over which it is given and the volume of lung irradiated are other factors. Radiographic changes are rare at a dose rate of 20 Gy (2000 rad) over 2–3 weeks, but are usual with doses of 60 Gy (6000 rad) or more over 5–6 weeks.

The radiological changes correspond to the pathology. The

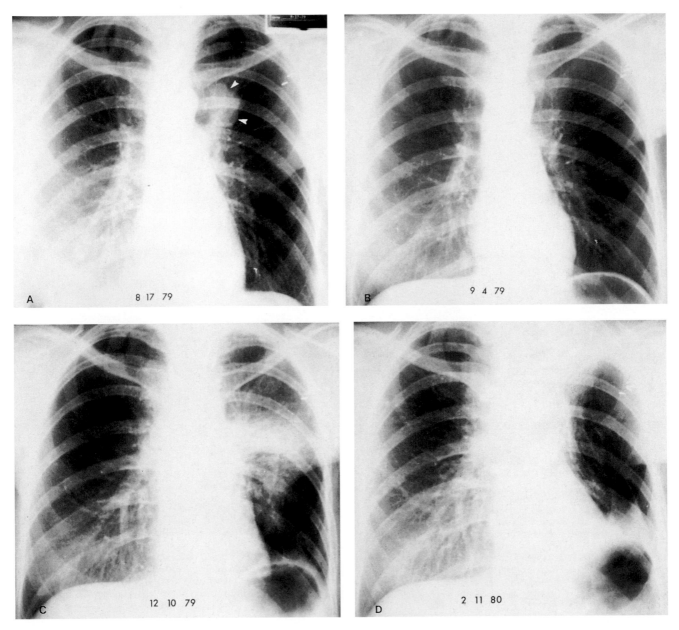

Fig. 18.40 Radiation pneumonitis in a woman of 32 one year after a left mastectomy for carcinoma. Surgical clips overlie the left axilla. **A.** Medial left upper zone opacity (arrowhead) is caused by metastasis to left internal mammary lymph nodes. **B.** 18 days later, following radiotherapy, the left upper mass has gone. **C.** 16 weeks after treatment there is extensive consolidation in the left mid and upper zones. **D.** Five months after treatment there is gross left upper lobe fibrosis, the mediastinum has shifted to the left and the left hemidiaphragm is elevated. The patient remained asymptomatic throughout this time.

acute or exudative phase is not usually evident until a month or more after treatment, and may take up to six months to appear.

Consolidation, usually with some volume loss, occurs. It is not segmental or lobar, but corresponds to the shape of the radiation portal. An air bronchogram may be visible. The patient is usually asymptomatic, but may have a pyrexia or cough. Fibrosis then occurs, and is usually complete by 9–12 months (Figs 18.38, 18.39). Fibrosis, if extensive and severe enough, may cause displacement of fissures, the hila or mediastinum, and compensatory hyperinflation of the less affected lung (Fig. 18.40). Very dense fibrosis may produce an air bronchogram (Fig. 18.41).

A *pleural effusion* as a result of irradiation is rare, and is more likely to be due to the malignant disease being treated. Pericardial effusion may occur as a late complication of irradiation. Necrosis of ribs or a clavicle may be seen on the chest X-ray following radiotherapy (Fig. 18.42) and radiation-induced sarcomas are well recognized although rare.

The diagnosis of *radiation pneumonitis* and *fibrosis* is usually easy, based on the history and characteristic shape, but occasionally apical fibrosis following treatment of breast cancer may resemble tuberculosis.

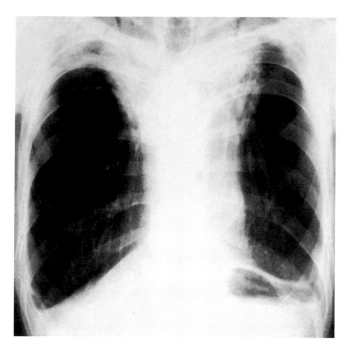

Fig. 18.41 Massive radiation fibrosis. Patient with Hodgkin's disease treated with mediastinal irradiation and chemotherapy (MOPP–bleomycin). Note gross bilateral upper lobe fibrosis with extensive air bronchogram.

REFERENCES AND SUGGESTIONS FOR FURTHER READING

Trauma

Ball, T., McCrory, R., Smith, J. O., Clements, J. L., Jr. (1982) Traumatic diaphragmatic hernia: errors in diagnosis. *American Journal of Roentgenology*, **138**, 633–637.

Batra, P. (1987). The fat embolism syndrome. *Journal of Thoracic Imaging*, **2(3)**, 12–17.

Brooks, A. P., Olson, L. K., Shackford, S. R. (1989) Computed tomography in the diagnosis of traumatic rupture of the thoracic aorta. *Clinical Radiology*, **40**, 133–138.

Cochlin, D. L., Shaw, M. R. P. (1978) Traumatic lung cysts following minor blunt chest trauma. *Clinical Radiology*, **29**, 151–154.

Crass, J. R., Cohen, A. M., Motta, A. O., et al (1990) A proposed new mechanism of traumatic aortic rupture: the osseous pinch. *Radiology*, **176**, 645–649.

George, P. Y., Goodman, P. (1992) Radiographic appearance of bullet tracks in the lung. *American Journal of Roentgenology*, **159**, 967–970.

Goarin, J. P., LeBret, F., Riou, B., et al (1993) Early diagnosis of traumatic thoracic rupture by transesophageal echocardiography. *Chest*, **103**, 618–619.

Hartley, C., Morritt, G. N. (1993) Bronchial rupture secondary to blunt chest trauma. *Thorax*, **48**, 183–184.

Mirvis, S., Keramati, B., Buchman, R., et al (1988) MR imaging of traumatic diaphragmatic rupture. *Journal of Computer Assisted Tomography*, **12**, 147–149.

Morgan, P. W., Goodman, L. R., Aprahamian, C., et al (1992) Evaluation of traumatic aortic injury: does dynamic contrast-enhanced CT play a role? *Radiology*, **182**, 661–666.

Parkin, G. J. S. (1973) The radiology of perforated oesophagus. *Clinical Radiology*, **24**, 324–332.

Raptopoulos, V., Sherman, R. G., Phillips, D. A., et al (1992) Traumatic aortic tear: screening with chest CT. *Radiology*, **182**, 667–673.

Richardson, P., Mirvis, S. E., Scorpio, R., et al (1991) Value of CT in determining the need for angiography when the findings of mediastinal hemorrhage on chest radiographs are equivocal. *American Journal of Roentgenology*, **156**, 273–279.

Rollins, R. J., Tocino, I. (1987) Early radiographic signs of tracheal rupture. *American Journal of Roentgenology*, **148**, 695–698.

Schild, H. H., Strunk, H., Weber, W., et al (1989) Pulmonary contusion: CT vs plain radiograms. *Journal of Computer Assisted Tomography*, **13**, 417–420.

Sefczek, D. M., Sefczek, R. J., Deeb, S. L. (1983) Radiographic signs of acute traumatic rupture of the thoracic aorta. *American Journal of Roentgenology*, **141**, 1259–1262.

Somers, J. M., Gleeson, F. V., Flower, C. D. R. (1990) Rupture of the right hemidiaphragm following blunt trauma: the use of ultrasound in diagnosis. *Clinical Radiology*, **42**, 97–101.

Valliers, E., Shamji, F. M., Todd, T. R. (1993) Post pneumonectomy chylothorax. *Annals of Thoracic Surgery*, **55**, 1006–1008.

Wiot, J. F. (1975) The radiologic manifestations of blunt chest trauma. *Journal of the American Medical Association*, **231**, 500.

The postoperative chest and intensive care

Carter, A. R., Sostman, H. D., Curtis, A. M., Swett, H. A. (1983) Thoracic alterations after cardiac surgery. *American Journal of Roentgenology*, **140**, 475–481.

Goodman, L. R. (1980) Postoperative chest radiograph: 1. Alterations after abdominal surgery. *American Journal of Roentgenology*, **134**, 533–541.

Goodman, L. R. (1980) Postoperative chest radiograph: 11. Alterations after major intrathoracic surgery. *American Journal of Roentgenology*, **134**, 803–813.

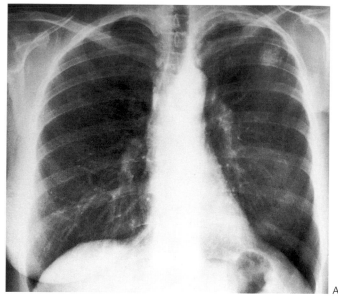
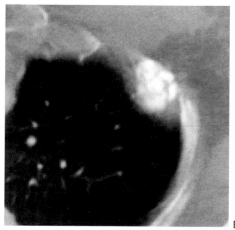

Fig. 18.42 Radiation-induced osteonecrosis. **A.** Chest radiograph obtained 15 years after left mastectomy and radiation therapy demonstrates a dense opacity projected over the left second rib. **B.** On CT there is a calcified mass arising from the second rib. Long-term follow-up showed no evidence of progression.

Goodman, L. R., Kuzo, M. D. (eds) (1996) Intensive care radiology. *Radiological Clinics of North America*, **34**, 1.

Spirn, P. W., Gross, G. W., Wechsler, R. J., Steiner, R. M. (1988) Radiology of the chest after thoracic surgery. *Seminars in Roentgenology*, **23**, 9–31.

Thorsen, M. K., Goodman, L. R. (1988) Extracardiac complications of cardiac surgery. *Seminars in Roentgenology*, **23**, 32–48.

Radiation injury of the lung

Boushy, S. F., Belgason, A. H., Borth, L. B. (1970) The effect of radiation on the lung and bronchial tree. *American Journal of Roentgenology*, **108**, 284–292.

Davis, S. D., Yankelevitz, D. F., Henschke, C. I. (1992) Radiation effects on the lung: clinical features, pathology and imaging findings. *American Journal of Roentgenology*, **159**, 1157–1164.

Huvos, A. G., Woodward, H. Q., Cahan, W. B., et al (1985) Post irradiation osteogenic sarcoma of bone and soft tissue: a clinico-pathologic study in 66 patients. *Cancer*, **55**, 1244–1255.

Ikezoe, J., Takashima, S., Morimoto, S., et al (1988) CT appearance of acute radiation-induced injury in the lung. *American Journal of Roentgenology*, **150**, 765–770.

Libshitz, H. I., Shuman, L. S. (1984) Radiation-induced pulmonary change: CT findings. *Journal of Computer Assisted Tomography*, **8**, 15–19.

Polansky, S. M., Ravin, C. E., Prosnitz, I. R. (1980) Lung changes after breast irradiation. *American Journal of Roentgenology*, **139**, 101–105.

Rowinsky, E. K., Abeloff, M. D., Wharam, M. D. (1985) Spontaneous pneumothorax following thoracic irradiation. *Chest*, **88**, 703–708.

Wencel, M. L., Sitrin, R. G. (1988) Unilateral lung hyperlucency after mediastinal irradiation. *American Research into Respiratory Disease*, **137**, 955–957.

19

THE CHEST IN CHILDREN

Donald Shaw

TECHNIQUES

Plain Radiographs These remain the basis for evaluation of the chest in childhood. In the neonate, satisfactory films can be obtained in incubators using modern mobile X-ray apparatus. The baby lies on the cassette and the film is exposed. Although automatic triggering of the exposure can be made using variations of temperature at the nostril and of electrical impedance across the chest in the differing phases of respiration, an experienced radiographer will usually be able to judge the end of inspiration. An adequate inspiration will be with the right hemidiaphragm at the level of the eighth rib posteriorly. Films in expiration frequently show a sharp kink in the trachea to the right and varying degrees of opacification of the lung fields, with apparent enlargement of the heart. Films should be well collimated, the baby positioned as straight as possible and lordotic films avoided, especially if the heart size is of particular interest. As much monitoring equipment as possible should be removed. Magnification radiography in the neonate allows better evaluation of the lung granularity in hyaline membrane disease, but the construction of most incubators makes this technique difficult and its vogue has passed.

Computed radiography is proving of particular use in intensive care, and the ability of data manipulation to show better supportive apparatus such as tubes is useful.

Children over five years can usually cooperate sufficiently to stand for a PA film like adults. Below this age some form of chest stand is needed in which an assistant, preferably the mother, can hold the child in front of a cassette with a suspended protective lead apron behind which she stands. With proper collimation, the dose to the mother is small and her position allows the child to be held straighter than from a position to the side. The difference between a PA and an AP projection in the small child is usually negligible. High kilovoltage techniques with added filtration and the use of a grid allow evaluation of the trachea and major bronchi, which is important in stridor, in investigating mediastinal masses and to assess isomerism in congenital heart disease.

Fluoroscopy Limitation of radiation exposure is vital in childhood, but quick fluoroscopic examination of the chest can frequently prove extremely useful, in particular in the evaluation of differing lung radiolucencies in suspected foreign body aspiration. With obstructive emphysema, the affected lung will show little volume change in respiration and the mediastinum will swing contralaterally in expiration. Prior to the advent of computed tomography, fluoroscopy had been advocated for the detection of dubious lung metastases.

A *barium swallow* is a useful adjunct to the evaluation of pediatric lung disease, especially when there is stridor, or mediastinal masses or vascular anomalies are suspected.

Tomography Conventional tomography generally gives poor results in children and has been superseded by computed tomography, particularly in the detection of pulmonary metastases, especially in Wilms tumor and bone sarcomas. Intrathecal contrast media are generally no longer used as adjuncts to CT scanning of paravertebral masses.

High-resolution CT scanning has effectively replaced bronchography in the diagnosis of bronchiectasis though occasional opacification of the bronchial tree is indicated for local bronchostenotic lesions. Experience is growing in the evaluation of parenchymal disease such as the various alveolitides. Spiral scanning will overcome many of the problems with movement in childhood.

Angiography Angiography is infrequently used in extracardiac chest pathology. It provides valuable information, however, in arteriovenous malformation and pulmonary sequestrations. *Digital vascular imaging* has proved a less invasive technique in such cases. *Embolization of bronchial arteries* has been used in bronchiectatic severe hemorrhage.

Radionuclide Scanning Perfusion studies with technetium-99m macroaggregates are well established in adults, but, in children, combination with a ventilation scan using krypton-81 m is a more useful technique for investigating the unilateral small lung, differing radiolucency, suspected bronchiectasis and hypoplasia or aplasia of the pulmonary vasculature.

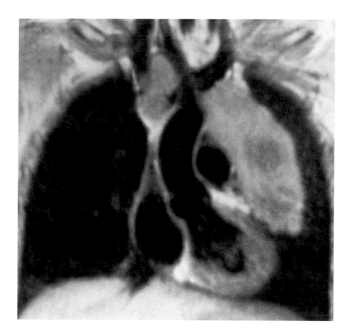

Fig. 19.1 Coronal MRI scan (T₁-weighted) in a child with a mediastinal mass. Note how the heart and great vessels are readily differentiated by low signal due to blood flow from the glandular masses due to Hodgkin's disease.

Ultrasound Ultrasound has proved useful in confirming the diagnosis of pleural and pericardial effusions and in indicating appropriate sites for aspiration of fluid. Mass lesions, particularly when close to the chest wall and in the mediastinum, can be evaluated.

MRI Experience in the use of this method is increasing. The advantages of an inherently higher contrast resolution are partly offset by image degradation, particularly due to respiratory movement. The longer scanning times, often associated with a noisy environment, may require the child to have a general anesthetic or at least to be heavily sedated. Evaluation of mediastinal structures, however (Fig. 19.1), has proved successful, particularly in cases of tumor, aberrant pulmonary vessels and extrinsic compressive lesions of the airways. Extension into and involvement of the spinal canal and spinal cord is also well assessed (Fig. 12.43). MRI has proved particularly useful in the differentiation of physiologically prominent thymic shadows from shadows caused by a pathological process such as lymphoma. As elsewhere in the body, MRI is of value in the evaluation of musculoskeletal lesions, particularly rib and shoulder girdle tumors.

As yet, parenchymal lesions cannot be investigated with as good a resolution as can be achieved by CT, the preferred technique for evaluation and enumeration of pulmonary metastases and detection of calcified lesions.

SPECIFIC FEATURES OF THE CHEST RADIOGRAPH IN CHILDREN

The Thymus The normal thymus is a frequent cause of widening of the superior mediastinum during the first years of life. The lateral margin often shows an undulation—the thymic wave—which corresponds to the indentations of the ribs on the inner surface of the thoracic cage. Particularly on the right, the thymus may have a triangular 'sail-like' configuration. The thymus may involute in times of stress, and a decrease in size can be induced by steroids. At times, the differentiation of physiologic thymus from pathology in the anterior mediastinum can be difficult. Ultrasound examination will usually differentiate cystic lesions from the homogenous normal thymic tissue. Occasionally the normal thymus can act as a significant space-occupying lesion in the superior mediastinum and in such cases differentiation may be helped by computed tomography or MRI.

The Cardiothoracic Ratio In toddlers, the cardiothoracic ratio can at times exceed 50% and care should be exercised in overdiagnosis of cardiomegaly.

Kink of the Trachea to the Right This is a frequent feature of a chest film taken in less than full inspiration. This is a physiologic buckling and does not represent a mass lesion.

The Soft Tissues These may be prominent in children, and the anterior axillary fold crossing the chest wall can at times mimic a pneumothorax. Similarly, skin folds can at times cast confusing shadows. Plaits of hair over the upper chest can mimic pulmonary infiltrations.

Pleural Effusions Whereas in adults an early sign of pleural effusion is blunting of the costophrenic angles, in childhood it is more common to see separation of the lung from the chest wall with reasonable preservation of the clarity of the costophrenic angles, and accentuation of the lung fissures.

THE SMALL LUNG

Discovery of a small lung on a radiograph can be elucidated by ventilation and perfusion radionuclide lung scans using krypton-81 and technetium-99m macroaggregates. The complete absence of V–Q in one lung in the presence of an ipsilateral opaque hemithorax, with mediastinal shift to the affected side, is highly suggestive of a diagnosis of pulmonary aplasia or of extreme pulmonary hypoplasia.

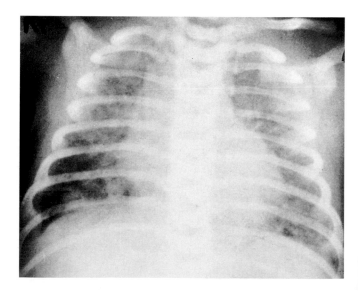

Fig. 19.2 Wet lung, or transient tachypnea of the newborn. Patchy parenchymal shadowing on the first day of life.

The complete absence of perfusion in a small lung, with a decreased ventilation, is typical of congenital absence of the pulmonary artery. Both perfusion and ventilation are shown to be decreased in the presence of a small hemithorax, as may be seen in *Macleod syndrome*, with postinfective maldevelopment, with aplasias of single lobes and with pulmonary hypoplasia. A segmental perfusion defect in a fully ventilated lung is associated with pulmonary sequestration.

RESPIRATORY DISTRESS IN THE NEWBORN

Transient Tachypnea of the Newborn, or Wet Lung Disease (Fig. 19.2)

The amount of fluid in the newborn lung varies, but typically is quickly cleared after birth. Some babies, however, show a transient respiratory distress due to excess lung fluid. Predisposing conditions include prematurity, a diabetic mother and cesarean section. The radiographs show diffuse parenchymal patchy shadowing with perihilar streakiness. The prognosis in this condition is good and there is usually progressive clearing, complete within two or three days.

Hyaline Membrane Disease (Fig. 19.3)

In this condition a deficiency of the pulmonary surfactant leads to alveolar collapse. Conditions which predispose to this include prematurity, cesarean section and perinatal asphyxia. In mild hyaline membrane disease, the radiological appearances consist of a mild granularity throughout the lung fields. As the condition

becomes more severe, an air bronchogram becomes apparent. In the most severe cases the lungs are virtually opaque, with loss of differentiation of the cardiac and thymic and diaphragmatic contours. Uncomplicated hyaline membrane disease is a symmetric condition.

Bronchopulmonary Dysplasia (Fig. 19.4)

Severe hyaline membrane disease is typically treated by artificial ventilation of the lungs. If ventilation needs to be prolonged (especially if high pressures and high inspiratory oxygen tensions are required), damage can occur to the lungs. The hyaline membrane present in the alveoli becomes organized and fibrous tissue develops within the lungs. As a consequence, areas of the lungs collapse, with compensatory emphysema developing in residual aerated alveoli. This leads to a coarse reticulation and at times to variable amounts of segmental collapse, and occasionally to considerable areas of localized emphysema. Whereas hyaline membrane disease, if uncomplicated, and transient tachypnea of the newborn will quickly resolve, bronchopulmonary dysplasia can lead to severe respiratory distress lasting months and may end in respiratory failure and death.

Pulmonary Interstitial Emphysema (Fig. 19.5)

In this condition gas enters the interstitial tissues of the lungs and gives rise to multiple small lucencies throughout the lung fields. Some of these lucencies are due to air passing from the interstitial tissue into the relatively large lymphatics of the newborn lungs. A lung affected by interstitial emphysema is frequently larger than

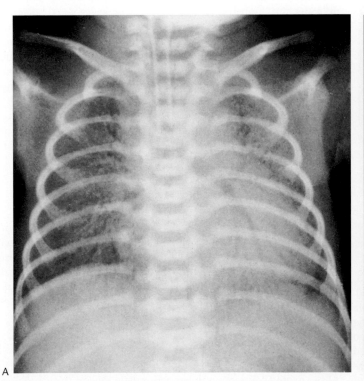 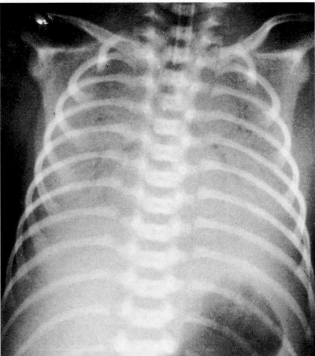

Fig. 19.3 Hyaline membrane disease. **A.** Mild changes aged 1 day—fine reticulonodular shadowing with accentuation of the air bronchogram. Endotracheal tube. **B.** More advanced changes aged 3 days—marked opacification with loss of diaphragmatic and cardiac contours.

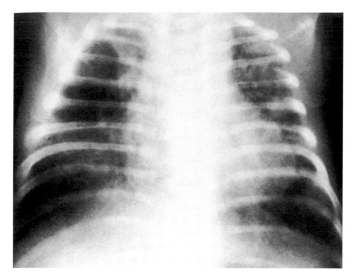

Fig. 19.4   Bronchopulmonary dysplasia. Patchy shadowing from areas of loss of volume and fibrosis, with areas of compensatory emphysema, especially in the right upper lobe.

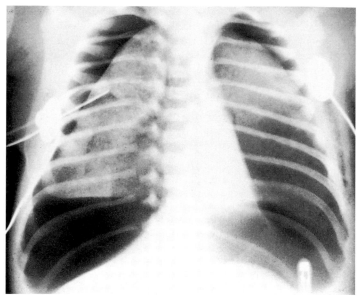

Fig. 19.6   Bilateral pneumothoraces in hyaline membrane disease. Right intercostal drain.

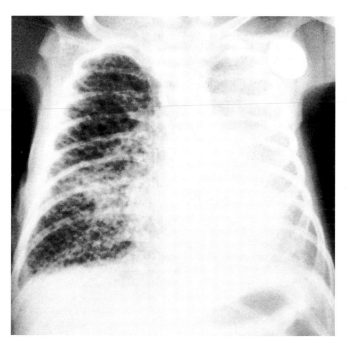

Fig. 19.5   Pulmonary interstitial emphysema. Fine reticular shadowing in the right lung with deviation of the mediastinum contralaterally. Hyaline membrane disease in the left lung.

the contralateral one and may lead to deviation of the mediastinum. If bilateral, venous return to the heart can be impeded. Interstitial emphysema is a frequent precursor of *pneumothorax* (Fig. 19.6) and pneumo-mediastinum. At times, the child being artificially ventilated for hyaline membrane disease will undergo marked deterioration, with the appearance of a bloodstained tracheal aspirate. This is frequently due to *pulmonary hemorrhage* and is accompanied by a marked increase in the opacification of the lungs as the alveoli become filled with hemorrhagic edema. If the child's condition stabilizes, the edema is usually quickly

resorbed, but such a hemorrhage can frequently be a terminal event. It is important in the evaluation of neonatal respiratory distress to be adequately acquainted with the obstetric and maternal history. If there is a history of prolonged rupture of the membranes, patchy shadowing seen in the newborn lungs may well be due to *intrauterine pneumonia*. If there has been intrauterine respiratory distress, *aspiration of meconium* can lead to respiratory embarrassment. The lungs typically show bilateral, symmetric, rather coarse shadowing, with frequent overdistension, complicated from time to time by pneumothorax and pneumomediastinum. Resolution of meconium aspiration can be prolonged. The *Mikity–Wilson syndrome* is essentially a radiological appearance consisting of diffuse interstitial infiltrations giving rise to a multicystic appearance. Onset is usually accompanied by apnea and cyanosis in premature babies, later in the first week of life. Episodes of aspiration probably account for at least part of the syndrome, and if resolution does not occur, the condition can at times progress to bronchopulmonary dysplasia.

Pleural Effusions

In the newborn these may be part of hydrops fetalis or of congestive cardiac failure. Chylothorax is the most common condition, causing a large pleural effusion; such effusions most frequently occur in the right pleural cavity when unilateral and can lead to respiratory distress with deviation of the mediastinum. With repeated pleural aspiration the effusion usually disappears over a period of a week or two.

Congenital Lobar Emphysema

Gross overinflation of an upper and middle lobe in this condition leads to infantile respiratory distress with contralateral deviation of the mediastinum, and compression of the other lobes of the

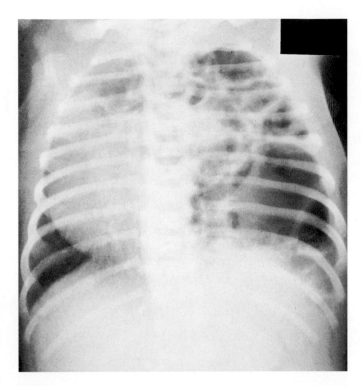

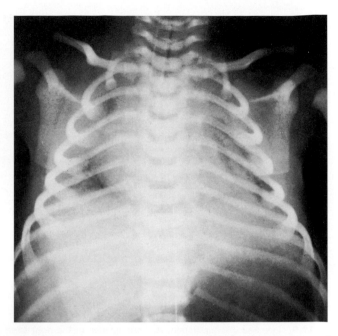

Fig. 19.8 Pulmonary hypoplasia. The rib cage shows the typical triangular configuration. An umbilical aortic catheter is present.

Fig. 19.7 Diaphragmatic hernia. Stomach and intestine occupy the left hemithorax with deviation of the mediastinum to the right.

same lung. Excision is often necessary. A similar but less florid appearance can be produced by a persistent ductus arteriosus obstructing the left upper lobe.

Cystic Adenomatoid Malformation

This rare congenital cystic anomaly can lead to deviation of the mediastinum and compression of adjacent normal lung, leading to neonatal distress, or may present as repeated localized pneumonia. The cysts, which may be filled with fluid in the neonatal period, are usually obvious.

Congenital Diaphragmatic Hernia (Fig. 19.7)

This is most frequently through the posterolateral part of the diaphragm, more frequently on the left. The hemithorax is filled with stomach or gut and as the newborn baby swallows gas, distension leads to respiratory embarrassment with contralateral deviation of the mediastinum. Surgical correction is urgently required; otherwise the condition is frequently fatal. The ipsilateral lung is usually hypoplastic. Congenital heart disease is an important association.

Pulmonary Hypoplasia (Fig. 19.8)

This condition is frequently lethal, and is often associated with prenatal obstructive uropathy or renal aplasia. The lungs are small and the thoracic configuration triangular. Hypoplastic lungs are seen in several *skeletal dysplasias* such as asphyxiating thoracic dystrophy.

At times it is difficult to differentiate whether respiratory distress is due to lung disease or to congenital heart disease. However the clinical findings and the response to oxygenation and artificial ventilation will frequently allow such differentiation. Real-time cardiac ultrasound considerably facilitates diagnosis of structural anomalies of the neonatal heart, but at times resort must be made to formal cardiac catheterization.

Extracorporeal Membrane Oxygenation

Support by this technique is of particular use in congenital diaphragmatic hernia and in severe oxygenation problems in small babies as a temporary measure. Plain radiography will show the typically rather dense, infrequently ventilated lungs and importantly the position of the arterial and venous catheters and the presence of complications such as air leaks, pleural effusions and hemorrhagic collections.

CONGENITAL PULMONARY SEQUESTRATION (Fig. 19.9)

This is an abnormality of development in which a portion of the lung shows separation from the normal bronchial tree and blood supply, though retaining some characteristics of lung tissue. Cases can be divided into intralobar, lying within the lung, and extralobar, in which the sequestrated segment develops enclosed in its own pleura (when it is termed by some 'an accessory lung'). In intralobar sequestration there is a non-functioning portion of the lung, usually lying posteriorly in the left lower lobe. The right lower lobe is the next most common situation, and other lobes are rarely affected. Typically the segment is not connected with the normal bronchial tree, and when communication is established it is usually in association with infection. The radiological appearances are of a soft-tissue mass in the posterior part of the lower

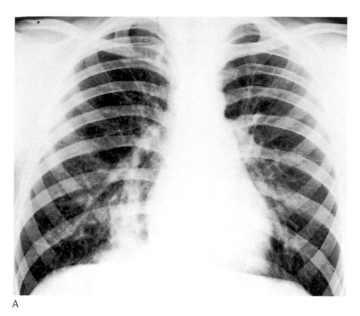

A

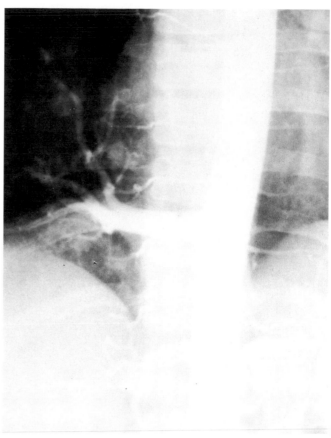

B

Fig. 19.9   Pulmonary sequestration. **A.** Consolidation in the right lower lobe was associated with absent bronchial filling on bronchography. **B.** Angiography demonstrated a large feeding artery arising from the right of the descending thoracic aorta.

lobe, usually on the left contiguous with the diaphragm. If connection has been established with the bronchial tree, air-containing cystic masses with or without air–fluid levels will be seen. Bronchographic contrast medium rarely enters the lesion. The bronchial tree is spread round the mass and is typically complete in the number of its divisions. Extralobar sequestrations are much less common, and usually interposed between the inferior surface of the left lower lobe and the diaphragm. They are frequently associated with other congenital anomalies and found incidentally during neonatal autopsies. Left-sided congenital diaphragmatic hernia may be associated.

Intralobar sequestrations typically derive their arterial blood supply from the aorta, usually the descending thoracic aorta, occasionally the abdominal aorta. Usually the venous drainage is via the pulmonary venous system, but occasionally via the inferior vena cava or azygos system. In contrast to the intralobar variety, venous drainage of extralobar sequestration is usually via the inferior vena cava, azygos or portal venous systems. The arterial supply is frequently from the abdominal aorta or one of its branches. The diagnosis of sequestrated segment should be borne in mind whenever an unusual abscess, cavity or cystic lesion is seen, particularly at the left base, and in all cases showing recurrent infection in one part of the lung.

CONGENITAL BRONCHIAL ATRESIA

This abnormality consists of an atresia of a lobar or smaller segment of bronchus, and particularly affects the apical posterior segment of the bronchus of the left upper lobe. Mucous secretions inspissated within the patent airways distal to the atresia can produce an elliptic mass. Peripheral to this, collateral air drift causes overinflation. Fluoroscopy will show expiratory air trapping in the involved segments and the vascular supply is diminished.

Although the lesion may be associated with infection, it is usually discovered on routine chest radiography.

PULMONARY ARTERIOVENOUS FISTULAE

Arteriovenous fistulae are commonly asymptomatic, but some patients will show cyanosis, clubbing and polycythemia and others will present with hemoptysis. About half of the patients with arteriovenous fistulae in the lungs (Fig. 19.10) will show such abnormal communications elsewhere in the skin and other organs (Rendu–Osler–Weber syndrome). Although the large fistulae typically present rounded homogenous masses with enlarged serpiginous vessels radiating to the hilum, there is a high incidence of multiple lesions in the lungs and, if resection is contemplated, careful angiographic evaluation of both lungs should be carried out preoperatively. Digital vascular imaging has facilitated this.

MUCOVISCIDOSIS

(*Cystic fibrosis of the pancreas*) Chronic suppuration in the lungs is an important feature of this condition, in which many organ systems are involved. The lungs appear normal at birth but poor clearance of bronchial secretions leads to obstruction, particularly of the smaller bronchi. In infancy this can lead to overdistension of the lungs, resulting in flattening of the diaphragms, sternal bowing and increased dorsal kyphosis. Infiltration of the bron-

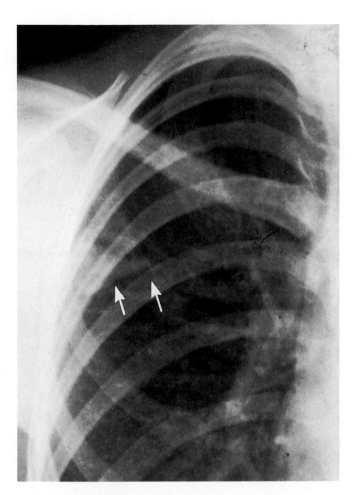

Fig. 19.10 Arteriovenous malformation. Peripheral serpiginous dilated blood vessels in the right upper lobe.

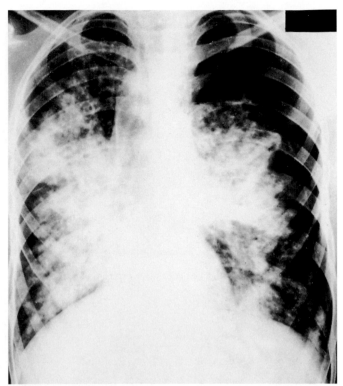

Fig. 19.11 Advanced cystic fibrosis (mucoviscidosis). Gross peribronchial shadowing with confluent pneumonic shadowing. There is a left pneumothorax with slight displacement of the mediastinum to the right.

chial walls by lymphocytes and plasma cells is seen radiologically as peribronchial thickening, particularly noticeable in bronchi seen end-on. Small discrete opacities are seen in later childhood in the periphery of the lung fields, due to small peripheral abscesses. When these burst into the bronchioles they remain as small thin-walled air spaces. Segmental bronchiectasis is seen consequent upon segmental collapse and consolidation. The upper lobes are more frequently involved in the bronchiectasis associated with cystic fibrosis than in other forms. Parabronchial abscesses can give rise to a more specific form of bronchiectasis, with characteristic rounded shadows arising close to the medium-sized bronchi with a widespread irregular distribution throughout the lung fields (Fig. 19.11). Pulmonary suppuration can lead to hilar lymph node enlargement. The hilar shadows may also be enlarged in the later stages of the disease, when pulmonary hypertension arises as a complication. In later childhood peripheral areas of emphysema arise as a result of the fibrotic changes occurring more centrally.

Pneumothorax is an important complication in the later stages of the disease and can lead to dramatic deterioration. The emphysematous changes are usually associated with a relatively narrow heart shadow, but cardiac enlargement in cor pulmonale is usually a sign of a poor prognosis. Although the infections

associated are usually staphylococcal, *Pseudomonas* or other Gram-negative infections, superinfection with tuberculosis and *Aspergillus* can occur. In the latter this may be associated with total collapse of the lung or extensive variable areas of consolidation, sometimes with considerable parenchymal destruction. Repeated suppuration can lead to severe hemorrhage, and bronchial artery embolization has been used to control such life-threatening episodes.

Pleural disease is an uncommon feature, but is recognized as a late complication, when it can compromise selection for heart-lung transplantation, in which preoperative CT evaluation has proved useful.

LANGERHANS CELL HISTIOCYTOSIS
(*Histiocytosis X*)

In childhood, bone and central nervous system manifestations are frequently more prominent than lung involvement. Fine widespread nodularity can at times resemble miliary tuberculosis (Fig. 19.12), but often shows a reticular pattern which may progress to 'honeycomb' lung and complicating pneumothoraces.

BRONCHIOLITIS

This is often associated with the respiratory syncytial virus or pertussis. The lungs appear overinflated, with streaky peribronchiolar shadows. More confluent consolidation may complicate a frequently grave clinical condition.

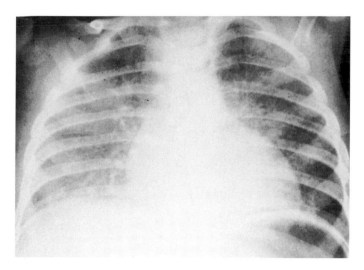

Fig. 19.12 Histiocytosis X. Fine nodularity in both lung fields.

INHALED FOREIGN BODIES (Fig. 19.13)

The variety of objects which children manage to aspirate is wide but peanuts are very common. There is a tendency to enter the more vertical right main bronchus. Complete obstruction will lead to peripheral collapse but partial obstruction can lead to obstructive emphysema. Films in expiration as well as inspiration, supplemented if necessary by fluoroscopy, will show mediastinal shift away from the obstructive emphysema on expiration. Bronchoscopy should be performed on strong clinical grounds even if the radiographs are normal.

TRAUMA

Contusion of the lung can occur without rib fracture. Patchy resulting hemorrhagic consolidation can cavitate or resolve uneventfully.

HYDROCARBON ASPIRATION

Petrol or kerosene (paraffin), if accidentally swallowed, can enter the trachea and may cause patchy basal lung shadowing, sometimes with delayed onset and sometimes with pneumatocele formation (Fig. 19.14).

IMMUNE COMPROMISE

A wide variety of common viruses, such as measles, or less common organisms such as *Pneumocystis* or cytomegalovirus, cause extensive pulmonary shadowing in leukemia or in children with immune deficiency or undergoing chemotherapy. At times biopsy may be necessary to establish the diagnosis, although *Pneumocystis* frequently has a typical appearance with gross opacification (Fig. 19.15) and an air bronchogram.

In *acquired immune deficiency syndrome* (AIDS) in childhood, in addition to those infections common to the immune-

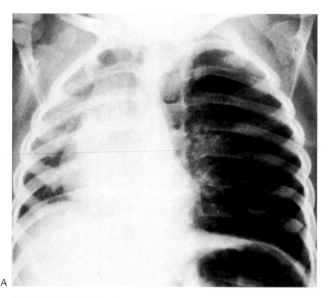

A

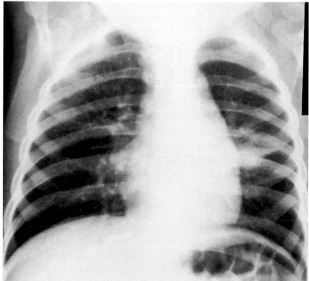

B

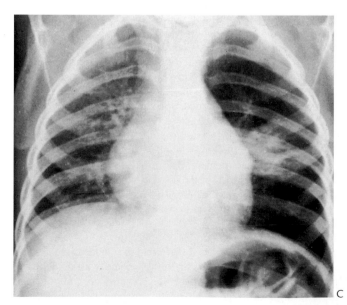

C

Fig. 19.13 Foreign body inhalation. **A.** Obstructive emphysema from a foreign body in the left main bronchus. **B,C** Same child later; loss of volume in the left lung with patchy collapse in the apex of the left lower lobe; in inspiration (**B**) the mediastinum is slightly to the left; in expiration (**C**) the volume to the left lung changes little with the mediastinum swinging to the right.

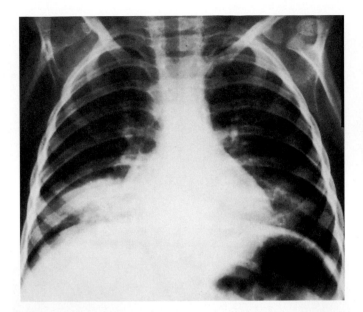

Fig. 19.14 Kerosene (paraffin) aspiration. Basal shadowing with early left basal pneumatocele.

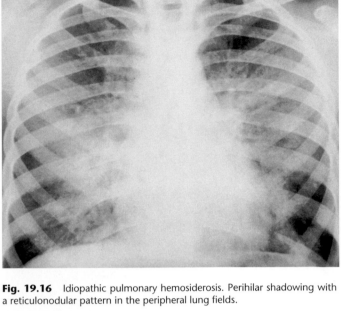

Fig. 19.16 Idiopathic pulmonary hemosiderosis. Perihilar shadowing with a reticulonodular pattern in the peripheral lung fields.

IDIOPATHIC PULMONARY HEMOSIDEROSIS
(Fig. 19.16)

This serious condition, frequently fatal in early adulthood, starts in childhood with repeated pulmonary hemorrhage, at first revealed as patchy shadowing with intervening clearing, but progressing to permanent linear and reticular shadowing.

ASTHMA

Prolonged episodic bronchospasm reveals itself radiologically as overdistension of the lungs with a low flat diaphragm, sternal bowing, peribronchial shadowing seen as 'rings' end-on or 'tramlines' longitudinally, with occasional patchy shadowing. *Aspergillus* colonization can lead to extensive parenchymal shadowing.

Pneumomediastinum is most usually associated with asthma in childhood; extension results in subcutaneous emphysema, particularly in the neck. Pneumothorax may also, uncommonly, complicate asthma.

TUBERCULOSIS

This is described in Chapter 15. In childhood, miliary tuberculosis is still too frequently seen, especially in immigrants. It can be congenital. A fine nodularity is evenly distributed throughout both lung fields (Fig. 19.17). At times, mediastinal lymph node enlargement is also apparent.

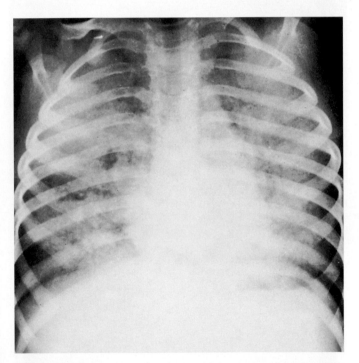

Fig. 19.15 *Pneumocystis* pneumonia. Widespread alveolar shadowing.

compromised, a widespread nodularity in the lung fields can represent lymphocytic infiltration.

BRONCHIECTASIS

Bronchiectasis is much less commonly seen now and is usually associated with some immune compromise. It may also follow local damage to the airways such as a retained foreign body or following severe infections.

PNEUMONIA

Many childhood pneumonias are viral in origin, with non-specific features of patchy consolidation, overdistension and prominent hilar shadows (Fig. 19.18), because of the relatively narrow peripheral airways in the young.

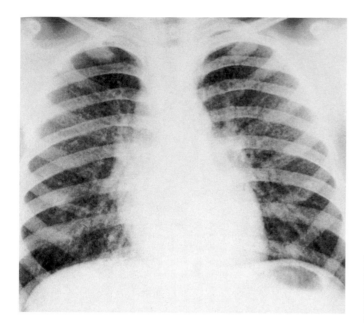

Fig. 19.17 Miliary tuberculosis. Fine nodularity throughout both lungs.

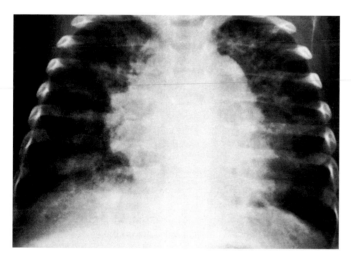

Fig. 19.18 Measles. Hilar lymph node enlargement with streaky shadowing radiating into the central lung fields.

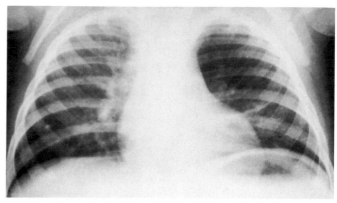

Fig. 19.19 Pneumatocele. Previous left staphylococcal pneumonia.

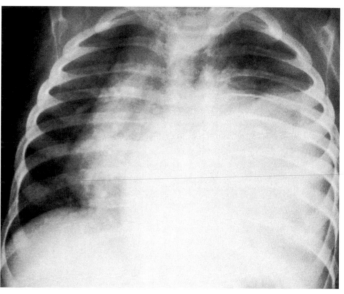

Fig. 19.20 Neuroblastoma. A large left posterior mass deviates the mediastinum to the right, with thinning and separation of the adjacent posterior ends of the ribs.

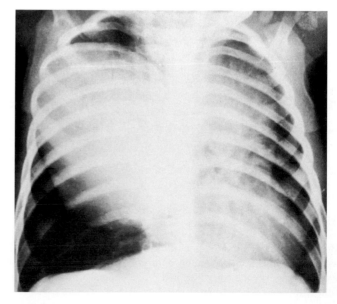

Fig. 19.21 Foregut duplication cyst with obstructive emphysema of the right lung.

An important complication is obliterative bronchiolitis. Decreased vascularity of the affected areas leads to radiolucency, and relative failure of lung growth is associated with air trapping (*Macleod* or *Swyer–James syndrome*).

Staphylococcal pneumonia, in its earlier stages non-specific in appearance, can develop highly characteristic pneumatoceles (Fig. 19.19) showing as thin-walled radiolucencies which can at times rapidly enlarge and lead to pneumothorax. Their resolution is frequently slow, with persistence long after pneumonic consolidation has resolved.

INTRATHORACIC MASSES

Neurogenic tumors such as neuroblastoma (Fig. 19.20) and ganglioneuroma are typically posterior, frequently deforming ribs.

Calcification within the tumor and pleural effusions may be present.

Foregut duplication and bronchogenic cysts are common middle mediastinal masses (Fig. 19.21) and can cause bronchial or esophageal compression. Vertebral anomalies are frequent. Ectopic gastric mucosa may be demonstrated by technetium-99m in some of these cysts.

Cystic hygromas usually have a component in the neck as well as extension into the upper chest. Ultrasound is useful to demonstrate their characteristic massively cystic appearance.

Hilar lymph node enlargement occurs more obviously in pneumonia in childhood and is a feature of lymphoma and metastatic malignancies.

REFERENCES AND SUGGESTIONS FOR FURTHER READING

Avery, M. E., Fletcher, B. D., Williams, R. G. (1981) *The Lung and its Disorders in the Newborn Infant*, 4th edn. (Major Problems in Clinical Pediatrics.) Philadelphia: W.B. Saunders.

Carty, H., Shaw D., Brunelle, F., Kendall, B., (eds) (1994) *Imaging Children*. London: Churchill Livingstone.

Chernick, V., Kendig, E. L. (1990) *Disorders of the Respiratory Tract in Children*, 5th edn. Philadelphia: W.B. Saunders.

Felman, A. H. (1987) *Radiology of the Pediatric Chest. Clinical and Pathological Correlations*. New York: McGraw-Hill.

Griscom, N. T., Wohl, M. E. B., Kirkpatrick, J. A. (1987) Lower respiratory infections; how infants differ from adults. *Radiologic Clinics of North America*, **16**, 367–387.

Kaufmann, H. J. (ed) (1967) *Progress in Paediatric Radiology. Vol. 1. Respiratory Tract*. Basel: Karger.

Phelan, P. D., Landau, L. I., Olinsky, A. (1982). *Respiratory Illness in Children*, 2nd edn. Oxford: Blackwell.

Silverman, F., Kuhn, J., (eds) (1985) *Caffey's Pediatric X-ray Diagnosis*, 8th edn. Chicago: Year Book.

Singleton, E. B., Wagner, M. L. (1971) *Radiologic Atlas of Pulmonary Abnormalities in Children*. Philadelphia: W. B. Saunders.

Swischuk, L. E. (1989) *Imaging of the Newborn Infant and Young Child*, 3rd edn. Baltimore: Williams & Wilkins.

Wesenberg, R. L. (1973) *The Newborn Chest*. Hagerston, M. D.: Harper & Row.

20

THE NORMAL HEART: METHODS OF EXAMINATION

M. J. Raphael and R. M. Donaldson
With contributions from Richard W. Whitehouse, Jeremy P. R. Jenkins and E. Rhys Davies

PLAIN FILMS

The plain chest film, although it rarely provides a specific diagnosis of cardiac abnormality, is sufficiently important to be considered an integral part of the complete clinical assessment of the patient suspected of suffering from heart disease. It may indicate the nature of the functional derangement, and also its severity. To do this it should show the overall heart size, and evidence of selective chamber enlargement. It must also be of sufficient quality to enable the lung vessels to be studied. The standard cardiac series has consisted in the past of a low-kilovolt (kV) chest film to show lung parenchyma, a penetrated postero-anterior chest film to see detail within the heart, and a left lateral film with barium in the oesophagus to show left atrial size. Today, a high-kV posteroanterior chest with an antiscatter system represents an excellent single frontal film compromise, enabling intracardiac details and lung vessel anatomy to be seen on one film. Combined with a high-quality lateral film, so that the left lower-lobe bronchus may be identified, a two-film cardiac study is adequate for routine purposes, although calcification is difficult to perceive.

There is no place for routine oblique films in the examination of the heart. They are impossible to standardize and rarely give information which cannot be obtained more satisfactorily by other means.

FLUOROSCOPY

Image amplification fluoroscopy is easily performed but has only a limited place in the examination of the heart. Screening will show the relationship of any abnormal shadows to the heart. It is excellent for recognizing and locating intracardiac calcification, and may be of slight value in studying prosthetic valves.

Even in experienced hands it is of only limited value in the study of left ventricular aneurysm. The recognition of hilar dance in left to right shunts, and of systolic expansion of the left atrium in the diagnosis of mitral incompetence, are now of purely historical interest.

TOMOGRAPHY

Whereas conventional tomography has virtually no place in present-day cardiac radiology, CT is of value in the investigation of the heart and great vessels.

CARDIAC COMPUTED TOMOGRAPHY

Richard W. Whitehouse

Technical Considerations Conventional CT scanners now have image acquisition times of 1–2 s for 360° scans and as little as 0.6 s for partial scans. Even so, a significant proportion of the cardiac cycle will occur during this time, resulting in blurring of the cardiac image. Ultrafast CT, using a scanner designed to obtain images in 50 or 100 ms acquisition times by magnetically deflecting the X-ray beam around an anode in an X-ray tube which partially encircles the patient can produce rapid sequential images of cardiac function within one cardiac cycle. This equipment is commercially available but expensive, and so clinical availability is limited.

Dynamic spatial reconstruction, a technique using multiple X-ray tubes and image intensifier chains to produce 'real time' multiple cross-sections with similar image acquisition times to ultrafast CT is not commercially available.

The role of conventional CT for cardiac imaging is in practice losing ground to ultrasound, MRI, and isotope studies, all of which have had greater development of functional cardiac measurements in addition to imaging. Conventional CT does, however, produce

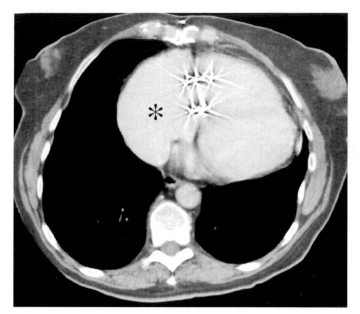

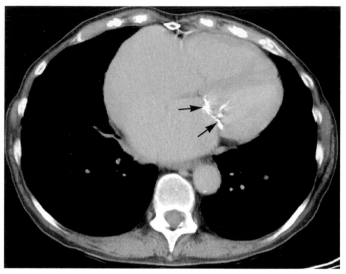

Fig. 20.3 Mitral valve ring calcification (arrow) (spiral scan). (Courtesy of Dr R. Sawyer.)

Fig. 20.1 Ebstein anomaly treated with a tricuspid valve replacement. Note the markedly enlarged right atrium (*).

satisfactory images of cardiac anatomy, particularly with contrast enhancement to demonstrate chamber anatomy and the great vessels. CT is established for morphological diagnosis, particularly in congenital heart disease (Fig. 20.1), intracardiac masses, and pericardial disease. Electrocardiographic gating of CT data acquisition can be used to improve the relationship of conventional CT images to phases of the cardiac cycle but is not widely used in practice.

Normal Appearances The relationships of the cardiac chambers, their sizes, and concordance can be demonstrated by sequential scanning during rapid bolus injection of contrast medium (Fig. 20.2). The chamber wall thicknesses can be estimated on contrast-enhanced scans but not on unenhanced scans where the attenuation of blood is similar to muscle. Cardiac valve structure

and motion cannot be well seen due to motion blurring, but calcification in the valve rings can be demonstrated (Fig. 20.3). Calcification in coronary arteries can be demonstrated, but ultrafast CT is required to reliably measure its location and extent (the value of spiral CT for identifying coronary artery calcification is currently under assessment (Fig. 20.4)). The absence of coronary artery calcification on ultrafast CT effectively excludes significant coronary artery stenosis.

Myocardial Infarction Chamber wall thickness on contrast-enhanced ungated CT is effectively measured in diastole as the cardiac cycle is relatively longer in diastole than systole. Thinning of the left ventricular myocardium and interventricular septum may be seen after myocardial infarction. Intracardiac thrombus adherent to the endocardium may also be evident as non-enhancing filling defects (Fig. 20.4).

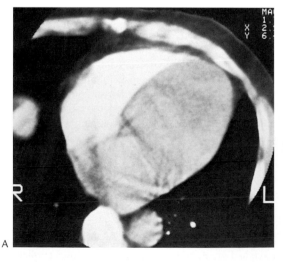

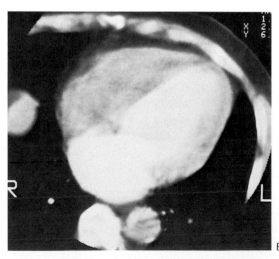

Fig. 20.2 Normal intracardiac anatomy. Sequential scans at the same level demonstrate transit of contrast medium through (**A**) right ventricle and (**B**) left atrium and ventricle.

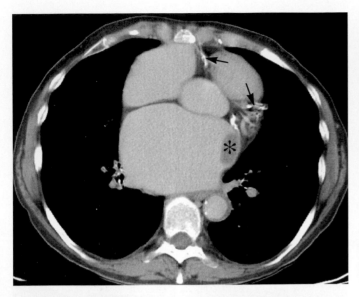

Fig. 20.4 Coronary artery calcification (arrows) and thrombus (*) in the dilated left atrium are both evident. (Courtesy of Dr R. Sawyer).

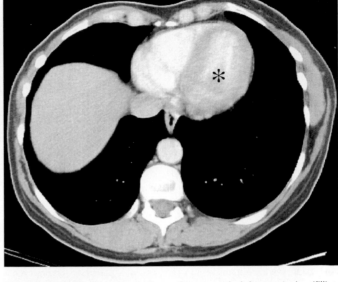

Fig. 20.6 Normal contrast-enhanced scan with left ventricular 'filling defect' due to papillary muscle (*).

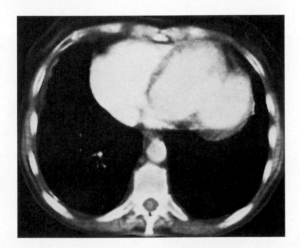

Fig. 20.5 Left ventricular aneurysm. Contrast enhancement demonstrates neck of apical and posterior aneurysm communicating with left ventricular cavity.

Cardiac Masses The normal papillary muscles are commonly seen as filling defects in the left ventricle on contrast-enhanced CT, and should not be mistaken for tumour or thrombus (Fig. 20.6). The commonest intracavitary cardiac tumor is a *myxoma*, usually found in the left atrium. Cystic areas within the tumor are common. *Rhabdomyomas* may occur in children with *tuberous sclerosis*; these occur in the cardiac muscle of any chamber, and may be multiple. Primary cardiac *sarcoma* is rare. Metastatic disease may occasionally occur, particularly from melanoma, lymphomas, and carcinoma of the bronchus.

Left Ventricular Aneurysms Left ventricular aneurysms are found at postmortem in 3.5–20% of patients who have had a myocardial infarction. Aneurysms are defined as local areas of total lack of left ventricular wall motion or paradoxical wall motion. The size of a left ventricular aneurysm, its relationship to the remaining left ventricle and the presence of thrombus within it can be demonstrated on CT (Fig. 20.5).

Coronary Artery Bypass Grafts Graft patency can be demonstrated by contrast enhancement and clearance in the graft on CT, with similar accuracy as for selective coronary angiography, but significant stenosis without occlusion may not be identified. Sections at more than one level may be necessary to decide on patency or occlusion of a graft. Metallic surgical clips will cause streak artefacts, interfering with the assessment of the grafts; non-opaque surgical materials should therefore be used if this method of follow-up is anticipated.

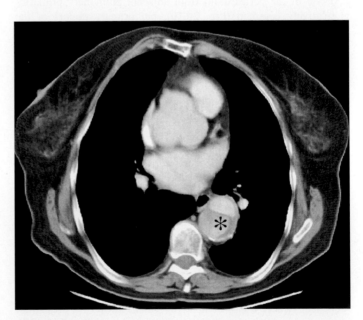

Fig. 20.7 Dilated aortic valve and coronary sinuses giving an enlarged clover leaf shape to the aortic root. (Patient with Marfan's syndrome, note the chronic dissection of the descending aorta (*) and the pectus carinatum deformity.)

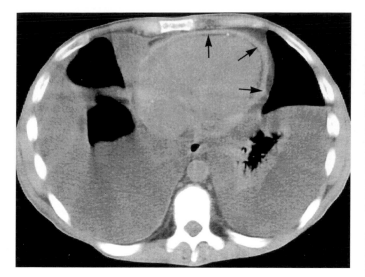

Fig. 20.8 Pericardial thickening (arrows) in a patient in chronic renal failure.

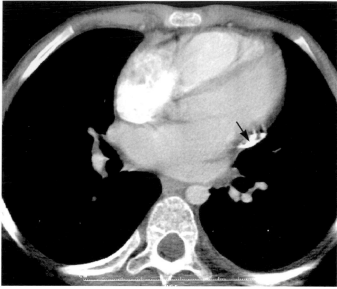

Fig. 20.9 Chronic constrictive pericarditis with focal pericardial calcification (arrow). (Courtesy of Dr R. Sawyer.)

Valve Disease Valve motion is too rapid for conventional or spiral CT to 'freeze'. Gross dilatation of the aortic valve may be demonstrated (Fig. 20.7), and valve calcification is easily seen. Tricuspid valve regurgitation will allow reflux of intravenous contrast medium (injected into the upper limb) into the inferior vena cava and hepatic veins, where it can be identified before contrast reaches this region from the normal lower-body circulation.

Pericardial Disease Pericardial thickening (Fig. 20.8), effusion and calcification (Fig. 20.9) can be identified on CT, separated from the myocardium by the thin epicardial fat layer. Tumor invasion of the pericardium from adjacent pulmonary primaries is relatively common (Fig. 20.10), but primary tumors of the pericardium are rare.

MAGNETIC RESONANCE IMAGING

Jeremy P. R. Jenkins

Cardiac MRI is now an established, although still advancing, technique providing information on morphology and function of the heart and cardiovascular system in both health and disease. Its attractions include a wide topographical field of view with visualization of the heart and its internal morphology and surrounding mediastinal structures, the capability of multiple imaging planes, and a high soft-tissue contrast discrimination between flowing blood and myocardium without the need for contrast medium or invasive technique. The multiplanar facility, including oblique sections, allows true long- and short-axis views of the heart (as used in echocardiography) and long-axis images of the thoracic aorta to be obtained routinely (Fig. 20.11).

The use of *ECG gating* of the radiofrequency (RF) pulse sequence, typically *spin echo T_1 weighted*, allows for sequential images to be acquired at different times during the cardiac cycle, providing images of the internal morphology of the heart and great vessels with high spatial resolution. ECG gating initiates the RF pulse sequence to a constant point in the cardiac cycle, thus

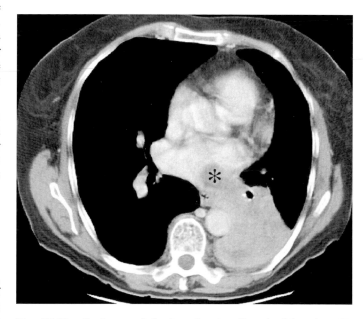

Fig. 20.10 Carcinoma of the bronchus invading the left atrium (*), transgressing the pericardium.

controlling the effects of heart motion and reducing flow-related artefacts. A *sequential* ECG-gated multislice T_1-weighted spin echo sequence gives contiguous anatomic sections but with each image at a different phase of the cardiac cycle. This is a rapid way, within a single R–R ECG interval, of obtaining anatomic detail over a wide area (Fig. 20.12). Using *incremental* ECG-gated multislice imaging, each section can be obtained at a different spacing throughout the cardiac cycle at a designated anatomical level (see Fig. 20.13). Newer magnet systems permit multislice with multiphase images to be collected at the same time, allowing the whole heart to be assessed. The typical spacing between

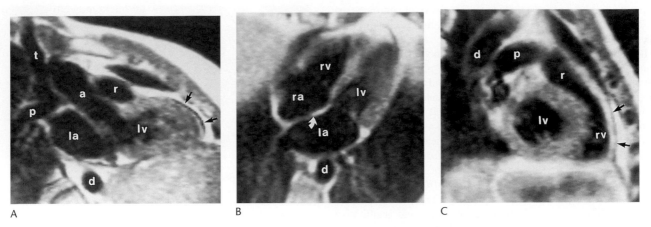

Fig. 20.11 **A**. Long-axis two-chamber view of the heart on a compound oblique ECG-gated spin-echo T$_1$-weighted image (TE = 26 ms). **B**. Four-chamber view on a compound oblique gated image using similar parameters. **C**. Short-axis view of the left ventricle using compound oblique planes with similar parameters. a, ascending aorta; d, descending aorta; la, left atrium; lv, left ventricle; r, outflow tract of right ventricle; ra, right atrium; rv, right ventricle; p, main pulmonary arteries; t, trachea; straight arrows, pericardium; curved arrow, interatrial septum.

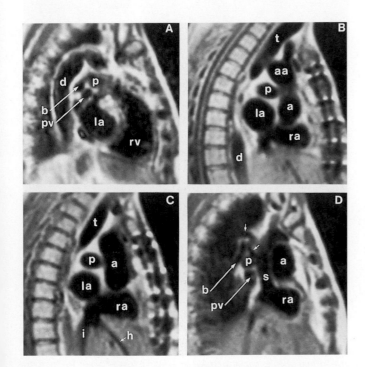

Fig. 20.12 Four sagittal multisection gated spin echo images (TE 24 ms) **A** left to **D** right of the midline demonstrating normal anatomy, and the localized low- and high-signal artefacts from metallic sternal sutures following coronary artery bypass graft surgery. Same key as in Fig. 20.11, and including: aa, aortic arch; b, bronchus; h, hepatic vein; i, inferior vena cava; pv, pulmonary vein: s, superior vena cava; small arrows in D, azygos vein. (Adapted with permission from Jenkins & Isherwood 1987.)

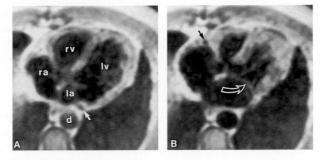

Fig. 20.13 Two transverse gated spin echo images (TE 24 ms), **A** end-diastole and **B** end-systole. Same key as in Fig 20.5, and including: curved arrow, closed mitral valve leaflets; straight arrow in A, left circumflex artery; straight arrow in B, right coronary artery

images is 25–50 ms (limited by a signal-to-noise ratio (SNR) constraint on some magnet systems). These images can be interpolated, stacked in order, and put into a cine display mode. This technique allows visualization of the beating heart, which helps to assess cardiac wall motion and also to evaluate blood flow. A fluctuation in myocardial signal, related to varying levels of phase-encoded noise in images obtained at different phases of the cardiac cycle, makes it difficult to evaluate changes in signal intensity from the walls. ECG gating, although relatively easy to instigate, reduces flexibility in the repetition time (TR) of the sequence which is controlled by the R–R interval of the ECG. A gated T$_2$-weighted spin echo sequence can be performed by increasing the TR to twice the R–R interval, and the TE to greater than 60 ms.

The *gated spin echo technique* clearly demonstrates internal cardiac anatomy and adjacent major vessels due to the intrinsic contrast from the flow void effect (Figs 20.11–20.13). The reasons why some images are not diagnostic are poor cooperation by the patient, an irregular heart rate, or a low-amplitude R-wave below the threshold sensitivity of the triggering device. In addition, difficulty in correct triggering can occur due to peaked T-waves, simulating the R-wave. Blood (which acts as a conductor) flowing in the aorta interacts with the magnetic field, producing a voltage which causes artefacts on the ECG. The myocardium and its endocardial surface can be delineated, although the latter may be obscured by signal from slow-flowing blood within the chamber during certain phases of the cardiac cycle. The interatrial and interventricular septa can be visualized, together with the papillary apparatus and the moderator band in the ventricles. The relatively thin and mobile cardiac valves are not consistently seen. The pericardium consists of fibrous tissue, and produces a linear low signal anterior to the right ventricle (see Ch. 21). Portions of the proximal coronary arteries can often be detected (see Figs 23.58 and 23.60).

MRI can provide both anatomic and functional information about the heart. Using spin echo techniques, global and regional right and left ventricular function as represented by stroke volumes and ejection fractions can be accurately obtained. Data from MRI are more accurate than those derived from left ventricular angiography, where the calculation is based on the assumption that the left ventricle is ellipsoid in shape. Volume measurement by MRI is independent of cavity shape, with the area from contiguous spin echo sections integrated over the chamber of interest. *Gradient echo imaging* (also called *cine or cine flow MRI*), using gradient-refocused echoes (e.g. even-echo rephasing) and a low flip angle (typically 30–60°), can also provide a qualitative and quantitative assessment of valvular function and blood flow in vivo (see Ch. 23).

In spin echo imaging, the blood pool is usually demonstrated as a signal void. In contrast, the blood pool in gradient echo imaging has a high signal, with myocardium and stationary tissues retaining an intermediate mid-gray signal (Figs 20.14 and 20.15). High-contrast discrimination can thus be achieved between the blood pool and myocardial/vessel wall using either technique. The gradient echo sequence allows shorter timing intervals between scans (TR can be lower than 30 ms on some magnet systems) giving approximately 25 frames/acquisition with a typical R–R interval of 800 ms (the number of scans obtained is approximately the R–R interval divided by the TR). A further advantage of gradient echo imaging is its sensitivity to the disturbed flow and consequent signal loss associated with stenotic and regurgitant valves, shunts and vessel narrowings. The extent of signal loss associated with diseased valves or areas of stenosis is related to the severity of the lesion and correlates well with pressure gradient measurements at angiography (see Ch. 23). In addition, with gradient echo imaging both flow direction and a measurement of velocity can be derived by the use of 'phase mapping'. *Phase mapping* requires two sets of even-echo rephased scans to be obtained simultaneously. One set is phase-encoded, using a gradient profile to encode for flow in a selected direction. The two sets are subtracted producing a *velocity map* (see Fig. 25.102). The phase shift induced by flowing blood is proportional to its velocity, and is detected as either a dark or light gray signal, depending on the direction of flow. Stationary tissue does not demonstrate any phase shift, and thus remains mid-gray. Shortening of the TE of the gradient echo sequence (a reduction of the echo time of 3 ms has been achieved) allows reclamation of signal from areas of incoherent or turbulent flow (see Fig. 23.54). Flow velocity measurements can then be made.

Gradient echo imaging can also be used to provide quantitative evaluation of regional wall motion and systolic wall thickening to assess extent of regional myocardial ischemia and infarction. A more sensitive method of quantifying myocardial motion and contraction is based on a novel technique termed 'cardiac tagging'. Specified regions of the myocardium during diastole can be labeled by selective RF saturation of multiple thin grid lines which 'tag' points in the myocardium. This tagging is followed by incremental multislice spin echo imaging, which allows sampling during the contractile phase of the cardiac cycle. The tagged regions appear as strips of low signal intensity, and their pattern of displacement reflects the intervening myocardial motion. This

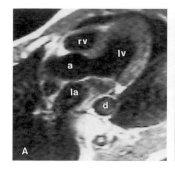
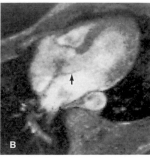

Fig. 20.14 Compound oblique gated images through the cardiac long-axis plane. **A.** Spin echo (T$_E$ 26 ms) scan. **B.** Gradient echo (T$_E$ 26 ms) scan. Same key as in Fig. 20.5, and including: arrow, mitral valve leaflet. (Adapted with permission from Mitchell et al 1989.)

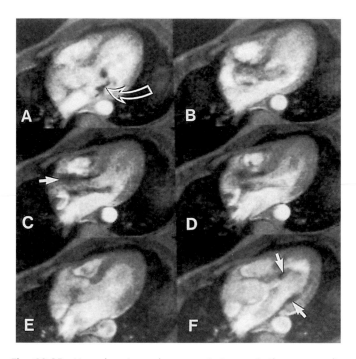

Fig. 20.15 Normal anatomy shown on six images in the same cardiac long-axis plane at 100 ms intervals through the cardiac cycle using the gradient echo sequence (T$_E$ 26 ms), with **A** 30 ms to **F** 530 ms after the R-wave of the ECG. Curved arrow in A, signal loss distal to the mitral valve at end-diastole; straight arrow in C, peripheral signal loss distal to aortic valve in mid-systole; straight arrows in F, signal loss adjacent to the mitral valve leaflets in diastole. (Adapted with permission from Mitchell et al 1989.)

technique allows easy evaluation of dyskinetic areas of the myocardium. In addition to the translational and rotational movement of the heart, more complex motions such as cardiac twist have been demonstrated. Further work with this method has provided a three-dimensional picture of myocardial motion and contraction.

In contrast to other techniques, including two-dimensional echocardiography (2DE) and angiography, anatomic information is easily defined on MRI. This is particularly valuable in the assessment of suspected congenital heart defects and abnormalities of the great vessels. The advantages of MRI over 2DE are a wider topographical window and a superior contrast resolution. In obese patients, provided they fit into the magnet bore, good resolution images can be obtained. 2DE can be limited by body habitus, and difficulties may arise in demonstrating the aortic arch, the descending thoracic aorta, and the epicardial border of the left ventricular free wall.

Chemical Shift Imaging This technique, which can separate and quantify the water and fat protons in vivo, is able to detect and study the composition of atheromatous plaques.

Echo Planar Imaging (EPI) This is a different MRI technique that offers virtual real-time, i.e. 'snapshot', imaging. It employs very short data acquisition times (milliseconds), and involves repeated sampling of the transverse magnetization in the presence of large, rapidly-switched field gradients, and requires specialized hardware and software. It offers great potential for the examination of the rapidly beating heart and the coronary arteries.

Magnetic Resonance Spectroscopy (MRS) This technique can monitor the metabolism of intact organs non-invasively. Much of the work on MRS in the heart has been concerned with the assessment of myocardial ischemia, and metabolic alterations have been demonstrated in these circumstances. Several major technical problems, including spatial resolution and localization, are currently being investigated, and must be solved before its clinical role can be established.

Safety Aspects of Cardiac MRI Patients with pacemakers or pacing lines in situ should be excluded from the MRI unit and should not enter the 5 gauss (0.5 millitesla) line of the fringe field. Cardiac pacemakers can be damaged or change operation on exposure to switching magnetic field gradients. Although all pacemakers exhibit a torque when placed in the main field, this is unlikely to result in movement of the pacemaker within the chest or abdominal wall, due to the presence of surrounding fibrosis.

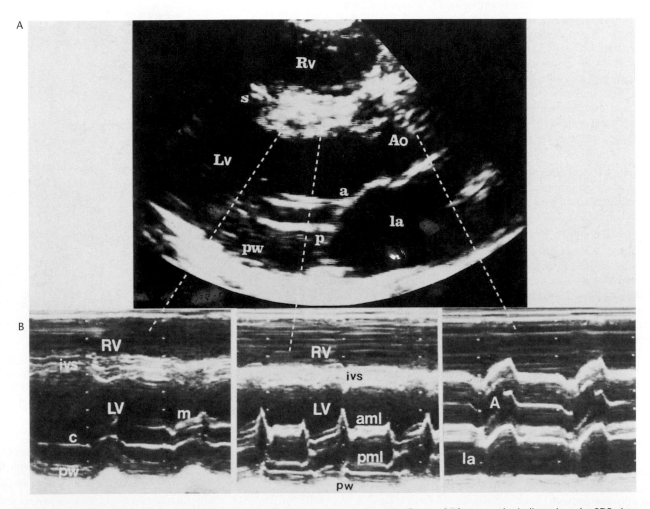

Fig. 20.16 **A**. 2DE picture of a normal heart, long-axis view. **B**. M-mode pictures corresponding to the beam angles indicated on the 2DE picture, made simultaneously on a modern machine. **Left-hand panel**: The beam goes through the left ventricular cavity below the level of the mitral valve. Both anterior and posterior walls of the left ventricle can be identified, together with their endocardial surfaces, and they move inwards together. Note that the cavity diameter can be measured in diastole and systole, as can the wall thickness. Without 2DE control the exact level at which the beam intersects the left ventricular cavity would be uncertain. **Middle panel**: The characteristic M-shaped movement indicates that the beam is intersecting the anterior leaflet of the mitral valve. In addition, the posterior leaflet of the mitral valve can be identified as moving in the opposite direction in diastole. **Right-hand panel**: The box-shaped opening movement of the aortic valve leaflets can be seen, which confirms that the beam is going through the aortic root. The left atrium can be identified lying behind the aorta, and its long diameter can be measured. Key to Figs 20.16–20.40: RV, right ventricle; LV, left ventricle; Ao (or A), aorta; LA, left atrium; PW, posterior wall; a (or aml), anterior leaflet mitral valve; p (or pml), posterior leaflet mitral valve; c, chordae tendinae; ivs (or s), interventricular septum; PA, pulmonary artery; RA, right atrium; L.ax, long-axis view; S.ax, short-axis view; e, endocardium; t, tricuspid valve; ias, interatrial septum; ED, end-diastole; ES, end-systole; AV, aortic valve; MV, mitral valve.

Patients with prosthetic heart valves (excluding the old Starr–Edwards valve replacement (pre-6000 model)) can be safely scanned without danger of valve displacement or significant image artefact (see Fig. 25.103). A localized loss of signal is to be expected close to prosthetic valves, so other imaging techniques are required to evaluate these implants. Surgical clips, including sternal wires, used in coronary artery bypass grafting and other cardiac surgery are not a significant problem, producing only local artefacts.

CARDIAC ULTRASOUND

1. Two-dimensional Echocardiography Ultrasonic imaging of the heart or 'echocardiography' is based on pulsed echo techniques, and allows the anatomy and movements of intracardiac structures to be studied non-invasively with ease and reproducibility. The ultrasound beam is automatically scanned to build up a two-dimensional real-time moving image which is recorded on videotape. The echo signal indicates the presence and location of the structure in the sound beam.

Some details of intracardiac anatomy and pathology are much better documented by ultrasound than by X-ray or other imaging methods. The structures shown by 2DE depend on the transducer position and the direction of oscillation. 2DE images are effectively tomograms, showing structures in a 'slice' of the heart. The most common planes used in adult echocardiography are shown in Figs 20.16–20.19.

2. M-mode Echocardiography Any one of the directions of the sound beam may be sampled to print out the pattern of distance of the reflecting structure over time, in order to record the motion of these structures. The technique is useful for measuring dimensions and certain functional changes (Fig. 20.16).

3. Doppler Echocardiography Doppler echocardiography registers the shift in frequency that results from reflection of the transmitted sound from moving materials such as blood. The application of pulsed and continuous-wave Doppler principles to 2DE permits blood flow direction, and velocity to be derived. Using the 2DE image as a map, a sampling box can be positioned electronically by the operator adjacent to an abnormal valve, or tracked along the septum to observe turbulent flow. A flow profile of the direction or average flow velocity may be derived, and this provides insight into the physiological burden of valvular heart disease or intracardiac shunts.

The direction and velocity of the blood are calculated by an equation that relates them to the direction and magnitude of the Doppler shift in the frequency of the sound and the angle between the direction of the sound and the blood flow. If such Doppler analysis is confined to the returning series of sound waves corresponding to a given distance from the transducer, it is called the pulsed-wave method.

Pulsed-wave Doppler (PD) echocardiography allows localization of the signal in the heart, but is limited by its inability to record the movements of the blood at very high speed. The alternative method requires two tranducers; one transmits sound continuously, and the reflected sound is received simultaneously by the other. This continuous-wave method (CW) cannot identify the origin of the signals returning from all points along the path of the sound beam, but it can record the high blood velocities typical of the jets associated with stenotic valves (see Fig. 23.9). Both PD

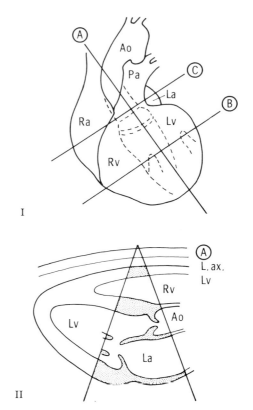

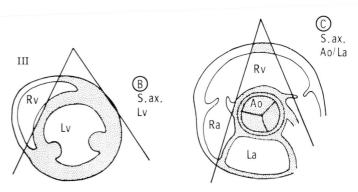

Fig. 20.17 2DE scanning of the heart. **I.** The heart shown diagrammatically with the standard scanning planes indicated. A. The long-axis view. B. Short-axis view through the cavity of the left ventricle below the level of the mitral valve. C. Short-axis view more cranially than in B. For key see Fig. 20.10. **II.** Long-axis view. **III.** Short-axis views.

and CW Doppler echocardiograms are recorded with a spectral display of velocity (or frequency) plotted against time with the strength of the signal at each velocity recorded as a level of gray shading (see Fig. 23.10).

4. Color Flow Doppler Mapping (CFM) In CFM of the Doppler signal, the pulsed-wave signal with respect to blood velocity and direction of flow throughout the imaging plane is color coded, and produces a color map over the two-dimensional image (see Figs 23.7 and 23.8). The direction, velocity, and nature of flow may be related to the cardiac structures.

PD and CW Doppler do not display flow images. They produce flow information from a very small area of interest indicated by the operator. Color flow mapping automatically gathers Doppler

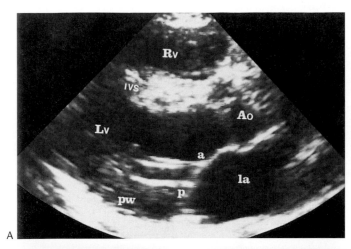

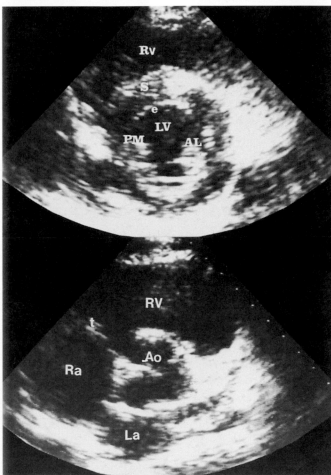

Fig. 20.18 2DE standard views corresponding to Fig. 20.17. **A.** Long-axis view. This is useful for orientation of the cardiac structures and good for acquired disease of the mitral and aortic valves. It is also useful in left ventricular disease. **B. Top:** A short-axis cut through the left ventricle. The size and shape of the left ventricular cavity and wall thickness are demonstrated. **Bottom** Short-axis cut at the level of the aortic valve. As the transducer is angled cranially from the left ventricle the beam leaves the papillary muscles and intersects the mitral valve, which has a characteristic 'fish-mouth' appearance. More cranial angulation intersects the aortic valve and also reveals the right ventricular outflow and in children the pulmonary valve and pulmonary artery and its bifurcation.

shift information from multiple sample volumes along each 2DE scan line. Mean velocities are calculated from the Doppler shift, and color coded. electronically for display of direction and velocity.

5. Exercise Echocardiography Imaging after exercise or dobutamine stimulation may be used to demonstrate the development of new or worsening of regional wall motion abnormalities as a result of ischemia. It is technically difficult, requiring digital image acquisition and analysis, and involves subjective interpretation.

6. Invasive Echocardiography Although echocardiography is primarily a non-invasive technique, it has been used in a variety of invasive procedures including:

1. *Transesophageal echocardiography (TEE)* Conventional 2DE is limited in certain situations because of poor depth penetration or interference from anterior structures reducing the access window. TEE allows high-quality color flow images in all cases. The technique requires the passage of an esophagoscope with an ultrasound transducer at its tip and this can be, to some degree, angled and advanced to different levels to visualize the aorta and the heart in multiple projections. Both 2DE and CFM are available in current equipment. Current indications for TEE in the heart include the assessment of prosthetic valve dysfunction, endocarditis, intracardiac thrombus and masses, cardiac sources of embolization, and intraoperative monitoring of left ventricular function. It is valuable in demonstrating dissections of the thoracic aorta, particularly in the ascending aorta.

2. *Contrast echocardiography*, which requires intravenous injection to visualize flow.

3. *Intracardiac echocardiography*, to supplement angiographic studies.

4. *Intravascular ultrasound*, where the transducer is mounted on a small intravascular probe. This technique is excellent for demonstrating the walls of vessels, whereas angiography demonstrates only the lumen.

5. *Myocardial perfusion imaging*, which may be performed with ultrasound contrast agents.

7. Three-dimensional Echocardiography This technique provided enhanced appreciation of spatially oriented data. A major hindrance to its widespread application is the time required for image acquisition and processing. However, it sets the stage for the next major advance in echocardiographic imaging.

Summary

Standard 2DE provides decisive information on intracardiac anatomy in the vast majority of neonates and small children with congenital heart disease and in over 70% of adults with acquired heart disease. The limiting factor is usually the ultrasound window, and in these patients TEE will usually give the required information, though it does require esophagoscopy. Functional information is usually obtained initially using CFM, which will reveal areas of abnormal flow, such as intracardiac shunts and leaking valves, but it should be realized that the information is semiquantitative at best. Valvar stenoses may be quantified using

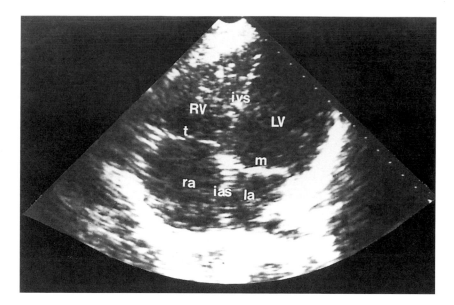

Fig. 20.19 2DE, the four-chamber view. To obtain this view the transducer is rotated as well as angled so that all four chambers can be identified simultaneously, together with both atrioventricular valves. This view gives one of the best demonstrations of the left ventricle and the ventricular septum, and also of the atrioventricular valve. In acquired heart disease it enables structural abnormality to be seen. In congenital heart disease this view is excellent for identifying the opening of the valves into their respective ventricles. 'Drop-out' of echoes in the interatrial septum are common in this view, but by obtaining the view subcostally, more conclusions about the interatrial septum may be drawn.

CW Doppler sampling, which is required to demonstrate the very high flow rates caused by a valvar stenosis.

ISOTOPES IN CARDIOLOGY

Isotope imaging generally is dealt with elsewhere, and in this section a resumé of the cardiac application is attempted. Isotopes have been used to study ventricular function and myocardial perfusion.

Ventricular Function Studies

Radionuclide techniques for monitoring global and regional ventricular functions fall into two major categories: (1) *first-pass studies*, in which the injected bolus dose is monitored during its first passage through the heart and great vessels; and (2) *gated equilibrium studies*, in which the tracer mixes with the blood pool before data collection. Both of these nuclear studies can be performed at the patient's bedside using a mobile γ-camera; each technique has its own strengths and weaknesses (Table 20.1).

Following injection, the labeled radioactive tracer localizes in the heart, releasing energy in the form of γ-photons which traverse overlying tissues and interact with the imaging device (single-crystal or multicrystal γ-camera). A collimator permits only photons arising from specific areas of the heart to interact with the camera. The imaging device converts the γ-photon energy into an electrical signal that can be processed; an on-line computer records the information and permits the optimal visual or quantitive display of the data.

For cardiac nuclear imaging a number of heart cycles have to be averaged to provide data for accurate interpretation of structure and function. In first-pass studies, data are usually summed without regard to physiological signal; in the gated equilibrium technique the start of each cardiac cycle is identified from a physiological marker (the R-wave of the electrocardiogram), and data from each cycle are added in the correct temporal sequence ('gated'). Gated nuclear imaging is inaccurate if the cardiac rhythm is very irregular.

First-pass Method The first-pass method of radionuclide angiography consists of rapidly injecting a bolus of isotope (⁹⁹ᵐTc pertechnetate) into the antecubital vein and obtaining images as the bolus passes through the right heart, lung fields, and left heart chambers. A multidetector γ-camera with high count rate characteristics (up to 250 000 counts per second) should be used, its disadvantage being its lack of mobility. The representative cycle can be played in cine format for quantitive evaluation of wall motion; superimposed end-diastolic and end-systolic perimeters are generated to evaluate regional wall motion further (Fig. 20.20).

Although single-crystal γ-cameras can also be used for this method, the count density obtained with them is limited and may hinder the accuracy of the values obtained. They have the advantage of mobility.

Gated Equilibrium Studies (multiple gated acquisition, MUGA) (Fig. 20.21) An isotope which remains fixed within the vascular space (such as ⁹⁹ᵐTc-labeled human serum albumin or red blood cells) is administered intravenously. This isotope permits the recording of data for up to 4 h, thus allowing the acquisition of multiple images in various projections and also the study of the ventricular response to interventions. After equilibrium, the counts are synchronized in relation to a portion of the cardiac cycle using the R-wave of the ECG, and the cardiac cycle is divided by the computer into a fixed number of frames. This synchronization is called 'gated' imaging. Frame durations of 40–50 ms are usually adequate. Most studies require 6–10 min to

Table 20.1 Comparison of the two methods of radionuclide angiography

	First-pass	Equilibrium
Radiopharmaceutical	^{99m}Tc pertechnetate (readily available). Bolus required	^{99m}Tc-labeled red blood cells or human serum albumin (preparation takes 15–20 min)
Camera	High count rate capability (multicrystal)	Conventional
Camera positioning	Before injection of agent any projection (RAO possible)	After administration of agent. Left anterior oblique projection of choice
Imaging time	30 s	3–10 min
Measurement per injection	One	Multiple repeat measurements
Advantages	1. Minimal background activity 2. Temporal separation—optimal views of chambers 3. Visualization of inferior and anterior wall motion abnormalities slightly superior 4. Analysis of lung flow possible 5. Measurement of cardiac output 6. Quantification of shunts	1. Permits repeat studies after intervention over long periods 2. Estimation of severity of valvar regurgitation

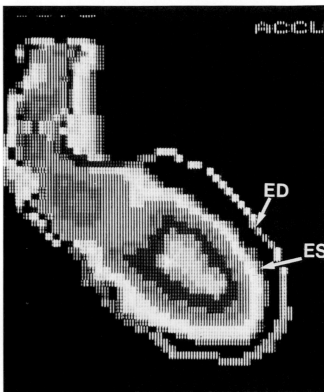

Fig. 20.20 Normal first-pass radionuclide ventriculography. Diastole and systole can both be identified, the shape of the ventricle determined, and the pattern of contraction seen.

obtain adequate counts for data analysis. Derived data are then processed by the computer to determine the variables of left ventricular contraction as with first-pass data.

Quantitive Data Analysis

Ejection Fraction Semi-automatic methods for measuring the cardiac ejection fraction have been in clinical use for many years. After data accumulation, the region of interest (i.e. the left ventricle) is identified, and the computer generates a time/activity curve with a cyclic rise and fall in counts (Fig. 20.22). The counts are proportional to the volume of the chamber. The difference between peak counts at end-diastole to trough counts at end-systole reflects the stroke counts; stroke counts divided by end-diastolic counts (after appropriate background correction) determine the ejection fraction. This time/activity curve is independent of geometric assumptions inherent in the area–length technique utilized in contrast ventriculography and echocardiography.

Regional Wall Motion Analysis The images are viewed in a cine film format on a continuous loop for evaluation of wall motion abnormalities; by color coding and by recycling the images over and over again a better perception of the ventricular function is obtained. The subjective interpretation of the images is complemented by the quantitive data; normal (see Figs 20.20 and 20.21) and abnormal (Fig. 20.23) systolic wall motion in different areas of the ventricle can be assessed fairly accurately by this method. Wall motion can also be studied from display of parametric data derived by computer analysis of the gated cardiac cycle. The cardiac cycle is divided into its various temporal frequency components, each frequency characterized by a specific amplitude and phase. The amplitude image represents the amount of contraction. The analysis of ventricular emptying and relaxation is derived from the phase image (see Fig. 20.22); the degree of regional phase delay is generally related to the severity of contraction abnormalities and occurs in segments of the ventricle with no movement (akinetic) or in those moving paradoxically in systole (dyskinetic).

NUCLEAR TECHNIQUES FOR THE STUDY OF MYOCARDIAL PERFUSION AND INFARCT IMAGING

Assessment of Myocardial Perfusion

The use of thallium-201 myocardial scintigraphy for myocardial perfusion imaging has found wide acceptance in routine practice. Since thallium-201 uptake has been shown to be mainly dependent on myocardial blood flow and to a lesser degree on local cell metabolism, it can be used to assess the extent of

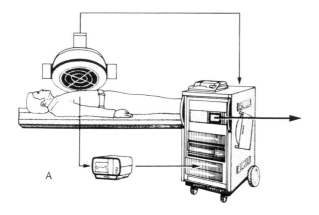

Multiple Gated Studies (MUGA)

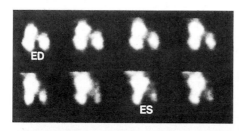

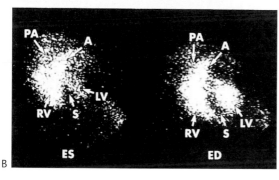

Fig. 20.21 Gated equilibrium radionuclide ventriculography. The γ-camera is positioned in the left anterior oblique position to obtain separation of right and left ventricles; data acquisition is synchronized ('gated') by the computer to the ECG signals.

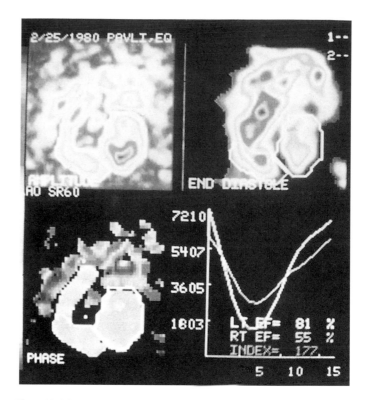

Fig. 20.22 Quantitative data analysis of the normal cardiac cycle (amplitude and phase analysis) made from a gated equilibrium scan. The phase image demonstrates uniform (normal) contraction. From the time activity curve, the ejection fraction of both ventricles (LT EF, RT EF) is calculated and expressed as a percentage.

hypoperfusion and hence ischemic disease in the walls of the heart. Since the physical half-life of the isotope is 73 h, transient myocardial ischemia can be detected by comparing the uptake data at the time of exercise with those obtained 3–4 h later at rest. The thallium is injected at maximal exercise. Ten minutes after the exercise the patient is placed beneath the detector of the γ-camera, and thallium scintigrams are made successively in the left anterior oblique 45° and anterior orientations (Fig. 20.24). Late imaging is performed in the same sequence after 3–4 h. An area with reduced thallium uptake early after exercise may be due to either transient uptake abnormalities (ischemia) or a previous myocardial infarction (scar). While in an acute ischemic area the uptake defect decreases or disappears with time (Fig. 20.24), the activity remains diminished or absent in an infarcted zone. The visual interpretation of these images depends on observer experience, image quality, ratio of myocardial to background activity, and the medium in which the images are presented. To

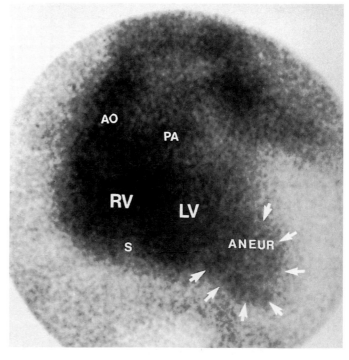

Fig. 20.23 Gated equilibrium scan in the left anterior oblique position. An apical left ventricular aneurysm has been demonstrated (arrows).

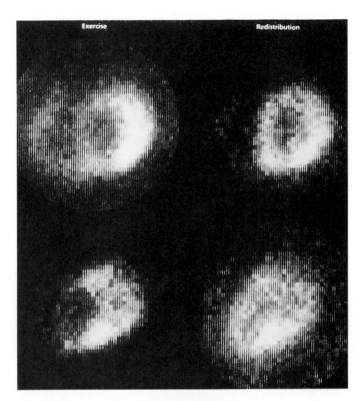

Fig. 20.24 Thallium-201 myocardial perfusion scanning. **Top**: Left anterior oblique views. **Bottom**: Lateral views of the same patient. Note the activity defect which is present in the septal aspect of the left ventricle on exercise but which fills in during the redistribution phase, seen on both views. The reversibility of the perfusion defect suggests that the myocardium is ischemic but not necrotic. Note that the wall of the right ventricle is also demonstrated during exercise. The use of ^{201}Tl is one of the few ways of demonstrating abnormalities of right ventricular perfusion.

improve the reliability of the diagnosis, computer programs have been developed for the quantitative analysis of these images. The sensitivity and specificity of exercise thallium-201 myocardial imaging appear to be in the range of 85–95%, a moderate but definite improvement on the exercise ECG.

Prognostic information provided by exercise thallium-201 imaging includes extent of stress perfusion abnormalities, extent of redistribution, and indirect signs of severe stress left ventricular dysfunction. In addition to conventional planar techniques, *single-photon emission tomography* (SPECT) allows more precise assessment of resting and exercise myocardial perfusion abnormalities.

In patients who cannot perform physical exercise, pharmacological stress testing (with dobutamine, dipyrimidole, or adenosine) in conjunction with myocardial perfusion imaging provides an alternative means of evaluation to standard exercise imaging.

New Agents Radiopharmaceuticals containing technetium-99, such as Sestamibi (^{99m}Tc-MIBI), have a shorter half-life (6 h) than thallium. This allows larger doses of isotope to be injected, and the higher-energy photons produce better-quality images, particularly useful in very obese patients. Like thallium-201, the initial myocardial accumulation of Sestamibi is proportionate to regional blood flow. It is of value in detecting ischemia but less accurate in assessing viability.

Assessment of Myocardial Viability This is critically important in patients with multiple infarctions, ongoing ischemia, and left ventricular dysfunction. In such patients, prediction of the degree of recovery of function with revascularization is crucial in deciding whether revascularization should be attempted. In two situations myocardium may appear non-viable, but is only non-contractile:

1. *Stunned myocardium.* Acute reversible ischemia, not persistent enough to cause necrosis, may result in temporary failure of mechanical function, which may recover with time.
2. *Hibernating myocardium.* This results from chronic severe ischemia when residual myocardial perfusion is enough to support cellular life and membrane function but not contractile function, which may recover when adequate perfusion is restored.

Although *positron emission tomography* (PET) using [^{18}F]-fluorodeoxyglucose is considered to be the 'gold standard' in identifying continued metabolic activity in non-contractile myocardium in which function is likely to return, thallium-201 SPECT is a more cost-effective and relatively simple procedure requiring a standard reinjection of thallium-201 before the resting scan. By combining the information from scintigraphic images with the coronary arteriogram, a logical and individualized plan for revascularization can be developed.

Infarct Imaging Agents A variety of technetium-labeled phosphates are taken up by irreversibly damaged myocardium; a positive concentration gradient is therefore achieved between infarcted and normal tissue. The main application of these radiopharmaceuticals is the serial evaluation of infarct size (usually overestimated by this method), in the differentiation between old and recent infarction (particularly in patients with bundle branch block on the ECG), and in the visualization of right ventricular infarction. The infarct may be detected as a positive focus 12 h to 1 week after infarction.

Positron Emission Tomography of the Myocardium

E. Rhys Davies

Conventional single-photon emission CT (SPECT) studies using ^{201}Tl (a potassium analog) and ^{99m}Tc agents are invaluable indicators of myocardial function. Positron emission tomography (PET) studies with ^{82}Rb (a generator-produced potassium analog) and ^{18}FDG (a glucose analog) are proving to have several technical advantages. ^{82}Rb, as well as being widely available, has a short half-life, enabling rapid and serial studies to be done. Typically a baseline study followed by a pharmacological stress study are done, and high sensitivity and specificity are reported for myocardial ischemia. The cyclotron-produced radionuclides that are used in the same way are ^{13}NH$_3$ and H$_2$^{15}O. If myocardial metabolism is being studied, the radiopharmaceutical of choice is ^{18}FDG. Although ^{18}FDG is an analog for glucose transport and phosphorylation, it is not metabolized and therefore accumulates in the cells, giving a clear depiction of viable myocardium. It is generally accepted that ^{201}Tl techniques are less accurate than this because they tend to overestimate the extent of damaged myocardium. Further discussion of PET will be found in Chapter 59.

ANGIOCARDIOGRAPHY

Angiocardiography is the X-ray imaging of the heart following the injection of radiopaque contrast medium. Selective angiocardiography, the positioning of the contrast medium injection, through a cardiac catheter, selectively in relation to the lesion to be demonstrated, is invariably employed. Selective angiocardiography is always combined with cardiac catheterization so that intracardiac pressures and, if necessary, oxygen saturations can be measured. The aim is to delineate not only the types of abnormality which may be present but also their severity, so hemodynamic assessment is essential in other than coronary artery disease.

Modern angiocardiography apparatus utilizes primarily digital imaging. For cine radiography, the most frequently used technique, biplane 512 matrix filming at 50 frames/s is commercially available. Apart from its image quality, instantaneous frame replay and stenosis quantification provide advantages. Pulsed digital fluoroscopy also reduces radiation dose to both the operator and patient.

Selective angiocardiography requires the site of contrast injection to be chosen for the best display of the lesion suspected by clinical, echocardiographic, or hemodynamic assessment. Contrast is injected downstream of leaking valves (cine angiography is still the best method of assessing the severity of regurgitation), upstream of obstructions, and in the chamber or vessel originating a shunt. The volume of contrast and its delivery rate is usually individually tailored to the problem to be investigated. For problems involving abnormal structure of the heart, where anatomic delineation is important, a volume of 1 ml/kg body weight should be delivered within 2 s, and the inevitable ectopic beats accepted for the sake of the high density of contrast which may be obtained. For functional cardiac studies such as left ventriculography in acquired heart disease, a slow injection should avoid ectopic beats, and a low density of opacification will be accepted. Here, 8–16 ml/s over 3 s, depending on the size and activity of the left ventricle and the quality of the X-ray equipment, will be adequate. A rate- and volume-controlled injector is essential.

The choice of projection will also be influenced by the problem to be studied. For congenital heart disease, compound angulated views to profile the various parts of the cardiac septa are the rule, and are much used in coronary arteriography. Thus, tube mounts with a compound angulation facility to both rotate around the patient and angle along the patient are required.

Contrast Medium The standard ionic contrast media have pronounced effects on both the heart and the circulation. Passage of the contrast medium through the coronary circulation produces profound, though transient, changes in the ECG. These may be associated with demonstrable impairment of ventricular contraction and a rise in the left ventricular filling pressure, and associated left ventricular dilatation. The fall in blood pressure which is associated with angiocardiography is mediated in part by the impairment of ventricular contraction associated with the perfusion of the coronary arteries by the contrast and in part by the peripheral vasodilatation which the contrast medium produces. Subsequently there is an increase in cardiac output due to hemodilution. Injection of contrast medium into the pulmonary artery may be associated with a rise in pulmonary artery pressure.

The low osmolar contrast media are associated with much less subjective discomfort and significantly less hemodynamic abnormality than the standard media, though their viscosity and lack of anticoagulant properties are disadvantages. It seems likely that, in spite of their cost, these will be the agents of the future.

Angiocardiography is usually good at anatomic delineation of lesions but much less satisfactory in determining their severity and the degree of hemodynamic disturbance that they have produced. Angiocardiography can demonstrate an obstruction, be it valvar or subvalvar (or even supravalvar), but the severity of the obstruction must be assessed by the pressure gradient. This may be obtained by passing a catheter across the obstruction or by having catheters on either side. In the right heart the gradient across the pulmonary artery can usually be obtained by passing a catheter into the pulmonary arteries beyond the pulmonary valve and withdrawing it to the right ventricle. For tricuspid valve gradients it is customary to employ a double-lumen catheter because the overall pressures are low, pressure differences are very low, and balancing the pressure recording system is critical. In the left heart an aortic gradient may be obtained by crossing the aortic valve retrogradely to the left ventricle from the aorta or by measuring aortic and left ventricular pressures separately, the latter from a trans-septal catheter. Mitral gradients may be obtained by measuring an indirect left atrial pressure from a wedged pulmonary artery catheter, and by a catheter in the left ventricle.

When the significance of a gradient is not clear it may be necessary to measure the cardiac output (gradient depends not only on the severity of the obstruction but the flow across it), and it may be necessary to increase the cardiac output by exercise to confirm the presence of a significant gradient.

The measurement of valvar regurgitation at angiocardiography is difficult whatever measure is adopted. Aortic regurgitation is best assessed by cine aortography in the left anterior oblique projection and mitral regurgitation by cine left ventriculography in the right anterior oblique projection. Quantification of the appearances is not really satisfactory but gives a general guide to the severity of the condition. An attempt may be made to assess pulmonary and tricuspid incompetence by cine angiography, but the significance of the findings is never clear in view of the presence of the catheter across the valve.

The number and size of shunts may be demonstrated by angiocardiography, but the degree of shunting requires either measurements of oxygen saturation changes or other more complex methods to measure shunt volumes.

Pulmonary vascular resistance, an important measurement in the management of congenital heart disease, requires knowledge not only of the pressure in the pulmonary artery and in the left atrium but also of the flow across the lungs.

The present method of studying left ventricular function, a key factor in the surgical management of patients with acquired heart disease, consists of studying the size of the left ventricle and the proportion of its content which it ejects with each beat (ejection fraction (%), $EF = (SV/EDV) \times 100$, where SV is the systolic volume and EDV is the end-diastolic volume). This can be obtained by measuring the volume of the ventricle on cine angiograms, based on the assumption that the left ventricle is an ellipsoid of revolution, but most radiologists use visual assessment based on experience. Though the ejection fraction is the best method available for measuring ventricular function, it is widely influenced by factors outside the heart itself, and may ultimately be replaced.

The era of catheterization and angiocardiography in every patient with heart disease considered for surgery has already drawn to a close. Any patient with acquired heart disease in whom the number and severity of the valvular lesions can be estimated on the basis of the clinical examination and echocardiography, and in whom coronary artery disease is not suspected, can be operated on without this invasive investigation. An increasing number of patients with more complex congenital heart diseases are being subjected to surgery on the basis of the clinical and 2DE examinations without angiocardiography. In some areas of anatomic delineation, particularly in the congenital abnormalities of the atrioventricular valves and their connections, 2DE is demonstrably superior to angiography. In two areas, however, angiocardiography is still vital. In the investigation of coronary disease there are no simple non-invasive methods available. In disorders of the pulmonary circulation associated with congenital heart disease standard 2DE does not easily get beyond the main pulmonary artery, and to a lesser extent the same difficulty applies beyond the aortic valve; in these areas angiocardiography (or MRI) is still indicated in the absence of transesophageal echocardiography.

NORMAL ANATOMY

Although the basic anatomy of the heart and its vessels is well known from the dissecting room, the appearances of these structures in situ in the closed thorax may well appear unfamiliar when demonstrated by radiological methods. The normal superior vena cava (Fig. 20.25) forms the right border of the superior mediastinum. It is not normally visible as a discrete shadow. It may be visibly enlarged when distended, as in right heart cardiac failure.

A *persisting left superior vena cava* (which usually drains to the coronary sinus and thence to the right atrium) may be recognized as a low-density shadow in the left superior mediastinum (Fig. 20.26).

The *inferior vena cava* is commonly recognized on good-quality lateral views of the chest by its straight posterior border rising from the diaphragm to join the back of the heart in the middle of the right atrium. It may also be seen in the frontal view in the right pericardiophrenic angle (Fig. 20.27), and may be visibly distended in heart failure.

The *azygos vein* rises in the posterior mediastinum on the right side and passes forward to join the superior vena cava before it enters the right atrium. Occasionally the normal azygos vein may be seen as a small 'end-on' shadow in the angle between the right main bronchus and the trachea. When an azygos lobe is present, its fissure points to the azygos vein. The azygos vein may be quite large in the absence of pathology, when it may be confused with a paramediastinal mass. Contrast studies will serve to identify the shadow as vascular. It may be pathologically enlarged when the right heart filling pressure is increased from both cardiac and non-cardiac causes as in superior vena cava or portal obstruction. It reaches its largest size, however, when there is congenital interruption of the infrahepatic part of the inferior vena cava so that the distal inferior vena cava drains directly into the azygos vein which returns all the blood from the lower half of the body (Fig. 20.28). This arrangement always suggests the possibility of left isomerism or polysplenia.

A *left hemiazygos vein*, if present, may also be enlarged for similar reasons.

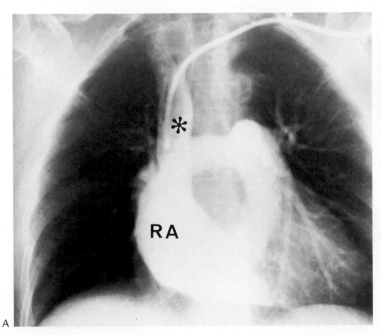
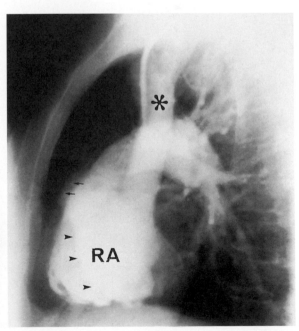

Fig. 20.25 Normal right atrial angiogram. The injection has been made from a catheter in the superior vena cava. **A**. Frontal view. **B**. Lateral view. The asterisk indicates the superior vena cava, and arrowheads mark the front border of the right atrium in the lateral view, overlapped by the right ventricle. Arrows indicate the front border of the right atrial appendage. The superior vena cava forms the right border of the superior mediastinum, and the right atrium forms the border of the heart. Only the right atrial appendage forms part of the front border in the lateral view.

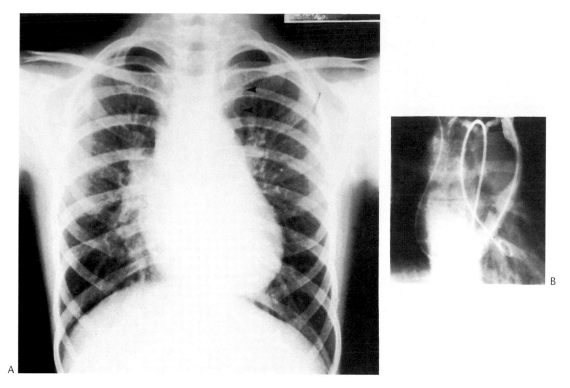

Fig. 20.26 **A**. Persisting left superior vena cava. This appears as a low-density shadow (arrowed) to the left of the superior mediastinum on the plain film. **B**. The matching angiogram shows it to descend to the left of the aortic arch.

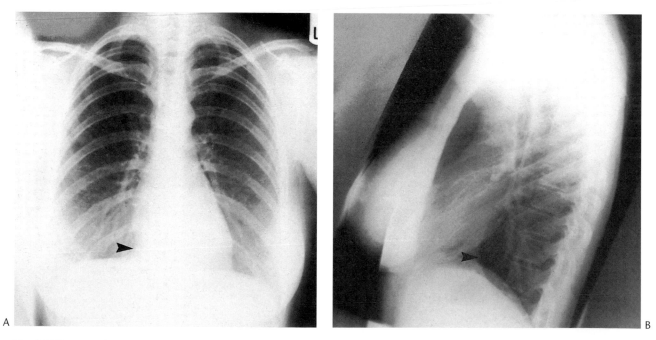

Fig. 20.27 Normal inferior vena cava (arrowed) seen in **A** frontal and **B** lateral views.

The **right atrium** (see Fig. 20.25) is a globular chamber forming the right heart border in the frontal view. Its broad-based appendage passes forward and to the left from its upper anterior aspect, to sit on the front of the heart. The appendage is the only part of the right atrium seen anteriorly in the lateral view. The posterior wall of the right atrium is marked in the lateral chest film by the entrance of the inferior vena cava (Fig. 20.29).

When the right atrium is enlarged, it protrudes the right heart border to the right and increases its radius of curvature, as the spherical chamber increases its diameter (Fig. 20.30). A big right

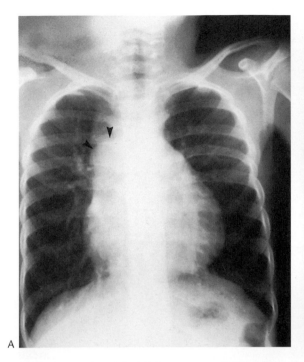
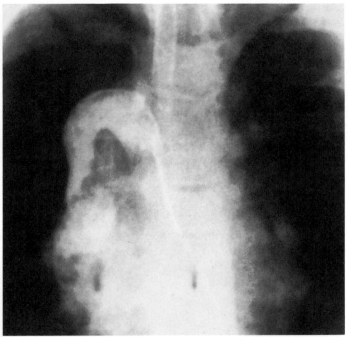

Fig. 20.28   Interruption of the inferior vena cava. **A**. The enlarged azygos vein (arrow) may resemble the aortic arch. **B**. Contrast studies in the same case show the azygos continuation of the inferior vena cava arching over the right main bronchus, to enter the right atrium.

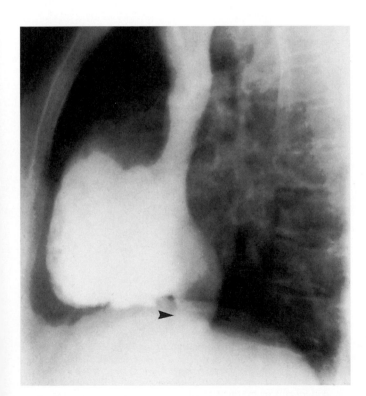

Fig. 20.29   Right atrial angiocardiogram, lateral view. Contrast medium has been injected into the superior vena cava and has refluxed down the inferior vena cava (arrow), showing it entering the back of the right atrium.

atrial appendage can fill in the space, seen in the lateral view, between the front of the heart and the back of the sternum.

Right atrial enlargement can occur in relation to acquired

tricuspid valve disease, both stenosis and incompetence, and in congenital anomalies of the tricuspid valve, both stenosis and incompetence, and more particularly in Ebstein's anomaly. The right atrium can also be enlarged when it carries a high flow as in atrial septal defect.

The morphological characteristics by which the right atrium is distinguished as right, in complex congenital heart disease, are the presence of the limbus of the fossa ovalis on its septal aspect and its broad-based and squat atrial appendage.

The **right ventricle** (Fig. 20.31) is a chamber of complex shape. In the frontal view it appears triangular. The tricuspid valve enters from its right-hand posterior aspect, and the ventricular apex lies at the left inferior part. At the top of the right ventricle the pulmonary valve sits on the top of the muscular conus or infundibulum which separates it from the tricuspid valve. Seen from the side the right ventricle is flattened with a meniscal cross-section produced by the large interventricular septum (really part of the left ventricle) bulging into the right ventricle. The right ventricle does not contribute to the cardiac outline in the frontal view but forms most of the front of the heart in the lateral view. In the normally shaped chest only the lower half of the normal heart is in contact with the sternum.

Selective enlargement imposes the triangular shape of the right ventricle on the heart in the frontal view (Figs 20.32 and 20.33). A bulge may be seen on the left heart border above the apex but below the expected position of the left atrial appendage where the large right ventricle, usually its infundibulum, forms part of the left heart border. Alternatively the bulge may be the large right ventricle lifting up a normal left ventricle. In the lateral view, selective right ventricular enlargement may be recognized by the bulging forward of the front of the heart, increasing the area of contact with the sternum. A similar filling-in may also result if the right atrial appendage is very large. Right ventricular enlargement

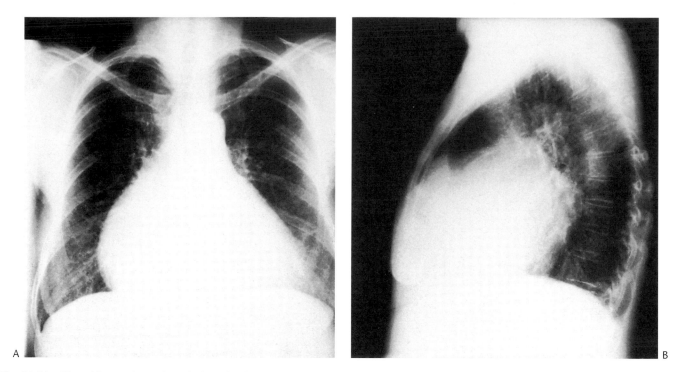

Fig. 20.30 Tricuspid stenosis. **A**. The right heart border has bulged to the right and its radius of curvature has increased. **B**. In the lateral view, the gap between the front of the heart and the sternum is filled in.

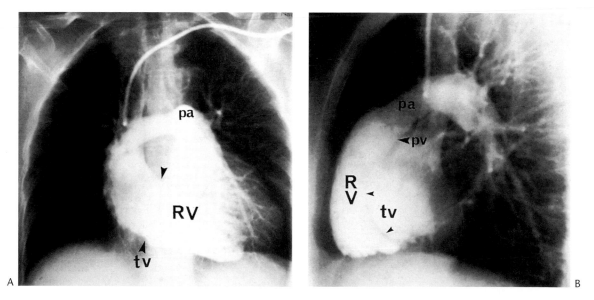

Fig. 20.31 Normal right ventricular angiocardiogram, superior vena cava injection. **A**. Frontal view. **B**. Lateral view. The right ventricle does not contribute to the cardiac silhouette in the frontal view except at the upper left border where its infundibulum reaches to the left border of the heart. It forms the front of the heart in the lateral view. These angiocardiograms indicate the position of the tricuspid valve, which because of its oblique lie is not seen in the profile in either frontal or lateral views but its approximate position is indicated by the arrows. The pulmonary bay may be seen to be formed by the left border of the main pulmonary artery beyond the pulmonary valve and before it divides into right and left pulmonary arteries. The triangular shape of the right ventricle in the frontal view is obvious with the pulmonary artery sitting on its infundibulum. The flat shape in the lateral view is also obvious.

may also occur as a result of pulmonary hypertension or pulmonary valve disease (usually pulmonary incompetence), tricuspid valve disease, or left-to-right shunts.

The right ventricle is characterized morphologically by its muscular conus, which separates its entry from its exit valves, by its coarsely trabeculated septal aspect, and by the direct attachment of part of its valve to the septum, either by chordae tendinae or by a papillary muscle of the conus.

The **left atrium** (Fig. 20.34) has an oval shape when seen from the front, and is flattened when seen from the side. The four

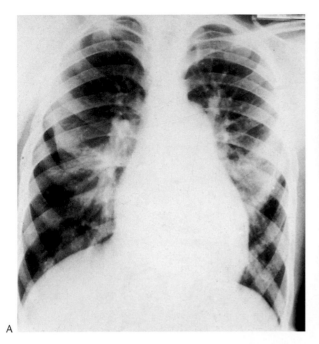
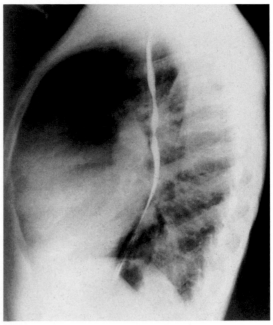

Fig. 20.32 Right ventricular enlargement due to atrial septal defect. **A.** Frontal view. Note the triangular shape of the heart with an indeterminate apex and a bulge of the left mid-heart border. There is also a convex pulmonary bay and pulmonary plethora (see below). **B.** Lateral view. This shows that there is slight bulging forward of the sternum but, in addition, there is an increased area of contact between the front of the heart and the sternum.

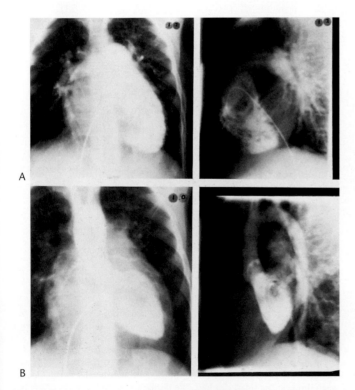

Fig. 20.33 Biventricular angiography in atrial septal defect. Same patient as Fig. 20.32. **A.** Frontal and lateral right ventricular angiograms. **B.** Frontal and lateral left ventricular angiograms. Note that the left border of the heart is now formed by the markedly enlarged right ventricle which also accounts for the increased contact of the heart with the sternum in the lateral view. The left ventricle, which has been pushed back by the large right ventricle, no longer contributes to the cardiac silhouette in the frontal view.

pulmonary veins enter its posterior aspect, two on each side. The left atrium forms the upper posterior border of the heart, although this border cannot clearly be seen as it is not in contact with air-containing lung. The position of the border can be identified on good-quality films, as the air-containing left main bronchus lies in contact with the back of the heart; so does the esophagus, and when this is opacified with barium it marks the back wall of the left atrium. The left atrial appendage is a narrow, finger-like protrusion from the left upper anterior border of the left atrium, passing forward round the upper left heart border to be buried in the epicardial fat. In the normal heart, neither the body of the left atrium nor its appendage makes any significant contribution to the cardiac silhouette in the frontal view.

Left atrial enlargement (Fig. 20.35) may involve the appendage or the body or both. The enlarged appendage may be identified, first by the straightening of the normally concave left heart border, then by the appearance of a discrete bulge below the pulmonary conus and above the left ventricle. Enlargement of the left atrial body may occur to the right, where it first appears as a double shadow through the heart, progressing to form the right heart border. When gross it extends to the left. Enlargement may also occur posteriorly, displacing the left main bronchus and barium-filled esophagus backward. As most left atrial enlargement is associated with mitral valve disease, the subject is considered again in Chapter 23, but enlargement may occur in any process causing either pressure or volume load to be transmitted to the left atrium, particularly left ventricular disease. The left atrium is the most sensitive chamber for the detection of chamber enlargement.

The morphological characteristics of a left atrium are the opposite of those of the right. It lacks a limbus to the fossa ovalis, and its appendage is long finger-like and narrow based.

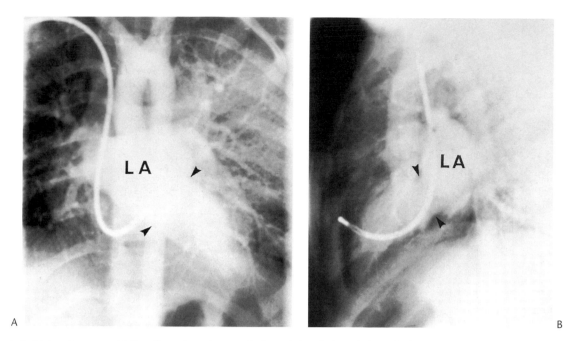

Fig. 20.34 Left atrial angiogram and follow-through angiogram. **A**. Frontal view. **B**. Lateral view. The left atrium forms a flattened structure, which is the upper posterior border of the heart in the lateral view, but does not contribute to the cardiac silhouette in the frontal view. The arrows indicate the position of the mitral valve which is not seen in profile.

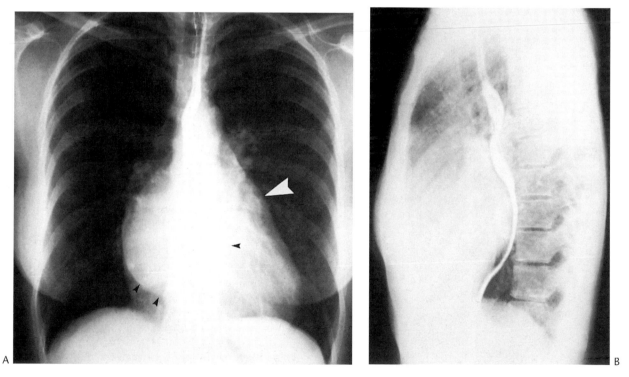

Fig. 20.35 Selective left atrial enlargement. **A**. Frontal view. The left atrial appendage produces a localized bulge on the left heart border (white arrow) below the pulmonary bay. The double shadow (paired arrows) of the left atrium is seen through the heart shadow. The displacement of the aorta to the left is indicated by the single arrow. Note that the right atrial shadow continues below the diaphragm as it is anchored by the inferior vena cava. **B**. Lateral view. Note the localized posterior displacement of the barium-filled esophagus, which returns to its normal position at the site of the mitral valve.

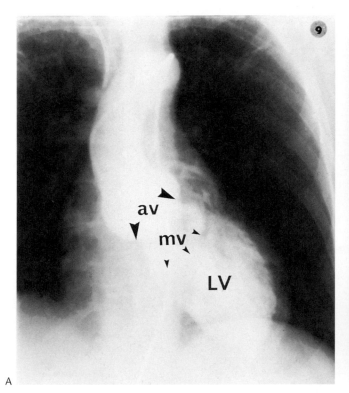
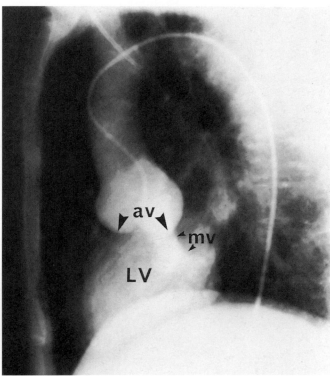

Fig. 20.36 Left ventricular angiocardiograms. **A**. Frontal view. The left ventricle forms the left border of the cardiac silhouette, and its apex forms the apex of the heart. The aortic valve lies approximately in the middle of the heart shadow. The mitral valve can be identified by the non-opaque blood entering and, with contrast medium, trapped under the posterior leaflet (small arrows). **B**. Lateral view. The left ventricle forms the lower part of the posterior border of the heart. The aortic valve lies approximately in the middle of the heart shadow. The anterior leaflet of the mitral valve (small arrows) is suspended from the non-coronary cusp of the aortic valve. The mitral valve lies obliquely and is not seen in profile in these views but its approximate position has been indicated. The aorta, beginning at the aortic valve, extends to the right of the superior mediastinum and then passes to the left of the esophagus and trachea to reach the posterior mediastinum, and turns downward as the descending aorta. On the right the aorta is concealed by the superior vena cava, and its most posterior part forms the aortic knob of the frontal chest X-ray.

The left ventricle (Fig. 20.36) is a carrot-shaped structure whose base is formed by the fibrous skeleton of the aortic and mitral valves. The long axis of the ventricle points from the base, downward, forward, and to the left to the apex of the left ventricle, which in turn almost invariably forms the apex of the heart. The left ventricle forms the left border of the heart in the frontal view and the lower posterior border, below the level of the mitral valve, in the lateral view.

Left ventricular enlargement is recognized in two ways. Left ventricular hypertrophy produces a rounding of the cardiac apex. Left ventricular dilatation (Fig. 20.37A) imposes its shape on the heart in the frontal view, with elongation of the cardiac apex either to the left or to the left and downward, often combined with the rounding of the apex. Left ventricular enlargement may sometimes be identified in the lateral view when the soft tissue shadow of the left ventricle protrudes behind the line of the barium-filled esophagus, or more than 2 cm behind the back of the right atrium as indicated by the entrance of the inferior vena cava (Fig. 20.37B).

Left ventricular enlargement may occur in any pressure or volume overload of the left ventricle. Pressure overload results from hypertension, coarctation, aortic heart disease, or any form of congenital aortic obstruction. Volume overload may be caused by mitral or aortic regurgitation or left-to-right shunt. Left ventri-

cular enlargement may also result from diseases of heart muscle such as ischemia or cardiomyopathy.

The morphological characteristics of the left ventricle are the lack of a muscular conus separating the entry and exit valves, which are in fibrous continuity, a smooth septal aspect, and a mitral valve which is not attached directly to the ventricular septum.

The **aorta** (see Fig. 20.36) begins at the aortic valve, which lies just above the middle of the heart shadow in both frontal and lateral views. The aortic valve lies within the heart mass and does not usually cast a discrete shadow. Rarely a faint small double shadow may be seen through the heart in the frontal view, rather resembling that of the left atrium, though seen to be continuous with the ascending aorta. The normal ascending aorta does not form a discrete shadow in the right superior mediastinum, being covered by the superior vena cava. When dilated and elongated in old age or hypertension the ascending aorta bulges to the right. Only the frontal wall of the ascending aorta is easily identified in the lateral view, the posterior wall not being in contact with gas-containing lung is imperfectly seen. The arch of the aorta passes in front of the trachea and then backward to the left of the trachea and esophagus. It can usually be seen indenting the left side of the trachea, in correctly penetrated films, and also the barium-filled esophagus. In cases of doubt those signs indicate the side of the

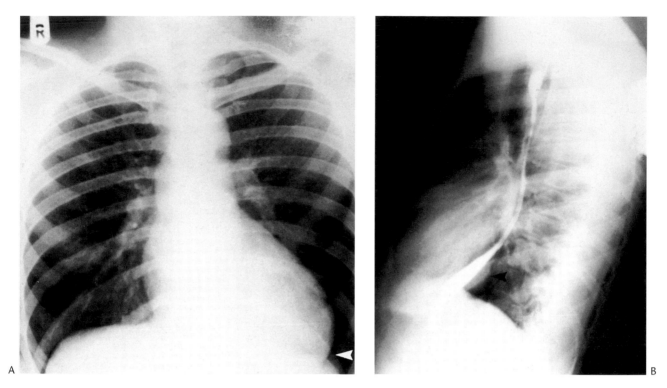

Fig. 20.37   Selective left ventricular enlargement in aortic incompetence. **A**. Frontal view shows that the left ventricle has enlarged along its long axis, taking the apex of the heart to the left and downward (white arrow). **B**. Lateral view shows the left ventricle extending behind the line of the barium-filled esophagus (arrow).

aortic arch. The shadow of the aortic knob is formed by the most posterior part of the aortic arch. The left border of a descending aorta can usually be identified in adult patients as a straight line passing downward and toward the midline, lying to the left of the spine and in continuity with the arch of the aorta.

The **main pulmonary artery** (see Fig. 20.31), that part of the pulmonary artery between the pulmonary valve and the bifurcation into the right and left pulmonary arteries, forms the floor of the pulmonary bay and lies on the left between the aortic arch and the heart proper. In the normal adult the floor of the pulmonary bay tends to be straight. In children and young women, a convexity, indicating a prominent main pulmonary artery, may still be normal.

CARDIAC SIZE

The plain film is an important indicator of cardiac size. The detection of cardiac enlargement is an important aspect of its use. The customary method of assessment is the measurement of the cardiothoracic ratio (Fig. 20.38). In adult caucasian patients this should not exceed 50% (two standard deviations above the mean), but in colored patients up to 55% may still be normal.

The cardiothoracic ratio is increased in the elderly; this may be due to an infolding of the ribs, reducing the thoracic component of the ratio, or due to heart disease. The cardiothoracic ratio may be increased in the neonate (see p. 564).

The transverse diameter of the heart may be measured directly on a radiograph taken at 1.8 m. An upper limit of 16 cm for men and 15 cm for women is usual. The advantage of a single

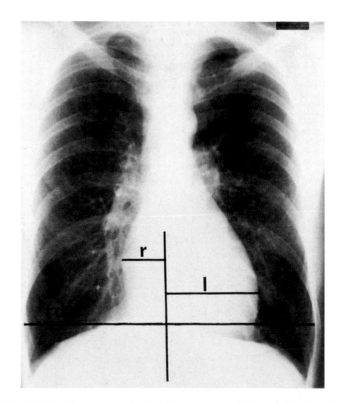

Fig. 20.38   The assessment of cardiac enlargement. The cardiac diameter should be the maximum cardiac diameter (r + 1). The transverse thoracic diameter is measured in various ways; here it is measured as the maximum internal diameter of the thorax.

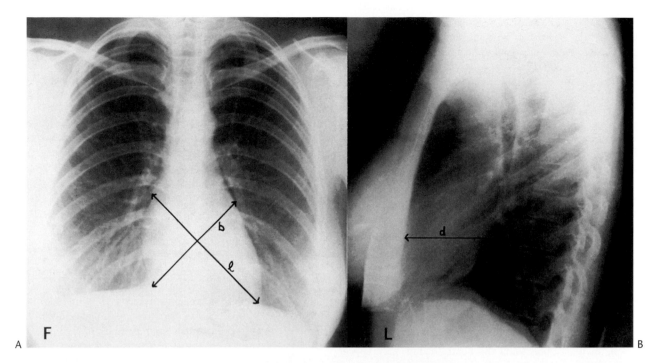

Fig. 20.39 Measurement of cardiac volume. The volume of the heart may be measured on the assumption that the heart is an ellipsoid, and if the lengths of its three axes can be determined, its volume = $l \times b \times d \times \pi/6 \times 1/m^3$ (where m is the magnification factor).

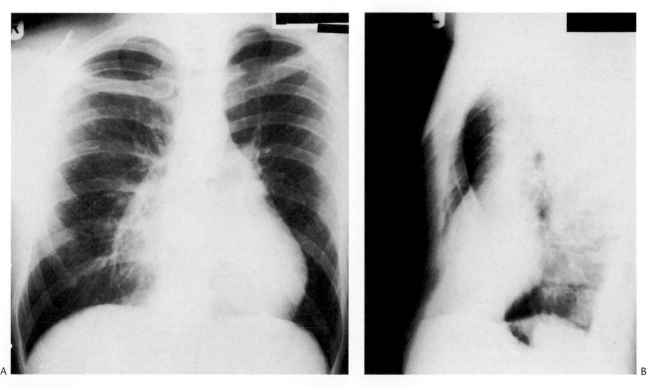

Fig. 20.40 Depressed sternum. **A**. Frontal view. The heart is displaced to the left. Its left border is straight and there is a prominence in the position of the main pulmonary artery. There is an ill-defined shadow to the right of the vertebral column. The clue to those appearances is given by the visualization of the intervertebral discs at the level of the lower thoracic spine where normally they would disappear. **B**. Lateral view. This demonstrates the enormous sternal depression. This patient was thought to have a normal heart.

measurement is that it may be compared in serial films. A difference of 2 cm is held to be a significant change. This applies only when the heart is originally normal, and physiological differences of almost that size may be encountered. In significantly enlarged hearts much less change in diameter will be significant.

The measurement of cardiac volume (Fig. 20.39), on the assumption that the heart may be represented as an ellipsoid, is not routinely performed, other than in Scandinavia.

In the neonate, the heart may be relatively larger compared to the thorax than in the adult, and a cardiothoracic ratio of up to 60% is not necessarily abnormal. Considerable care should be taken before diagnosing cardiomegaly radiologically, as much unnecessary investigation may follow. The neonatal chest is also difficult to study radiologically as the heart shape tends to be non-specific because of the right ventricular preponderance which is present at birth. The mediastinal structures are frequently concealed by a large thymus so that identification of the side of the aortic arch and of the pulmonary bay may be difficult or impossible.

DEPRESSED STERNUM

Analysis of the size and shape of the heart may be made difficult or impossible in the presence of skeletal deformities, of which depressed sternum (Fig. 20.40) is the most common. The presence of odd murmurs, apparently related to the deformity but resembling those of heart disease, may complicate the clinical examination. In the frontal view the heart shadow may appear overtly enlarged. Its left border is often straightened and the main pulmonary artery may appear prominent. The right border of the heart may bulge to the right if the heart is compressed against the spine, but most commonly it is not seen to the right of the sternum when the heart, as is usual, is displaced to the left. The central pulmonary vessels may appear prominent, and this together with the slightly odd murmurs may raise the possibility of an atrial septal defect. Ill-defined shadowing, often extensive, is frequently seen in the right pericardiophrenic angle, which the unwary might take for a pulmonary lesion. It does not show an air bronchogram. The easy visibility of the vertebral bodies and their intervertebral disks through the heart shadow of the standard frontal film always raises the possibility that the appearances of the heart are due to depressed sternum. If downward-sloping anterior ribs are present, this virtually confirms the diagnosis.

The appearances on the lateral view are often rather unimpressive, varying from a slight reduction in the anteroposterior diameter of the chest from flattening of the sternum to gross sternal depression with compression of the heart against the spine. The 'straight back syndrome', whose chief radiological feature is obvious from its name, also leads to a narrowing of the anteroposterior diameter of the chest, with squashing of the heart between sternum and spine, and similar, though less marked, cardiac appearances to those of depressed sternum, in the frontal view. It may be associated with prolapse of the mitral valve.

REFERENCES AND SUGGESTIONS FOR FURTHER READING

Anderson, R. H., Becker, A. E. (1982) *Cardiac Anatomy: an Integrated Text and Colour Atlas*. Edinburgh: Churchill Livingstone.

Brown, K. A. (1991) Prognostic value of thallium 201 myocardial imaging: a diagnostic tool comes of age. *Circulation* **88**, 363–381.

Carr, D. H. (1988) *Contrast Media*, Edinburgh: Churchill Livingstone.

Daniel, W. G., Mugge, A. (1995) Trans oesophageal echocardiography. *New England Journal of Medicine*, **332**, 1268–1278.

Donaldson, R. M., Westgate C. (1985) *A Guide to Cardiac Ultrasound*. London: King & Wirth.

Elliott, L. P., Bargeron, L. M., Soto, B., Bream P. R. (1980) Axial cine-angiography in congenital heart disease. *Radiologic Clinics in North America*, **18**, 515–546.

Feigenbaum, H. (1986) *Echocardiography*, 5th edn. Philadelphia: Lea & Febiger.

Fowler, N. O. (ed.) (1983) *Non-invasive Diagnostic Methods in Cardiology*. Philadelphia: F.A. Davis.

Germano, G., Van Train, K., Garcia, L., et al (1992) *Quantitation of Myocardial Perfusion with SPET: Current Issues and Future Trends in Nuclear Cardiology, The State of the Art and Future Directions*. St Louis: Mosby Year Book, pp. 77–88.

Grossman, W. *Cardiac Catheterisation and Angiography*. Philadelphia: Lea & Febiger.

Hatle, K., Angelson, B. (1985) *Doppler Ultrasound in Cardiology. Physical Principles & Clinical Applications*. Philadelphia: Lea & Febiger.

Higgins, C. B. (ed.) (1983) *CT of the Heart and Great Vessels*. Mount Kisco, New York: Futura.

Maddah J., Schelbert, H., Brunken, R. (1994) Role of thallium 201 and PET imaging in evaluation of myocardial viability and management of patients with CAD and LV dysfunction. *Journal of Nuclear Medicine*, **35**, 707–715.

Netter, F. H. (1969) *The Ciba Collection of Medical Illustrations*, Vol. 5. *The Heart*. London: Ciba.

O'Rourke, R. F. (1988) Value of Doppler echocardiography for quantifying valvular stenosis or regurgitation. *Circulation*, **78**, 483–485.

Raphael, M. J., Allwork, S. P. (1974) Angiographic anatomy of the left ventricle. *Clinical Radiology*, **25**, 95–105.

Raphael, M. J., Allwork, S. P. (1976) Angiographic anatomy of the right heart. *Clinical Radiology*, **27**, 265–272.

Simpson, I. A., de Belder, M. A., Kenny, A., et al (1995) How to quantitate valve regurgitation by echo Doppler techniques. *British Heart Journal*, **73**, 1–9.

Underwood, R., Firmin, D. (1987) *An Introduction to Magnetic Resonance of the Cardiovascular System*. London: Current Medical Literature.

Walton, S., Ell, P. J. (1983) *Introduction to Nuclear Cardiology*. London: Current Medical Literature.

Zaret, B., Wackers, F. J. (1993) Nuclear cardiology. *New England Journal of Medicine*, **329**, 775–783.

CT

Collins, M. A., Pidgeon, J. W., Fitzgerald, R. (1995) Computed tomography manifestations of tricuspid regurgitation. *British Journal of Radiology*, **68**, 1058–1060.

Link, K. M., Lesko, N. M. (1994). Cardiac imaging. *Radiological Clinics of North America*, **32**(3).

Wegener, O. H. (1992). *Whole Body Computed Tomography*. Oxford: Blackwell Scientific.

MRI

Blackwell, G. G., Cranney, G. B., Pohost, G. M. (1992) *MRI: Cardiovascular System*. New York: Gower Medical.

Boxt, L. M. (ed.) (1996) Cardiac MR imaging. *Magnetic Resonance Imaging Clinics of North America*, **4**, 191–432.

Brown, J. J., Scott, A. M., Sandstrom, J. C., Perman, W. H. (1990) MR spectroscopy of the heart. *American Journal of Roentgenology*, **155**, 1–11.

Davis, C. P., McKinnon, G. C., Debatin, J. F., Wetter, D., Eichenberger, A. C., Duewell, S., von Schulthess, G. K. (1994) Normal heart: evaluation with echo-planar MR imaging. *Radiology*, **191**, 691–696.

de Roos, A., van Voorthuisen, A. E. (1989) Magnetic resonance imaging of the heart—morphology and function. *Current Opinion in Radiology*, **1**, 166–173.

Edelman, R. R., Li, W. (1994) Contrast-enhanced echo-planar MR imaging of myocardial perfusion: preliminary study in humans. *Radiology*, **190**, 771–777.

Edelman, R. E., Hesselink, J. R., Zlatkin, M. B. (eds) (1996) Cardiovascular system. Part VI. In: *Clinical Magnetic Resonance Imaging*, 2nd edn. Philadelphia: W. B. Saunders, Chapts 52–55, pp. 1615–1793.

Gutierrez, F. R., Brown, J. J., Mirowitz, A. (1993) *Cardiovascular Magnetic Resonance Imaging*. St Louis: Mosby Year Book.

Hartnell, G. G., Meier, R. A. (1995) MR angiography of congenital heart disease in adults. *Radiographics*, **15**, 781–794.

Henkelman, R. M. (1990) Technologic advances in magnetic resonance imaging and spectroscopy for cardiovascular applications. *Current Opinion in Radiology*, **2**, 542–546.

Jarvinen, V. M., Kupair, M. M., Hekali, P. E., Poutanen, V.P. (1994) Right atrial MR imaging studies of cadaveric atrial casts and comparison with right and left atrial volumes and function in healthy studies. *Radiology*, **191**, 137–142.

Jenkins, J. P. R., Isherwood, I. (1987) Magnetic resonance imaging of the heart: a review. In: D. J. Rowlands (Ed.) *Recent Advances in Cardiology 10*, Edinburgh: Churchill Livingstone, pp. 219–247.

Mansfield, P., Morris, P. G. (1982) *NMR Imaging in Biomedicine*. New York: Academic Press.

Miller, S. W. (1996) *Cardiac Radiology—The Requisites*. St Louis: Mosby.

Mirowitz, S. A., Lee, J. K. T., Gutierrez, F. R., Brown, J. J., Eilenberg, S. S. (1990) Normal signal-void patterns in cardiac cine MR images. *Radiology*, **176**, 49–55.

Mitchell, L., Jenkins, J. P. R., Watson, Y., Rowlands, D. J., Isherwood, I. (1989) Diagnosis and assessment of mitral and aortic valve disease by cine-flow magnetic resonance imaging. *Magnetic Resonance in Medicine*, **12**, 181–197.

Nayler, G. L., Firmin, D. N., Longmore, D. B. (1986) Blood flow imaging by cine magnetic resonance. *Journal of Computer Assisted Tomography*, **10**, 715–722.

Rees, S. (1990) Magnetic resonance studies of the heart (the George Simon Lecture). *Clinical Radiology*, **42**, 302–316.

Sakuma, H., Caputo, G. R., Steffens, J. C., O'Sullivan, M., Bourne, M., Shimakawa, A., Foo, T. K., Higgins, C. B. (1994) Breath-hold MR cine angiography of coronary arteries in healthy volunteers: value of multiangle oblique imaging planes. *American Journal of Roentgenology*, **163**, 533–537.

Shellock, F. G., Kanal, E. (1994) *Magnetic Resonance Bioeffects, Safety and Patient Management*. New York: Raven Press.

Zerhouni, E. A., Parish, D. M., Rogers, W. J., Yang, A., Shapiro, E. P. (1988) Human heart: tagging with MR imaging—a method for non-invasive assessment of myocardial motion. *Radiology*, **169**, 59–63.

21

THE PERICARDIUM

M. J. Raphael and R. M. Donaldson
With a contribution from Jeremy P. R. Jenkins

NORMAL ANATOMY

The pericardial sac consists of two layers separated by a potential space which is lubricated by a few milliliters of pericardial fluid. The parietal pericardium is a tough fibrous sac, enclosing the heart and attached to the central tendon of the diaphragm below. The visceral pericardium is closely applied to the surface of the heart. The two layers are fused next to the heart at the entry of the pulmonary veins to the left atrium posteriorly and at the entry of the inferior vena cava to the right atrium inferiorly. The two layers extend up the aorta, to fuse about half-way between the aortic valve and the origin of the innominate artery; they extend along the main pulmonary artery, fusing with it before its bifurcation, and along the superior vena cava.

Radiographic Appearances

The pericardium has the same radiographic density as the heart. In spite of this it may be identified on the frontal film if there is a substantial amount of epicardial fat, which produces a low-density linear shadow, with a normal-density shadow of the pericardium appearing as a thin white line outside it.

The epicardial fat line is often best identified in the lateral view, and enables an estimate of the thickness of the pericardium to be made (see later).

The pericardial outline may be obscured by the pericardial fat pads, which may develop in the cardiophrenic angles as ill-defined low-density triangular shadows with their vertices in the cardiophrenic angles. The outline of the heart with its pericardium is often identifiable through them. The nature of these shadows is usually obvious from the lateral view, where they have a characteristically ill-defined triangular shape with the base of the triangle abutting on the anterior chest wall. Rather similar appearances may be produced by pleural thickening over the base of the middle lobe or lingula. Only rarely do these appearances lead to difficulties in differentiation from tumors or hernias occurring in the regions of the anterior cardiophrenic angles.

Ultrasound

The parietal pericardium produces strong echoes in both M-mode and cross-sectional echocardiography (CSE). In the absence of pericardial disease the strong echoes are continuous with the posterior wall of the left ventricle. The pericardium cannot be identified anteriorly unless it is abnormal.

CT Scanning

Using modern high-speed machines the anterior and caudal part of the pericardium, where it is surrounded externally by the mediastinal fat and internally by epicardial fat, can be identified in almost all patients without the use of contrast medium. The normal pericardium appears as a fine line, 1–2 mm thick, in front of the lower part of the right and left ventricles and right atrium. Patchy areas of apparent pericardial thickening up to a few millimeters in thickness may be identified over the right ventricle in the apparently normal patient, and are thought to be movement artefacts. The normal pericardium cannot usually be identified posteriorly.

MRI Scanning

The pericardium is well visualized on cardiac MRI (see below).

Angiocardiography

Opacification of the right atrium by contrast medium injection into it or the vena cava, and frontal filming, will demonstrate the combined thickness of the pericardium and the wall of the right atrium, which is normally less than 3–4 mm. Later filming, as the contrast medium passes through the chambers of the heart, may also be helpful in detecting displacements and deformities of these chambers resulting from pericardial disease.

Pneumopericardium

The inner aspect of the pericardium may be outlined by gas introduced during pericardiocentesis, and the thickness of the pericardium determined.

DISEASES OF THE PERICARDIUM

CONGENITAL DEFECTS

These are rare and may be partial or complete, and usually involve the left side of the pericardium. Partial defects are usually asymptomatic, but may produce symptoms if the left atrial appendage herniates through the defect and then strangulates. They may be associated with non-specific murmurs. Complete absence of the pericardium is not usually associated with specific clinical features. In both conditions, the plain films suggest the diagnosis.

In partial defects there is a bulge on the left heart border, usually in the position of the left atrial appendage and appearing to suggest that this structure is enlarged. However, there is no other radiological evidence of left atrial enlargement and no clinical features to suggest this, though the non-specific murmurs may be confusing. Rarely the pulmonary artery may appear enlarged if it herniates through the defect and this (Fig. 21.1), combined with non-specific murmurs, may suggest a diagnosis of pulmonary stenosis.

CT scanning reveals partial absence of the left pericardium and prominence and altered rotation of the main pulmonary artery.

Angiocardiography in the levophase of a pulmonary artery injection will confirm that the abnormal shadow is the left atrial appendage or an otherwise normal main pulmonary artery. In view of the danger of strangulation, it has been suggested that the left atrial appendage should be amputated and the pericardial defect closed.

Complete defects of the left pericardium (Fig. 21.1) produce a characteristic appearance, with the whole heart displaced to the left with a prominent pulmonary artery shadow, perhaps a prominence of the left atrial appendage and with a slightly prominent left ventricular border. Gas-containing lung may be interposed between the heart and the left diaphragm if there is no connection between the pericardium and the diaphragm.

The diagnosis is usually made with confidence from the plain film and the absence of other features of heart disease. CT scanning may demonstrate the absence of the left pericardium and the altered axis of the main pulmonary artery to the left, and thus confirm the diagnosis. If there is still doubt, an artificial pneumothorax will allow gas to enter the pericardium and confirm its absence.

PERICARDIAL EFFUSION

This is the commonest abnormality of the pericardium to be encountered in routine radiological practice. The presenting features may be pain, when the cause is inflammatory, or malignant disease, or the clinical features of tamponade. Tamponade is characterized by shortness of breath, hypotension, pulsus paradoxus, and distended neck veins, and depends on the rapidity of fluid collection; over a liter may be present without symptoms if it collects slowly, whereas 200–300 ml collecting rapidly may cause symptoms. The fluid in the indistensible pericardial sac compresses the heart and obstructs the entry of blood through the vena cavae, leading to a fall in cardiac output.

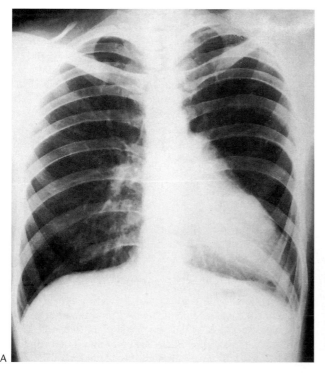
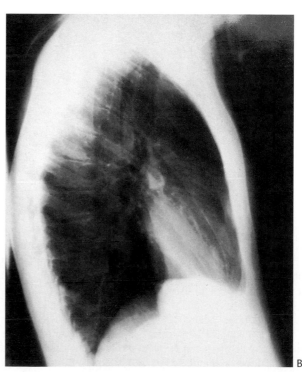

Fig. 21.1 Congenital absence of the left pericardium. **A.** Frontal view. Note that the heart is displaced to the left and there is a prominence in the position of the main pulmonary artery. Note also that the outline of the left diaphragm is clear as far as the spine. **B.** Lateral view. This is unremarkable.

The commonest disease of the pericardium, pericarditis, does not produce radiological abnormality unless an effusion is present.

Radiological Appearances

The plain film appearances depend on the amount of fluid and its distribution. If there is sufficient fluid the heart shadow will be enlarged, and in larger effusions, grossly so. It may have a globular or non-specific shape, but in large effusions there is very often a rather localized bulge in the left upper cardiac border which may lead to confusion (Fig. 21.2). Although the heart shadow appears enlarged, there are no features on the film to suggest selective chamber enlargement.

The accumulation and dispersal of fluid produces rapid changes in the heart size on serial films, and when these occur they always suggest pericardial fluid as the cause.

Displacement of the epicardial fat stripe inwards, when this can be identified, also points to a pericardial effusion. This is usually better seen on the lateral view, though in our experience it is rare (Fig. 21.2).

Screening of the heart to show diminished pulsation and changes in shape from erect to supine posture is of historical interest only.

The obstruction of venous return to the right heart rather than the left heart leads to a reduction in flow and pressure through the lungs, so that abnormalities of the pulmonary vasculature are striking by their absence.

These features lead to one of the characteristic appearances of a pericardial effusion: a large heart with clear lungs rather than congested lungs, which usually occur in heart disease. The other feature to suggest a pericardial effusion is a rapid change in heart size over serial films.

Other Investigations

Once a pericardial effusion is suspected, *echocardiography* is the next step (Fig. 21.3). The CSE shows an echo-free space surrounding the heart, and if the effusion is large the whole heart can be seen swinging in it. CSE allows visualization of the aspiration needle during pericardiocentesis and thus avoids penetration of the myocardium. Several signs of cardiac tamponade have been described, such as right ventricular diastolic collapse, but the sensitivity of these is poor. Doppler examination shows an exaggerated inspiratory increase in tricuspid flow velocity, but again this feature is rather non-specific.

CT scanning is also very helpful in medium and large pericardial effusions, showing a continuous layer of fluid surrounding the heart. The layer may be of either high or low density but this characteristic does not help in distinguishing the nature of the fluid.

Angiocardiography is now only rarely required, but right atrial angiography in the anteroposterior view will show an increase in the combined thickness of the right atrial wall and the pericardium to more than 4 mm. However, it does not distinguish fluid from thickening. It would also show elevation of the floor of the right ventricle due to inferior fluid, and will show any localized fluid collecting over the left ventricle.

Aspiration The nature of the pericardial effusion may be obvious on the basis of known clinical features, otherwise fluid may be aspirated and examined. *Gas* (or *contrast agent*) may be introduced into the pericardium at aspiration to outline the inside of the pericardium and indicate its thickness. A thin smooth pericardium suggests a transudate; a thick pericardium, an infec-

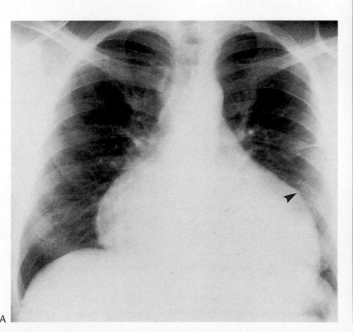
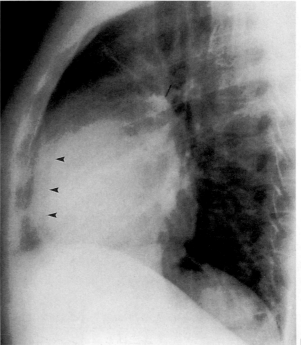

A   B

Fig. 21.2 Pericardial effusion. A chest film taken 6 months previously was normal. **A.** Frontal chest film. The heart silhouette has dramatically increased in size. There is an ill-defined bulge (arrow) above the cardiac apex. The lungs show no features of cardiac failure, which might be expected if this were a dilated heart. **B.** Lateral chest film. Epicardial fat is clearly identified (arrows), displaced away from the edge of the cardiac silhouette and indicating the presence of a pericardial effusion.

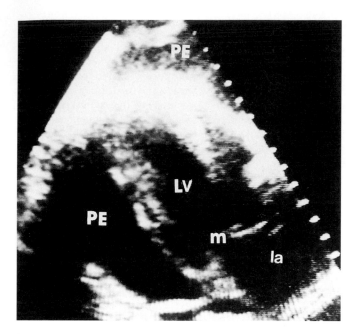

Fig. 21.3 Pericardial effusion, CSE study. In this long-axis view, a large echo-free space of pericardial effusion (PE) is seen both behind and in front of the left ventricle (LV). la, left atrium; m, mitral valve.

tion; and localized masses on the inside of the pericardium, a tumor. The heart structures are often clearly identified when there is gas in the pericardium.

A pneumopericardium may also result from chest or abdominal trauma or after cardiac surgery.

Etiology

The following conditions may be associated with a pericardial effusion.

Malignant Disease Secondary malignant disease, usually from the breast, commonly produces a pericardial effusion and may lead to tamponade.

Inflammatory Disease Bacterial, tuberculous or viral infections may all lead to an exudative pericardial effusion.

Heart Disease A pericardial effusion may result from cardiac failure or may be associated with myocardial infarction when this is complicated by *Dressler syndrome*.

Endocrine Diseases The best known of these is myxedema, which frequently has a substantial though often asymptomatic pericardial effusion.

Collagen Diseases All the collagen diseases may be associated with a pericardial effusion, but in systemic lupus erythematosis it may be quite large.

Uremia A large pericardial effusion may be a feature of uremia though it rarely leads to tamponade.

Hemopericardium This may result from trauma, from rupture of the heart in the course of myocardial infarction, or a dissecting aneurysm leading into the pericardium.

CONSTRICTIVE PERICARDITIS

In this condition there is impairment of filling of the chambers of the heart, almost always involving mainly the right heart, and due to thickening and hence rigidity of the pericardium. Viral and tuberculous pericarditis are the commonest causes leading to constriction, but hemopericardium may lead to constriction, as may collagen disease involving the pericardium.

The patient presents with edema and may have hepatomegaly and ascites. Shortness of breath is not a feature. The diagnosis of heart disease may not be obvious as there are no murmurs, and the neck veins may be so distended that pulsations are not visible, and the heart itself may not be enlarged. The diagnosis of constriction presents two problems: recognizing that the cause of symptoms is heart disease, and distinguishing constriction of the pericardium from a restrictive cardiomyopathy.

Radiological Appearances

On plain film examination, the heart may be normal in size (Fig. 21.4A) or may be non-specifically enlarged. Straightening of the right heart border with a smoothing-out of its contour from superior to inferior vena cava may be seen (Fig. 21.4A). There may be pleuropericardial adhesions roughening the outline of the heart. About half the cases have pericardial calcification, seen over the front and sides of the heart but not at the back where fluid cannot collect at the insertion of the pulmonary veins into the left atrium (Fig. 21.4B). Calcification may be seen on the plain film but is often better demonstrated by fluoroscopy, which is not only more sensitive but is also able to locate calcification to the pericardium. Calcification also develops in the atrioventricular groove and may encircle the heart. Calcification, however, does not invariably mean constriction.

Due to constriction over the right heart, the lungs are usually clear though there may be a pleural effusion. In those unusual cases where constriction in the atrioventricular groove obstructs left atrial emptying, pulmonary oedema may develop. Not all calcified pericardiums are constricted.

Investigations

These are usually devoted to confirming the presence of constriction, and distinguishing this condition from restrictive cardiomyopathy. The CSE shows normally functioning chambers and may identify pericardial calcification by the dense echoes it produces. In the absence of calcification or pericardial fluid, the CSE may not demonstrate any abnormality of the pericardium. The *CT scan* will usually identify thickening of the pericardium and suggest a diagnosis of constrictive pericarditis (Fig. 21.5), but neither it nor the *MRI scan* can do other than show that the pericardium is abnormal, and this does not necessarily mean constriction is present. The demonstration of a normal pericardium (Fig. 21.6) virtually excludes the diagnosis of constrictive pericarditis.

Cardiac Catheterization and Angiocardiography Right and left ventricular catheterization and simultaneous pressure records are required to establish a diagnosis of constriction. When constriction is present, the diastolic pressures in the right and left ventricle are identical. Thickening of the pericardium can be

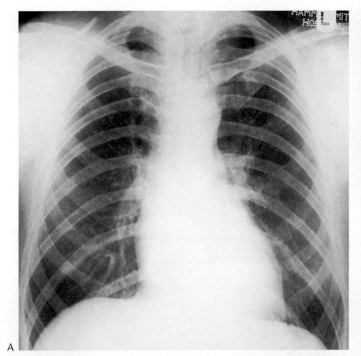

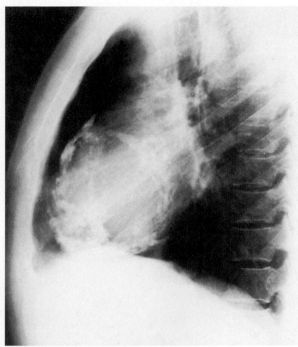

A

B

Fig. 21.4 Constrictive pericarditis. **A.** Frontal view. In this slightly light film the heart and lungs appear normal, apart from some possible straightening of the right heart border. **B.** Lateral view. This shows extensive pericardial calcification spreading over the front of the right ventricle and also encircling the heart in the atrioventricular grooves. There is no calcium at the back as fluid cannot collect there.

demonstrated by a right atrial injection, showing an increase in the thickness of the combined right atrial wall and pericardium above the normal 4 mm (Fig. 21.5C). The demonstration of thickening does not, however, inevitably point to constriction.

TUMORS OF THE PERICARDIUM

These are relatively rare, the only common tumor encountered is the benign *spring-water cyst* (synonym *pleuropericardial cyst*, *pericardial coelomic cyst*). These cysts are unilocular and thin walled and attached to the pericardium either intimately or by a pedicle, and are in some ways similar to pericardial diverticula, except that these communicate with the pericardial cavity. They are most commonly found in the pericardiophrenic angle, more often on the right than the left, though they can occur in any part of the lower half of the mediastinum. The smaller cysts may take up a rather 'tear-drop' shape and lie in an elongated fashion in the lower end of the oblique fissure, though the large ones are almost always spherical. On fluoroscopy they may be seen to change shape with respiration.

In the majority of cases the diagnosis is usually obvious on the plain radiograph, when they appear as rounded, sharply defined cystic shadows anteriorly in the pericardiophrenic angle (Fig. 21.7). Rarely a Morgagni hernia, which may be filled only with omentum in the elderly, may cause confusion. Barium study will distinguish the two.

Secondary malignant involvement of the pericardium is common, producing a pericardial effusion and possibly tamponade. The breast is a common primary site.

MRI OF THE PERICARDIUM

Jeremy P. R. Jenkins

The normal pericardium, demonstrated using ECG-gated T_1-weighted spin echo sequences, is a thin (less than 2 mm) line of low signal intensity between the high signal of pericardial fat and either the intermediate signal of myocardium or high signal of epicardial fat (Fig. 21.8). A variation in the clarity and thickness of the low-intensity line is observed during different phases of the cardiac cycle and in different anatomic regions. The low-intensity line is thicker in systole than in diastole and is best seen overlying the anterior part of the right ventricle. The variation in the thickness of this low-intensity line can be partly explained by a phase discontinuity artefact due to the shearing action between the visceral and parietal pericardium, produced in turn by the to-and-fro movement of the myocardium. This shearing action is most pronounced at the surface of the right ventricle, producing a loss of signal from the pixels spanning the pericardium. The normal pericardial space also contains a small amount of fluid (up to 25–50 ml) and on T_1-weighted images this may make the pericardium appear slightly thicker. The variation in clarity of the low intensity line and its apparent absence over certain parts of the heart on MRI are due to chemical shift and motion artefacts.

MRI has been found to be a useful complementary procedure to CSE in the study of patients with suspected pericardial abnormalities. Pericardial effusions, thickening and tumors can be differentiated. MRI is the best modality for the characterization of pericardial fluid collections and the assessment of extrinsic invasion and compression of the pericardium.

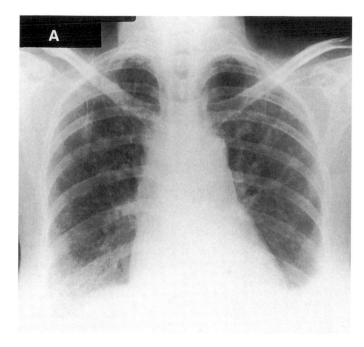

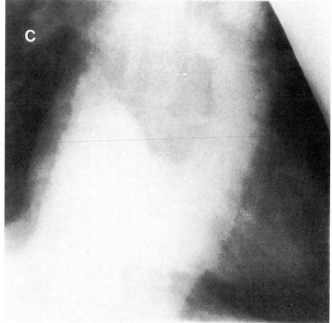

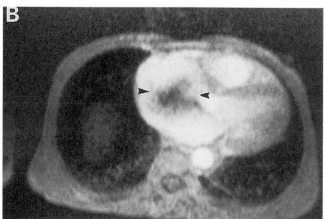

Fig. 21.5 Constrictive pericarditis. **A**. Frontal view. The heart is normal in size with some straightening of the right heart border. There are bilateral pleural effusions, larger on the left. There is also abnormal pulmonary shadowing due to active tuberculosis. This was the cause of the constriction. **B**. CT scan of the heart without contrast medium, same patient. Low-attenuation areas of pericardial fluid (F) surround the heart. The pericardium remains of normal thickeness over the right ventricle (single arrow) but is grossly thickened over the left ventricle (multiple arrows). **C**. Right atrial angiogram, same patient. The increased thickness between the opacified right atrium and the outer aspect of the cardiac shadow is clearly visible. This indicates pericardial thickening but does not necessarily indicate constriction.

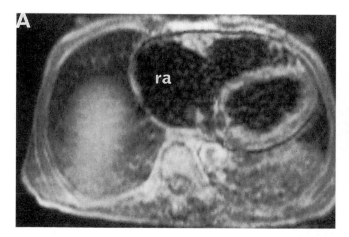

Fig. 21.6 Restrictive cardiomyopathy. **A**. MRI scan, spin echo technique. The pericardium is clearly seen as a dark stripe outlined by the high signal from epicardial and pericardial fat and surrounding the front and left side of the heart. It is of normal thickness, virtually excluding the diagnosis of constrictive pericarditis, which, if present, would require surgery. Note the large right atrium (ra), compatible with tricuspid regurgitation. **B**. FEER (field even echo rephasing) sequence. Flowing blood is seen as a high signal. Note the signal drop-out from turbulent flow (arrows) produced by tricuspid regurgitation.

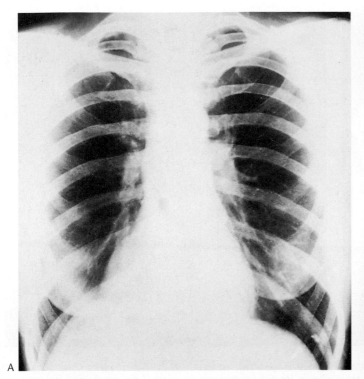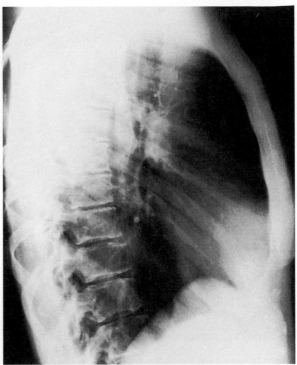

Fig. 21.7 Pericardial cyst. **A.** Frontal chest radiograph. there is a sharply defined abnormal shadow in the right pericardiophrenic angle. **B.** Lateral view. This is seen to lie anteriorly; this is one of the characteristic sites for a pericardial cyst.

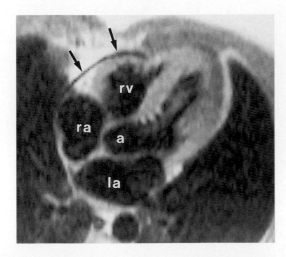

Fig. 21.8 Long-axis oblique gated T_1-weighted spine echo image (TE 26 ms) of the left ventricle and aortic outflow tract demonstrating the pericardium (arrowed) as a low signal overlying the right ventricle. a, ascending aorta; la, left atrium; ra, right atrium; rv, right ventricle.

Pericardial Effusion

MRI correlates well with CSE in the assessment of size and distribution of pericardial effusions. It is more useful, however, in detecting small fluid collections and in differentiating between exudative and transudative effusions. Cross-sectional echocardiography should, nevertheless, be used as the initial screening technique for the diagnosis and evaluation of pericardial effusions, reserving MRI for a problem-solving role when CSE results are inconclusive or there is a need for further tissue characterization (Fig. 21.9).

The differentiation of an exudative from a transudative pericardial effusion is based on the signal intensity appearance relative to the myocardium. A transudative effusion has a lower signal, similar to that of normal pericardial fluid, whereas as exudative collection has a higher signal than that of myocardium (see Fig. 23.59). Hemorrhagic effusions can be differentiated from other fluid collections by their medium-to-high signal intensity due to altered blood on T_1-weighted spin echo images. Non-hemorrhagic effusions usually give low signal on T_1-weighted spin echo images, whereas those associated with uremia, trauma and tuberculosis give a heterogeneous signal, related to a higher protein content. Effusions are usually differentiated from pericardial thickening by their morphological appearances rather than by changes in signal intensity (cf. Figs 21.10 and 23.59). Pericardial fluid, thickened fibrous pericardium and calcification all give a nonspecific low signal on MRI. CT, as might be expected, remains superior in the differentiation of fibrous and calcified tissue, and in the detection of pericardial calcification. In gradient echo images the pericardial space and any effusion are usually demonstrated as areas of high signal similar to moving blood.

Constrictive Pericarditis

Thickening of the pericardium associated with constrictive pericarditis can be diagnosed and differentiated from restrictive

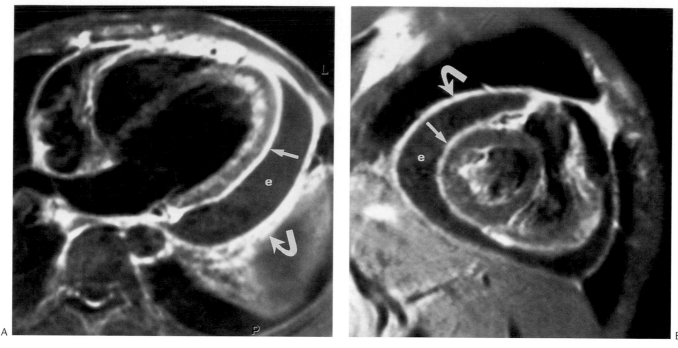

Fig. 21.9 Inflammatory pericarditis on **A** transverse and **B** parasagittal ECG-gated T_1-weighted spin echo (SE 750/15) images following intravenous administration of gadolinium chelate. There is a large low-signal pericardial effusion (e) with marked enhancement of the parietal (curved arrow) and visceral (straight arrow) pericardia.

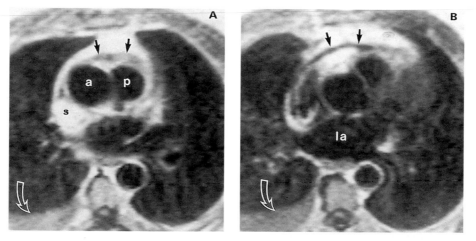

Fig. 21.10 Constrictive pericarditis with a thickened pericardium (straight arrows) and a right pleural effusion (curved arrow) on two transverse T_1-weighted spin echo images (TE 26 ms). Same key as in Fig. 21.8, and including: p, pulmonary artery; s, superior vena cava.

cardiomyopathy by MRI. In restrictive cardiomyopathies the thickness of the pericardium is normal but there may be small pericardial effusions, whereas in constrictive pericarditis the pericardium is thickened (up to 5 mm or more) (Fig. 21.10). MRI assessment of myocardial wall thickness and cardiac function can also provide useful information. In constrictive pericarditis, in addition to pericardial abnormality, the end-diastolic volume is small, with a small compressed right ventricle and normal to increased systolic myocardial wall thickening. In restrictive cardiomyopathy there may be abnormal myocardial wall thickness and systolic thickening.

Pericardial Tumors

Pericardial cysts can be readily differentiated from pericardial fat pads and Morgagni hernias on the basis of signal intensity and morphological appearances. A pericardial cyst has a low and high signal appearance on T_1-and T_2-weighted spin echo images, respectively, whereas fat gives a high signal on both. A Morgagni hernia will show a defect in the diaphragm in connection with the peritoneal space and may contain liver or bowel. Infiltration of the pericardium by extrinsic tumor can be inferred from absence or loss of the pericardial low-intensity line.

REFERENCES AND SUGGESTIONS FOR FURTHER READING

Higgins, C. B. (ed.) (1983) *CT of the Heart and Great Vessels*. NY: Futura, Mount Kisco.

Jefferson, K., Rees, S. (1980) *Clinical Cardiac Radiology*, 2nd edn. London: Butterworths.

Schiller, N. B. (1980) Echocardiography in pericardial disease. *Medical Clinics of North America*, 64, 253.

Shabbetai, R., Mangierdi, L., Bhargava, V. et al (1979) The pericardium and cardiac function. *Progress in Cardiovascular Diseases*, 22(2), 107–134.

Underwood, R., Firmin, D. (1987) *An Introduction to Magnetic Resonance of the Cardiovascular System*. London: Current Medical Literature.

MRI

Blackwell, G. G., Cranney, G. B., Pohost, G. M. (1992) *MRI: Cardiovascular System*. New York: Gower.

Globits, S., Higgins, C. B. (1996) Adult heart disease. In Edelman, R. E., Hesselink, J. R., Zlatkin, M. B. (eds) *Clinical Magnetic Resonance Imaging*, 2nd edn. Philadelphia: W.B. Saunders, ch. 54, pp. 1711–1756.

Gutierrez, F. R., Brown, J. J., Mirowitz, A. (1993) *Cardiovascular Magnetic Resonance Imaging*. St Louis: Mosby Year Book.

Link, K. M. (1990) Noninvasive evaluation of the pericardium and myocardium. *Current Opinion in Radiology*, **2**, 586–594.

Miller, S. W. (1996) *Cardiac Radiology—The Requisites*. St Louis: Mosby Year Book.

White, C. S. (1996) MR evaluation of the pericardium and cardiac malignancies. *Magnetic Resonance Imaging Clinics of North America*, **4**, 237–251.

22

THE PULMONARY CIRCULATION

M. J. Raphael and R. M. Donaldson

The pulmonary circulation begins at the pulmonary valve, which sits on the infundibulum of the right ventricle. The valve cannot be identified specifically on the plain film but can be identified by cross-sectional echocardiography (CSE). It may very rarely calcify in middle-aged patients when the valve is congenitally abnormal or the seat of bacterial endocarditis, or in the presence of pulmonary hypertension.

The main pulmonary artery beyond the pulmonary valve may be identified on the frontal film, as its left border forms the floor of the pulmonary bay. This is the concavity of the left mediastinal shadow, below the knob-like shadow of the arch of the aorta, and above the shadow of the heart. In the normal adult the floor of the pulmonary bay is straight. In children and young women (Fig. 22.1A), a slight convexity is within normal limits.

Enlargement of the main pulmonary artery produces a convexity of the floor of the pulmonary bay. The main pulmonary artery is enlarged in left to right shunts, in pulmonary hypertension and in the post-stenotic dilatation of pulmonary valve stenosis; enlargement may be extreme in certain situations such as when the Eisenmenger reaction occurs in rare association with an atrial septal defect, and in the pulmonary hypertension associated with bilharzia.

The main pulmonary artery divides after a variable distance into the right and left pulmonary arteries (Figs 22.1B and 22.2). The left pulmonary artery appears as the continuation of the main, passing backwards. It gives off the left upper-lobe branches as it passes above the left main bronchus and then arches downwards as the branch to the left lower lobe before dividing into the branches to the basal segments. The left pulmonary artery and its descending branch are silhouetted against the lung and can be identified on the plain film, as forming part of the left hilum and its continuation into the left lower lobe.

The right pulmonary artery appears as a sharply angled branch of the main pulmonary artery and passes to the right in the mediastinum. It divides within the mediastinum, and its upper-lobe branch leaves the mediastinum above the right hilum to supply the upper lobe. The descending branch of the right pulmonary artery is the vessel first to be identified, as it forms the lower part of the right hilum where it is outlined against the lung (Fig. 22.1A and B).

In the lateral view the right and left pulmonary arteries may be distinguished. The left pulmonary artery lies above and posterior to the radiolucency of the carina 'end-on'; the right pulmonary artery in front and slightly below (Fig. 22.2).

In the lungs the arteries lie within the parenchyma roughly following the bronchial branching pattern. The short descending branches of both the right and left lower-lobe arteries can usually be identified before they break up into the branches to the basal segments. The vessels to each lobe can be identified even though the branching pattern is variable. The arteries branch and taper smoothly out from the hilum, and can be followed as discrete shadows to the outer third of the lung (Fig. 22.1A and B).

The pulmonary arterioles, capillaries and pulmonary venules, contribute to the lung radiopacity but cannot be identified as discrete structures.

The pulmonary veins form an inconstant arrangement (Fig. 22.1C). The pulmonary veins of the upper lobe collect into the superior pulmonary vein, those of the lower lobe into the inferior pulmonary vein. The two veins on each side join the four corners of the left atrium.

The pulmonary veins may be distinguished from the arteries on the plain film (Fig. 22.3) by their course and position. The lower lobe veins run horizontally to reach the left atrium and are usually visible and distinguishable from the more vertically running branches of the descending branch of the pulmonary artery. The upper lobe veins when visible, lie lateral to the upper lobe arteries, and run vertically to pass through the hilar shadow to reach the left atrium.

The hilar shadow has a concave outer aspect, formed by the superior pulmonary vein above, and descending branch of the pulmonary artery below.

The upper lobe veins may not be visible on the erect film for two reasons: they are collapsed in the erect position as the normal left atrial pressure is inadequate to distend them, and they carry little blood as the normal pulmonary artery pressure is inadequate

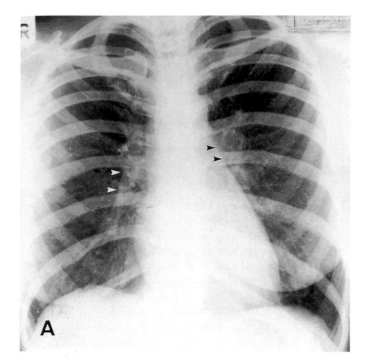

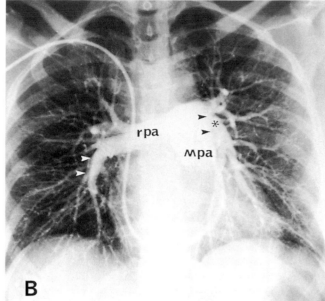

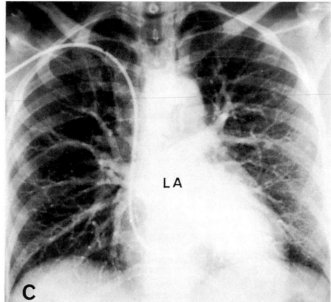

Fig. 22.1 A young woman with sudden onset of chest pain. **A.** Frontal film. The pulmonary artery beyond the pulmonary valve produces a slight convexity of the pulmonary bay (black arrows). The normal straight outer border of the descending right pulmonary artery may also be seen (white arrows). **B.** Pulmonary angiogram, arterial phase, same patient. The main pulmonary artery (mpa), beyond the pulmonary valve (black arrows), forms the floor of the pulmonary bay. The right pulmonary artery (rpa) appears as a branch of the main. It crosses the mediastinum and divides within it, so the arteries to the right upper lobe come out from the mediastinum above the hilum. The descending branch of the right pulmonary artery can be identified (white arrows) after it leaves the mediastinum and emerges to become silhouetted against the lung. The descending branch of the left pulmonary artery (asterisk) may also be seen silhouetted against the lung as it forms the left hilar shadow. **C.** Pulmonary angiogram, venous phase, same patient. The pulmonary veins are seen joining the left atrium (LA). They converge to form four pulmonary veins, the superior and inferior pulmonary veins on each side, joining the four corners of the atrium.

to perfuse the apices of the lungs. The normal upper lobe vessels in the first interspace are rarely more than 3 mm in diameter.

The diameter of the descending branch of the right pulmonary artery does not normally exceed 15 mm in women and 16 mm in men. Normally it has a rather straight outer border. A convex outer border suggests that the vessel is abnormally large, a concave outer border that it is abnormally small. These features are probably more helpful than measurements in evaluating pathology in the pulmonary circulation.

Rarely, the superior and inferior pulmonary veins may join each other, forming a confluence, before entering the left atrium. This confluence can form a discrete rounded or oval shadow on the plain film (Fig. 22.4), on either side, and particularly so when there is an increase in pulmonary vein pressure. This shadow may

resemble a tumor, but its nature is usually obvious because of its characteristic site right next to the left atrium, and once suspected can be confirmed by demonstrating its relationship to the pulmonary vein.

ABNORMALITIES OF THE PULMONARY CIRCULATION

The concept of pulmonary vascular resistance is derived by an analogy from electricity. In the lung, PVR (pulmonary vascular resistance) is defined as P/F. P is the pressure across the pulmonary vascular bed between the arteries and the veins, i.e. the pressure gradient (voltage, sic) in millimeters of mercury and F is the blood flow (equivalent to current) through the lungs in

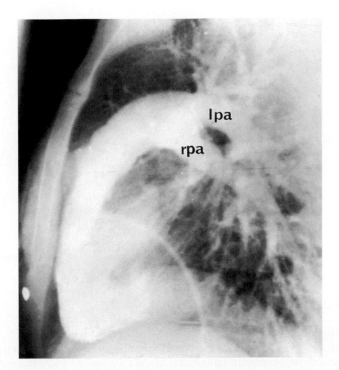

Fig. 22.2 Lateral angiogram to show the pulmonary arteries. The left pulmonary artery (lpa) lies above and behind the 'end-on' carina; the right pulmonary artery (rpa) lies below and in front.

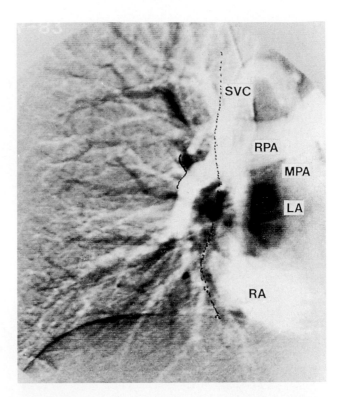

Fig. 22.3 Digital subtraction pulmonary angiogram. The use of computer techniques allows pulmonary arteries and veins to be displayed separately but simultaneously, in the same examination. The arterial phase appears in white, the venous phase in black; the right edge of the mediastinum has been dotted in. It is formed by the superior vena cava (SVC) above (the injection catheter, imperfectly subtracted due to movement misregistration, may be seen) and the right atrium (RA) below. The concavity of the outer aspect of the right hilum has been marked in ink. It is formed by the superior pulmonary vein above, descending vertically to reach the left atrium (LA) below the hilum, and the descending branch of the right pulmonary artery (RPA) below. The upper-lobe artery is seen emerging from the mediastinum above the hilum and lying medial to the upper-lobe pulmonary vein. The lower-lobe vessels are less clearly seen, due to misregistration. MPA, main pulmonary artery.

liters per minute. The normal pulmonary vascular resistance is one-sixth that in the systemic circulation so that the normal pulmonary artery pressure (20/10 mmHg) is one-sixth that of the systemic circulation. The pulmonary artery pressure is easy to measure, and, as pulmonary venous pressure is usually small, is taken to indicate the pressure gradient, unless there is evidence of pulmonary venous hypertension.

In normal lung a marked increase in flow is accompanied by an increase in pulmonary artery pressure even though pulmonary vascular resistance is normal, so-called hyperkinetic pulmonary hypertension. When the increase in flow is reversed, pressure will fall to normal. An increase in pulmonary artery pressure may also occur if there is a rise in pressure in the pulmonary veins. This pressure will be transmitted directly back through the pulmonary vascular bed to the pulmonary artery, so-called passive pulmonary hypertension.

When a rise in pulmonary artery pressure is due to obstruction of the vessels within the lung the condition is termed pulmonary hypertension. It may be due to obstruction or destruction of the pulmonary capillary bed, to obstruction or vasoconstriction of the smaller arteries and arterioles or to obstruction of the larger arteries.

CONGENITAL HEART DISEASE

Changes in the pulmonary circulation in congenital heart disease will be fully dealt with in Chapter 25, but the general patterns of abnormality are considered briefly here. Congenital heart disease may also show abnormalities and have pulmonary changes similar to those in acquired heart disease.

Pulmonary Plethora

This is the characteristic appearance of the lung vessels in the presence of increase in pulmonary flow, usually from a left to right shunt, rarely from an increase in cardiac output. The main pulmonary artery is enlarged, producing a convex pulmonary bay. The pulmonary arteries and veins are increased in size and can be followed into the outer third of the lung. Upper and lower lobe flows are equalized. Pulmonary edema in association with large shunts may be superimposed on the appearances of pulmonary plethora.

If gross pulmonary plethora is present and an enlarged pulmonary artery cannot be identified, it may be normally situated but concealed by the thymus, absent as in truncus arteriosus, or misplaced in the mediastinum as in transposition of the great arteries.

In the neonate the appearances of pulmonary plethora may be mimicked by an underexposed film. The following may produce the appearances of pulmonary plethora:

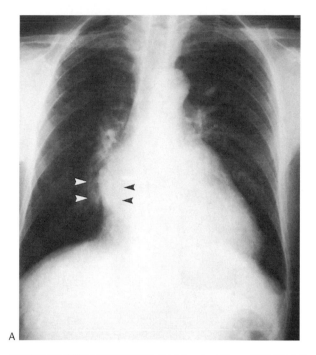

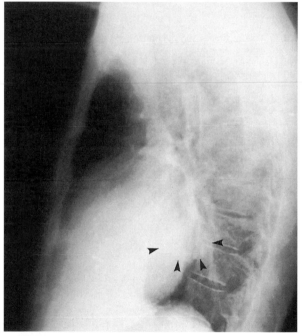

Fig. 22.4 Confluence of the pulmonary veins. In this patient with mitral valve disease, there is a large sharply demarcated rounded shadow at the right corner to the left atrium (arrows). The nature of the shadow is suggested by its sharp definition and characteristic site, with pulmonary veins entering it. **A.** Frontal view. **B.** Lateral view.

1. *Left to right shunts*
   a. Without cyanosis:
        Atrial shunts
        Ventricular shunts
        Aortopulmonary shunts

   b. With cyanosis:
        All the following lesions are characterized by mixing of arterial and venous blood within the heart:
            Transposition of the great arteries
            Total anomalous pulmonary venous drainage
            Truncus arteriosus
            Common atrium
            Single ventricle
            Double-outlet right ventricle
2. *Increased cardiac output*
   Pregnancy
   Anemia
   Thyrotoxicosis
   Beriberi
   Systemic arteriovenous fistulas
   Chronic liver disease
   Polycythemia
   Paget's disease

PULMONARY ARTERY PRUNING

High-pressure left to right shunts are associated with obstructive changes in the smaller pulmonary arteries and arterioles which lead to an increase in pulmonary vascular resistance and a rise in pulmonary artery pressure, ultimately to systemic levels, and hence to a reduction and then reversal of a shunt, the *Eisenmenger reaction*. The characteristic but not invariable appearance in this situation is of a large main, and large central pulmonary arteries which taper down rapidly to very small vessels over a few orders of branches, giving a 'pruned tree' appearance. Unless the appearances are gross the level of the increase of pulmonary vascular resistance cannot be judged by the plain film appearances.

In long-standing Eisenmenger reaction patients, calcification may develop in the main and central pulmonary arteries. The Eisenmenger reaction is a common complication of large ventricular septal defects and large patent ductus arteriosus defects, but is rare in atrial septal defects. Rise in pulmonary vascular resistance may also occur in association with similar communications in transposition of the great arteries or in syndromes allied to ventricular septal defect such as double-outlet right ventricle and single ventricle.

Pulmonary Oligemia   Reduced blood flow from obstruction proximal to the main pulmonary artery may lead to characteristic appearances. The main pulmonary artery is small and often displaced medially (as in the tetralogy of Fallot) producing an empty or concave pulmonary bay. The pulmonary vessels are small and the lungs are hypertranslucent. These appearances can be mimicked in the neonate by overexposure of the film, and are then difficult to assess, and the pulmonary bay itself may be obscured in the neonate by a large thymus.

Asymmetrical Perfusion   The plain film may demonstrate abnormal asymmetrical perfusion. There is a normal perfusion gradient from above downwards (see p. 000) and the reverse perfusion gradient of pulmonary venous hypertension is considered below. Differences in perfusion on the two sides, as evidenced by difference in the size and extent of the blood vessels on the two sides are a common feature of congenital heart disease, either as a result of revascularization surgery such as Blalock or Waterston shunt operations, or with congenital abnormalities of perfusion, scattered throughout the lungs, are always strongly suggestive of complex pulmonary atresia (see below).

Bronchial Circulation An increase in the bronchial circulation, which usually develops as a response to severe obstruction of the pulmonary circulation, leads to an enlargement of the bronchial arteries. The enlargement may be suspected by a curious spotty appearance of the lungs, spreading out from the hilum. Pulmonary oligemia can often be seen in association with this appearance of the bronchial circulation.

PULMONARY VENOUS HYPERTENSION

Impairment of function of the valves or chambers of the left heart commonly leads to a rise in pressure in the left atrium which is transmitted back into the (valveless) pulmonary veins, producing pulmonary venous hypertension. This increase in pressure leads to the distension of the normally collapsed upper-lobe veins. These veins may be recognized on the erect plain film (Fig. 22.5), as enlarged and rising up toward the apex of the lung. They may enlarge alone or there may be some enlargement of the arteries which accompany them, so that the vessels above the hilum appear larger than those below. The positive identification of *upper-lobe blood diversion* almost invariably indicates disorder of the left side of the heart, though basal emphysema may rarely produce similar appearances without the explanation being obvious. Rarely, local lung disease involving the upper lobes may

prevent its radiological recognition. However, it is common to see the changes of pulmonary edema (see later) indicating severe functional impairment of the left heart, without recognizing upper-lobe blood diversion.

The explanation for the development of upper-lobe blood diversion is not clear. It has been suggested that perivascular edema surrounding the lower-lobe veins in the erect position leads to their compression and produces the redistribution of flow to the upper lobe.

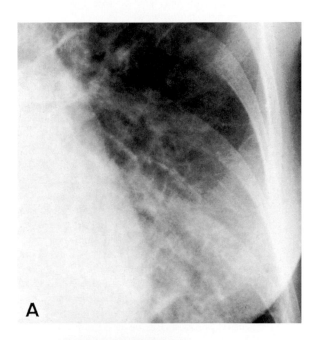

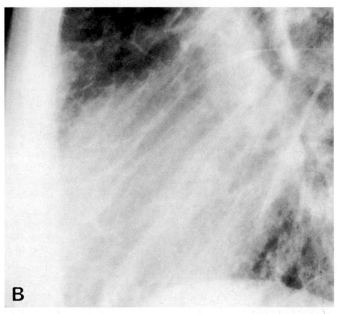

Fig. 22.5 The end result of long-standing severe pulmonary venous hypertension. There has been a closed mitral valvotomy through the left sixth rib. There is very marked upper-lobe blood diversion, with very large upper-lobe pulmonary veins and almost no veins visible in the lower lobes. There is also severe pulmonary arterial hypertension, with gross enlargement of the main and central pulmonary arteries with peripheral tapering. In addition, note the characteristic densities of pulmonary ossific nodules.

Fig. 22.6 Pulmonary interstitial edema. **A.** Localized frontal view of the left base. **B.** Localized lateral view of the front of the chest. The horizontal basal peripheral line shadows are the B lines, probably due to edema of the interlobular septa. The lines running in apparently random directions are the A lines. In the lateral view, the B lines can be seen running horizontally at the back of the sternum, together with A lines. In addition, the fissures are thickened, indicating fluid within them.

As the pulmonary venous pressure rises above 25 mmHg it exceeds the plasma osmotic pressure and enters the threshold for *pulmonary edema*. This appears initially as *interstitial lines* (Fig. 22.6). *B lines* are horizontal basal peripheral non-branching fine lines visible on the frontal and lateral film. They are thought to be due to edema of the interlobular septa through which the lymphatics pass. *A-lines* are irregular lines spreading out from the hilum and thought to be due to edema of the intercommunicating lymphatics. They are less frequently seen but have the same import as the B-lines. They may also be seen behind the sternum rising up the chest on the lateral view.

Interstitial Edema This is mainly seen in association with a rise in left atrial pressure from any cause; mitral valve disease— either stenosis or incompetence, or obstruction at the mitral valve from a left atrial myxoma—leads to a rise in left atrial pressure which is transmitted back to the pulmonary veins. *Left ventricular failure*, either from aortic disease, hypertension or disease of heart muscle, may be associated with the rise in left ventricular and hence left atrial pressure and pulmonary edema. The non-failing left ventricle of *hypertrophic cardiomyopathy* may become so stiff that the high pressure required to distend it in diastole is transmitted back to the left atrium and leads to pulmonary venous hypertension. Rarely the obstruction may lie in the pulmonary veins in unusual forms of *constrictive pericarditis* or in *pulmonary veno-occlusive disease*. In this last condition the plain film illustrates the characteristic appearances of interstitial and alveolar edema but there is no overt upper lobe blood diversion or evidence of left heart disease. Unless a lung biopsy is taken, the diagnosis becomes one of exclusion. Interstitial lines are also a feature of a number of primarily lung diseases (see Section 2).

Once the left atrial pressure rises beyond the level at which the distended lymphatics can clear edema fluid from the lungs, overt **alveolar pulmonary edema** develops (Fig. 22.7). The classical appearance of this is of a confluent alveolar shadowing developing in both lungs and having a perihilar or 'bat's wing' appearance. The densest shadow appears around the hilar regions spreading off to an ill-defined periphery and sparing the bases of the lungs. Less commonly it may be localized to one lung, or part of the lung when its typical situation is in the right upper lobe. It may develop in the lung bases, or it may appear as a rather granular shadowing throughout the lungs without any overt perihilar concentration, or even as a peripherally distributed abnormal shadowing. Its association with a large heart, its rapid onset, rapid change with diuretic therapy, and often its extent, together with lack of fever, usually serve to differentiate it from infection.

Other features which may be seen in pulmonary edema are blurring of the outline of the slightly distended hilum and blurring of the outlines of the central pulmonary vessels, due to perivascular edema. Similar blurring may be seen around bronchi taken end on in the frontal chest X-ray, the so-called 'endobronchial cuffing'. These features go to support the diagnosis of pulmonary edema.

The development of **pleural effusion** is common in the evolution of pulmonary edema and may go to support the diagnosis. Pleural effusions may be of considerable size, and have their characteristic appearances in the costophrenic angles; however, when very small they may appear as the lamellar shadow of a small parietal effusion lying against the outer wall of the thorax deep in the costophrenic angles. Fluid in the fissures of the lung

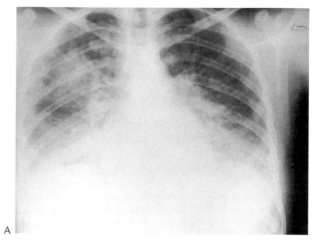

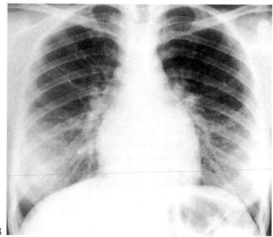

Fig. 22.7 Acute pulmonary edema in mitral stenosis. The heart shadow is not large but shows the features of selective left atrial enlargement, compatible with mitral valve disease. **A.** On admission there was extensive bilateral pulmonary shadowing, primarily perihilar, and associated with loss of definition of the outline of the hila and vessels. **B.** Within 1 day this shadowing had cleared. The extensive nature of the shadowing, its perihilar rather than segmental distribution, and the rapidity with which its appearance changed, are the features which point to the diagnosis of pulmonary edema.

may be recognized as thickenings of the fissures in both the frontal and lateral view and may go to support the diagnosis. Although pleural fluid may take any distribution it is relatively common for quite large effusions to collect in the fissures in the pulmonary edema of cardiac failure, where they may appear to resemble tumor masses on the frontal film. The nature of these 'disappearing tumors' is quite clear when a lateral view is taken.

Once diuretic therapy has begun, the relationship between rise in pulmonary venous pressure and radiological demonstration of pulmonary edema is lost.

A sustained rise in left atrial pressure leads not only to distension of the upper-lobe veins but also to constriction of the lower-lobe veins and then the arteries, so that flow through the lungs is virtually confined to the upper lobes. These appearances are most commonly seen in long-standing mitral valve disease, the 'stag's antlers' appearance (see Fig. 22.5).

Initially, pulmonary venous hypertension is associated with a rise in pulmonary artery pressure equivalent to the rise in the

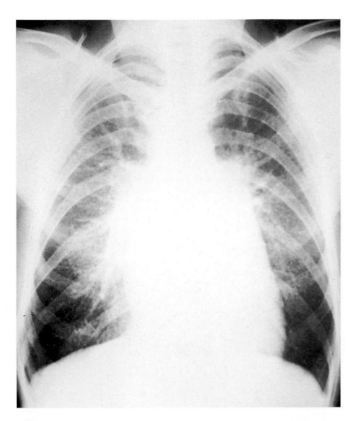

Fig. 22.8 Pulmonary hemosiderosis secondary to long-standing mitral valve disease. The fine granular background pattern to the lung is typical of hemosiderosis. In addition, note changes suggestive of mitral valve disease: straightening of the left heart border and some upper-lobe blood diversion.

pressure in the pulmonary veins, so that the pressure gradient across the lungs is normal, so-called passive pulmonary hypertension.

Ultimately, obliterative changes in the pulmonary arterioles develop, leading to superimposed active pulmonary arterial hypertension, which is thought to be some form of protective reaction to the lungs. This can be seen on the plain film (see Fig. 22.5) when enlargement of the main pulmonary artery and the central pulmonary arteries develops, the changes being particularly marked in the upper lobe. When such changes are present, they indicate pulmonary arterial hypertension, but their absence does not exclude it.

Long-standing pulmonary venous hypertension may be associated with the development of **hemosiderosis** (Fig. 22.8), which appears on the plain film as a series of fine punctate calcifications scattered throughout the lungs.

Very long-standing severe pulmonary venous hypertension may also be associated with the development of **pulmonary ossific nodules** (see Fig. 22.5). These are small areas of bone formation in the lungs, never larger than 1 cm in diameter, the diameter of the secondary lobule. They often appear to have a trabecular structure.

PULMONARY ARTERIAL HYPERTENSION

This is considered to be present when the pulmonary artery pressure is over 30 mmHg systolic (and the pulmonary venous

pressure is normal). In the absence of a shunt the pulmonary artery pressure can rise above the systemic levels.

When the pressure in the pulmonary artery approaches systemic levels a number of consequences develop. The right ventricle is unable to increase its output against this high pressure, so that any fall in peripheral vascular resistance, such as that produced by exercise, leads to a fall in systemic blood pressure and may lead to syncope. This is the mechanism of hypotension and death associated with angiocardiography which produces a profound peripheral systemic vasodilatation. Low, fixed, cardiac output may lead to an anginal type of chest pain. Shortness of breath may be a feature. The high pulmonary artery pressure leads ultimately to right ventricular failure with dilatation and peripheral edema. This clinical picture will of course be modified according to the nature of the underlying causative lung disorder.

Radiographic Appearances The plain film (Fig. 22.9) characteristically shows a large and often triangular heart. The main pulmonary artery and central pulmonary arteries are usually large, and may be very large, but taper rapidly to the periphery. Rarely the pulmonary vessels or heart may appear normal but it is rare for the main pulmonary artery to be inconspicuous.

The pulmonary artery systolic pressure may be accurately measured by continuous wave Doppler echocardiography from the velocity of the tricuspid regurgitant signal (see Fig. 23.19). Lung scanning usually shows normal perfusion and ventilation though rarely small peripheral perfusion defects may be seen.

PULMONARY EMBOLISM

This may lead to a variety of clinical pictures according to the size and number of the emboli and the underlying state of the circulation.

Acute Massive Pulmonary Embolism

This occurs when one or more large pulmonary emboli, usually consisting of detached thrombus from the larger veins of the lower limb, impact in the central pulmonary arteries. It leads to the rapid onset of severe pulmonary obstruction, but this is usually associated with only a modest rise in pulmonary artery pressure, as right ventricular dilatation and failure quickly ensue. The clinical onset is usually with some shortness of breath, hypotension and tachycardia and perhaps chest pain. A history suggestive of deep-vein thrombosis of the legs may be present. The physical signs of a loud P2 on auscultation and the ECG evidence of right ventricular strain may suggest the diagnosis, but the clinical picture could fit with myocardial infarction, concealed haemorrhage or other cause of shock.

Radiographic Appearances The plain film may be helpful in this situation if it is of good quality and if the patient is otherwise fit (Fig. 22.10A). There may be a moderate increase in the heart size. The characteristic feature is the demonstration of localized areas of underperfusion of the lung. These may be brought into relief by an apparent increase in perfusion of other segments. Large areas of one or both lungs may be affected. Increased density of the main pulmonary artery associated with peripheral cut-off vessels, though well recognized, is exceptionally rare. Comparison with previous radiographs may be helpful in recognizing changes in the pulmonary vascular supply to the lungs. The characteristic changes are usually not recognized in

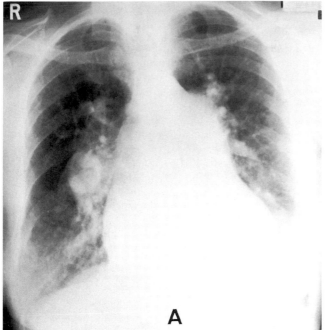

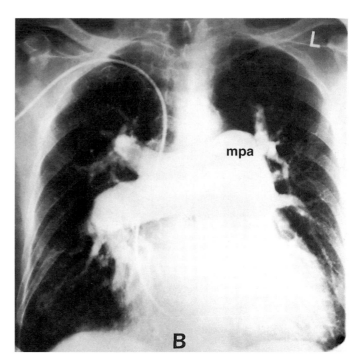

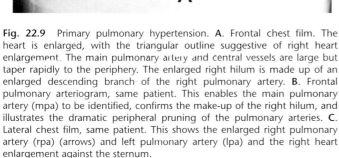

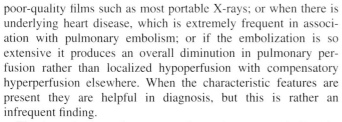

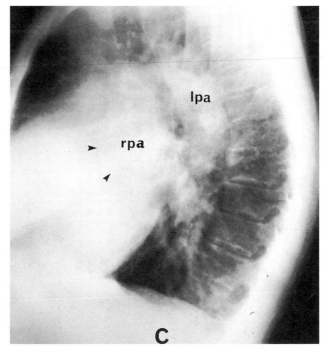

Fig. 22.9 Primary pulmonary hypertension. **A.** Frontal chest film. The heart is enlarged, with the triangular outline suggestive of right heart enlargement. The main pulmonary artery and central vessels are large but taper rapidly to the periphery. The enlarged right hilum is made up of an enlarged descending branch of the right pulmonary artery. **B.** Frontal pulmonary arteriogram, same patient. This enables the main pulmonary artery (mpa) to be identified, confirms the make-up of the right hilum, and illustrates the dramatic peripheral pruning of the pulmonary arteries. **C.** Lateral chest film, same patient. This shows the enlarged right pulmonary artery (rpa) (arrows) and left pulmonary artery (lpa) and the right heart enlargement against the sternum.

poor-quality films such as most portable X-rays; or when there is underlying heart disease, which is extremely frequent in association with pulmonary embolism; or if the embolization is so extensive it produces an overall diminution in pulmonary perfusion rather than localized hypoperfusion with compensatory hyperperfusion elsewhere. When the characteristic features are present they are helpful in diagnosis, but this is rather an infrequent finding.

The investigation of acute massive pulmonary embolism is, according to the facilities available, the time of day at which the clinical picture develops and the clinical certainty of the clinician. The situation clinically may be so precarious and the diagnosis so certain that little more than an ECG and a plain X-ray may be taken before beginning treatment with anticoagulants. The fatal pulmonary embolus is often not the one which brought the patient to medical attention, but one which follows soon after; if this can be prevented the patient should recover completely (Fig. 22.11). If the diagnosis is in doubt, it is usually quicker in most departments to organize emergency pulmonary angiography than pulmonary scanning, and this should be the investigation of choice (see Fig. 22.10B).

Subacute Pulmonary Embolism

When the emboli are smaller and fewer so that acute cor

pulmonale does not develop immediately, changes have time to develop in the lungs. As the lungs have a second, bronchial, circulation, pulmonary infarction rarely develops. This is usually when a large vessel is occluded and there is impairment of the bronchial circulation, a feature which commonly occurs in association with heart failure. The usual sequence of events following occlusion of a pulmonary artery (Fig. 22.12) is that the unperfused lung ceases to aerate properly, and this is associated with some reduction in volume. This is commonly seen on the plain film as an elevation of the diaphragm on the affected side. Over the next few days this hypoventilation may lead to areas of

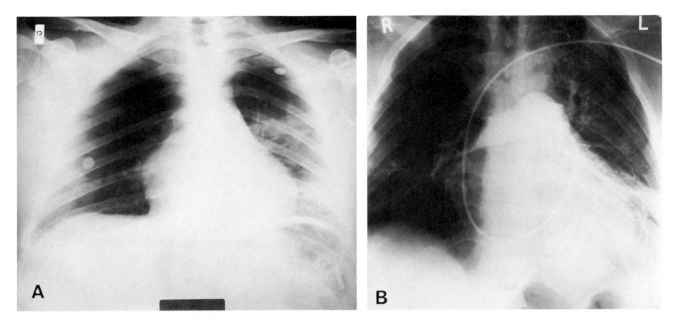

Fig. 22.10 Acute massive pulmonary embolism. **A.** Frontal chest film (portable). The right lung and the left upper zone are hypertransradiant due to oligemia, and there is overperfusion of the left mid and lower zones. **B.** Pulmonary arteriogram, same patient. The leading edge of an embolus is seen impacted in the right pulmonary artery, producing virtually complete obstruction. Another embolus is seen in the supply to the left upper lobe which is also impaired. Only the left lower lobe fills adequately with contrast medium.

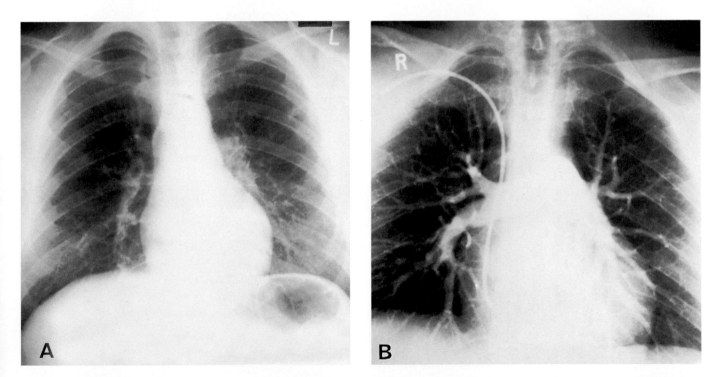

Fig. 22.11 The pulmonary embolism of Fig. 22.10, 4 months later, after effective treatment. **A.** Frontal film. This is now entirely normal **B.** Pulmonary arteriogram. The pulmonary emboli have completely resolved.

collapse which usually re-expand if the patient survives. Infarction itself may develop to some degree in the affected vascular segment of which the obstructed artery forms the apex and the pleural aspect the base. The infarction may be barely visible but may lead to a hemorrhagic pleural effusion, and this may be seen as a small fluid collection in the costophrenic angle.

The infarction very rarely appears as the characteristic triangular shadow described in older textbooks. More commonly it appears as an area of rather nondescript consolidation whose chief characteristic is that it is associated with a pleural surface. This may only be apparent on the lateral view, and includes the surfaces of the fissures as well as the periphery of the lungs.

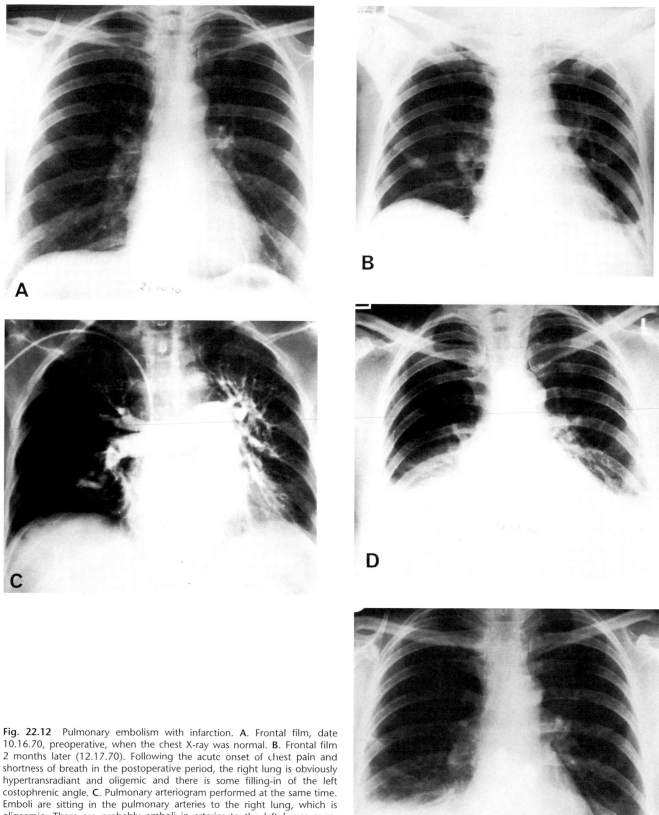

Fig. 22.12 Pulmonary embolism with infarction. **A**. Frontal film, date 10.16.70, preoperative, when the chest X-ray was normal. **B**. Frontal film 2 months later (12.17.70). Following the acute onset of chest pain and shortness of breath in the postoperative period, the right lung is obviously hypertransradiant and oligemic and there is some filling-in of the left costophrenic angle. **C**. Pulmonary arteriogram performed at the same time. Emboli are sitting in the pulmonary arteries to the right lung, which is oligaemic. There are probably emboli in arteries to the left lower zone. **D**. Frontal film, 12.23.70. Patchy basal consolidation and pleural fluid have appeared, indicating the development of infarction. **E**. Frontal film 2½ weeks later following effective treatment. The infarction at the left base, which was reversible, has cleared. On the right, more extensive infarction is still visible, and line shadows of pulmonary scarring are developing.

These infarctions are usually partial and reversible in the course of time. They may disappear entirely or may heal to a linear scar. However, if the infarction is large and there is impairment of bronchial perfusion, it may be irreversible, and heal ultimately by scarring and fibrosis in the lungs.

The plain film appearances of pulmonary embolism with infarction are largely confined to the lung bases, the right side being more commonly involved than the left.

Pulmonary embolism with infarction is associated with a sudden onset of chest pain, with hemoptysis and with progressive increase in shortness of breath, as emboli arrive progressively and occlude the lung bed. A normal chest X-ray, even if of good quality, does not exclude the diagnosis, which may be clinically difficult. It should be suspected in any case of what appears to be a chest infection which does not respond to antibiotics, or in which the shortness of breath seems excessive. It should be considered with any patient with chest pain and clinical indications of possible deep-vein thrombosis. It may also be suspected in any patient, particularly in patients with heart failure, in whom the possibility of complicating pulmonary embolism arises, and in whom shortness of breath appears to be out of proportion to the underlying condition. It is in the subacute pulmonary embolism that isotope lung scanning plays its major role.

Isotope Lung Scanning

Modern methods of isotope imaging of the lung using a large-crystal γ camera have enormously improved diagnositic accuracy in pulmonary embolism. Technetium-labeled albumin macro-aggregates or microspheres injected intravenously will impact in the lung in the absence of any right to left shunt, either cardiac or extracardiac. The distribution of these microspheres may be recorded by the γ camera. A normal perfusion isotope lung scan excludes the diagnosis of pulmonary embolism from venous thrombus. If the perfusion lung scan shows the characteristic wedge-shaped localized perfusion deficits then pulmonary embolism becomes a possibility. Perfusion deficits can be caused by localized lung pathology such as infections or areas of emphysema or they can be part of a pattern of diffuse obstructive airways disease of the chronic bronchitis type. Multiple perfusion deficits involving part of the lung which appear normal on the chest X-ray increase the suspicion of pulmonary embolism. At this stage it is desirable to perform a ventilation scan; much the most effective is the inhalation of krypton-81m until equilibrium is reached and then recording the ventilation pattern with a γ camera (Fig. 22.13). When the localized deficiencies of perfusion can be matched with deficiencies of ventilation the likely underlying cause is some form of lung disease, and if a chest film appears normal, then obstructive airways disease is most likely (Fig. 22.14). When the ventilation remains normal yet a localized perfusion deficit is present, pulmonary embolism is highly likely;

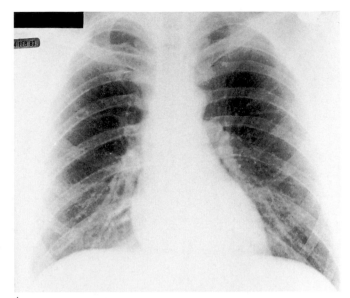

A

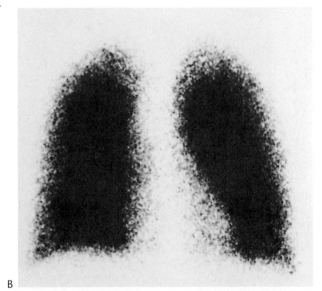

B

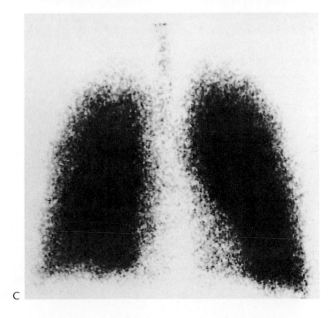

C

Fig. 22.13 Normal lung scan in a patient with acute chest pain. **A**. Frontal film. Normal. **B**. Frontal perfusion scan. This shows even perfusion over the whole of both lungs. **C**. Krypton-81m ventilation scan. This shows even ventilation over both lungs. Note the activity in the trachea which can be recognized in this type of ventilation scan. The even and matched distribution of radionuclide with perfusion and ventilation excludes the diagnosis of pulmonary embolism.

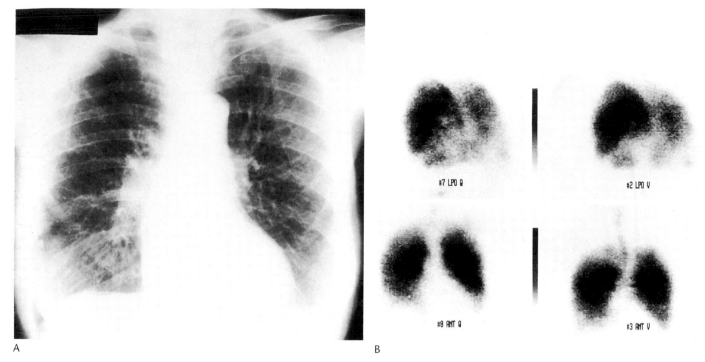

Fig. 22.14   Chronic obstructive airways disease. **A.** Frontal film. Apart from a slight 'streakiness' of the lung markings, which always raises the possibility of obstructive airways disease, the appearances are normal. **B.** Computer reconstructions of perfusion and ventilation scans. Perfusion is on the left and ventilation on the right. Note that in the left posterior/oblique (LPO) view there is a very large but matched defect of perfusion at the left base. The matching suggests that this is due to obstructive airways disease and not to pulmonary embolism.

if the mismatch is definite and the perfusion deficits typical (Fig. 22.15), then the diagnosis may be taken as proven and treatment instituted.

Pulmonary Angiography

If the ventilation/perfusion findings are not typical or a full study cannot be performed, then it is desirable to proceed to angiography. Pulmonary angiography is usually performed by passing a catheter from a vein in the elbow through the heart to the main pulmonary artery. The pulmonary artery pressure can be recorded and then a pulmonary angiogram performed. A bolus of 50 ml at 25 ml/s is usually satisfactory, and a large film format rapid film changer with rapid early and slow delayed films gives whole lung cover and adequate definition.

Venous angiography using a catheter in a peripheral vein and a larger bolus may give adequate visualization of the pulmonary arteries, and this technique has now been upgraded by the use of digital subtraction angiography so that a fine catheter placed in the superior vena cava using a mechanical injector to give a large bolus of contrast gives adequate opacification of each lung in turn. This technique is best suited to the recognition of large central emboli.

The right lung is usually well seen in the frontal view; the direct posterior inclination of the left pulmonary artery means that it, and its proximal branches, may be too foreshortened and a right posterior oblique which is usually obtained by raising the left shoulder towards the overhead tube, will unfold them. With sophisticated apparatus the anteroposterior film may be taken with cranial angulation of the X-ray tube to reduce the fore-

shortening of the central pulmonary vessels within the mediastinum.

Pulmonary emboli can usually be directly demonstrated as sharply demarcated intraluminal filling defects in the contrast-filled pulmonary arteries (see Figs. 22.10B and 22.12C). When these are seen the diagnosis is certain. The presence of emboli reduces blood flow in the affected vessel so that parts of the lung may appear underperfused, but similar appearances may be produced by abnormal lung and are only suggestive rather than specific. Reabsorbed pulmonary emboli from previous episodes may appear as irregular narrowings of vessels without the demonstration of the intraluminal filling defects. Normal pulmonary arteries down to the usual limits of the pulmonary arteriogram vessels of about 2–3 mm exclude recent pulmonary embolus.

Pulmonary emboli may be macerated and pushed peripherally by the pulmonary artery catheter or lysed rapidly by the local infusion of streptokinase, which may be necessary if the patient is in extremis as in massive pulmonary embolism. More usually the simple prevention of further pulmonary emboli by anticoagulant therapy is enough to save the patient's life and to promote the complete reabsorption of emboli. This takes place over a period of several weeks, and the subsequent pulmonary arteriogram may appear entirely normal (see Figs 22.10B and 22.11B). Further venous emboli may be prevented by the percutaneous insertion of a vena cavae filter device if anticoagulant therapy proves ineffective.

CT Scanning

Modern high-speed CT will often show emboli as far as lobar or segmental arteries.

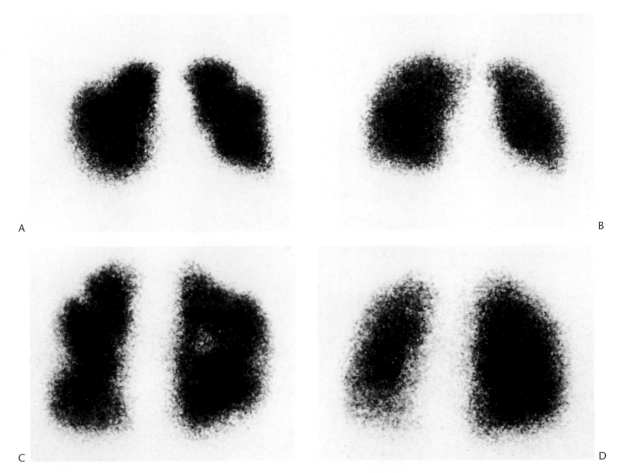

Fig. 22.15 Acute pulmonary embolism. **A,B.** Frontal perfusion and ventilation scans. **C,D.** Posterior perfusion and ventilation scans. Note the multiple wedge-shaped deficits on both the frontal and posterior perfusion scans but the entirely normal distribution of the radionuclide in the frontal and posterior ventilation scans. These appearances are typical of acute pulmonary embolism. The plain film was normal.

CHRONIC PULMONARY THROMBOEMBOLISM

Established and irreversible pulmonary hypertension may develop as the result of continuing release of small emboli to the circulation. The patient presents with the clinical features of pulmonary hypertension and right heart failure though in the history there may rarely be episodes of recurrent chest pain and hemoptysis and a history of deep-vein thrombosis in the legs. This form of pulmonary embolism is characterized, commonly, by the presence of widespread small-vessel disease in the lung and with associated localized obstructions of larger vessels.

The *plain film* will show the large main pulmonary artery which is usually seen in pulmonary hypertension and also enlargement of central vessels and peripheral pruning. This is of a patchy nature with some vessels remaining obviously enlarged and others small or absent and associated with hypertranslucent areas of the lungs (Fig. 22.16A).

The *isotope lung scan* will show widespread perfusion deficits with normal ventilation. Cardiac catheterization will reveal a pulmonary artery pressure which is markedly raised and may reach systemic levels, and pulmonary angiography shows several large vessels blocked proximally and with no distal perfusion of that segment of the lung, whereas other vessels are obviously enlarged and perfusing the remaining part of the lung. The disease may be so advanced that only one lobe of a lung appears to be adequately perfused (Fig. 22.16B). All such patients who present with non-specific right-heart failure possibly secondary to pulmonary hypertension should be investigated with a lung scan which will differentiate large-vessel thromboembolic disease from small-vessel primary pulmonary hypertension. The distinction has become one of therapeutic importance with successful attempts to perform pulmonary thromboendarterectomy which may permanently lower the pulmonary artery pressure.

Chronic pulmonary thromboembolism may also occur as a complication of bilharzia. The plain film changes are often exceptionally gross with very extreme dilatation of the main and central pulmonary arteries and with marked pruning peripherally (Fig. 22.17).

Pulmonary hypertension may also result from tumor emboli, and the usual source is choriocarcinoma.

Fat Embolism   Fat embolism following major bone trauma may be associated with respiratory systems and a miliary or perihilar shadowing in the lungs. Fat globules may be seen in the sputum. However, the respiratory symptoms are more usually due to cerebral embolization occurring at the same time.

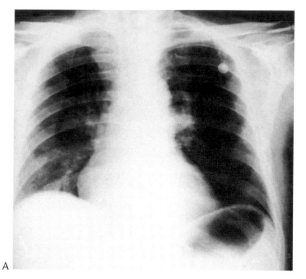

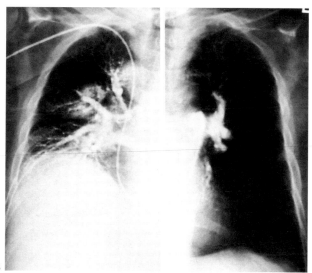

Fig. 22.16 Chronic pulmonary thromboembolism of the large-vessel variety. **A.** The frontal film shows a hypertransradiant left lung with areas of hypertransradiancy mixed with areas of increased perfusion in the right lung. **B.** The pulmonary arteriogram of this patient shows obstructions of many of the large branches of the left pulmonary artery with irregularity and rapid tapering of the arteries of the right lung, leading to patchy perfusion.

OTHER CAUSES OF PULMONARY ARTERIAL HYPERTENSION

Chronic Bronchitis

Chronic bronchitis is defined as excessive sputum production associated with hypertrophy of the mucus glands of the bronchi. Acute infective exacerbations are extremely common. Super-added bronchospasm is also extremely frequent. In addition, infection of the abnormal bronchial mucosa leads to airways obstruction, and in long-standing severe cases to hypercapnia and hyoxia with cyanosis, which in turn lead to a rise in pulmonary artery pressure, and also to right-heart failure with peripheral edema, the so-called 'blue bloater' type of patient.

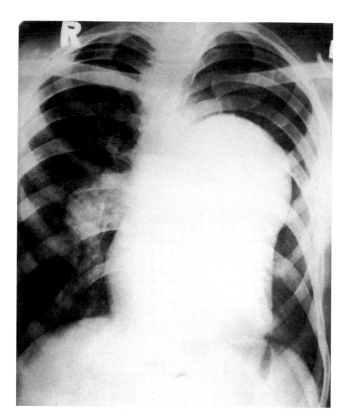

Fig. 22.17 Bilharzial pulmonary hypertension. Note the enormous enlargement of the main pulmonary artery. Some of the largest main pulmonary arteries are seen in this condition.

Between acute attacks the plain film may look relatively normal, though the lungs are often overinflated. The heart appears small but the main and central pulmonary arteries often appear rather large. There may be evidence of emphysema with bullae and diaphragmatic adhesions, and there may be scars of previous infections within the lung. In the acute phase the diaphragms rise and the lungs are no longer overdistended. The heart shadow increases in size and the main and central pulmonary arteries also enlarge. The increase in vessel size may occur out to the periphery of the lungs so that the appearances almost resemble those seen in a shunt. There may be fresh pulmonary consolidation. If the patient recovers, these changes reverse and the appearances revert to those before the infection (Fig. 22.18).

Special investigations to make the diagnosis of chronic bronchitis are rarely indicated though its presence may complicate the interpretation of lung scans, if these have been performed to exclude pulmonary embolism. Perfusion deficits are common but they are usually associated with ventilation defects, and in experienced hands the exclusion of pulmonary embolism is not difficult.

Emphysema

Emphysema, the destruction of the terminal air spaces of the lung, often complicates chronic bronchitis but may occur alone. The usual pattern is of a dyspneic but not cyanosed patient, the so-called 'pink puffer'. Rarely, emphysema, especially when gross,

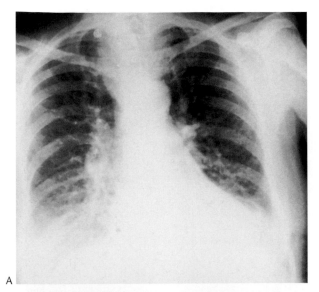

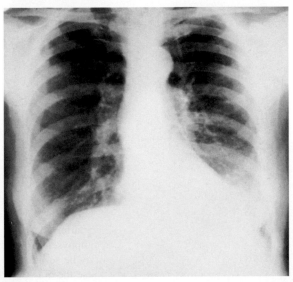

Fig. 22.18 Chronic obstructive airways disease with an acute exacerbation. **A.** The heart is large and the pulmonary vessels increased in size and apparently in number, almost resembling a shunt. **B.** Six weeks later, after resolution of the acute episode, both the heart and the pulmonary vessels have reduced in size. Note, however, that the central vessels still remain quite large.

may lead to hypercapnia and pulmonary hypertension and cor pulmonale.

Cystic Fibrosis With modern treatment many patients are surviving the inevitable severe respiratory infections to reach adolesence or beyond. In some of these patients, characteristic cor pulmonale and pulmonary hypertension may develop with a large main and central pulmonary vessels against a background of overinflated lungs with the characteristic features of cystic fibrosis.

Other Conditions Pulmonary hypertension and right-heart failure may be associated with severe *kyphoscoliosis* of the thoracic spine, particularly when it occurs in the high thoracic region. Hypercapnia and hypoxia may occur. The problem is

primarily one of hypoventilation due to a combination of respiratory muscle difficulty and underdevelopment of lung. In severe kyphoscoliosis the chest deformity is often so gross that no effective conclusions about the state of the lungs can be drawn from the usual plain films.

The *Pickwickian syndrome* consists of somnolence in an extremely obese patient. Polycythemia is present, and there may be right ventricular hypertrophy with right ventricular failure and associated pulmonary hypertension.

Ondine's curse is *idiopathic hypoventilation*. It occurs in young adult males and presents with lack of energy, somnolence, headache, shortness of breath on exertion and polycythemia. The sufferers often stop breathing intermittently when they are asleep, and this produces cyanosis. There may be pulmonary hypertension. The lungs are normal. A rather similar syndrome may occur in children with *hypertrophy of the adenoids*.

Pulmonary hypertension may also develop in patients who live at high altitudes.

CALCIFICATION OF PULMONARY ARTERIES

Calcification in pulmonary arteries can occur as a result of atheroma of the arterial wall, or in thrombus within arteries. Atheroma is almost always due to long-sustained severe pulmonary hypertension, and thus calcification may occur in the pulmonary arteries in those conditions in which this situation occurs. In addition, the majority of cases of pulmonary artery thrombosis occur in conditions where pulmonary hypertension is a major manifestation, and hence on occasions pulmonary artery atheroma and thrombosis occur together. The characteristic appearance of pulmonary artery calcification is that of curvilinear calcifications, demonstrable by films of appropriate penetration, in the position of what are obviously enlarged central pulmonary arteries, and in addition there is peripheral pruning. Differentiation of pulmonary artery calcification from the so-called 'egg shell calcification' of hilar glands is usually not in doubt.

PULMONARY ARTERY THROMBOSIS

Thrombosis of the main pulmonary artery or its branches is an uncommon complication of a variety of lung, heart and blood diseases. It may occur in association with parenchymal lung disease, with rheumatic or congenital heart disease, in association with sickle-cell anemia, polycythemia, or even trauma to the lung. It may be found at postmortem or demonstrated unsuspectedly by pulmonary angiography. There are no specific symptoms or signs, the occurrence being just part of the natural history of the underlying disease process.

The *radiological appearances* depend on the extent of the thrombosis. Where a lobar or segmental artery alone is involved, the plain chest X-ray will probably not reflect any change. Where a main pulmonary artery is entirely thrombosed, the hilar shadow is thought to be dense and rather sharply defined, and slightly large. There will be a marked reduction of the peripheral lung markings. It may be difficult to recognize these changes if the appearances of the lung are disorganized by the underlying precipitating disease.

The appearances at *pulmonary angiography* will vary according to the extent of the obstruction. Occlusion of a lobar or segmental vessel will be manifest by non-filling of this vessel, but without the classical leading edge of an embolus sign. Thrombosis of the main pulmonary artery will be revealed by a failure of any peripheral filling, and often by the demonstration of a filling defect within the main pulmonary artery, the thrombus itself. Again, contrast medium will probably not trickle past the intra-luminal mass, pointing to this as an intrinsic thrombosis rather than an ill-fitting embolus.

ANEURYSM OF THE PULMONARY ARTERIES

Dilatations of the pulmonary arteries are common in situations of altered pulmonary hemodynamics. They may occur in association with increased flow, as in atrial septal defect; with increased pulmonary artery pressure, as in long-standing mitral valve disease; or when these factors are combined, particularly in patent ductus arteriosus. These dilatations may be visualized radio-graphically, but rarely exert a specific influence over the course of the underlying disease. Aneurysms of the pulmonary arteries, dilatations associated with abnormalities of the wall of the pulmonary artery, are rare. They may be due to syphilis, atheroma, mycotic embolization or other local disease of the arterial wall, or to trauma. These aneurysms may be asymptomatic, or may lead to recurrent chest pain and hemoptysis, presumably by peripheral embolization of the aneurysmal contents. It is this latter group of aneurysms which presents problems in differential diagnosis, because they are unilateral and also have therapeutic implications.

Radiological Appearances In virtually all cases in which radiological examination of the chest has been performed, the aneurysm has been recognized as a rounded shadow in the hilum. It may grow to a large size, and be visible in the lateral view extending anterosuperiorly from the hilum. Curvilinear calcification may be demonstrated in its wall. Secondary lung abnormalities may be seen. In the cases where aneurysmal dilatation is associated with alterations of pulmonary hemodynamics due to heart disease, the pulmonary artery dilatations are commonly bilateral, and evidence of underlying cardiopulmonary abnormalities will usually be obvious. The chief differential diagnosis on plain film radiography is from a localized aortic aneurysm, which usually affects an older age group and has a male sex preponderance. Bronchogenic carcinoma, or more rarely other lung or mediastinal masses, may also be considered in the differential diagnosis.

The diagnosis is confirmed by contrast examination. Any apparent increase in wall thickness is likely to be due to clot lining the aneurysm. Obstructions of peripheral arteries in relation to the aneurysms may be evidence of embolization. In the investigation of hilar mass by angiography it is important that filming should be carried on into the levophase so that if a mass fails to fill from the pulmonary artery it may be possible to determine its relationship to the opacified aorta.

SCIMITAR SYNDROME

The degree of hemodynamic abnormality associated with anomalous insertion of the pulmonary veins depends on the number of pulmonary veins which are abnormally draining, and the site into which they insert. Total anomalous pulmonary

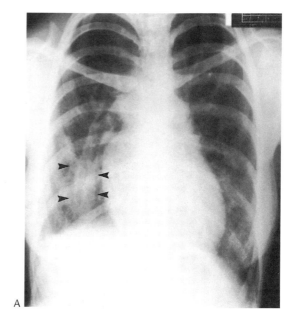

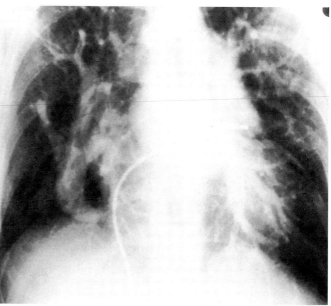

Fig. 22.19 Scimitar syndrome, the heart normally situated. **A.** In the frontal film the scimitar is indicated by arrows. **B.** It can be clearly identified in the levophase of the pulmonary angiogram. Almost the entire right lung drains anomalously to this vessel, which is passing below the diaphragm.

venous drainage usually presents as a cardiac emergency. The majority of forms of partial anomalous venous drainage are associated with atrial septal defect, and are considered in that section. The occurrence of an abnormal pulmonary vein draining the right lower lobe and inserting below the diaphragm, usually into the inferior vena cava, may occur in the absence of significant heart disease and may be considered separately. The condition may present with recurrent respiratory infection involving the right lower lobe of the lung and physical findings may reveal some crowding of the ribs of the right hemithorax and the presence of adventitial sounds in the right lung. The murmur

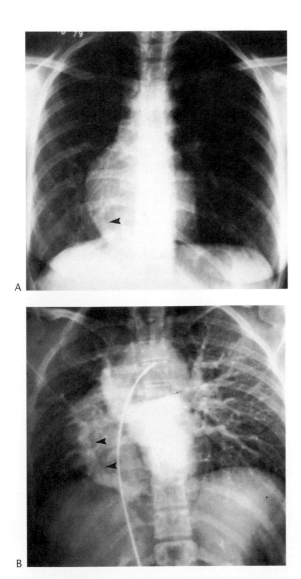

Fig. 22.20 Scimitar syndrome associated with dextroposition of the heart. **A.** In the plain film the scimitar shadow (single arrow) is overlapped and largely concealed by the misplaced heart. **B.** In the venous phase of the pulmonary angiogram, it can be clearly identified (paired arrows) passing below the diaphragm.

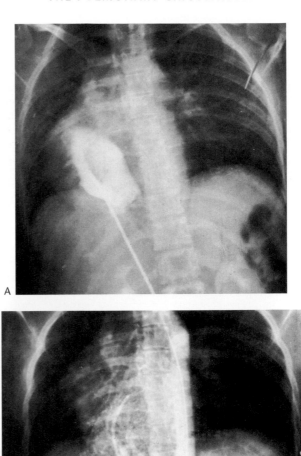

Fig. 22.21 Scimitar syndrome. **A.** A venous catheter has been passed from the inferior vena cava into the abnormal vein. **B.** Aortogram shows a systemic blood supply (arrow) ascending from the lumbar aorta through the diaphragm to supply part of the right lower lobe.

of any associated atrial septal defect may also be heard as the condition commonly occurs in association with atrial septal defect.

Radiological Appearances   The characteristic findings are those which give the syndrome the name; the abnormal pulmonary vein is visible as an inverted scimitar-shaped shadow of soft tissue density in the right lower zone terminating at or below the diaphragm. The shape is so characteristic that when seen the diagnosis of the nature of the abnormal shadow is rarely in doubt (Fig. 22.19). Where the right lower lobe is hypoplastic, as it may be when drained by an anomalous vein, and particularly when supplied by a systemic artery, the diagnosis may be complicated by displacement of the heart and mediastinal structures to the right, *dextroposition* of the heart. This may be so marked as to obscure the characteristic scimitar shadow unless good-quality

overpenetrated films are taken (Figs 22.20 and 22.21). The condition is not of course a true dextrocardia as the apex of the heart still remains pointing to the left. Scimitar syndrome is one of the several causes of dextroposition of the heart.

The appearances of the scimitar are pathognomonic. Investigation is only indicated to elucidate the presence of any associated intracardiac malformation or prior to surgery to determine which parts of the lung are drained by the abnormal vein, and how the arterial supply of the abnormal part of the lung is derived. For this reason the preoperative assessment consists not only of selective pulmonary angiography filmed into the levophase to demonstrate the scimitar and its drainage, but also descending aortography to determine any element of systemic supply to the abnormal lung (Fig. 22.21B). When the condition presents in the neonatal period it may lead to very severe symptoms and be difficult to treat.

RIGHT PULMONARY ARTERY–LEFT ATRIAL COMMUNICATION

This congenital malformation usually occurs as an isolated abnormality unassociated with other cardiac abnormalities. The communication is usually a saccular aneurysm of the descending branch of the right pulmonary artery which opens into the left atrium, though pulmonary venous abnormalities may also occur. Patients may present at any time from infancy to middle age. Symptoms are usually those of cyanosis and exertional dyspnea. Emboli occur only rarely. About half of all patients have rather non-specific murmurs.

Over 75% of patients (Figs 22.22 and 22.23) have an abnormal density, visible at chest radiography and fluoroscopy, at the right heart border, below and behind the right hilum, and this is the aneurysmal dilatation of the pulmonary artery. A cardiac catheter may be passed through the fistula to the left atrium. Pulmonary angiography will opacify the aneurysm and demonstrate its communication with the left atrium.

PULMONARY ARTERIOVENOUS MALFORMATIONS

These are direct communications between the smaller pulmonary arteries and veins. The right-to-left shunt produced leads to dilatation of the terminations of these vessels. The lesions may be multiple in one-third of cases and may show progressive enlargement. Also in one-third of cases they are associated with telangiectasis elsewhere—*Osler–Weber–Rendu disease.*

The pulmonary lesions may be asymptomatic, or lead to dyspnea or hemoptysis. The right-to-left shunt may be complicated by polycythemia, cyanosis and cerebral abscess. These may worsen as the lesions increase in size.

Radiological Appearances   If the lesions are large and have led to dilatation of the peripheral pulmonary artery and vein, a soft tissue density will be seen (Fig. 22.24A) which may change size if studied fluoroscopically during extremes of respiration. Tomography should be done to confirm the vascular nature of the lesion by demonstrating the supplying vessels, and reveal other small lesions not suspected on the standard chest X-ray. Their vascular nature may be apparent on enhanced CT.

The definitive investigation is pulmonary angiography, which is claimed to be both easy and helpful in this condition, as the high flow through the lesions aids in the opacification. It demonstrates enlargement of feeding arteries and draining veins and the direct connection between the two (Fig. 22.24B). There is no enlargement of the main pulmonary artery in uncomplicated arteriovenous malformations. Investigation should be performed if the condition is suspected prior to surgery, as if its nature is known, only a limited resection is required; also unsuspected lesions may be demonstrated. Embolization may alleviate symptoms.

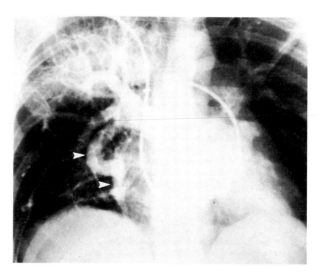

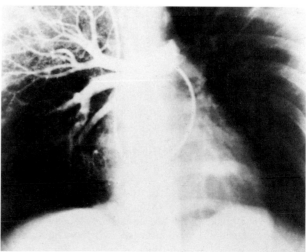

Fig. 22.23 Right pulmonary artery to left arterial communication. Pulmonary angiograms. In the venous phase the dilated right pulmonary artery (white arrows) has been opacified and is seen to be draining into the left atrium.

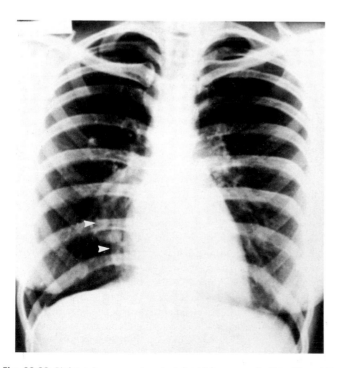

Fig. 22.22 Right pulmonary artery to left atrial communication. The white arrows indicate the abnormal density at the right heart border.

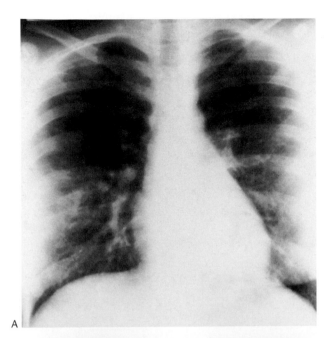

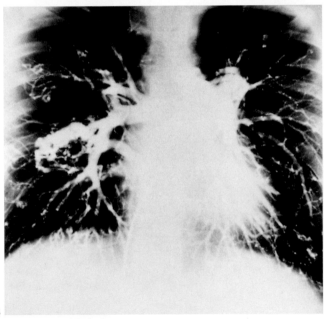

Fig. 22.24 Pulmonary arteriovenous malformations. **A.** Frontal chest film. Abnormal pulmonary shadows, typically elongated, can be identified in the right mid zone. **B.** Pulmonary arteriogram. The pulmonary arteriovenous malformations in the right mid zone, associated with premature venous filling, can be identified. Additional abnormal pulmonary vessels are clearly visible in the right upper zone and throughout the left lung.

PULMONARY VARIX

Localized dilatations of the pulmonary veins may occur with acquired or congenital heart disease, or may occur in asymptomatic patients, unassociated with cardiac abnormality. They are usually recognized as rounded or lobulated shadows often near the hila on the chest X-ray and which may be taken for some unrelated cause. Some may be seen to change size with respiration on fluoroscopy. Tomography may demonstrate the draining vein

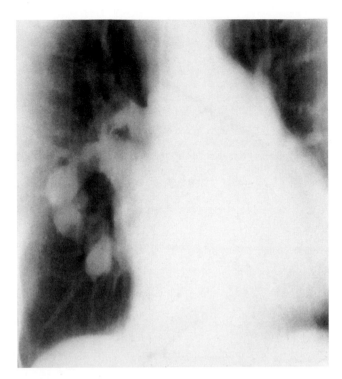

Fig. 22.25 Pulmonary varix. The anteroposterior tomogram shows the multiple rounded densities associated with the pulmonary veins which are typical of pulmonary varices. The venous nature of these was confirmed by angiography.

(Fig. 22.25), thus suggesting the diagnosis. Confirmation of the nature of the abnormal shadow is obtained by selective pulmonary angiography. The shadows show delayed filling with contrast after pulmonary artery injection and impaired drainage of the isolated vein. The appearances differ angiographically from those of arteriovenous malformation, which shows early shunting and enlarged drainage veins. The difference is due to the bypassing of the capillary bed in arteriovenous malformations.

REFERENCES AND SUGGESTIONS FOR FURTHER READING

Alderson, P. O., Martin, E. C. (1987) Pulmonary embolism; diagnosis with multiple imaging modalities. *Radiology*, **164**, 297–312.

Auger, W. R., Fedullo, P. F., Moser, K. M., Buchbinder, M., Peterson, K. L. (1992) Chronic major vessel thromboembolic pulmonary artery obstruction. Appearance at angiography. *Radiology*, **182**, 393–398.

Fazio, F., Lavender, P., Steiner, R. E. (1978) Krypton 81 m ventilation and 99Tcm perfusion scans in chest disease. *American Journal of Radiology*, **130**, 421–428.

Ferris, E. J., Holder, J. C., Lim, W. N. et al. (1984) Angiography of pulmonary emboli: digital studies and balloon occlusion cine angiography. *American Journal of Radiology*, **142**, 369–373.

Gomes, A. S. (1991) Pulmonary angiography. In Marcus, M. L., Schelbert, H. R., Skorton, D. J., Wolf, G. L. (eds) *Cardiac Imaging. A Companion to Braunwald's Heart Disease*, pp. 149–161. Philadelphia: W.B. Saunders. .

Goodman, P. C. (1984) Pulmonary angiography. *Clinics in Chest Medicine*, **5**, 465–477.

Grossman, Z. D. et al (1984) Digital subtraction angiography of the pulmonary arteries for the diagnosis of pulmonary embolism. *Radiology*, **150**, 843–844.

Harris, P., Heath, D. (1978) *The Human Pulmonary Circulation*. Edinburgh: Churchill Livingstone.

Jefferson, K., Rees, S. (1980) *Clinical Cardiac Radiology*, 2nd edn. London: Butterworths.

Morrell, N. W., Seed, W. A. (1992) Diagnosing pulmonary embolism. Editorial. *British Medical Journal*, **304**, 1126–1127.

Moser, K. M., Auger, W. R., Fedullo, P. F. (1990) Chronic major-vessel thromboembolic pulmonary hypertension. *Circulation*, **81**, 1735–1743.

Nicod, P., Peterson, K., Levine, M. et al (1987) Pulmonary angiography in severe chronic pulmonary hypertension. *Annals of Internal Medicine*, **107**, 565–568.

Novelline, R. A., Balterowich, A. H., Athanasoulis, C. A., Waltman, A. C., Greenfield, A. J., McKusick, K. A. (1978) The clinical course of patients with suspected pulmonary embolism and a negative pulmonary arteriogram. *Radiology*, **126**, 561–567.

Perlmutt, L. M., Braum, S. D., Newman, G. E., Oke, E. J., Dunnick, N. R. (1987) Pulmonary arteriography in the high risk patient. *Radiology*, **162**, 187–189.

Raphael, M. J. (1970) Pulmonary angiography. *British Journal of Hospital Medicine*, 377–390.

Rees, S. (1981) Arterial connection of the lung. *Clinical Radiology*, **32**, 1–15.

Stein, P. D., Athanasoulis, C., Alavi, A. et al (1992) Complications and validity of pulmonary angiography in acute pulmonary embolism. *Circulation*, **85**, 462–468.

Stein, P. D., Athanasoulis, C., Greenspan, R. H., Henry, J. W. (1992) Relation of plain chest radiographic findings to pulmonary arterial pressure and arterial blood oxygen levels in patients with acute pulmonary embolism. *American Journal of Cardiology*, **69**, 394–396.

23

ACQUIRED HEART DISEASE

M. J. Raphael and R. M. Donaldson
With a contribution from Jeremy P. R. Jenkins

VALVULAR HEART DISEASE

RHEUMATIC FEVER

This condition, now decreasing in incidence in the West, but still a major problem in developing countries, results from an abnormal response to group A streptococcal infection. The major clinical feature, flitting pains in the large joints, comes on about 2–3 weeks after a sore throat. There is no radiological evidence of joint destruction. Clinical evidence of carditis may be present and there may be radiological cardiomegaly, due either to carditis or to pericardial effusion. The acute phase usually regresses to an asymptomatic or quiescent phase lasting for many years, as chronic valve damage develops. The mitral is the commonest valve to be affected, followed by the aortic and then tricuspid valves. A history of rheumatic fever can be elicited in about half the patients with rheumatic valve disease. A similar valve disease may be seen after chorea.

MITRAL VALVE DISEASE

Mitral Stenosis

Much the commonest cause of obstruction at the mitral valve is rheumatic fever. Stenosis develops by fusion of the leaflet commissures, thickening of the valve leaflets and shortening and thickening and adherence of the chordae tendineae, all of which restrict valve opening. Until the orifice is critically narrowed, symptoms are few, then shortness of breath on exertion develops. Overt cardiac failure may not appear until the onset of atrial fibrillation. The clinical diagnosis is usually obvious, once the characteristic apical diastolic murmur is heard; however, a similar murmur may be heard in torrential aortic incompetence (the Austin–Flint murmur), in atrial septal defect (the patient, if elderly, may also be in atrial fibrillation), and in other forms of mitral obstruction (left atrial myxoma, and congenital obstructions). The murmur may be inaudible in low-output states or with tachycardia.

Radiographic Appearances   The plain film signs are those of selective left atrial enlargement, which may vary from trivial to gross (Figs 23.1 and 23.2). Enlargement of the left atrial appendage is almost universally present as part of the left atrial enlargement and always suggests rheumatic mitral disease (as opposed to non-rheumatic). This enlargement may vary from a simple straightening of the left heart border to a very gross local protrusion (Fig. 23.3).

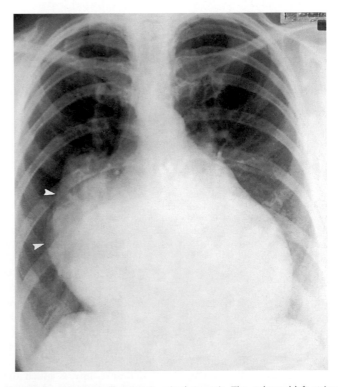

Fig. 23.1   Left atrial dilatation in mitral stenosis. The enlarged left atrium (arrows) extends beyond the right heart border. Note that the border of the right atrium can be identified where it is joined by the inferior vena cava coming up through the diaphragm.

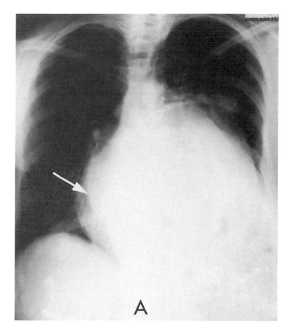

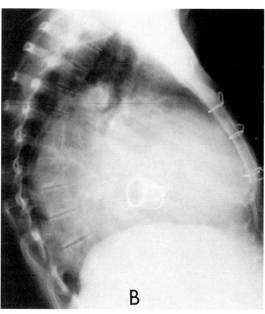

Fig. 23.2 Gross left atrial enlargement in association with a prosthetic mitral valve. **A**. Frontal view. The double shadow of the left atrium, seen to the right of the spine, is indicated by an arrow. Note that the left atrium has so lifted up the left bronchus that it now goes upward. **B**. Lateral view. The prosthetic valve is more clearly seen. Again, the left bronchus goes upward. The right bronchus can also be seen in its normal position.

Mitral Valve Calcification This indicates longstanding and usually severe mitral valve disease (Fig. 23.4). It is not commonly seen on the plain film. It is best seen in the lateral view between the left atrium and the left ventricle, and is more rarely seen in the frontal view on an adequately penetrated film, in the position of the mitral valve. Image amplification fluoroscopy is much the best way of detecting such calcification, locating it to the mitral valve, and identifying its movement toward the apex of the heart in diastole. It must be distinguished from the characteristically

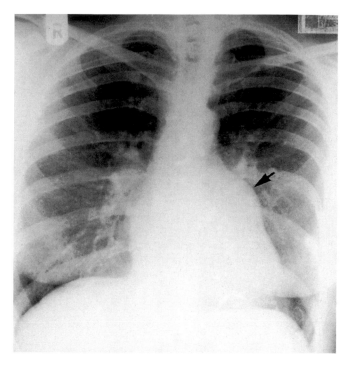

Fig. 23.3 Rheumatic mitral stenosis. This frontal film shows marked enlargement of the left atrial appendage (arrow).

'C'- or 'J'-shaped calcification which may occur in the mitral valve ring in the elderly. This may also be associated with a murmur but is of little hemodynamic importance (Fig. 23.5). Calcification in the mitral ring is also seen around the attachments of prosthetic valves which have been in position for several years.

Calcification may occur in the left atrium in longstanding mitral valve disease with atrial fibrillation (Fig. 23.6).

Marked *changes in the pulmonary circulation* resulting from the chronically raised left atrial pressure may be present (see Ch. 22). Upper-lobe blood diversion is seen in its most florid form, and is brought into prominence by lower-lobe vascular constriction. Enlarged main and central pulmonary arteries and peripheral pruning indicate pulmonary arterial hypertension. Longstanding interstitial edema with acute alveolar pulmonary edema may be seen. *Hemosiderosis* and ossific nodules are mainly seen in rheumatic valve disease.

A very large or aneurysmal left atrium (one which reaches to within an inch, or 2.5 cm, of the chest wall) may be associated with segmental or lobar collapse from bronchial compression usually on the right (Fig. 23.7). The consolidation of pulmonary infarction may occur. Tracheobronchial calcification is also common in rheumatic mitral valve disease.

Cardiac Ultrasound The distinctive motion in the two-dimensional echocardiography (2DE) image of the mitral valve leaflets is due to their tethering by chordal and commissural fusion (Fig. 23.8). An estimate of mitral valve area can be obtained from Doppler recordings of mitral valve flow, with considerable reliability (Fig. 23.9). The discrete jet of mitral stenosis is clearly visualized by color flow mapping (Fig. 23.10). The presence of left atrial thrombus can also be documented (Fig. 23.11); the left atrial appendage, however, can only be visualized by trans-esophageal echocardiography.

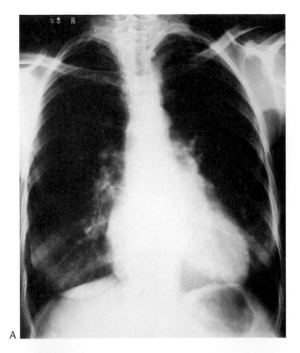

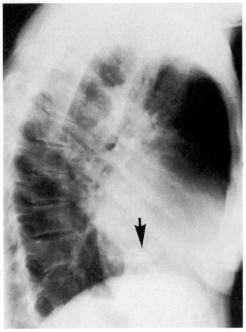

Fig. 23.4 Calcified mitral valve in rheumatic mitral stenosis. The calcification is best seen in the lateral view (arrow).

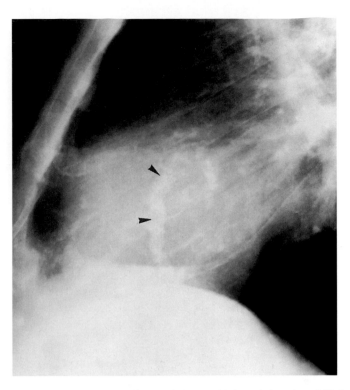

Fig. 23.5 Calcification in the mitral ring. In this lateral view the calcified mitral valve ring (arrows) appears as a characteristic C-shape; it may take a J-shape.

Rheumatic Mitral Incompetence

Rheumatic mitral incompetence results from destruction of cusp tissue, mainly at the free edges, so that these do not meet and seal off the orifice, and also shortening of the chordae which hold the valve in the open position. The clinical presentation is with shortness of breath, and the hallmark of the condition is the apical pan-systolic murmur radiating to the axilla. Symptoms may be precipitated by the development of atrial fibrillation. The murmur may be confused with that of non-rheumatic mitral incompetence or ventricular septal defect. When there is a murmur of associated mitral stenosis, or additional aortic valve disease, and a history of rheumatic fever, the diagnosis is obvious. Many patients have been diagnosed as having rheumatic fever when a murmur is first heard in childhood following an atypical febrile illness, and may turn out to have congenital heart disease. The commonest result of rheumatic mitral valve disease is a valve which is both stenosed and incompetent, failing to open properly in diastole, and failing to adequately seal the mitral orifice in systole. The valve cannot be both severely stenosed and severely incompetent as stenosis limits the degree of incompetence that can develop.

Radiographic Appearances The plain film findings resemble those of mitral stenosis though the heart, particularly the left atrium, is in general larger, and the left atrium may be very large or aneurysmal in mitral incompetence. It is not usually possible to identify specifically associated left ventricular enlargement due to mitral incompetence. If present, left ventricular enlargement is usually due to aortic valve disease. It is not possible to diagnose mitral incompetence by fluoroscopic demonstration of systolic expansion of the left atrium.

Cardiac Ultrasound The echocardiographic assessment of mitral incompetence consists mainly in determining its etiology. The severity of the regurgitation cannot be assessed by the appearances of the valve itself. Mitral regurgitation caused by chronic rheumatic carditis is usually associated with thickened, deformed and often calcified cusps. Regurgitation through the mitral valve can be determined and quantified into mild, moderate and severe by Doppler color flow mapping (Fig. 23.12).

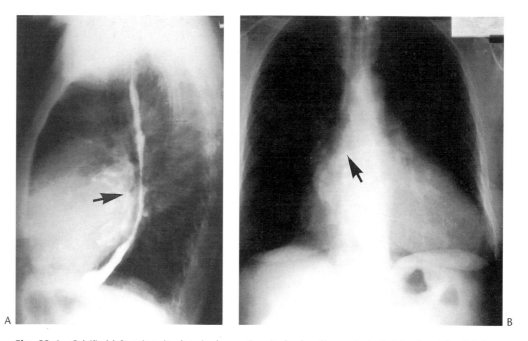

Fig. 23.6 Calcified left atrium in chronic rheumatic mitral valve disease. In both lateral and frontal views curvilinear calcification (arrow) is identified in the position of the wall of the left atrium.

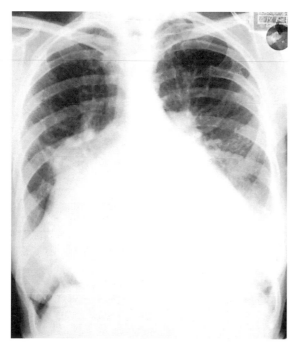

Fig. 23.7 Lobar collapse in association with left atrial enlargement. In this patient, with a very large left atrium, there is segmental collapse of the middle and part of the lower lobe on the right, due to bronchial compression.

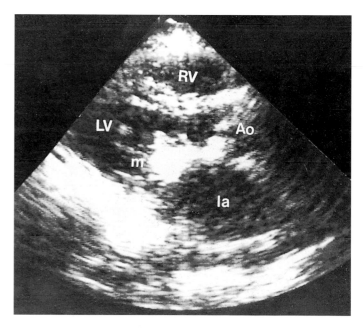

Fig. 23.8 Rheumatic mitral stenosis. The 2DE image shows marked fibrosis and tethering of the mitral (m) leaflets due to chordal and commissural fusion. Ao, aorta; la, left atrium; RV, right ventricle; LV, left ventricle.

Non-rheumatic Mitral Incompetence

Two patterns of abnormality are commonly seen. In the commoner variety, *myxomatous degeneration of the valve leaflets* allows redundant valve tissue to balloon into the left atrium in systole, and the same process may lead to elongation of the chordae. The ballooning of the valve produces an audible systolic click, and if chordal elongation is severe enough to impair apposition of the leaflets, mitral incompetence results.

Chordal rupture may also precipitate mitral incompetence by producing a flail leaflet (or part of a leaflet) so that apposition fails. This condition often progresses jerkily with groups of chordae rupturing and producing mitral incompetence, followed by compensatory left ventricular dilatation and then another episode of rupture.

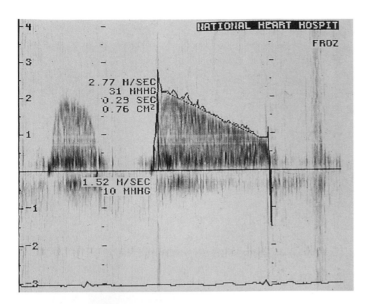

Fig. 23.9 Doppler flow study in mitral stenosis. Left ventricular inflow guided by color flow mapping. The mitral valve area is derived from the mean pressure drop (mean gradient) across the mitral valve. This shows severe mitral stenosis (mitral valve area around 0.76 cm²).

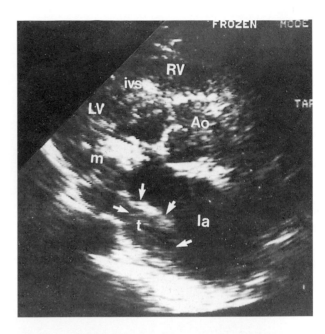

Fig. 23.11 Mitral stenosis. The 2DE image demonstrates a large left atrial (la) cavity and the presence of atrial thrombosis (arrows). There is fibrosis and calcification of the mitral leaflets. Other lettering as in Fig. 20.16.

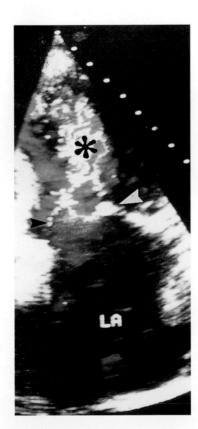

Fig. 23.10 Color flow mapping, apical view. The mitral leaflets are thickened and fibrosed (arrows). The abnormal (increased) flow velocity across the valve causes aliasing and a flame shaped jet of turbulent flow (*). The discrete jet of mitral stenosis is shown by CFM. LA, left atrium.

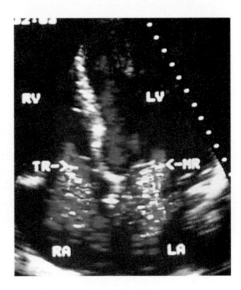

Fig. 23.12 Color flow Doppler mapping in combined mitral and tricuspid regurgitation. The extensive red coloring in the left atrium (LA) indicates marked mitral regurgitation (MR), the lesser coloring in the right atrium (RA) indicates a lesser but still significant degree of tricuspid regurgitation (TR). Other lettering as in Fig. 20.16.

Both types of mitral involvement may lead to cardiac failure which may be steadily or intermittently progressive and may lead to death. There is a characteristic mid- or late-onset systolic murmur which may be initiated by a click. Atrial fibrillation is rarer than in rheumatic carditis. The differential diagnosis includes other causes of a late systole murmur combined with left ventricular hypertrophy on the ECG, i.e. aortic stenosis and hypertrophic cardiomyopathy. Mitral incompetence in the course of ischemic heart disease is considered below.

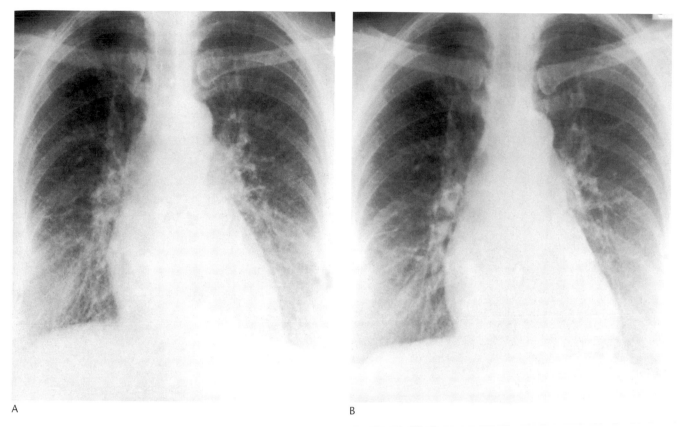

A   B

Fig. 23.13 Acute non-rheumatic mitral regurgitation. **A**. Frontal view in the acute phase. The heart size is virtually normal, even in the presence of high left atrial pressure as evidenced by the preferential dilation of the upper-lobe vessels and interstitial edema. **B**. Frontal film 2 weeks later. This shows clearing of the edema though upper-lobe blood diversion can still be seen.

Radiographic Appearances The plain film appearances are very different from those in rheumatic mitral incompetence. In the acute phase the heart may be virtually normal in size and shape even in the presence of pulmonary edema or other evidence of a high left atrial pressure (Fig. 23.13). If the patient survives to enter the chronic phase, the heart enlarges with a left ventricular configuration. Left atrial enlargement is slight and the left atrial appendage is very rarely enlarged. Calcification does not occur. In the proposed mitral valve associated with Marfan syndrome, aortic root dilatation may be present.

Rarer causes of non-rheumatic mitral incompetence are those associated with a *left atrial myxoma* damaging the mitral valve, with *bacterial endocarditis* involving the mitral valve, with *cardiac trauma* damaging the mitral valve, with *ischemic heart disease* involving the papillary muscles and with *cardiomyopathy* leading to mitral incompetence. Congenital causes are dealt with in Chapter 26.

Cardiac Ultrasound 2DE is very useful in the diagnosis of non-rheumatic and mitral incompetence. It shows virtually all cases of prolapse of the mitral valve leaflet (Fig. 23.14) and also the flail mitral leaflet associated with chordal rupture. The essential feature is that the anterior and posterior leaflets do not oppose properly in systole, usually because one or the other has prolapsed back into the left atrium. Doppler sampling and Doppler color flow mapping again serve to localize and quantify the valvar regurgitation (see Fig. 23.12).

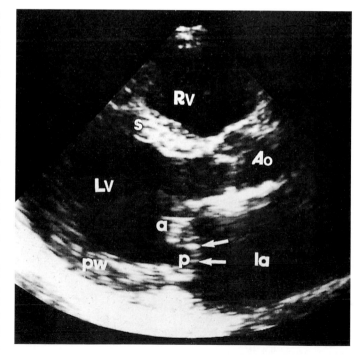

Fig. 23.14 Mitral valve prolapse. The 2DE image shows striking bowing of the posterior (p) mitral leaflet into the left atrium (la) (arrows). Other lettering as in Fig. 20.16.

Cardiac Catheterization and Angiocardiography Investigation is indicated for the diagnosis in those rare cases where it is in doubt, even after echocardiography.

Severity Catheterization and angiocardiography are better able to assess the severity of the valve lesion than echocardiography. When severity is in doubt, or with associated lung disease as a possible cause of dyspnea, and specially when more than one valve is abnormal, hemodynamic and angiographic investigation may be indicated. Additionally, they may help when it is not clear whether valve disease or impaired left ventricular function is the cause of the patient's symptoms, particularly after valve replacement.

Associated Coronary Artery Disease Coronary arteriography is routinely performed before surgery in patients with chest pain, ischemic changes on the ECG, or when they are aged over 55 years. The severity of mitral valve obstruction is assessed by measuring the gradient across the mitral valve between simultaneously recorded indirect left atrial (wedge) pressure (or direct left atrial pressure recorded by a transeptal catheter) and the left ventricular pressure obtained by retrograde catheterization of the left ventricle across the aortic valve. The flow across the valve must also be measured by determining the cardiac output. If the gradient is low at rest, in patients clinically suspected of having significant mitral obstruction, it is usual to increase the cardiac output by exercise and check the gradient again.

Mitral incompetence is assessed by **cine left ventriculography** in the right anterior oblique projection. This projection brings the mitral valve into profile, and separates the left ventricle from the left atrium. The severity of mitral regurgitation is estimated by the rapidity with which contrast passes across the mitral valve from the left ventricle to the left atrium to opacify the left atrium. Rapid passage of large quantities of contrast indicate that regurgitation is severe. In non-rheumatic mitral incompetence this feature can be misleading as the atrium is commonly small and opacifies rapidly with only slight regurgitation. In this situation, pulmonary artery and left atrial pressures, if normal, suggest that regurgitation is not severe. The angiographic appearances of the mitral valve are of interest but rarely of significance. The normal mitral valve is flung widely open in diastole, allowing an ill-defined broad front of non-opaque blood to enter the opacified left ventricle. If the valve is stenosed it is outlined by opaque blood on its ventricular aspect and non-opaque blood on its atrial aspect, producing a domed valve if examined in profile (Fig. 23.15) or appearing as a filling defect under the aortic valve if seen 'en face'.

The regurgitation of rheumatic mitral disease usually appears as one or more discreet jets of contrast passing through the mitral valve directly back into the left atrium (Fig. 23.16). Non-rheumatic mitral regurgitation appears as a jet of contrast escaping under the flail mitral valve and passing in a circular fashion around the wall of the left atrium.

A prolapsing mitral valve can be seen to balloon backward into the left atrium during ventricular systole, but it must be distinguished from the various crevices which appear in the left ventricle in the mitral valve area, by the fact that it must disappear entirely in ventricular diastole. When regurgitation occurs with a prolapsing valve, the prolapse may be demonstrated as developing in ventricular systole by angiography, and the regurgitation may be seen to start only when prolapse has fully developed (Fig.

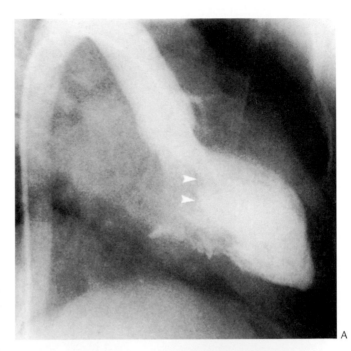

A

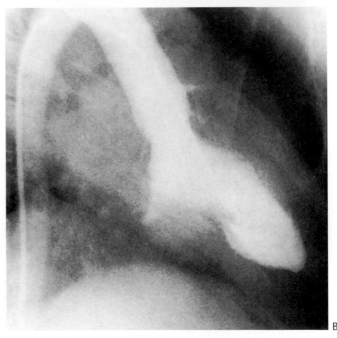

B

Fig. 23.15 Left ventriculography in mitral stenosis. **A**. Right anterior oblique diastole. The stenosed valve is outlined by non-opaque blood on its atrial side so that it domes (arrows) into the ventricle in diastole. **B**. Right anterior oblique systole. The mitral valve has closed normally.

23.17). Thus angiography demonstrates that the prolapse itself is responsible for the click and the late onset of mitral incompetence. This explains the mid or late systolic onset of the systolic murmur which characterizes the condition.

Left Ventricular Function This may be assessed from the cine left ventriculogram by the size of the ventricle and the degree of emptying that occurs with each beat, although in the presence of atrial fibrillation, assessment may be difficult.

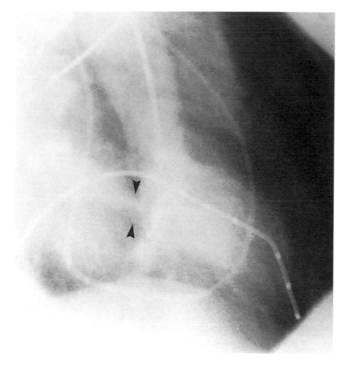

Fig. 23.16 Rheumatic mitral regurgitation. Left ventriculography in the right anterior oblique (RAO) projection, systole. A discrete jet of mitral regurgitation (arrowed) passes through the closed mitral valve into the left atrium.

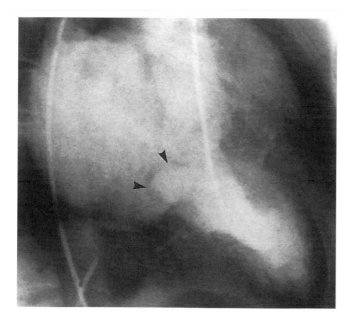

Fig. 23.17 Prolapse of the mitral valve. Systolic left ventriculogram in RAO projection. Part of the mitral valve, probably the middle scallop of the posterior leaflet, is clearly visible (arrows) prolapsing back into the left atrium.

Coronary Arteriography This will exclude or demonstrate associated atheromatous coronary artery disease. It may also demonstrate blood vessel formation in left atrial thrombus, which is a not uncommon finding when it is performed for the investigation of longstanding rheumatic heart disease.

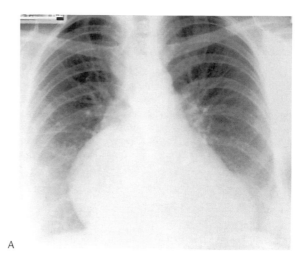

A

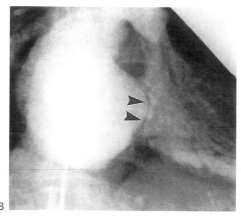

B

Fig. 23.18 Tricuspid stenosis developing in the course of rheumatic valvular heart disease. **A.** The frontal chest film shows a bulge of the large right atrium to the right. **B.** The right atrial angiogram in RAO projection confirms the enlargement of the right atrium and demonstrates its cause, a stenosed tricuspid valve (arrows).

TRICUSPID VALVE DISEASE

This most commonly occurs late in the course of rheumatic heart disease. Tricuspid stenosis or tricuspid incompetence may be due to involvement of the valve by the rheumatic process, or tricuspid incompetence may be functional. Tricuspid disease may be suspected clinically when the jugular venous pressure is raised and its form abnormal, and the liver is enlarged and pulsatile, when the murmurs closely resemble those of mitral valve disease.

The *plain film* shows enlargement of the right atrium, bulging the heart shadow to the right (Fig. 23.18). Right atrial enlargement can usually be distinguished from left atrial enlargement due to mitral disease, by the entry of the inferior vena cava, which limits its extent below.

The development of the characteristic murmur in a patient with a known carcinoid syndrome indicates the well-recognized development of tricuspid stenosis in this condition. It may be associated with a large right atrium on the plain film.

Bacterial endocarditis on the tricuspid valve is a common complication of *intravenous drug abuse*. The majority of the infections are staphylococcal, the main clinical and radiological manifestations appear in the lungs with extensive areas of

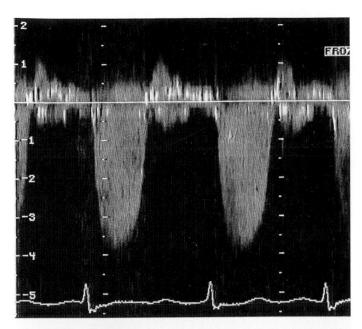

Fig. 23.19 Tricuspid regurgitation and pulmonary hypertension. Apical view showing retrograde high-velocity flow into the right atrium (away from the transducer) in systole as a result of tricuspid regurgitation. The maximum retrograde flow is 4.5 m/s. The estimated pulmonary artery systolic pressure (using the modified Bernouilli equation) = 4.5 × (maximum velocity)^2.

consolidation often progressing rapidly to cavitation. In those patients who survive and develop significant tricuspid incompetence, right atrial enlargement may be detected on serial chest films.

Cardiac Ultrasound   2DE visualizes the tricuspid valve, and in the majority of cases it is able to show thickening of the valve when it is stenosed. Vegetations on the leaflets are visualized by 2DE in cases of bacterial endocarditis. The Doppler modality is useful in assessing tricuspid stenosis; color flow mapping is particularly effective in visualizing the retrograde systolic flow into the right atrial cavity in tricuspid regurgitation (see Fig. 23.12). An indirect estimate of pulmonary artery systolic pressure can be obtained from the Doppler-derived trans-tricuspid valve gradient (Fig. 23.19). Measurement of the systolic pulmonary artery pressure is helpful in assessing the patient's symptoms and the effect of disease of the left side of the heart on the pulmonary circulation.

Cardiac Catheterization and Angiocardiography   These may be difficult to perform and interpret in tricuspid valve disease. Tricuspid stenosis is measured by simultaneous recording of right ventricular and right atrial pressures. As the pressures in diastole are low and the pressure gradients, even when significant, are small, pressures must be measured very carefully.

Right atrial angiography may reveal the large right atrium and thickened, domed, tricuspid valve leaflets, confirming that the tricuspid valve is abnormal. Right ventriculography will show tricuspid incompetence, but the significance of the findings must be assessed carefully as some regurgitation may occur through the tricuspid valve during right ventriculography simply because the catheter, passed through the tricuspid valve, holds it open.

AORTIC VALVE DISEASE

The aortic valve may be stenotic or incompetent or both.

Aortic Stenosis

This may occur as a congenitally stenotic valve or may develop in adult life either on the basis of a congenital bicuspid valve or from inflammatory commissural fusion which develops in the course of rheumatic heart disease.

Calcific Aortic Stenosis   This usually develops on the basis of a congenitally bicuspid valve, which may be detected in its mobile, prestenotic phase by its ejection click, there being no murmur. With deposition of calcium on the abnormal valve, beginning in

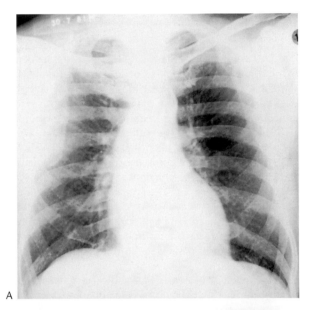

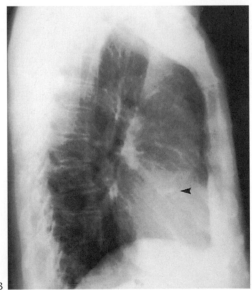

Fig. 23.20 Aortic stenosis. **A**. Frontal film, showing rounding of the left ventricular apex indicative of left ventricular hypertrophy, and also poststenotic dilatation of the ascending aorta. **B**. Lateral film, showing calcification (arrowhead) in the position of the aortic valve.

the fourth decade, mobility (and the click) is lost, and stenosis develops. Valve calcification is invariable as it is the stenosing process (not as in mitral stenosis a result of the stenosis). Calcification makes the cusps rigid and impedes the flow of blood.

Presentation is with shortness of breath, angina or syncope. The diagnosis is made on the basis of the slow rising plateau pulse, the ejection systole murmur and thrill and the presence of left ventricular hypertrophy in the ECG.

Plain films may show rounding of the left ventricular apex indicative of left ventricular hypertrophy, poststenotic dilatation of the ascending aorta, and, on the lateral film, calcification in the position of the aortic valve (Fig. 23.20).

In older patients, when the aorta has become unfolded and slightly dilated, localized poststenotic dilatation may be difficult to detect. Significant aortic stenosis may be present with a virtually normal heart shadow though it is rare not to detect some evidence of ventricular enlargement in either the frontal or lateral view.

Cardiac Ultrasound 2DE shows a thickened immobile aortic valve with dense echoes indicative of calcium deposition. It may also show thickened ventricular walls and permit the detection of various forms of subvalvular or supravalvular stenosis. Doppler studies require the utilization of continuous-wave measurements because of the high blood flow velocities reached in the aortic root in aortic stenosis. By recording the maximal velocity of blood flow in the ascending aorta, it is possible to recognize left ventricular outflow tract obstruction and also estimate severity with great reliability (Fig. 23.21).

The clinical diagnosis is usually obvious when the characteristic murmur is heard, though rarely hypertrophic cardiomyopathy and non-rheumatic mitral regurgitation may have similar murmurs and also show left ventricular hypertrophy on the ECG.

In serious doubt, fluoroscopy will show valve calcification or exclude it. Note that the amount of calcium correlates only very roughly with the severity of the aortic stenosis.

Difficulty may be encountered when congestive cardiac failure has developed and cardiac output is so low that the characteristic murmur is not audible; the clinical picture may then resemble congestive cardiomyopathy; the presence of valve calcification on the lateral plain film may be the first indication of the diagnosis.

Rheumatic Aortic Stenosis This is due to commissural fusion immobilizing the cusps. Calcification is frequently visible on image amplification fluoroscopy but is rarely more than a few flecks and is almost never seen on the plain film. Left ventricular hypertrophy may be seen on the plain film but poststenotic dilatation is rare. A history of rheumatic fever and evidence of mitral valve involvement either clinically or on echocardiography point to the diagnosis.

Aortic Incompetence

This is most commonly due to damage to the aortic cusps by *rheumatic fever* or *endocarditis*, and it may occur in association with aortic stenosis. More rarely it may be due to primary disease of the aortic wall when this is involved by aortitis of any etiology (syphilis being the best known) or due to an aortic root aneurysm occurring either alone or as part of Marfan syndrome. *Dissecting aneurysm* reaching to the ascending aorta and valve ring may also

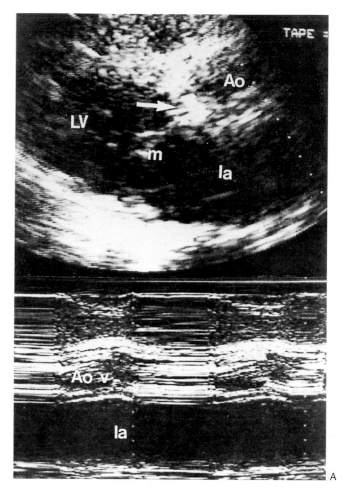

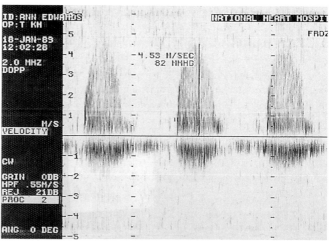

Fig. 23.21 Aortic stenosis. **A**. 2DE study visualizing a thickened immobile valve with dense echoes indicative of calcium deposition (arrow). **B**. Continuous-wave Doppler sampling from the aortic jet of a patient with aortic stenosis. The peak velocity of over 4 m/s indicates a predicted pressure gradient of 82 mmHg. Lettering as in Fig. 20.16.

precipitate aortic incompetence. The diagnosis is made clinically on the basis of the collapsing pulse and the detection of an early diastolic murmur.

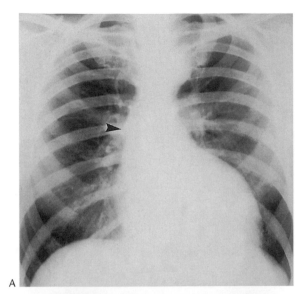

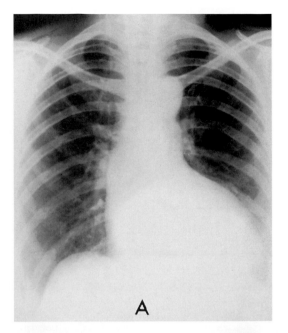

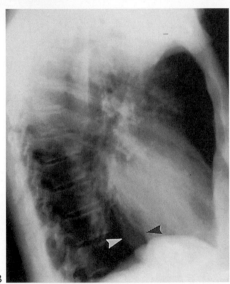

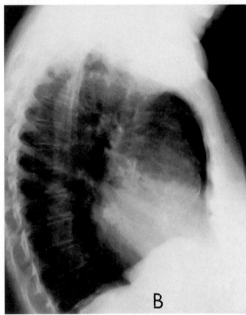

Fig. 23.22 Gross left ventricular dilatation from chronic aortic incompetence. **A**. The axis of the heart is elongated to the left with rounding of the apex. There is slight prominence of the ascending aorta (black arrow). **B**. The body of the left ventricle (white arrow) can be seen bulging behind the line of the right atrium (black arrow).

Fig. 23.23 Aortic incompetence due to syphilitic aortic root aneurysm. **A**. Frontal view, showing left ventricular dilatation extending to the left and only a slight prominence in the position of the ascending aorta, with a barely visible rim of calcium. **B**. Lateral view, showing a large saccular aortic root aneurysm clearly outlined by calcification.

Radiographic Appearances The appearances will vary depending on whether the aortic incompetence is chronic or of acute onset. In the chronic form the plain film shows a large heart with left ventricular configuration, and the heart size is commensurate with the severity of the aortic incompetence (Fig. 23.22). The aorta is often large in both the ascending part and the arch. Calcification of the aortic valve is not a feature of pure aortic incompetence but may be seen if aortic incompetence is combined with stenosis on a calcified, congenitally abnormal, valve. Aortic root abnormalities may show a localized aortic deformity, or what may appear to be simply a large ascending aorta bulging to the right of the mediastinum, or less often to the left. Sometimes the frontal film appears normal, but an abnormal forward bulge of the root of the aorta may be seen on the lateral view (Fig. 23.23). Rarely no aortic abnormality may be detectable.

In *acute aortic incompetence*, usually due to bacterial endocarditis or aortic dissection, there may be congestive cardiac failure with a virtually normal-sized heart, when this has not had time to dilate.

The diagnosis of aortic incompetence is usually obvious once the early diastolic murmur has been heard. Only in acute aortic incompetence may this be inaudible.

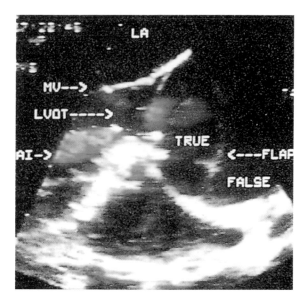

Fig. 23.24 Transesophageal echocardiography in aortic dissection. True and false lumens, and the intimal flap, are all visualized. Colorflow Doppler indicates significant aortic incompetence. Labelling as in Fig. 20.16.

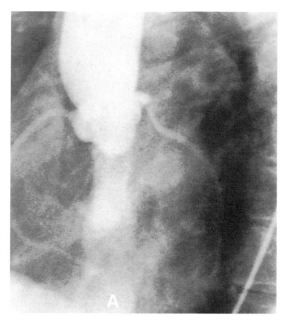

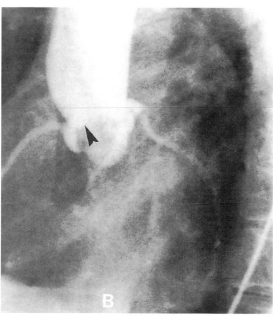

Fig. 23.25 Aortography in aortic stenosis Left anterior oblique (LAO) projection **A.** Diastole. The aortic valve appears largely normal and there is slight aortic regurgitation. **B.** Systole. The domed aortic valve (arrow) is clearly seen, and passing through its center is a negative jet of non-opaque blood, indicating the size of the orifice.

Cardiac Ultrasound   2DE may show an abnormal aortic valve and a large hyperdynamic left ventricle. Abnormalities of the aortic root may also be picked up by 2DE, which may recognize aortic root abscess and vegetations in endocarditis. Pulsed Doppler and Doppler color flow mapping are sensitive in distinguishing the severity of the aortic regurgitation, although precise volumetric measurements are not possible at present.

Transesophageal echocardiography is of particular value when aortic dissection is suspected. Aortic incompetence, often of acute onset, may be due to disease of the wall of the aorta such as the aortic root aneurysm which occurs often in association with Marfan syndrome, or dissections which have spread to involve the root of the aorta. It is claimed to be the definitive technique for studying dissections of the aorta non-invasively (Fig. 23.24).

CT Scanning   CT has been extensively utilized in the recognition of both dissections and aortic aneurysms.

Magnetic Resonance Imaging   More recently, MRI has been used for the same purpose. Both CT and MRI are able to make a diagnosis of aneurysmal dissection but neither is able to demonstrate reliably the hemodynamic consequences of involving the aortic valve or the anatomic consequences of involving the coronary arteries, for which catheterization and angiography are required.

Cardiac Catheterization and Angiocardiography (Fig. 23.25)
The severity of aortic stenosis is assessed by measuring the gradient across the aortic valve, and knowing the cardiac output. The left ventricular pressure may be obtained if the valve can be crossed retrogradely, or measured by a trans-septal approach. The aortic pressure is obtained by retrograde catheterization.

The angiographic visualization of the aortic valve is by retrograde root aortography using cine radiography in the left anterior oblique projection.

The normal aortic valve has three sinuses of Valsalva with three

valve cusps which close in diastole so that no contrast leaks pass them into the left ventricle; in systole they fly open against the side of the aorta where they usually cannot be seen. The lowermost sinus of Valsalva seen on the aortogram is always the non-coronary.

Aortic Stenosis   In lone calcific aortic stenosis, calcification can almost invariably be seen and may be extremely gross. Even in rheumatic aortic stenosis, small flecks of calcification are commonly seen on good-quality angiograms. The stenosed valve (Fig. 23.25) may be domed or simply show restricted opening. It is usually thickened so that the cusps are well seen. The densely calcified valves are almost immobile during the cardiac cycle. The aortic root is often pinched in rheumatic aortic disease.

The severity of aortic stenosis can only be estimated angiographically when a discrete negative jet of non-opacified blood is seen. In the absence of a recognizable negative jet at root aortography (or positive jet at left ventriculography), no positive conclusions can be drawn, as the density of calcification correlates only very roughly with the severity of the stenosis. A small negative jet indicates severe stenosis.

Aortic Incompetence Aortic incompetence is categorized from the left anterior oblique cine aortic root angiogram in four grades:

1. A small puff of contrast enters the left ventricle in diastole and is cleared immediately in systole
2. The left ventricle is outlined with contrast in diastole but it is still cleared away in systole
3. Progressively increasing opacification of the left ventricle occurs with each beat
4. Massive immediate opacification of the left ventricle occurs.

Unfortunately there is no close correlation between this radiological assessment and the degree of aortic incompetence quantified by measurement of the regurgitant flow by ventricular volume studies.

In disease of the aortic cusps the appearances of the aortic regurgitation are largely non-specific except when there is a pinhole jet of regurgitation through a valve cusp. This always raises the possibility of cusp perforation. Patients with rheumatic aortic incompetence may show evidence of 'doming' of the valve with commissural fusion. In acute bacterial endocarditis the nature of the pathological process may be suspected by recognizing paravalvar abscesses tracking into the septum (it is these that produce heart block, and indication for immediate surgery) or between the left ventricle and the left atrium.

When aortic wall disease is suspected, investigation is always indicated. Dissections may be diagnosed by the tracking of contrast between the aortic wall and the elevated flap of intima (see Ch. 26). Angiography will reveal contrast tracking between the intima and the media in dissecting aneurysms. Occasionally the characteristic intimal flap will not be seen, but evidence of aortic wall thickening will suggest further diagnostic efforts. Aortic root aneurysms will be seen as rather symmetrical fusiform dilatations of the aortic root involving the valve ring and often the cusps of the aortic valve (the so-called triple sinus aneurysm) but the dilatation usually stops short of the origin of the innominate artery. In Marfan syndrome, small intimal dissections may not be seen at aortography, and attacks of acute chest pain probably represent small dissections even in the presence of a non-diagnostic arteriogram.

ISCHEMIC HEART DISEASE

CORONARY ARTERIOGRAPHY

This is the radiological visualization of the coronary arteries (and left ventricle) by direct selective injection of contrast medium. It is the most sensitive and accurate method of studying disease in the coronary arteries, and the effects of this disease on the heart, and a description of the technique and findings, must be considered first.

Technique Two approaches are available to cannulate the coronary arteries. The more popular is the percutaneous femoral Seldinger technique using preshaped catheters, different for each coronary artery and for the left ventricle. Different configurations have been described by Judkins and Amplatz.

The earlier technique, that of Sones, required an arteriotomy of the right brachial artery and used a single, soft-tipped catheter which was buckled against the aortic valve and introduced into each coornary artery in turn, and into the left ventricle.

Filming Digital imaging with up to 60 frames/s using a 512 matrix is now available, and is the modality of choice. It allows image processing, instantaneous replay and computer analysis.

Normal Coronary Anatomy The left coronary artery (Fig. 23.26) comes off its sinus of Valsalva, which is on the left and slightly posterior. The main stem, of variable length, passes to the left and divides into two.

The *anterior descending coronary artery* passes forward over the surface of the heart in the anterior interventricular groove (which marks the interventricular septum) and reaches to, and beyond, the apex of the heart to reach the inferior interventricular groove on the undersurface. Parallel *septal branches* descend from the anterior descending artery into the septum, and diagonal branches to the free wall (as opposed to the septum) of the left ventricle pass to the left. The *circumflex artery* passes to the left in the left atrioventricular groove (which marks the atrioventricular valvar plane, separating the atrial from the ventricular part of the heart). It gives off forward-running obtuse marginal branches to the left ventricular free wall, and normally terminates above the crux.

The *right coronary artery* (Fig. 23.27) comes off its sinus of Valsalva, in front and only slightly on the right, and passes forward and to the right to reach the right atrioventricular groove, in which it encircles the right side of the heart. Its first branch, the conus branch, is to the conus of the right ventricle; its second, which runs posteriorly, is the sinus node artery to the sinus node in the interatrial septum. Then come right ventricular branches. The usual, dominant, right coronary artery reaches the crux (the junction of the atrioventricular plane and the interventricular plane on the undersurface of the heart). Immediately before the crux it gives off the posterior descending coronary artery, which runs forward in the inferior interventricular groove to supply the posterior septum. At the crux the right coronary artery loops into the myocardium, giving off the atrioventricular node artery at the apex of the loop before emerging back onto the surface of the heart. The right coronary artery then continues in the left atrioventricular groove, supplying posterolateral left ventricular branches to the left ventricular free wall.

Normal Variants Variation of balance of the coronary arteries can make interpretation of the angiogram difficult. The common variation is left dominance. The circumflex branch of the left coronary artery is very large and extends around the back of the heart in the left atrioventricular groove until it reaches the crux, where it supplies the posterior descending and atrioventricular nodal branches. The right coronary artery is consequently small and supplies only the right ventricle, and may appear abnormal.

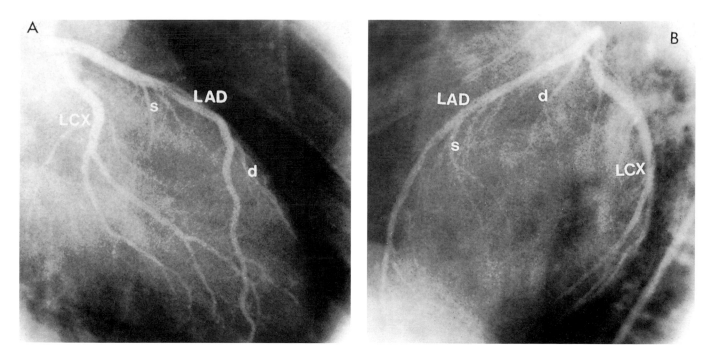

Fig. 23.26 Left coronary artery. **A**. RAO view. **B**. LAO view. The main stem, whose length can vary, passes to the left and divides into the anterior descending (LAD) and circumflex (LCX) branches. s, septal branch; d, diagonal branch.

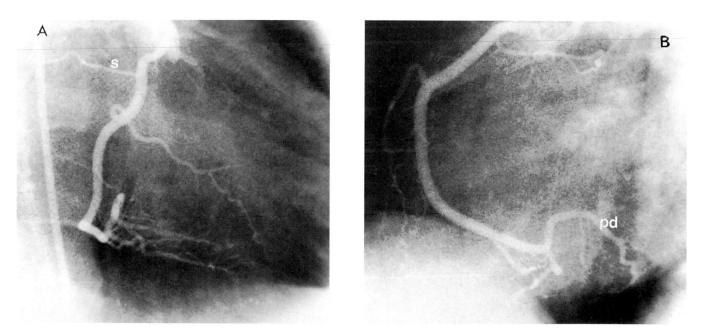

Fig. 23.27 Right coronary artery. **A**. RAO view. **B**. LAO view. The usual dominant right coronary artery gives off the posterior descending (pd) branch immediately before the crux of the heart. s, sinus node artery.

The circumflex rarely may be so large as to entirely replace the right coronary artery, or the right coronary artery may be so large that there is virtually no circumflex. Both may be large, and the anterior descending artery very small.

Congenital Anomalies These abound in the coronary circulation. The circumflex may arise from the right coronary artery or from the right sinus of Valsalva; rarely the anterior descending artery may do this. The circumflex branch and anterior descending artery may have separate origins from the left coronary sinus of Valsalva. These anomalies lead to difficulties in catheterization but do not in themselves produce symptoms. Origin of the left coronary artery from the right sinus of Valsalva or of the right coronary artery from the left sinus of Valsalva may lead to symptoms if the artery is compressed.

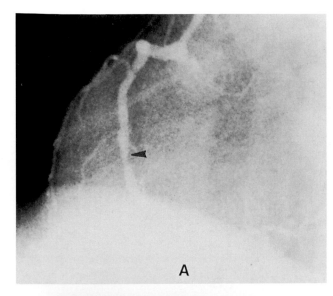

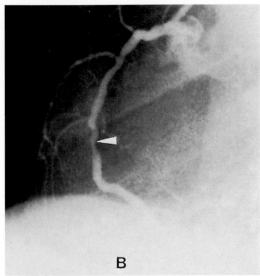

Fig. 23.28 Coronary artery disease, right coronary artery, LAO view. **A**. Atheromatous lesion in the mid third of the right coronary artery appearing as an irregularity of outline (arrow). **B**. Same patient 14 months later, visualizing a severe stricture (arrow).

Coronary Disease

The normal coronary artery is a smoothly outlined, gently tapering structure at angiography. *Atheroma* appears as an irregularity of outline (Fig. 23.28A). When atheromatous plaques spread around the artery to form a stricture this can be identified and its severity evaluated (Fig. 23.28B). Angiography understates the extent of atheroma and the severity of stricture. Complete occlusions may be detected and the patency of the vessel beyond the complete occlusion identified as it opacifies by collateral flow (Fig. 23.29).

Spasm   During coronary arteriography, spasm may also be seen. Catheter-induced spasm usually occurs as a smoothly tapered narrowing, usually in the right coronary artery, at the catheter tip. It is not usually associated with symptoms, and may be relieved by nitroglycerin. Spontaneous or drug (ergot preparations) induced spasm often begins at a rather minor atheromatous plaque and may progress to occlusion of the whole artery, often with the

development of the patient's symptoms and ECG changes. It is usually relieved by nitroglycerin.

Kawasaki Disease   This condition is now being increasingly diagnosed in children presenting with fever, a rash and mucocutaneous symptoms. The coronary arteries are frequently involved with aneurysm formation, which may lead to clotting and thrombosis.

Left Ventriculography

The normal left ventricle is a carrot-shaped structure with the aortic and mitral valves at its base (Fig. 23.30). It contracts concentrically, with its anterior wall apex and inferior wall all moving equally inward. Ischemic heart disease (Fig. 23.31) produces localized abnormalities of wall movement (see Fig. 23.30)—hypokinesia (reduced movement), akinesia (no movement) and dyskinesia (paradoxical movement). Wall movement abnormalities are associated with overall impairment of function which can be seen on the angiogram as ventricular dilatation and poor emptying. Emptying is measured as the *ejection fraction* ((stroke volume/diastolic volume) × 100), the proportion of the ventricle which empties with each beat, and in the normal heart it is two-thirds. Significantly impaired function would be represented by an ejection fraction of under 50%, proceeding to the very severest impairment, 10–20%.

ANGINA PECTORIS

This is an episodic pain occurring almost anywhere above the diaphragm and thought to be due to transient myocardial ischemia. Classical angina is a crushing chest pain, often radiating to the left arm, brought on by exercise, and relieved by rest or trinitrin. The ECG becomes abnormal during pain with ST segment depression. This condition is almost invariably associated with obstructed coronary arteries.

Diagnosis of angina pectoris may be difficult when the pain develops in a bizarre site, such as the jaw, or when its relationship to exercise and relief by rest is unclear, as may occur in the many mixed patterns of angina which may be encountered.

The *plain film* is normal in patients with uncomplicated angina pectoris unless there has been a previous myocardial infarction.

Prinzmetal's Variant Angina   This is an anginal pain, often coming on spontaneously, and associated with ST segment elevation on the ECG. The coronary arteries develop spasm during the pain but show no atheromatous narrowing when the patient is symptom-free.

Thallium Scanning   When performed during the ischemic episode this may show a perfusion deficit which fills in at rest, supporting the idea that a localized area of myocardium becomes ischemic, and that this is the cause of symptoms. Unfortunately, thallium scanning is neither sensitive nor specific enough to be a particularly useful test in excluding the diagnosis of coronary artery disease, though if its results are very positive it does support the diagnosis.

MYOCARDIAL INFARCTION

When ischemia is severe enough to lead to death of muscle the syndrome of myocardial infarction results. The clinical features

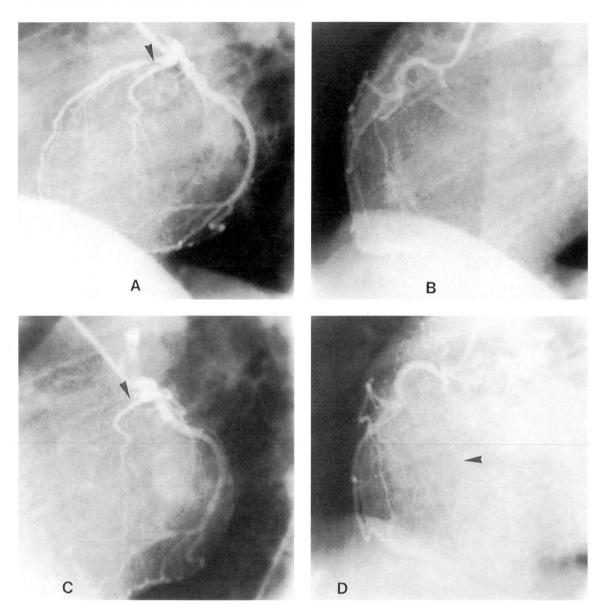

Fig. 23.29 Progression of coronary disease. LAO views. **A**. Left coronary artery. There is a critical narrowing at the origin of the anterior descending branch (arrow). **B**. Right coronary artery. **C,D** seven months later following an anterior infarction (see Fig. 23.31). The left coronary artery has become completely occluded (C, arrow) and fills via collaterals from the right coronary artery (D, arrow).

depend on the size of the infarction, the presence of arrythmias and the development of the mechanical complications of myocardial infarction.

Radiographic Appearances The *plain films* are initially ward unit portable films done anteroposterior, at short distance and often with low-power apparatus. They are thus usually of poor quality and with distorted geometry and with the heart size difficult to assess. The size of the heart will depend on the size of the current infarct and the effects of any previous infarctions. It may be small if the present infarct is the only one and is small, and large if the present infarct is large or there have been previous infarcts. The pulmonary vessels will reflect the hemodynamic disturbance, with upper-lobe blood diversion, and interstitial and alveolar edema, reflecting progressively more severe disturbance

with higher left atrial pressure. Persisting pulmonary edema or a large heart is a bad prognostic feature.

In the convalescent phase a number of features may be seen. Ill-defined basal shadows beginning within a day or two of infarction and developing into broad basal line shadows are probably areas of collapse due to diaphragmatic splinting from pain (Fig. 23.32).

Dressler's Syndrome Dressler's syndrome of pleuritis pneumonitis and pericarditis comes on after 10 days with chest pain and fever (Fig. 23.33). Small effusions may be seen in the costophrenic angle, with ill-defined basal shadows resembling pulmonary infarcts, but the prompt response to aspirin or steroids usually makes the diagnosis obvious. Rarely a pericardial effusion may be so large as to cause tamponade. Dressler syndrome may remit and relapse.

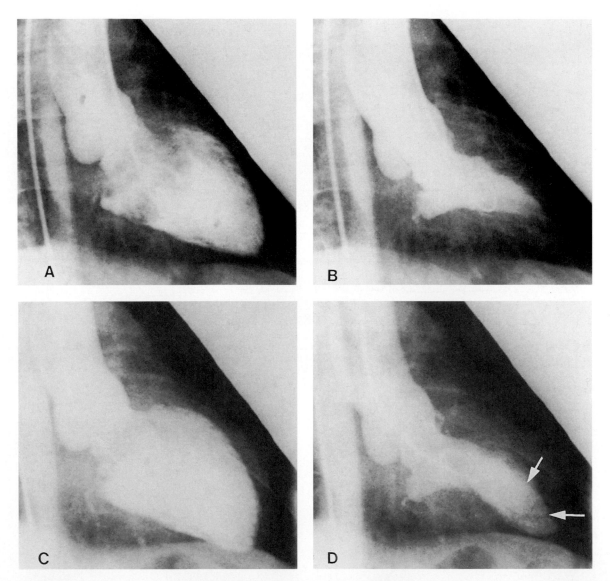

Fig. 23.30 Progression of coronary disease. Left ventriculogram (RAO views) (same patient as Fig. 23.29). **A,B** Initial study visualizes normal left ventricle, which is shaped like an upside-down carrot (with the aortic and mitral valves in its base) and contracts concentrically. **C;D**. Seven months later, following anterior infarction and occlusion of the left anterior descending coronary branch (see Figs 23.29C and 3.31). The left ventriculogram shows localized abnormality of wall movement in the anteroapical wall of the heart (arrows).

With recovery, departmental films may be taken. *Coronary calcification* may be identified by its parallel line appearance, usually best seen in the lateral view, in the position of the anterior descending or right coronary artery. It is much better seen at image amplification television fluoroscopy. Calcification may also be seen in old infarcts as a curvilinear density in the position of the wall of the left ventricle. Multiple infarctions produce congestive failure, 'ischemic cardiomyopathy'. The heart is large with a left ventricular configuration, though all chambers are involved to some extent. Pulmonary edema may be seen in untreated cases.

Ventricular Aneurysm This aneurysm may develop about 2 months after a large infarction. Patients may present with congestive cardiac failure, angina, arrythmias, or may be asymptomatic. A variety of appearances may be seen, varying from an apparently normal heart shadow (rarely) through to left ventricular enlargement, and to a localized bulge of the apex of the heart (Fig. 23.34). The lungs will reflect the effects of treatment on the hemodynamic disturbance. In some cases, curvilinear mural calcification may be seen, which always suggests an aneurysm and one of longstanding (Fig. 23.35). The diagnosis may be confirmed by *isotope ventriculography*, either first-pass or multiple-gated studies, 2DE, which also shows thrombus (Fig. 23.36), or *CT scanning*, which demonstrates the aneurysm and may also show intraventricular clot. *Left ventriculography* and *coronary arteriography* are usually performed preoperatively.

Perforation of the Ventricular Septum Perforation of the ventricular septum following anterior myocardial infarction is marked by clinical deterioration and the development of a systolic murmur. The heart is usually large, and the lungs show gross

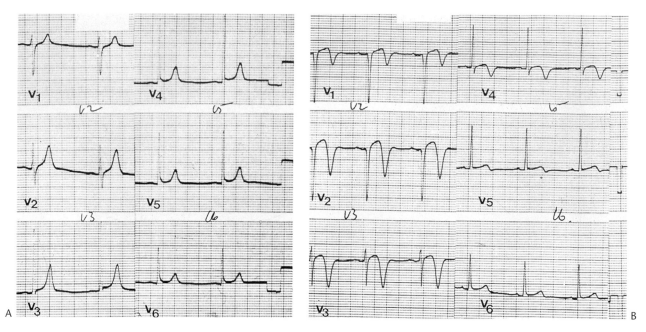

Fig. 23.31 Electrocardiographic tracings corresponding to Figs 23.29 and 23.30. **A**. Normal ECG obtained at the time of the initial angiographic assessment (precordial leads V1–V6). **B**. The ECG shows an evolving anterior infarction following occlusion of the left anterior descending vessel (see Fig. 23.29C).

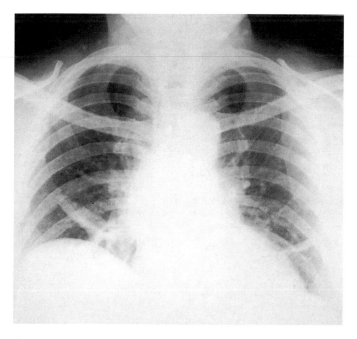

Fig. 23.32 Myocardial infarction. The chest X-ray demonstrates broad basal line shadows, probably areas of collapse due to diaphragmatic splinting from pain.

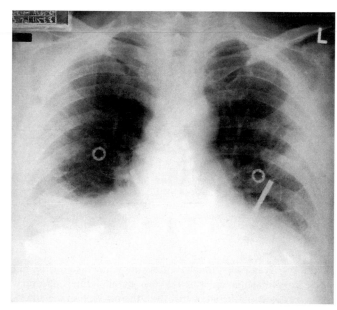

Fig. 23.33 Postmyocardial infarction (Dressler) syndrome. Small effusions are seen in both costophrenic angles, together with ill-defined basal shadows resembling pulmonary infarcts.

pulmonary edema. Echocardiography shows not only the large and dyskinetic left ventricle but usually reveals the site of the perforation (Fig. 23.37). The abnormal jet can be visualized by Doppler color flow mapping, and this technique will also differentiate septal perforation from the clinically similar postinfarction mitral regurgitation.

Left ventriculography and coronary arteriography are usually

attempted preoperatively if the patient's clinical condition permits. Pulmonary plethora may be seen in those few patients who survive long enough to develop it.

Postinfarction Mitral Incompetence   This may be trivial if there is slight ischemia of the papillary muscle, or catastrophic if the papillary muscle necroses and ruptures. This event is marked

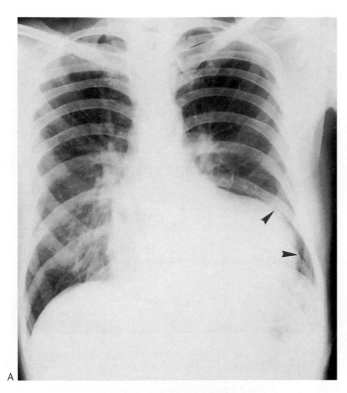

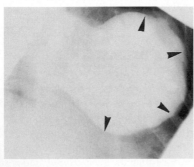

Fig. 23.34 Ventricular aneurysm. **A**. The chest radiograph shows an enlarged heart with a localized bulge. **B**. The aneurysm is clearly defined in the left ventriculogram, which visualizes a large anteroapical dyskinetic area (arrows).

by sudden clinical deterioration and the development of a systolic murmur. The heart may be moderately enlarged, but left atrial enlargement is not seen. There is usually gross pulmonary edema. 2DE may demonstrate the size and function of the left ventricle in the presence of a flail mitral leaflet. The mitral regurgitation is visualized by Doppler color flow mapping. Coronary angiography is usually performed preoperatively.

CORONARY ARTERY SURGERY

The standard surgical procedure for the treatment of ischemic heart disease is saphenous vein aortocoronary bypass graft. The vein is attached end to side to the ascending aorta above, and end to side to the coronary artery below, beyond the obstruction. Distal variations are used with Y-grafts or jump grafts.

The indication for surgery, and hence the indications for preoperative coronary arteriography, are:

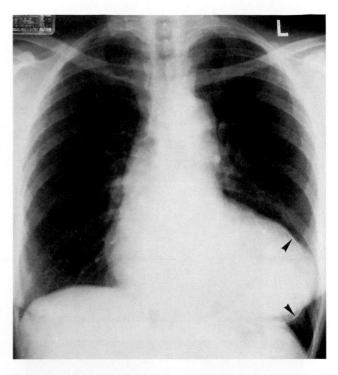

Fig. 23.35 Ventricular aneurysm. Cardiac enlargement and apical calcification (arrows) in a patient with a longstanding left ventricular aneurysm.

1. Angina unresponsive to medical treatment
2. Postinfarction ischemia, either anginal, or on exercise testing
3. Mechanical complications
4. Before valve surgery in patients with chest pain or aged over 50 years.

Coronary arteriography is also used postoperatively to study the state of the grafts and the state of the native coronary circulation, in cases where angina recurs. Blocked grafts, strictured grafts and progress in the disease of the native circulation are all causes of unsuccessful relief of ischemia.

NON-SURGICAL INTERVENTIONS

Percutaneous Transluminal Coronary Angioplasty This technique is a significant advance in the management of coronary artery disease. It consists of using a large-diameter guide catheter to introduce a small balloon dilatation catheter into the coronary artery and through the stricture to dilate it (Fig. 23.38). The main indications for the procedure should be similar to those for coronary bypass surgery, as this may be needed to manage the complications. Severe single-vessel non-occlusive strictures remain the classical indication for the procedure, and respond well with a high success rate (>90%) initially and a low complication rate (3% emergency surgery). About one-third of strictures will recur and can be redilated. The indications are currently more relaxed, with multivessel disease being attempted, and in certain situations one vessel will be dilated, that causing the symptoms, the so-called culprit lesion, in the presence of other blocked vessels, though this is obviously more hazardous. Acute complications of coronary angioplasty, complex lesions, and

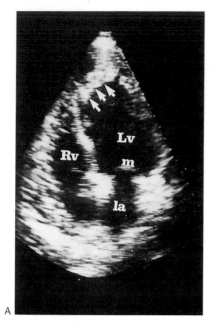

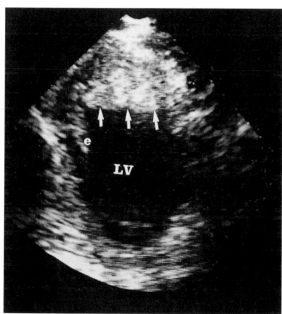

Fig. 23.36 Ventricular aneurysm. The 2DE study (apical and short-axis views) visualizes an anteroapical thinned-out aneurysmal area with mural thrombus (arrows). e, endocardium; lettering as in Fig. 20.16.

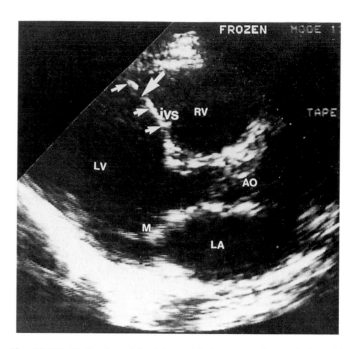

Fig. 23.37 Perforation of the interventricular septum in association with anterior myocardial infarction. The 2DE study reveals an anteroseptal (ivs) thinned-out segment corresponding to the infarction (small arrows) and reveals the site of the perforation (long arrow). Other lettering as in Fig. 20.16.

HEART MUSCLE DISEASE

When heart failure occurs without recognizable mechanical cause the fault is presumed to be in the heart muscle itself. Heart muscle disease occurring in recognized association is so described, e.g. alcoholic heart disease. When there is no recognizable cause the condition is termed cardiomyopathy. Three varieties are recognized, *congestive* (dilated), *hypertrophic* and *restrictive*.

CONGESTIVE (DILATED) CARDIOMYOPATHY

The hallmark of this condition is dilatation of the left ventricle with impairment of emptying, i.e. a reduction in the ejection fraction. Asymptomatic dilatation may be present for years, symptoms only developing when congestive cardiac failure supervenes.

Presentation may be with congestive cardiac failure often manifesting as an attack of bronchitis, as an arrythmia or rarely with chest pain or even embolism from clot in the left ventricle. The clinical findings of a third sound gallop and an abnormal ECG indicate left ventricular disease.

The usual differential diagnosis is from other forms of congestive cardiac failure, particularly ischemic heart disease, left ventricular aneurysm, silent aortic stenosis or even silent mitral stenosis. Ventricular dilatation may be associated with slight mitral regurgitation and a systolic murmur, and occasionally it may be difficult to distinguish between congestive cardiomyopathy with some mitral regurgitation and mitral regurgitation leading to severe cardiac failure.

Radiographic Appearances The *plain film* almost always shows cardiac enlargement, which may be purely left ventricular

recurrent strictures may now be managed by intracoronary stenting (Fig. 23.39)

Thrombolytic Therapy   A great deal of research has demonstrated that the immediate exhibition of thrombolytic therapy in acute myocardial infarction (preferably in under 4 h) will result in lysis of the causative thrombus in about 60% or more of blocked arteries. The effect of this is to limit the extent of infarction, improve ventricular function long term, and lower mortality compared to controls. Thus, in the absence of contraindications, and if the infarction is taken early enough, intravenous thrombolytic therapy is the treatment of choice.

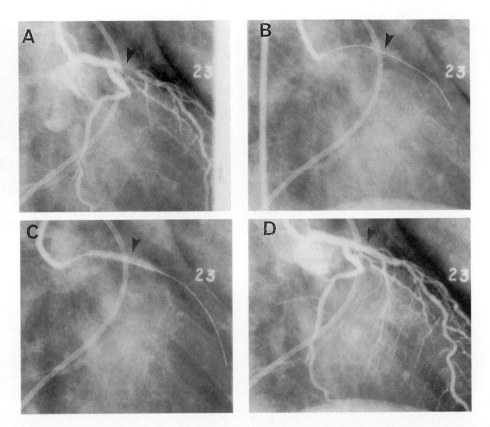

Fig. 23.38 Percutaneous transluminal coronary angioplasty. **A**. The guide catheter has been engaged in the left coronary ostium and a preprocedure angiogram serves to demonstrate a severe proximal stenosis of the anterior descending coronary artery (arrow). **B**. The steerable guide-wire has been passed through the guide catheter into the left coronary artery. It has entered the anterior descending coronary artery and crossed the stenosis (arrow). **C**. The balloon catheter has been passed over the guide-wire and into the stenosis, and inflated (arrow). The two studs indicate the position of the balloon before inflation. **D**. After the balloon catheter and wire have been removed, a postprocedure angiogram shows that the stenosis has been almost entirely relieved (arrow).

(Fig. 23.40), or the heart may be globular in shape if all chambers are involved. Very rarely, left ventricular enlargement may only be seen in the lateral view. The lungs will show evidence of raised left atrial pressure in the untreated patient. Patients usually respond to treatment with considerable clinical improvement, a reduction in heart size (rarely to normal) and the clearing of the lungs. Relapse, however, is usual, and response to treatment less satisfactory with each relapse.

Myocardial perfusion imaging is used to assess viability and to exclude 'hibernating myocardium' (see Ch. 20). Isotope ventriculography usually demonstrates the dilated and poorly but concentrically contracting left ventricle. It will also exclude the surgically treatable possibility of left ventricular aneurysm.

2DE (Fig. 23.41) will demonstrate the large and overall poorly contracting left ventricle and exclude silent aortic and mitral stenosis.

Cardiac catheterization and angiocardiography are only indicated when the diagnosis is still in doubt. The dilated, poorly but concentrically contracting cavity of the left ventricle is usually obvious (Fig. 23.42); mitral and aortic stenosis and left ventricular aneurysm can all be excluded. In those cases complicated by mitral regurgitation the severity of this may be assessed, and taken together with the degree of impairment of left ventricular contraction it is usually possible to distinguish between congestive cardiomyopathy and mitral regurgitation. The coronary arteries may also be studied at the same time.

HYPERTROPHIC CARDIOMYOPATHY

In this condition there is inappropriate hypertrophy of the myocardium occurring in the absence of any recognized stimulus. The hypertrophy is usually asymmetrical, and often concentrated in the upper septum, though all types of distribution of hypertrophy may be seen. The excessive muscle apparently contracts well.

The condition may present as sudden death; with shortness of breath due to difficulty in filling the hypertrophied stiff left ventricle; with angina; or with arrythmias. The pulse is characteristically jerky, and the apex beat left-ventricular with an atrial beat. Auscultation reveals a late systolic murmur and a fourth heart sound. The ECG usually shows gross left ventricular hypertrophy.

The *plain film* findings range from an apparently normal heart through a heart showing obvious left ventricular hypertrophy, often with a rather chunky outline to it (Fig. 23.43), to a globular heart with all chambers being involved. Evidence of raised left atrial pressure may be seen in the lungs.

The differential diagnosis usually lies between ischemic heart disease, fixed aortic stenosis, non-rheumatic mitral regurgitation and hypertrophic cardiomyopathy.

Cardiac Ultrasound 2DE will provide diagnostic information by visualizing the localized 'asymmetric' or generalized septal

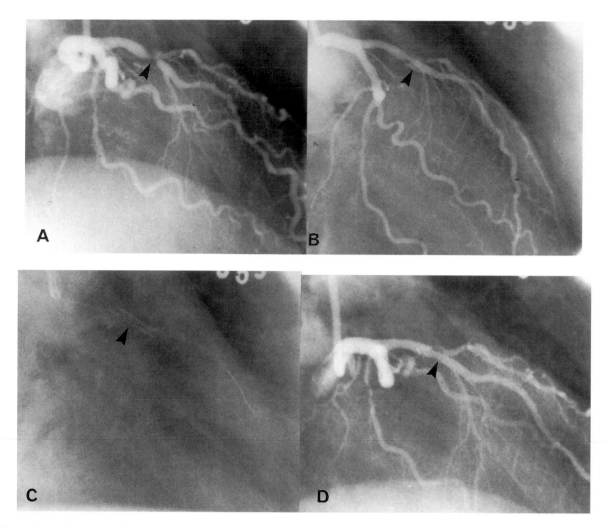

Fig. 23.39   **A**. Control angiogram showing the severe stricture of the anterior descending coronary artery (arrow). **B**. After balloon angioplasty, a large intimal flap (arrow) is visible. **C**. Insertion of a metallic stent (arrow). **D**. Final angiogram showing the good lumen after stenting. No intimal flap is now visible.

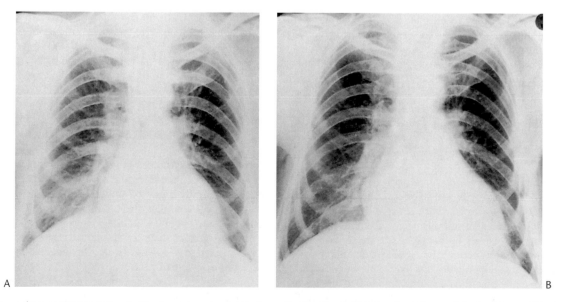

Fig. 23.40   Congestive cardiomyopathy. **A**. The heart is only slightly large. **B**. Significant dilatation involving mainly the left ventricle has developed 16 months later.

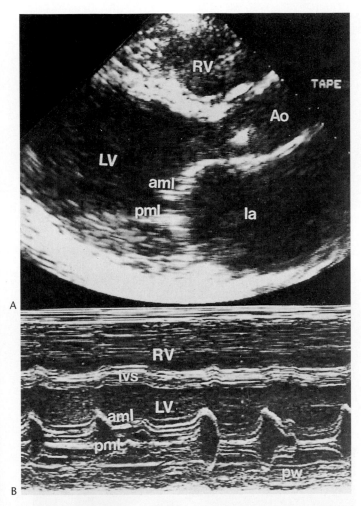

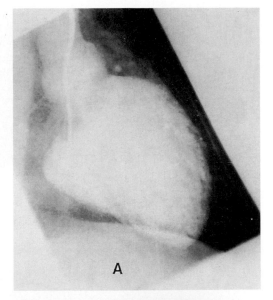

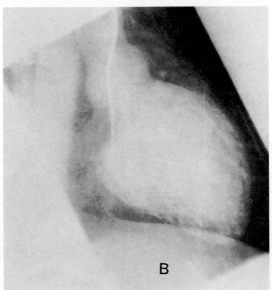

Fig. 23.41 Congestive cardiomyopathy. 2DE demonstrates a large left ventricular cavity with poor wall movement, together with limited opening of the mitral valve leaflets (aml, pml) due to the low cardiac output. Other lettering as in Fig. 20.16.

Fig. 23.42 Congestive cardiomyopathy. Left ventricular cine angiogram (RAO view) corresponding to Fig. 23.40B. Diastolic **A** and systolic **B** frames demonstrate a large ventricular cavity with generalized reduction in wall motion.

hypertrophy, the obstruction to the left ventricular outflow, the small left ventricular cavity and abnormal mitral valve movements (Fig. 23.44). A Doppler study will estimate outflow tract gradient.

Cardiac Catheterization This may reveal a high filling pressure and a variable intracavity gradient which may be provoked by postectopic beats. Angiocardiography reveals a range of abnormalities from a left ventricular one indistinguishable from normal to one which is of normal size but empties excessively and with prominent papillary muscles and septum (Fig. 23.45), through to the grossly distorted ventricle almost resembling a myocardial tumor.

RESTRICTIVE CARDIOMYOPATHY

Mild forms of this may be encountered in patients being investigated for non-specific chest pain and found to have a high end-diastolic filling pressure in the left ventricle with no other abnormality.

The most florid example is seen in the condition of *endomyo-cardial fibrosis*, which is usually identified in Africans, but is seen sporadically in Europeans under the name of *Leoffler's endocarditis*. The pathological process is the laying down of fibrous tissue on the inner aspects of the ventricles beginning at the apices and spreading to involve the inlet valves.

On the left side this leads to difficulty in filling the ventricle (but not of contraction or emptying) and mitral incompetence. On the right side there is a high filling pressure in the right ventricle and tricuspid incompetence, and there may be a pericardial effusion. In left-sided involvement the heart tends to be normal in size unless mitral regurgitation is severe. With right-sided involvement the heart shadow is large and globular.

Cardiac ultrasound will show a small heart with good systolic

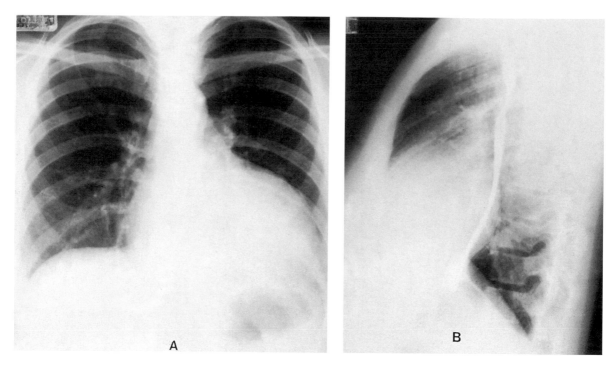

Fig. 23.43 Hypertrophic cardiomyopathy. **A**. Frontal film. The heart shadow is markedly enlarged with an elongation of its axis to the left and rounding of the apex but with a rather bulky and irregular outline. **B** Lateral film. The enlarged left ventricle bulges back beyond the line of the barium-filled esophagus. In this patient the cavity of the ventricle (see Fig. 23.45) is normal in size, and the bulk of the heart shadow is due to an enormous increase in thickness of the wall of the heart.

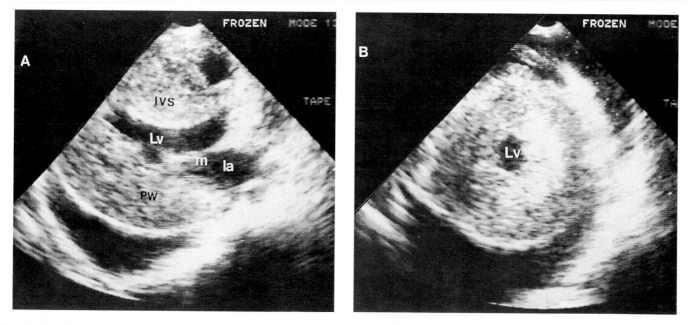

Fig. 23.44 Hypertrophic cardiomyopathy. 2DE visualizes the massive septal and posterior wall hypertrophy, almost obliterating the ventricular cavity. **A**. Long-axis view. **B**. Short-axis view. Lettering as in Fig. 20.16.

function and rapid early diastolic filling, and impaired compliance is seen using Doppler techniques.

Findings of *angiocardiography* are characteristic, with amputation and smoothing off of the apices of the ventricles and atrioventricular valvar regurgitation.

SPECIFIC HEART MUSCLE DISEASE

Abnormalities of heart muscle leading to a clinical syndrome similar to that of congestive cardiomyopthy may occur in a large variety of conditions.

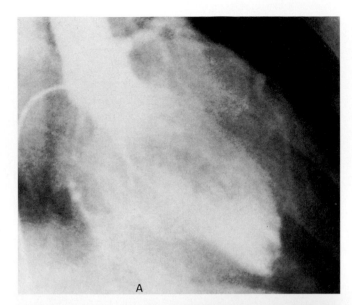

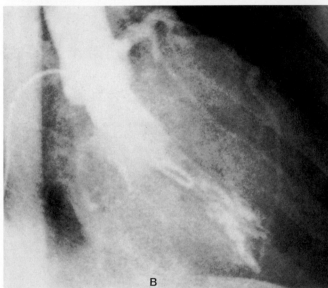

Fig. 23.45 Hypertrophic cardiomyopathy. Left ventricular cine angiogram (RAO views). **A.** Diastolic frame. **B.** Systolic frame. Note the systolic obliteration of the ventricular cavity which results from the massive muscle hypertrophy.

Infections and Collagen Disorders

Viral Myocarditis This may be suggested when congestive cardiac failure occurs in relation to an obvious viral pyrexia (usually coxsackie virus), particularly when there is a high, rising, antibody titre. However, cardiomyopathy may apparently begin with an influenza-like illness, or myocarditis may have no antecedent pyrexia. Endocardial biopsy, showing inflammatory cells eroding myocardial fibers, is the most satisfactory diagnostic tool, and may indicate appropriate treatment.

Bacterial Myocarditis A toxic myocarditis may occur with severe bacterial infections, and is a well-known complication of the exotoxin of diphtheria. Myocarditis may also occur in the course of bacterial endocarditis.

Parasites *Chagas's disease* due to infection by *Trypanosoma cruzi*, leads to a patchy fibrotic destruction of the myocardium causing left ventricular failure after a long latent period. The esophagus may be involved, producing appearances similar to those of achalasia. The disease is confined to Latin America.

Collagen Diseases Collagen diseases including rheumatic fever may involve the heart in their acute phase, leading to arrythmias or congestive cardiac failure. Systemic lupus erythematosus usually produces a pericardial (and pleural) effusion. It may also produce sterile vegetations (Libman–Sacks) on the mitral and aortic valves.

Myocardial Infiltrations

Hemochromatosis The deposition of iron in heart in this condition leads to congestive cardiac failure, and is the cause of death of about one-third of patients.

Sarcoidosis Involvement of the heart by sarcoidosis is rare, but may precede the appearance of sarcoidosis elsewhere in the body by several years. The usual manifestation is an arrythmia, but congestive cardiac failure may occur and rarely there may be mitral incompetence from papillary muscle involvement.

Amyloid Heart Disease Amyloid may involve the heart alone or as part of a generalized disorder. There is severe cardiac failure, with low cardiac output and a low-volume pulse. The patient is often murmur-free. Cardiac ultrasound shows a myocardium that looks like 'ground glass' and moderate impairment of systolic function.

Glycogen Storage Disease This condition usually presents in the neonatal period with characteristic muscle weakness, but rarely the heart failure may appear first. The condition may be suspected by echocardiography or left ventriculography, which shows a moderate cavity dilatation associated with gross wall thickening.

Metabolic Disorders

Thyroid Disease Both forms of thyroid disease may lead to cardiac abnormalities. Myxedema usually produces a pericardial effusion, but there may be involvement of the heart muscle with cardiac dilatation. Thyrotoxicosis usually produces atrial fibrillation and should be suspected when this condition develops in the absence of mitral valve disease. Cardiac dilatation may also occur if thyrotoxicosis leads to high-output cardiac failure.

Acromegaly There is generally held to be a specific dilated cardiomyopathy in association with acromegaly, but there is also a very high instance of hypertension and coronary artery disease.

Beriberi This condition, due to a deficiency of thiamine, leads to a high-output, or much more rarely a low-output, cardiac failure. It usually responds to thiamine.

Drugs and Poisons

Alcoholic Heart Disease Alcoholic heart disease may be manifest by arrythmias or overt congestive cardiac failure. A history of excessive intake of alcohol, and improvement when alcohol is forsaken, suggest the specific diagnosis.

Drugs β-blocking drugs in large doses may lead to cardiac dilatation or overt cardiac failure. It is not clear whether this only occurs in the presence of heart disease or could occur in a normal heart. The anthracycline antimitotic agents may lead to irreversible congestive cardiac failure. The effect is critically dose related.

Other Conditions

Congestive cardiomyopathy may develop in a variety of heredo-familial neuromuscular disorders and may be the cause of death. Congestive cardiomyopathy may also develop after pregnancy (*postpartum cardiomyopathy*). It usually responds to treatment but may relapse with subsequent pregnancies.

MISCELLANEOUS CONDITIONS

TUMORS OF THE HEART

Secondary Tumors   Commonly originating from breast or bronchus, these tumors are much commoner than primary tumors. They are often silent and only recognized at necropsy. Involvement of the pericardium leading to pericardial effusion and tamponade is much commoner. Cardiac ultrasound may show tumor embolization in the right heart.

Primary Tumors   Primary tumors of the heart are rare, and the majority are benign, consisting mainly of *myxomas* (50%), rhabdomyomas and fibromas. The clinical manifestations often depend on the site of origin. Intracavity tumors are often pedunculated and cause obstruction whereas intramural tumors may infiltrate, leading to arrythmias or cardiac failure.

MYXOMAS

The vast majority of these occur in the left atrium, orginating from a pedicle attached to the left side of the interatrial septum. Three groups of symptoms may occur:

1. *Obstructive.* Presentation is with shortness of breath. Examination reveals the physical signs of mitral valve disease, though with normal rhythm. The physical signs may vary from day to day or with the position of the patient.

2. *Embolic.* Parts of the tumor may embolize, producing stroke or limb ischemia. On occasion the first diagnosis of myxoma has been histologic examination of an embolectomy specimen.

3. *Systemic.* Fever, anemia, a raised erythrocyte sedimentation rate, and sometimes finger clubbing may suggest the possibility of infective endocarditis, though blood cultures are sterile and splenomegaly does not occur.

Radiographic Appearances   The plain film appearances may vary from a normal chest X-ray to an enlarged heart with selective left atrial enlargement, and the left atrial appendage may also be enlarged (Fig. 23.46). If obstruction is severe, upper-lobe blood diversion or pulmonary edema may be seen. Very rarely, myxomas may be calcified, and such calcification may be visible moving up and down in the atrium at fluoroscopy.

Cardiac Ultrasound   Correctly performed, 2DE should invariably identify the tumor in the left atrium (the commonest site) (Fig. 23.47) or anywhere else in the heart. The mobility of the pedunculated tumor descending into the mitral valve in ventricular diastole is very typical. In cases where the echo window is

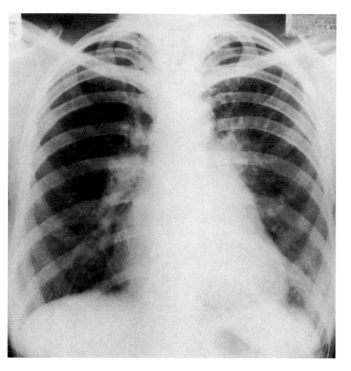

Fig. 23.46   Left atrial myxoma. The chest X-ray shows selective enlargement of the left atrium; the left atrial appendage is also enlarged.

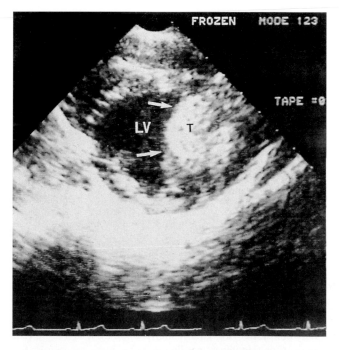

Fig. 23.47   Myocardial tumor. The 2DE image (short-axis view) demonstrates the presence of an intracavitary echo-dense mass (T) (arrows). LV, left ventricle.

poor, the *transesophageal echocardiogram* will almost invariably be diagnostically decisive.

Both *CT scanning* and *MRI* have been used to visualize myxomas and other cardiac tumors. With the introduction of the

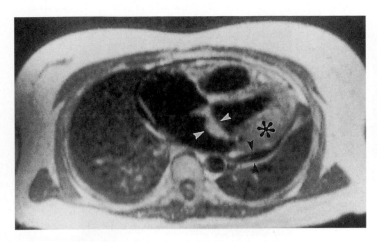

Fig. 23.48 Myocardial tumor. Spin echo MRI scan shows the expansion of the free wall of the left ventricle by a tumor (asterisk) and its spread onto the mitral valve, which is seen to be grossly thickened (white arrows). The tricuspid valve is seen at this level to be of normal thickness. There is a small pericardial effusion (black arrows).

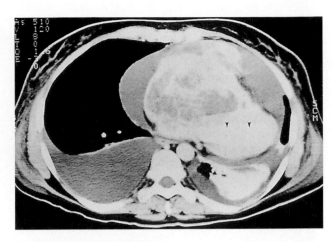

Fig. 23.49 Malignant angiosarcoma—CT scan with contrast. The tumor mass appears as an irregular filling defect in the right atrium and ventricle. The left ventricle is displaced posteriorly (arrows). A large pericardial effusion surrounds the heart.

transesophageal echogram, they have little role in diagnosis, but may be able to elucidate the extent of tumors (Figs 23.48 and 23.49).

Cardiac catheterization and angiocardiography are no longer indicated with adequately performed echocardiography. Occasionally, cavity opacification may be required to determine the extent of a tumor, and coronary angiography may be valuable, not only in demonstrating the coronary anatomy prior to surgery, but also in showing a pathological circulation which is not an infrequent feature of myxomas but is also seen in left atrial thrombus in longstanding rheumatic mitral disease, and also in malignant cardiac tumors.

TRAUMA TO THE HEART

Trauma to the heart may be either penetrating or blunt.

Penetrating Injuries These usually lead to hemopericardium and tamponade, and require emergency drainage and possibly open surgery. Penetrating wounds may also damage the coronary arteries, producing myocardial infarction or disrupt the valves of the heart.

Blunt Trauma These may lead to myocardial contusion, producing a similar clinical finding to myocardial infarction. The coronary arteries may be injured, leading to the syndrome of myocardial infarction. The valves may be disrupted, producing incompetence.

False Aneurysm This may result from trauma to the heart. They are characterized by an unusual origin from the left ventricle and a narrow neck. They require surgery as they may rupture.

ENDOCARDITIS

Bacterial (or rickettsial) infections may settle on abnormal valves on either side of the heart, or in congenital heart lesions such as the right ventricle opposite a ventricular septal defect; or on a patent ductus arteriosus. The resultant infection produces a protracted and, unless treated, fatal febrile illness.

Vegetations are best assessed by 2DE, where they appear as rapidly oscillating masses that are either attached to or replace normal valve tissue. These masses can be localized to the individual leaflet, and the size and mobility of the lesion readily assessed.

An extremely small vegetation may be missed by 2DE; improper gain settings may result in a false-positive diagnosis. Furthermore, severely fibrotic, calcified or redundant valves may be incorrectly diagnosed as bacterial vegetation, and many patients have normal echocardiograms in the presence of confined infective endocarditis. The presence of a visible mass in the clinical setting of infective endocarditis does not always require surgical intervention; approximately 50% of the patients with this situation have been successfully treated medically.

Excavating *abscesses* may be identified by angiography or by 2DE on transesophageal echocardiography.

MRI OF ACQUIRED HEART DISEASE
Jeremy P. R. Jenkins

Valvular Heart Disease

Accurate measurement of left and right ventricular stroke volumes using spin echo images allows small discrepancies to be highlighted. In the absence of a shunt this indicates a regurgitant fraction. In the presence of dysfunction of two or more valves, gradient echo imaging can be used (see Ch. 20). The area of signal loss in the high-signal blood pool proximal to an abnormal valve relates to the degree of regurgitation (Fig. 23.50). The severity of valvular stenosis can also be assessed by the length of signal loss distal to the valve (Fig. 23.51). Good concordance has been observed between this signal loss and pressure gradients measured at angiography or by Doppler ultrasound. Aortic sclerosis, with thickened and abnormal aortic valve leaflets on 2DE but no pressure gradient at angiography, produces loss of signal distal to the valve (using TE values of 22–28 ms) but to a

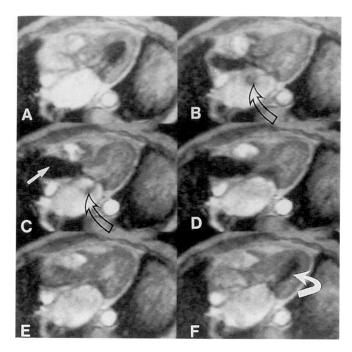

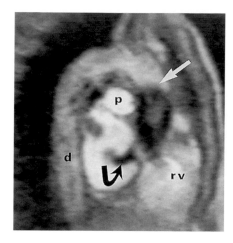

Fig. 23.52 Aortic sclerosis (no pressure gradient across the valve) on an oblique gated gradient echo image (T_E 22 ms) through the aortic arch at peak systole, where the signal loss (maximum length 5 cm) distal to the aortic valve is confined to the ascending aorta (straight arrow). Note the coincidental mitral regurgitation (curved arrow). Key as in Fig. 23.51.

Fig. 23.50 Aortic and mitral stenosis and mitral regurgitation demonstrated on six oblique gated images in the cardiac long-axis plane using the gradient echo sequence (T_E 26 ms) with timings at 100 ms intervals from **A** 30 ms to **F** 530 ms after the R-wave of the ECG. Straight arrow, signal loss distal to the aortic valve in systole from aortic stenosis; curved open arrows, signal loss proximal to the mitral valve in systole from mitral regurgitation; curved solid arrow in F, signal loss distal to the mitral valve in diastole due to mitral stenosis. (Reproduced with permission from Mitchell et al 1989.)

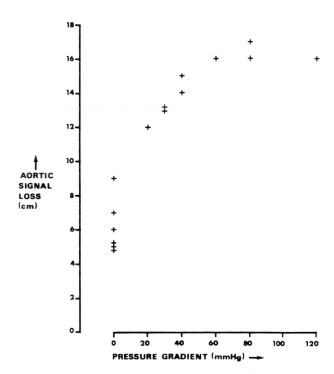

Fig. 23.53 Graph of peak aortic valve pressure gradient against maximum length of signal loss distal to the valve on gradient echo imaging. (Reproduced with permission from Mitchell et al 1989.)

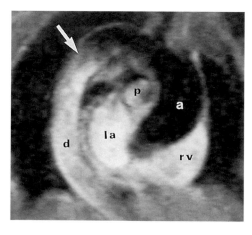

Fig. 23.51 Arotic stenosis on an oblique gated echo image (T_E 22 ms) through the aortic arch during peak systole. Note signal loss, with a maximum measured length of 16 cm, extending to the descending aorta (arrowed), due to turbulent flow distal to the stenosed aortic valve (on cardiac catheterization the pressure gradient across the valve was 80 mmHg). a, ascending aorta; d, descending aorta; la, left atrium; p, pulmonary artery; rv, right ventricle.

lesser degree than with stenosis of the valve (Fig. 23.52). The length of signal loss, which does not reach the aortic arch in sclerosis, allows differentiation between the two conditions (Fig. 23.53). By using shorter TE values the signal can be reclaimed in the area of disturbed flow, allowing peak blood flow velocity measurements to be made (Fig. 23.54). A pressure gradient can then be calculated by the modified Bernoulli equation (viz $G = 4v^2$, where G is the pressure gradient in millimeters of mercury and v is the peak velocity through stenosis in meters per second) as used in Doppler ultrasound.

It is important that the normal appearances on gradient echo imaging where partial signal losses can be observed adjacent to valves in different phases of the cardiac cycle be appreciated and not mistaken for valvular dysfunction (see Fig. 23.56).

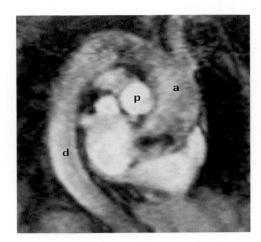

Fig. 23.54 Aortic stenosis on an oblique gated gradient echo (T_E 12 ms) image through the aorta at peak systole. Note reclamation of signal in the aorta using the shorter echo time which can allow direct measurement of flow velocity. (Same patient as in Fig. 23.51.)

Ischemic Heart Disease

Several reports, using both animal and human data, have shown that MRI is accurate in the estimation of acute myocardial infarct size. On T_2-weighted spin echo images a high signal is produced from the infarcted myocardium. This area is less well visualized as a low signal on T_1-weighted scans but shows marked enhancement following intravenous gadolinium–diethyltriammine pentaacetic acid (gadolinium–DTPA) with improved conspicuity as compared with T_2-weighted spin echo imaging (Fig. 23.55). Unenhanced T_1-weighted spin echo scans are, however, useful in demonstrating wall thinning and other complications of infarction, including left ventricular aneurysm, pericardial effusion, cardiac chamber enlargement and septal rupture producing a ventricular septal defect. The accuracy in the detection of myocardial infarction on MRI was 87%, using the criteria of abnormal high signal and reduced wall thickening. In acute infarction, some reduction in systolic wall thickening can usually be demonstrated on MRI within 24 h of the onset of chest pain. No differences in signal intensity have been found between reperfused and non-perfused infarcted myocardium. There is conflicting evidence as to whether the contrast agent gadolinium–DTPA can aid in this separation.

Gradient echo imaging allows dynamic scanning with qualitative and quantitative assessment of ventricular function, including an accurate measure of myocardial mass, together with evaluation of the end-diastolic and end-systolic wall thickness (Fig. 23.56). The distinction between flowing blood and thrombus is more consistently demonstrated using gradient echo images than on conventional ventional spin echo scans. On gradient echo imaging there is a high contrast between the high signal from flowing blood and the low signal from thrombus (Fig. 23.57). In addition, the cine-loop display improves identification of the dyskinetic segment of the infarcted segment. Viable myocardium can be distinguished from scar or chronic infarction by assessment of systolic wall thickening. The former shows some thickening of the myocardium in systole, whereas the latter can be identified as an area of absent systolic thickening and diastolic wall thinning.

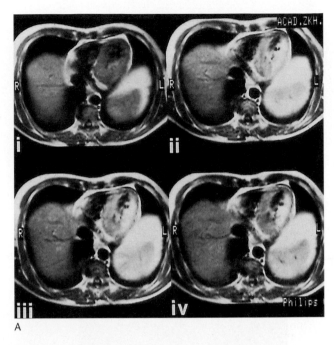

A

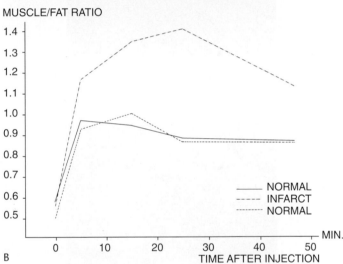

B

Fig. 23.55 **A**. Acute myocardial infarction of 7 days duration on transverse gated T_1-weighted images (i) before and (ii–iv) after gadolinium–DTPA. (ii) was performed immediately postinjection, (iii) 10 min and (iv) 20 min later. The posterolateral wall infarct shows marked enhancement and is clearly delineated. Note the lesser degree of enhancement of the normal myocardium in the early postcontrast phase. **B**. Graph of signal intensity versus time in the same patient, demonstrating maximal contrast between the infarcted region and two areas of normal myocardium approximately 20–30 min after gadolinium–DTPA administration. (Reproduced with permission from de Roos et al 1988; prints kindly supplied by Dr A. de Roos.)

In the evaluation of coronary artery bypass grafts, the accuracy in the detection of graft patency is 90% using the spin echo technique. The grafts appear as small areas of signal voids due to flowing blood, with errors in diagnosis due to surgical clips in situ and small size of grafts (Fig. 23.58). A disadvantage of the spin echo technique is that the presence of a signal void infers patency, indicating some, but not necessarily effective, blood flow down the graft. Gradient echo imaging not only enables graft

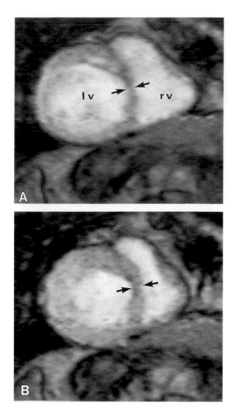

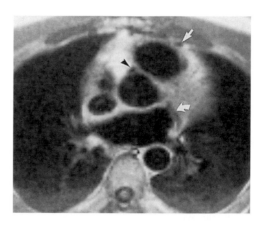

Fig. 23.58 Patent left anterior descending coronary artery bypass graft (straight arrow) is demonstrated on a transverse gated spin echo image (TE 26 ms). The native right coronary (arrowhead) and left circumflex (curved arrow) arteries are also visualized. (Reproduced with permission from Jenkins et al 1988.)

Fig. 23.56 Chronic myocardial infarction producing marked septal wall thinning (arrowed) on two gated short-axis gradient echo images (TE 26 ms) **A**. End-diastole. **B**. End systole. lv, left ventricle; rv, right ventricle.

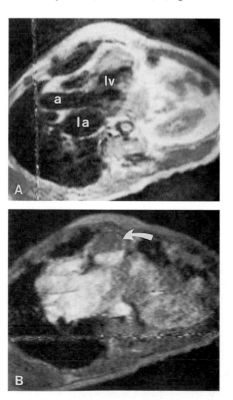

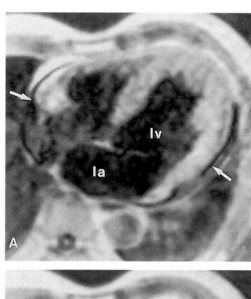

Fig. 23.57 Thrombus (arrowed) in a left ventricular aneurysm on two gated long-axis scans. **A**. Spin echo (TE 26 ms). **B**. Gradient echo (TE 28 ms). Key as in Fig. 23.51.

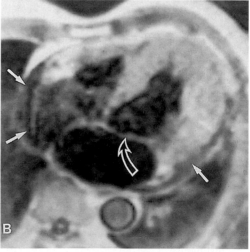

Fig. 23.59 Hypertrophic cardiomyopathy on transverse gated spin echo images (TE 40 ms). **A**. End-diastole. **B**. End-systole. The myocardium is markedly thickened, with an associated pericardial effusion (straight arrows). Key as in Fig. 23.51. (Adapted with permission from Jenkins & Isherwood 1987.)

patency to be more accurately detected but is also able to measure the flow velocity through the graft.

Heart Muscle Disease

Cardiomyopathies   Whilst MRI can clearly demonstrate ventricular hypertrophy and wall thickness, it is unlikely to replace 2DE in the routine evaluation of these changes. A clear distinction between the hypertrophic and congestive groups of cardiac muscle disease can be observed with MRI, with delineation of the extent and distribution of muscle involvement (Fig. 23.59). In the unusual form of apical hypertrophic cardiomyopathy, MRI is useful in showing the extent of involvement. Gradient echo imaging can be used to evaluate the functional consequences of hypertrophic cardiomyopathy as well as defining any associated myocardial ischemia.

Cardiac Sarcoidosis.   MRI appears to be the most sensitive imaging technique in the detection of cardiac involvement by sarcoidosis. Infiltration of the left ventricular myocardium and interventricular septum can be demonstrated as patchy high signals on T_2-weighted spin echo images, allowing correct localization for myocardial biopsy and histological confirmation.

Amyloid Infiltration.   In amyloid heart disease, MRI has demonstrated a thickened atrial septum and myocardium with reduced wall thickening during systole.

Cardiac Transplant.   MRI is of limited value in the detection of acute and chronic cardiac transplant rejection, based on currently used tissue characterization parameters including intravenous gadolinium–chelate. Acute rejection induces an increase in the myocardial wall thickness, predominately of the left ventricle. Myocardial wall thickening, best evaluated by gradient echo imaging, could in principle be used to detect rejection. This parameter, however, is more readily and repeatably assessed on 2DE.

Cardiac Masses

Whilst 2DE is the mainstay technique used in the diagnosis of left ventricular thrombi and other mass lesions (including right atrial myxoma), a significant number of patients cannot be adequately assessed by this method due to body habitus or proximity of the lesion to the cardiac apex. In a recent study, only 15 of 25 (60%) patients with *left ventricular thrombus* secondary to chronic anterior myocardial infarction were diagnosed correctly by 2DE—six (24%) were inadequate 2DE studies compared with none on MRI or CT. On spin echo imaging some abnormal signal, due to slow flow, can be noted in the blood pool of the ventricular chambers, mimicking thrombus formation. The introduction of gradient echo imaging has overcome this disadvantage; the blood pool is shown consistently as a high signal fluctuating with time against the constant intermediate mid-gray signal of thrombus (see Fig. 23.57). In addition, functional information can be gained in the demonstration of the dyskinetic segment adjacent to the thrombus.

MRI can distinguish some mass lesions such as lipomas and

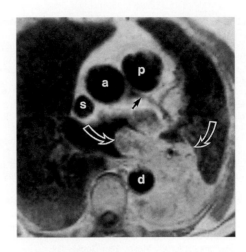

Fig. 23.60   Enhancing bronchial carcinoma (curved arrows) invading the left lower lobe bronchus, left atrium and descending aorta on a transverse gated T_1-weighted post-gadolinium–DTPA spin echo image (TE 26 ms). Note the associated lower-lobe collapse, which is difficult to differentiate from the tumor. The left coronary artery (straight arrow), with its anterior descending and circumflex branches, is shown. Key as in Fig. 23.51; s, superior vena cava.

fibromas, which give high (similar to surrounding fat) and low (due to a paucity of mobile protons) signals, respectively. Cystic lesions usually give a high signal on T_2-weighted spin echo scans, greater than those of adjacent fat. Some difficulty, however, may occasionally be encountered on MRI in differentiating between cystic and solid lesions, a distinction that can easily be made on 2DE. Lymphomas give a higher signal, and myxomas a signal similar to myocardium on spin echo imaging. Myxomas can be diagnosed by their characteristic appearance and position. The use of gadolinium–chelate enables enhancing tumor to be separated from non-enhancing thrombus (Fig. 23.60). Calcified intracardiac lesions cannot be clearly visualized and a heavily calcified mass may be missed due to the low signal obtained from such tissue. The use of gradient echo imaging can improve the sensitivity in the detection of such lesions. CT, however, is the technique of choice in the assessment of cardiac calcification. In patients suspected of having an atrial myxoma, sufficient information is usually gained on 2DE making MRI unnecessary. MRI does have a role in the further assessment of suspected intracardiac filling defects suspected on 2DE, and in clearly defining normal structures such as a prominent moderator band in the right ventricle or fat pad in the atrioventricular groove. Comparative studies of transoesophageal ultrasound and MRI in the evaluation of cardiac masses are needed.

On MRI, intra- and extracardiac masses can be directly visualized, together with their relationship to surrounding structures. Paracardiac masses are best evaluated by spin echo imaging because of its high soft-tissue contrast resolution and discrimination. MRI can complement 2DE in defining the extent of metastatic disease, with its wider topographical view more easily delineating thoracic and abdominal involvement.

REFERENCES AND SUGGESTIONS FOR FURTHER READING

Blackwell, G. G., Cranney, G. B., Pohost, G. M. (1992) *MRI: Cardiovascular System*. New York: Gower.

Boxt, L. M. (ed). (1996) Cardiac MR imaging. *Magnetic Resonance Imaging Clinics of North America*, **4**, 191–432.

de Roos, A., Matheijssen, N. A., Doornbos, J., van Dijkman, P. R. M., van Voorthuisen, A. E., van der Wall, E. E. (1990) Myocardial infarct size after reperfusion therapy: assessment with Gd-DTPA-enhanced MR imaging. *Radiology*, **176**, 517–521.

Donaldson, R. M., Raphael, M. J. (1982) Missing coronary artery. *British Heart Journal*, **42**, 62–70.

Edelman, R. R., Li, W. (1994) Contrast-enhanced echo-planar MR imaging of myocardial perfusion: preliminary study in humans. *Radiology*, **190**, 771–777.

Globits S, Higgins C. B (1996) Adult heart disease. In Edelman, R. E., Hesselink, J. R., Zlatkin, M. B. (eds) *Clinical Magnetic Resonance Imaging*, 2nd edn, ch. 54, pp. 1711–1756. Philadelphia: W.B. Saunders.

Gutierrez, F. R., Brown, J. J., Mirowitz, A. (1993) *Cardiovascular Magnetic Resonance Imaging*. St Louis: Mosby Year Book.

Hartnell, G., Cerel, A., Kamalesh, M. et al (1994) Detection of myocardial ischaemia: value of combined myocardial perfusion and cineangiographic MR imaging. *American Journal of Roentgenology*, **163**, 1061–1067.

Hurst, J. J. (1990) *The Heart*, 7th edn. New York: McGraw-Hill.

Jenkins, J. P. R., Isherwood, I. (1987) Magnetic resonance imaging of the heart: a review. In Rowlands, D.J. (ed.) *Recent Advances in Cardiology 10*, pp. 219–247. Edinburgh: Churchill Livingstone.

Jenkins, J. P. R., Love, H. G., Foster, C. J., Isherwood I., Rowlands, D. (1988) Detection of coronary artery bypass graft patency as assessed by magnetic resonance imaging. *British Journal of Radiology*, **61**, 2–4.

Julian, D., Camm, A. J., Fox, K. M., Hall, R. J. C., Poole-Wilson, P. A. (eds) (1989) *Diseases of the Heart*. London: Baillière Tindall.

King, S. B. IIIrd., Douglas, J. S., Jr (1985) *Coronary Arteriography and Angioplasty*. New York: McGraw-Hill.

Lund, J. T., Ehmand, R. L., Julsrud, P. R., Sinak, L. J. (1989) Cardiac masses: assessment by MR imaging. *American Journal of Roentgenology*, **152**, 469–473.

Miller, G. (1989) *Invasive Investigation of the Heart*. Oxford: Blackwell.

Miller, S. W. (1996) *Cardiac Radiology—The Requisites*. St Louis: Mosby.

Mitchell, L., Jenkins, J. P. R., Watson, Y., Rowlands, D. J., Isherwood, I. (1989) Diagnosis and assessment of mitral and aortic valve disease by cine-flow magnetic resonance imaging. *Magnetic Resonance in Medicine*, **12**, 181–197.

Raphael, M. J., Hawkin, D. R., Allwork, S. P. (1980) The angiographic anatomy of the coronary arteries. *British Journal of Surgery*, **67**, 181–187.

Rees, S. (1990) Magnetic resonance studies of the heart. (The George Simon Lecture.) *Clinical Radiology*, **42**, 302–316.

Saeed, M., Wendland, M. F., Sakuma, H. et al (1995) Coronary artery stenosis: detection with contrast-enhanced MR imaging in dogs. *Radiology*, **196**, 79–84.

Reiber, J. H. C., Serruys, P. W. (1988) *New Developments in Quantitative Coronary Arteriography*. Dordrecht: Kluwer.

Sakuma, H., Caputo, G. R., Steffens, J. C. et al. (1994) Breath-hold MR cine angiography of coronary arteries in healthy volunteers: value of multiangle oblique imaging planes. *American Journal of Roentgenology*, **163**, 533–537.

Sakuma, H., O'Sullivan, M., Lucas, J. et al (1994) Effect of magnetic susceptibility contrast medium on myocardial signal intensity with fast gradient-recalled echo and spin-echo MR imaging: initial experience in humans. *Radiology*, **190**, 161–166.

Stanford, W., Galvin., J. R., Skorton, D. J., Marcus, M. L. (1990) The evaluation of coronary bypass graft patency: Direct and indirect techniques other than coronary arteriography. *American Journal of Roentgenology*, **156**, 15–22.

24

CONGENITAL HEART DISEASE

Peter Wilde

The incidence of congenital heart disease in live births is estimated at between 0.5 and 1.0% in various large series. Many of these recorded abnormalities are relatively simple, with only a small proportion of cases having very complex abnormalities. The common congenitally *bicuspid aortic valve* (2% incidence in the population) is not included in these figures, nor is the increasingly recognized *patent ductus arteriosus* in premature infants.

This relatively low incidence means that many radiologists will see only a small number of congenital heart disease cases each year, particularly if they are not working in a center with special pediatric or cardiac interests. It is not possible for a general radiologist or even a general pediatric radiologist to be familiar with the detailed radiology of all forms of congenital heart disease. It is essential, however, that all radiologists are sufficiently well informed in this field to be able to recognize possible cardiac problems and guide further investigation. They should also be able to assist in basic medical management and be aware of the changing patterns of disease seen in the natural history or surgical management of many of these conditions.

Over the last two decades the progress in treatment of congenital heart disease has been spectacular and, in particular, operative management has led to the survival of many patients who would previously have died from their congenital malformations. In many cases surgery is able to achieve complete or nearly complete anatomic correction of the abnormality, and in many other cases a high level of palliation can be achieved. An increasing number of patients will return for routine radiological assessment following surgery.

The treatment of congenital heart disease is generally undertaken in large specialist centers, and in these there will usually be a team approach to diagnosis and management. The best centers will have close cooperation between cardiac physicians, surgeons and radiologists. The specialist radiologist will be able to offer a range of investigations, particularly echocardiography and angiocardiography, and increasingly MRI. More recently the radiologist has also had a role to play in the management of cases requiring interventional treatment, particularly balloon dilatation of stenotic

valves and vessels and less commonly the embolization and occlusion of abnormal communications and channels.

Radiologists may deal with congenital heart disease at various stages and in various ways. These include:

1. Recognition that congenital heart disease is present. A preliminary diagnosis or general diagnosis is frequently possible from the *chest radiograph*, but it is rare that the plain film will give a precise, accurate and reliable diagnosis of the intracardiac abnormality.

2. Detailed diagnosis by *echocardiography* with the possible addition of *cardiac catheterization, angiography,* and other techniques.

3. Detailed evaluation of investigation results, usually at a joint case conference in which the full clinical picture is assessed and management is discussed.

4. Management, which can be continued medical management, palliative surgery, corrective surgery, *or interventional catheter techniques.* The radiologist may well have an important role in the interventional techniques, as well as in monitoring management by the use of plain chest radiography and other non-invasive imaging techniques.

5. Follow-up, usually done jointly between the specialist centre and the referring center. In many major centers there is now a clinic for 'grown-up congenital heart disease' (GUCH) patients who need to be managed throughout their adult life.

The two most obvious ways in which cardiac surgery has changed in recent years are the increasing number of total anatomic corrections that are possible and the decreasing age at which these operations are performed. In many large units a high proportion of congenital heart abnormalities are now completely corrected before the age of 1 year or even in the first few weeks of life. In some cases early palliative surgery precedes later definitive surgery. This has a particular effect on the practice of cardiac radiology, because the classical appearances of longstanding congenital heart abnormalities on the chest radiograph are becoming increasingly uncommon and their practical importance less.

Cardiac surgery is considered to include the heart and great vessels, and can be divided into two major types: closed heart surgery and open heart surgery. In *closed heart surgery* the operation is performed while the heart continues to function, and for this reason most closed heart operations are limited in terms of intracardiac repair. This type of procedure is most commonly carried out for abnormalities of the aorta and pulmonary arteries and palliation of other conditions. The procedures include *repair of coarctation*, insertion of a *systemic-to-pulmonary shunt*, or *banding of the main pulmonary artery*.

Open heart surgery requires that the cardiac function must cease. During this time the patient is maintained on cardiopulmonary bypass or is cooled to low temperatures to facilitate a safe period of cardiac standstill. In this situation it is vital that the cardiac surgeon has full knowledge of the nature of the abnormality or abnormalities before undertaking the operation, so that the time taken for the repair is kept to an absolute minimum. This reduces the risks of operative mortality and morbidity, which increase progressively with the length of time the heart is taken out of circulation.

The practice of preoperative assessment has changed considerably in recent years. Nowadays the *clinical*, *radiographic*, and, particularly, *echocardiographic* data are frequently adequate to make a complete diagnosis of the intracardiac abnormality. *Cardiac catheterization* and *angiography* are still required in a significant number of patients with a full echo diagnosis, because additional details may be required for precise management decisions to be made. In some cases this detail is of a hemodynamic nature. It is often necessary to measure the pulmonary vascular resistance in patients with large left-to-right shunts to exclude the possibility of irreversible pulmonary damage. Certain pressure gradients and absolute intracardiac pressures are also needed if they are not obtained by Doppler echocardiography.

It is sometimes necessary to clarify anatomic detail by *angiocardiography*, often with a view to excluding known pitfalls that may be encountered by the surgeon. For example, coronary anatomy cannot adequately be assessed by echocardiography while it can be clearly assessed using cine angiography. The pulmonary artery anatomy is often crucial to the management of many patients, and it is often not possible to visualize the left and right pulmonary arteries beyond their origins by echocardiography due to surrounding intrapulmonary air. Other fine details of anatomy are often obtained by cardiac catheterization and angiography, such as the assessment of small or multiple ventricular septal defects (unless high-quality Doppler color flow mapping is available) and the visualization of systemic-to-pulmonary collaterals or shunts. There will also be cases where the echo study has been technically difficult for one reason or another and the angiogram is essential.

Finally, the cardiac catheterization procedure is sometimes accompanied by an interventional procedure. These include *Rashkind balloon septostomy* for transposition of the great arteries (now sometimes performed under echocardiographic control), *dilatation of the pulmonary valve or coarctation*, and, more recently, *ductal closure, occlusion of abnormal communications*, and *vascular stenting*. These techniques are developing rapidly but require expert knowledge of intracardiac anatomy to ensure their success.

CLASSIFICATION AND DESCRIPTION OF CONGENITAL HEART DISEASE

A number of different attempts have been made to classify congenital heart disease, but whichever approach is adopted there is a large array of differing conditions which must be recognized.

The first and most important requirement is for accurate description of what is being seen. It is therefore vital to recognize the morphological appearance of each cardiac chamber and each great vessel wherever possible so that abnormal connections are unambiguously described. It is frequently helpful to use the phrase *morphologically left ventricle* to describe a ventricular chamber which has all the characteristics of the left ventricle irrespective of where it is in the patient and irrespective of which connections it makes. It is, for example, possible to have a morphologically left ventricle that lies on the right side of the body or to the right of the other ventricle.

The morphological features of important structures are described in detail in Chapter 20, and are here briefly reviewed.

Right Atrium The appearance of the atrial appendages has long been fundamental in the accurate determination of atrial morphology and is particularly suited to angiocardiography or, on occasion, the pathological or surgical examination. It is not possible to determine this information from plain films, and it can be difficult to achieve using echocardiography. The right atrial appendage is broad based and triangular in shape. The inferior vena cava almost always enters the right atrium, and though this rule is not invariable, it is a clinically important guide. The site of drainage of the inferior vena cava can be demonstrated by angiocardiography or echocardiography. The latter technique can also be very helpful in assessing the anatomy of the atrial septum to determine morphology; the septum secundum lies to the right of the septum primum and its lower margin forms the upper edge of the foramen ovale. This is frequently patent in early life, but even in later life the closed fossa ovale remains as a marker of the right side of the atrial septum.

Left Atrium This chamber can be defined most precisely by its atrial appendage, which is long and narrow, usually curling around the left side of the heart. The left atrium cannot reliably be defined by the presence of pulmonary veins as these can often be anomalous.

Right Ventricle This is rhomboid in shape and shows heavy bands of trabeculation throughout the chamber. There is often a prominent band crossing the main cavity of the ventricle, the 'moderator band'. The trabecular pattern is particularly suited to demonstration by angiocardiography, but can sometimes be deduced using echocardiography. In the assessment of trabecular pattern by any technique it is important to look comparatively at both ventricles because the typical patterns may be a little distorted in some complex cases.

The papillary muscles arise from multiple groups in the right ventricle, and there is usually some attachment of chordae to papillary muscle or muscles on the septum, which itself is heavily trabeculated. The atrioventricular valve of the right ventricle is by definition the tricuspid valve, and is inserted slightly more toward the apex of the heart than the atrioventricular valve of the left ventricle (mitral valve). This particular feature is very well demonstrated by echocardiography. There is normally an outflow muscular tube known as the conus or infundibulum which leads up to the exit semilunar valve. The semilunar valves (pulmonary and aortic) are named in accordance with the appropriate great artery, so the exit valve of the right ventricle is not necessarily the pulmonary valve.

Left Ventricle This is the ventricular chamber with a more symmetrical oval shape and fine lattice-like trabeculation. The basal half of the interventricular septum is smooth, without any trabeculation. There are normally two large papillary muscles in this ventricle, both of which arise from the free wall and not from the interventricular septum. Both papillary muscles give attachment to chordae from both mitral valve leaflets.

The atrioventricular valve entering the left ventricle is by definition the mitral valve, and the insertion of the mitral valve is further toward the base of the heart than the atrioventricular valve of the right ventricle, the tricuspid valve. In the left ventricle there is usually fibrous continuity between the inflow and outflow valves, although this is not always the case. The fibrous continuity is well demonstrated on the two-dimensional long-axis echo-cardiographic view, where the anterior leaflet of the mitral valve is seen arising from the posterior wall of the aortic root.

The Pulmonary Artery This is the great artery which bifurcates into two branches after a short distance, each branch supplying one lung. If two great arteries are present then it is often easier to define the aorta first. It is also important to distinguish true pulmonary arteries arising from the pulmonary trunk from abnormal aortopulmonary vessels.

The Aorta This is the great artery which supplies branches to the head and neck. The aorta cannot be defined in terms of its connection to the heart (in transposition of the great arteries the aorta arises from the right ventricle) or the presence of coronary branches (anomalous coronary vessels can arise from the pulmonary artery).

CLASSIFICATION OF CARDIAC ABNORMALITIES

In recent years a reasonably standardized approach has been achieved in the description of congenital cardiac abnormalities. Although this is not necessarily used in the description of very simple abnormalities, it is invaluable in the description of complex abnormalities as it avoids confusion or ambiguity. The approach is one with five major descriptive steps:

1. Situs
2. Cardiac connections
3. Looping
4. Positions
5. Malformations.

These will be described in turn.

Situs The abdominal and thoracic viscera are asymmetrical, and for this reason normal situs can be recognized by obvious features such as the liver and inferior vena cava lying on the right side and the spleen and heart lying on the left side. The very high association with the inferior vena cava draining into the right atrium has led to the development of the term *visceroatrial situs*. This essentially means that the atrial situs in almost all cases conforms

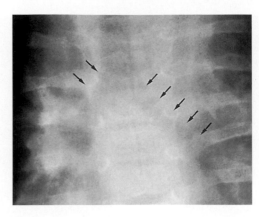

Fig. 24.1 Plain radiograph of the mediastinum showing normal bronchial anatomy. Arrows indicate the length of left and right bronchi.

to the situs of the upper abdominal viscera, irrespective of the situs or position of the remainder of the heart. A transverse upper abdominal ultrasound scan will allow definition of the visceroatrial situs by showing variations in position of the inferior vena cava, aorta, and sometimes the azygos vein.

It is also important to recognize the presence of asymmetry in the lungs, which is usually apparent in the form of *bronchial situs*. The right main bronchus is shorter, wider, and more vertically orientated than the left main bronchus, which is usually at least 1.5 times as long as the right from bifurcation to first major branch (Fig. 24.1). The bronchial situs nearly always corresponds to the visceroatrial situs. Special filtration techniques of chest radiography may be needed for the assessment of bronchial situs.

From time to time, situs abnormalities will occur, and it is important to describe variations accurately:

a. *Situs solitus.* This describes the normal situation with normal visceroatrial situs (liver, inferior vena cava and right atrium on the right side) and normal bronchial situs. The 'position' of the cardiac mass and/or cardiac apex is not directly related to visceroatrial situs and may not correspond with it. The apex can occasionally be directed toward the right side even with normal visceroatrial situs, this sometimes being described as *isolated dextrocardia* or dextrorotation of the heart (Fig. 24.2).

b. *Situs inversus.* In this condition there is complete reversal of the visceroatrial situs and the bronchial situs. The condition is not necessarily associated with any other cardiac abnormality. An example of this is shown in Figure 24.3. Meticulous technique in the use of radiographic side markers is of paramount importance. If films are marked up after processing, then cases of total situs inversus are almost certainly going to be marked wrongly. Once again the cardiac apex may not lie in the expected position. Thus, in most cases of situs inversus the cardiac apex lies on the right side, but occasionally it will lie on the left (*isolated levocardia*).

c. *Situs ambiguous.* This describes a situation in which the left- and right-sided nature of abdominal or thoracic organs and the atria are not clearly distinct. A number of variations of this can be recognized. The first of these is most easily understood as 'bilateral right-sidedness'. In this condition there is a mid-line liver running across the upper abdomen (Fig. 24.4), the spleen is absent, the stomach is usually centrally positioned, and the

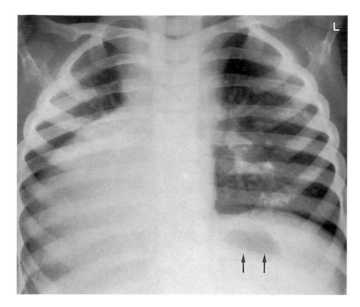

Fig. 24.2 Chest radiograph of a patient with visceroatrial situs solitus (gastric bubble arrowed) and isolated dextrocardia.

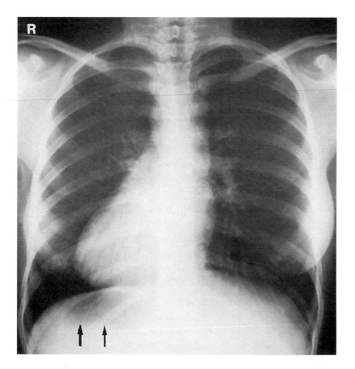

Fig. 24.3 Chest radiograph of a patient with total situs inversus (gastric bubble arrowed).

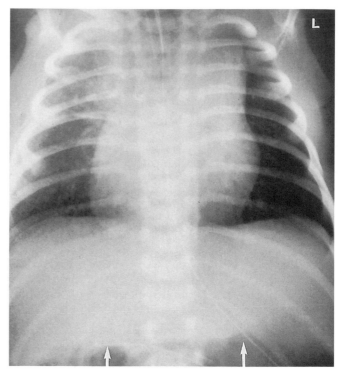

Fig. 24.4 Chest radiograph of an infant with situs ambiguous showing a centrally positioned cardiac apex and transverse liver (arrowed). There were complex intracardiac anomalies.

bronchial anatomy shows right-sided morphology of both major bronchi. Both atrial chambers have right-sided characteristics and, not surprisingly, there is a frequent association with abnormalities of pulmonary venous drainage. Often many other cardiac abnormalities are also associated with this condition. '*Bilateral left-sidedness*' is also associated with a mid-line liver, often smaller, but there is frequently polysplenia and bilateral left atrial morphology, and the two main bronchi both show left morphology.

There is, by definition, abnormal systemic venous drainage. Again, there is an association with major cardiac abnormality. The final form of situs ambiguous is one in which the morphological characteristics of the various structures are very hard to determine, and a left- or right-sided nature cannot easily be determined. In this case again many cardiac anomalies can be associated.

Cardiac Connections Once the cardiac chambers have been identified in morphological terms it should be possible to state which vessel or chamber is connected to which. For example, in transposition of the great arteries it can be stated that the aorta arises from the morphologically right ventricle and the pulmonary artery arises from the morphologically left ventricle. In this situation there is said to be *ventriculoarterial discordance*. From time to time there will be *atrioventricular discordance*, which will occur when the morphologically right atrium drains into the morphologically left ventricle and vice versa.

In some cases the connections will not be completely distinct, as, for example, in the *tetralogy of Fallot*, where the aorta partially overrides onto the right ventricle from its position above a large ventricular septal defect. Complete overriding of great arteries can occur in the presence of a ventricular septal defect, most typically in *double-outlet right ventricle*.

If there is a large ventricular septal defect lying between the atrioventricular valves there can also be partial or total override of the mitral or tricuspid valve. Double-inlet ventricle is thus a recognized occurrence. Although it is a simple matter to state that an atrioventricular valve is related to one or other or both ventricles, the diagnosis of the exact relationship may not be easy.

The complex curving nature of the interventricular septal anatomy and the limitations of all the imaging techniques make precise diagnosis very difficult in some cases. Surgical or pathological inspection does not provide an unequivocal diagnosis in every case either. In spite of these difficulties, it should be the aim of any intracardiac examination in complex congenital heart disease to obtain a clear idea of the basic relationships of the chambers, with any difficulties in description or nomenclature being stated clearly.

Looping (or topology) This term relates to the ventricular loop which has been formed during cardiac development. If the heart is well enough developed to have two ventricles, each with an inlet and an outlet, and an interventricular septum lying between them, then it will be possible to define the loop. D-loop and L-loop configurations are stereoisomers (mirror images) of each other, the difference between the two types of loop being analogous to the difference between the left hand and right hand. Each hand is uniquely different, being defined by the relationship of the fingers and thumb with the palm and back of the hand. Whichever position a hand is in, it can always be distinguished as a right or left hand. Looping is also independent of cardiac situs or position.

The normal *ventricular D-loop* can be understood most simply using the analogy of the *right hand rule* devised by Van Praagh. In this description the morphological right ventricle is likened to a right hand. The inflow is represented by the thumb, the outflow is represented by the fingers, and the interventricular septum will lie on the palmar side of the hand. This can be appreciated by placing one's right hand near another person's heart. If, however, the morphologically right ventricle is configured in such a way that the relationship of inflow, outflow, and interventricular septum can only be represented by a left hand, this infers that the ventricle is actually a stereoisomer of a normal D-loop ventricle, and is an L-loop ventricle.

L-looping is most frequently seen in association with transposition of the great arteries in the condition known as anatomically corrected transposition or commonly just '*corrected transposition.*'

Position Although the position of the heart in the chest is the first thing to be seen on a chest radiograph, the absolute position is of secondary importance in describing the fundamental nature of the congenital heart abnormality. The position is of course of practical importance in planning surgical procedures. If one imagines that the heart is a model made out of extremely flexible elastic material, then it is easy to see that the position of even a completely normal heart can be considerably distorted by twisting, stretching, or turning various chambers into different positions, while the heart still maintains absolutely normal situs, cardiac connections, and ventricular looping. Similarly, the presence of particular situs, connection, or looping arrangements does not necessarily indicate what the final cardiac position will be.

A complex positional variation is the '*criss-cross*' heart. In this abnormality there is, in addition to any other abnormalities of situs or connection, an additional twist of the ventricular mass. This results in the ventricles lying in unexpected positions given the particular situs and connection. Sometimes the ventricles adopt a superoinferior relationship, but occasionally their positions can be completely reversed. The simplest example to understand would occur in a heart with normal situs and connections; in this case, twisting of the ventricular mass could lead to the

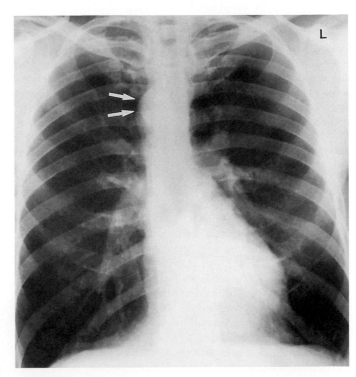

Fig. 24.5 Chest radiograph showing an isolated right-sided aortic arch (arrows indicate aortic knuckle).

morphologically left ventricle lying anterior to the posteriorly displaced morphological right ventricle.

It is important to note the position of the *aortic arch* relative to the trachea. The normal aortic arch is left sided, but some congenital abnormalities are associated with a higher than normal incidence of right-sided arch. There are a number of variations in aortic branching patterns which will be considered later. The recognition of a right-sided aortic arch is of course important for surgical planning. A right-sided arch may also occur in isolation (Fig. 24.5).

Malformations This refers to the specific deformities or abnormalities within the heart, such as *stenotic or atretic valves*, *abnormal communications*, and *narrowed vessels*. These malformations are often the most obvious abnormality, and they are commonly used as the overall descriptive term for a particular abnormality (e.g. *ventricular septal defect*, *pulmonary atresia*, or *coarctation of the aorta*). Some malformations are a little more complex, for example atrioventricular septal defects, and in some cases there are multiple associated malformations as in tetralogy of Fallot (ventricular septal defect and pulmonary stenosis).

In many cases the malformations are the only abnormality, and in this situation the full description of situs, connection, looping, and position is omitted for simplicity in general discussion, the implicit assumption being made that all these other aspects are normal. This is acceptable in normal practice, provided that the full descriptive nomenclature is used as soon as the congenital heart abnormality is anything other than straightforward.

Malformations also occur commonly in association with the more complex abnormalities, and in fact they are frequently associated with major abnormalities of situs, looping, or connection.

HEMODYNAMIC AND FUNCTIONAL PRINCIPLES

A thorough understanding of the radiology of congenital heart disease must include not only structural abnormalities but also functional abnormalities. Normal cardiac anatomy and physiology must be understood before the developmental, functional, and pathological consequences of the abnormalities can fully be appreciated.

Developmental Aspects

Development of Chambers and Vessels The blood flowing through a chamber or vessel is a powerful stimulus for the growth of the cavity. Conversely, if there is no flow then the structure will be hypoplastic or absent. It is the chamber size that is affected by flow, not usually the wall thickness (hypertrophy). This is seen most dramatically in the condition of *hypoplastic left heart*, in which the left ventricle fails to develop beyond a tiny size because there is aortic and/or mitral atresia that prevents normal flow through the left ventricle and aorta. It is also seen in some cases of *pulmonary atresia* when the low pulmonary blood flow predisposes to very small pulmonary arteries. The converse is also true, high flow leading to a large cavity size, as is seen in right heart dilatation with an atrial septal defect.

The pressure generated by a chamber stimulates the development of the muscular wall rather than the size of the cavity. Thus, in pulmonary atresia with an intact ventricular septum there is a high-pressure obstructed ventricle with very low flow through it. In this situation the chamber is usually very small but very hypertrophied. In tetralogy of Fallot, the right ventricle is subjected to high pressure and high flow (most of which passes down the aorta), and thus the chamber shows both dilatation and hypertrophy. Some surgical procedures are directed at increasing flow through structures in order to encourage their growth.

Physiological Changes at Birth In fetal life the right-sided cardiac pressures and the pressure in the pulmonary artery remain high because the postnatal low-resistance pulmonary capillary bed has not yet developed. At birth, the first breath of the infant initiates the rapid decrease in pulmonary vascular resistance, which in turn leads to a rapid decrease in right-sided cardiac pressures. This causes the interatrial foramen to close by acting like a valve, and will also stimulate closure of the patent ductus arteriosus. Ductal closure is a complex phenomenon, and may take some hours or days or even weeks in premature infants. It is important to realize, however, that the consequential drop in pulmonary artery pressure can take several hours or days to be complete, and this will have important consequences on the clinical and radiological presentation of certain conditions in early life.

Signs and symptoms of left-to-right shunts will tend to increase in the early days and weeks of life as the pulmonary resistance falls (Fig. 24.6). On the other hand, some conditions (e.g. pulmonary atresia) are *'ductus dependent'*, and the closure of the ductus in early life will lead to progressive pulmonary oligemia and consequent cyanosis.

Pathological Circulations

Left-to-right Shunt In the normal postnatal situation the pressure in the right ventricle and pulmonary artery will be much lower than that on the left side because of the lower vascular resistance in the lungs. If any communication between the left and right side of the heart exists, there will be a left-to-right shunt. This can be measured by catheter oximetry, or non-invasively by radionuclide studies and Doppler techniques. The ratio of pulmonary to systemic flow (often called the Q_P/Q_S ratio) can vary from less than 2:1 (a small shunt) to 4:1 (a moderate shunt) or as much as 10:1 or over (a very large shunt). It is generally

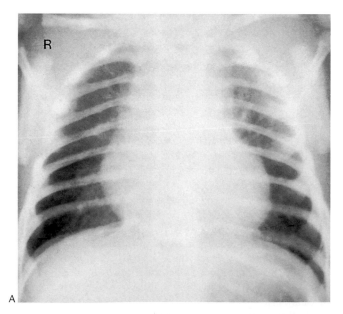
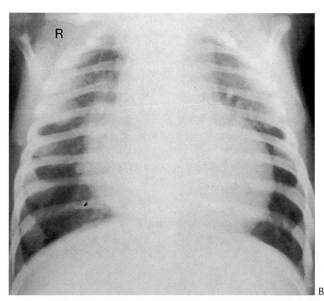

Fig. 24.6 A. Chest radiograph of an infant aged 1 day. The heart is only slightly enlarged and the child was asymptomatic. **B.** Chest radiograph of the same infant after 1 month. The heart size has increased and the pulmonary vasculature is now plethoric. The child had developed feeding difficulties, and a ventricular septal defect was diagnosed.

held that a shunt of 2:1 or less is difficult to detect on the chest radiograph by either pulmonary plethora or increased heart size.

If the left-to-right shunt is at the *atrial level* then the pressure in the left and right ventricles will not necessarily be affected. The right ventricle can tolerate a significantly increased flow of blood by increasing its cavity size and contractility while maintaining normal or slightly raised pressures. On the chest X-ray the lung fields will be *plethoric* (generalized enlargement of all the vessels), and the dilated right-sided chambers will manifest themselves as an increased heart size (Fig. 24.7). If this situation exists for many years the continuing large flow in the lungs can gradually damage the pulmonary circulation, and will eventually lead to a right-sided pressure increase and ultimately equalization of left- and right-sided pressures. Thus, simple atrial septal defects do not often cause trouble in childhood or early adult life but may cause pulmonary hypertension or heart failure in middle age or later.

If the *ventricular septal defect* is small this will increase the flow through the lungs but will not necessarily raise the pressure on the right side. It is highly probable that small ventricular septal defects will close in the early years of life.

If there is a large ventricular septal defect, then the left and right ventricles will immediately be at the same pressure, and the lower resistance of the lungs will induce a large left-to-right shunt. In this situation the combination of increased flow and increased pressure in the lungs will produce progressive pulmonary vascular damage at a much earlier age than would occur with atrial mixing. Irreversible pulmonary damage will occur in this situation, and ultimately the right-sided pressure elevation will cause reversal of the shunt with the development of cyanosis (*Eisenmenger syndrome*). The development of this condition is associated with a reduction in the left-to-right shunt with consequent reduction in the heart size and decreased pulmonary plethora. Thus the chest radiograph that is 'improving' or has

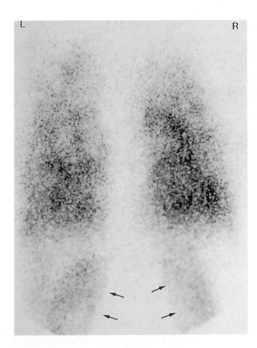

Fig. 24.8 Posterior view of a ^{99m}Tc microsphere lung scan in a patient with Eisenmenger syndrome. Renal uptake (arrowed) is due to right-to-left shunting in the heart.

returned to 'normal' may actually be showing the development of progressive irreversible damage. A similar situation can occur with any other high-pressure mixing situation such as might occur with a large *patent ductus arteriosus* or other *aortopulmonary connection*. The right-to-left shunting is occasionally demonstrated by radionuclide techniques (Fig. 24.8).

Circulation in Transposition Complete transposition of the great arteries with no other intracardiac abnormality is incompatible with life unless there is mixing of the two circulations at some point. It is useless to have a large amount of well-oxygenated blood returned to the left atrium if it is subsequently redirected to the left ventricle and then to the pulmonary artery and lungs again. There is usually a small amount of shunting across the foramen ovale, which sustains life in the early postnatal period, but it is essential to improve mixing at an early stage. In line with the principles outlined above, the obligatory shunting is best at an atrial level where the pressure is low, and it is thus common practice to perform a *Rashkind balloon septostomy* as soon as possible in cyanosed infants with transposition of the great arteries. This procedure ruptures the thin septum primum covering the foramen ovale, which facilitates increased atrial shunting (which must of course be in both directions). Although the total amount of shunting from left to right and right to left must be equal, there is overall much more blood flowing in the pulmonary circuit than the systemic circuit, so that the small proportion of this oxygenated pulmonary flow which passes across the atrial septum will be adequate to sustain the systemic requirements. The vessels in the lungs will consequently be enlarged.

Patients with complete transposition frequently have other communications between pulmonary and systemic circuits, common examples being ventricular septal defects and patent ductus

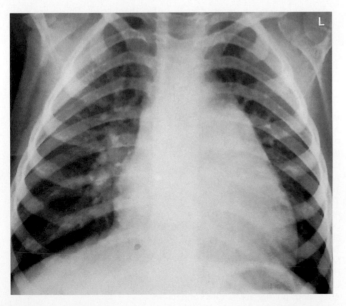

Fig. 24.7 Chest radiograph of a child with a moderately large atrial septal defect. The main pulmonary artery segment is large, and the lung vessels are large.

arteriosus. These communications will be advantageous in increasing the mixing but disadvantageous in that they will predispose to high pulmonary pressures which might permanently damage the lungs.

Common Mixing Circulation This can occur with a number of different conditions. A *common atrium* or *total anomalous pulmonary venous drainage* to the right atrium will produce this at the atrial level. An *atretic tricuspid valve* will lead to obligatory right-to-left shunting into the left atrium and consequent common mixing. At the ventricular level a very *large ventricular septal defect* or any of the 'single ventricle' variants will produce common mixing. At the great arterial level there will be common mixing in *pulmonary atresia* and *common truncus arteriosus*.

In all these situations the aorta and pulmonary artery will both be supplied with partially desaturated blood. The lungs will be at little disadvantage if they receive adequate flow (unless they are subjected to an excessively high pressure/flow combination) but the systemic supply will be significantly affected and the patient will be cyanosed, the degree depending on the particular hemodynamic details. If there is very rapid circulation through the lungs, then there will be a high proportion of saturated blood returned to the common mixing pool, and the cyanosis will be slight (as in truncus arteriosus). If pulmonary blood flow is low, then the common mixing pool will be very desaturated (for example in pulmonary atresia).

Pulmonary Atresia In many congenital cardiac abnormalities there is complete obstruction of the pulmonary artery or valve which may be associated with atresia or narrowing in the right ventricular outflow tract. In this situation no blood will enter the pulmonary circulation in the normal way, and the only flow in the pulmonary circuit will be that produced by *ductal flow* or by *systemic to pulmonary collaterals*, the latter being small or absent at birth.

In patients in this category, closure of the patent ductus arteriosus at birth can lead to rapid progressive cyanosis, and it is therefore necessary to increase the blood supply to the lungs. In the short term this is done by *medical therapy* to keep the patent ductus open, but as soon as practicable a *systemic-to-pulmonary shunt* is performed to improve the blood flow into the lungs. Patients surviving this early stage without surgical palliation will go on to develop *aortopulmonary collateral communications*. These vary considerably, and can enter the lungs in many sites. Some of these vessels may be of bronchial artery origin, but it is not always clear what their morphological origins are. Supply is most frequently from the descending aorta, but subclavian, internal mammary, and intercostal arteries may give rise to collaterals.

Left-sided Obstruction *Coarctation of the aorta* and *aortic valve stenosis* are two common obstructive lesions which, if severe, can lead to left-sided heart failure in early life. This will be radiographically manifest as enlargement of pulmonary vessels (due to pulmonary venous hypertension, not plethora), possible interstitial or alveolar pulmonary edema, and cardiomegaly. Obstruction at the *mitral* or *left atrial* level is less common, but will give the pulmonary changes with less cardiomegaly because the left ventricle is not working against the obstruction.

Right-sided Obstructions Severe obstruction to the outflow into the lungs is usually a less serious problem than severe systemic outflow obstruction but it can still have important effects.

Right ventricular failure can be caused by *very severe pulmonary stenosis*, but commonly this does not occur because a ventricular septal defect will also be present (e.g. tetralogy of Fallot) which will allow decompression of the elevated right-sided pressures by right to left shunting.

Birth Asphyxia Obstetric problems which lead to severe birth anoxia can have serious cardiac effects. These are most commonly manifest as heart failure with cardiomegaly and pulmonary changes. If resuscitation is achieved successfully, the chest radiograph may revert to normal over a few days.

IMPORTANT CONGENITAL CARDIAC ABNORMALITIES

A number of conditions will be discussed in detail, and are presented in order of frequency of occurrence as shown in Table 24.1. The data are taken from the Bristol Registry of Congenital Heart Disease, and represent all live births presenting with congenital heart disease to the center in the period from 1977 to 1987. These figures have not changed significantly in recent decades and are essentially in line with published data from other centers.

The following conditions with a reported incidence of less than 1% are also discussed:

- Truncus arteriosus
- Ebstein's anomaly
- Sinus of Valsalva fistula
- Double-outlet ventricle
- Great arterial anomalies
- Coronary anomalies
- Arteriovenous malformations
- Cardiac tumors.

Systemic venous anomalies are also discussed. These are quite commonly associated with other forms of congenital heart disease,

Table 24.1 Incidence of congenital cardiac abnormalities[a]

Condition	Incidence (%)
Ventricular septal defect	36.1
Atrial septal defect	8.2
Patent ductus arteriosus	7.9
Pulmonary stenosis	6.9
Coarctation of the aorta	5.9
Aortic stenosis	5.7
Tetralogy of Fallot	4.6
Transposition of the great arteries	3.8
Atrioventricular septal defect	3.6
Pulmonary atresia	2.6
Single ventricle	2.2
Tricuspid atresia	1.5
Mitral valve abnormalities	1.4
Hypoplastic left heart syndrome	1.4
Cardiomyopathy	1.3
Anomalous pulmonary venous connection	1.2
Total	94.3

[a] Bristol Registry of Congenital Heart Disease, 1977–1987.

occurring in 10% of cases with diagnosed congenital heart disease.

VENTRICULAR SEPTAL DEFECT (VSD)

This abnormality is the commonest of all, and can occur alone or be associated with other simple or complex congenital heart conditions. The interventricular septum has a complex curved shape, and defects can occur in any part of it. Various descriptive classifications have been proposed but the following classification (or a modification of it) is generally accepted.

Perimembranous Defect   This is the commonest type of VSD, involving the membranous septum and adjacent muscular tissue below the aortic root and close to the upper margin of the tricuspid valve annulus. Sometimes this can be large and extend round toward the outlet part of the septum.

Muscular Defects   These can be grouped as follows:

1 *Inlet* or basal muscular defect lying in the muscular septum between the mitral and tricuspid valves.

2. Mid-muscular or *apical* defect between the main right and left ventricular chambers, sometimes called an apical trabecular defect.

3. *Outlet* defect. This involves either the high anterior trabeculated part of the septum or the band of muscle immediately below the pulmonary valve forming the conus of the right ventricle (the term 'conal' defect is sometimes used in the latter situation).

It is possible for single or multiple VSDs to be present at any site throughout the large and complex shape of the interventricular septum. In diagnosis and investigation of this condition it is not only important to confirm the presence of interventricular communication but to localize the exact site and size of the communication and to determine if there are any additional communications. The latter point is essential if corrective surgery is to be successful.

If defects are of the large inlet or outlet type, it may be possible to override the inlet or outlet valves. The overriding aorta in the tetralogy of Fallot is a good example of this. The term *malalignment VSD* is sometimes used in this situation. Extreme forms of malalignment will result in such conditions as double-inlet or double-outlet ventricle. These will be considered elsewhere.

The *Gerbode defect* is a communication through the small portion of the basal septum that separates the left ventricular outflow tract from the right atrium (the atrioventricular septum). This defect is very rare and must be diagnosed with care, because it can easily be confused with a perimembranous defect and coexistent tricuspid regurgitation.

Many other congenital heart defects are associated with a VSD, and these will be considered in the appropriate sections. Of particular importance is the association of VSD with *coarctation of the aorta*, which can produce a particularly severe form of infantile cardiac failure. The remainder of this description will deal with the various forms of 'simple VSD', i.e. unassociated with other anomalies.

Clinical Presentation   The presentation of this condition depends on the overall size of the interventricular communication. The condition does not normally present in the first few days of life unless the interventricular septal defect is very large. This is because the pulmonary vascular resistance drops markedly in the first days and weeks of life and thus prevents the early development of pulmonary plethora. The characteristic systolic murmur may take even longer to develop. Thus, even with large VSDs the patient may be asymptomatic, with a normal chest radiograph at birth. A large VSD will present after a few days or weeks, with breathlessness and feeding difficulties, and the chest X-ray will usually show moderate enlargement of the heart with prominence of the main pulmonary artery, the hilar pulmonary arteries and the peripheral pulmonary arteries (see Fig. 24.6). In severe cases there will be cardiac failure also.

With smaller VSDs, the presentation can be much later in life and may occur with the detection of an asymptomatic murmur. In these cases the chest X-ray can range from normal (if the communication is very small) to mild or moderate cardiac enlargement with mild or moderate pulmonary plethora.

It is not an easy matter in pediatric practice to distinguish ventricular septal defect from other left-to-right cardiac shunts (e.g. patent ductus arteriosus, aortopulmonary communication, or even a large atrial septal defect) on the basis of the chest X-ray alone, particularly in the young infant. Distinction becomes easier with increasing age, due to the differing natural histories of the conditions, but this is obviously of little immediate value in individual infants or children. It is important to point out, however, that a large VSD with a big shunt presenting early in life will inevitably lead to severe pulmonary damage and pulmonary hypertension in the first few years of life. It is thus essential to recognize the abnormality and treat the condition as soon as possible. *Echocardiography* is vital in the differential diagnosis of these conditions, and must be performed as soon as the condition is clinically or radiographically suspected.

Non-invasive Imaging   The diagnosis of VSD can usually be confirmed on *two-dimensional echocardiography* (Fig. 24.9). It is most important that the full extent of the interventricular septum is examined in any case of suspected VSD. The examination will include, as an absolute minimum, the *parasternal long- and short-axis views* and the *apical four-chamber views* (Fig. 24.10). (NB. Orientation of echocardiographic images is variable, and pediatric cardiologists often present images in the 'inverted' position with the apex of the scan sector at the bottom of the

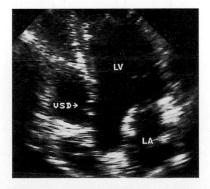

Fig. 24.9 Two-dimensional echocardiogram taken from the apex in a child with a small perimembranous ventricular septal defect (VSD). The margins of the defect act as distinct echogenic structures. LV, left ventricle; LA, left atrium.

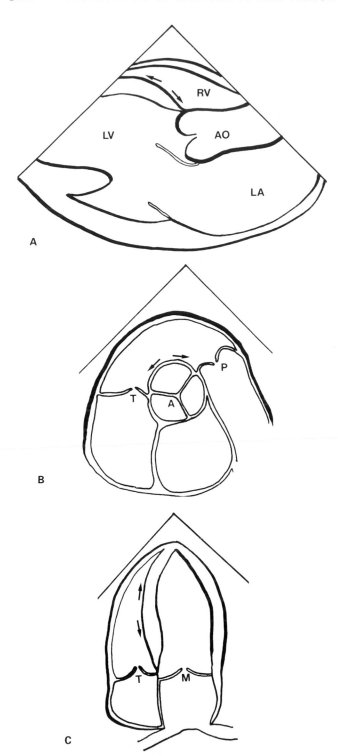

image. In this Chapter the conventional adult orientations are used as these are likely to be more familiar to the radiologist.) Each view will include a sweep along the heart in the particular plane being examined. Sometimes the defect is easier to identify because the edges of the septal hole act as strong ultrasonic reflectors and highlight the defect. In some parts of the septum the trabecular pattern will produce multiple reflections which can obscure small defects. In some cases of perimembranous VSD there is associated tissue in or near the defect which can partially obstruct it, the growth of this probably being one of the mechanisms of spontaneous closure of moderate or small defects. Sometimes there is prominent bulging of this tissue into the right ventricle, the so-called '*aneurysmal perimembranous VSD*'.

It may be necessary to use *Doppler flow assessment* to detect the presence of small defects, using the turbulent jet passing through the defect as a marker. Careful searching along the right ventricular surface of the septum with the pulsed Doppler sample volume will usually reveal any abnormal jet. In this situation the addition of *color flow mapping* has been very valuable in speeding and simplifying the detection of small or multiple ventricular septal defects (Fig. 24.11). Color flow imaging will also show the direction of the jet, which is particularly important if a continuous-wave Doppler beam is to be aligned with the jet to measure the peak jet velocity and calculate the pressure drop across the VSD. This is an important non-invasive method for deducing the right ventricular pressure.

Mild tricuspid regurgitation is frequently associated with perimembranous VSDs, and Doppler techniques are particularly useful in detecting this, though care must be taken to avoid confusion with the VSD jet itself.

MRI has been used with success to demonstrate VSDs, but at present the technique is only sufficiently accurate to detect large defects, and cannot be used reliably to detect small defects in uncommon positions. Conventional *CT scanning* is not of practical use in the detection of VSDs.

Defects cannot be visualized with any clarity using *nuclear medicine* techniques, but first-pass studies are occasionally useful in calculating pulmonary-to-systemic flow ratios, and in conjunction with echocardiography they can produce a non-invasive assessment of a VSD.

Fig. 24.10 **A.** Diagram showing a parasternal long-axis echocardiogram. The arrows indicate the region for seeking a ventricular septal defect on Doppler examination. LV, left ventricle; RV, right ventricular outflow tract; AO, aortic root; LA, left atrium. **B.** Parasternal short-axis echocardiogram at the level of the aortic root. The arrows indicate the area which should be examined just below the aortic valve to detect a perimembranous ventricular septal defect. T, tricuspid valve; A, aortic valve; P, pulmonary valve. **C.** Apical four-chamber echocardiogram. The arrows indicate where a muscular ventricular septal defect might be sought using Doppler techniques. T, tricuspid valve; M, mitral valve.

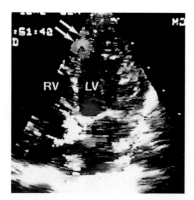

Fig. 24.11 Color flow Doppler study taken in an apical four-chamber view. The arrows indicate the orange flow pattern (toward the transducer) of an apical muscular defect. LV, left ventricle; RV, right ventricle.

Cardiac Catheterization and Angiography Cardiac catheterization is still frequently undertaken if there is any doubt about the intracardiac anatomy or about the nature of the pulmonary vascular resistance. Cardiac angiography must be performed in such a way that the interventricular septum is completely examined in its entirety. There is no such thing as 'the view that profiles the septum'; rather, there are many views which profile different parts of the septum, and they must be used in a logical fashion not only to locate the site of the known VSD but to confirm or exclude the possibility of additional VSDs.

If biplane cine angiocardiography is available, the best two views to select for initial examination of the septum are:

1. 65° left anterior oblique (LAO) with a 20–25° cranial tilt
2. 30° right anterior oblique (RAO).

These two views will demonstrate the majority of the perimembranous, inlet, and mid-muscular septum (LAO view) and the high anterior and conal septum (RAO view). The outflow region will not be demonstrated adequately by the LAO view because the region will be obscured by contrast medium in the ventricle and aorta.

If the VSD demonstrated by these views is small and clearly localized then no additional view is necessary. If the VSD is large, however, it may be obscuring additional defects, and its dimension in the foreshortened plane may not be apparent. If multiple defects are shown, at least one additional view may be necessary to localize the defects precisely. With biplane studies the following additional two views may be helpful:

1. 55° LAO view with a 10–15° caudal tilt
2. 40° RAO view with a 15° caudal tilt.

The LAO view will distinguish high from low defects in this view, whereas the previous cranial tilt will distinguish basal from apical defects. The RAO view will profile the portion of the septum between the inflow and outflow portions.

A full series of four views is not of course mandatory, and the potential hazards of radiation and contrast medium must always be considered. Nevertheless, it is not in the patient's best interests if the study is completed with inadequate localization for proper surgical management. If single-plane studies are being performed, the first two views are essential, and two ventricular injections are necessary.

The study of a VSD should not be concluded before consideration of the possible coexistence of a *patent ductus arteriosus*. A moderate or large VSD will give rise to simultaneous aortic and pulmonary opacification, and with some overlapping of structures it is not always possible to exclude a patent ductus with certainty. A separate aortogram (RAO 30°, LAO 60°) is thus required.

The most common VSD is in the membranous or perimembranous region, and often occurs with some form of associated fibrous tissue which is often closely related to the tricuspid valve (Fig. 24.12). In some cases the VSD is aneurysmal, with a bulging structure being pushed toward the right ventricle with each systolic contraction of the left ventricle, and this can occasionally cause obstruction in the outflow tract of the right ventricle. Often a large VSD can be virtually occluded

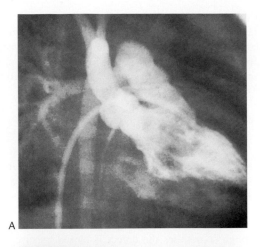

A

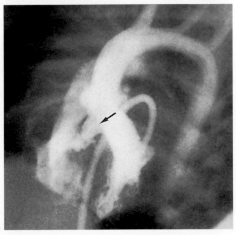

B

Fig. 24.12 **A**. Left ventricular cine angiogram taken in a right anterior oblique view. There is simultaneous filling of the aorta and pulmonary artery, indicating the presence of a ventricular septal defect which is not profiled in this projection. **B**. Simultaneous view of the same angiogram but shown in the cranially angled LAO view. An aneurysmal perimembranous VSD is profiled (arrowed).

with such a large membranous aneurysm. Large VSDs in this region can also be associated with *aortic regurgitation* due to prolapse of the aortic root into the defect, and this is another reason for performing an aortogram in the complete assessment of a VSD.

Surgical Treatment Treatment of a VSD is most commonly surgical, but small defects may be left for some years (as long as there is no significant pulmonary hypertension) to see if spontaneous closure occurs. During this period, precautions must be taken against the development of infective endocarditis.

It has been common practice in the past to place a *band around the pulmonary artery* as a palliative operation in small infants with large VSDs, so that a definitive closure of the VSD can take place at a later age (often 3 or 4 years). This approach is rapidly giving way to earlier and earlier primary closure of the VSD, which is now done under the age of 1 year in many cases, and in some cases in the first few weeks of life. *Primary closure* is a more complex operation in the very small infant but has the advantage that the pulmonary artery anatomy is not distorted and a second operation is not required. If banding is undertaken, a cardiac angiogram is usually necessary to assess the pulmonary artery anatomy prior to definitive closure, because reconstruction of the pulmonary artery will need to be planned carefully. Angiography of the main pulmonary artery is best performed in the following two views:

1. Steep LAO view (65°) with a 15° caudal angulation
2. Steep cranially tilted (30° if possible) anterior view.

The former view shows the origins of both left and right pulmonary arteries in most cases, and the latter view avoids the foreshortening of the main pulmonary artery seen in the normal anterior view.

Closure of the VSD is usually performed using a prosthetic patch, although sometimes the defect is closed by direct suture. Wherever possible the surgeon will close the defect from an approach via the right atrium and tricuspid valve. This avoids the need for any incision into the ventricle, but underlines the need for accurate diagnosis, because the entire septum cannot be inspected from this approach.

Recent studies using color flow Doppler show that in the early postoperative period there is often leakage through the patch, which soon ceases as the patch endothelializes. The patch itself is usually easy to see in two-dimensional imaging as it is very echogenic.

ATRIAL SEPTAL DEFECT (ASD)

This abnormality can be divided into two major categories, the *ostium* primum ASD (which will be considered separately under the heading of 'Atrioventricular septal defects') and the *ostium secundum* ASD, which is the more common type. The ostium secundum defect is usually at the level of the foramen ovale and does not involve the tissues of the septum primum or the atrioventricular valves. A third form of ASD is less common and is known as the *sinus venosus defect*. This is very high in the atrial septum near the insertion of the superior vena cava. This type of defect is often associated with some form of partially anomalous pulmonary venous drainage.

ASD must be distinguished from *patent foramen ovale*. The latter condition is a normal finding in small infants, because in the first few weeks or months of life the flap valve mechanism across the foramen ovale has not finally fused shut. In abnormalities where the atrial chambers are enlarged, this can cause stretching of the foramen ovale, which can sometimes regress after appropriate treatment. In practical terms, the patent foramen ovale is distinguished from a true ASD by the persisting interatrial pressure difference in the former condition. This can be detected in some adults as an incidental finding, particularly when using color flow Doppler mapping (Fig. 24.13).

The low-pressure shunting that occurs with ASD is usually accommodated very well by the right ventricle, and patients with an isolated ASD very rarely present with significant problems in the early years of life. Presentation later in childhood or adolescence is quite common, when mild abnormalities are detected on routine medical examination or chest X-ray. The *chest X-ray* is usually normal if the pulmonary-to-systemic flow ratio is less than 2:1, but if it exceeds this level there will be pulmonary plethora and cardiac enlargement (see Fig. 24.7). The cardiac enlargement is

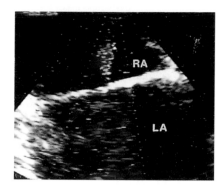

Fig. 24.13   Color flow Doppler study taken from the subcostal position in an adult with mitral valve disease. The patent foramen ovale is seen as an orange jet (toward the transducer). This was an incidental finding. LA, left atrium; RA, right atrium.

mainly due to right atrial and right ventricular dilatation, both these chambers taking increased flow.

From time to time, ASD will present in the middle-aged or elderly, when heart failure or pulmonary hypertension can finally develop and cause symptoms for the first time. In patients with significant pulmonary arterial hypertension (usually the elderly untreated patients), the chest X-ray will show dramatic appearances of centrally dilated pulmonary arteries and peripheral pulmonary vascular 'pruning' (Fig. 24.14). There is a risk of these patients with pulmonary hypertension having a paradoxical embolus from a systemic venous thrombosis. These patients may be inoperable.

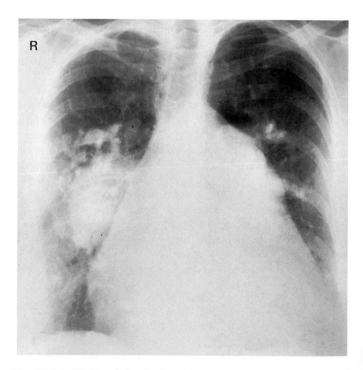

Fig. 24.14   Chest radiograph of an elderly women with an ASD and severe pulmonary hypertension. The main pulmonary artery and hilar pulmonary arteries are very large, with peripheral vascular attenuation.

ASD occurs quite commonly in association with many other cardiac abnormalities, and in some conditions it is an obligatory communication that sustains life, as in the case of tricuspid atresia or total anomalous pulmonary venous drainage.

Non-invasive Diagnosis *Echocardiography* is the cornerstone of diagnosis in this condition. Two-dimensional imaging will show the defect in almost all cases (Fig. 24.15). The typical *secundum defect* is best seen from the subcostal view, which places the interatrial septum at a significant angle to the examining beam and reduces the chance of an artefactual false-positive diagnosis. The latter can occur in the apical view when the interatrial septum lies parallel to the beam and reflects poorly, causing 'drop-out' and an apparent defect. The characteristic dilatation of the right-sided chambers is well seen, and the dominance of the right ventricular volume overload will often be seen as 'paradoxical' septal motion (Fig. 24.16). This is an abnormal anterior movement of the interventricular septum during ventricular systole.

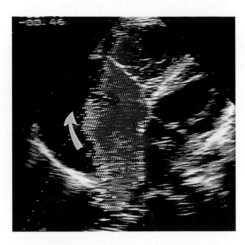

Fig. 24.17 Color flow Doppler study in a patient with a secundum ASD septal defect in the same orientation as in Fig. 24.15. Flow through the defect toward the tricuspid valve is in red (toward the transducer).

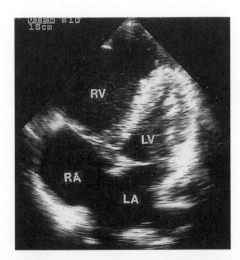

Fig. 24.15 Modified apical four-chamber echocardiogram of a patient with a secundum ASD. The right-sided chambers are considerably enlarged. LA, left atrium; RA, right atrium; LV, left ventricle; RV, right ventricle.

The *ostium primum defect* (also known as partial atrioventricular septal defect) is also well seen, as is atrioventricular valve anatomy. The less common *sinus venosus defect* is harder to visualize, as it lies high in the atrium near the termination of the superior vena cava. Transesophageal studies are often used to demonstrate this difficult lesion. All studies of ASD must be accompanied by a thorough examination of the pulmonary and systemic venous connections, as these are quite often abnormal.

Doppler studies will often complete the diagnostic information. *Color flow mapping* is particularly helpful in the diagnosis of the defect and any venous anomalies (Fig. 24.17). A short accceleration time in pulmonary artery flow can sometimes point to the presence of pulmonary hypertension, as will a high-velocity jet of tricuspid regurgitation. Pulmonary-to-systemic flow ratios can be calculated using Doppler techniques, but these are very time-consuming and are prone to error. Simpler and more accurate non-invasive assessment of the degree of left-to-right shunting can be achieved by first-pass *radionuclide studies*.

Cardiac Catheterization and Angiography A comprehensive echocardiographic diagnosis will often eliminate the need for invasive investigation, but there will be occasions when there is a need for catheterization, either to calculate the shunt ratio accurately or to confirm or exclude some anatomic detail. A left atrial injection of contrast medium is occasionally helpful, but usually angiography is used to assess abnormal venous anatomy or to assess left ventricular function. ASD is of course commonly associated with other forms of congenital heart disease which might require cardiac catheterization for diagnosis.

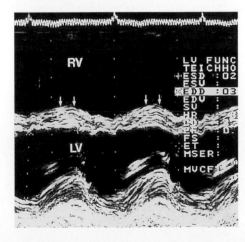

Fig. 24.16 M-mode echocardiogram of a patient with an ASD and right ventricular volume overload. There is 'paradoxical' motion of the interventricular septum (arrowed). LV, left ventricle; RV, right ventricle.

Treatment The condition requires surgical closure in patients with a significant shunt. *Surgical treatment* is relatively straightforward, and so surgery for ASD is often also carried out in patients with relatively mild symptoms, because the operation has a very low mortality and complications in later life can be avoided. *Transcatheter occlusion* of ASD is being developed, and may become practical in the near future.

PATENT DUCTUS ARTERIOSUS (PDA)

The patent arterial duct is a vital part of the fetal circulation, and this communication usually closes within the first few days of life. The ductus arteriosus often remains open rather longer in premature infants, but in the majority of cases it still closes spontaneously. If there is a persistent failure of closure of the duct, then the consequences will depend on the size of the communication. A tiny residual PDA can remain undiagnosed throughout life as it will produce minimal effects. A large PDA will have similar effects to a large VSD, with pressure and volume overloading of the pulmonary circulation. In most diagnosed cases the PDA is closed surgically to avoid the risk of endocarditis, whether or not there is a large shunt. PDA is commonly associated with many other congenital cardiac abnormalities, and no investigation of congenital heart disease is complete without diagnosis or exclusion of a coexisting PDA.

The clinical sign of a continuous murmur is classically associated with a PDA, but *coronary artery fistulas* and a *ruptured sinus of Valsalva* can also give a continuous murmur, and must be distinguished from PDA by echocardiography or angiography.

The *chest X-ray* will show pulmonary plethora if the shunt is large, and there will be mild to moderate cardiac enlargement. The normally smooth outline of the aortic knuckle and upper descending aorta will often be interrupted by the 'bump' of the ductus, but this is often difficult to detect in young infants in whom the normal aorta is hard to visualize. In an older child or adult it is probably true to say that the presence of a well-defined aortic knuckle leading into a straight and uninterrupted descending aorta will almost certainly exclude the presence of a PDA. Later in life there may be some *calcification* present in a PDA. The ascending aorta and aortic arch carry greater flow than normal in this condition, and consequently the aortic knuckle is sometimes enlarged, but this cannot be regarded as a reliable sign.

The presence of a ductal communication can often be lifesaving in neonates with pulmonary atresia. The physiological closure of the ductus will lead to increased cyanosis, and the use of *prostaglandin therapy* is directed toward maintaining ductal patency until a definitive palliative or corrective operation can be performed. In this situation the anatomy of the ductus arteriosus is different to normal, with the angulation of the communication being opposite to normal. This is due to the abnormal ductal flow, being from aorta to pulmonary artery in fetal life.

Non-invasive Imaging *Echocardiography* will show clearly the persistent communication on two-dimensional scanning in many cases. The best view for demonstration of the PDA is a modification of the parasternal short-axis view, sometimes called the '*ductus cut*'. The imaging plane in this view is orientated anatomically through the main pulmonary artery, the left pulmonary artery, the ductus itself and the descending aorta. A PDA can also be imaged from other views, particularly the suprasternal view, which will show the same structures (Fig. 24.18). The images can sometimes be misleading if there is particular prominence of the diverticulum at one or both ends of the ductus arteriosus. The aortic and pulmonary diverticula can both be large even when there is no actual continuity, and thus visualization of complete continuity of the duct on the images is essential for a reliable diagnosis.

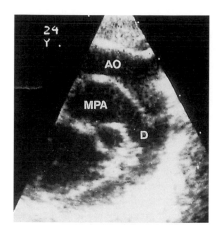

Fig. 24.18 Suprasternal echocardiogram of a patient with transposition of the great arteries and a PDA (D). The great arteries lie parallel in this condition. AO, aorta; MPA, main pulmonary artery. (Courtesy Dr R. Martin.)

Doppler echocardiography is of great value in the diagnosis of this condition. Careful positioning of the pulsed Doppler sample volume in or near the duct will reveal the characteristic continuous turbulent signal of ductal flow. This can also be shown on continuous-wave Doppler (Fig. 24.19), and of course the flow can be mapped clearly using *color flow imaging*. In older patients, imaging of the duct itself often proves difficult, and in this situation Doppler evaluation is of particular importance and is sometimes the only definite sign of the abnormality. Hemodynamic circumstances will affect the nature of ductal flow. In particular, if there is pulmonary hypertension with equal pulmonary and systemic pressures, then ductal flow will be much reduced, and Doppler techniques will be of limited use. In this situation, angiography can also be difficult. There are a number of conditions that will cause unusual flows in the pulmonary arteries, for example pulmonary hypertension or pulmonary valve stenosis, and so the accurate diagnosis of PDA depends on detection of flow in the communication itself, not just an abnormal flow pattern in the pulmonary arteries.

Aortopulmonary window is a rare condition that can present similarly to a large PDA. There is usually a large direct communication from the ascending aorta to the pulmonary artery. Echo-

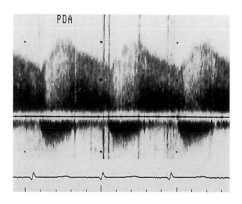

Fig. 24.19 Continuous-wave Doppler study taken from the parasternal position. Continuous flow through the PDA is shown above the baseline—toward the transducer. (Courtesy Dr R. Martin.)

cardiographers must be certain that the condition is not overlooked, and color flow Doppler techniques will doubtless make this easier.

CT scanning and *nuclear medicine* studies have relatively little part to play in the assessment of the condition. *MRI* has an increasing role in the diagnosis of the condition, particularly in larger and adult patients in whom echocardiography may be difficult.

Cardiac Catheterization and Angiography Angiography is a reliable method of diagnosing the condition, and a well-placed aortic injection will show the abnormality. This is often achieved with an arterial catheter, but frequently the venous catheter can be passed via the right heart chambers to the pulmonary artery and then to the aorta via the actual patent ductus. Passage of the catheter through the communication can of course be diagnostic in itself but it is important to advance the catheter well down the descending aorta below the diaphragm to avoid confusion with a position in a lower-lobe pulmonary artery. This method does not show the size of the duct itself, and on occasion a catheter can be passed across the obstructed lumen of a recently closed ductus.

Standard cardiac oblique views, RAO 30° and LAO 60°, are usually best for the demonstration of the abnormality. Ideally, both views are recorded because each has its own advantages. The RAO view clearly separates the main pulmonary artery from the ascending aorta, and is excellent for the detection of very small shunts, but the view may foreshorten the duct itself. The LAO view will usually profile the duct well, but sometimes the superimposition of a large main pulmonary artery and the aorta can obscure detail. Angiographers must be careful not to miss an *aortopulmonary window*, as it can often be out of profile if inappropriate projections are selected and may not be shown at all if the ascending aorta is not opacified.

It is important not to overlook a PDA in the presence of other important left-to-right shunts. In the case of a *large VSD*, a left ventricular injection will produce almost simultaneous opacification of the aorta and pulmonary artery. In these circumstances, the ductal communication can often be hard to diagnose with certainty, and a separate aortic injection is necessary to exclude the condition. *Coarctation of the aorta* is commonly associated with a PDA.

There are variations in the site of the ductus arteriosus which depend on variations in the development of the sixth arch. The ductus can be right-sided, and may occasionally form part of a vascular ring. There may be a bilateral ductus arteriosus in rare cases. Very rarely the ductus itself may become aneurysmal.

Treatment In the majority of cases there is *spontaneous closure*, but in a few children there is a clinical need to close the communication. This is sometimes performed through a left thoracotomy incision, which allows the communication to be ligated and sometimes also divided. *Simple ligation* can sometimes be inadequate, with persistent communication being detectable in later life in a proportion of cases.

In recent years, transcatheter occlusion has become usual. The *Rashkind duct occluder* is a device that takes the form of two small stainless steel 'umbrellas' mounted 'back to back', with foam material fixed to the spokes of each umbrella. In appropriately selected cases the folded device can be loaded into a catheter delivery system, whence it can be introduced into the ductus arteriosus via the right heart chambers. The umbrellas stabilize the device between the aorta and main pulmonary artery (Fig. 24.20). Alternative devices are spiral coils which lie

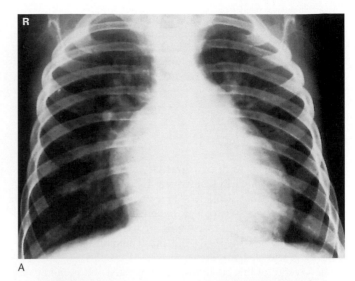

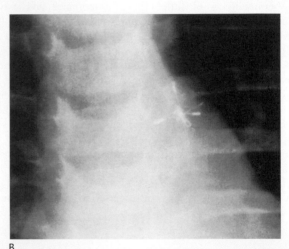

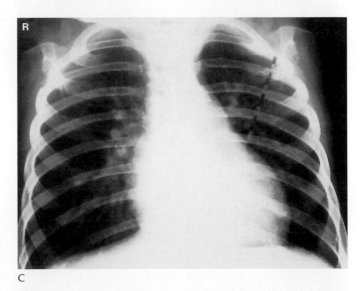

Fig. 24.20 **A.** Chest radiograph of a child with a PDA immediately before closure. The heart is large, and there is pulmonary plethora. **B.** Localized view of the Rashkind duct occluder in position in the same patient. **C.** Chest radiograph in the same patient 24 h after ductal occlusion. The heart has decreased considerably in size.

between aortic and pulmonary diverticula and encourage thrombosis around any communications. The techniques are still new, and can be complicated by accidental displacement of the device, but as experience grows this is likely to be the treatment of choice for most cases of persistent PDA that require closure. There is a small but significant recurrence rate with the devices.

PULMONARY STENOSIS

The most common form of pulmonary stenosis is *isolated pulmonary valve stenosis* in which there is fusion and thickening of the pulmonary valve leaflets. There may also be *infundibular stenosis* with right ventricular hypertrophy causing increased contractility and systolic narrowing of the outflow tract. *Distal pulmonary stenosis* involving the main pulmonary artery or its branches is also recognized.

The severity of this condition varies greatly, and in mild cases the abnormality is of little clinical importance and may not present until late in life or not at all. Many cases of mild pulmonary stenosis present at routine medical examination with a heart murmur or with an abnormal chest radiograph or electrocardiogram.

More severe cases may present with tiredness and breathlessness, and the most severe cases may be associated with cyanosis and heart failure. In cases of moderate to severe stenosis, it is not reduction of cardiac output but the strain on the right side of the heart which causes problems. The *chest X-ray* often shows a prominent main pulmonary artery which is caused by post-stenotic turbulence and consequent dilatation, and the proximal left pulmonary artery is also dilated in many cases because it lies in a direct line with the main pulmonary artery (Fig. 24.21). The right pulmonary artery is not usually so dilated because it

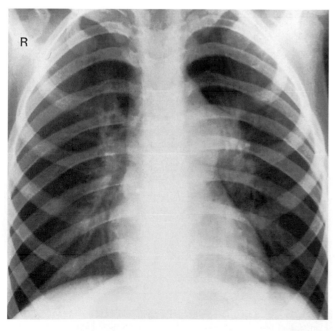

Fig. 24.21 Chest radiograph of a child with pulmonary valve stenosis. The main pulmonary artery and left pulmonary artery are considerably enlarged, but pulmonary vascularity is otherwise normal.

branches quite sharply from the main pulmonary artery and turbulence from the stenotic valve is not carried down into it. Peripheral pulmonary vascularity is normal or slightly oligemic. In cases where infundibular stenosis predominates, the main pulmonary artery may not be recognized as abnormally dilated on the chest X-ray because the turbulence caused by the obstruction is not carried into the main pulmonary artery.

Non-invasive Imaging Diagnosis is usually possible by *echocardiography*, particularly if a Doppler examination with continuous-wave techniques is available. Two-dimensional imaging can be difficult, as the pulmonary valve lies partially behind the left sternal border, but turning the patient well to the left and keeping the transducer close to the sternum will frequently give a satisfactory short-axis view. Good-quality images are needed to distinguish simple leaflet fusion from a thickened and dysplastic valve. *Doppler studies* are the key to diagnosis, not only detecting the high-velocity flow through the stenotic valve but also to quantify the severity of the lesion. Infundibular stenosis (often dynamic with marked systolic narrowing) and pulmonary artery stenosis can both be diagnosed using echocardiography. The pressure drop or 'gradient' across the stenotic valve can be estimated using continuous-wave Doppler measurements.

Cardiac Catheterization and Angiography Contrast medium injection into the right ventricle will nominally give an excellent demonstration of pulmonary valve anatomy, the best two views being the lateral projection and a steeply cranially tilted (20–25°) anterior view. The cranial tilt is necessary to minimize the foreshortening of the infundibulum and main pulmonary artery segment. Passage of the catheter across the valve will of course allow measurement of the pressure drop caused by the stenosis.

Treatment Treatment has changed considerably in recent years. Mild forms of pulmonary stenosis (up to a pressure drop of approximately 40 mmHg) do not normally require surgery. More severe cases have traditionally had *pulmonary valvotomy* performed surgically, but recent interventional techniques have been very successful, and in most cases of pulmonary valve stenosis a *balloon dilatation* technique is now the treatment of choice (Fig. 24.22). Excellent results are obtained using this approach (Fig. 24.23). Occasionally the valve is too dysplastic (thickened, deformed, and irregular) for balloon valvuloplasty to be indicated. Successful balloon valvuloplasty requires careful measurement of the pulmonary valve annulus from the preliminary angiogram and selection of an appropriate-sized balloon, usually slightly larger than the annulus itself. Pulmonary regurgitation may develop or increase after the procedure but it is rarely a problem.

COARCTATION OF THE AORTA

In this condition there is a characteristic shelf-like narrowing of the aorta which usually occurs just beyond the origin of the left subclavian artery. The severity of this narrowing can vary considerably and it is this severity which determines the age of presentation.

Severe coarctation of the aorta can present in the first few days or weeks of life with cardiac enlargement and cardiac failure (Fig. 24.24). Physiological closure of the PDA presents a potential hazard in severe coarctation in infancy, as it may impair renal and other vital perfusion.

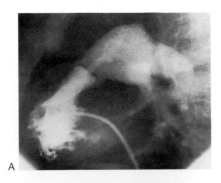

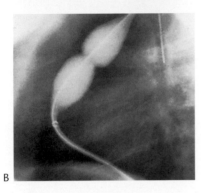

Fig. 24.22 A. Lateral view of a right ventricular angiogram in a child with pulmonary valve stenosis. The doming of the stenotic valve and the central jet of contrast medium are seen. There is poststenotic dilatation of the main pulmonary artery. **B.** Lateral view of pulmonary valve dilatation in the same patient. The indentation in the balloon indicates that the valve is not yet fully dilated.

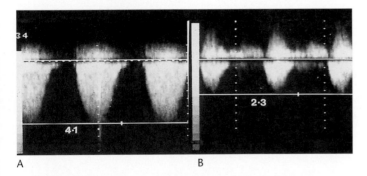

Fig. 24.23 Continuous-wave Doppler traces taken from a patient immediately before and after pulmonary valve dilatation. Peak velocity is indicated (in m/s), and can be used in the modified Bernoulli equation (pressure (in mmHg) = 4 × velocity (in m/s^2)) to show a predilatation pressure drop of 67 mmHg reduced to 21 mmHg.

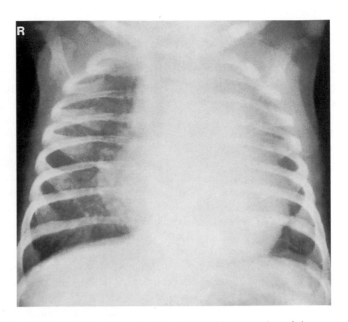

Fig. 24.24 Chest radiograph of an infant with coarctation of the aorta. There is cardiomegaly and evidence of left heart failure.

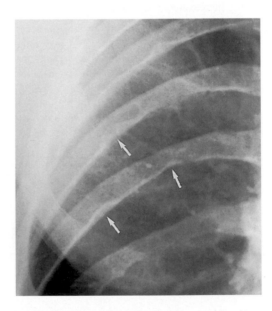

Fig. 24.25 Localized view of the ribs showing notching (arrowed) in an adult patient presenting with coarctation of the aorta.

Lesser degrees of coarctation may present later in life with abnormal physical signs or abnormality on the chest X-ray. The classic late appearances on the chest X-ray are a small or irregular contour of the upper descending aorta and rib notching, caused by the prominent intercostal collateral vessels which are bypassing the narrowing (Fig. 24.25). Rib notching is rare in the first 5 years of life, and it is increasingly common for the condition to be detected and treated before this age. There is an association with abnormalities of the aortic valve, in particular a *bicuspid aortic valve*, which can develop in later life to a stenotic aortic valve.

Coarctation of the aorta has numerous variations in severity, but the site of the coarctation itself can also vary. Occasionally the narrowing can occur between the left common carotid and the left subclavian artery, and in this situation the rib notching is likely to be unilateral, being generated only on the right side from the right subclavian distribution into the right intercostal vessels. Sometimes there is quite severe hypoplasia of the aortic arch, particularly between the left common carotid artery and the left subclavian artery.

Interruption of the aortic arch is the most severe variant of the condition. In this condition both carotid arteries and sometimes one or both subclavian arteries arise from the ascending aorta before the interruption. The PDA supplies the lower half of the body, which becomes severely compromised as the ductus arteriosus closes. There may be a substantial gap between the two parts of the aorta.

Non-invasive Diagnosis   In experienced hands, *echocardiography* is reliable in the diagnosis of the condition, but it becomes increasingly problematic in older patients because of difficult ultrasonic access from the suprasternal notch, the best site for imaging. Care must be taken to avoid misdiagnosis due to the aorta passing out of the plane of the scan. An associated PDA must always be sought. Doppler studies can help by demonstrating the abnormal persistent diastolic flow through the narrowing, but this also depends on good ultrasonic access. The 'gradient' across the coarctation can, in theory, be measured using Doppler techniques, but practical experience has shown this to be somewhat unreliable. *MRI* can be used very successfully to demonstrate coarctation (Fig. 24.26), both with regard to the coarctation itself and also the presence of any major collateral vessels.

In some cases the anatomy of the bypassing collaterals needs to be assessed for surgical planning. This is hard to achieve by echocardiography, and *angiography* is often necessary, although MRI is proving increasingly successful.

Cardiac Catheter and Angiography   Catheter access for an ascending aortic injection of contrast medium to demonstrate the aortic arch and coarctation can sometimes be a problem. A severe coarctation can prevent an arterial catheter from crossing from below, and in older patients without an ASD or VSD, access to the left side of the heart from the right heart chambers may not be possible. Left-sided access may be achieved by trans-septal puncture or by the brachial arterial approach, but these offer a higher risk of complications than usual.

Alternative angiographic approaches may be used. A pulmonary artery injection may be followed through to the left side, and,

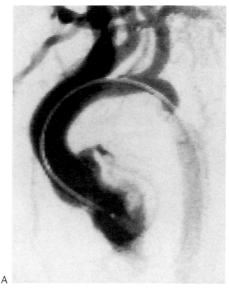

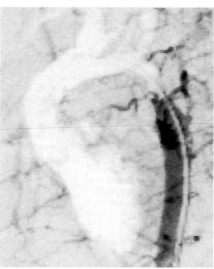

Fig. 24.27   **A.** Digital subtraction study of a left ventriculogram in the LAO projection. A severe coarctation of the aorta is seen in the typical position. **B.** Late image from the study shown in part A shows delayed filling of the descending aorta by collaterals.

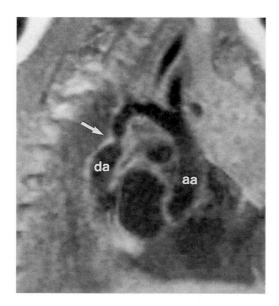

Fig. 24.26   Oblique sagittal gated spin echo MRI scan of a child with coarctation of the aorta (arrowed). aa, ascending aorta; da, descending aorta. (Courtesy of the Trustees of the Bristol MRI Centre.)

with good equipment, excellent details of the coarctation and collateral vessels may be achieved. Digital subtraction angiography offers the opportunity for even better contrast enhancement in this situation (Fig. 24.27). Peripheral or central venous contrast injection causes considerable dilution of contrast medium, and images are not usually of satisfactory quality.

Treatment   There is a long-term risk of severe systemic hypertension in the upper body, and this is the indication for repair even in asymptomatic patients. In severely ill infants the operation is often carried out as an emergency, frequently following ultrasound diagnosis alone.

Surgical repair is carried out by various techniques, which include the incorporation of the left subclavian artery as a flap (Fig. 24.28) or direct anastomosis of the aorta after resection of the narrow segment. Occasionally, prosthetic patch material is

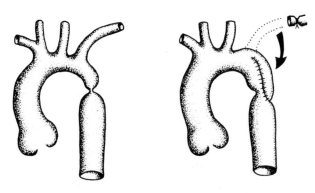

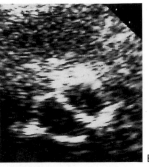

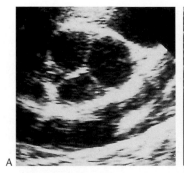

Fig. 24.28 Diagram showing the subclavian flap repair for coarctation of the aorta. (Reproduced from Jordan & Scott 1989, with permission.)

Fig. 24.29 **A.** Short-axis echocardiogram of a normal aortic valve showing three leaflets. **B.** Short axis echocardiogram of a bicuspid aortic valve.

incorporated into the repair. It should be noted, however, that surgical correction of coarctation carries a small but definite risk of paraplegia developing as an operative complication in older patients. Recent attempts at correction using *balloon dilatation* have been attempted, but it has not yet been established as a definitive technique for primary treatment. Balloon dilatation has been more successful in the treatment of a proportion of patients who develop restenosis after initial surgical repair. Repair of aortic interruption is, of course, more complex, and it carries a higher mortality.

AORTIC STENOSIS

Congenital aortic stenosis has a variety of forms, varying from a simple malformation in which the leaflets of the aortic valve remain partially fused, to a complex dysplastic valve which may be bicuspid or even unicuspid. There are also various forms of *subaortic stenosis*, ranging from a simple diaphragm to more complex tubular narrowing or obstructive fibrous tissue in the left ventricular outflow tract. Distinctly different is the dynamic narrowing of the left ventricular outflow tract caused by *hypertrophic cardiomyopathy*.

Supravalvular aortic stenosis occurs above the sinuses of Valsalva and is less common but can nevertheless be considered under the heading of congenital aortic stenosis. This most commonly occurs in *Williams syndrome*, in which there is severe hypoplasia of the ascending aorta above the sinuses of Valsalva. The condition may be associated with vascular abnormalities elsewhere, including peripheral pulmonary artery stenosis and renal artery stenosis. Associated features are a typical *'elfin facies'* and vitamin-D hypersensitivity. In suitable cases, surgery can enlarge the aorta at the point of stenosis.

The degree of obstruction in aortic stenosis is extremely variable, and the severity will determine the mode of presentation. *Severe cases* present in infancy with heart failure and left ventricular dilatation with impaired function. Severe aortic stenosis presenting in early infancy carries a high mortality, and early operation is required to divide the fused commissures. *Milder degrees* of aortic stenosis carry a better prognosis and can be operated on electively in childhood. Recently a number of critical cases have been detected by fetal echocardiography.

The condition can be recognized on *chest X-ray* if there is a dilated ascending aorta due to poststenotic dilatation, but this is usually seen in older children only. Heart failure and cardiomegaly may be recognized in infancy, and in this situation there is little to distinguish the X-ray from that of severe coarctation or other forms of left ventricular failure.

Congenital bicuspid valves are not normally stenotic but they can lead to 'acquired' calcific aortic stenosis in adult life. They are present in up to 2% of the 'normal' population. The abnormality can be recognized clearly on *two-dimensional echocardiography* (Fig. 24.29). There is an association between coarctation of the aorta and congenital bicuspid aortic valve. There is also an increased incidence of 'left dominant' coronary circulation with bicuspid aortic valve.

Non-invasive Diagnosis The diagnosis of aortic stenosis can be made easily with *echocardiography*. *Good-quality* images of the left ventricle and aortic valve are usually possible from standard views. It is important to examine the subaortic and supra-aortic regions as carefully as the valve itself (Fig. 24.30). The most typical type of aortic stenosis shows thin (or only slightly thickened) leaflets that 'dome' in systole due to the narrow opening between the fused commissures. The presence of left ventricular hypertrophy should be noted as well as the overall contractility of the left ventricle. The aortic valve gradient can be measured using *continuous-wave Doppler studies*, the peak velocity of flow across the valve being used to calculate the peak

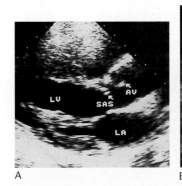

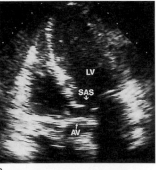

Fig. 24.30 **A.** Parasternal long-axis echocardiogram showing an obstructive subaortic membrane. **B.** Apical four-chamber echocardiogram of the same case showing the obstructive subaortic membrane. LV, left ventricle; AV, aortic valve; SAS, subaortic stenosis.

pressure drop using the modified Bernoulli formula. *Color flow Doppler examination* will show the stenotic jet, any subaortic obstruction, and any coexisting aortic regurgitation.

The detail of qualitative and quantitative information available from echocardiography means that surgery can often be performed on the basis of a good ultrasound study.

Cardiac Catheterization and Angiography   This is still an important technique, and is used to measure valve 'gradient' and left ventricular pressures. Left ventricular angiography will allow assessment of ventricular function as well as assessing the function of the mitral valve. A supra-aortic injection is usually performed to detect or exclude coexistent aortic regurgitation.

Left ventriculography is best performed in RAO 30° projection and LAO 60° with 20° cranial tilt.

The cranial tilt allows better profiling of the left ventricular outflow tract to exclude subaortic stenosis. Aortography is best performed in the same projections but without the cranial tilt.

Treatment   Minor degrees of stenosis can be observed for many years till there are signs of deleterious left ventricular effects. Echocardiography is useful as a routine check for early signs of left ventricular dilatation or impairment. Valve replacement is not practical in small infants and children as there are no suitable prostheses. Thus, severe cases in early life are usually treated by *surgical valvotomy*. This can be very successful, but will almost always be followed by *valve replacement* in later life. Transfer of the pulmonary valve to aortic position with the implantation of a homograft replacement in the pulmonary position is another surgical option. The introduction of *balloon valvuloplasty* has altered the management of some cases of congenital aortic stenosis, and the procedure has been life-saving in some critically ill infants. There are potential complications with the technique, however, one of which is the development of severe aortic regurgitation.

The surgical treatment of a localized diaphragm and a tubular hypoplasia of the outflow tract are substantially different and vary from case to case. Interventional techniques have played little part as yet in the treatment of subaortic stenosis.

TETRALOGY OF FALLOT

This abnormality is a complex of four related abnormalities which are part of a fundamental malformation of the heart. A large ventricular septal defect (1) is associated with malalignment of the great arteries, such that the aortic root overrides the ventricular septal defect (2) and is thus partly related to the right ventricle. There is associated stenosis of the right ventricular outflow tract (infundibulum) and pulmonary valve (3), together with a variable degree of hypoplasia of the pulmonary valve annulus and pulmonary arteries. The infundibular stenosis may have a dynamic component to the obstruction, being maximal in late systole. Finally there is right ventricular hypertrophy (4), which develops as a response to the systemic pressure in the right ventricle. In some cases the hypertrophied muscle bundles in the right ventricle can produce an additional intraventricular obstruction.

This abnormality is expressed in different ways, which depend mainly on the severity of the pulmonary stenosis. In mild cases of pulmonary stenosis the abnormality behaves much like a simple ventricular septal defect, with possible benefit caused by the restriction of blood flow into the lungs (as in pulmonary artery banding). These patients form the *acyanotic* end of the spectrum. More typically, presenting cases are *cyanosed* because the pulmonary stenosis is sufficiently severe to restrict pulmonary blood flow. These children will present in childhood with varying degrees of cyanosis and fainting spells on exertion, which are usually caused by increasing infundibular obstruction to pulmonary flow with increasing cardiac work.

The most severe end of the spectrum is represented by critical pulmonary stenosis and severe pulmonary artery hypoplasia with very little flow into the lungs through the pulmonary valve. In this situation life must be sustained by alternative flow into the pulmonary vascularity, and this occurs by *ductal flow* or by *aortopulmonary collaterals* that develop in early life. The severe cases in this spectrum will present shortly after birth with progressive cyanosis as the ductus arteriosus closes. These babies will need urgent palliation by systemic shunting to maintain pulmonary blood flow or early primary correction.

Approximately 25% of patients with tetralogy of Fallot (or pulmonary atresia and ventricular septal defect—a closely related condition) have a *right-sided aortic arch*. This type of right arch is usually associated with mirror imaging branching (i.e. left brachiocephalic, right common carotid, and right subclavian in order of branching).

The chest X-ray is often not classical (see Fig. 24.37A), but in the classic developed appearance there will be concavity in the left heart border in the region of the hypoplastic main pulmonary artery, upward prominence of the cardiac apex due to the distortion by the large right ventricle, pulmonary oligemia, and in some cases a right-sided aortic arch (Fig. 24.31). While these signs are almost diagnostic, many cases of tetralogy of Fallot have a nearly normal chest film.

Non-invasive Imaging   *Echocardiography* is very useful in diagnosing the condition, and will show the ventricular septal defect, the overriding aorta, and the right ventricular hypertrophy very clearly. The pulmonary valve and pulmonary artery anatomy is often more difficult to assess by ultrasound, as these areas lie deeply and are partially surrounded by air, but it is still possible to

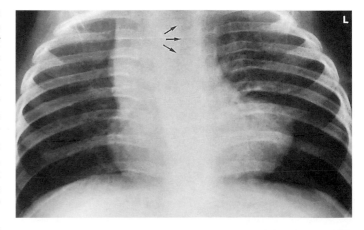

Fig. 24.31 Chest radiograph of an infant with tetralogy of Fallot. The trachea is indented by the right-sided aortic arch (arrowed), the cardiac apex is angled upward, and the lung fields are oligemic.

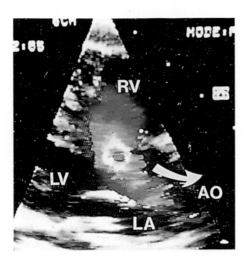

Fig. 24.32 Color flow Doppler study in a child with tetralogy of Fallot. In this parasternal long-axis view here is right-to-left flow from the right ventricle (RV) to the aorta (AO). The majority of the flow is encoded blue (away from the transducer), but the fastest moving central flow shows aliasing (orange). LV, left ventricle; LA, left atrium.

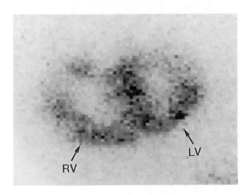

Fig. 24.33 Thallium-201 scan in the left anterior view. In this adult patient with long-standing tetralogy of Fallot without complete correction there is marked right ventricular hypertrophy, with activity equalling that in the left ventricular wall.

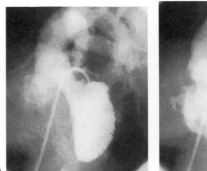
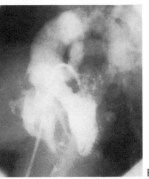

Fig. 24.34 **A.** Cranially angled LAO left ventriculogram of a child with tetralogy of Fallot. There is early passage of contrast to the right ventricle across the VSD. Aortic override is seen. **B.** Later image from the same study. The right ventricle is now well filled. The hypoplastic pulmonary arteries can be seen.

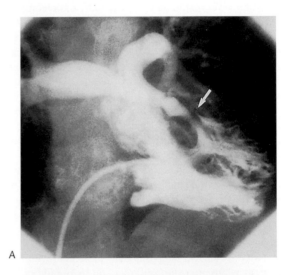

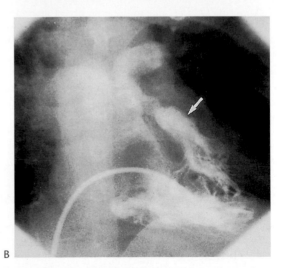

Fig. 24.35 **A.** Cranially angled anterior view of a right ventriculogram of a patient with tetralogy of Fallot. Severe infundibular stenosis is seen in systole (arrowed). The hypoplastic pulmonary annulus and main pulmonary artery can be seen. **B.** Diastolic image from the same study. The right ventricular infundibulum is now much wider (arrowed).

measure the proximal parts of the vessels in many cases. The right ventricular outflow gradient and the pulmonary valve gradient can both be estimated using *Doppler techniques*, but there are many possible inaccuracies due to the many levels at which obstruction can occur. Right-to-left shunting across the VSD can be seen on color-flow Doppler examination (Fig. 24.32). Coronary anatomy cannot usually be assessed noninvasively.

Other non-invasive imaging techniques have little to add in most cases, but there are occasional applications, for example the occasional use of *thallium-201 scanning* to demonstrate the degree of right ventricular hypertrophy (Fig. 24.33).

Cardiac Catheterization and Angiography This is often required in addition to echocardiography because precise assessment of anatomy is essential in surgical planning. The size of the pulmonary valve annulus as well as the size and anatomy of the more distal pulmonary arteries must be determined.

Left ventricular angiography should be performed in views similar to those selected for a simple VSD (Fig. 24.34), but a steeper LAO view (e.g. 70°) is sometimes helpful, due to the rotation of the heart produced by the large right ventricle. Right ventriculography is best performed in a very steep LAO (e.g. 80–90°) and a cranially tilted (20°) anterior view to show the right ventricular outflow and pulmonary valve (Fig. 24.35). An aortogram performed in 30° RAO and 60° LAO oblique views will show a PDA, aortopulmonary collaterals, aortic arch anatomy, and brachiocephalic and coronary anatomy.

The most common *coronary artery variant* occurring with tetralogy of Fallot is the anomalous origin of the left anterior descending coronary artery from the right coronary artery. This vital artery runs over the surface of the right ventricle just where the surgeon might make the incision to enlarge the right ventricular outflow tract, and so it is extremely important to detect this in advance, either by good-quality opacification of the aortic root or occasionally by selective coronary arteriography.

Treatment   Surgical treatment will depend on the severity of the condition, but the long-term aim will be total correction by closure of the VSD (using an oblique patch) and reconstruction of the right ventricular outflow tract and pulmonary arteries. In the latter situation a transannular patch may be incorporated into the repair to widen the outflow. In most cases the pulmonary valve function is destroyed by the reconstruction of the right ventricular outflow tract, but the pulmonary regurgitation that follows appears to be of little clinical significance.

In severe cases presenting in early life a palliative shunt may be performed if the child is too small or too ill for definitive repair. This is usually achieved with a *Blalock shunt* from the subclavian artery to the pulmonary artery. The classic procedure involves division of the subclavian artery and forming an end-to-side anastomosis with the ipsilateral pulmonary artery. The more recent 'modified Blalock' shunt uses an interposed prosthetic graft which allows continued patency of the subclavian artery (Fig. 24.36).

Postoperative appearances on the chest X-ray may be characteristic. Not only should the pulmonary oligemia revert to normal, but the right ventricular outflow tract and main pulmonary artery may look unusually large, due to the presence of an outflow patch (Fig. 24.37). In cases palliated with a Blalock shunt there may be a difference in pulmonary blood flow in the two lungs, particularly if anatomic abnormalities prevent satisfactory central connection between the two pulmonary arteries. The Blalock shunt itself may cause troublesome narrowing of the pulmonary artery into which it is inserted and this can be recognized on angiography (Fig. 24.38).

Interventional techniques do not as yet have a major part to play in the treatment of this condition although some centers have used *balloon dilatation* to palliate the pulmonary stenosis.

TRANSPOSITION OF THE GREAT ARTERIES (TGA)

D-loop Transposition   The common form of this abnormality is D-loop transposition, in which the atrial and ventricular anatomy is normal. There is a simple reversal of connection of the great arteries, with the aorta arising from the morphologically right ventricle and the pulmonary artery arising from the morphologically left ventricle. The exact orientation of the great arteries varies, but the most common arrangement is with the aortic valve arising from a high anterior position from the right ventricle, and

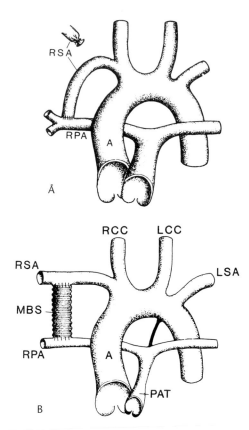

Fig. 24.36   **A.** Diagram showing the classic Blalock shunt. A, aorta; RPA, right pulmonary artery; RSA, right subclavian artery. **B.** Diagram showing a modified Blalock shunt. MBS, modified Blalock shunt; RCC, right common carotid artery; LCC, left common carotid artery; LSA, left subclavian artery; PAT, pulmonary artery trunk. (Both diagrams reproduced from Jordan & Scott 1989, with permission.)

the pulmonary valve arising from the lower posterior position above the left ventricular outflow tract. There is loss of the normal arrangement where the right ventricular outflow twists around the left ventricular outflow. The two great arteries run parallel upward from their respective chambers (Fig. 24.39). This leads to the formation of a relatively narrow pedicle which can frequently be recognized on the chest X-ray.

These infants usually present in the first few weeks of life with cyanosis and breathlessness. Cyanosis depends on the exact degree of mixing at the atrial or ventricular level. Although the condition can be diagnosed simply by echocardiography, cardiac catheterization is commonly performed so that the Rashkind balloon septostomy can be performed at the same time. In this technique an inflated balloon is used to rupture the thin part of the septum primum covering the foramen ovale in order to improve the atrial mixing and thus allow a higher proportion of oxygenated blood to pass from the left atrium to the right atrium and right ventricle, and then to the systemic circulation. This procedure has been performed under echocardiographic control (Fig. 24.40).

The *chest X-ray* is often, but not always, characteristic. The heart is slightly enlarged and rounded, and there is pulmonary plethora. The pedicle remains narrow because the main pulmonary artery is behind the aorta (Fig. 24.41). The condition may give

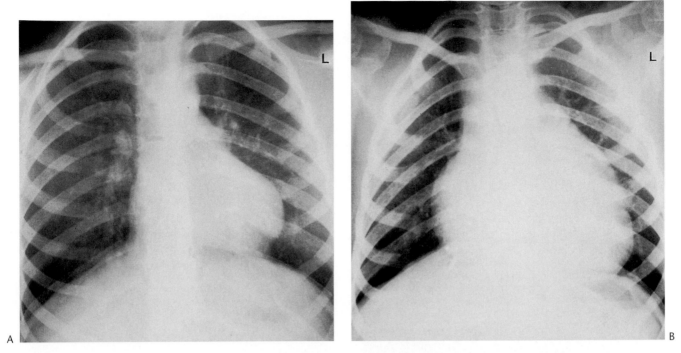

Fig. 24.37 **A.** Preoperative chest radiograph of a child with classic tetralogy of Fallot. The appearances of mild oligemia and mild pulmonary artery hypoplasia do not allow definitive diagnosis from this film. **B.** Postoperative chest radiograph of the same patient. The left heart border is much more prominent, mainly due to the right ventricular outflow patch.

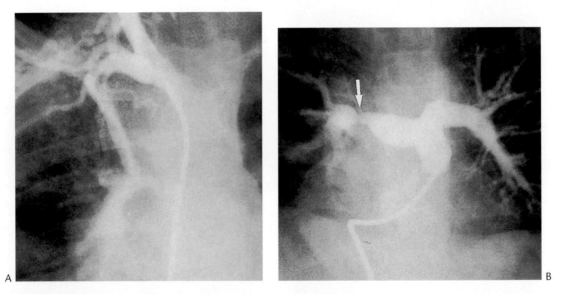

Fig. 24.38 **A.** Anterior view of a selective angiogram of a right Blalock shunt. The right pulmonary artery is opacified. **B.** Anterior view of a pulmonary arteriogram in the same patient. There is a severe stenosis at the site of insertion of the Blalock shunt.

a similar appearance on chest X-ray to truncus arteriosus, where there is again loss of the normal twisting arrangement of the main pulmonary artery around the aorta. There are many associated conditions, the most common of which are *VSD*, *PDA* (see Fig. 24.18), *coarctation of the aorta*, and *pulmonary* (or *subpulmonary*) *stenosis*, the last being particularly important as it can be difficult to treat surgically.

L-loop Transposition This abnormality of the great arteries is distinctly different to the more usual D-loop TGA, but it still conforms to the morphological definition of transposition (or ventriculoarterial discordance). This condition is also known as 'anatomically corrected transposition' or just 'corrected transposition'. The cardiac apex is normally directed to the left, but the morphologically left ventricle lies anterior and to the right

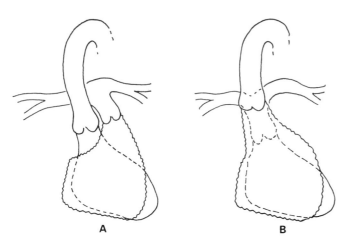

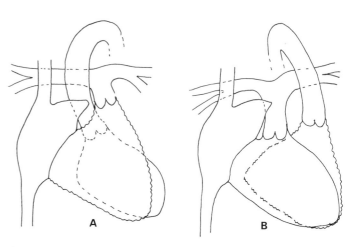

Fig. 24.39 **A.** Diagram showing normal great arterial connections in the anterior view. The morphological left ventricle (smooth outline) lies posteriorly to the morphological right ventricle (wavy outline) as shown by the interrupted line. **B.** Diagram showing connections in D-transposition of the great arteries in the anterior view. Compare with part A. The great arteries have an anteroposterior relationship, which gives the narrow pedicle.

Fig. 24.42 **A.** Normal cardiac connections in the anterior view. The morphological left ventricle (smooth outline) lies posterior to the morphological right ventricle (wavy outline) as shown by the interrupted line. **B.** Connections in L-transposition of the great arteries ('corrected transposition'). The morphological right ventricle (wavy line) lies behind the morphological left ventricle (smooth line) as shown by the interrupted line. The aorta has a leftward origin, which accounts for the long curved left heart border seen in some cases.

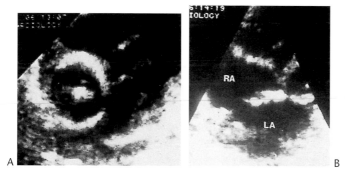

of the posterior ventricle, which is of right morphology. Visceroatrial situs is normal, which means that there is atrioventricular discordance as well as ventriculoarterial discordance (Fig. 24.42). Thus the abnormal connections result in a *physiologically corrected circulation*. Patients with this abnormality will usually have symptoms only if there is an associated abnormality, and the symptoms, treatment, and prognosis will all depend on the nature of the additional malformations. Common associations are *VSD* and *conduction abnormalities*.

Fig. 24.40 **A.** Subcostal echocardiogram showing a Rashkind balloon being drawn from the right atrium (RA) to the left atrium (LA). to rupture the atrial septum. **B.** Echocardiogram of the same patient, taken immediately afterward, showing an ASD created by the balloon septostomy. (Courtesy Dr R. Martin.)

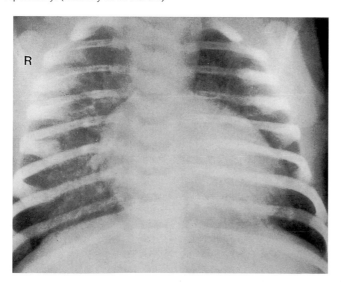

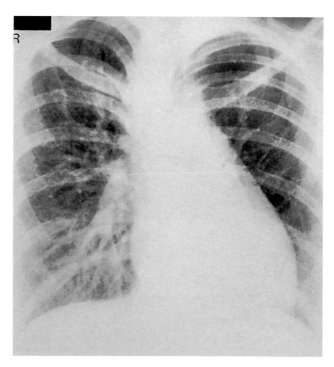

Fig. 24.41 Chest radiograph of an infant with D-transposition of the great arteries. The pedicle (mediastinum) is narrow, and there is cardiomegaly and pulmonary plethora.

Fig. 24.43 Chest radiograph of a patient with L-transposition of the great arteries. There is a long smooth curve to the left heart border due to the abnormal leftward origin of the aorta.

The *chest X-ray* may show a characteristic long curve to the left heart border due to the abnormal leftward origin of the aorta (Fig. 24.43) but this is not reliable in all cases as the positions of the great arteries are somewhat variable. A significant proportion of these patients have chest X-rays indistinguishable from normal.

Non-invasive Imaging *Echocardiographic* diagnosis is relatively straightforward in both types of TGA, but care must be taken to identify correctly the two parallel great arteries as they may not lie in typical positions. The aorta can be identified specifically if the vessel is traced up to the brachiocephalic artery origins. It is essential to avoid the pitfall of assuming which great artery is which simply by position. Two-dimensional imaging will show the smaller left ventricle in D-loop TGA, which pumps to the pulmonary circuit, and the reversed curve of the interventricular septum will usually be apparent (Fig. 24.44). Associated conditions must be sought. In the case of L-loop TGA, the reversal of the morphologically left and right ventricles can be demonstrated by the reversed insertions of the antrioventricular valves (Fig. 24.45).

Cardiac Catheterization and Angiography Angiography will show clearly the abnormal connections (Fig. 24.46) and will also

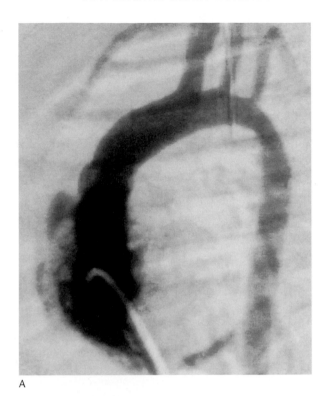

A

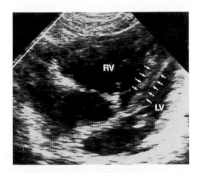

Fig. 24.44 Subcostal echocardiogram of a patient with D-transposition of the great arteries. The morphological right ventricle (RV) is much larger than the morphological left ventricle (LV), and the interventricular septum (arrowed) is curved toward the left ventricle.

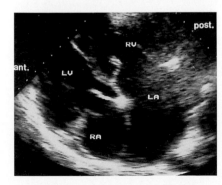

Fig. 24.45 Modified apical four-chamber view in a patient with L-transposition of the great arteries. The morphological left ventricle (LV) lies anteriorly and the morphological right ventricle (RV) lies posteriorly, as shown by the insertions of their respective atrioventricular valves. The tricuspid valve in the right ventricle is inserted more apically than the mitral valve. ant., anterior; post., posterior; RA, right atrium; LA, left atrium. (Compare the valve insertions with the diagrams in Figs 24.10C and 24.50A.)

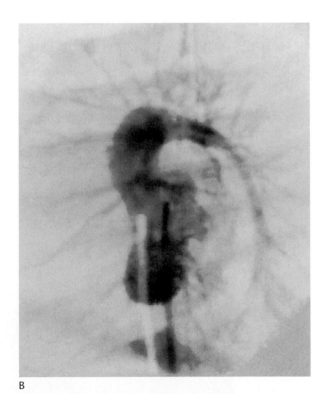

B

Fig. 24.46 **A.** Digital subtraction angiogram of a right ventricular injection recorded in the anterior oblique projection. The anteriorly placed morphological right ventricle gives rise to the aorta, indicating D-transposition of the great arteries. **B.** Digital subtraction left ventriculogram of the same patient and in the same projection. The pulmonary artery arises from the morphological left ventricle.

be useful for clarifying details of anatomy concerning associated anomalies. It is again important to assess *coronary anatomy* for surgical planning, particularly when the great arterial switch procedure is being contemplated. Left ventriculography is probably best for assessment of possible VSDs, even though the cavity is usually at a lower pressure than the right ventricle. This is because of the relatively simpler contours of the morphological left ventricle. It is also essential to examine the left ventricular outflow to exclude obstruction, and this is best achieved using a 20° cranially tilted LAO 60° projection which profiles the outflow well. Right ventriculography in standard oblique views (LAO 60° and RAO 30°) will confirm the diagnosis, show right ventricular function, and demonstrate the coronary arteries. An aortic injection may be helpful to exclude a PDA and to show coronary anatomy in more detail.

Treatment Initial palliation by *Rashkind septostomy* is frequently performed in the neonatal period as described above. Definitive surgical treatment is of two types. The more traditional approach has been to use an *atrial baffle operation* (Mustard or Senning) in which the venous returns are redirected at atrial level so that systemic venous return is directed to the left ventricle and pulmonary artery with pulmonary venous return being directed to the right ventricle and aorta via an intra-atrial conduit (Fig. 24.47). This operation provides a satisfactory physiological circulation but it leaves the right ventricle performing the systemic pumping function, and this can from time to time cause problems in later life. There are also problems with stenosis developing in the surgically formed systemic venous pathways, particularly in the earlier Mustard procedure in which a large prosthetic patch is incorporated into the atrial repair (Fig. 24.48). The Senning procedure makes better use of the native tissues.

Although the atrial baffle procedure is not commonly performed today, there are many adolescents and adults with this operative anatomy who may need further investigation or surgery.

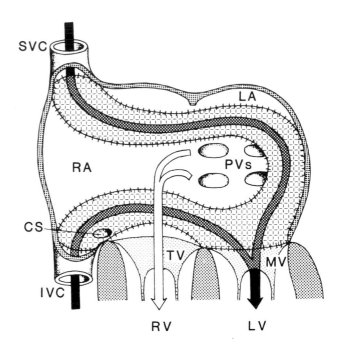

Fig. 24.47 Mustard procedure for D-transposition of the great arteries. A prosthetic intra-atrial conduit leads the systemic venous return from the superior vena cava (SVC) and inferior vena cava (IVC) to the left ventricle (LV) through the mitral valve (MV). Flow from the pulmonary veins (PVs) passes over the conduit to reach the right ventricle (RV) through the tricuspid valve (TV). RA, right atrium; LA, left atrium, CS, coronary sinus.

A more recent approach has been to use the *great arterial switch operation*. This is complicated by the need to transpose the coronary arteries as well as the great arteries themselves (Fig. 24.49). This procedure has superseded the atrial baffle procedure, with low operative mortality. The great arterial switch operation

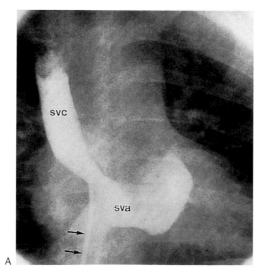
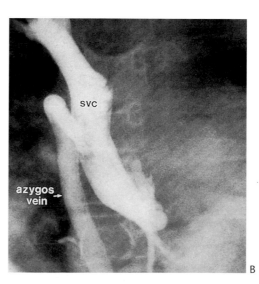

Fig. 24.48 **A.** Anterior view of an angiogram performed with the venous catheter (arrowed) passed to the superior vena cava (svc) in a patient with a previous Mustard operation. Contrast medium flows to the systemic venous atrium (sva) before its passage to the left ventricle. **B.** Similar angiogram to that in part A, but there is severe postoperative narrowing at the point of entry of the superior vena cava to the systemic venous atrium. Flow bypasses the obstruction through a dilated azygos vein.

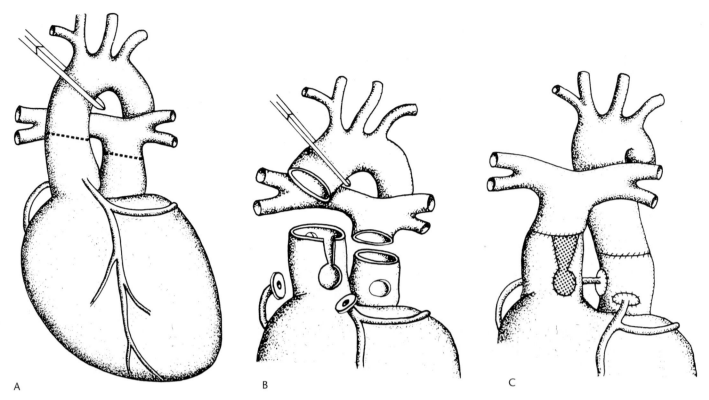

A   B   C

Fig. 24.49 **A.** Cross-clamping of the aorta prior to the great arterial switch procedure for D-transposition of the great arteries. **B.** Division of the great arteries and excision of the origins of the coronary arteries with a small 'button' of aortic wall. **C.** Re-anastomosis of the great arteries and coronary arteries. Systemic arterial blood flows into the coronaries from the newly created 'aortic root', previously the main pulmonary artery. (Reproduced from Jordan & Scott 1989, with permission.)

cannot be performed in patients where the morphologically left ventricle has become accustomed to functioning at low pressure over a long period. The procedure should thus be performed in the first few days or weeks of life or later in life in those patients with a large VSD and equalization of the ventricular pressures. In cases where the left ventricle has adapted to a low pressure, some surgeons have 'trained' it by performing pulmonary artery banding some time before a 'switch' procedure.

If there is D-loop TGA with a large VSD, the *Rastelli procedure* may be indicated. In this operation the VSD is closed with an oblique patch, directing left ventricular flow to the aorta through the VSD. An external conduit, sometimes with a prosthetic or homograft valve, is used to connect the right ventricle to the main pulmonary artery. In this way, normal circulation is effectively reconstituted.

ATRIOVENTRICULAR SEPTAL DEFECT (AVSD)

This group of conditions has also been known as *atrioventricular canal defect*. All the variations of the condition have the same fundamental cardiac abnormality. The base of the interventricular septum in the region of the membranous septum is normally in continuity with the atrial septum primum. This central portion of the cardiac structure is missing in all types of atrioventricular septal defect. The *partial* type of AVSD results in only an interatrial communication, and leads to the so-called 'ostium primum' ASD. The total AVSD leads to interventricular and interatrial communications with a large common atrioventricular valve. There is also an '*intermediate*' type in which the interventricular communication is relatively small, due to partial tethering of the common atrioventricular valve to the septal crest.

Figure 24.50 shows the difference between the normal heart, partial AVSD and complete AVSD, comparing them with a secundum ASD.

The atrioventricular valves are commonly malformed and produce regurgitation of varying degrees. This is not invariably present, but when it is, it will lead to exacerbation of any symptoms produced by left-to-right shunting. In the case of the partial defect (ostium primum ASD) the anterior leaflet of the mitral valve has a cleft, which can be an important cause of regurgitation.

There is an increased association of this condition with Down's syndrome. The presentation varies, depending on the precise nature of the abnormality, but tends to be earlier and more severe than with conventional ASDs and VSDs of similar size. There is no specific abnormality that can be detected on chest X-ray to differentiate these conditions from the more usual type of ASDs or VSDs, although the cardiac enlargement, pulmonary plethora, and cardiac failure are often all more prominent. The presence of only 11 pairs of ribs may be a clue to an underlying Down's syndrome etiology.

Non-invasive Diagnosis *Echocardiography* is the key to diagnosis in this range of conditions. The atrioventricular valve anatomy can clearly be seen (Fig. 24.51), and the presence of a

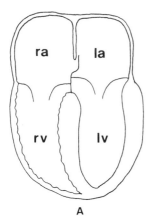
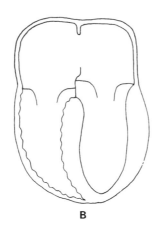
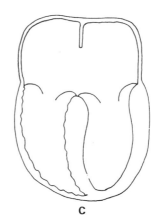
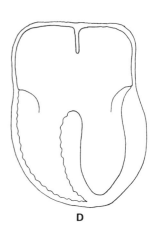

A   B   C   D

Fig. 24.50 **A**. Normal relationships of the interventricular and interatrial septa with the atrioventricular valves. The atrioventricular valves are inserted into the septum primum (thin line). ra, right atrium; las left atrium; rv, right ventricle; lv, left ventricle. **B**. Ostium secundum ASD. The atrioventricular valves and left ventricular outflow tract are normal. **C**. Ostium primum ASD. The septum primum is absent and the atrioventricular valves are inserted in a low position into the crest of the muscular interventricular septum. **D**. Total AVSD. A large common valve separates the atrial cavities from the ventricular cavities. There is an ostium primum ASD and a large VSD in continuity.

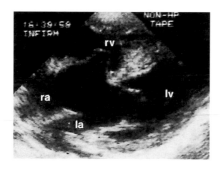

Fig. 24.51 Subcostal echocardiogram showing an ostium primum ASD defect lying between the left atrium (la) and the right atrium (ra). There is no ventricular septal defect between the left ventricle (lv) and the right ventricle (rv).

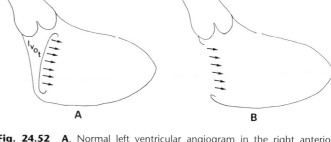

A   B

Fig. 24.52 **A**. Normal left ventricular angiogram in the right anterior oblique projection. Diastolic inflow does not wash out contrast medium lying below the aortic root in the left ventricular outflow tract (lvot). **B**. Left ventricular angiogram performed in a patient with an AVSD. The normal left ventricular outflow region is missing due to the absent septum primum, and so the contrast medium in the subaortic region is washed out by the incoming mitral flow. This produces the frequently misinterpreted 'goose-neck' appearance.

ventricular component to the defect is usually obvious. There is often considerable enlargement of the right-sided cardiac chambers, and the right atrium may be particularly large if there is accompanying atrioventricular valve regurgitation. *Doppler studies* will clearly demonstrate the presence of atrioventricular valve regurgitation, and this is particularly well seen on *color flow studies*. This regurgitation is more commonly seen through the mitral valve in ostium primum ASD, and the regurgitant jet is often directed across the interatrial defect to the right atrium.

Cardiac Catheterization and Angiography Angiography is also capable of demonstrating the anatomy clearly. The most obvious abnormality seen on angiography is the absence of the usual left ventricular outflow tract. The mitral valve hinges directly from beneath the aortic root (Fig. 24.52), and when open creates a distinct appearance that has been likened to a 'goose-neck', a misleading term that is open to misinterpretation; it does not indicate narrowing of the left ventricular outflow tract in systole but merely reflects the washout of contrast medium during ventricular diastole as the abnormally positioned mitral valve is open.

Views can be the same as for assessing a straightforward VSD, but the large right-sided chambers may necessitate a more steeply angled LAO view to profile the basal septum. A conventional LAO view will show the common valve well as the non-opaque atrial blood passing through it, but a cranial tilt will aid in exclusion of additional defects and can help in detecting small interventricular communications in the 'intermediate' type. Both the cleft mitral valve and variable degrees of mitral prolapse are well shown on angiography. Atrioventricular valve regurgitation is well assessed by angiography, but it should be remembered that the catheter may have been passed into the left ventricle through the valve and so might itself produce regurgitation.

Treatment Surgery in this condition is somewhat more complex than with conventional ASDs or VSDs as the repair usually involves some form of reconstruction of the atrioventricular valves as well as patch closure of one or both septal defects. There is no place for interventional therapy in this condition at present.

PULMONARY ATRESIA

The presence or absence of a VSD with pulmonary atresia will markedly affect the expression of the condition.

Pulmonary Atresia with VSD In these circumstances the anomaly is essentially the same as a very severe form of tetralogy of Fallot. The obstructed outflow of the right ventricle, together with the usual override of the aorta, means that the right ventricle can empty into the aorta, although it must do this at the same systemic pressure as the left ventricle. Flow thus continues through the right ventricle, and the chamber remains large and its walls become hypertrophied due to the systemic pressure in it. The pulmonary arteries are often very small, and they receive their blood supply from the PDA initially and then subsequently through aortopulmonary collateral vessels of various sorts.

The *chest X-ray* shows a slightly enlarged heart, often with a slightly upturned apex due to the right ventricular enlargement; the pulmonary bay is small and the lung fields are oligemic. There is a right aortic arch in about 25% of cases (Fig. 24.53). In older patients the multiplicity of aortopulmonary collaterals can give a complex vascular pattern, particularly near the hilar regions, and this can sometimes be mistaken for pulmonary plethora. Palliation with various types of shunt is often required in early life, and this may give rise to uneven vascularity in the lungs (Fig. 24.54).

Angiography is commonly required in the diagnosis of this condition because successful definitive surgery depends on careful planning of a reconstructed outflow from the right ventricle to the pulmonary arteries, which themselves often need reconstruction. It is usually not possible to determine all the details of the anatomy of the hypoplastic pulmonary arteries and the collaterals

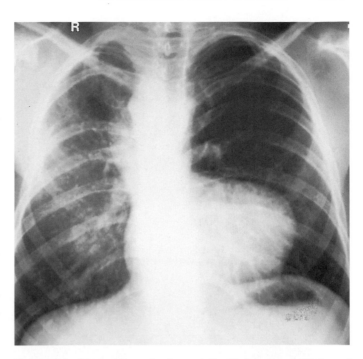

Fig. 24.54 Chest radiograph of an adult with long-term palliation of pulmonary atresia. There is a right-sided aortic arch and an upturned cardiac apex. The vascularity in the right lung is more prominent due to the presence of a right-sided shunt.

using echocardiography. A good-quality aortogram, together with a series of selective angiograms to different collaterals, is usually required. In difficult cases where there is very poor collateral flow to the pulmonary arteries it may be helpful to perform a wedged pulmonary venous injection to opacify the hypoplastic pulmonary arteries. It is important that comprehensive selective angiography is carried out as there may be many sites of origin of collaterals, both from the aorta and the brachiocephalic arteries.

Surgery may be similar to that required for a severe form of the tetralogy of Fallot, but this is only possible if there is a reasonably sized pulmonary artery. In some cases, complex reconstructions of hypoplastic pulmonary arteries are attempted, but often long-term palliation with multiple shunting procedures is the only option. In some cases a central pulmonary artery is reconstructed by 'unifocalization' of the distal pulmonary vessels. If the main pulmonary artery is of good size, the VSD may be closed and an external conduit, usually with a valve, is placed from the right ventricle to the pulmonary artery, *the Rastelli procedure* (Fig. 24.55).

Pulmonary Atresia with Intact Ventricular Septum In this situation there is no outlet for the right ventricle, and thus no way that it can decompress. The cavity is usually very small but often generates very high pressures (suprasystemic), especially if there is a small but functionally competent tricuspid valve. Under these circumstances the unusual problem of abnormal coronary communications can occur. Blood may shunt from right to left through the abnormal vessels, and this can cause myocardial ischemia and sometimes infarction. The *chest X-ray* will show a small pulmonary segment and pulmonary oligemia, but the cardiac contour will show a more rounded left ventricular contour

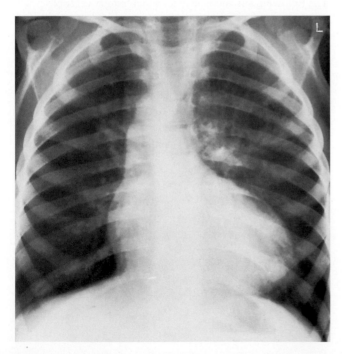

Fig. 24.53 Chest radiograph of a child with pulmonary atresia and a VSD. There is a right-sided aortic arch indenting the trachea which accentuates the concave pulmonary bay. The left heart border does not show an upturned apex as seen in Fig. 24.54.

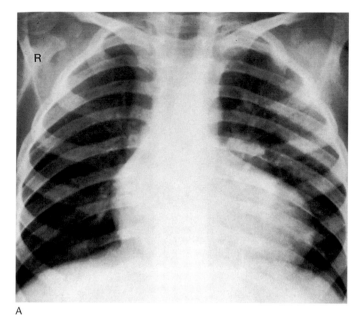

R

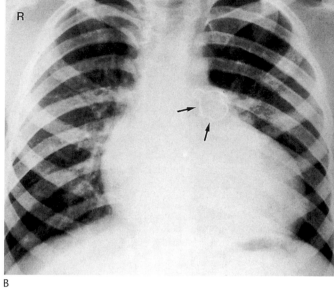

R

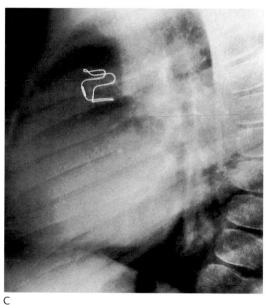

C

Fig. 24.55 **A**. Chest radiograph of a child with pulmonary atresia and a left-sided aortic arch. **B**. Chest radiograph of the same patient following closure of the VSD and insertion of an external valved conduit (arrowed) from the right ventricle to the main pulmonary artery. **C**. Lateral view of part B, showing the metallic frame of the prosthetic valve in the conduit.

(as this chamber takes all the cardiac flow), often similar to that seen in tricuspid atresia. Imaging techniques are particularly important in this condition as the size and function of the right ventricle must be estimated in great detail.

Palliative shunting may be needed in early life, but a successful surgical correction is dependent on the degree of underdevelopment of the right ventricular cavity. If the right ventricle is extremely hypoplastic, then the condition must be considered as a form of 'single ventricle', but if there is reasonable development of the right ventricular cavity, a full correction might be possible, although this is often a high-risk procedure. Patients with very severe pulmonary valve stenosis are considered in a similar way.

Single Ventricle (primitive ventricle)   There are many complex variants in this category and they must all be assessed carefully on their individual merits. The conditions are commonly referred to as 'single ventricle', but this is not always an easy description to understand, because often a second small or rudimentary ventricular chamber is present; but according to accepted morphological classifications the small chamber may not be entitled to the name 'ventricle'. The second small chamber often acts, via a VSD, as an outlet chamber.

The following situations may lead to a 'single ventricle':

1. *Double-inlet ventricle*—both atrioventricular valves enter the same ventricle (Fig. 24.56), or there is considerable override of one valve across a VSD

2. *Common inlet valve*—a single large atrioventricular valve enters a large ventricular chamber

3. *Atresia of one atrioventricular valve, mitral or tricuspid*—may be indistinguishable from situation 2

4. *Very large VSD* with little residual septal tissue, effectively a single chamber.

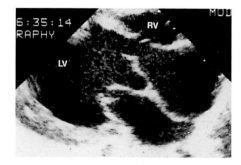

Fig. 24.56 Left parasternal echocardiogram of a patient with 'single ventricle'. Both atrioventricular valves enter the large left ventricle (LV) from two distinct atria. Outflow to the aorta is via a restrictive VSD and a small outflow chamber of right ventricular type (RV).

Multiple abnormalities are common, and nothing must be taken for granted in the assessment of the cases. Great arterial connections may be abnormal and must be assessed carefully. Atrial anatomy may be abnormal and there may be a single common atrium. The positions of the chambers may be distorted or twisted, and this must also be taken into careful consideration. Other malformations such as pulmonary stenosis, coarctation, or PDA may well be present.

In all these cases there is common mixing of the pulmonary and systemic venous return in the heart, and the clinical presentation depends particularly on the presence or absence of *pulmonary stenosis*. If pulmonary stenosis is present, the patient may be cyanotic with pulmonary oligemia, and if absent, the patient may have heart failure and pulmonary plethora.

There is no 'typical' *chest X-ray*, but the heart is often enlarged, with the pulmonary vascularity depending on the presence of other abnormalities. The size and position of the great arteries will help to determine the overall cardiac configuration. *Angiography* and *ultrasound* must be used, as appropriate for the circumstances, but in these complex cases it is often useful to assess the anatomy by both techniques to ensure maximum diagnostic accuracy. Work with *MRI* suggests that this modality may become the technique of choice for 'unscrambling' these complex cases, particularly in older patients where detailed echo studies are more difficult.

In the presence of only one useful ventricle, surgical options are often palliative, using shunts or pulmonary artery banding, but reconstructive surgery using the single ventricular chamber is increasingly carried out. This is normally achieved by the use of the *Fontan procedure* or one of its variants such as total cavopulmonary connection (TCPC). This operation uses the single ventricle to pump systemic blood to the aorta whilst redirecting systemic venous return to the lungs without the use of a second ventricle. This is often achieved by the direct anastomosis of the right atrial appendage to the main pulmonary artery. The details of the technique will vary with individual cases, but the success of the procedure depends on a well-functioning systemic ventricle and low pulmonary vascular resistance. Occasionally, *cardiac transplantation* can be offered to these patients.

TRICUSPID ATRESIA

In this condition there is no tricuspid orifice, the valve having either fused leaflets or a mass of obstructive tissue in the expected valve plane (Fig. 24.57). There is obligatory flow of the systemic venous return across an ASD to the left atrium and the left ventricle. The left ventricle is large as it carries both pulmonary and systemic venous return. Some of the blood in the left ventricle then crosses a VSD to reach the right ventricle and the pulmonary artery, while the remainder passes out in the normal way through the aortic valve.

The VSD is often restrictive (small size with a pressure drop across it and a low-pressure right ventricle), and there may be associated pulmonary stenosis. The right ventricle is often so underdeveloped that the condition is considered as one of the 'single ventricle' group. There is often relatively low pulmonary blood flow, although this is not invariable, and the condition may be expressed in various ways, depending on the state of the VSD and right ventricular outflow.

The *chest X-ray* commonly shows pulmonary oligemia, a small pulmonary bay, and a moderately large heart with a rounded

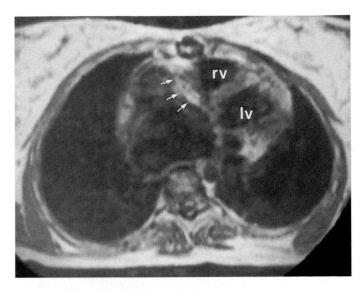

Fig. 24.57 Transverse gated spin echo MRI scan of a patient with tricuspid atresia. A wedge-shaped segment of tissue (arrowed) lies in the expected position of the tricuspid valve. rv, right ventricle; lv, left ventricle. (Courtesy of the Trustees of the Bristol MRI Centre.)

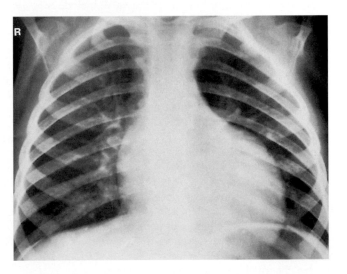

Fig. 24.58 Chest radiograph of a patient with tricuspid atresia. There is pulmonary oligemia, a small pulmonary artery, and a prominent rounded left ventricular curve to the left heart border.

contour due to the downward and leftward enlargement of the left ventricle (Fig. 24.58). *Echocardiography* will show the anatomy clearly, with Doppler studies adding information about flow across the interatrial septum and the pressure drops across the VSD and the pulmonary valve.

Cardiac angiography will show the anatomy well. Left ventriculography should be modified by the use of a shallower than usual LAO projection (e.g. 40–50° LAO) to take account of the alteration of the position of the interventricular septum by the large left ventricle and small right ventricle.

Surgical treatment will depend on the details of the individual case. If the VSD is relatively small and the right ventricle is poorly developed, then correction can only be achieved by the use of a Fontan or TCPC procedure.

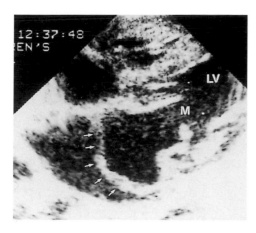

Fig. 24.59 Subcostal echocardiogram of a patient with cor triatriatum. A prominent membrane runs across the left atrium (arrowed). M, mitral valve; LV, left ventricle.

MITRAL VALVE ABNORMALITIES (including supramitral ring and cor triatriatum)

Obstructive lesions in or near the mitral valve include *congenital mitral stenosis*, *supramitral ring*, and *cor triatriatum*. The first resembles rheumatic stenosis, with fusion of the valve leaflets and doming of the valve. A supramitral ring is an obstructive diaphragm lying very close to the mitral valve on the left atrial side. Cor triatriatum is a condition in which there is an obstructive membrane in the left atrium, which divides it into high- and low-pressure portions with a small and restrictive communication between the two (Fig. 24.59).

The *chest X-ray* is similar in all cases, showing a normal-sized heart with increased pulmonary vessel size, due to pulmonary venous hypertension similar to that seen in the obstructed form of totally anomalous pulmonary venous drainage. There will often be pulmonary edema. *Echocardiography* will show the obstructive detail well, often better than angiography. Doppler studies may indicate the degree of obstruction.

Mitral regurgitation can form part of a complex abnormality such as AVSD, but it can also occur alone. In the latter case there may be abnormal papillary muscle formation such as a single papillary muscle giving a 'parachute' mitral valve. The chest X-ray will show signs of pulmonary venous hypertension and possibly pulmonary edema. The heart will be larger than with obstructive mitral lesions because of the ventricular volume overload.

HYPOPLASTIC LEFT HEART SYNDROME (aortic atresia)

At the most severe end of the spectrum of aortic stenosis lies aortic atresia. If there is no flow through the aortic valve the left ventricle itself will not develop, being only a rudimentary slit-like cavity. The aortic atresia may also be associated with mitral atresia. This abnormality is known as hypoplastic left heart syndrome.

In this condition the right ventricle performs the entire systemic pumping function, with the systemic blood supply being directed through the ductus arteriosus. The brachiocephalic branches are supplied retrogradely, and the ascending aorta is diminutive in

size, carrying only reverse flow from the PDA and aortic arch sufficient to fill the coronary arteries. The condition is almost uniformly fatal, and this probably explains why the condition appears relatively low on the list of incidence of congenital heart disease. Many cases probably die before being recognized at a pediatric cardiology referral center. Patients with hypoplastic left heart are often born in good condition but deteriorate very rapidly in the first few days of life as the life-sustaining ductus closes.

In the case of hypoplastic left heart, the diagnosis can almost always be made by *echocardiography*. The key feature to identify is the diminutive ascending aorta and the single functional ventricle, because these are the features associated with the uniformly poor prognosis *Cardiac catheterization* may be required if high-quality echocardiography is unavailable. In this situation the best approach is to perform a normal catheter study from the venous approach, and pass the angiographic catheter to the pulmonary artery or, if possible, through the PDA to the descending aorta. An *angiogram* performed from either of these positions will immediately show the retrograde flow down the diminutive ascending aorta, and the diagnosis will be confirmed. The condition can now be recognized by *antenatal echocardiography*.

Some experimental approaches to surgery are being investigated at present, with radical multistage reconstructions being attempted in a few specialized centers. Some surgical successes have been achieved with *neonatal heart transplantation* in a small number of specialized centers.

CARDIOMYOPATHY

Hypertrophic Cardiomyopathy Hypertrophic cardiomyopathy with left ventricular outflow obstruction can occur in infants and children, and is thought to be dominantly inherited in a proportion

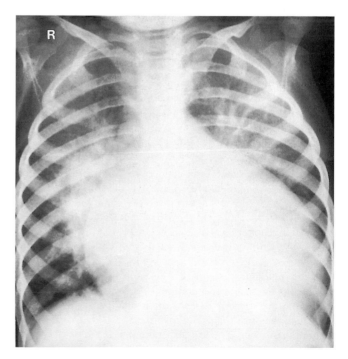

Fig. 24.60 Chest radiograph of a child with a severe dilated cardiomyopathy. There is marked cardiomegaly and left heart failure.

of cases. There are also associations with *Noonan's syndrome* and *maternal diabetes*, but in the latter circumstance the condition tends to resolve, whereas it tends to be progressive in the remainder. There is an association with arrhythmias and sudden death in a minority of cases. Diagnosis is classically made on the *echocardiogram*, which may show asymmetrical hypertrophy of the interventricular septum and obstruction of the left ventricular outflow tract by anterior motion of the mitral valve.

Dilated Cardiomyopathies Dilated cardiomyopathies (alternatively called *endocardial fibroelastosis*) occur occasionally in infancy, and are most commonly related to intrauterine infections. Occasionally they are due to inherited factors or are secondary to valvular or coronary anomalies. The etiology of the conditions is often hard to determine. The chest X-ray will show a large heart with pulmonary signs of cardiac failure (Fig. 24.60), and other imaging modalities will be capable of demonstrating the poor ventricular function. This is particularly clearly seen on two-dimensional echocardiography, which will also demonstrate the characteristic endocardial thickening. Occasionally the condition can be detected by fetal echocardiography. Surgery has little to offer in this condition apart from transplantation.

Endomyocardial fibrosis is a tropical condition in which there is endocardial thickening which leads to cavity obliteration.

ANOMALOUS PULMONARY VENOUS CONNECTION

This abnormality of cardiac connection can take various forms.

Partial Anomalous Pulmonary Venous Connection (PAPVC)
This can occur when one or more individual pulmonary veins drain to the right side of the atrial septum, either into the right atrium itself or into the superior or inferior vena cava. This abnormality is commonly associated with ASD, in particular the sinus venosus type of defect, and it is important to check pulmonary venous connections when performing echocardiographic or angiographic examination for ASD assessment. The anomalous veins can often be redirected correctly at surgery, providing the surgeon is aware of the problem.

Sometimes an anomalous pulmonary vein can drain down to the inferior vena cava below the diaphragm, more commonly on the right side (Fig. 24.61). This vein can sometimes be identified on the chest X-ray as a curved vessel in the right lower zone, widening as it approaches the right cardiophrenic angle (Fig. 24.62). This is sometimes referred to as the *scimitar syndrome*. The condition is frequently associated with hypoplasia of the right lung, and sometimes there is a shift of the heart to the right.

Total Anomalous Pulmonary Venous Connection (TAPVC)
This is a more serious condition which can take three forms, *supracardiac*, *cardiac*, or *infracardiac*. In all three types the major pulmonary veins come to a confluence behind the left atrium but do not communicate directly with it (Fig. 24.63). In the case of *supracardiac TAPVC* there is a large ascending vein on the left side, which is a remnant of the embryological left superior vena cava. This connects into the left brachiocephalic vein, which then passes down the right-sided superior vena cava into the right atrium (Fig. 24.64). The *cardiac* type of abnormality drains into the right side of the heart, usually via the enlarged coronary sinus. In the case of *infracardiac TAPVC* the confluence of pulmonary veins drains downward in a descending vein which passes

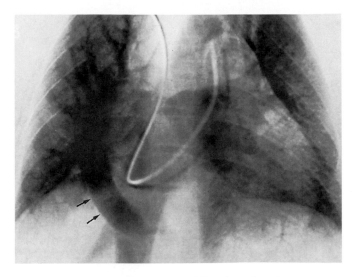

Fig. 24.61 Digital angiogram of a follow-through pulmonary artery injection in a patient with partial anomalous pulmonary venous drainage. A large vein (arrowed) is seen draining from the right lung to the inferior vena cava below the diaphragm.

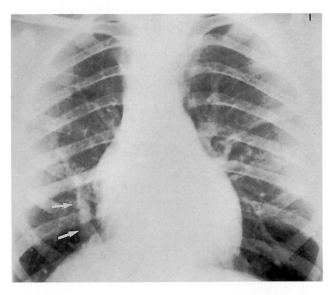

Fig. 24.62 Chest radiograph of the same patient as in Fig. 24.61. The anomalous vein (scimitar sign) is seen in the right lower zone (arrowed).

through the diaphragm, often obstructed at this point, into either the portal venous system or the inferior vena cava. The portal venous system is usually at a higher pressure than other venous systems, and this fact may also contribute to the 'obstruction' in this condition (Fig. 24.65). The pulmonary venous blood then returns to the right atrium through the inferior vena cava.

In all of these conditions there is total cardiac mixing at the right atrial level, and the patient remains partially cyanosed. In the case of supracardiac or cardiac TAPVC the *chest X-ray* shows that the heart is enlarged and there is pulmonary plethora, which is obligatory due to the need for a higher pulmonary flow in the mixed circulation (Fig. 24.66). The supracardiac TAPVC will often show wide mediastinum due to the left-sided ascending vein, and in long-established cases the classic *cottage loaf* heart

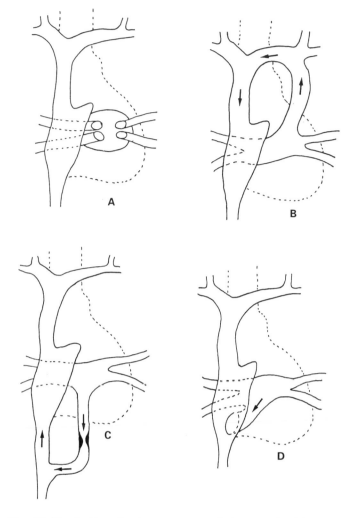

Fig. 24.63 **A**. Normal pulmonary venous drainage to the left atrium. **B**. TAPVC of the supracardiac type draining to a left-sided ascending vein and then to the left brachiocephalic vein. **C**. TAPVC of the infracardiac type showing obstructed drainage to the inferior vena cava. **D**. TAPVC of the cardiac type draining to the coronary sinus.

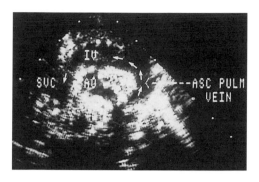

Fig. 24.64 Coronal suprasternal echocardiogram showing TAPVC of the supracardiac type draining as shown in Fig. 24.63B. IV, brachiocephalic vein or innominate vein; SVC, superior vena cava; AO, aorta. (Courtesy Dr R. Martin.)

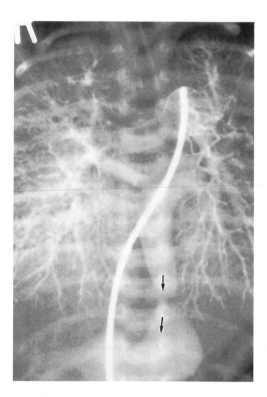

Fig. 24.65 Follow-through pulmonary arteriogram of a child with obstructed TAPVC of the intracardiac type draining past an obstruction at the diaphragmatic level (arrows) to a dilated vein connecting to the inferior vena cava.

will be evident. This will become less common because these cases are now usually diagnosed and treated in infancy. The infracardiac type of abnormal drainage will often be associated with little or no cardiac enlargement, and the obstruction of the pulmonary circulation will lead to interstitial edema and heart failure. The findings of a normal heart size with severe heart failure usually indicate infracardiac TAPVC (Fig. 24.67).

Non-invasive Diagnosis The three types of TAPVC may be diagnosed by *echocardiography*, the abnormal venous confluence being visible behind the left atrium. The abnormal course of drainage can usually be traced. The left atrium is usually small, and there is right-to-left flow across the atrial septal communication. The flow in the venous confluence and drainage channels can often be shown using *Doppler color flow mapping*.

PAPVC can be diagnosed by the visualization of the individual veins draining to the right atrium, but the diagnosis can be more difficult if the site of drainage is to the inferior or superior vena cava rather than to the right atrium.

Cardiac Catheterization and Angiography Angiography will also show these features, but it may not be necessary if high-quality ultrasound results are available. A large and rapid injection of contrast medium to the main pulmonary artery will opacify the pulmonary venous system well. The anterior view is the clearest for demonstrating the venous pathways. Infants presenting with this condition are often seriously ill, and the morbidity of catheterization and angiography is significant.

The delineation of the individual pulmonary veins in PAPVC can be more difficult and may require separate injections to the left and right pulmonary arteries in oblique views. Sometimes the direct injection of contrast medium to the suspected abnormal

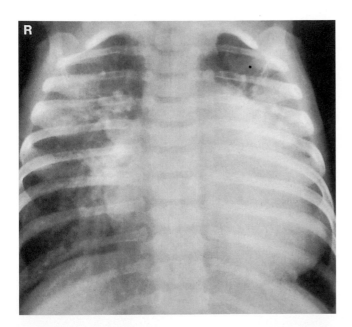

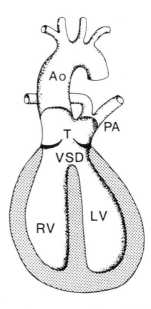

Fig. 24.66 Chest radiograph of a child with TAPVC of the cardiac type draining to the coronary sinus. There is marked cardiomegaly and pulmonary plethora but the upper mediastinum is not wide because the drainage is directly to the heart.

Fig. 24.68 Anatomy of truncus arteriosus. RV, right ventricle; LV, left ventricle; T, common truncus arteriosus; PA, pulmonary artery; Ao, aorta. (Reproduced from Jordan & Scott 1989, with permission.)

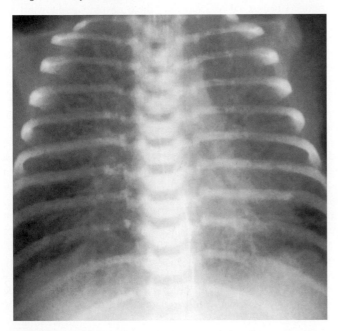

Fig. 24.67 Chest radiograph of a child with obstructed TAPVC of the infracardiac type. The heart borders are obscured by diffuse interstitial edema but there is no significant cardiomegaly.

veins can be diagnostic, but this approach can be surprisingly difficult to interpret as the contrast medium is rapidly diluted and the atrial anatomy is often unclear. In either case, oblique views are preferable to posteroanterior and lateral views as they will separate the two atria more effectively.

Treatment Surgery is directed toward reanastomosing the pulmonary venous confluence with the left atrium, dividing the abnormal connection and closing the ASD that is present. In spite

of its apparently straightforward nature the operation carries a higher than average mortality. Surgical treatment of PAPVC usually consists of closing the associated ASD with a patch that incorporates all the pulmonary veins into the left atrium, but surgery may not be necessary at all for this condition.

TRUNCUS ARTERIOSUS

In this condition a single great artery arises from the heart, due to a failure of division of the embryonic common truncus arteriosus. The common truncus arises from above a large VSD (Fig. 24.68) and the pattern of division of the common truncus varies. A single common pulmonary artery with a well-developed main pulmonary artery segment may arise from the common truncus before it divides into left and right pulmonary arteries—*type 1 truncus arteriosus*. In *type 2 truncus arteriosus* the length of the main pulmonary artery segment is negligible, but the two pulmonary arteries arise close together just above the truncal valve. In *type 3 truncus arteriosus* the left and right pulmonary arteries arise independently from the main truncus at a higher level, usually one from each side of the main artery. Type 3 truncus is the least common form. Various intermediate forms have also been classified. Pulmonary atresia with large aortopulmonary collateral vessels has sometimes been called pseudotruncus, but this is misleading as the condition is developmentally quite different.

In all cases there is common mixing across the VSD, and the flow in the pulmonary arteries is very large, because it originates directly from the common truncus which is at systemic pressure. In many cases a fully developed main pulmonary artery segment does not develop in its usual position, and so the *chest X-ray* shows marked pulmonary plethora with a relatively narrow mediastinal shadow (as in transposition of the great vessels). With truncus arteriosus there is also an increased incidence of *right-sided aortic arch*. In many patients the heart is moderately enlarged and there may be cardiac failure. *Echocardiographic*

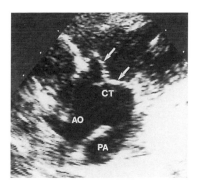

Fig. 24.69 Modified subcostal echocardiogram in truncus arteriosus. CT, common truncus; AO, aorta; PA, pulmonary artery. The truncal valve is arrowed.

diagnosis is relatively straightforward (Fig. 24.69), which is helpful, as it is difficult to perform good angiography on these patients due to the very fast blood flow through the heart, which dilutes the contrast medium. The patients are often very ill, and catheterization with angiography produces significant morbidity. There may still be difficulties in obtaining good detail of the truncal branching pattern, and MRI shows great promise in such cases.

Palliation by banding of the pulmonary artery is sometimes carried out, but the preferred operation is a complete correction with closure of the VSD. This will allow the left ventricle to empty through the truncal valve, and a separate prosthetic or homograft valved conduit must be placed from the right ventricle to the pulmonary arteries (Fig. 24.70).

EBSTEIN'S ANOMALY

This condition is an anomaly of the tricuspid valve. It has often

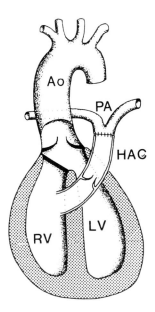

Fig. 24.70 Correction of common truncus arteriosus using the Rastelli procedure. RV, right ventricle; LV, left ventricle; Ao, aorta; HAC, homograft aortic conduit; PA, pulmonary artery. (Reproduced from Jordan & Scott 1989, with permission.)

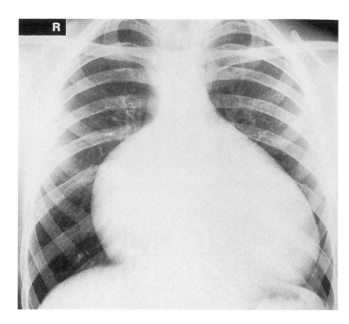

Fig. 24.71 Chest radiograph of a child with severe Ebstein's anomaly. There is marked globular cardiomegaly and pulmonary oligemia.

been described as a displacement of the tricuspid valve toward the apex of the right ventricle which produces a larger right atrium and a smaller right ventricle. This is in effect what is present, although the more precise descriptions of cardiac morphologists detail a condition in which the tricuspid annulus is normally positioned and the valve leaflets are larger and more redundant than normal, being adherent to the right ventricular walls, particularly the septum, for some distance into the ventricular cavity.

The result of this anomaly is a larger right atrium than normal (the so-called 'atrialized' portion of the right ventricle) and a relatively small right ventricle which is relatively ineffective in pumping blood to the lungs. There is often associated infundibular narrowing. The function of the tricuspid valve itself is variable, sometimes being normal, but often showing significant regurgitation. The clinical presentation varies considerably, severe cases presenting in infancy with right heart failure and poor forward flow to the pulmonary artery. The *chest X-ray* in these cases may show massive globular cardiomegaly with pulmonary oligemia (Fig. 24.71). The mildest expression occurs in some adults who present with mild signs or symptoms and a virtually normal chest X-ray.

Ultrasound studies show the abnormal tricuspid valve as a very prominent feature (Fig. 24.72) and many of the functional aspects can be derived from Doppler studies. The need for catheterization depends on the clinical severity and the quality of the echocardiogram.

SINUS OF VALSALVA FISTULA

In this condition there is usually enlargement of one of the sinuses of Valsalva in the aortic root, commonly the right sinus. This may rupture into the right ventricle and produce a left-to-right shunt. There will be continuous flow from the higher-pressure aorta to the right ventricle, and the murmur may be mistaken for a patent

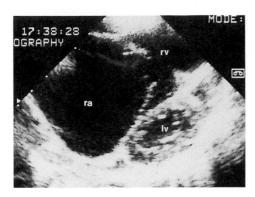

Fig. 24.72 Subcostal echocardiogram in a child with Ebstein's anomaly. This view shows the marked right atrial enlargement (ra) and the prominent tricuspid valve. In spite of the displacement of the valve, the right ventricle (rv) is still larger than the left ventricle (lv).

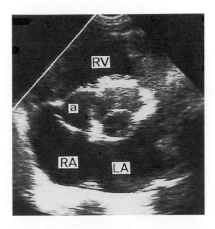

Fig. 24.73 Parasternal short-axis echocardiogram showing a sinus of Valsalva aneurysm (a). RV, right ventricle; RA, right atrium; LA, left atrium.

ductus arteriosus, a coronary fistula or the recognized association of VSD with aortic regurgitation.

The *chest X-ray* may show typical features of a left-to-right shunt, but the aneurysmal sinus itself is rarely visible on the cardiac contour. *Echocardiography*, particularly with color flow Doppler mapping, will show the abnormality (Fig. 24.73). An aortic root *angiogram* will also show the lesion.

It is important to distinguish this condition from the *perimembranous ventricular defect*. The communications are in very similar positions, one above and one below the aortic valve. Besides visualization of the defect, differentiation can be achieved using continuous-wave Doppler studies, which will show that there is prominent continuous flow through the aortoventricular defect, which is due to the persistent differential pressure between the two chambers.

The principles of surgical repair are relatively straightforward, but it may be complicated by aortic regurgitation due to the distortion of the aortic valve by the abnormality and the repair.

DOUBLE-OUTLET VENTRICLE

Double-outlet right ventricle is the most usual type of double-outlet ventricle. Once again each case must be assessed individually, but accurate anatomic assessment is vital. Corrective

surgery is usually possible, but this depends on detailed knowledge of the intracardiac anatomy. There are usually two well-developed ventricles with a VSD, and so the positions of the great arteries and the septal defect must all be determined accurately. A double-outlet right ventricle with a large subaortic VSD can be corrected by closing the VSD with an oblique patch, allowing the left ventricle to empty to the aorta through the VSD. If the VSD is subpulmonary, a more complex procedure is required to redirect flow to the appropriate great arteries. The latter condition with a subpulmonary defect is often termed a *Taussig–Bing anomaly*.

The chest radiograph will give clues about the nature of the anomaly, but echocardiography and cardiac angiography are both very important diagnostic techniques for the determination of the precise intracardiac anatomy.

GREAT ARTERIAL ANOMALIES (including vascular rings)

Anomalous Right Subclavian Artery The commonest major variation in the aortic arch and its branching is the anomalous right subclavian artery occurring with a normal left-sided arch. The right subclavian artery is the last brachiocephalic branch of the aorta, arising from the descending portion of the arch. The anomaly causes inconvenience for surgeons and those performing right brachial artery catheterization, but it does not normally produce symptoms. The vessel runs obliquely behind the

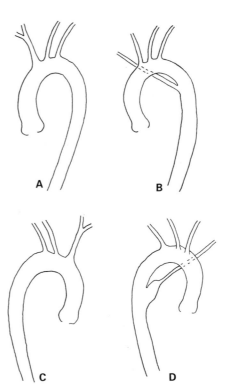

Fig. 24.74 **A.** Normal left aortic arch branching. **B.** Left aortic arch with an anomalous origin of the right subclavian artery. **C.** Right aortic arch with 'mirror image' branching, This is the commonest type associated with cyanotic congenital heart disease. **D.** Right aortic arch with an anomalous origin of the left subclavian artery arising from a posterior diverticulum. This is the commonest type of right aortic arch to occur as an isolated abnormality.

esophagus, and its indentation can be recognized on the barium swallow.

Right-sided Aortic Arch There are two common forms of right-sided aortic arch. The first is the so-called *mirror image type*, with the brachiocephalic branches being the mirror image of normal. This type is the most usual form of right arch to be found in association with the various types of cyanotic heart disease (25% incidence in tetralogy of Fallot and pulmonary atresia). The second form of right arch is that with an *anomalous origin of the left subclavian artery*. This is almost the mirror image of the anomalous right subclavian type, but the anomalous vessel often arises from a prominent *diverticulum* which can make a prominent indentation in the posterior part of the esophagus. This type is the most likely to be found as an isolated anomaly (approximately 0.1% of the population). Common aortic arch variations are shown in Figure 24.74.

Double Aortic Arch This anomaly is more serious as it can form a vascular ring that compresses the trachea or major bronchi and causes stridor in infancy. It can be diagnosed occasionally on the chest X-ray or barium swallow by evidence of bilateral compression on the trachea or esophagus. Echocardiography may also be useful in making the diagnosis, but it can be difficult to identify with confidence the two separate arches. MRI can show the condition clearly, and may become the investigation of choice in the future (Fig. 24.75). At present, angiography is essential for definitive confirmation.

Anomalous Origin of the Left Pulmonary Artery (pulmonary artery sling) This is another important cause of stridor in infancy. The left pulmonary artery arises as a branch of the right pulmonary artery and runs posteriorly to the right of the trachea, reaching its destination in the left hilum as it passes leftward behind the trachea. This is one of the few conditions where an abnormal vascular structure runs anterior to the esophagus (between the esophagus and trachea). This can occasionally be recognized as an abnormal soft-tissue structure on the lateral chest X-ray between the esophagus and trachea. This condition is difficult to treat surgically as there may be distortion and narrowing of the trachea or bronchii.

Diagnosis may involve barium swallow and bronchography, but once again echocardiography and MRI may add more information, and arteriography will produce the definitive diagnosis.

There are very many other vascular anomalies, some of which can cause tracheal compression. Sometimes a vascular ring is formed by *rudimentary vascular bands* which are not demonstrated angiographically, and this possibility must always be considered. Any vascular ring can potentially cause major airway obstruction, and thus stridor in infancy is a serious problem which must always be investigated thoroughly, usually with angiography (see Appendix B).

CORONARY ANOMALIES

There are many variants of coronary anatomy, and most cause no problems. The most common is the *'left dominant'* system in which the posterior descending artery arises from the circumflex artery rather than the right coronary artery, this occurring in

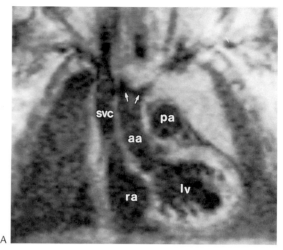

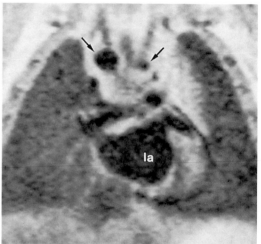

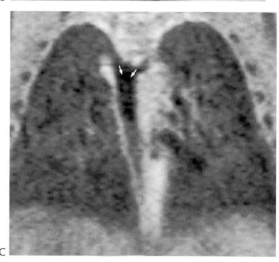

Fig. 24.75 **A**. Coronal gated spin-echo MRI scan from a child with a double aortic arch. The ascending aorta (aa) bifurcates at its upper end (arrows). lv, left ventricle; pa, pulmonary artery; svc, superior vena cava; ra, right atrium. **B**. A more posterior coronal section from the same study. The large right and small left arches are shown in cross-section (arrows) with brachiocephalic arteries arising from them. **C**. A yet more posterior coronal section of the same study, showing confluence of the two arches to form the descending aorta. The findings were confirmed at surgery with no angiography being necessary. (Courtesy of the Trustees of the Bristol MRI Centre.)

5–10% of the normal population. Numerous other variants in the course of the vessels have been documented. There is one anomalous course with theoretical clinical consequences, namely the left coronary artery which runs between the aorta and main pulmonary artery where it may be compressed, but it has been hard to document this problem precisely.

Clinically important abnormalities include *anomalous origin* of one or both coronary arteries *from the pulmonary artery*. This leads to desaturated coronary perfusion and/or reversed coronary flow, and can cause myocardial ischemia, myocardial infarction, or sudden death in infancy. Surviving infants can have marked cardiomegaly due to severe ischemic cardiomyopathy.

Coronary fistulas to cardiac chambers or the pulmonary artery occur occasionally and often present asymptomatically with a continuous murmur. Ninety percent drain to the right side of the heart, most often from the right coronary artery, and function as a left-to-right shunt. The shunt itself is often less of a worry in younger patients than the other potential complications such as coronary ischemia (the 'steal' phenomenon) or endocarditis. In later life the systemic-to-pulmonary shunting may become symptomatic. The fistulous communications can dilate to aneurysmal proportions with the development of unusually positioned bumps on the heart border seen on *chest X-ray*. The aneurysmal fistulas may calcify, and in theory they can rupture, but this latter has rarely been reported. These lesions may be diagnosed or suspected on *ultrasound examination*, but *angiography* is essential for precise evaluation. The communications are commonly closed surgically to prevent complications, but, more recently, interventional occlusion techniques have been employed to close them (Fig. 24.76).

Kawasaki's disease is not a congenital abnormality but is acquired in childhood. It is probably infective in origin and has systemic features which give it the alternative name of *'mucocutaneous lymph node syndrome'*. A relatively mild illness in young children may be followed by the development of aneurysmal dilatation of the proximal coronary arteries. These can often be seen on *echocardiography* and there is generally no indication for angiography, because there is no specific therapy for the coronary abnormalities apart from general medical measures and observation. The coronary dilatations can resolve in many cases, but in a minority they can dilate and rupture or become stenotic.

ARTERIOVENOUS MALFORMATIONS (systemic and pulmonary)

Both types of arteriovenous malformation are uncommon.

Systemic Arteriovenous Malformations These abnormalities may cause local problems but can also produce high-output cardiac failure. A shunt through an *aneurysmal vein of Galen* in the skull is a possibility that must always be remembered when considering heart failure of unknown cause in infancy. An intracranial bruit is often a key sign, and a left ventricular or aortic injection must be followed to the skull to exclude this condition if it is seriously considered.

Pulmonary Arteriovenous Malformations These can sometimes be obvious on the chest X-ray, but this is not always the case as they may be obscured by other structures or they may be of the complex (plexiform) type with no large vessel or aneurysm present. These abnormalities can produce profound central cyanosis, and they require angiography for definitive diagnosis.

In some situations, systemic or pulmonary arteriovenous malformations are amenable to closure by transcatheter embolization, but frequently surgical treatment is necessary.

CARDIAC TUMORS

It is debatable whether cardiac tumors can be described as congenital abnormalities, but they occur occasionally in the newborn and have even been detected antenatally. The commonest tumor in children is the *rhabdomyoma*. This is usually histologically benign, a hamartoma, but can sometimes cause fatal obstruction within the heart. They are commonly multiple and are frequently associated with *tuberous sclerosis*. Surgery is best avoided as they do not grow with the heart and so become less of a problem as the child becomes older.

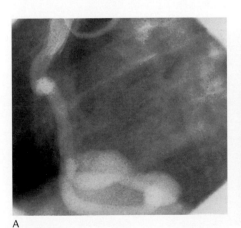
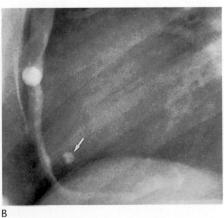
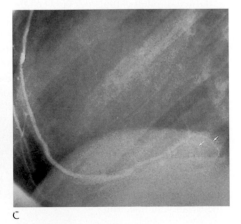

A   B   C

Fig. 24.76 **A**. Selective right coronary arteriogram in the L→L AO projection in a child with an aneurysmal fistula to the right ventricle. **B**. Angiogram, from the same patient, in the same projection immediately after embolization with a detachable balloon (arrowed). **C**. Angiogram in the same projection taken 1 year later. The fistula remains closed, the right coronary artery has decreased in size, and the distal myocardial branches are now seen (arrowed). (Courtesy of Dr G. Hartnell.)

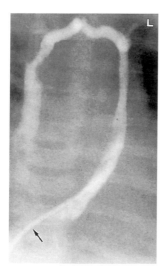

Fig. 24.77   Bilateral superior vena cava. A venous catheter (arrowed) has been used for an angiogram in the left superior vena cava which drains to the coronary sinus. There is a large intercommunicating vein between the left and right vena cavae.

Teratomas and *fibromas* are occasionally diagnosed. The *myxoma* is a commoner tumor in the older child and has well-known features, particularly when it occurs in its commonest site, the left atrium. The presentation may be with a murmur, malaise and pyrexia, obstructive symptoms and signs, or with a systemic embolus. All tumors, but particularly the left atrial myxoma, are well suited to diagnosis by *echocardiography*, and the latter condition should always be treated by urgent surgical removal.

SYSTEMIC VENOUS ANOMALIES

Bilateral Superior Vena Cava   A bilateral superior vena cava is the commonest systemic venous anomaly, being present in about 10% of patients with congenital heart disease. Many of these are small left-sided connections, only about half being large enough to be of hemodynamic significance. In a proportion of cases there is an intercommunicating vein between the two venae cavae at the root of the neck (Fig. 24.77). The left superior vena cava usually drains into the coronary sinus. It is not normally of clinical importance, but is surgically important, as the venous connections need to be correctly placed in instituting cardiopulmonary bypass, and in some complex procedures the presence of a left-sided superior vena cava is a positive benefit for construction of the final repair.

The condition cannot be diagnosed easily on the plain chest radiograph but is generally recognizable on a good-quality *echocardiogram*. The condition is often signalled by an unusually large coronary sinus entering the right atrium. *Angiography* will provide a definitive diagnosis, and this can be performed via the inferior vena cava (during cardiac catheterization) or by a left subclavian vein injection.

Interruption of the Inferior Vena Cava   An uncommon anomaly is interruption of the inferior vena cava just before it reaches the heart. The venous drainage from the lower body continues into the azygos system, draining into the superior vena cava through the azygos vein on the right side. The hepatic veins usually drain directly to the right atrium. The abnormality rarely produces symptoms but can be very inconvenient if catheterization is being performed via the inferior vena cava. It is often associated with ambiguous cardiac situs.

FETAL ECHOCARDIOGRAPHY

The routine 16–18 week antenatal ultrasound scan has now expanded considerably to include assessment of a wide range of organs. The heart can be clearly visualized at this stage with good equipment, and the 'routine' examination should include assessment of the '*four-chamber view*'. More detailed cardiac scanning starts with this view and includes other assessments as described below. This detailed cardiac assessment is only available in certain specialist centers at present, but the technique is becoming more widely available as experience develops.

Protocol for Fetal Cardiac Scanning

• The transverse section of the fetal chest shows a four-chamber view with normal orientation of the cardiac apex to the left (Fig. 24.78). (The left side should be determined using the

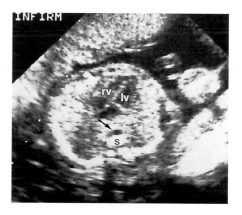

Fig. 24.78   Transverse echocardiogram of a 20-week-old fetus showing the 'four-chamber view'. rv, right ventricle; lv, left ventricle; s, spine. The descending aorta is arrowed.

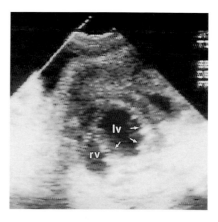

Fig. 24.79   Fetal echocardiogram in a fetus with a left ventricular cardiomyopathy due to critical aortic stenosis. The left ventricle (lv) is much larger than the right ventricle (rv), was visibly less contractile, and showed endocardial fibroelastosis (arrowed) as an echogenic endocardium.

overall orientation of the fetus, not by comparison with adjacent organs, which might also be malpositioned.)

- The fetal heart should occupy about a third of the area of the thorax.
- Both ventricles should be of similar size (Fig. 24.79). Both atria should be of similar size.
- Mitral and tricuspid valves should be seen, in their normal offset relationship, the tricuspid valve being positioned slightly closer to the cardiac apex than the mitral valve.
- The valve of the foramen ovale should be visible as a thin mobile structure on the left side of the atrial septum.
- Adjustment of the transverse section should show normal connections of the pulmonary artery and aorta. M-mode tracings of cardiac valve movements can often be recorded (Fig. 24.80).

The schedule described above is possible in most cases and can be used to exclude most major structural abnormalities, depending on the experience of the operator. If abnormalities are detected, decisions regarding future management can be made, and these include termination of pregnancy, treatment of the mother with drugs (fetal cardiac failure), and referral to a specialist center for delivery. Defects with minor anatomic derangements such as small VSD or isolated stenosis of the pulmonary valve cannot be detected reliably. Counseling of parents is a valuable part of the procedure.

The technique can be extended further. The long- and short-axis planes of the heart can be shown to confirm the anatomy and connections of the great arteries. The aortic arch can usually be visualized. Systemic and pulmonary venous connections can

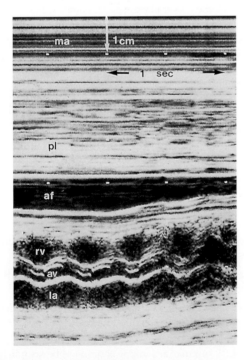

Fig. 24.80 M-mode echocardiogram across the normal aortic valve of a 20-week-old fetus. ma, maternal abdomen; pl, placenta; af, amniotic fluid; rv, right ventricle; av, aortic valve; la, left atrium. Depth and time markers are shown, indicating that the heart rate is 150 beats/min and the aortic root diameter is 4 mm.

often be seen. Doppler studies can be used to confirm normal flow through valves and vessels, and this can sometimes demonstrate pathology such as a regurgitant valve.

Heart rate and rhythm, as well as more detailed assessment of ventricular function, can be derived from the fetal M-mode examination. The normal fetal heart rate is well in excess of 100 beats/min (usually 150–180 beats/min at 18 weeks' gestation). Persistent bradycardia below 100 beats/min is associated with a high chance of structural cardiac abnormality. Transient periods of bradycardia (30–60 s only) are of no prognostic significance.

Most patients scanned are mothers who have had a previous child with congenital heart disease. In this group there is a two- to three-fold increase in the chance of congenital heart disease in the fetus. This should be seen in the context of overall incidence, and even in these mothers the chance of congenital cardiac abnormality being present is still only 2–3%. Thus the great majority of scans are normal and are reassuring for the parents. There is a small but increasing group of parents with congenital heart defects in whom the risk of congenital heart disease in the fetus is slightly greater at 3–4%.

Referrals are also made in cases when a less experienced operator suspects an abnormality in a routine scan or a scan performed for another reason. It is not surprising to find that detailed cardiac scanning will reveal a much higher incidence of abnormality in this group, hence the importance of checking the four-chamber view as part of the protocol in the 'routine' antenatal scan. Detailed cardiac scans may also be helpful when other congenital abnormalities have been detected.

If a cardiac abnormality is detected it is essential to discuss the findings with the obstetrician and pediatric cardiologist so that proper advice can be given to the mother. In some cases of major abnormality, such as hypoplastic left heart syndrome, termination might be considered, but in other cases careful management of the pregnancy and early cardiological attention for the infant might be considered more appropriate. In many cases, detailed discussion of possible surgery and the prognosis will need to be discussed with the parents and pediatric cardiology or surgery specialists.

SUMMARY OF CHEST X-RAY APPEARANCES IN CONGENITAL HEART DISEASE

Particular points should be considered in the assessment of the chest film in the case of known or suspected congenital heart disease.

1. Note abdominal and cardiac *situs* at the start. If possible, assess the bronchial situs. Beware the handwritten side-marker: the radiographer may have been fooled too!

2. Note the overall *cardiac size*. It is generally unhelpful to read too much into this unless comparing serial films. Consider only normal, moderately enlarged or very enlarged.

3. Look at the *mediastinum*. Is the pulmonary artery segment absent, small, normal, or enlarged? Is the aortic arch visible, is it normal in appearance, on which side is it? (Note tracheal indentation and descending aorta as part of this.) If a thymic shadow is present, then assessment can be difficult, particularly in the youngest infants.

4. Look at the *pulmonary vascularity*. First decide if the vessels are clearly visible or not. If not, consider heart failure (interstitial

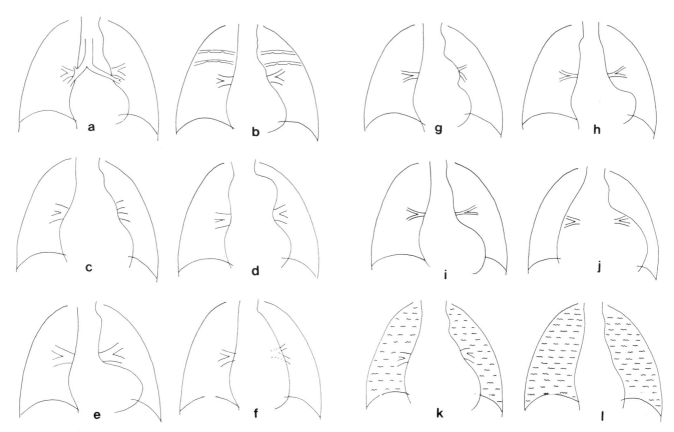

Fig. 24.81   a. Normal cardiac contour and normal pulmonary artery size. Normal bronchial anatomy is superimposed. **b**. Normal heart size and pulmonary vessels with a small and irregular aortic knuckle and rib notching. Established coarctation in an older child or adult. **c**. Cardiomegaly and large pulmonary vessels. Left-to-right shunt, particularly ASD or VSD. Also consider PDA and partially or totally anomalous pulmonary venous connection of the cardiac type (draining directly to the heart). A left-to-right shunt alone rarely gives massive cardiomegaly. **d**. Cardiomegaly and large pulmonary vessels with a very wide upper mediastinum. Totally anomalous pulmonary venous connection of the supracardiac type. A large thymus will widen the mediastinum also. **e**. Moderate cardiomegaly and large pulmonary vessels with a small pulmonary artery segment. Pulmonary arteries must be anatomically abnormal, so consider D-transposition of the great arteries and truncus arteriosus. The latter is more likely if the aortic arch is right sided. **f**. Large smooth curve to the left heart border. L-transposition of the great arteries with an abnormal leftward position of the aorta. The appearance may also be due to other complex malpositions. L-loop TGA may occasionally have a virtually normal chest X-ray. **g**. Prominent main pulmonary artery with normal or small pulmonary vessels. Pulmonary valve stenosis. The left pulmonary artery also may be dilated. The dilatation is not prominent in subpulmonary stenosis and is not invariably present in valvar stenosis. **h**. Upturned cardiac apex, right-sided aortic arch, and small pulmonary vessels. This is almost diagnostic of tetralogy of Fallot, but can be seen in pulmonary atresia with a VSD and in a few cases of double outlet right ventricle (similar hemodynamics). **i**. Small pulmonary artery and pulmonary vessels with a large rounded left heart border. Tricuspid atresia. The condition is variable, and there can be normal or occasionally increased vascularity depending on the hemodynamics of the VSD and pulmonary valve. Sometimes pulmonary atresia can give this appearance. **j**. Very large heart with normal or small pulmonary vessels. Ebstein's anomaly, dilated cardiomyopathy (including anomalous coronary origin from the pulmonary artery), and pericardial effusion. There may be associated left heart failure with cardiomyopathy. **k**. Cardiomegaly with large pulmonary vessels and pulmonary edema. Left to right shunt with failure, left heart obstruction (aortic stenosis or coarctation), severe mitral regurgitation (alone or with other conditions), and cardiomyopathy. **l**. Small heart with pulmonary edema. Obstruction before the heart. Totally anomalous pulmonary venous connection of the obstructed intracardiac type, cor triatriatum, or congenital mitral stenosis. Pulmonary conditions must be distinguished.

or alveolar pulmonary edema), complex collateral vasculature, or pulmonary disease. These are not always easy to distinguish. If vessels are distinct, are they:

- Definitely oligemic
- Normal to oligemic
- Normal
- Normal to plethoric
- Definitely plethoric.

(Abnormal vascular distribution within the lung is generally unhelpful in infants and small children unless very marked, e.g. unilateral plethora with a shunt.)

5. Is there any characteristic *unusual shape* to the heart contour that suggests a particular diagnosis?

6. Is there any *evidence of previous surgery* (e.g. thoracotomy, sternal wires or implanted prosthesis)?

7. *Note skeletal or other abnormalities* (e.g. 11 pairs of ribs suggests Down syndrome, which in turn suggests AVSD.

Figure 24.81 summarizes major patterns to be seen in a number of well-recognized congenital cardiac abnormalities. The recognition of these patterns will not lead to a definitive diagnosis in many cases but it will usually help to classify the type of abnormality present, often allowing the radiologist to highlight key functional and anatomic features which will be of vital importance in further diagnosis and management of the patient.

SUMMARY OF IMAGING TECHNIQUES IN CONGENITAL HEART DISEASE

Plain Chest Radiograph

- Essential in initial assessment but not often fully diagnostic
- Essential in continuing management of patients
- Standard supine anteroposterior film in small children and infants
- Standard erect posteroanterior and lateral films in older children and adults
- Localized view for bronchial anatomy.

Fluoroscopy

- Rarely needed for diagnostic purposes
- An essential part of diagnostic and therapeutic catheter techniques.

Barium swallow

- Occasionally helpful in the assessment of vascular anomalies
- Otherwise superseded by other techniques.

Echocardiography

This is the most important non-invasive diagnostic technique. *Two-dimensional imaging* uses three main echocardiographic windows (left parasternal, apical, and subcostal) to examine the heart in three main planes (long axis, short axis, and four chamber). Modified views are also used as well as the suprasternal approach for assessing the great vessels.

M-mode imaging (one-dimensional imaging) is useful for accurate measurement of distances and timing within the heart.

Doppler echocardiography can be used in imaging congenital heart disease. *Pulsed Doppler interrogation* allows measurement of flow at a specific point selected within an image, but is limited in its ability to record high-velocity flow accurately, with aliasing being a common problem. Continuous-wave Doppler interrogation can be used to measure the highest velocities but has no depth resolution along the beam. The high velocities in pathological flows can be used to deduce pressure drops by means of the modified Bernoulli equation. *Color flow mapping* is similar to pulsed Doppler examination, but the image as a whole is analysed, flow toward and away from the transducer being coded in different colors. Color flow mapping is also limited in its ability to record high-velocity flow accurately.

Transesophageal echocardiography can produce very high-resolution images, and is particularly suited to larger patients in whom good-quality imaging is hard to achieve. Pediatric-sized transducers are now available. The technique has increasingly important applications in the operating theatre and intensive care unit.

Nuclear Medicine

Myocardial perfusion imaging is rarely indicated.

Ventriculography, particularly using first-pass studies, is occasionally useful for measuring pulmonary-to-systemic flow ratios. The normal decay of activity in the right ventricle as the activity moves on to the lungs is interrupted by additional peaks of activity as left-to-right shunting occurs. In complex cyanotic cases it can occasionally be useful to compare pulmonary and systemic blood flow by using *radionuclide-labeled microparticles*.

Computed Tomography

Normal scan times are too slow to allow accurate recording of intracardiac detail although newer 'spiral' scanners are shortening scan times. In addition to this, contrast medium is needed to outline cardiac chambers. The technique is sometimes useful for the assessment of mediastinal masses, which may be close to the heart. A few very sophisticated fast scanners are in use in some specialist centers. These use an accelerator to produce an electron beam which can be moved very fast around the patient to give scan times of 50 ms or less.

Magnetic Resonance Imaging

This technique is in its infancy as far as the study of congenital heart disease is concerned but it holds enormous promise. Temporal and spatial resolution are limited at present, but as equipment and techniques improve and become more widely available, MRI will probably equal or even exceed echocardiography as the most important non-invasive cardiac imaging technique.

The advantages of cardiac MRI can be summarized as follows:

1. Short scan times or gating can 'freeze' cardiac motion.
2. Scans can be taken in transverse, coronal, or sagittal planes, and complex combinations of these planes can also be achieved.
3. Cardiac chambers and walls can be distinguished clearly without the use of contrast media.
4. Blood flow patterns can be recognized. It may soon be possible to quantify stenotic and regurgitant lesions as well as volume flow (cardiac output, shunts, etc.)
5. Three-dimensional reconstructions of complex anatomy will soon be possible.

Cardiac Angiography

It will be some time yet before cardiac angiography is superseded as one of the mainstays of cardiac imaging. As non-invasive techniques replace catheter techniques in more and more cases, there is a parallel increase in interventional therapies, which need the full resources of a catheterization and angiography laboratory.

Many angiograms are still performed using 35 mm cine film recording techniques from the image intensifier. Equipment suspensions must allow a full range of oblique views, as well as cranial and caudal angulation, so that appropriate structures can be profiled. Biplane cine techniques are commonly in use in pediatric cardiology as they allow more views to be taken for smaller doses of contrast medium to the patient. *Digital recording* of images has now reached a stage where it is potentially better than cine film recording. Manipulation of contrast and other image detail is possible, and radiation doses can be reduced significantly. Only the best (and most expensive) digital equipment is adequate, however, because image acquisition at 25 frames per second on a 512×512 matrix is a minimum requirement. This type of system requires a very large storage capacity, and this has been one of the main factors limiting the development of cardiac digital studies. Digital recording of the radiographic image is the key requirement, subtraction of the digital image being only of secondary importance. Intravenous injections of contrast medium have not proved adequate, so digital techniques do not dispense with intracardiac catheters.

Contrast Medium   A major load can be put on the circulation of a sick child by contrast medium. and thus great care must be taken with its use. Nevertheless, it must be used properly, and inadequate volumes or rates of injection which produce poor angiograms are of no benefit to the patient. Wherever finances permit, non-ionic media should be used, and iodine concentrations of 350–400 mg/ml are necessary. Lower concentrations may be possible with good-quality digital equipment. Contrast medium should be administered fast enough to prevent unnecessary dilution, and catheter size must be selected appropriately for the anticipated injection. New non-ionic dimers are now being introduced which are isotonic at high iodine concentrations.

The following is a guide to contrast medium doses for use with non-ionic media of 370 mg iodine/ml, when using conventional cine film technique:

• Start with 1 ml/kg, suitable for a normal ventricle in a neonate

• Reduce by 25–50%, for hypoplastic chambers or a small aorta
• Increase by 50–100%, for large chambers with large flow or shunts
• Also reduce progressively with increasing weight, as follows:
  2–10 kg, no change
  10–20 kg, reduce by 20%
  20–30 kg, reduce by 30%
  30–50 kg, reduce by 40%.

The contrast medium must be delivered in 1.5–2 cardiac cycles to avoid excessive dilution. Thus, neonates with heart rates of 150–180 beats/min will need it delivered in 0.5–0.7 s. This may not be possible if a relatively large dose is to be delivered through too small a catheter. If a child weighing 4 kg with a very large VSD and a heart rate of 180 beats/min is to be studied by left ventriculography, a dose of 8 ml of contrast medium should be delivered at 16 ml/s. This may not be achieved through a 5 French catheter, and a 6 French size must be used.

Total dose limits are hard to state with accuracy, as they depend on the condition of the child and the sequence of the injections; 4 ml/kg is a safe limit for divided doses of 370 mg iodine/ml non-ionic medium, provided the child is reasonably well and not dehydrated. With care and proper hydration this arbitrary limit can be exceeded. As with all diagnostic radiology, the potential benefits must be weighed against the potential hazards in any individual cases.

REFERENCES AND SUGGESTIONS FOR FURTHER READING

Anderson, R. H., MacCartney, F. J., Shinebourne, E. A., Tynan, M. J. (1987) *Paediatric Cardiology*. Edinburgh: Churchill Livingstone.

Elliott L. P. (1991) *Cardiac Imaging in Infants, Children and Adults*. J. B. Lippincott, Philadelphia.

Freedom, R. M., Culham, J. A. G., Moes, C. A. F. (1984) *Angiocardiography of Congenital Heart Disease*. London: Macmillan.

Jordan, S. C., Scott, O. (1989) *Heart Disease in Paediatrics*, 3rd edn. London: Butterworths.

Sutton, M. St J., Oldershaw, P. (1989) *Textbook of Adult and Pediatric Echocardiography and Doppler*. Oxford: Blackwell.

Meire H., Cosgrove D., Dewbury K., Wilde P., (1993) *Clinical Ultrasound*, vol. 4. *Cardiac Ultrasound*. Edinburgh: Churchill Livingstone.

25

ARTERIOGRAPHY AND INTERVENTIONAL ANGIOGRAPHY

David Sutton and Roger Gregson
With contributions from P. L. Allan and Jeremy P. R. Jenkins

Historical

It is a remarkable fact that the history of arteriography began only a few weeks after the discovery of X-rays. Roentgen announced his discovery of X-rays in December 1895, and the first arteriogram was produced within a month, when Haschek and Lindenthal in Vienna published the picture of the arteries of an amputated hand in January 1896 (Haschek & Linderthal 1896).

Realizing the enormous potential of Roentgen's work they had immediately begun experimenting with the injection of radiopaque substances into the arteries of amputated limbs. Even by today's standards of rapid communication this was an outstanding achievement.

Unfortunately the absence of a safe intravascular contrast medium for in vivo work and the prolonged exposures then necessary (about 60 min) meant that this work could not be put into clinical practice.

It was to be another 27 years before the first successful in vivo arteriograms were achieved (Sicard & Forestier 1923; Berberich & Hirsch 1923; Brooks 1924). Soon afterwards, Moniz carried out his classical work on cerebral angiography which was first published in 1928 (Moniz 1931), and in 1929 Dos Santos described lumbar aortography (Dos Santos et al 1931).

Cardiac catheterization was first carried out by Forssman in Germany in 1929 (Forssman 1929) and in 1936 Amiaille first opacified the heart chambers by catheterization. In 1937 Castellanos, Pereiras and Garcia described the use of right-heart angiocardiography in the diagnosis of congenital heart disease, and in 1941 Farinas (Farinas 1941) first described retrograde catheter angiography.

Although all the basic work had now been done, it was not till the 1950s that arteriography became widely used in medicine. This was because arteriography was still an investigation which required surgical intervention, and Scandinavian workers did not develop percutaneous techniques of arteriography till the 1940s. The percutaneous technique of catheterization was not developed till

1953 (Seldinger 1953). It was these innovations which, together with the development of organic iodinated contrast media, set the stage for the more widespread use of angiography.

TECHNIQUES OF IMAGING ARTERIES

The majority of arterial investigations continue to be carried out by direct percutaneous needle puncture, or by percutaneous catheterization of arteries followed by conventional cut film radiography or by digital subtraction angiography. These will be discussed below.

Other imaging techniques, however, have made important and increasing contributions to the study of arterial pathology, and the prospect of safe non-invasive angiography as a routine is now closer than ever.

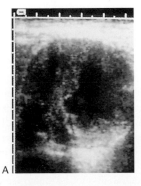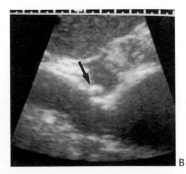

Fig. 25.1 Abdominal aortic aneurysm shown by ultrasound. **A**. Transverse section showing irregular intramural thrombus. The aneurysm diameter measures 5 cm. **B**. Coronal section. The right renal artery is clearly shown proximal to the upper end of the aneurysm (arrow). The coronal plane is essential for clear visualization of this area.

Ultrasound   This has long been used to demonstrate aneurysms of the abdominal aorta and is the simplest and cheapest method of diagnosing such lesions and measuring their size (Fig. 25.1). It is also an ideal method for monitoring the clinical progress of aortic aneurysms, and it can be used to diagnose and assess peripheral aneurysms as well.

The method can also be used to assess arterial stenosis and thrombosis of accessible vessels such as the internal carotid origins. The use of Doppler ultrasound for this and other purposes greatly extends the scope of ultrasound, and is discussed below.

Radionuclide Angiography   Though resolution is too poor to compare with conventional angiography, the method will readily show aortic aneurysms (Fig. 25.2) or major arterial occlusions. It has also been used to show the patency of arterial grafts; and was particularly useful in dealing with patients with known iodine sensitivity, which precludes the use of conventional contrast media.

Computed Tomography   This is a non-invasive method of demonstrating major vascular lesions such as thoracic or abdominal aneurysms. It is usual, however, to inject an intravenous bolus of contrast medium prior to the examination to show intraluminal clot and other abnormalities, a procedure which is minimally invasive compared with direct arteriography. With this technique, large aneurysms are well shown and their dimensions accurately measured (Fig. 25.3). Dissecting aneurysms can be diagnosed (Fig. 25.4) and the anatomy of a coarctation demonstrated. The patency of coronary or other arterial grafts can also be shown by CT.

The advent of spiral and double-helical CT scanners has greatly enhanced the usefulness of CT angiography, and makes it possible to produce images comparable to those of direct arteriography, which it can now replace for many purposes. Spiral CT angiography also makes possible 3D images of high quality (Figs 25.5 and 25.6). The rapid acquisition time of spiral CT enables a whole vascular territory to be imaged within a single 30 s breathhold. This can be timed to coincide with the arterial or venous phase following a peripheral intravenous injection of contrast. Images can be examined from many different viewing angles, unachievable by conventional angiography. Metallic prostheses and aneurysm clips present no hazard as with magnetic resonance angiography (MRA). Further examples of spiral CT angiography are shown in Ch. 56.

Magnetic Resonance Imaging   This is an ideal non-invasive method for demonstrating lesions of the major vessels. The absence of an intraluminal signal from rapidly flowing blood provides a high degree of contrast between lumen and vessel wall and its surrounding tissues (Fig. 25.7). Thrombus and hematoma can be easily differentiated by their relatively high signal (see Fig 25.36), and major branches can be identified. Nevertheless, ultrasound, as an equally non-invasive and radiation-free method of routine screening for such lesions as abdominal aortic aneurysms, remains the method of choice in the abdomen and limbs. It is also much cheaper and more readily available than MRI. The latter, however, is now of considerable importance in the brain and thorax and in the difficult and problem cases which are not readily resolved by ultrasound, e.g. some cases of suspected dissecting aneurysm. Recent advances in technique have also greatly improved the resolution and potential of MRA, which is now replacing direct invasive angiography in many areas (see below and Ch. 56).

Venous Arteriography   This was used in the past as a method

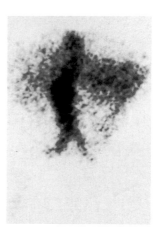

Fig. 25.2   Nuclear angiogram showing aneurysm of the abdominal aorta. This method gives a good idea of the lumen but not of the wall of clot.

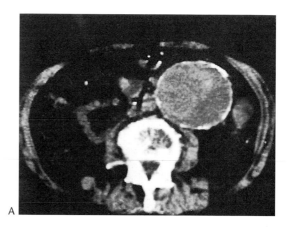

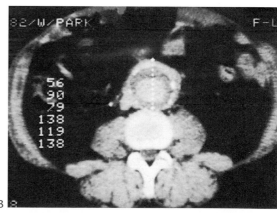

Fig. 25.3   **A** CT scan of the lower abdomen shows a huge abdominal aneurysm with a diameter of 8.5 cm and a calcified wall. **B**. CT scan of the lower abdomen in another patient after intravenous contrast medium shows the lumen of a medium-sized aneurysm with a wall of clot. The diameter as measured by the electronic cursor is 5.6 cm. The wall is thickened and irregular and enhances with contrast medium, features of so-called 'inflammatory' aneurysms or perianeurysmal fibrosis.

of showing major vessels such as the aorta without the hazards of direct arteriography. A large intravenous bolus of contrast medium was used, and substraction films of the appropriate area obtained to acquire images of the aorta and great vessels. These were often

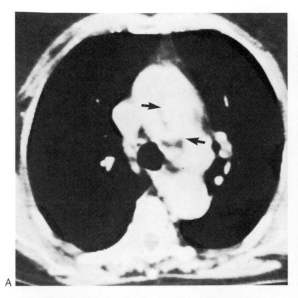
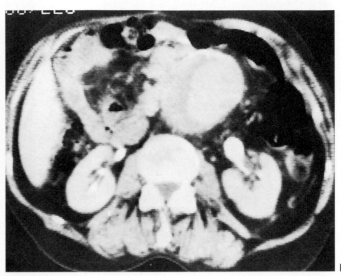

Fig. 25.4 **A**. Dissecting aneurysm shown by CT after contrast medium; both the true and false lumen are opacified but are separated by displaced intimal flaps (arrows) in the dilated ascending aorta (W512 L60). **B**. Dissection involving the abdominal aorta, which shows fusiform aneurysmal dilatation. Contrast in both the true and false lumens is separated by intimal flap (W512 L38).

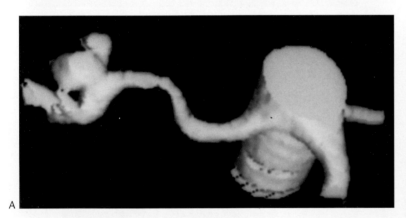
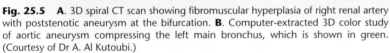
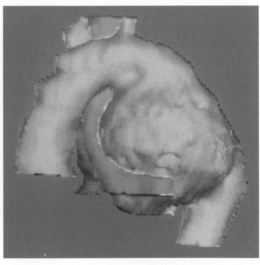

Fig. 25.5 **A**. 3D spiral CT scan showing fibromuscular hyperplasia of right renal artery with poststenotic aneurysm at the bifurcation. **B**. Computer-extracted 3D color study of aortic aneurysm compressing the left main bronchus, which is shown in green. (Courtesy of Dr A. Al Kutoubi.)

adequate for the demonstration of major lesions though the resolution was not comparable with that obtained by direct arteriography. This method was the forerunner of the more sophisticated DSA technique.

Digital Subtraction Angiography This is similar to the technique just described but uses the image intensifier and computers to obtain rapid digital information as the bolus of contrast medium passes through the arteries. The computer is able to subtract the bones and other tissues, leaving only the vessels filled with contrast medium in the analog images obtained (Figs. 25.8 and 25.9).

Using intravenous injections this method can be performed on an outpatient basis, and has been widely used as a screening procedure for such lesions as carotid stenosis and thrombosis and renal artery stenosis. DSA has also proved useful as a less invasive technique for left ventriculography and for postoperative

angiography. Thus, it has been used to check the patency of grafts, in the follow-up of angioplasty, and in the postoperative assessment of aneurysms.

The technique is also now widely applied to direct arteriography, where it has largely replaced conventional cut film angiography. Here its main function is to reduce the dose and volume of contrast medium used for intra-arterial injections and to permit the use of smaller and safer catheters. Catheters as small as 3 French are now routinely used, sometimes on an outpatient basis.

Carbon Dioxide DSA Intravenous injection of CO_2 was first used in the 1950s to demonstrate pericardial effusions by outlining the right auricle. CO_2 was later used for intra-arterial injection, though contrast was poor. The advent of DSA vastly improved the visibility of the gas, so that images can now be obtained comparable with conventional iodinated contrast films. CO_2 is highly soluble

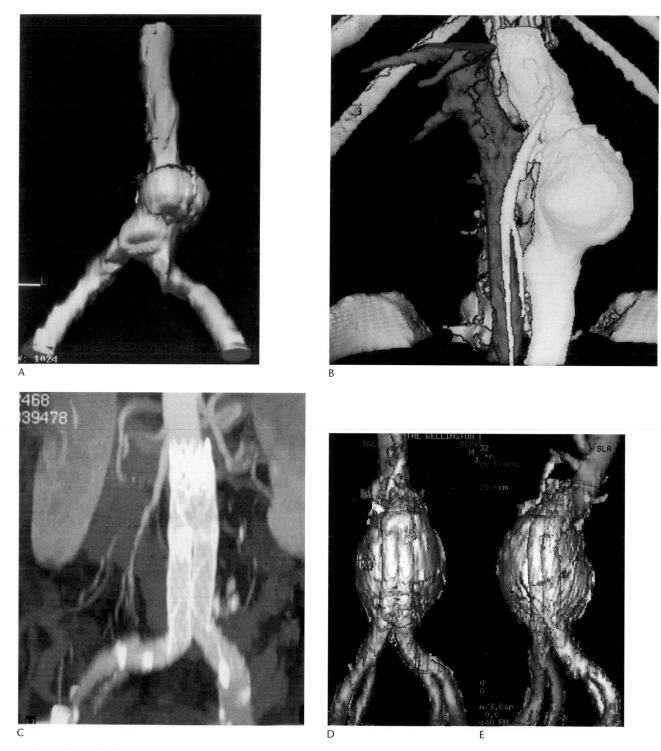

Fig. 25.6 **A**. 3D spiral CT scan showing biloculated false aneurysm complicating lower end of aortic graft. **B**. Spiral CT. 3D reconstruction showing abdominal aortic aneurysm. The inferior vena cava and hepatic veins are also well shown. **C**. Spiral CT. 3D surface shaded study of prosthesis replacing aortic aneurysm. **D,E**. AP and oblique views of double aorta-iliac grafts in situ after transfemoral insertion through a large abdominal aortic aneurysm. 3D-CT color coded. The images can be computer rotated to view from any angle. (Courtesy of Dr A. Al Kutoubi).

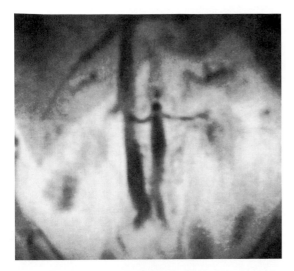

Fig. 25.7 Coronal MRI scan showing abdominal aorta and renal arteries, inferior vena cava, hepatic and right renal veins.

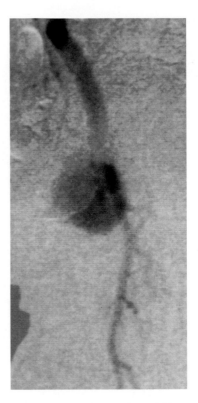

Fig. 25.9 Intravenous DSA image showing femoral false aneurysm following cardiac catheterization.

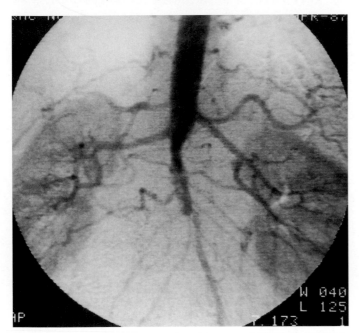

Fig. 25.8 Intravenous DSA image showing aortic thrombosis.

in unsaturated blood serum, and is therefore injected as a bolus to fill the area of interest, where it is normally rapidly absorbed, the volume and rate depending on the blood flow to the target. Because of the low viscosity, small (3 French) catheters can be used. Kerns et al (1995) from the University of Florida regard the method as a viable and safe alternative to iodinated contrast, though the question of possible neurotoxicity precludes its use for cerebral angiography. The method has obvious value in patients with documented or suspected sensitivity to iodinated contrast media, and in high-risk renal failure patients.

DIRECT ARTERIOGRAPHY

Two basic techniques are widely used for direct arteriography:

1. Percutaneous needle puncture
2. Percutaneous arterial catheterization.

The sites for arterial puncture and arterial catheterization are illustrated in Figure 25.10.

PERCUTANEOUS NEEDLE PUNCTURE

In the past the method was applied to most vessels in the body, though percutaneous catheterization has now taken over many of the areas where it was once so widely used (e.g. carotid angiography). Investigations practised for different areas include or have included:

1. Head and neck:
   a. Common carotid arteriography
   b. Vertebral arteriography
2. The upper limb:
   a. Subclavian arteriography
   b. Axillary arteriography
   c. Brachial arteriography
3. The abdomen:
   Lumbar aortography
4. The lower limb:
   Femoral arteriography.

For most practical purposes, direct needle puncture has long ago been superseded by percutaneous catheterization in the head and

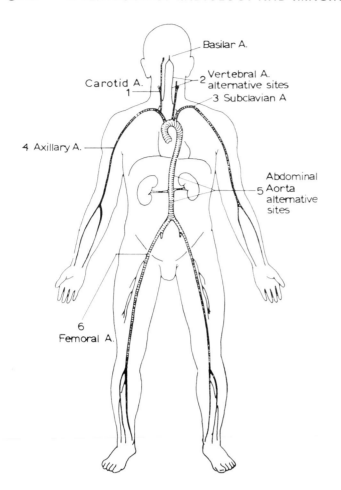

Fig. 25.10 Sites of arterial puncture: 1, carotid artery; 2, vertebral artery, showing alternative sites; 3, subclavian artery; 4, axillary artery; 5, abdominal aorta showing alternative sites; 6, common femoral artery. Sites of percutaneous catheterization: 6, common femoral artery; 4, axillary artery; 1, carotid artery (rarely used).

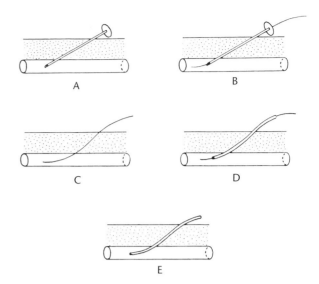

Fig. 25.11 Technique of percutaneous catheter insertion using the Seldinger–Sutton needle. **A.** Needle inserted into artery. **B.** Guide passed through needle into artery. **C.** Needle withdrawn leaving guide in artery. **D.** Catheter passed over guide into artery. **E.** Guide withdrawn leaving catheter in artery.

neck, upper limb and abdomen, though it is still widely used for femoral arteriography, and to a lesser extent for lumbar aortography. It may also still be used as a back-up method in the other areas when catheterization fails or is impractical for technical reasons.

PERCUTANEOUS ARTERIAL CATHETERIZATION

Percutaneous arterial catheterization is based on the original work of Seldinger in Stockholm (Seldinger 1953). The use of a special needle and guide-wire permits the percutaneous introduction of a catheter into a superficial and palpable vessel such as the femoral artery. The basic technique is illustrated in Figure 25.11. The most useful sites for the insertion of catheters into the arterial tree are:

1. The femoral artery in the groin
2. The axillary artery in the axilla.

Catheters have also been inserted from the brachial artery just above the elbow, from the radial artery just above the wrist, from the common carotid artery in the neck, and from the abdominal aorta using a translumbar approach. In practice, the femoral and

axillary arteries permit investigation of most areas, and the other sites of insertion are little used except in special circumstances.

Selective and Superselective Arterial Catheterization

This is a refinement of the standard technique in which specially shaped catheters are introduced into branches or sub-branches of the aorta. Arteries which are frequently catheterized include most major branches of the abdominal aorta (renal, celiac axis, superior and inferior mesenteric arteries), major branches of the aortic arch (subclavian, innominate, and left common carotid arteries and their major branches, including the vertebrals, and internal and external carotid arteries). Superselective catheterization is frequently performed on branches of the celiac axis, including the splenic, hepatic, and gastroduodenal arteries, and on branches of the external carotid such as the internal maxillary.

Most catheterizations are now performed with relatively small catheters, usually of 5 French gauge, or less.

TECHNIQUE OF ARTERIAL PUNCTURE

The technique used for arterial needle puncture is similar for most of the arteries used.

The common femoral artery is readily palpable in the groin, and is usually punctured just below Poupart's ligament. The axillary artery is palpable with the arm held in abduction and is punctured in its lower part. The common carotid artery was punctured with the neck slightly extended, though as noted above this is now rarely done.

In all the above cases the artery is palpated and fixed by the index and middle fingers of the right handed operator's left hand whilst the needle is inserted with the right hand.

For lumbar aortography the abdominal aorta is approached from the left lumbar region with the patient lying prone. A preliminary X-ray film with markers is usually taken to localize the vertebral

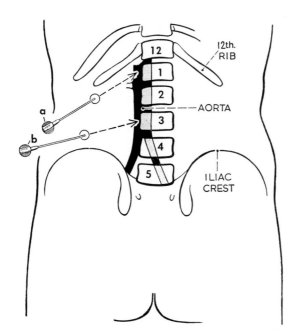

Fig. 25.12 Lumbar aortography—site of puncture. **a**. High puncture. **b**. Low puncture.

levels. Depending on the purpose of the investigation, the aorta is punctured either at L1 (for renal angiography, aortic thrombosis, or abdominal aneurysms) or below the renals at L3 (for low aortic or iliac or peripheral vascular disease) (Fig. 25.12).

Successful puncture of an artery is marked by rapid pulsation of arterial blood through the needle into the transparent plastic connecting tubing. This is the signal for immediate flushing of the system with saline, which is then sealed off by the tap between tubing and syringe. Saline flushing is continued intermittently throughout the procedure except during the contrast medium injections. The aim is to keep the needle and tubing free of blood (except momentarily) so that no stasis or clotting can occur in the system.

TECHNIQUE OF PERCUTANEOUS CATHETERIZATION

A simplified Seldinger technique routinely used by the author is illustrated in Figure 25.11, and consists of the following consecutive steps:

1. The artery (usually the femoral and less commonly the axillary) is punctured by a thin-walled needle as described above.

2. Once the needle tip is firmly in the vessel lumen the connecting tubing is detached, allowing blood to spurt back (Fig. 25.11A). The guide-wire is then immediately passed through the needle into the vessel, and its tip advanced 5–8 cm along the lumen (Fig. 25.11B). Holding the guide-wire firmly in position, the needle is then withdrawn along it and off the guide-wire (Fig. 25.11C). Meanwhile, firm manual pressure is maintained with gauze swabs at the puncture site to prevent oozing of blood and hematoma formation.

3. The catheter, with a two-way tap attached to its hind end, is now passed along the guide-wire and into the artery. The guide-wire is longer than the catheter and protrudes from its back end

once the catheter tip reaches beyond its front end (Fig. 25.11D). It can then be removed, leaving the catheter safely in the artery (Fig. 25.11E). Saline can now be perfused through the catheter exactly as with needle puncture.

The catheter can now be pushed along the artery to any desired level. In tortuous or atheromatous arteries it may be necessary to use special guides with more flexible tips in order to advance catheters through difficult areas.

Saline infusion of the catheter is maintained either by slow hand injection or by an automatic drip system. Unless contraindicated for clinical reasons, heparinized saline is routinely used to counteract any tendency to clot formation in or around the catheter tip.

RADIOGRAPHIC APPARATUS

Arteriography requires rapid serial films of the area under investigation to capture the flow of the contrast medium through the arteries and in some cases through the capillary bed and drainage veins as well. In some areas (e.g. the lower limb), four serial films taken within 5–8 s may be adequate; in others (e.g. the aortic arch), films taken at a rate of three or four per second for 4 s may be necessary. In certain conditions such as large arteriovenous fistulas or angiomas, multiple rapid serial films will also be required to define the full anatomy of the lesion.

Many types of commercial serial film changers are on the market, and choice will depend on local availability and preferences. For most purposes the versatile Puck changers, allowing speeds of three films per second, are adequate.

Fine-focus high-power X-ray tubes are essential for rapid serial films and to facilitate magnification techniques. Subtraction techniques are also widely used in angiography.

Arteriography is now more widely practised using DSA. This has many advantages, including lower doses and volumes of contrast medium and automatic electronic subtraction. Resolution is less than can be obtained with the best film techniques but is adequate for most practical purposes.

Injections of contrast medium can be performed by hand for many forms of angiography, but pressure injection using specialized apparatus is essential for thoracic aortography, abdominal flush aortography, and angiocardiography. It is also essential for DSA using intravenous injection.

ANESTHESIA

Most angiographic procedures can be carried out under local anesthesia, but basal sedation may be necessary with the more complex investigations. Some drugs such as pethidine are more likely than others to produce a hypotensive reaction and must therefore be used with caution, particularly if arterial stenosis is suspected. Hypotension can precipitate thrombosis in such patients.

General anesthesia is usually necessary with children, and may be required with difficult or very nervous patients or those unable to cooperate. Besides prolonging the investigation and increasing its cost, it undoubtedly adds to the hazards, since, apart from the added complications of general anesthesia, the patient is unable to react to misplaced injections or other mishaps. With a conscious patient, symptoms and untoward reactions are at once apparent, and the procedure can be stopped immediately.

CONTRAST MEDIA

The earliest vascular contrast media mentioned above were far from ideal. They included lipiodol injected into veins in small quantity (Sicard & Forestier 1923) ad strontium bromide (Berberich & Hirsch 1923) and sodium iodide (Brooks 1924), which were the first contrast agents injected into arteries. Thorium dioxide (Thorotrast) was used by Moniz (Moniz 1931) and became the standard medium in the 1930s. Unfortunately it was retained indefinitely by the reticuloendothelial system, and being radioactive gave rise to delayed malignancy. Abdominal films taken years after injection showed a characteristic stippling in the spleen resembling miliary calcification.

Organic iodide preparations stemmed from the work of Swick (1929), who developed uroselectan (Iopax) (containing one atom of iodine per molecule) as a reliable agent for intravenous urography. Later, organic iodines were developed, first with two and then with three atoms of iodine per molecule. The standard media widely used in the 1970s and 1980s are listed in Table 25.1.

It is estimated that over 50 million doses of iodinated contrast media per annum are currently used worldwide in radiological practice, and they represent a major item in the operating expenses of most radiological departments.

The ideal contrast medium should be completely non-toxic and completely painless to the patient in the high concentrations used for angiography. A further advance toward this ideal was the introduction in the 1980s of *low-osmolality* contrast media. These agents are relatively painless, compared with their high-osmolar predecessors, and are claimed to produce fewer toxic side-effects. Both these benefits are related to the low osmolality, which is closer to that of normal plasma than was that of their predecessors. At an iodine concentration of 280 mg/ml the osmolality measures about 480 mmol/kg H_2O. This compares with 1500 mmol/kg H_2O for the equivalent Conray (high-osmolar) preparation and 300 mmol/kg H_2O for plasma (Table 25.2).

Further low-osmolality contrast media introduced in recent years include the non-ionic monomers Ultravist (iopromide) from Schering; Iopentol (Nycomed, Oslo), and Iomeron (iomeprol) from Bracco (Italy). Also recently introduced are Isovist (iotrolan) by Schering, a dimeric non-ionic low-osmolar contrast medium, and Visipaque (iodixanol)—also an isotonic non-ionic dimer—from Nycomed.

Osmolality is proportional to the ratio of iodine atoms to the number of particles in solution. In the older hyperosmolar contrast media, this ratio was 3:2, whereas the new low-osmolar agents have a ratio of 3:1 and do not ionize in solution. Ioxaglate, which is a monoacid dimer, does ionize in solution but has a similar iodine: particle ratio (6:2 or effectively 3:1) and therefore enjoys the same benefits of low osmolality. To date the only drawback to the new media is that they cost a good deal more than their predecessors, and this remains an important factor inhibiting their more widespread use.

Dosage

Peripheral and Smaller Arteries   As a general principle, the dose of contrast medium injected is related to the flow rate in the vessel being injected. Small vessels with low flow rates require small amounts at low pressures, while large vessels with high flow rates require larger volumes at high pressures. The recommended doses for different smaller arteries are listed in Table 25.3, and in most arteries the recommended dose can safely be repeated after a short interval. In each case the injection is made in about 1–2 s.

Of the high-osmolar contrast media, we regarded Urografin 310 as the best for cerebral angiography and Triosil 370 as preferable for coronary angiography, since there is experimental evidence that these agents are less toxic than other high-osmolar products at these sites. The quantity used for coronary artery injections varies

Table 25.1   Intravascular contrast media

Product	Formula	Iodine content (g/ml)	viscosity (mPa s) at 37°C
Hypaque 45	Sodium diatrizoate 45% w/v	0.27	2.1
Hypaque 65	Sodium diatrizoate 25% w/v and N-methylglucamine salt of diatrizoic acid 50% w/v		8.4
Hypaque 85	As Hypaque 65 but mixture is: (1) 28.33% w/v; and (2) 56.67% w/v	0.44	12.2
Urografin 290	Mixture of the sodium and the methylglucamine salts of diatrizoic acid in the proportion 10:66	0.44	8.4
Urografin 370		0.37	8.5
Urografin 310 (Angiografin)	Meglumine amidotrizoate 65%	0.306	5.1
Conray 280	Meglumine iothalamate 60% w/v	0.28	4.0
Conray 325	Sodium iothalamate 54% w/v	0.375	2.7
Conray 420	Sodium iothalamate 70% w/v	0.42	5.4
Cardio-Conray	Meglumine iothalamate 52%, sodium iothalamate 26% w/v	0.40	8.6
Triosil 280	Meglumine metrizoate 59% w/v (with Ca)	0.28	4.0
Triosil 370	Meglumine metrizoate (with Na and Ca)	0.37	8.5
Triosil 350	Sodium metrizoate 52% w/v (with meglumine, Ca or Mg)	0.35	3.4
Triosil 440	Sodium metrizoate 66% w/v (with meglumine, Ca or Mg)	0.44	6.6

Table 25.2   Low-osmolality contrast media

Product	General formula	Iodine atoms: particles in solution	Iodine content (mg/ml)	Viscosity (mPa s) at 37°C
Iopamidol (Niopam), non-ionic		3:1	200 300 370	2.0 4.7 8.6
Iohexol (Omnipaque), non-ionic	Similar to above but with different radicles R_1, R_2 or R_3	3:1	240 280 300 350	3.3 4.8 6.1 10.6
Ioxaglate (Hexabrix), ionic		6:2 [= 3:1]	320	7.5

Table 25.3   Recommend doses of Conray 280 or equivalent (smaller arteries)[a]

Artery	Dose (ml)
Femoral	20
Subclavian (or axillary)	20
Carotid	10
Vertebral	8
Renal	10
Inferior mesenteric	15
Intercostal	3
Bronchial	5

[a]Using standard cut film techniques (doses can be reduced by two-thirds for DSA).

from 4 to 8 ml, depending on the state of the patient and the flow rate in the individual vessel.

As already explained, the new low-osmolar contrast media are preferable to the older high-osmolar products, and should be used routinely whenever cost is not a major inhibiting factor.

Larger Arteries

1. *Arch aortography.* For injections into the aortic arch, which has the highest flow rate in the body, 40 ml of high-concentration contrast medium is injected by a pressure machine at 20 ml/s. Triosil 370 or 440 and Conray 420 were high-osmolar products widely used for this purpose, though they have been now largely replaced by the new low-osmolar agents such as iopamidol 370, iohexol 350 or Hexabrix 320.

2. *Abdominal aortography.* Whether performed by catheter or by lumbar injection, 30 ml of a high concentration contrast medium (Conray 420, Hypaque 350, Hexabrix 320 or iohexol 350), delivered in 1.5–2 s, is regarded as a safe dose for high aortic injection, i.e. above the renal arteries, and provided both kidneys are functioning normally. However, if there is severe renal impairment or only one kidney functioning, caution should be observed, and the dose reduced to a maximum of 20 ml. A similar precaution is necessary if there is an aortic thrombosis present which would result in a higher dose to the kidneys.

For a low aortic injection, i.e. below the renal arteries, 25 ml injected in 1.5 s is usually adequate.

The normal celiac axis and superior mesenteric arteries both have high flow rates and can tolerate injections of 30 ml of Hypaque 350 or equivalents at one injection. Some workers recommend doses as high as 50 ml where it is desirable to show the portal circulation. Speed of injection, however, is relatively low at 8 ml/s.

As already noted, doses can be substantially reduced for arterial DSA.

CONTRAST MEDIUM REACTIONS

Reactions to the intravascular injection of contrast media, whether intravenous or intra-arterial, are not uncommon (about 12% in one major intravenous series using high-osmolar contrast media). Fortunately, the vast majority are trivial or of minor importance. Reactions can be classified as mild, intermediate, or severe. The latter are potentially fatal but formed less than 0.25% of the series just quoted.

The mechanism of these reactions is debated, though many factors have been postulated, including anxiety, histamine and serotonin release, antigen–antibody formation, activation of the complement and coagulation systems, and interruption of the blood–brain barrier.

Mild reactions include sneezing, mild urticaria, nausea and vomiting, conjunctival injection, mild pallor or sweating, limited urticaria or itchy skin rash, feelings of heat or cold, tachycardia or bradycardia, and arm pain following intravenous injections. Recovery is rapid and requires no treatment except reassurance.

Intermediate reactions include widespread urticaria, bronchospasm and laryngospasm, angioneurotic edema, moderate hypotension, faintness, headache, severe vomiting, rigors, dyspnea, chest or abdominal pain. Immediate treatment is required but response is rapid.

Severe reactions are rare but can be fatal. They include cardiopulmonary collapse with severe hypotension, pulmonary edema, refractory bronchospasm and laryngospasm. Also seen are myocardial ischemia, tachycardia, bradycardia, other arrhythmias, cardiac arrest, severe collapse, loss of consciousness, and edema of the glottis.

The mortality from hyperosmolar intravenous contrast medium injections is estimated at 1 case per 40 000 injections. Arterial injections probably carry a similar risk.

The risk from the newer low-osmolar media appears to be significantly lower for minor and intermediate reactions (about 3% as against 12%); it also appears to be significantly lower for severe reactions, but is not yet accurately quantified for fatal reactions, where the evidence remains inconclusive.

Risk Factors   *Major risk factors* associated with the use of contrast media include:

1. Allergy, especially asthma
2. Extremes of age (under 1 year and over 60 years)
3. Cardiovascular disease
4. History of previous reactions to contrast medium.

Minor risk factors include diabetes mellitus, dehydration, impaired renal function, hemoglobinopathy and dysproteinemia. *Drug risks* include β-blocker therapy (predisposes to bronchospasm and other severe reactions), adrenal suppression (patients on steroids require additional steroids before contrast administration), and interleukin-2 therapy (may cause contrast hypersensitivity).

Previous minor reactions to contrast medium are not a contra-indication to a repeat examination, but patients with previous severe reactions should be examined by other means. Patients with previous intermediate reactions should be carefully assessed and the examination abandoned or, if essential, only repeated under careful control. This implies pretreatment for 3 days with oral prednisone (50 mg) 8-hourly. Ephedrine (25 mg) and diphenhydramine (50 mg) are also given 1 h before the examination, and only a low-osmolar contrast medium should be used.

Pretesting for allergy with small doses of contrast medium was once widely performed but has now been abandoned as completely unreliable. Fatalities have occurred after previous negative test doses, and test doses have themselves resulted in fatalities.

Treatment   Emergency drugs and equipment should be immediately available wherever contrast media are used. Intermediate and severe reactions usually involve hypotension, which is treated by elevation of the legs and may require rapid intravascular fluid. Oxygen may also need to be administered, and it is essential to distinguish a vasovagal reaction (characterized by hypotension with bradycardia) from an allergic or anaphylactoid reaction (characterized by hypotension with tachycardia). The former requires atropine, 0.6–1.2 mg i.v., whilst the latter requires epinephrine.

Iodism The radiologist should be aware that free iodine present in contrast media will interfere with the performance of radioactive iodine tests of thyroid function. Salivary gland enlargement ('iodine mumps') may follow several days after the injection, and hyperthyroidism may be induced. Minor skin rashes may also be seen several days after contrast medium administration.

Nephrotoxicity Intravascular contrast media may have a nephrotoxic effect. The pathogenesis is debated but may be multifactorial due to vasconstriction, a direct toxic effect on tubular cells, and cast formation in tubules with intrarenal obstruction. Acute renal failure due to nephrotoxicity is claimed to occur in 5% of patients with chronic renal failure but in less than 1% of patients with normal function. Clinically the patient may be asymptomatic with rapid recovery, may show non-oliguric renal dysfunction, or, rarely, show severe oliguric renal failure.

Risk factors include large doses of contrast medium, dehydration, diabetes mellitus, pre-existing renal insufficiency and multiple myeloma. Caution in administering contrast media is desirable in diabetic patients with impaired renal function, in multiple myeloma patients with Bence–Jones proteinuria, and in hyperuricemic patients. Dehydration is definitely contraindicated in patients at risk.

PHARMACOANGIOGRAPHY

This refers to the use of vasoactive drugs to modify blood flow to target organs. The procedure was once very popular but is now rarely used.

Vasodilators These drugs were used to reverse vasospasm, to increase the size of arterioles and collaterals, and to improve the visualization of the venous return. They will also enhance the outline of non-vascular lesions such as cysts, by contrast with the enhanced parenchyma. They were once widely used in arterioportography for better visualization of the portal circulation. They were also used in peripheral arteriography to improve visualization of poorly filling distal vessels.

The vasodilators used were Priscoline (tolazoline) for the splanchnic, femoral, and brachial arteries, prostaglandin E_1 in the femoral artery, and bradykinin in the renal and superior mesenteric arteries.

In healthy patients, Priscoline was given as a 25 mg bolus in the splanchnic vessels, and as a 12 mg bolus into limb vessels. It must be used with caution in cardiac patients as it can produce hypotension and cardiac arrhythmias.

Vasoconstrictors These can help to distinguish tumor from normal circulation since the latter reacts to them but the former does not and thus stands out more clearly. Epinephrine was once widely used for this purpose in both renal and splanchnic arteriography. It is administered as a 3–6 μg bolus into the renal artery, and as a 5–8 μg bolus into splanchic vessels. Vasopressin and angiotensin have also been used as vasoconstrictors.

Epinephrine increases blood pressure and peripheral resistance and must therefore be used with great caution in patients with cardiac disease, where it may be contraindicated.

Hyperventilation can be used in cerebral angiography to produce similar effects, since normal cerebral vessels react to hyperoxemia and hypocapnia by vasoconstriction while tumor vessels are unaffected. Hyperventilation was performed by the anesthetist in cerebral angiograms conducted under general anesthesia.

COMPLICATIONS

Many complications have resulted from arteriography, and these are summarized in Table 25.4. This formidable list of complications emphasizes that arteriography should not be undertaken lightly and that it is best performed by radiologists with considerable training and experience in this field. The complication rate is also significantly lower at centers where large numbers of arteriograms are routinely performed than at centers where they are only occasionally seen.

A full discussion of the complications of arteriography will be found in specialist monographs, but attention is drawn below to some of the more important complications.

Damage to Arterial Walls This may result from a traumatic needle or catheter puncture. Local subintimal stripping may result, particularly if contrast medium or saline is accidentally injected subintimally (Figs 25.13 and 25.14). In small vessels this can result in actual occlusion and thrombosis (see below). The use of short bevelled needles, together with skill and experience, is the main means of preventing these accidents.

Perivascular injection of contrast medium can also occur (Fig. 25.15), but is relatively harmless apart from local pain and discomfort to the patient being examined under local anesthesia.

Thrombosis of Arteries As just noted, this can result from

Table 25.4 Complications of contrast arteriography

A. *General*
   1. Contrast reactions
      a. Severe life-threatening
      b. Intermediate
      c. Minor (coughing, sneezing, mild, urticaria)
   2. Embolus
      a. Catheter clot
      b. Cholesterol
      c. Cotton fibre
      d. Air
   3. Septicemia
   4. Vagal inhibition

B. *Local*
   1. Puncture site
      a. Hemorrhage and hematoma
      b. False aneurysm
      c. Arterio-venous fistula
      d. Perivascular or subintimal contrast injection
      e. Local thrombosis
      f. Local infection
      g. Damage to adjacent nerves
   2. Damage to target or other organs due to
      a. Excess of contrast
      b. Catheter clot embolus
   3. Fracture and loss of guide-wire tip
   4. Knot formation in catheters
   5. Embolization accidents (see below)
   6. Angioplasty accidents (see below)

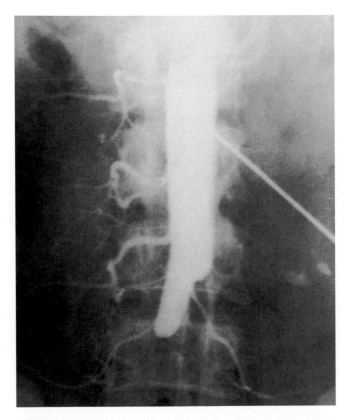

Fig. 25.13 Subintimal injection of contrast medium at lumbar aortography. Most of the contrast medium lies in the wall of the aorta and right common iliac artery. A small amount is intraluminal and outlines lumbar arteries. Contrast medium in the aortic wall persists on serial films.

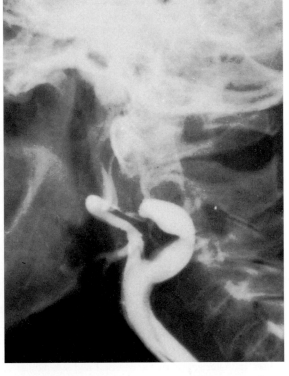

Fig. 25.14 Subintimal injection of contrast medium at needle common carotid arteriogram. Contrast medium persists in the arterial wall on serial films. Note linear translucencies caused by displaced intima.

trauma to the arterial wall at arterial puncture, or from subintimal stripping from injections of contrast medium or saline with formation of a local dissecting aneurysm. Another well-documented mechanism is formation of clot at the end of a catheter. This is then stripped off as the catheter is withdrawn through the puncture hole and forms a focus for local thrombosis. Another causative or contributory factor is a severe hypotensive reaction (see below). Whatever mechanism or combination of mechanisms is responsible, there is also a direct relationship with the experience of the operator and with the adequacy of the patient's cardiovascular system. Patients with cardiovascular insufficiency and severely atheromatous vessels are at greater risk, and should only be examined by experienced operators.

Systemic Heparinization This is generally recommended to counter catheter clot formation and thrombosis. As soon as the catheter has been passed into the aorta, 3000 units of heparin are injected. The procedure is useful in prolonged catheterization procedures, and rarely causes any problem. If there is excessive oozing from the puncture site at completion, heparinization can be reversed by injecting 10 mg of protamine sulfate per 1000 units of heparin used.

Allergy The minor allergic contrast reactions (see above) rarely give rise to concern, and patients can be reassured that sneezing, coughing, or urticaria will rapidly subside. However, radiologists must be aware of the danger of the very rare major hypersensitivity

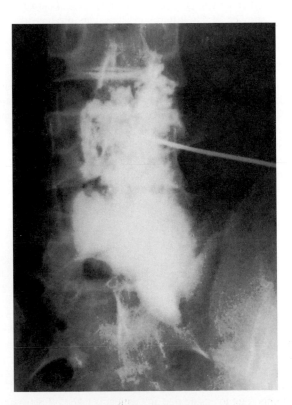

Fig. 25.15 Perivascular injection of contrast medium at lumbar aortography.

reaction, and be prepared for its prompt treatment. This requires dexamethasone 10–20 mg i.v., and if necessary artificial respiration with positive pressure and oxygen. For edema of the glottis, 0.5 mg of epinephrine subcutaneously or intramuscularly is recommended, together with slow intravenous injection of an antihistamine. Arrangements should also be ready beforehand for the emergency treatment of such catastrophies as cardiac arrest, ventricular fibrillation, and collapse with circulatory insufficiency.

Hypotension Severe hypotensive reactions may occur with any arteriographic procedure, but particularly with complex or prolonged investigations. Blood pressure should be monitored, and it should be remembered that patients with vascular disease, particularly atheromatous stenosis, may have lesions in many vessels and that hypotension can precipitate a thrombosis. Coronary infarction or hemiplegia from a carotid thrombosis are potential complications.

Hypotension has also been recorded several hours after a major procedure and the patient must be monitored on the ward for several hours after arteriography.

Catheter Clot Embolus Clot may form in and around the tip of a catheter, particularly during a prolonged procedure, and such a clot may be detached by a contrast medium injection. The main danger is with catheters lying in or proximal to the cerebral vessels, when detached clot may be directed to the brain. Left ventriculography, coronary arteriography, arch aortography, and 'headhunter' catheterization of the cerebral and subclavian vessels are all procedures which carry this risk. The use of small catheters and speedy and skilled angiography help to minimize the risk, as does systemic heparinization.

Cholesterol Embolization This may occur spontaneously in patients with severe atheromatous disease. It may also occur after surgery, and is occasionally precipitated by arterial catheterization. A large shower of cholesterol crystals can produce disastrous results, particularly if vital organs are involved. Postmortem studies suggest that minor degrees of cholesterol crystal embolism are commoner than is generally appreciated.

Air Embolus Undoubtedly air embolus has been a cause of fatalities in the past, particularly when large steel syringes were used for major injections. Air could easily enter a large opaque syringe and could be injected without the operator being aware of the mishap, especially if the nozzle was horizontal or pointing upwards. Even with the translucent plastic syringes now in general use, great care must be taken not to include air when loading with contrast medium or saline solution, and all injections should be made with the nozzle pointing down.

Hematomas and False Aneurysms The occurrence of these at the puncture site should be relatively uncommon, provided small needles are used and the tips of larger catheters are well tapered. They are seen most frequently with hypertensive patients. After an arterial puncture, firm manual pressure transmitted through gauze swabs should be maintained on the puncture site till all oozing has stopped. The puncture site should also be inspected before the patient leaves the department (an hour or two later) and the following morning, and the patient warned to report immediately if there is any further swelling or oozing.

False aneurysms (pulsating hematomas) will require surgical treatment.

It is important to ensure that any patient is taken off anticoagulant drugs before arteriography and that the prothrombin time has fallen to normal before the investigation.

Damage to Nerves Transaxillary catheterization carries the particular risk of damage to branches of the brachial plexus since the artery is closely related to its distal part. This can result in severe disability. Most of the reported cases were due to nerve compression by hematomas or false aneurysms, though direct damage by needle puncture may be responsible in some cases. Transaxillary catheterization should only be undertaken by senior and experienced angiographers, and observation for signs of hematoma or nerve damage should be maintained for 24 h after the investigation. If symptoms of paresis appear and progress, they are usually due to compression by a hematoma, and urgent surgical decompression of the neurovascular sheath is essential if permanent paralysis is to be prevented.

Femoral nerve palsy is a much rarer complication of femoral artery puncture though transient pain or paresthesia in the cutaneous distribution of the femoral nerve is not uncommon, usually resolving within 24 h.

Vagal Inhibition This may occur after a major contrast medium injection, and has been encountered after intravenous urography and intravenous cholangiography. It is characterized by collapse of the patient with bradycardia. This helps to distinguish it from circulatory collapse in acute allergy, which is usually associated with tachycardia. The distinction is of vital importance, since the latter is often treated with epinephrine, a drug which is contra-indicated in vagal inhibition, where atropine is the drug of choice and may be life-saving.

Damage to Organs Since angiography often targets vital organs, including the heart, brain, kidneys, and bowel, it is not surprising that damage to such organs can result, followed by death or serious morbidity. In most cases the cause has been arterial thrombosis from the causes mentioned above, or organ damage from an excessive dose of contrast medium.

Non-fatal brain damage has resulted in hemiplegia, both transient and permanent. Cortical blindness—occasionally permanent, but fortunately in most cases transient—has resulted from vertebral angiography.

Spinal cord damage is a rare and tragic complication of arteriography, usually due to an excessive dose of contrast medium entering a main artery of supply to the spinal cord. Thus, paraplegia has been recorded after both lumbar and abdominal aortography, presumably from injection of the artery of Adamkewicz which supplies the cord from D8 downward and arises from one of the upper lumbar or lower intercostal arteries.

Tetraplegia has resulted from vertebral angiography and from thyroid axis angiography. In the latter case, an excess of contrast medium has entered the deep cervical artery which supplies the cervical cord. It has been suggested that such cases should be treated by replacement of cerebrospinal fluid with isotonic saline and by systemic steroids, though others doubt the value of this.

Coronary Angiography This carries the special dangers of vagal inhibition, ventricular fibrillation, cardiac systole, and myocardial infarction. All of these are potentially fatal unless immediate treatment is at hand.

Embolization and Angioplasty These carry special hazards which are discussed below.

INTERVENTIONAL VASCULAR RADIOLOGY

Interventional vascular radiology has developed from diagnostic angiography, and now plays a central role in the management of patients with vascular disease. Because these therapeutic angiographic procedures are often simple, effective, and efficient with a low morbidity and mortality, they have increased the number of treatment options available to patients by enabling a percutaneous endovascular procedure to be performed instead of a conventional surgical one. They have also increased the range of treatment available by offering procedures to patients who are either unfit for surgery or whose symptoms do not merit its risks.

Interventional vascular radiology includes transluminal angioplasty, therapeutic embolization, vascular infusion therapy, and the insertion and retrieval of intravascular foreign bodies. The scope and complexity of these procedures, however, continues to grow.

TRANSLUMINAL ANGIOPLASTY

The technique of percutaneous transluminal angioplasty (PTA) was initially performed in 1964 by Dotter and Judkins, who used coaxial catheters to dilate arterial stenoses. However, it was the development of the polyvinyl chloride balloon catheter by Gruntzig and Hopff in 1974 that led to the widespread use of this technique, which is the commonest interventional vascular procedure performed in the world today.

The basic technique of PTA involves passing a guide-wire and catheter across a stenosis or through an occlusion in a blood vessel. A balloon catheter is then positioned across the diseased segment and dilated up to the same size as the adjacent lumen, in order to increase the blood flow through the artery or vein (Figure 25.16).

The mechanism of how PTA works was originally thought to be due to compression and redistribution of the soft atheromatous material along the arterial wall, but histopathological studies with electron microscopy have now shown that the balloon splits the atheromatous plaque producing clefts in the intima, which extend into the media but not the adventitia. Platelets then aggregate on the damaged surface, and healing of the intima and media occurs over several weeks by the formation of intimal hyperplasia and fibrosis with retraction of the plaque, resulting in an improved arterial luminal diameter.

In patients with vascular disease, atherosclerosis is by far the commonest cause of the variety of arterial stenoses and occlusions in patients treated by PTA, but other pathological conditions such as fibromuscular dysplasia, arteritis, intimal hyperplasia, radiation damage, and trauma are also amenable to treatment with PTA.

Angioplasty in Peripheral Vascular Disease

Many patients undergoing investigation for peripheral vascular disease with symptoms of intermittent claudication, rest pain, ischemic ulceration, and gangrene are suitable for PTA. This can be performed in symptomatic patients as an alternative to a surgical bypass graft or in combination with surgery to improve the inflow or outflow in the adjacent arteries. It is also used to treat patients with intermittent claudication, whose symptoms limit their lifestyle but are not severe enough to require reconstructive surgery, and to try and prevent amputation in patients with rest pain, ulceration, and gangrene who are unfit for surgery (*limb salvage angioplasty*).

PTA is therefore indicated in symptomatic patients with arterial stenoses or short occlusions in the lower limbs on angiography. The contraindications include the presence of fresh thrombus in the arteries, which should be treated by either thrombolysis or aspiration

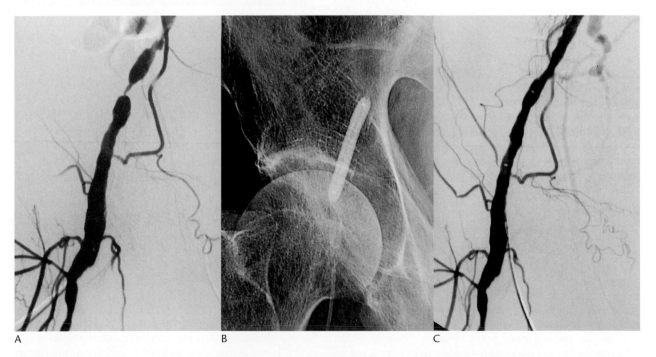

A   B   C

Fig. 25.16   A. Arteriogram showing 75–90% stenoses in the right external iliac artery and occlusion of the right superficial femoral artery before angioplasty. **B**. Balloon catheter in the external iliac artery during the angioplasty. **C**. Angiographic result in the external iliac artery after angioplasty.

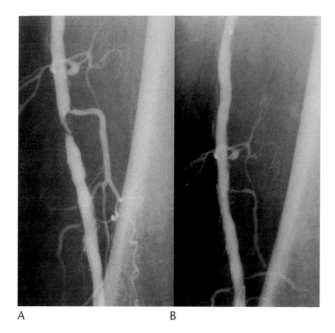

Fig. 25.17 A. A suitable lesion for PTA—arteriogram showing 75% stenosis in the distal left superficial femoral artery. **B**. Arteriogram after angioplasty.

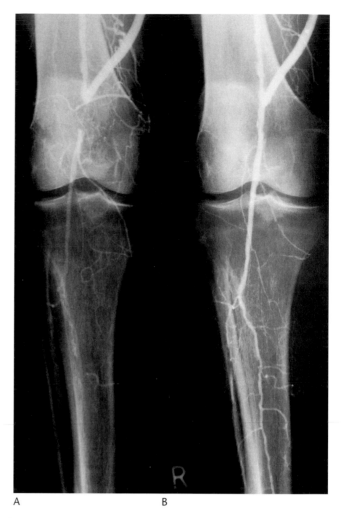

Fig. 25.18 A. Arteriogram showing a short 2 cm occlusion in the right popliteal artery, below the distal anastomosis of a femoropopliteal vein graft. **B**. Arteriogram after angioplasty.

thrombectomy, a total aortic occlusion, and long occlusions in the iliac, femoral, or popliteal arteries, although even these can now occasionally be treated successfully. The ideal lesion for PTA is a short, smooth, central 50–90% stenosis in a large artery, such as the common or external iliac artery in a patient with normal distal arteries, because the technical and clinical success rates are very high (Fig. 25.17). Patients undergoing PTA should be started on treatment with an antiplatelet drug, such as *aspirin* or *dipyridamole*, 24 h before the procedure, and this should be continued for at least 3–6 months after the procedure and possibly for life. Increased exercise and stopping smoking should also be encouraged. During the procedure, patients should receive 3000–5000 units of heparin intra-arterially. After the procedure some patients are treated with *warfarin*.

Iliac artery stenoses and short occlusions up to 5–7 cm in length are usually approached from below following a retrograde catheterization of the ipsilateral common femoral artery. This can be punctured even if there is no femoral pulse, with the help of palpation, fluoroscopy, ultrasound, or DSA. Iliac artery lesions can also be approached across the aortic bifurcation following catheterization of the contralateral common femoral artery or following catheterization of the axillary or brachial artery, usually in the left arm. Stenoses in the internal iliac, common femoral, proximal superficial, and deep femoral arteries are often approached across the aortic bifurcation. Distal superficial femoral and popliteal artery stenoses and short occlusions up to 10–15 cm in length are usually approached from above following an antegrade catheterization of the ipsilateral common or superficial femoral artery (Fig. 25.18). Femoral artery lesions can also be approached from below following catheterization of the ipsilateral popliteal artery. Stenosis of the lower abdominal aorta and tibial artery stenoses and short occlusions up to 3–5 cm in length are also suitable for PTA.

The size of the balloon should be similar to the size of the artery undergoing PTA, because a balloon that is too small produces an inadequate dilatation and a balloon that is too big can rupture the artery. The size of the balloon used in iliac artery PTA is usually about 6–10 or 12 mm in diameter, and in superficial femoral and popliteal PTA it is usually 4–6 mm in diameter. The tibial arteries require 2–3 mm diameter balloons, and the aorta either a large single 12–16 mm diameter balloon or two 8–10 mm diameter balloons. Lesions at the aortic bifurcation also require the simultaneous use of two 6–10 mm diameter balloons (the kissing balloon technique). The balloons are usually 4 cm in length, but range from 2 to 10 cm long.

The initial technical success of the procedure is usually based on hemodynamic pressure measurements and/or angiographic appearances, depending upon the site of the PTA. The intra-arterial pressure is measured above and below the lesion before aortic or iliac artery PTA. A pressure gradient of 15–20 mmHg or greater at rest is a significant drop, but a pressure gradient of up to 10 mmHg at rest is not. In patients without a significant drop in pressure, injection of a vasodilator such as *papaverine*, *tolazoline*, or *glyceryl trinitrate* through the catheter simulates the effect of exercise. An increase in the pressure gradient to more than 20 mmHg then indicates that the stenosis is significant and requires angioplasty. The ideal hemodynamic result following PTA is no residual pressure gradient at all, but this is not always attainable.

The intra-arterial pressure is not usually measured in femoral, popliteal, or tibial PTA, because the measurements are not so accurate in these smaller arteries with the catheter positioned in an antegrade direction. Arteriography is performed before and after angioplasty in femoral, popliteal, and tibial PTA, and the ideal angiographic result is no residual stenosis at all, but slight narrowing of the arterial lumen is often acceptable. Endovascular ultrasound and angioscopy have also been used to assess the initial technical success of PTA.

The technical success rate in iliac artery PTA is 90–95% for stenoses and 80–90% for occlusions, with a patency rate of 65–95% at 2 years and 50–85% at 5 years. The technical success rate in femoral and popliteal artery PTA is 85–95% for stenoses and 60–90% for occlusions with a patency rate of 45–85% at 2 years and 20–70% at 5 years. In comparison, the patency rate for aorto-bifemoral bypass surgery is 70–85% at 5 years with an operative mortality of 2–5%, and the patency rate for femoropopliteal bypass surgery is 40–80% at 5 years with an operative mortality of 1–2%. The procedure-related mortality of angioplasty is negligible at 0.2%.

The complication rate for PTA is 2–3%, with complications occurring at the arterial puncture site, the angioplasty site, distal to the site of the angioplasty, and in the systemic circulation.

Complications at the arterial puncture site are similar to those in diagnostic arteriography, and include *hemorrhage* and *hematoma* formation, *subintimal dissection*, and *thrombosis*, the development of a *false aneurysm* or an *arteriovenous fistula*, *nerve trauma*, and *local infection*. A false aneurysm can be treated by a compression technique, which involves using the ultrasound probe to occlude the neck of the false aneurysm in order to thrombose it, while maintaining flow in the adjacent artery.

Complications at the angioplasty site include *subintimal dissection*, *thrombosis*, and *perforation*. Subintimal dissection may produce occlusion of the artery, particularly in an antegrade direction where the flow of blood tends to open the flap, whereas in a retrograde direction the flow of blood tends to close the flap. Subintimal dissection can be treated by further angioplasty or the insertion of a vascular stent. Perforation of the femoral or popliteal artery within an occlusion is not usually significant, but rupture of an iliac artery produces a retroperitoneal hemorrhage, which can be fatal. Arterial rupture can be treated by inflation of the angioplasty balloon at the site or the insertion of a vascular stent. Acute occlusion at the site of the angioplasty due to thrombosis is one of the indications for thrombolysis. Rupture of the balloon also occasionally occurs, but is not usually significant.

Complications distal to the site of the angioplasty include *arterial spasm* and *embolization*. Spasm in the popliteal and tibial arteries can be treated with *nifedipine*, *isosorbide dinitrate*, or *tolazoline*, which is best given prophylactically. Distal embolization of thrombus or atheromatous debris can be treated by aspiration thromboembolectomy or thrombolysis.

Sytemic complications include a vasovagal reaction, hypotension, myocardial infarction, cerebral–vascular accident, cholesterol crystal embolization, renal failure, and septicemia.

Restenosis and chronic reocclusion are detected on follow-up with duplex ultrasound, and can be treated by repeat angioplasty or the insertion of a vascular stent.

Subclavian, axillary, and brachial artery stenoses and short occlusions up to 3–5 cm in length are also suitable for PTA in patients with an ischemic arm or a subclavian steal syndrome, and are usually approached following catheterization of the femoral artery. Subclavian and axillary artery lesions can also be approached from below following catheterization of the brachial artery. The technical success rate in subclavian artery PTA is 80–95%, with a patency rate of 75% at 4 years. There is a risk of carotid or vertebral artery embolic complications.

Coronary Angioplasty

Coronary artery PTA and other cardiac interventional vascular procedures such as balloon valvoplasty of the pulmonary, aortic and mitral valves, atrial septostomy, balloon dilatation of aortic coarctation, and closure of a patent ductus arteriosus are discussed in Chapters 23 and 24.

Carotid Angioplasty

Innominate, common carotid, internal carotid, and vertebral artery stenoses, but not occlusions, can be treated by PTA in patients with transient ischemic attacks or vertebrobasilar insufficiency, and are usually approached following catheterization of the femoral artery. The technical success rate is 90–95%, and the long-term results are awaited from the clinical trials in progress.

Renal Angioplasty

Many patients with hypertension undergo investigation in the search for a treatable cause for their raised blood pressure, but only 4–5% have renovascular hypertension due to renal artery stenosis, which may be due to either atherosclerosis or fibromuscular dysplasia.

Renovascular hypertension is the main indication for renal artery PTA, but its use in patients with deteriorating renal failure due to renal artery stenosis or even occlusion is becoming increasingly important. Renal artery stenoses and short occlusions up to 1–2 cm in length are usually approached from below following catheterization of the femoral artery, but can be approached from above following catheterization of the left axillary or brachial artery, if there is a very acute angle between the aorta and renal artery. The size of balloon used in renal artery PTA is usually about 4–6 mm in diameter.

The technical success rate in renal artery PTA is 90% for stenoses and 50% for occlusions. Long-term results show that 95% of patients with fibromuscular dysplasia benefit from PTA, with 60% cured of their hypertension and 35% improved, whereas 70% of patients with non-ostial atheroma benefit from PTA, and of these only 30% are cured and 40% improved. About 40% of patients with deteriorating renal function show a decrease in serum creatinine levels following renal artery PTA. The complication rate for renal artery PTA is at least 10%, and this includes renal infarction. Restenosis and ostial atheroma can be treated by the insertion of a vascular stent.

Renal Transplant Artery Stenoses   These are also suitable for PTA, and are usually approached across the aortic bifurcation following catheterization of the contralateral femoral artery. Stenoses on the *venous side of an arteriovenous fistula* occur in patients on hemodialysis, and can be treated by PTA.

Mesenteric Angioplasty

Celiac and superior and inferior mesenteric artery stenoses, but not occlusions, can be treated by PTA in patients with mesenteric ischemia, and are usually approached from below following catheterization of the femoral artery, but can be approached from above following catheterization of the left axillary or brachial artery.

ADJUNCTIVE TECHNIQUES TO ANGIOPLASTY

There are also a number of other devices and techniques available for use in the treatment of patients with peripheral vascular disease. These have been developed to improve the initial technical success and long-term patency rates of PTA, and include mechanical rotational devices, atheroma removal devices, and intravascular stents.

Mechanical Rotating Devices   The mechanical rotating devices are used to recanalize complete occlusions, where conventional catheter and guide-wire combinations have failed. The recanalized channel still requires balloon dilatation, if the recanalization is successful. The *rotational transluminal angioplasty catheter system* (ROTACS) is a low-speed battery-driven catheter, which rotates at about 100 rpm and produces a recanalization rate of 80%. The *Kensey catheter* is a high-speed electric motor driven catheter, which rotates at 10 000–20 000 rpm and produces a recanalization rate of 70–90%, with a long-term patency rate of 50–70% at 2 years. The *Rotablator* is a very high-speed gas turbine driven catheter, which rotates at 100 000–200 000 rpm and produces a recanalization rate of 90%, but a long-term patency rate of only 25–40% at 2 years. These high-speed devices produce microparticles with distal embolization.

Atheroma Removal Devices   The atheroma-removing devices are also used to recanalize complete occlusions, where conventional catheter and guide-wire combinations have failed, but can be used to treat stenoses. Subsequent balloon dilatation is again required.

The *transluminal endarterectomy catheter* (TEC) cuts through the atheroma, which is then aspirated through the catheter by a vacuum, producing a technical success rate of 80–90%. The *Simpson atherectomy catheter* slices off the atheroma, which is then collected in a small chamber, producing a technical success rate of 80–90%.

The small capacity of the chamber limits its use to eccentric stenoses. Both these devices have high restenosis rates of 15–45%.

Laser-assisted Angioplasty   This technique uses a hot-tip metal probe or a sapphire-tipped hybrid probe, coupled to a continuous- or pulsed-wave argon or neodymium–yttrium aluminum garnet (Nd–YAG) laser generator, to recanalize complete occlusions. The recanalized channel is produced by direct heat from the hot-tip metal probe, which reaches a temperature of about 400°C, or direct heat and laser energy from the sapphire-tipped hybrid probe, which allows 10% of the laser energy to exit directly through a window in the tip of the probe. Balloon dilatation of the recanalized channel is required. Laser-assisted angioplasty has a primary recanalization rate of 70–90% with a long-term patency rate of 60–70% at 2 years, but a high risk of arterial perforation of up to 20%.

Intravascular Stents   These are used to maintain the lumen of a vessel by a mechanical supporting effect on its wall. Intravascular stents are mainly used in the iliac, coronary, and renal arteries, but have been used in the aorta, and in the femoral popliteal, subclavian, and carotid arteries. The types of vascular stent available include the flexible Wallstent and Strecker stent and the rigid Palmaz stent. The indications for their use are to prevent an acute occlusion developing after an intimal flap has been produced by angioplasty, to abolish the pressure gradient across a significant residual stenosis after angioplasty, and to treat recurrent stenoses and following recanalization of an occlusion in the iliac, coronary, or renal arteries (Fig. 25.19). The long-term patency rate in the iliac arteries is 90–95% at 2 years.

Intravascular stents have also been used to treat stenoses in the iliac, subclavian, and hepatic veins, and in renal dialysis shunts.

The Palmaz and Gianturco Z stents and the Wallstent are used in the endovascular grafts that have been developed for the treatment of abdominal aortic aneurysms. The Palmaz or Gianturco Z stents seal the top end of the Dacron graft in the neck of the aneurysm and the bottom end in the common iliac artery, whereas the Wallstents prevent kinks and twists in the limbs of the graft itself. The three basic types of endovascular graft available for abdominal aortic aneurysms are an aorto-aortic system, an aortobi-iliac system and an aorto-uni-iliac system, which necessitates the use of an occluding device in the contralateral common iliac artery and a femorofemoral cross-over Dacron graft. These large-caliber systems require a femoral arteriotomy for insertion at present, but smaller-caliber systems can be used percutaneously for iliac and popliteal artery aneurysms and femoral artery occlusions.

Vena Caval Filters   There are a large number of permanent and temporary filters available for insertion into the inferior vena cava, and these include the Greenfield titanium filter, the Cardial steel filter, the Gianturco–Roehm bird's nest filter, the Gunther tulip filter, the Simon nitinol filter, the LGM Venatech filter, and the Antheor filter. The indications for the insertion of an inferior vena caval filter are patients with recurrent pulmonary emboli despite good anticoagulation, pulmonary emboli or deep-vein thrombosis in patients with a contraindication to anticoagulation, deep-vein thrombosis in patients with pulmonary arterial hypertension, and as prophylaxis against pulmonary emboli in high-risk patients.

Inferior vena caval filters are ideally positioned below the renal veins following catheterization of the femoral or internal jugular vein, but can be positioned in the suprarenal inferior vena cava if there is thrombus in the renal veins or infrarenal inferior vena cava. These filters reduce the rate of recurrent pulmonary emboli from 20 to 2%, and the associated mortality from 10% to less than 1%. The complications of insertion of a filter include thrombosis of the femoral or internal jugular veins, caval thrombosis, and central migration of the filter.

RETRIEVAL OF INTRAVASCULAR FOREIGN BODIES

A variety of diagnostic, monitoring, and therapeutic lines, catheters, wires, and other foreign bodies are introduced into the arterial or venous systems of an increasing number of patients during their clinical management. Occasionally, small or large fragments of these catheters or wires are broken off during their insertion or removal and are lost within the vascular system, usually on the venous side. Foreign bodies in the veins migrate centrally and may lodge in the right atrium, right ventricle, and main pulmonary arteries or their branches, whereas foreign bodies in the arteries are carried peripherally and tend to lodge at a vessel bifurcation.

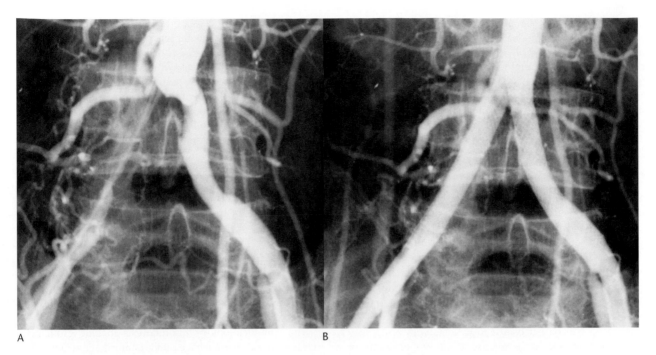

Fig. 25.19 **A**. Arteriogram showing a short 4 cm occlusion in the right common iliac artery. **B** Arteriogram after insertion of Wallstents in both common iliac arteries.

Intravascular foreign bodies produce a high complication rate of 70% with a mortality rate of 40% if they are not removed. These complications may occur immediately or be delayed for weeks, months, or years, and include cardiac arrhythmias, myocardial perforation, endocarditis, pulmonary emboli, septicemia, and mycotic aneurysms.

A venous foreign body is retrieved following catheterization of the femoral or internal jugular vein and an arterial foreign body via the femoral artery. A vascular sheath, large enough to accommodate the foreign body, is placed in the femoral vein or artery. The foreign body is then grasped by a loop snare, stone retrieval basket, or biopsy forceps, and withdrawn into the sheath for removal, but may initially need to be dislodged by a catheter to get it into a better position.

VASCULAR INFUSION THERAPY

The purpose of vascular infusion therapy is to deliver a smaller dose of the drug to an organ system, at a higher concentration than can be obtained by systemic administration, via a catheter selectively positioned in the artery supplying that particular vascular bed. The drugs that have been used in therapeutic pharmacoangiography include vasoconstrictors, vasodilators, and cytotoxic and fibrinolytic drugs.

Vasoconstrictors   Vasoconstrictive drugs, such as vasopressin, epinephrine, and norepinephrine can be used in the treatment of *acute gastrointestinal hemorrhage*. After localizing the site of the bleeding by selective arteriography, an intra-arterial infusion of vasopressin at 0.1–0.2 units/min for 20 min is used to control it, by causing vasoconstriction of the blood supply to the gastrointestinal tract. If repeat arteriography after 20 min no longer shows extravasation of contrast medium, the infusion is continued for

12–24 h, and then the dose is reduced for a further 12–24 h, but if bleeding is still occurring, the dose is increased before being gradually reduced.

A vasopressin infusion into the left gastric artery is effective in controlling bleeding from esophageal mucosal tears and erosive gastritis in 80% of patients, although recurrent bleeding occurs in 20% of patients. An infusion into the superior or inferior mesenteric artery is also effective in controlling bleeding from colonic diverticula in 90% of patients, but once again there is recurrent bleeding in 30% of patients. This type of treatment is much less effective for chronic peptic ulcers and gastrointestinal tumors.

The complications of vasopressin include hypertension, cardiac arrhythmias, myocardial infarction, lower limb and mesenteric ischemia and infarction due to its vasoconstrictor effect as well as edema and electrolyte imbalance due to its antidiuretic effect.

Vasodilators   The use of vasodilators, such as isosorbide dinitrate or glyceryl trinitrate, nifedipine, and tolazoline, to prevent arterial spasm in patients undergoing popliteal, tibial and coronary artery PTA has already been discussed. Vasodilators, such as papaverine, tolazoline, reserpine, and the prostaglandins E_1 and $F_{2\alpha}$, have also been used in the treatment of Raynaud's disease, frostbite, trauma, and mesenteric ischemia.

Cytotoxic Drugs   A variety of cytotoxic drugs have been used as intra-arterial infusions in the treatment of both primary and secondary tumors. An infusion of *5-fluorouracil* and *mitomycin C* or *cisplatin* over 5 days into the hepatic artery in patients with hepatic metastases from colorectal carcinoma produces response rates ranging from 45 to 60%, after several cycles of chemotherapy, but an infusion of *cisplatin* and *vinblastine* in patients with hepatic metastases from breast carcinoma only produces a response rate of 20–30%. The use of *5-fluorouracil, adriamycin,* and *mitomycin C* produces a response rate of 60% in patients with hepatocellular carcinoma, but can also be used in combination with gelatin sponge fragments or Lipiodol to embolize the hepatic artery, resulting in response rates of up to 90%. Various other tumors including bronchial, renal, and bladder carcinoma, gynecological malignancies, and bone tumors have also been treated by selective intra-arterial infusions of these cytotoxic drugs. The commonest complication of this type of treatment is thrombosis of the artery supplying the tumor, as the catheters remain in position for several days.

Thrombolysis

Fibrinolytic therapy has been used in the treatment of various thrombotic diseases, such as acute myocardial infarction, acute lower limb ischemia, and acute pulmonary embolism. The technique of thrombolysis in lower limb ischemia was described in 1974 by Dotter, who used a catheter with its tip in the acute occlusion to deliver an intra-arterial infusion of a low dose of *streptokinase* into the thrombus, in order to reduce the hemorrhagic complications produced by the systemic fibrinolytic effect of the high-dose intravenous infusions that had been previously tried.

Thrombolysis can be performed in patients with acute critical lower limb ischemia as an alternative to an embolectomy or a surgical bypass graft, as these patients tend to have a poor clinical outcome.

The *indications* for intra-arterial thrombolysis are therefore distal arterial thrombosis or embolus involving the popliteal and tibial arteries, thrombosis of a surgical graft, thrombosis at the site of a recent angioplasty, and proximal arterial thrombosis involving the iliac and femoral arteries in a high-risk patient. Surgery is still indicated for proximal arterial embolus or thrombosis involving the aorta and iliac and femoral arteries, particularly if the ischemia is very severe. The *contraindications* to intra-arterial thrombolysis include a cerebral infarct within the previous 3 months due to the

risk of developing a cerebral hemorrhage, recent major surgery or trauma within the last month, active bleeding from any site, a clotting disorder, and muscle necrosis due to the risk of developing acute renal failure from the release of myoglobin.

Thrombolysis is usually performed at the time of the diagnostic arteriography with the tip of the catheter positioned in the thrombus. Iliac and proximal femoral artery occlusions are approached across the aortic bifurcation following catheterization of the contralateral femoral artery. Distal femoral and popliteal artery occlusions are approached following catheterization of the ipsilateral femoral artery. With the low-dose infusion technique, *streptokinase* at 5000 units/h, *urokinase* at 50 000 units/h, or *recombinant tissue plasminogen activator* at 0.5 mg/h is injected into the thrombus, and the degree of lysis monitored by arteriography over 24–48 h. Higher doses of these fibrinolytic drugs reduce the lysis time to 6–18 h. Any underlying stenosis revealed as the lysis progresses requires PTA. More recently, accelerated thrombolytic regimes have been developed to shorten the lysis time still further, and in pulse spray pharmacomechanical thrombolysis the fibrinolytic drug is injected throughout the thrombus via multiple holes or slits in the catheter, resulting in a lysis time of 1–3 h.

The complications of thrombolysis include groin hematoma, retroperitoneal hemorrhage, and hemorrhage from other sites, pericatheter thrombosis, distal embolization of thrombus, acute renal failure, and a cerebrovascular accident. Thrombolysis results in limb salvage in 70–80% of patients with a critically ischemic limb, an amputation rate of 5–10%, and a mortality rate of 10%.

Thrombolysis has also been used in the treatment of acute critical upper limb ischemia, renal artery occlusions, superior vena caval obstruction, and deep-vein thrombosis in the legs (Fig. 25.20). Small fragments of fresh thrombus can also be aspirated through a catheter with a large internal lumen, and larger amounts of fresh thrombus can be removed by high-speed mechanical rotating devices.

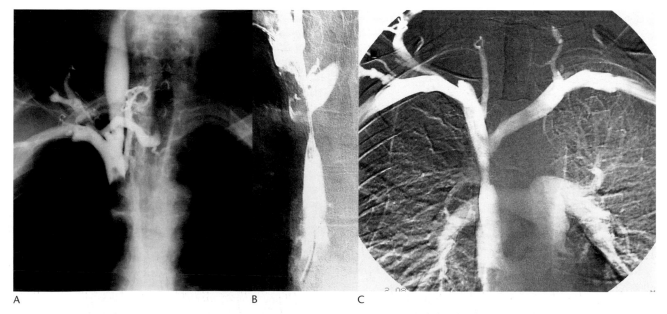

A   B   C

Fig. 25.20 Venograms showing complete occlusion of the superior vena cava due to thrombus **A** before thrombolysis and **B** a pulse spray catheter in the superior vena cava during the lysis with tissue plasminogen activator. **C**. Angiographic result in the superior vena cava and brachiocephalic veins after thrombolysis and the insertion of a Wallstent.

THERAPEUTIC EMBOLIZATION

The basic technique of therapeutic embolization involves the injection of embolic material through a catheter selectively positioned in an artery or vein to produce the formation of thrombus in that blood vessel resulting in the deliberate occlusion of the artery, vein, or vascular beds of an organ.

A large number of different solid and liquid materials have been used for therapeutic embolization over the last 30 years. The properties of the ideal embolic material are that it should be thrombogenic, but not toxic, and produce a permanent vascular occlusion. It should also be easy to inject through an angiographic catheter and available in a wide range of shapes and sizes that are both sterile and radiopaque.

The most commonly used embolic agents today include solid particulate materials, such as gelatin sponge fragments (Sterispon) and polyvinyl alcohol particles (Ivalon), mechanical devices, such as spiral metal coils and detachable balloons, and liquids, such as absolute ethyl alcohol and tissue adhesives. All these embolic materials produce a permanent vascular occlusion, except gelatin sponge, which only produces a temporary occlusion that recanalizes within a month. None of them, however, is the ideal embolic agent, and they are often used in combination to produce occlusions at various levels in the vascular tree. Gelatin sponge is not radiopaque, and has to be cut up into small 1–3 mm fragments, which are then suspended in contrast medium before injection. Polyvinyl alcohol is also not radiopaque, but is available in a range of sizes (150–250, 250–600, and 600–1000 µm diameter particles), which also need to be suspended in contrast medium before injection.

The metal coils are made of stainless steel, platinum, or tungsten and are available in a range of sizes and lengths with a spiral diameter of 1–20 mm or larger. The stainless steel coils have threads of wool, silk, or Dacron attached to them to increase their thrombogenicity. Metal coils are radiopaque and are delivered by being pushed through the catheter with a guide-wire. The detachable balloons are made of latex or silicone, and are available in 1 and 2 mm sizes, which can be inflated up to 4 and 8 mm in diameter. The balloons are not radiopaque and have to be filled with contrast medium before being detached from their microcatheter. Absolute ethyl alcohol and hypertonic 50% dextrose solution are mixed with contrast medium before injection, but the tissue adhesive Bucrylate is mixed with tantalum powder or ethiodol before injection, which makes it radiopaque and prolongs its polymerization time. Lyophilized dura mater fragments should no longer be used because of the potential risk of transmission of Creutzfeld–Jacob disease.

Embolization is generally performed as an alternative to a surgical procedure, particularly if the patient is unfit for surgery and the operation carries a high risk, but it may be the optimal method of treatment for the patient. Embolization is also performed in combination with surgery, generally to reduce the blood loss during an operation and thus shorten the procedure.

The indications for arterial embolization include the management of acute hemorrhage, the management of tumors, the treatment of arteriovenous malformations (AVMs), arteriovenous fistulas, and aneurysms as well as the ablation of function of an organ. The indications for venous embolization are the treatment of gastro-esophageal varices, the treatment of testicular variceles, and the ablation of function of the adrenal gland.

Embolization in the Management of Acute Hemorrhage

Embolization is used in the management of patients with bleeding from the gastrointestinal, genitourinary, and respiratory tracts, and in bleeding following trauma.

In patients with severe and continuing or recurrent bleeding from the upper or lower gastrointestinal tracts, mesenteric angiography should be performed when endoscopy and colonoscopy have failed to identify its site. It should also be performed after a positive radionuclide scan using either technetium-99m sulfur colloid or labeled red blood cells has demonstrated gastrointestinal hemorrhage. Active bleeding from mucosal ulcers, tumors, and following trauma of the stomach, duodenum, or rectum can be stopped by embolization of the left gastric, gastroduodenal, or superior rectal arteries in patients who are not suitable for surgery. The stomach, duodenum, and rectum all have a dual blood supply, unless there has been previous gastrointestinal surgery, and the risk of infarction and perforation is therefore low. Active bleeding from the small intestine, cecum, and colon has been treated by embolization, but the risk of infarction and perforation is high because of the single blood supply to these structures. A vasopressin infusion can be used to control bleeding in these patients.

Active bleeding from a false aneurysm in the pancreas due to recurrent pancreatitis or following trauma can be treated by embolization of the gastroduodenal or splenic arteries, and active bleeding from a false aneurysm in the liver due to hepatic metastases or following liver biopsy, blunt trauma, or hepatobiliary surgery can be treated by embolization of the appropriate branch of the right or left hepatic arteries.

In patients with severe and continuing or recurrent bleeding from the kidney or bladder, renal or pelvic angiography should be performed. Hematuria can be controlled by embolization of the kidney in patients with renal cell carcinoma who are unsuitable for surgery (Fig. 25.21). Active bleeding from a false aneurysm in the kidney following renal biopsy or trauma can be treated by embolization of the appropriate branch of the renal artery. Embolization is also the treatment of choice in patients with a renal AVM. Embolization of both internal iliac arteries is also used to control hematuria in patients with bladder tumors, who are unsuitable for surgery, and to treat patients with vaginal bleeding from gynecological tumors and post-traumatic internal hemorrhage following pelvic fractures.

Embolization of the bronchial arteries is also effective in controlling massive hemoptysis, and embolization of the internal maxillary arteries has been used in the treatment of life-threatening epistaxis.

Embolization of gastroesophageal varices is usually performed during a TIPPS procedure, but can also be done following a percutaneous transhepatic catheterization of the portal venous system.

Embolization in the Management of Tumors

Embolization is used in the management of patients with neoplastic disease as a preoperative technique to reduce blood loss during surgery, as a palliative technique to alleviate symptoms, and occasionally as a definitive procedure instead of surgery.

Preoperative embolization of a neoplasm is done to reduce blood loss during the surgery and to decrease tumor size, thus making the surgery much easier. This type of embolization was frequently

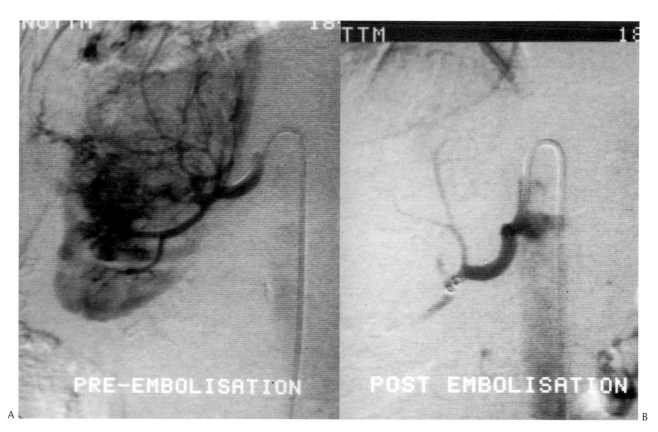

Fig. 25.21 **A**. Renal arteriogram showing a large renal cell carcinoma. **B**. After embolization of the right kidney with absolute ethyl alcohol, gelatin sponge fragments, and spiral metal coils.

performed several days before nephrectomy in patients with renal cell carcinoma, but this can in fact make the surgery more difficult as the inflammatory response that develops affects the tissue planes around the kidney. Preoperative embolization is still performed for renal cell carcinoma, but the timing of the procedure should ideally be only a few hours before the surgery. A balloon occlusion catheter can also be effectively used for this purpose. Other tumors that may require preoperative embolization include intracranial meningiomas, nasopharyngeal angiofibromas (Fig. 25.22), chemodactomas, primary bone tumors, and primary hepatic tumors.

Palliative embolization is performed to alleviate symptoms such as bleeding, pain, and the metabolic effects of endocrine tumors.

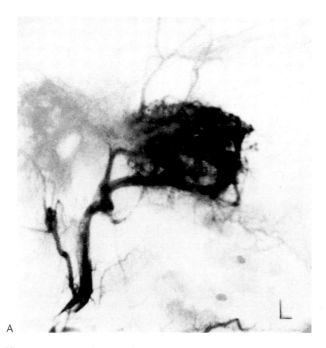

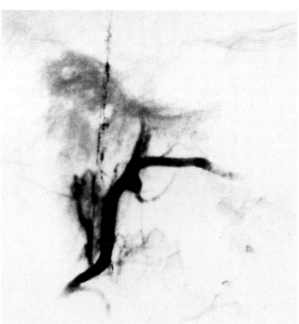

Fig. 25.22 Nasopharyngeal angiofibroma. **A**. Before embolization. **B**. After embolization.

This type of embolization is usually performed in patients with hepatic metastases. The liver has a dual blood supply and normally receives 75% of its blood from the hepatic portal vein and only 25% of its blood from the hepatic artery. Tumors, however, tend to receive 90% of their blood supply from the hepatic artery, but only 10% from the portal venous system. Hepatic artery embolization is therefore contraindicated if the portal vein is occluded.

Embolization of the hepatic artery is used to control hemobilia in patients with a false aneurysm from hepatic metastases, and to reduce pain from stretching of the liver capsule in patients with hepatomegaly from a primary tumor or hepatic metastases, by reducing the size of the liver. Embolization of the liver is also effective in controlling the symptoms of flushing and diarrhea produced by 5-hydroxytryptamine in patients with the carcinoid syndrome, by ablating the functioning capacity of the hepatic metastases. Symptomatic relief can also be produced in patients with hepatic metastases from insulinomas, glucagonomas, and vipomas.

Therapeutic embolization has been performed as the definitive procedure in the treatment of benign bone tumors, benign hepatic tumors, and ectopic parathyroid tumors in the mediastinum. Embolization of adrenal tumors by venous infarction has also been performed, in patients with both Cushing syndrome and Conn syndrome.

Embolization in the Treatment of Vascular Abnormalities

Embolization is used in the treatment of AVMs, arteriovenous fistulas, and aneurysms.

Patients with AVMs are difficult to treat surgically because the operative field is readily obscured by blood from the large number of arteries and veins in the malformation, the surgery often needs to be extensive to remove the malformation, and it has a tendency to recur if incompletely excised. Embolization alone is therefore often the optimal method of treatment, but it can also be used in a preoperative capacity. Small AVMs can be treated by embolizing the feeding arteries and the nidus of the lesion in one procedure, but large AVMs may require several procedures. AVMs with a significant arteriovenous component are most suited to embolization, but AVMs with a significant capillary–venous component can be treated by a direct venous approach. Post-traumatic arteriovenous fistulas and both true and false aneurysms can be embolized with large occluding devices such as balloons and metal coils (Fig. 25.23).

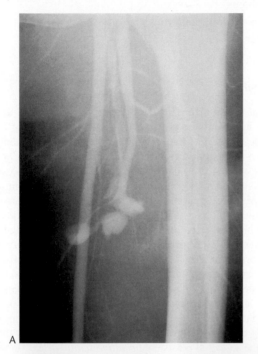

A

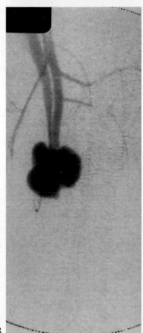

B

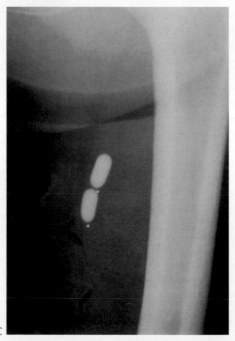

C

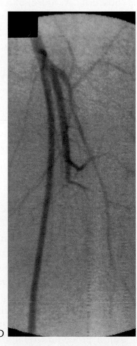

D

Fig. 25.23   **A,B**. Arteriograms showing an arteriovenous fistula between the left deep femoral artery and vein with false aneurysm formation due to a stab wound. **C,D**. After embolization with two balloons.

Patients with impaired fertility due to a left testicular varicele can also be treated by embolization of the left gonadal vein. Successful treatment results in an improved sperm count and quality.

Embolization to Ablate Organ Function

Embolization is used not only to ablate the functioning tissue in adrenal and parathyroid adenomas and hepatic metastases from carcinoid tumors, insulinomas and glucagonomas, but also the spleen in patients with hypersplenism. Embolization of the spleen is occasionally performed in patients who are unsuitable for surgery, and is best undertaken in several stages as there is a high risk of abscess formation in the infarcted splenic tissue. Embolization of the internal pudendal artery is also effective in treating patients with priapism. Gelatin sponge fragments should be used so that recanalization of the vessels can occur.

Complications of Embolization

The complications of embolization include the complications of both the arteriography and the use of contrast media, the postembolization syndrome, and the specific complications of the procedure.

The *post-embolization syndrome* usually occurs within 24–48 h of the procedure, and lasts for 3–7 days after the procedure. It is characterized by pain at the site of the embolization, nausea and vomiting, malaise, fever, leukocytosis, and raised inflammatory markers, and is more severe when a large volume of tissue has been embolized. The development of an *abscess* can, however, occur in the infarcted tissue, and it is important not to confuse this with the postembolization syndrome. Prophylactic antibiotics are therefore required in patients undergoing embolization of solid organs and strict aseptic technique is essential during the procedure. The presence of gas within the necrotic tissue is a normal finding after embolization and does not necessarily indicate the presence of a developing abscess. A more extensive volume of tissue infarction than planned may occur due to retrograde extension of thrombus in the embolized vessel, and *accidental tissue necrosis* may be produced in adjacent critical organs due to either reflux of solid embolic material into their arterial supply or permeation of liquid embolic material into their capillary bed.

Pulmonary embolization can occur when small particulate embolic material passes through arteriovenous communications in either vascular tissue or systemic AVMs, but this is not usually clinically significant. Similarly, systemic embolization can occur during the treatment of a pulmonary AVM. Large embolic devices such as metal coils and detachable balloons can be retrieved from the vascular system if they become misplaced. Release of metabolically active substances from functioning endocrine tissue occurs after embolization of hepatic metastases from carcinoid tumors and insulinomas.

Prophylactic pharmacological blocking agents are therefore required in these patients. Release of toxic radicals also occurs after embolization of any tissue, and this can lead to renal failure if large volumes of tissue are infarcted. Dehydration and the large doses of contrast medium used during an embolization also contribute to the development of renal failure.

The overall complication rate for most embolizations ranges from 3 to 10%, with a procedure-related mortality of 1–2%, but splenic embolization has a complication rate of nearly 20% and a mortality rate of 7%.

INDICATIONS FOR ARTERIOGRAPHY

VASCULAR LESIONS

The vascular lesions investigated by angiography will be discussed under the following headings:

1. Congenital
2. Aneurysms
3. Thrombosis and stenosis
4. Embolus
5. Angiomatous malformation
6. Arteriovenous fistula
7. Hemorrhage.

Congenital

Congenital anomalies of the arterial system are not uncommon. Those involving the aortic origin and the ascending aorta have been described in Chapter 24. The major coronary abnormalities are also discussed in the cardiac Chapter. *Anomalies of the great vessels* are noted in the neuroradiology (see Ch. 56), as are the commoner anomalies of the cerebral arteries. Anatomic variations of the peripheral arterial system are well described in anatomic texts, but some of those with clinical implications will be noted here.

The brachial artery occasionally divides into its radial and ulnar branches at a high level, and this had some practical importance when brachial arteriography was more widely practised. In the lower limb the popliteal artery sometimes divides into its anterior and posterior tibial branches above the knee joint. The femoral artery, which normally arises from the external iliac, may occasionally be replaced by a large branch of the dilated hypogastric artery passing through the greater sciatic notch and behind the femoral neck, the so-called persistent *primitive sciatic artery*. In these cases the true femoral artery is hypoplastic and may terminate in the profunda femoris. Congenital anomalies of the renal supply are very common, and some 25% of kidneys have an accessory artery supplying them. For this reason arteriography is performed on live renal donors to check that the proposed kidney is suitable for grafting. Occasionally three renal arteries are found, but four arteries are very rarely seen. Horseshoe and ectopic kidneys frequently have accessory arteries, often arising from the aortic bifurcation or iliac artery.

Anomalies of the arterial supply to the liver are also frequently seen. The classical anatomic description of the common hepatic artery arising from the celiac axis and dividing into right and left hepatic arteries is only seen in some 50% of cases. Some 20% have a right hepatic artery or an accessory right hepatic arising from the superior mesenteric artery. A further 20% have a left hepatic or accessory left hepatic artery arising from the left gastric artery. In about 2% of patents the common hepatic artery arises from the superior mesenteric.

Other major branches of the celiac axis, i.e. the splenic and left gastric arteries, may sometimes arise directly from the aorta.

The bronchial arteries which arise on the anterior surface of the aorta just below the level of the carina are double on the left in 60% of cases and on the right in 30%.

Coarctation of the Aorta   The condition has been described above, in Chapter 24. Poststenotic aneurysm occurs as a complication

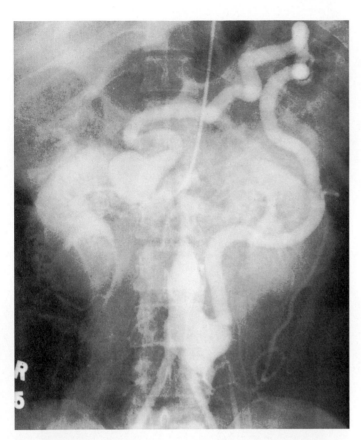

Fig. 25.24 Abdominal coarctation with involvement of the superior mesenteric origin. There is a collateral circulation through the artery of Drummond from the left colic branch of the inferior mesenteric to the middle colic branch of the superior mesenteric. Owing to the increased flow, aneurysms have developed at both ends of the collateral. (Courtesy of Dr R. Eban.)

in some 4% of cases (see Fig. 25.40). It should also be realized that the condition may also occur at more distal sites than the classic level in the distal arch, and can involve the lower thoracic or abdominal aorta. So-called abdominal coarctation usually affects the upper abdominal aorta, and may involve a short or long segment. Splanchnic vessels and the renal artery origins may also be involved in the lesion (Fig. 25.24).

Pseudocoarctation Pseudocoartation or lateral buckling of the aortic arch is an unusual condition which can simulate a rounded mass in the region of the aortic knuckle. There is a sharp kink in the aorta at the junction of the arch and descending aorta in the region of the ligamentum arteriosum. Buckling of the aorta may also occur in the mid-arch, and this is best identified in the lateral view.

Vascular Rings Such rings around the esophagus can be of many types, and the commonest lesions are illustrated in Appendix B. Study of the barium-filled esophagus is helpful in elucidating these lesions.

Hypoplasia of the Aorta This is sometimes encountered as a chance finding. It may be associated with Marfan syndrome, where there is a mesodermal defect and medial degeneration of the aorta. However, in Marfan syndrome the aorta will eventually dilate because of the medial defect, and dissecting aneurysms may develop, particularly in the ascending aorta.

Aneurysms

Aneurysms can be classified on an etiological basis as follows:

1. Congenital
2. Infective
3. Degenerative
4. Traumatic
5. Dissecting
6. Necrotizing vasculitis
7. Poststenotic.

Congenital Aneurysms These are commonest in the intracranial vessels, where they have in the past been termed 'congenital berry aneurysms'. While these aneurysms are basically due to a defect in the muscular coat at points of arterial bifurcation, it is clear from clinical experience that other factors such as age, atheroma, and hypertension are also important in their pathogenesis, as is

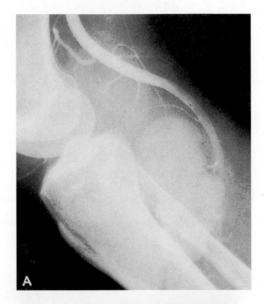

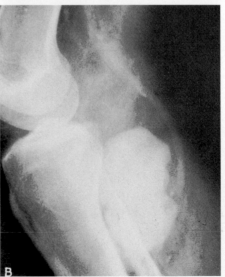

Fig. 25.25 **A,B**. Mycotic aneurysm in the lower popliteal artery.

the fact that they usually arise where the arteries lie in the subarachnoid space unsupported by surrounding soft tissues. They are discussed in more detail in Chapter 56. Congenital aneurysms have been described elsewhere in the body but are relatively rare, a fact which supports the importance of the local cerebral anatomy in their etiology.

Infective Aneurysms   Infective aneurysms may be classified as mycotic or syphilitic. *Mycotic aneurysms* are nearly always secondary

to bacterial endocarditis. They may involve any artery in the body, and we have encountered examples in the abdomen and pelvis, in the brain, and in the limbs (Figs 25.25–25.27). They can grow in size very rapidly and usually require urgent surgery to prevent rupture. Mycotic aneurysms are occasionally secondary to involvement of the arterial wall by an adjacent infection such as a pyogenic or tuberculous abscess.

Syphilitic aneurysms were once extremely common, but with the advent of antibiotics they are now rarely seen in developed

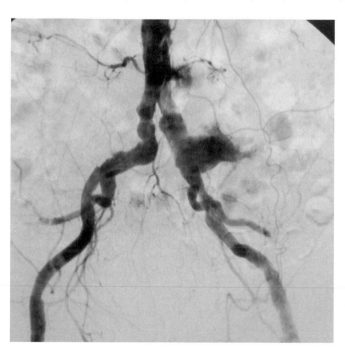

Fig. 25.26   Mycotic aneurysm of left common iliac artery in a patient with salmonella septicemia.

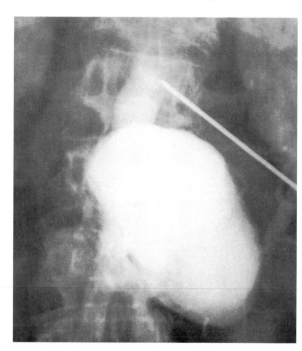

Fig. 25.27   Mycotic aneurysm at the origin of the inferior mesenteric artery.

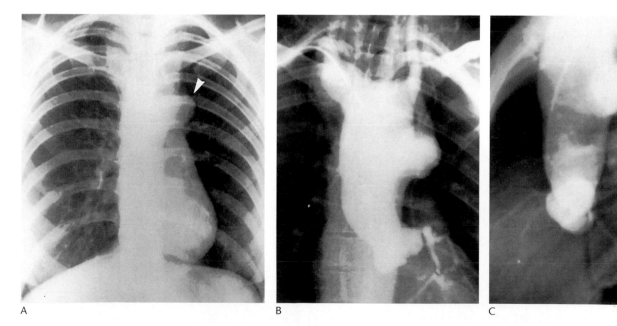

A   B   C

Fig. 25.28   A. Chest film showing aortic knuckle (arrow) apparently displaced downward by a supra-aortic mass. **B,C.** Angiograms showing that this is due to an aneurysm of the arch and innominate artery.

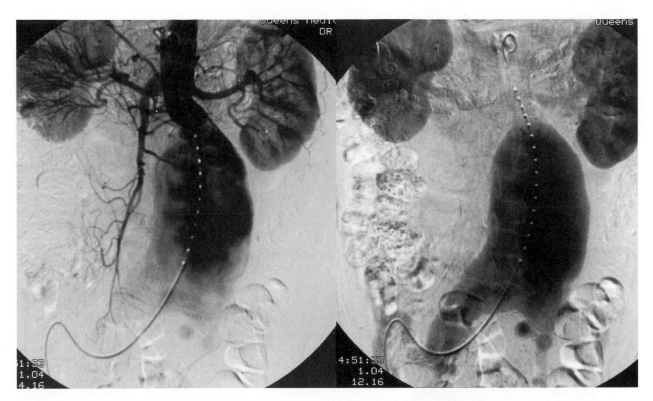

Fig. 25.29 Typical degenerative (atheromatous) abdominal aortic aneurysm extending into both iliacs.

countries. They can involve arteries in any part of the body but are commonest in the ascending aorta and arch, where they can reach a large size (Fig. 25.28). Angiography is usually required as a prelude to surgery with most mycotic aneurysms, though the diagnosis can be made with non-invasive imaging in most areas. CT or MRI will characterize large thoracic aneurysms, which can simulate mediastinal masses at simple radiography.

Degenerative Aneurysms   Degenerative aneurysms result from atheroma. They are commoner in males, and are seen most frequently in the abdominal aorta (Fig. 25.29). Other common sites are the iliacs and the popliteal arteries. They are also becoming more frequent in the thoracic aorta, where they have replaced syphilis as the main type of aneurysm in developed countries. Degenerative thoracic aneurysms affect mainly the descending aorta and distal arch, and rarely involve the ascending aorta. Atheromatous aneurysms may also occur in the splenic artery, in the renal artery, and in cerebral arteries, including the internal carotid and basilar arteries, where they can be fusiform or saccular. Atheroma is also thought to be a major contributory factor to the development of the smaller so-called 'congenital' berry aneurysms.

Degenerative aneurysms are often fusiform, resulting in generalized dilatation of the artery, but they may become saccular, particularly in the sites of election mentioned above. Such saccular aneurysms may rupture with disastrous or even fatal consequences. They may also form a nidus for intraluminal clot which can embolize to more distal vessels.

Imaging   *Simple radiography* often shows characteristic curved linear calcification in the wall of large aortic aneurysms or of atheromatous aneurysms at other sites.

Ultrasound is the simplest method of confirming a suspected diagnosis of abdominal aortic aneurysm (see Fig. 25.1) and monitoring any growth. It can also be used to diagnose popliteal and other peripheral aneurysms.

Nuclear angiography will show the lumen of an aneurysm well (see Fig. 25.2), but not the clot which may be between it and the outer wall.

CT has the advantage of showing both the lumen and the extent of any intraluminal clot. It can also show evidence of leakage and the important relationship of the renal arteries to the upper limit of an abdominal aneurysm. Direct measurement of the aneurysm in all planes is possible (see Fig. 25.3A). CT can also characterize the so-called 'inflammatory aneurysm' (see Fig. 25.3B) or perianeurysmal fibrosis. This has a thickened irregular and enhancing wall, probably due to slow periarterial hemorrhage, and should be differentiated from retroperitoneal fibrosis.

MRI can also easily define large aneurysms and their relationships as well as imaging them in all planes.

Traumatic Aneurysms   These can occur wherever an arterial wall is subject to injury (Fig. 25.30). Such aneurysms are commonest in the limbs, but can occur in the thorax, abdomen, and head and neck. They may follow direct penetrating injury from a knife, missile or foreign body, or they may result from closed injury. Trauma to the femoral artery in the groin is a well-recognized occupational hazard in the butchering trade.

Traumatic aneurysm of the aortic arch is a frequent and potentially fatal result of chest injury in automobile accidents. It can easily be missed, with disastrous results, if not specifically suspected and looked for, since many of these patients have multiple injuries. The shearing effect of an acute deceleration injury usually

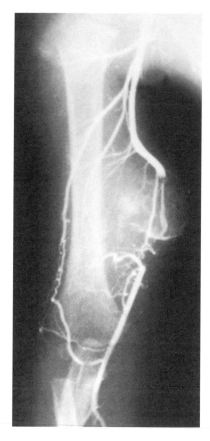

Fig. 25.30   Traumatic false aneurysm with rupture of the brachial artery in a child, following a fall while carrying a glass milk bottle.

involves the distal arch in the region of the ligamentum arteriosum. In most cases the injury is rapidly fatal, but some 20% of cases survive the acute episode by the formation of a periaortic hematoma and false aneurysm or because the adventitia has not yet ruptured.

It is vital to recognize these cases since secondary rupture will follow within 24 h in 30%, and within a week in most of the remainder. Only 2% will survive to chronic aneurysm formation, according to a study of 262 cases at the American Armed Forces Institute of Pathology.

Imaging   *Simple chest X-ray* may show broadening of the mediastinum, but this will be difficult to assess on portable or emergency films. *CT* may show periaortic hemorrhage.

Aortography will show the false aneurysm, usually near the isthmus (Fig. 25.31), but the signs may be more subtle, consisting merely of an intimal flap or mural irregularity at the site of the tear. A small ductus diverticulum may occur near this site but should be differentiated by its smooth wall and inferomedial position.

Dissecting Aneurysms   Dissecting aneurysms are mainly encountered in the aorta, and hypertension is the main predisposing cause. The incidence in the USA has been estimated at 5–10 cases annually per million population. Men are mostly affected, usually aged between 50 and 70 years. Only 5% of cases are under 40 years, and these are usually associated with rare causes such as Marfan syndrome or, in women, with pregnancy. Other rare associations are with coarctation, aortic stenosis, and bicuspid aortic valves.

Dissections usually commence in the aortic arch or ascending aorta and extend distally. De Bakey has classified them into three groups (Fig. 25.32). Type I commences in the ascending aorta and extends through the arch and descending aorta to the iliacs. Type II commences in the ascending aorta but does not extend beyond the arch. Type III commences in the distal arch and extends down to the iliacs.

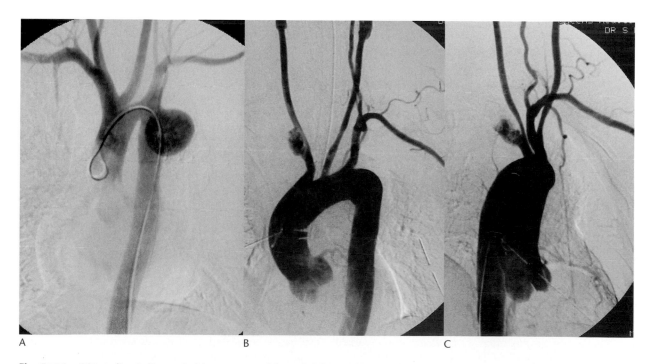

A   B   C

Fig. 25.31   DSA studies. **A**. Traumatic false aneurysm of the arch following RTA. **B,C**. Ruptured innominate artery following RTA.

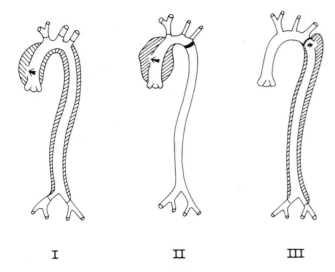

Fig. 25.32 Types of dissecting aneurysms (see text).

involving the ascending aorta (i.e. type III above); since the former are best treated surgically and the latter medically (see below).

The clinical features in classic cases are well known, and include sudden agonizing pain in the chest. It is important to realize, however, that many cases are atypical and easily missed or misdiagnosed, since symptoms may vary considerably depending on the aortic branches involved. Hemiplegia and vertebral symptoms may result from involvement of great vessels and their cerebral branches; paraplegia can follow occlusion of intercostal or lumbar arteries supplying the cord; in the abdomen the celiac axis and mesenteric arteries can be affected, giving rise to abdominal pain, mesenteric ischemia, or pancreatitis; renal artery occlusion may precipitate acute hypertension or anuria; the iliac vessels may be obstructed with lower-limb ischemia; retrograde spread of the dissection in the ascending aorta can lead to coronary involvement, causing cardiac ischemia or rupture into the pericardium with cardiac tamponade.

Dissecting aneurysms carry a grave prognosis: 30% are fatal within 24 h, and a further 50% of sufferers die in the next few days or weeks. Only 20% are likely to survive beyond 6 weeks, and half of these will die later from rupture of the aneurysm. Some of the late survivals are associated with a large re-entry of the dissection into the true lumen in the lower abdominal aorta, giving rise to the so-called 'double-bore' aorta. We have diagnosed cases of this type by aortography, where the true diagnosis was completely unsuspected by the referring physician.

The best prognosis rests with type III cases not involving the ascending aorta, and present opinion favors medical treatment in

Type II is the least common and is often associated with Marfan syndrome. It forms 10% of the cases, with types I and III representing 45% each.

From the surgical viewpoint a more practical classification is into two groups: type A, including all cases involving the ascending aorta (i.e. types I and II above), and type B, including those not

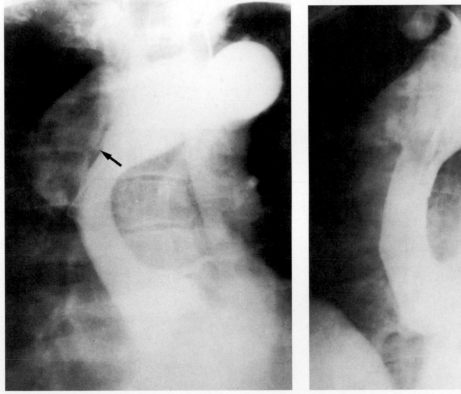

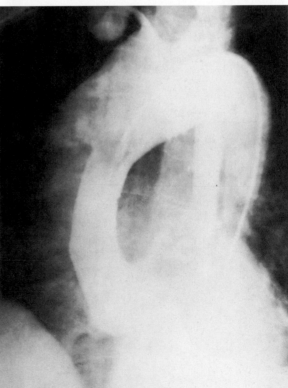

Fig. 25.33 Type I dissections; two cases. **A.** The dissection is compressing the true lumen of both the ascending and descending aorta. A small amount of contrast medium is seen entering the dissection through the tear in the intima of the ascending aorta (arrow). **B.** Contrast medium is entering the false lumen, separated by intimal flap in descending aorta.

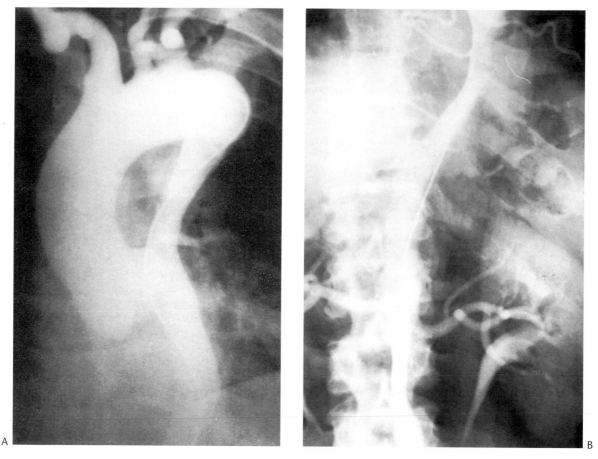

Fig. 25.34 Type III dissection. **A**. The dissection commences in the distal arch and compresses the descending aorta. **B**. Irregular compression of the lower thoracic and abdominal aorta. Both renal arteries fill well but the celiac and superior mesenteric arteries are not identified and appear compressed. They are probably perfused by the dissection, which shows faint opacification.

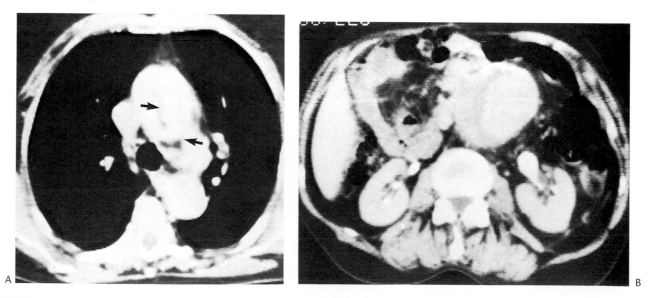

Fig. 25.35 **A**. Dissecting aneurysm shown by CT after contrast. Both true and false lumens are opacified but are separated by displaced intimal flaps (arrows) in the dilated ascending aorta (W512 L60). **B**. Dissection involving the abdominal aorta, which shows fusiform aneurysmal dilatation. Contrast medium in both true and false lumens separated by intimal flap (W512 L38).

these, since the survival rate is not significantly affected by surgery. However, surgery is recommended for types I and II or group A, which involve the ascending aorta. In one series of group A cases treated surgically, survival was 64% as against a medically treated survival rate of 22%. There is thus some urgency in establishing the diagnosis and case type as rapidly as possible.

Imaging   *Simple radiographs* of the chest may show widening of the mediastinum, though this may be difficult to assess on portable films. More characteristic is localized dilatation of the aortic knuckle and upper descending aorta, which may give rise to a prominent 'hump' sign due to lateral projection of the knuckle (Figs 25.33A and 25.34A). Lateral and anterior displacement of the trachea has also been described, and the descending aorta often bulges to the left and is sometimes lobulated. A recent chest film, if available, is most helpful, as a change in contour then becomes obvious. Medial displacement of the calcified intima at the aortic knuckle has been described but is rarely clear-cut, and a pleural effusion (hemothorax) is present in about 20% of cases. In patients with Marfan syndrome, localized bulging of the ascending aorta to the right may be recognized.

CT or *MRI* can both be used to confirm or refute a diagnosis of dissecting aneurysm. CT requires intravenous contrast enhancement, provided the patient's renal and cardiovascular state permits. In typical cases the dilated aorta is well shown, with the true and false lumens separated by a linear intimal flap (Fig. 25.35). MRI fulfills the same function without contrast (Figs 25.36, 25.100 and 25.102) and has the further advantage of easy sagittal and coronal imaging.

Aortography has been widely used in the past to confirm the diagnosis, and can provide much vital anatomic information, provided the patient is well enough for a thorough examination which may involve multiple areas. The transfemoral route is usually used, though the right transaxillary route can be used in cases where this is difficult. The catheter tip is passed into the aortic root so that the whole of the ascending aorta can be visualized and contrast medium can enter the false lumen if the tear is a proximal one (see Fig. 25.33). It also allows aortic insufficiency and regurgitation to be recognized.

Usually both the true and false lumens will fill with contrast medium, and the displaced intima appears as a linear band separating the two (see Fig. 25.33B). The intimal tear lies at the point where contrast medium enters the false from the true lumen (Fig. 25.33). In some cases only the true lumen fills, even with the catheter tip proximal to the tear (Fig. 25.34), implying that the false lumen contains blood clot or stagnant blood with no re-entry into the true lumen at a lower level. Such patients have a much better prognosis, and in one series had a 90% survival rate. In these cases only the true lumen is outlined by contrast, but it is compressed and distorted by the false lumen ('twisted tape' sign). This appearance is similar to that seen when injections are made with the catheter tip distal to the tear. Such injections are made deliberately with an abdominal series in order to show the lower limits of the dissection and involvement of the splanchnic and renal arteries (Figs 25.34B and 25.37).

The thoracic aorta is the commonest site for dissection but the lesion is occasionally encountered in more peripheral vessels. We have encountered examples in the abdominal aorta, the iliacs, and the renal arteries. Localized dissection in the internal carotid artery is also well documented. (See Ch. 56)

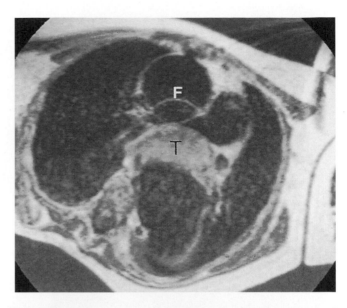

Fig. 25.36   Axial MRI section of thorax shows a dissecting aneurysm. In the ascending aorta both lumens are patent and separated by an intimal flap (F). In the descending aorta the false lumen contains thrombus (T). (Courtesy of Dr Peter Wilde and Bristol MRI Centre.)

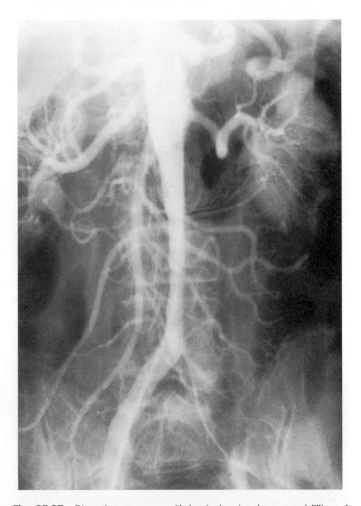

Fig. 25.37   Dissecting aneurysm. Abdominal series shows good filling of splanchnic and renal vessels but the lower abdominal aorta and left common iliac artery are obstructed. The latter forms the lower limit of the dissection.

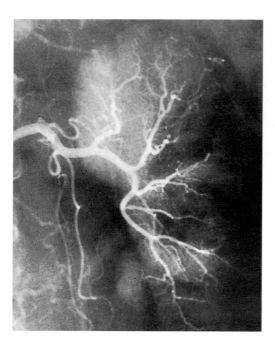

Fig. 25.38   Polyarteritis nodosa showing multiple microaneurysms.

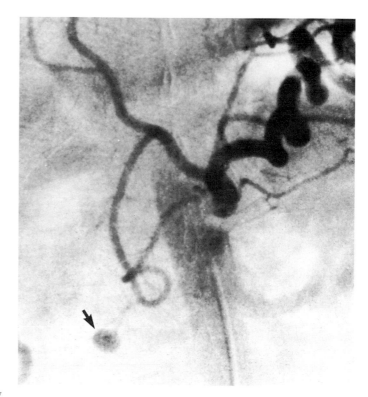

Fig. 25.39   Aneurysm of the pancreaticoduodenal arcade (arrow) secondary to acute pancreatitis (subtraction film).

Iatrogenic arterial dissection as a complication of angiography has been mentioned above. Such events are usually minor in degree and resolve spontaneously, particularly where they are produced by retrograde catheterization so that blood flow flattens rather than fills the intimal flap.

Necrotizing Vasculitis   The mysterious disease *polyarteritis nodosa* is associated with necrotizing vasculitis. The process involves the walls of small vessels, and as the disease progresses these weaken and aneurysms develop. The nodose lesions have a predilection for arterial bifurcations, but can occur anywhere along the artery. Any artery in the body may be involved, including the vasa vasorum, which accounts for the protean clinical manifestations.

The kidneys are very frequently involved and hypertension is seen in 70% of cases. Multiple small aneurysms may be identified at angiography and are characteristic, though not always seen (Fig. 25.38). The small aneurysms can rupture, giving rise to perirenal hematomas. Aneurysms of other splanchnic vessels can also rupture, leading to retroperitoneal or other abdominal hemorrhages. The demonstration of multiple small aneurysms is almost diagnostic, so that renal and visceral angiography is a valuable tool.

Other rarer causes of similar small aneurysms are *Wegener's granulomatosis* and *systemic lupus erythematosus*. *Atrial myxoma* embolization can also give rise to small peripheral aneurysms, as can necrotizing arteritis resulting from abuse of drugs, particularly *metamphetamine*. *Acute pancreatitis* may involve small vessels adjacent to the pancreas and lead to aneurysms which can rupture with serious consequences (Fig. 25.39).

Aneurysm of a coronary artery is a well-recognized complication of *Kawasaki disease*. This mysterious condition first characterized in Japan is now being increasingly diagnosed in America and Europe. It presents in young children with pyrexia, a rash, conjunctivitis, and later swollen hands and feet with sloughing of the palms and soles. Early diagnosis is vital since treatment with

γ-globulin in the first 10 days can prevent the development of aneurysms.

Poststenotic Aneurysms   These are probably due to turbulence and eddy flows affecting the vessel wall distal to the arterial stenosis. They are a well-recognized complication of coarctation, occurring in some 4% of cases (Fig. 25.40). They may also be seen in the subclavian artery in the thoracic inlet syndrome (see below), and in the renal artery with fibromuscular hyperplasia. They can also complicate atheromatous stenosis in any artery.

Stenoses and Thromboses

Congenital Stenoses   Congenital stenoses of major arteries as in thoracic and abdominal coarctation of the aorta have been described above. Abdominal coarctation may also involve the origins of splanchnic or renal arteries. Congenital stenoses have also been described in other vessels, including the pulmonary arteries.

Extrinsic Pressure   Pressure from tumors, cysts or other masses can also involve arteries and obstruct flow; in these cases the cause is usually obvious. Less commonly, localized arterial obstruction is due to a fibrous band, as may sometimes occur in the thoracic inlet syndrome, in renal artery stenosis or in the celiac compression syndrome. An anomalous tendon can obstruct the popliteal artery in popliteal entrapment, as can a developmental cyst in the popliteal wall (see below).

Arteritis   Arteritis of inflammatory or unknown etiology may also lead to arterial stenosis, as in Takayasu disease.

Atheroma   This is far and away the commonest cause of arterial stenosis and thrombosis in clinical practice, and, depending on the

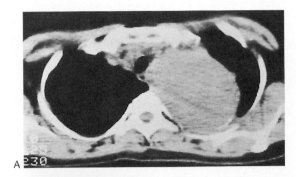

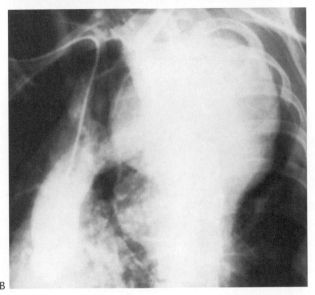

Fig. 25.40 **A**. CT of a large mediastinal mass presenting in a young woman. **B**. Transaxillary aortogram confirms giant poststenotic aneurysm and previously unrecognized mild coarctation.

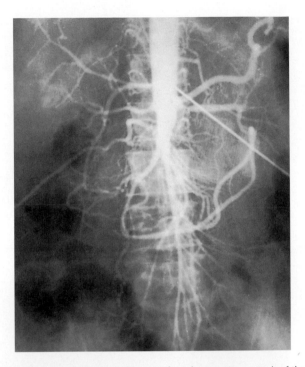

Fig. 25.41 Aortic thrombosis. There is also atheromatous stenosis of the left renal artery and filling of the inferior mesenteric from the artery of Drummond.

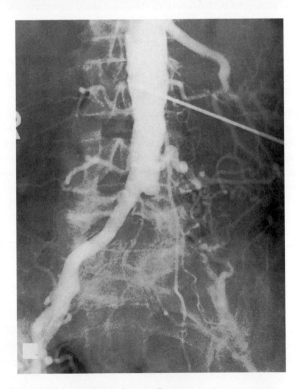

Fig. 25.42 Iliac thrombosis due to atheroma.

site, can give rise to a variety of clinical syndromes. It is found most often in males, though females are also frequently affected, particularly in the older age groups. Lesions of the greatest clinical importance involve:

1. Internal carotid and vertebral origins, giving rise to transient ischemic attacks and cerebrovascular insufficiency (see Ch. 56)
2. Coronary artery lesions causing cardiac ischemia (see Ch. 23)
3. Renal arteries, with resulting hypertension
4. The abdominal aorta
5. Iliac and femoral arteries.

Intermittent claudication is the cardinal symptom of stenosis and thrombosis of the aorta, iliacs, and femorals. Atheromatous stenosis also involves the major vessels to the upper limb, but is of less clinical significance because of the excellent collateral circulation.

Atheromatous stenosis of the abdominal aorta is frequently seen, as is its successor aortic thrombosis (Leriche syndrome). Lesions usually commence near the aortic bifurcation, and thrombosis extends upward, but usually stops short of the renal arteries (Fig. 25.41). Occasionally the origin of a renal artery is involved, with secondary hypertension ensuing.

The iliacs are among the commonest sites for atheromatous stenosis and thrombosis (Fig. 25.42), as are the femoral and popliteal arteries.

So-called 'primary popliteal thrombosis' occurs in young males, and though atheroma at a young age is occasionally responsible,

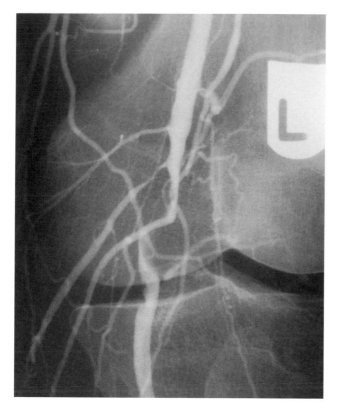

Fig. 25.43   Localized defect in the popliteal artery due to a popliteal cyst.

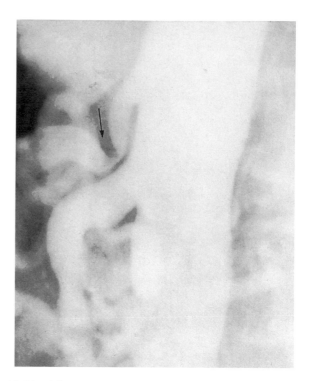

Fig. 25.44   Celiac stenosis shown by a lateral aortogram (arrow).

most cases are due to rare congenital anomalies, namely popliteal cysts and popliteal entrapment.

Popliteal Cysts   These usually present with calf claudication in men with an average age of 36 years. Angiography shows a healthy smooth-walled femoral artery and either a smooth narrowing suggesting external compression or a localized thrombosis in the popliteal artery (Fig. 25.43). The cyst secretes mucin, and lies in the wall of the artery. It is claimed to be due to developmental inclusion of mucin-secreting synovial capsular cells from the knee joint. Similar lesions have been described in other vessels including the iliac, radial, and ulnar arteries. The diagnosis has been made by CT of the popliteal artery, and could also be suggested by ultrasound or MRI.

Popliteal Entrapment   This also occurs mainly in young males, and may present in boys or adolescents either with calf claudication or, more commonly, acute popliteal thrombosis. The condition is due to an anomalous tendon of the medial head of gastrocnemius passing over and trapping the artery. Angiography shows either a characteristic linear external compression or thrombosis of the popliteal.

Celiac or Superior Mesenteric Stenoses   These stenoses resulting from atheroma are quite common, particularly at the origins of these arteries (Fig. 25.44). Other causes include fibromuscular hyperplasia and involvement by arteritis as in Takayasu disease, or by congenital coarctation or external celiac compression. Such lesions have been cited as causing dyspepsia and other gastrointestinal symptoms. However, it should be realized that the collateral circulation between the splanchnic vessels is so good

that even total occlusion of two of the three main vessels (celiac axis, superior and inferior mesenteric) can be easily tolerated (Fig. 25.45), and the inferior mesenteric is usually occluded in Leriche syndrome without referrable symptoms.

Celiac compression syndrome is the term used for gastrointestinal symptoms associated with narrowing of the celiac at its origin by external compression. This is due either to the median arcuate ligament of the diaphragm or to celiac plexus fibrosis. As implied above, this is more likely to be a chance association than a true syndrome.

Coronary stenosis and *thrombosis* due to atheroma and their investigation and treatment have been discussed in Chapter 23.

Renal Artery Stenosis   This is an important and sometimes remediable cause of renal ischemia and hypertension. Atheroma is the main etiological cause (Fig. 25.46), but in younger, mainly female, patients fibromuscular hyperplasia is also important (Fig. 25.47). This is a rare disease of unknown etiology leading to irregular beading of the vessel; it is further discussed below. Other rare causes of renal artery stenosis include extrinsic pressure by fibrous bands or sympathetic chain fibers, neurofibromatosis, and arterial stretching or compression by tumors. Aortic involvement by abdominal coarctation or by arteritis can also affect the renal artery, as can aortic thrombosis.

Whatever the cause of the renal ischemia, secondary hypertension may result, and the kidney can develop changes recognizable at both plain X-ray and urography. The affected kidney becomes smaller than normal but remains smooth in contour, unlike the irregular contour of the small kidney of chronic pyelonephritis. At urography, the excretion of contrast medium is slightly later than from the normal side, but as the investigation proceeds, contrast becomes denser on the affected side and shows small spindly calices.

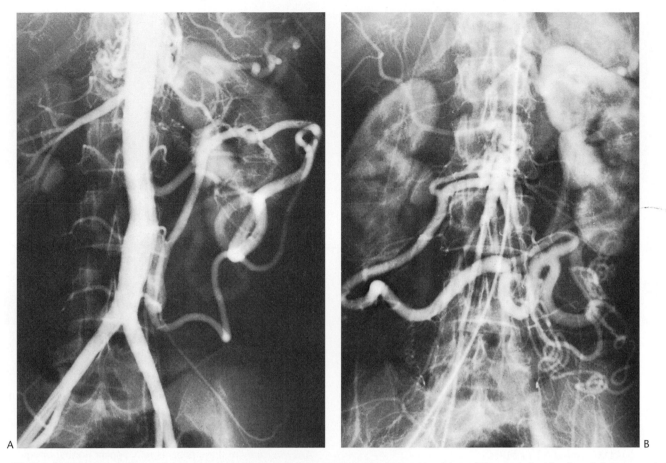

Fig. 25.45 **A**. Occlusion of celiac and superior mesenteric arteries. Separate origin of splenic artery. Artery of Drummond arising from inferior mesenteric. **B**. Artery of Drummond supplies the superior mesenteric origin and then the hepatic artery through pancreatic arcades.

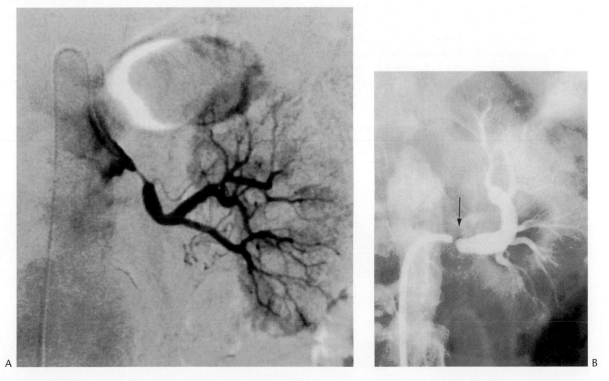

Fig. 25.46 **A**. Renal artery stenosis due to atheroma. **B**. Renal artery stenosis. Note poststenotic dilation of the renal artery.

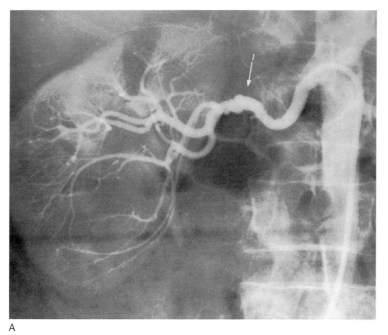

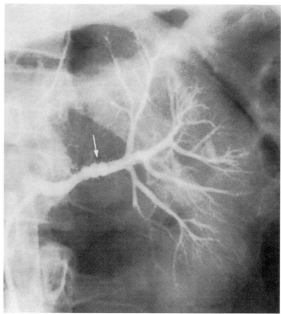

A

B

Fig. 25.47   A,B. Renal artery fibromuscular hyperplasia (arrows). See also Fig. 25.5A

The radiological treatment of renal artery stenosis by percutaneous angioplasty has been discussed above. The anatomy of renal artery stenosis is best shown by catheter arteriography, but screening for the condition can be accomplished on an outpatient basis by intravenous DSA; spiral CT or MRA.

Subclavian Stenosis   Compression of the subclavian artery at the root of the neck is seen in the thoracic inlet syndrome, and may be associated with various congenital anomalies. Some, such as cervical rib or an anomalous first rib, will be readily diagnosed on a plain film, but others, such as fibrous bands or compression by the scalenus anticus muscle, will only be manifest at angiography.

Clinically these patients may present with ischemic hands, with Raynaud's phenomenon, or with digital emboli. The latter derive from clot arising at the level of the lesion or in a poststenotic aneurysm. These are a frequent complication and are usually fusiform, though they can also be saccular (Fig. 25.48). Thrombosis of the subclavian artery can also result (Fig. 25.49).

Arteriography in these patients may appear normal or equivocal with the arm in neutral position, and Adson's maneuver may be necessary to confirm the lesion. This consists of fully abducting the arm with the head fully turned to the opposite side. These patients can also be investigated less invasively by intravenous DSA (Fig. 25.50).

Raynaud's Phenomenon   This frequently occurs in normal healthy individuals as an abnormal response to cold, In these cases it appears to be purely due to a spastic response of the small

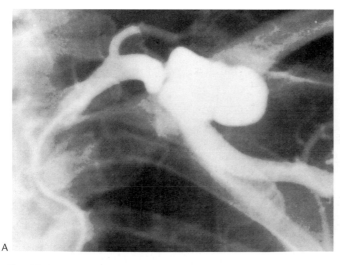

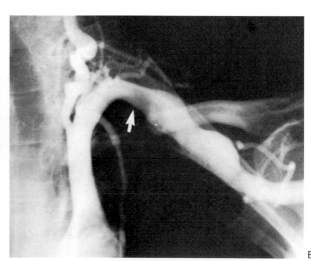

A

B

Fig. 25.48   Subclavian stenosis with poststenotic aneurysm formation. **A**. Saccular. **B**. Fusiform aneurysm.

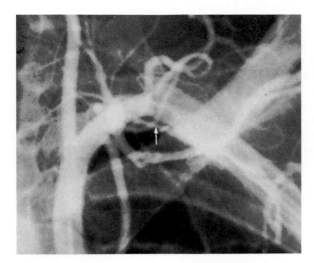

Fig. 25.49 Subclavian thrombosis (arrow).

Table 25.5 Digital ischemia and Raynaud's phenomenon

1. *Lesions of major vessels (often with small-vessel emboli)*
   Atheroma
   Takayasu's disease
   Non-specific arteritis
   African idiopathic aortitis
   Thoracic inlet syndrome
   Buerger's disease
   Fibromuscular hyperplasia
2. *Collagen disorder*
   Scleroderma
   Rheumatoid arthritis
   Polyarteritis nodosa
3. *Blood disorders*
   Polycythemia
   Sickle-cell disease
   Cryoagglutination
   The contraceptive pill
   PVC poisoning
4. *Specific conditions*
   Raynaud's phenomenon (spastic type)
   Vibrating tools
   Ergotism

vessels. Apart from this primary type, the condition may also be secondary to a variety of conditions which impair blood flow and includes major and minor vascular lesions. Table 25.5 lists the numerous diseases which have been associated with digital ischemia and Raynaud's phenomenon.

Atheromatous lesions in the subclavian, axillary, and brachial arteries are quite common, but are often asymptomatic because of the excellent collateral circulation at the root of the neck, shoulder, and elbow. Thus thrombosis of the first part of the subclavian artery is often encountered by chance during arch or headhunter angiography, when the vertebral artery on the affected side is demonstrated to supply the distal subclavian by reversed flow (subclavian steal—see Ch. 56). Atheromatous occlusions are also encountered in the distal vessels of the upper limb. In the digital vessels they can give rise to severe localized ischemia which may require amputation. In elderly men, most cases of localized digital ischemia are due to atheroma.

Generalized digital ischemia is usually due to a generalized disease such as scleroderma.

Buerger's Disease This has remained a controversial subject since the condition was first described in 1908. The diagnosis of Buerger's disease or 'thromboangitis obliterans' was once widely applied to a variety of vascular thromboses including the first cases of internal carotid thrombosis described by Moniz, as well as to the lower limb lesions originally described. As a healthy reaction to the overdiagnosis of Buerger's disease, Wessler et al (1960) pointed out that most of the cases examined by them were indistinguishable pathologically from atheromatous disease with thrombosis. This led some to the view that Buerger's disease was a myth and that most cases were in fact due to atheromatous disease.

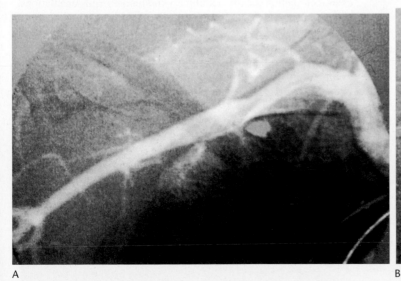

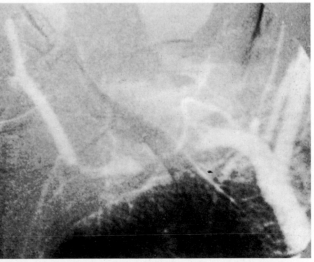

A   B

Fig. 25.50 Right subclavian artery shown by DSA. **A.** In neutral position there is slight fusiform aneurysmal dilatation, but no obvious stenosis. **B.** With Adson's maneuver there is marked obstruction.

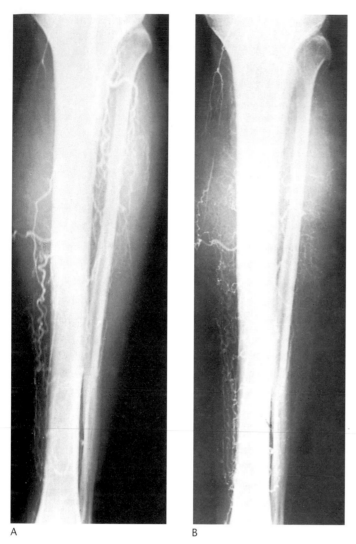

A   B

Fig. 25.51 Buerger's disease. Femoral arteriography showed normal smooth-walled femoral and popliteal arteries, but occlusion of the calf vessels with collaterals.

Angiographic studies show that whatever the pathological nature of the lesions, Buerger's disease does appear to be a separate clinical entity. It occurs in a much younger age group than typical atheromatous vascular disease, the patients being mainly in their twenties or early thirties. It also has a much higher male sex incidence than has atheroma, female patients being extremely rare; and there is a much stronger association with heavy cigarette smoking, the patients usually showing strong addiction, sometimes maintained despite the threat of amputation. Unlike atheroma, the major vessels (aorta, iliacs, and femorals) usually appear smooth walled and healthy, and the disease starts in the foot vessels and spreads retrogradely up the calf vessels. The typical angiographic appearance is of healthy femoral and popliteal arteries, with the calf vessels largely occluded and replaced by fine collaterals (Fig. 25.51). Long tortuous collaterals following the course of the occluded anterior and posterior tibial or peroneal arteries are sometimes seen and may represent hypertrophied vasa vasorum.

Spasm *Ergot poisoning* may occur in migraine patients who have overdosed themselves with ergotamine tartrate, of which there are several proprietary preparations. This results in peripheral vascular spasm, presenting as ischemic lower limbs. Such patients are easily misdiagnosed unless an adequate history is obtained, and we have been asked to perform angiography on several such patients without the referring physician suspecting the true diagnosis. The angiographic appearances are unusual but are diagnostic, consisting of spastic contraction of the vessels below the common femoral (the superficial femoral, popliteal, and peripheral vessels), which are uniformly narrowed, so that they appear more like narrow threads than normal vessels. Upper-limb vessel involvement has also been described, as has spasm of splanchnic and renal vessels. If the condition is correctly diagnosed, withdrawal of the offending drug brings a rapid reversal of the spasm.

Localized spasm of peripheral arteries may be induced at angiography, usually in small vessels with a prominent muscular coat, either by the guide-wire or catheter tip or by a local high concentration of contrast medium. It may be observed on the angiogram just distal to the tip of the catheter, and should not be mistaken for a local stenosis. Any doubt can be resolved by repeating the contrast injection with the catheter tip withdrawn to a more proximal position. *Beaded spasm* is a term used for an unusual appearance usually seen in the femoral and popliteal arteries and less commonly in other arteries such as the iliacs and splanchnics. The condition has also been referred to as 'standing' or 'stationary arterial waves' or 'arterial beading'. Its nature remains controversial but it is generally thought to represent a physical phenomenon due to arterial pressure waves. In our experience it has been seen most frequently in the femoral arteries of patients with Buerger's disease and high peripheral resistance from obliterated calf vessels. The regular and perfectly symmetrical nature of the beading has been likened to a chain of pearls, and helps to distinguish it from the asymmetrical and less regular beading of fibromuscular hyperplasia.

Fibromuscular Hyperplasia This is an unusual arterial disease first described in the renal arteries as a rare cause of renal artery stenosis and occurring mainly in young women. The diagnosis is made by angiography, which shows an irregular beaded appearance of the affected artery (see Fig. 25.47). The lumen of the artery, when examined pathologically, exhibits both stenoses and sacculations, and the latter may become aneurysmal. (See Fig. 25.5A)

The lesions are presumably congenital, though usually presenting in early adult life, and they have been described in many other arteries, though commonest in the renals. We have encountered examples in the iliac and splanchnic arteries as well as in the internal carotid artery, which is now a well-recognized site for the lesion.

It appears to be extremely rare in limb vessels, though we have previously reported a case in the brachial arteries of a middle-aged woman (Fig. 25.52).

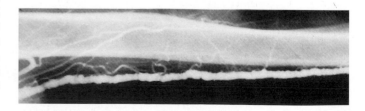

Fig. 25.52 Fibromuscular hyperplasia of the brachial artery in a woman of 50 years presenting with digital ischemia.

Arteritis

Takayasu's Arteritis   This is a rare condition first described in Japan in 1908 but now recognized to have a worldwide distribution. It manifests mainly in young women aged 20–30 years, and the incidence in the USA is 0.11%. The aorta is attacked by a granulomatous inflammation of the media proceeding to fibrosis and atheroma-like changes with involvement of the main branches, which can become thrombosed. The main pulmonary artery and its major branches may also be involved. The etiology is unknown, but an autoimmune mechanism has been postulated by some workers.

Clinical manifestations depend on the major aortic branches most affected and include upper-limb ischemia, ocular and cerebral symptoms, renovascular hypertension, coronary disease, and lower-limb ischemia. The *aortic arch syndrome* of progressive occlusion of the great vessels of the arch is a common complication (pulseless disease).

Angiography shows a surprising irregularity of the aorta, which resembles that of an elderly atheromatous person, together with stenoses or occlusions of the origins of the major branches.

Giant-cell Arteritis   This is a vasculitis affecting people above the age of 50 or 60 years and usually involving smaller or middle-sized arteries. It is not clear whether the cause is inflammatory or whether an autoimmune mechanism is involved. Temporal arteritis is common, as is involvement of intracerebral vessels, and blindness is a complication in some 10% of cases. Large-vessel vasculitis is very uncommon but is occasionally seen, and can give rise to lower-limb ischemia or an aortic arch syndrome. Angiography of the temporal artery may show irregular stenotic areas with intervening normal areas (skip lesions).

Embolus

Major embolus to the systemic arterial system is most commonly cardiac in origin, being seen in patients with atrial fibrillation and intra-atrial clot, or following clot formation in the left ventricle after cardiac infarction. Another cardiac cause is clot forming on prosthetic valves after cardiac surgery.

Embolus may also follow clot formation in a large aneurysm, which is then detached and carried distally.

The rare paradoxical embolus is carried from the venous system through a patent foramen ovale. This is present in one-third of the population but remains closed unless right atrial pressure exceeds left atrial pressure, as in chronic lung disease or pulmonary embolus, when clots may pass through to the left heart and systemic circulation.

Ulcerated atheromatous plaques in major vessels can also give rise to emboli from cholesterol showers or debris, which being smaller lodge in small peripheral vessels in the limbs and are usually less serious. However, when they affect the brain they can give rise to transient ischemic attacks or more serious strokes (see Ch. 56).

Finally, clot embolus is a well-recognized complication of catheter angiography, as previously described.

Of large emboli, 75% lodge at the aortic bifurcation, iliac bifurcation, or major vessels of the lower limb. The clinical diagnosis is usually obvious from the acute onset of pain, numbness, pallor, and coldness, with loss of peripheral pulses in the context of cardiac disease, aneurysm, or previous cardiac surgery. If, however, the onset is more insidious it may be difficult to differentiate from arterial thrombosis.

Angiography shows a sharp cut-off at the point of occlusion (Fig. 25.53) with sometimes a characteristic convex upper margin (meniscus sign). Larger emboli affecting the aortic, iliac, or femoral bifurcation are usually removed surgically with a Fogarty balloon catheter. They should be treated as surgical emergencies since a delay of more than 24 h leads to a significantly higher amputation rate. Smaller and more distal emboli and those in the arm have a better prognosis, but if the limb is at risk, treatment by intra-arterial thrombolysis may be attempted as described above. Mesenteric embolism should be suspected in patients with acute abdominal pain and coexisting atrial fibrillation, mitral stenosis, or a recent cardiac infarction.

Angiomatous Malformations

These lesions, also referred to as angiomas and congenital arteriovenous fistulas, represent direct communications between arterioles and venules without the interposition of a capillary bed. They are presumably congenital but often present in adults, probably due to increasing size after adult blood pressure is established. They are common in the cerebral circulation (see Ch. 56) but can present anywhere in the body. They should be distinguished from acquired communications between arteries and veins—arteriovenous fistulas—which are described below.

Figures 25.54, 25.55 and 25.56 show the angiographic appearances in lesions presenting in the hand, vulva, and bowel, respectively. In all cases there are hypertrophied arteries leading to the lesion and hypertrophied veins draining it, their size depending on the degree of shunt present. Both arteries and veins fill rapidly, and before contrast medium has passed through normal capillaries in the adjacent regions. Some smaller angiomas and those at very fine vessel level are more difficult to demonstrate and may require superselective angiography of the feeding vessels to show their full extent. Treatment by angiographic embolization has been discussed above.

Arteriovenous Fistula

This term is best limited to the condition where there is a single communication between an artery and a vein, and is mainly of traumatic origin, particularly following gunshot or other penetrating wounds. Occasionally it may result from a closed injury (Fig. 25.57). Traumatic fistulas may occur anywhere in the body, and we have encountered cases in all anatomic sites from the scalp to the foot.

Spontaneous arteriovenous fistula is also occasionally encountered, resulting from rupture of an aneurysm into an adjacent vein (Fig. 25.58). A site of election for this is the cavernous sinus, where rupture of an aneurysm can give rise to pulsating exophthalmos (see Ch. 56). Another well-documented site is the abdominal aorta, where rupture of an aneurysm into the inferior vena cava leads to aortocaval fistula (Fig. 25.59). These intra-abdominal cases can give rise to difficult diagnostic problems, and the larger shunts can give rise to high-output cardiac failure without the true cause being suspected.

So-called congenital arteriovenous fistulas are sometimes seen in infants and children, but it is usually difficult or impossible to exclude trauma in these cases.

Iatrogenic arteriovenous fistulas, apart from those deliberately induced for dialysis, can arise from many procedures, particularly orthopedic operations on the hip, ankle, and spine. Aortocaval and ilioiliac fistulas have followed lumbar disk operations when the rougeur has been passed through the anterior spinal ligament, and renal arteriovenous fistula is a common complication of renal biopsy. Arteriography has given rise to arteriovenous fistula at the site of puncture, usually of small arteries (brachial and vertebral), but it has also been recorded in the femoral artery. Because of the grossly hypertrophied drainage veins carrying arterial blood, a fistula may be very difficult to locate at surgery, and prior

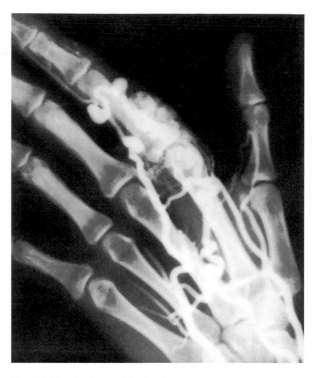

Fig. 25.54 Angioma of the hand.

angiography with localization of the fistula is essential. As with angiomas, the dilated feeding artery fills early, as do the dilated drainage veins, and large amounts of contrast medium with rapid serial films are necessary to clearly define the anatomy and the site of the fistula.

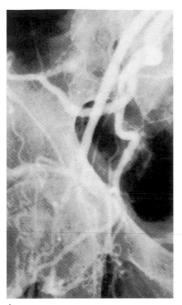
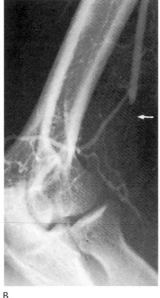

A
B

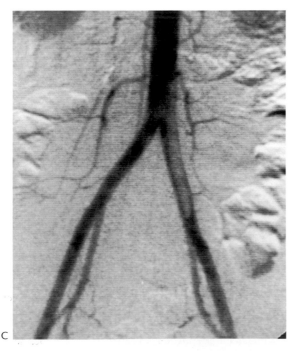
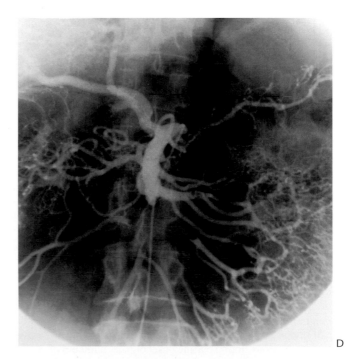

C
D

Fig. 25.53 **A**. Embolic occlusion of the common femoral artery. **B**. Embolic occlusion of the brachial artery (arrow). **C**. Embolus of the aortic bifurcation with clot defect extending into the left common iliac. DSA study. **D** Embolus of the superior mesenteric artery.

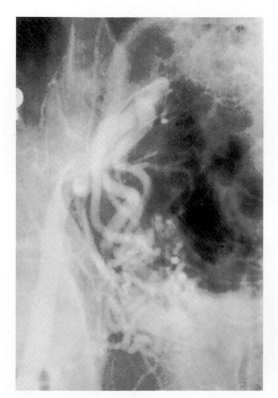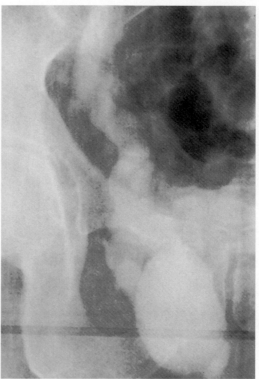

Fig. 25.55   Angioma of the pelvis, presenting as vulval swelling. Aneurysmal dilatation of draining vein.

A large arteriovenous fistula throws an extra burden on the heart because of the large amount of shunt, and can result in cardiac failure from high cardiac output unless successfully treated. As noted above, many fistulas, particularly smaller ones, are now treated successfully by embolization.

Hemorrhage

Arteriography can be extremely useful in the diagnosis and treatment of internal hemorrhage. Serious or life-threatening hemorrhage can be due to many causes, including trauma, peptic ulceration, ruptured aneurysms, neoplasms or inflammatory lesions involving blood vessels, radiation, and blood disorders. In many situations previously requiring surgical intervention, percutaneous catheterization and embolization as described above offers a simpler and safer alternative to surgery.

Upper Gastrointestinal Tract Hemorrhage   The common causes are esophageal varices, Mallory–Weiss tears, gastritis, gastric ulcer, and duodenal ulcer. Endoscopy is now widely used for both diagnosis and treatment, and angiography and embolization have played a diminishing role in recent years.

Hemorrhage from the small bowel is much less common and more difficult to diagnose. Scintigraphy, as described below, may be useful in demonstrating the site, and arteriography will occasionally demonstrate rare causes such as angioma (see Fig. 25.56). Other rare causes are jejunal diverticulum, Meckel's diverticulum, neoplasms and typhoid enteritis.

Lower Gastrointestinal Tract Hemorrhage   Radionuclide scintigraphy is the technique of choice for the investigation of acute lower gastrointestinal tract bleeding. Technetium-99m sulphur colloid or ^{99m}Tc-labeled red cells may be used to localize the approximate source of the hemorrhage, provided the patient is still bleeding (see Ch. 30).

Diverticulosis is the commonest cause and, rather surprisingly, most bleeding diverticula lie in the ascending colon, though diverticula are much less common here than in the sigmoid and descending colon. *Angiodysplasia*, the second commonest cause, also involves mainly the cecum or ascending colon, and these lesions can be multiple.

Colonoscopy is less successful in identifying these lesions than arteriography, which is often necessary. Bleeding from colonic diverticula can be controlled by vasopressin, though success may only prove temporary. Some cases have been controlled by embolization, though this requires difficult superselective catheterization. The alternative of emergency colectomy carries a high mortality, and even temporary control may permit a later elective colectomy. Angiodysplasias are often small and require high-quality angiograms for their demonstration, as bleeding is less severe than with diverticula. Arteriovenous shunting with early venous filling should raise suspicion (Fig. 25.60). These lesions are usually treated surgically.

NEOPLASMS AND MASS LESIONS

Arteriography was once widely used for the characterization of tumors, cysts, and other mass lesions but with the advent and constant improvement of the non-invasive techniques of ultrasound, CT, and MRI the method has become largely obsolete as a purely diagnostic tool. Where angiography is still used, its purpose is either to complement the non-invasive investigations by providing

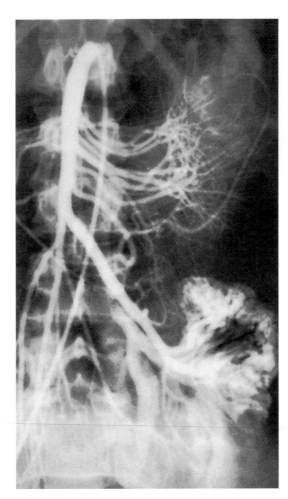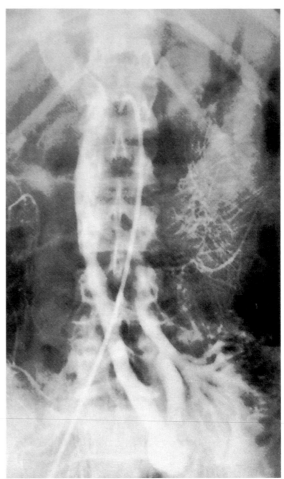

Fig. 25.56 Angioma of the small bowel with high-volume shunting into the portal system in a woman of 24 years with repeated attacks of melena. In the previous 10 years she had had four barium enemas and five barium follow-throughs with negative findings. Large angiomas like this are unusual in the bowel, small areas of dysplasia being more common.

anatomic information to the surgeon about the vascularity and blood supply of a tumor, or in some cases to permit embolization of inoperable tumors or of highly vascular tumors prior to surgery. In rare cases it may be used to help establish the correct diagnosis where ultrasound and CT have proved equivocal or inconclusive.

The value of angiography in tumor diagnosis arose from three facts. First, tumors often have circulations different from those in the tissues in which they arise. This results in abnormal or 'pathological' vessels being outlined by contrast and thus localizing and characterizing the neoplasm. Arteriovenous shunting with early opacification of drainage veins is a frequent feature of the more malignant neoplasms, which tend to be more vascular than benign tumors. Second, the growth of the tumor may displace and stretch the normal vessels at its margins, thus enabling less vascular tumors to be located. Third, tumors may actually involve adjacent arteries, leading to 'cuffing' or irregular narrowing of the affected arteries.

Renal Masses

Hypernephromas are usually highly vascular tumors, and the demonstration of typical pathological vessels in a renal mass is diagnostic (Fig. 25.61). Occasionally these tumors are so vascular as to simulate angiomatous malformations (Fig. 25.62). Conversely, they are also occasionally non-vascular, simulating cysts. However, such cases will sometimes show tortuous or irregular vessels entering the periphery of the mass, a feature not seen with cysts.

Renal cysts are typically rounded avascular masses best shown in the nephrogram phase. The cortex at the margin of the cyst is compressed and displaced, producing a pointed projection of opacified cortex, the so-called 'beak sign' (Fig. 25.63). Further, the normal arteries at the margins of the cyst are stretched and displaced.

Carcinoma of the renal pelvis is much less vascular than hypernephroma, but high-quality angiograms will show one or more abnormal fine tortuous vessels leading to the tumor, and similar appearances may be seen in carcinoma of the ureter.

Wilms' tumor (nephroblastoma) occurs in children below the age of 5 years, though occasionally presenting at an older age and even in an adult. These tumors can reach a very large size, and 10% are bilateral. At angiography they may show only limited neovascularity.

Angiomyolipoma (hamartoma) is a benign tumor, but the angiogram shows a vascular lesion which can be mistaken for a

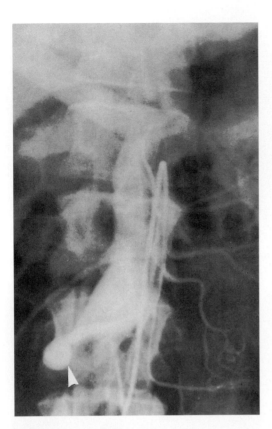

Fig. 25.57 Mesenteric–portal fistula (arrowed) shown by selective superior mesenteric injection. There is rapid filling of dilated superior mesenteric and portal veins. The lesion followed a crush injury to the abdomen.

carcinoma. Such tumors are common in tuberous sclerosis, when they may be multiple. *Xanthogranulomatous pyelonephritis* is a chronic inflammatory condition which can also produce a vascular angiogram resembling that of a malignant tumor.

Renal oncocytomas have been described as rare benign tumors resembling hypernephromas but well encapsulated and sometimes showing a 'spoke-wheel' pattern at angiography. The existence of this entity remains controversial, and they are considered by some to be low-grade hypernephromas.

Benign tumors of the kidney are rare but important in differential diagnosis. *Adenomas* are usually small and subcapsular in situation. A rare form of giant benign renal adenoma has been described which at angiography is well circumscribed and separate from adjacent normal renal tissue. There is no arteriovenous shunting or other feature to suggest malignancy.

The rare *renin-secreting juxtaglomerular cell tumor* is found in hypertensive patients. At angiography it shows as a small cortical defect in the nephrogram phase, resembling a small cyst. A few fine vessels to the tumor may be identified, as may the slight bulge in the surface of the kidney. Renin assay from the renal veins helps to confirm the diagnosis by demonstrating higher concentrations on the affected side.

Renal angiography has also been used in the past to confirm such benign conditions as *pseudotumors* (e.g. enlarged column of Bertin, dromedary hump, congenital polar enlargement, suprahilar and infrahilar lips, and areas of compensatory hypertrophy).

Renal Graft Angiography   Multiple arteries occur in 25% of

kidneys, and it is therefore necessary to perform angiography on live kidney donors to ensure that the proposed kidney has only one artery of supply. The grafted kidney is usually placed in the right iliac fossa with its artery anastomosed to the patient's internal iliac artery.

The commonest cause of failure of a transplant kidney is renal rejection, which can be early or delayed. Sometimes it is difficult to differentiate clinically between rejection of the graft and other complications affecting renal function.

A graft arteriogram will show whether the kidney is perfusing normally and will demonstrate such complications as stenosis at the anastomosis (Fig. 25.64). Generalized small-vessel occlusions, which are usually due to rejection, will be shown, as will thrombosis of the main artery or impaired perfusion. Kidney transplant arteriography can be performed by injection of a large bolus of contrast medium into the common iliac artery (20 ml of iopamidol 300 or equivalent of other contrast media). Selective angiography of the internal iliac artery will give better resolution, and intra-arterial DSA will permit low doses of contrast medium.

Hepatic Tumors

The primary investigation of liver masses is by ultrasound, with scintiscanning, CT, and MRI all able to provide further help in characterizing lesions. Angiography now has little place in such diagnostic studies, but it can still be used for therapeutic purposes such as intra-arterial chemotherapy or embolization or for the elucidation of the occasional problem case (see Ch. 34). Selective hepatic angiography can demonstrate both primary and secondary carcinoma of the liver. Such malignant tumors usually show a well-marked pathological circulation (Fig. 25.65), but are occasionally poorly vascularized and difficult to differentiate from benign masses. The latter tend merely to displace and stretch branches of the hepatic artery, though some are more vascular.

Hemangioma is the commonest benign tumor of the liver to show an abnormal circulation. These lesions are sometimes multiple, and can then be suspected as deposits at ultrasound or other non-invasive investigations. Differentiation is possible on the angiogram since the lesions, though vascular, show a typical sluggish circulation, with persistence of contrast medium in the venous phase (Fig. 25.66). This is quite unlike the rapid arteriovenous shunting seen in malignant tumors.

Hepatic adenomas may also occur, and have been described as a complication of hormonal treatment with contraceptive pills or with androgens. At angiography they are vascular tumors, but their vascular pattern is more regular than that of a malignant tumor, and they stand out as encapsulated tumors in the hepatogram phase (Fig. 25.67).

Pancreatic Tumors

Ultrasound, CT, and endoscopic retrograde cholangiopancreatography (ERCP) are now the methods of choice for the diagnosis of pancreatic tumors. Angiography, once widely used for this purpose, is now obsolete except for the elucidation of suspected small endocrine tumors.

Pancreatic *carcinoma* is relatively avascular, and tumors were recognized by displacement of vessels supplying the pancreas or by invasion of their walls with cuffing or occlusion.

Cystadenoma of the pancreas, however, can be highly vascular, and shows a florid pathological circulation (Fig. 25.68).

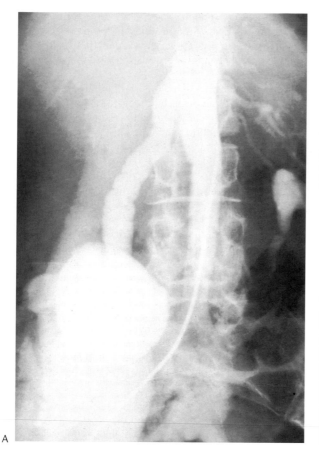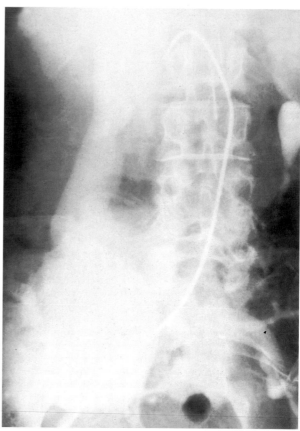

A   B

Fig. 25.58   Giant renal arteriovenous fistula, possibly due to rupture of an aneurysm associated with fibromuscular hyperplasia. The patient presented with heart failure and a pulsating mass clinically thought to be pelvic because of ptosed kidney. **A**. Arterial phase. **B**. Venous phase showing a dilated inferior vena cava.

Islet cell adenomas of the pancreas may be quite small and difficult to diagnose by non-invasive imaging techniques. At superselective angiography, however, they can be identified as a rounded blush of contrast in the venous or capillary phase (Fig. 25.69). Large islet cell adenomas are occasionally seen and can be highly vascular.

Pancreatic hormone-producing tumors can also be identified by venous blood sampling and assay from the pancreatic drainage veins. The samples are obtained by transhepatic portal vein catheterization as described below (see Ch. 35).

Adrenal Tumors

Angiography is no longer used for the diagnosis of adrenal tumors, and CT is now the primary imaging method (see Ch. 36).

Tumors of Bone and Soft Tissue

The newer imaging techniques, particularly CT and MRI, are now the investigations of choice for tumors involving bone and for soft-tissue tumors in all parts of the body. Angiography is now rarely undertaken in these cases except for embolization or other therapeutic purposes.

Malignant bone tumors are usually highly vascular, and the angiographic appearances are pathognomonic (Fig. 25.70). Prior to the advent of CT, angiography was widely used to demonstrate the extraosseous spread of such tumors (Fig. 25.71). Secondary deposits in bone vary in their vascularity, ranging from the highly vascular to the relatively non-vascular. Hypernephroma and thyroid metastases have been amongst the most vascular encountered, and such deposits in the soft tissues can simulate pulsating aneurysms.

Sarcoma of the soft tissues, when highly malignant, usually shows abundant pathological vessels (Fig. 25.72), but low-grade fibrosarcomas may be relatively non-vascular.

Chromaffinoma (chemodectoma)   These tumors are most frequently found at the carotid bifurcation, where they are known as *carotid body tumors*. They are extremely vascular and show a characteristic appearance at angiography (Fig. 25.73). Occasionally they are familial, when they can also be bilateral. Clinically they have been mistaken for local aneurysms, and, conversely, rare aneurysms at this site have been mistaken for carotid body tumors.

Another common site for chromaffinoma is the glomus jugulare at the base of the skull (*glomus jugulare tumor*). Here they are also very vascular, and the angiographic appearance is similar to that of the carotid body tumor. Careful superselective angiography of the external carotid feeding branches may be required to show their full extent or for embolization, which may be required prior to surgery or in inoperable cases (see Ch. 56). The *glomus*

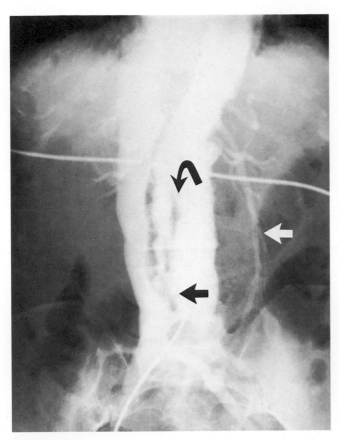

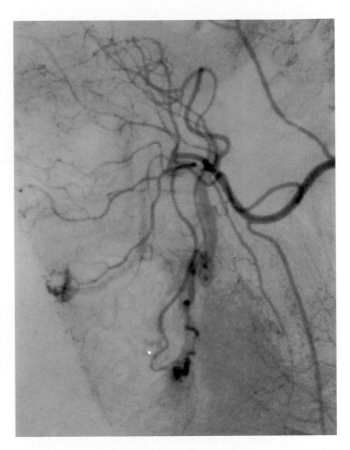

Fig. 25.59 Aortocaval fistula following spontaneous rupture of an abdominal aortic aneurysm. The superior mesenteric is displaced by the aneurysm containing mural thrombus (white arrow). The fistula into the inferior vena cava is marked by the black arrow. The curved arrow suggests an intimal flap in the aneurysm. (From Gregson et al (1983) by permission of the editor of Clinical Radiology.)

Fig. 25.60 Angiodysplasia of the cecum. Note early filling of drainage veins.

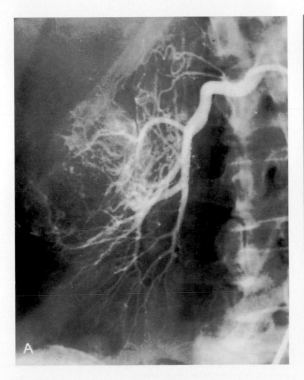

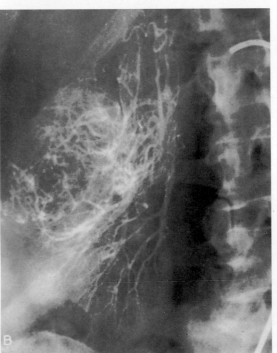

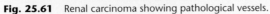

Fig. 25.61 Renal carcinoma showing pathological vessels.

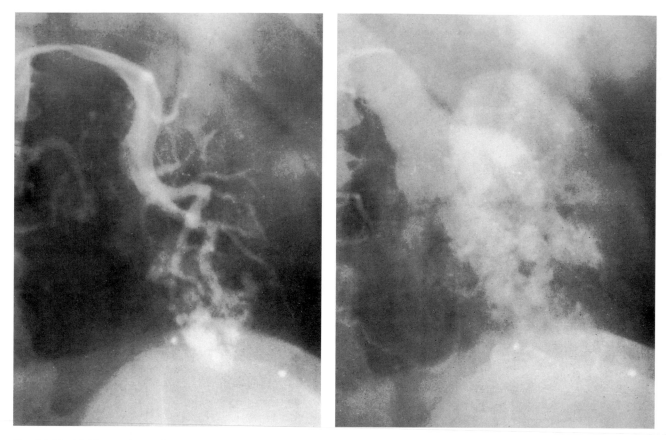

Fig. 25.62   Highly vascular renal carcinoma resembling angioma. Note the huge drainage vein in the nephrogram phase.

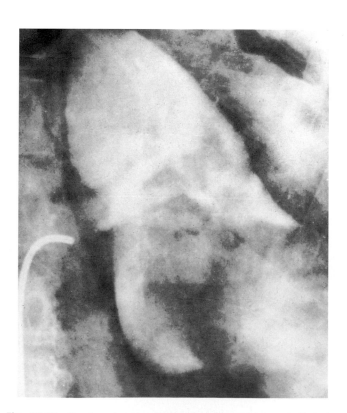

Fig. 25.63   Renal angiograms. Nephrogram shows large cyst displacing cortex ('beak sign').

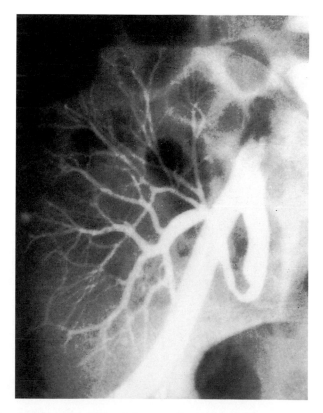

Fig. 25.64   Renal graft arteriogram. The patient developed secondary hypertension and a bruit. The arteriogram shows an unusual stenosis of the proximal segment of the graft artery.

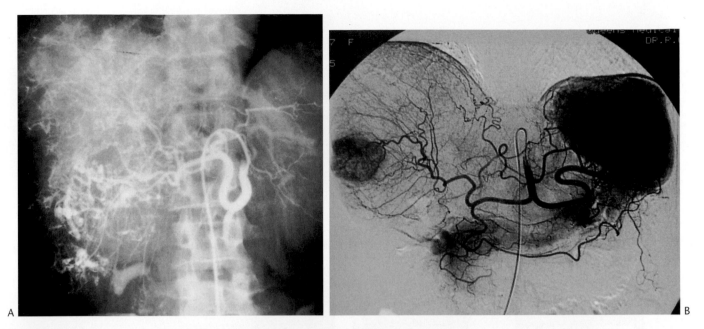

Fig. 25.65 **A**. Selective hepatic arteriogram. A large vascular tumor is shown in the lower part of the right lobe of the liver. Histology: primary hepatoma. **B**. Selective hepatic angiogram shows multiple vascular deposits from colonic carcinoma.

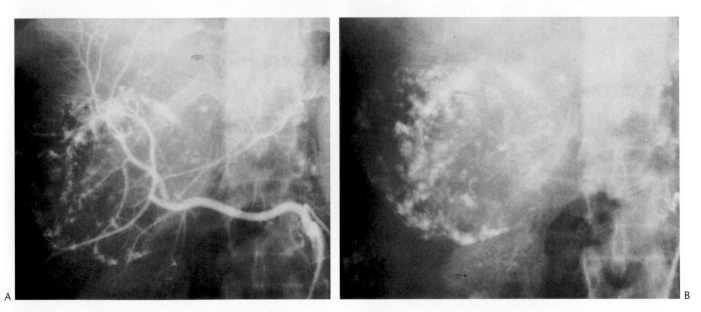

Fig. 25.66 **A**. Vascular lesion simulating tumor in the liver. Hemangioma. **B**. Note absence of drainage veins or arteriovenous shunting and persistence of contrast medium in the late phase.

tympanicum tumor lies in the middle ear, and will require high-quality subtraction films for its demonstration.

These tumors occur less commonly in other sites, but the angiographic appearances are similar. The *glomus vagale tumor* lies between the carotid body and glomus jugulare sites, while the *aortic body tumor* lies in the mediastinum above the aortic arch. Pelvic tumors are also described.

Nasopharyngeal Angiofibroma (juvenile angiofibroma) These highly vascular tumors present as swellings arising from the nasopharynx of adolescent boys. They may invade the antrum and produce swelling of the cheek. They are best shown by CT, which

is now the primary investigation of choice (Fig. 25.74), but they are also well shown by superselective angiography of the external carotid artery. Surgery, which may otherwise be hazardous, can be aided by prior embolization of the main feeding vessels.

Hemangiopericytoma These rare tumors of small blood vessels may occur anywhere in the body where there are capillaries, but are mainly seen in the soft tissues. They may be benign but they can also be highly malignant. In our experience the latter type are very vascular (Fig. 25.75), and malignancy may be related to the degree of vascularity. Specific diagnosis, however, depends on biopsy, and is made by the histopathologist.

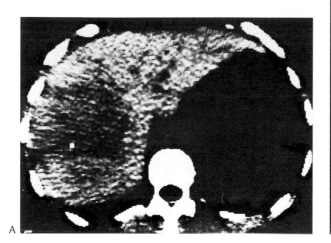

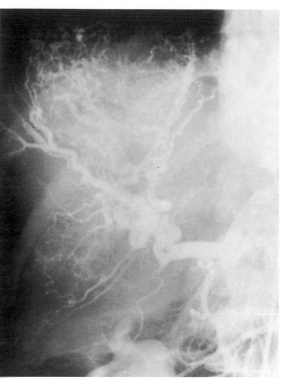

Fig. 25.67   Hepatic adenomas. **A**. CT image showing large low-density mass in right lobe of liver (WI34 L67). **B**. Angiogram showing a large vascular mass with a smaller mass in the lower part of the right lobe.

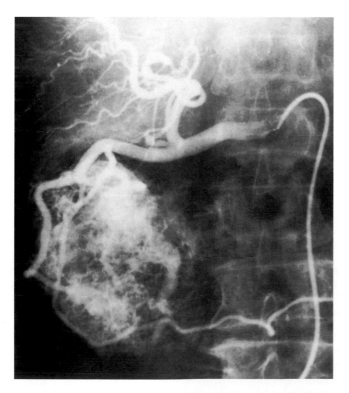

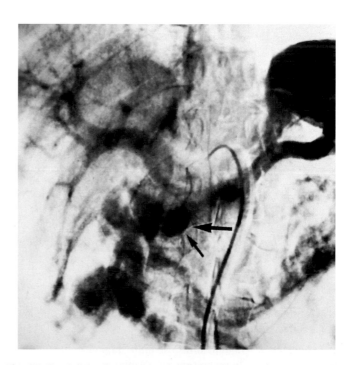

Fig. 25.68   Pancreatic cystadenoma showing florid pathological circulation in the head of the pancreas.

Fig. 25.69   Celiac axis angiograms (capillary and venous phase). Subtraction film. The well-defined blush in the pancreatic head (arrowed) was an insulinoma. (Courtesy of Dr R. Dick.)

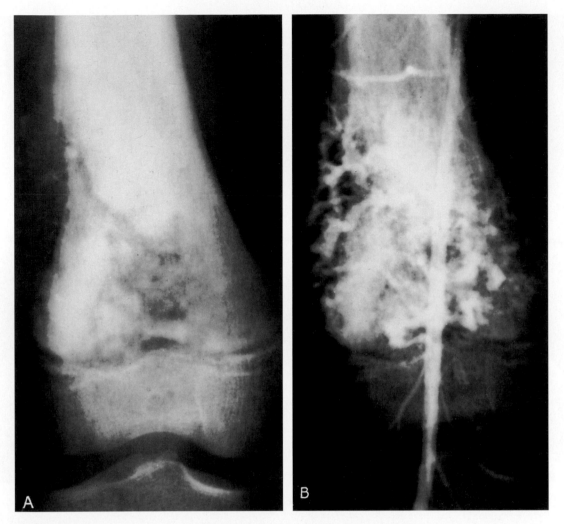

Fig. 25.70   Osteogenic sarcoma showing pathological vessels with arteriovenous shunting.

DOPPLER ULTRASOUND OF THE ARTERIES AND ABDOMINAL VESSELS

P. L. Allan

Doppler ultrasound techniques are based on the Doppler equation which was described by Christian Johann Doppler in 1842. The underlying principle is that when sound or light waves are moving between a transmitter and a receiver which are stationary in relation to each other then the receiver will register the same frequency as the transmitter emitted. If there is relative movement toward each other then the receiver will register a slightly higher frequency than was transmitted; conversely, if there is relative motion apart, then the receiver will register a slightly lower frequency. These small changes in frequency are known as Doppler shifts and can easily be measured by modern ultrasound equipment through direct comparison of the returning frequency with the transmission frequency.

The derivation of the Doppler equation used in medical ultrasound is

$$F_d = F_t - F_r = \frac{2F_t v \cos \theta}{c}$$

F_d is the frequency or Doppler shift; F_t is the transmitted frequency; F_r is the received frequency; v is the velocity of the reflector (usually blood in the vessels); θ is the angle between the direction of the ultrasound beam and the direction of flow of the blood; and c is the mean velocity of sound in the tissues, 1540 m/s. Using modern ultrasound equipment, the only variable which is unknown is the velocity of the reflecting blood cells, this can therefore be calculated as

$$v = \frac{F_d c}{2F_t \cos \theta}$$

The basic Doppler information is quite limited. It will show if there is moving blood present, which way it is going and how fast it is moving. Some information on the character of flow can be deduced, such as turbulent flow and decreased diastolic flow. Doppler shifts are given in units of frequency—kilohertz (kHz). The velocity of flow in meters or centimeters per second can only

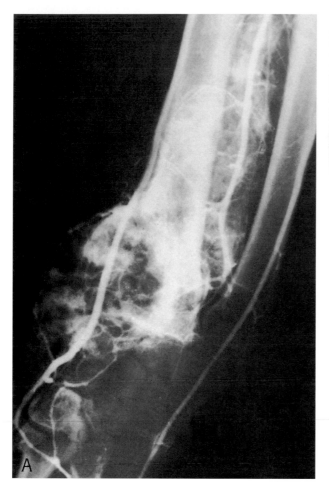

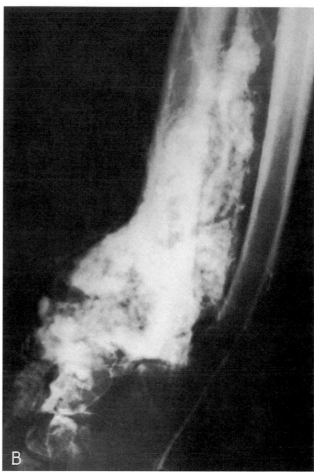

Fig. 25.71A and **B**   Malignant osteoclastoma. Note spread outside bone.

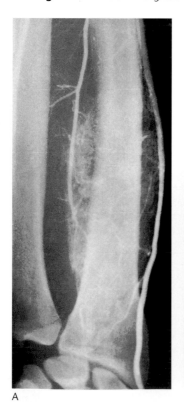

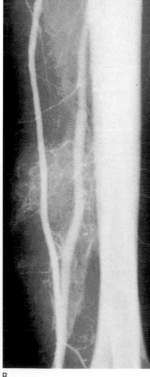

be calculated and displayed if an angle correction is applied using a cursor on the image of the vessel.

Types of Doppler Equipment

Continuous-wave Doppler (CW Doppler)   This is the simplest type of equipment. The probe contains two transducer crystals: one transmits continuously, the other receives continuously. The Doppler shift is calculated and 'displayed' as an audio signal. It is fortuitous that the conditions of medical Doppler result in Doppler shifts which are conveniently located within the range of human hearing. CW Doppler equipment is simple and cheap, but the main disadvantage is that any vessel in the line of the ultrasound beam contributes to the shift, and localizing the source of the shift is therefore not possible. This type of equipment is used in vascular clinics to locate arterial pulses, measure perfusion pressures, test for venous reflux, etc.

Duplex Doppler   These machines combine real-time imaging with pulsed Doppler. This allows the operator to identify a specific segment in a particular vessel and to place the gate, or sample volume, at a specific location so that the source of the Doppler signal is known. The time taken by the pulses of

Fig. 25.72   Malignant tumor of the forearm (rhabdomyosarcoma). **A**. Anteroposterior view. **B**. Lateral view.

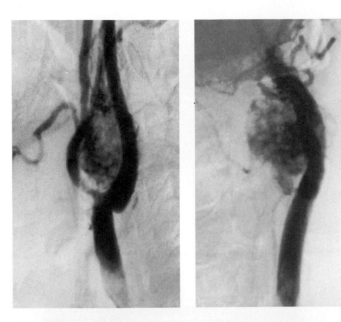

Fig. 25.73 Carotid body tumor.

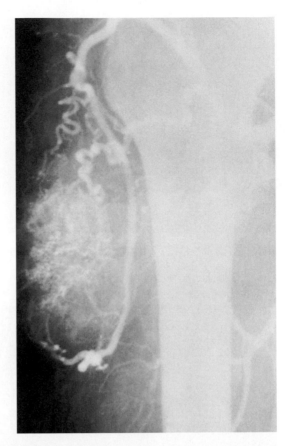

Fig. 25.75 Hemangiopericytoma. Patient presented with a lump in the thigh. The vascular tumor was highly malignant and metastasized rapidly.

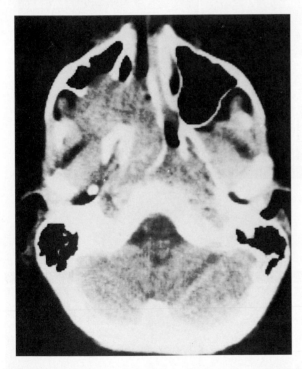

Fig. 25.74 Nasopharyngeal angiofibroma. CT image showing a large mass deforming the right antrum and nares (W256 L36).

supplying. For example, the internal carotid artery supplies the relatively low-resistance cerebral circulation and therefore has high diastolic flow in comparison to the external carotid artery, which supplies the higher-resistance circulation of the scalp and face, resulting in significantly lower diastolic flow (Fig. 25.76). The waveform characteristics can change significantly in response to physiological stimuli, as shown by the increased diastolic flow which is seen in the femoral arteries on exercising the leg muscles (Fig. 25.77).

Color Doppler   In duplex Doppler equipment, Doppler sampling is restricted to the small area of the sample volume. In color Doppler systems the pulses along each scan line are divided on return to the transducer, and some are used to provide imaging information and the rest are used to calculate the mean Doppler shift within small pixels of the image. This mean shift information is then coded on a color scale and displayed as a color map over the gray scale image. The choice of colors is arbitrary: usually shades of blue and red are used to represent flow toward and away from the transducer, with paler shades of the color representing higher velocities. The advantage of this technique is that areas of normal and abnormal flow can be identified and localized rapidly, although pulsed Doppler ultrasound is still required to obtain useful velocity information, such as peak systolic velocity (Fig. 25.78).

Power Doppler   The strength of the Doppler signal depends on the volume of blood reflecting the sound pulses and the velocity at which it is travelling. Small volumes of blood moving slowly

ultrasound to travel to and from the blood vessel means that, for deeper vessels, the pulse repetition frequency is limited, as the system has to wait for a pulse to return before transmitting the next pulse. This means that the magnitude of Doppler shifts which can be measured is limited, and detection of higher shifts in deeper vessels may not be possible in some circumstances. The Doppler information is transmitted as an audio signal and as a spectral display scrolling across the screen.

Vessels have different waveforms, or Doppler 'signatures', which depend on the size of the vessel and the type of capillary bed it is

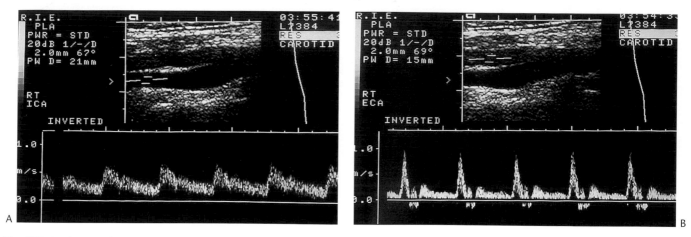

Fig. 25.76   The carotid bifurcation showing **A** high diastolic flow in the internal carotid artery compared with **B** the external carotid artery.

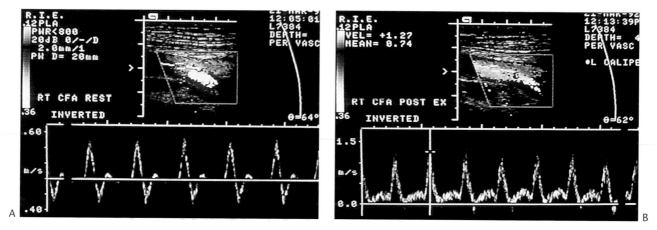

Fig. 25.77   The common femoral artery waveform **A** at rest and **B** after moderate exercise.

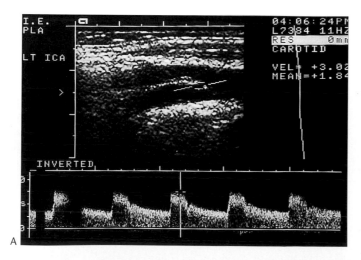

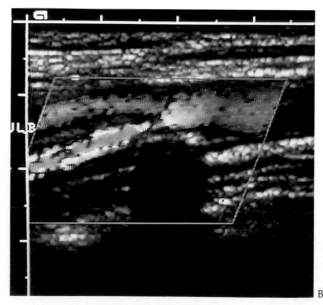

Fig. 25.78   A. Spectral Doppler image of the carotid bifurcation with a high velocity jet at the site of an hypoechoic plaque. **B**. Color Doppler image of a different patient with a calcified plaque in a similar location showing the high velocity jet in color.

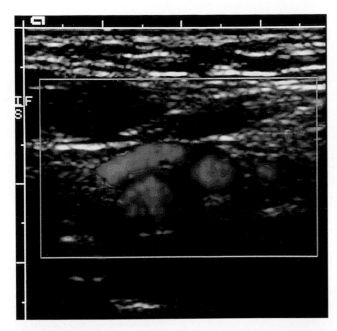

Fig. 25.79 Transverse view of the right carotid bifurcation using power Doppler ultrasound. It is not possible to distinguish the direction, or velocity of flow in the two branches of the artery from the more superficial internal jugular vein. The vertebral artery is seen on the right of the image.

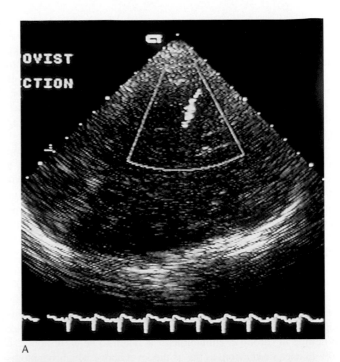

A

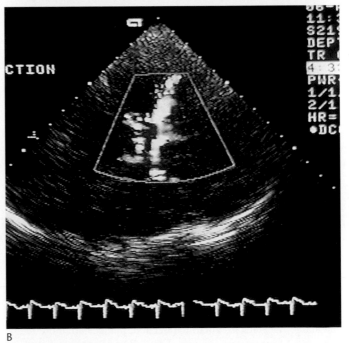

B

Fig. 25.80 Trans-cranial colour Doppler images of the circle of Willis **A** before and **B** after an injection of the echo-enhancing agent Levovist. Before the Levovist injection only the middle cerebral artery is seen; after the injection all the major components of the circle of Willis are visible.

produce a weak signal which is difficult to define from background noise. One way to improve this is to integrate all shift information together, thus increasing the overall power of the Doppler information and sensitivity of the system, but at the expense of losing directional and velocity information (Fig. 25.79). Power Doppler techniques are therefore good for showing areas of flowing blood, particularly when it is moving slowly, or in small vessels. Because of its higher sensitivity, it is more prone to movement artefact from respiratory motion, or bowel activity, but the technique has great potential for assessing tissue perfusion, or volume flow calculations when used in conjunction with ultrasonic echo-enhancing agents.

Echo-enhancing Agents

The signal-to-noise ratio for many Doppler applications is very poor. In order to improve this, several agents are being developed by pharmaceutical companies, and are just becoming available. The first compounds were too large to pass through the pulmonary capillaries, and were therefore restricted to use in the right heart, or for ultrasound hysterosalpingo-contrast sonography (HyCoSy). Subsequently, second-generation agents have been developed, which are less than 8–10 μm in diameter, and can therefore pass through the pulmonary capillaries into the systemic circulation. The first of these to be released commercially is based on small crystals of galactose, stabilized with palmitic acid, which trap small amounts of air in cavities (*Levovist*). The agent is injected into a peripheral vein. It can then be visualized as it passes through the systemic circulation and it continues to produce appreciable enhancement of the Doppler signal for up to 3–4 min after injection (Fig. 25.80). Insonating blood containing echo-enhancing agents in an appropriate manner can produce echoes at the second

and third harmonic frequencies, as well as the fundamental frequency; by tuning the receiver to the second harmonic frequency it is possible to filter out echoes returning at the fundamental frequency, and thus much of the noise and clutter associated with Doppler ultrasound. The information gathered from the second harmonic frequency therefore has a much better signal-to-noise ratio for signals returning from the echo-enhancing agent in the blood.

Measurement of a Stenosis

In simple hemodynamic terms, blood flows from regions of high energy to regions of lower energy; in practice this means from areas of greater pressure to areas of lower pressure. Energy is normally lost as blood travels from the heart to the capillaries, but if there are stenoses in the vessels this energy loss is increased and there is a reduction in the distal perfusion pressure, resulting in impaired tissue perfusion.

Stenoses can be assessed using two aspects of the ultrasound examination. Firstly, if the stenosis can be seen adequately, a direct measurement of the degree of stenosis may be made. This situation is usually restricted to larger arteries, such as the carotid or common femoral arteries; in addition, some information on the type of plaque may be apparent. Alternatively, the increase in velocity, which occurs as blood passes through a stenosis, can be used to help quantify the stenosis.

The difference between a hemodynamically significant stenosis and a clinically significant stenosis must be distinguished. A 50% diameter stenosis is said to be hemodynamically significant as the volume of blood flowing along the vessel starts to fall above this degree of stenosis. A clinically significant stenosis is more difficult to define: in carotid examinations it is taken to be at, or above, a 70% diameter reduction, as this is the level above which symptoms and signs are strongly associated with carotid disease. In the lower limbs and other territories it is less easy to define clinical significance as the presence of symptoms is highly dependent on the development and efficiency of any collateral channels that may be present.

Direct Measurement Two main measurements can be made: diameter reduction or cross-sectional area reduction. It is important to distinguish between the two, as a 50% diameter reduction is equivalent to a 75% area reduction; there is, therefore, the potential for significant misunderstanding in the interpretation of examination results if the terms are not defined. Area measurements are a little more accurate and take account of asymmetric distribution of plaque around the circumference of the vessel; however, they take a little longer to perform accurately. Diameters are a little easier to measure, but the vessel should always be examined both longitudinally and transversely in order to determine the most appropriate diameter to measure, usually the shortest.

In many cases the details of the plaque may be difficult to define, but in some cases the plaque will be seen clearly enough to identify certain characteristics which may be relevant to the patient's symptoms. Smooth, echogenic plaques are likely to be fibrotic and stable; whereas irregular, hypoechoic plaques are more likely to be unstable and act as a source of emboli from adherent thrombus, or plaque contents. Sometimes obvious ulceration may be seen.

Doppler Criteria These are usually based on peak systolic velocities, or ratios of the peak velocity at the stenosis to the peak velocity proximal to the stenosis. They are useful in situations where the residual vessel lumen cannot be visualized well enough to perform a direct measurement of the stenosis. In addition, examination of the spectral display may show changes in the waveform which are associated with stenoses or occlusions, such as spectral broadening, delayed acceleration and damping of the waveform.

Other Doppler-based indices have been developed to quantify changes in the waveform, these are the resistance index (RI), the

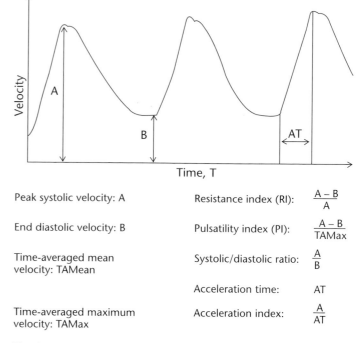

Peak systolic velocity: A

End diastolic velocity: B

Time-averaged mean velocity: TAMean

Time-averaged maximum velocity: TAMax

Resistance index (RI): $\dfrac{A - B}{A}$

Pulsatility index (PI): $\dfrac{A - B}{TAMax}$

Systolic/diastolic ratio: $\dfrac{A}{B}$

Acceleration time: AT

Acceleration index: $\dfrac{A}{AT}$

Fig. 25.81 Definition of indices used in Doppler ultrasound.

pulsatility index (PI), and the systolic–diastolic ratio (Fig. 25.81). These have the advantage that they can be used in situations where accurate angle correction, and thus velocity estimation, are not possible. The RI and PI reflect the degree of distal resistance, so that with increased peripheral resistance, as may occur with acute vascular rejection of a renal transplant, the RI tends toward a value of 1.0, whereas the PI tends toward values of 1.0 or more.

The acceleration time (AT) is the time taken, in seconds, for the peak systolic velocity to be reached. The acceleration index (AI) relates the acceleration time to the peak systolic velocity achieved. The application of these various indices will be discussed in relation to their value in specific clinical situations in the following sections.

Carotid and Vertebral Arteries

Disease in the carotid arteries is associated with cerebral vascular events, and for severe disease of more than 70% diameter reduction it has been shown that surgery is beneficial in symptomatic patients who have a stenosis of more than 70% diameter reduction, as subsequent significant vascular events occurred in 16.8% of the non-operative group, compared with only 2.8% of the operative group. The main indications for carotid ultrasound are therefore patients with transient ischemic attacks (TIAs) or reversible ischemic neurological deficits (RINDs), who may benefit from carotid endarterectomy surgery. It is not usually indicated in patients with established and completed strokes, unless these are milder, resolving strokes in younger patients who might be considered suitable for surgery. Patients with asymptomatic bruits will not normally be considered for surgery at present, but a trial of surgery in this group of patients has shown a reduction in subsequent stroke rate of 5.8% in patients with a 60%, or greater, stenosis compared with medical management; this finding may affect the future management of this type of patient. Other

Table 25.6 Diagnostic criteria for Doppler diagnosis of stenoses of 50 and 70% diameter reduction

Diameter stenosis (%)	Peak systolic velocity, ICA (m/sec)	Peak diastolic velocity, ICA (m/sec)	ICA/CCA systolic ratio
50	>1.5	>0.5	>2
70	>2.3	>0.75	>3

From Robinson et al (1988). Am. J. Roentgen. 151: 1045–1049
CCA, common carotid artery; ICA, internal carotid artery.

indications for carotid ultrasound include atypical symptoms which may be due to carotid disease; postendarterectomy patients; those in whom arteriography is technically impossible, or contraindicated; and the assessment of pulsatile cervical masses, including possible carotid body tumors.

The carotid vessels are scanned from low in the neck to high behind the mandible, the level and orientation of the bifurcation are noted, together with any obvious areas of disease. The vessels are then scanned using color Doppler ultrasound, and any abnormal areas of flow identified for subsequent assessment using spectral Doppler ultrasound. It should be remembered that there is normally a region of reversed flow in the carotid bulb and that this does not signify the presence of disease; in fact, its absence is strongly suggestive of a disturbance in blood flow. If no areas of significant disease are seen, it is common practice to take peak systolic velocity readings from the upper common, the internal carotid, and the external carotid arteries. If areas of disease are seen they are assessed by direct measurement, or by Doppler criteria such as peak systolic velocity and related measurements (see Fig. 25.78A). It is important to realize that the precise criteria vary depending on the type of equipment used and other technical factors relating to the examination: it is therefore important for each department to develop its own specific values which allow reliable identification of the key stenosis levels of 50 and 70% diameter reduction. The criteria used in our institution are listed in Table 25.6. Plaque morphology may be apparent in the carotids, and the presence of irregular, or ulcerated, hypoechoic plaques should be noted (Fig. 25.82), as these may be relevant to symptoms, even if the stenosis is not particularly great.

Carotid occlusion must be diagnosed with care on ultrasound. At high degrees of stenosis (>90% diameter reduction) there is only a small volume of blood flowing through the residual lumen and it is also flowing relatively slowly. The machine must therefore be reset to look for this low volume, slow flow and not the much higher velocities that might have been expected. The

greater sensitivity of power Doppler ultrasound is of value here and echo-enhancing agents will also contribute to confirming the diagnosis of occlusion, or identifying a small residual lumen, which is still potentially an operative candidate.

Pulsatile neck lumps can be identified rapidly with color Doppler ultrasound. They may be due to adjacent lymph nodes, cysts, or other masses. Carotid body tumors have a characteristic location between the internal and external carotid arteries, appearing as a predominantly hypoechoic mass splaying the arteries and relatively vascular on color Doppler ultrasound. Aneurysms of the carotid may occur spontaneously, as a result of penetrating neck trauma or hyperextension injuries (Fig. 25.83); ultrasound will show the nature of these masses and the involvement of the various carotid segments.

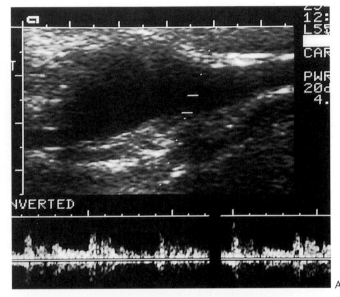

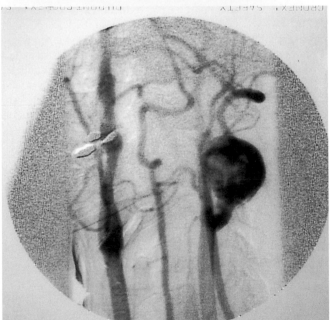

Fig. 25.83 An aneurysm of the internal carotid artery in a 25-year-old patient who suffered a whiplash injury in a road traffic accident.

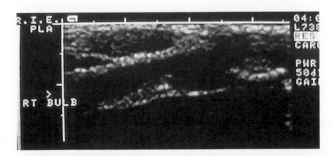

Fig. 25.82 An ulcerated plaque at the right carotid bifurcation.

Dissection of the carotid artery can occur as an extension of an aortic dissection, spontaneously within the carotid itself, or as a result of trauma. Ultrasound may show one of several appearances. Rarely two patent channels separated by a flap may be seen, and Doppler ultrasound will show significantly different flow patterns in the two channels. More frequently the false channel will thrombose, producing a characteristic, tapering stenosis or occlusion of the vessel. Recanalization of dissected vessels over a period of 6–8 weeks may be seen in 50–60% of cases.

Measurement of the *intima–medial thickness* (IMT) is feasible with today's high-resolution ultrasound machines. When the ultrasound beam is at right angles to the carotid walls, two white lines will be seen in normal vessels, particularly on the posterior wall. The first corresponds to the blood/intima boundary; the second to the outer media/adventitia region. Normally this is less than 0.8 mm, but several studies have shown that this increases significantly in patients with evidence of atheroma in other areas, such as the coronary arteries. The IMT increases slowly with age, but it may provide a useful tool in the assessment of patients with arterial disease in order to measure both the prevalence of disease and the progression, or regression, of disease over a period of time, depending on the treatment regimes employed.

The *accuracy of carotid Doppler ultrasound* has been well established over recent years. One study reviewed 16 spectral Doppler studies with a total of 2146 Doppler/arteriogram comparisons. duplex Doppler ultrasound had an overall sensitivity of 96%, a specificity of 86%, a positive predictive value of 89%, a negative predictive value of 94%, and an accuracy of 91% for the diagnosis of a stenosis diameter greater than 50%. Subsequently, further studies have confirmed the value of color Doppler ultrasound with similar or better levels of accuracy, and also its value in improving diagnostic confidence, clarifying difficult situations, and reducing examination times.

The Vertebral Arteries These can be visualized using color Doppler ultrasound. They may be examined in three segments of their course: most commonly in the vertebral canal as they pass cranially through the foramina transversaria; in the lower neck as they pass from the subclavian artery towards C6; and in the upper neck as they wind around the lateral masses of the atlas and enter the foramen magnum. There is often asymmetry in the diameter of the two vessels, in which case the left is usually the larger, and in up to 10% of individuals one of the vertebral arteries will have significant segments of atresia. The main items of information which can be gathered on these vessels include the fact that they are both present, the direction of flow in them, and whether the flow is normal or damped; occasionally a stenosis in the artery may be demonstrated. A stenosis, or absent segment, in one vessel is not of clinical significance as the basilar circulation can be maintained from the other artery. If reversed flow is demonstrated, it is a sign of an occluded, or severely stenosed, subclavian artery (subclavian steal syndrome) (Fig. 25.84). In some patients, exercise of the ipsilateral arm muscles may be required to produce reversed flow.

Transcranial Doppler Ultrasound

The use of ultrasound to examine the neonatal brain through the fontanelles and thin calvarial bones has been established for many years, but transcranial ultrasound in adults was limited by the marked attenuation of the ultrasound beam by the skull bones,

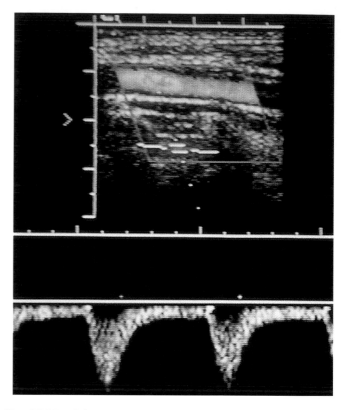

Fig. 25-84. Color Doppler image of the neck showing the common carotid artery (orange) with the vertebral artery between the lateral processes of the cervical spine. The blue of the vertebral artery shows that it is flowing in the opposite direction to the carotid; this is confirmed by the spectral display.

which can be up to 60 dB both on the way in and the way out. Transcranial Doppler ultrasound has been possible using pulsed Doppler ultrasound without imaging since 1982, but developments in transducers and imaging processing now mean that useful color Doppler images and spectra can be obtained in adults. The advantages include an ability to identify specific segments of the main cerebral arteries and to appreciate rapidly the direction of flow within these; in addition, more accurate and reproducible angle-corrected velocity estimations can be made.

The main access point for transcranial Doppler ultrasound is the thin squamous temporal bone in front of the ear. Careful scanning will locate the best acoustic window, although in 10% of subjects no suitable window will be found; problems are more likely in females, Blacks, and the elderly. The system is set to high sensitivity and, when the window is located, color Doppler ultrasound is used to identify the ipsilateral middle cerebral artery, which can then be traced centrally to locate the circle of Willis and its branches. A complete circle is only found in 25–30% of subjects, and many variations of the anatomy exist. The use of echo-enhancing agents has further improved the strength of the signal obtained, and these agents will certainly be of value in these examinations (see Fig. 25.80). The foramen magnum can be used to examine the upper vertebral arteries and the lower basilar artery; and the orbit can be used to examine the upper internal carotid artery and the anterior cerebral artery, although attention must be paid to the power output of the transducer as the beam will not be attenuated by bone at these sites.

The cerebral veins and the major venous sinuses are less easy to examine because of their orientation in relation to the scan plane and the slow flow within them.

The main indications for transcranial color Doppler ultrasound include monitoring of spasm and flow after strokes and subarachnoid hemorrhage, the assessment of intracranial collateral pathways, and the detection of significant stenoses (>65%) of the main cerebral arteries. It is also valuable in research into the changes in blood flow induced by drugs and physiological changes.

The Peripheral Arteries

The arteries of the limbs can be examined with ultrasound in patients with claudication in order to identify segments of stenosis, or occlusion. In the lower limb the arteries are followed from the groin distally to the calf, and segments of abnormal flow identified with color Doppler ultrasound. These can then be assessed using spectral Doppler ultrasound; the normal waveform is triphasic due to the relatively high distal resistance in the resting lower limb. A velocity of more than 4 m/s at a stenosis, or a fourfold increase in velocity in relation to the velocity above the abnormal segment, is compatible with a stenosis of 70% or more (Fig. 25.85). The main indication for ultrasound of the peripheral arteries is to identify patients who may benefit from angioplasty, and to distinguish these from patients who require distal bypass grafts.

The iliac arteries are more difficult to visualize in some patients but, with care and attention, they can often be examined adequately. If this is not possible, changes in the waveform at the groin, such as damping or spectral broadening, may indicate significant disease proximally.

There are three types of *bypass graft* procedure which may be used by surgeons: synthetic grafts, in situ and reversed autologous vein grafts; these can be monitored with color Doppler ultrasound. Graft occlusion occurring in the first 4–6 weeks after operation is usually due to technical factors, and failure after 2–3 years is usually caused by recurrent atheroma. Graft failure during the intervening period is usually the result of neointimal hyperplasia, which occurs most frequently at the origin of the graft, the distal insertion, or at the sites of inadequately ablated valves and communicating veins in cases of autologous vein grafts. Of all graft failures, 80% occur during this interim period. If problems with the graft can be identified on color Doppler ultrasound as part of a surveillance program before graft failure occurs, the secondary patency rate can be improved from 70% to 90%. The criteria used for assessing graft stenoses are similar to those for arterial stenosis: peak systolic velocities of more than 3.5 m/s are associated with stenoses of more than 70% diameter reduction (Fig. 25.86), as is a velocity ratio of more than 2.5. It should be remembered that a physiological stenosis will occur if there is a significant mismatch in caliber between the graft and the native artery; this should not be mistaken for a pathological stenosis. If the maximum graft velocity is less than 0.45 m/s there is a high association with subsequent graft failure (Fig. 25.87).

Arteriovenous fistulas may occur, particularly with in situ vein grafts, if any perforator veins or superficial communicating veins are missed at operation.

False Aneurysms These can occur after femoral catheterization, especially if larger catheters are used, or multiple catheter exchanges performed; anticoagulation following angioplasty is also a factor. Rates of occurrence from 0.6 to 6.0% have been reported. Color Doppler ultrasound provides a reliable method for the diagnosis of false aneurysms and monitoring their progress (Fig. 25.88). Many will thrombose spontaneously; a few will increase in size.

Thrombosis can be encouraged by ultrasound-guided compression. The transducer is used to press on the false aneurysm, and pressure is applied to stop flow in the lumen of the aneurysm and the channel linking it to the artery, but not within the artery itself. This pressure is maintained for 15 min, then released gradually. If

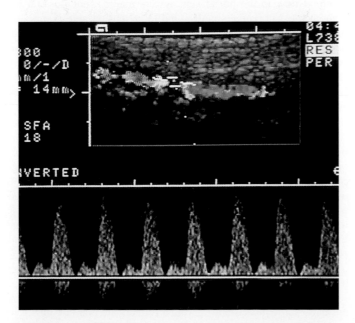

Fig. 25.85 A high-grade stenosis of the superficial femoral artery with a peak velocity of nearly 4 m/s.

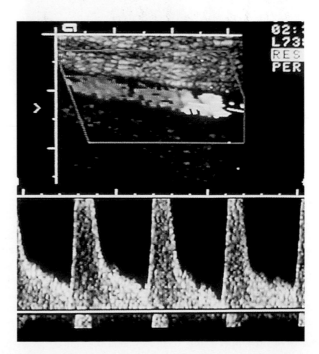

Fig. 25.86 An in situ vein graft showing a tight stenosis on color Doppler ultrasound with a peak velocity in excess of 5 m/s.

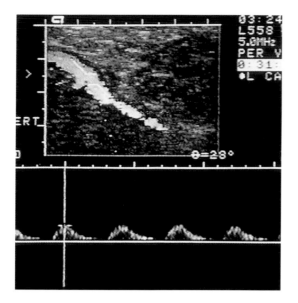

Fig. 25.87 Image of a graft insertion showing damped flow of low velocity (10 cm/s), which is strongly suggestive of a graft at risk of failure.

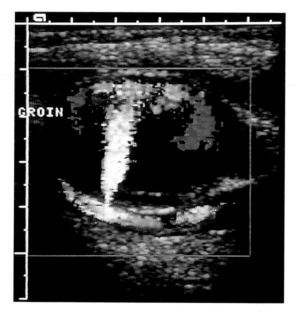

Fig. 25.88 A false aneurysm of the common femoral artery following arteriography. Color Doppler ultrasound shows the jet of blood leaving the artery.

flow is still present, pressure is reapplied for a further 15 min, and these cycles are repeated until thrombosis occurs. The procedure is uncomfortable and may be painful for the patient, so that some analgesia is often required. Most false aneurysms can be treated in this way, but the presence of infection and inability to apply adequate compression are contraindications; false aneurysms which are more than 7–10 days may take a little longer to thrombose.

Arteries of the Upper Limb Stenosis and occlusion of the arteries in the upper limb can be assessed with ultrasound. Compression syndromes can be investigated by imaging the subclavian artery

while moving the arm to different positions, and the point of compression accurately identified.

Dialysis Grafts Hemodialysis grafts may occlude, or develop a stenosis or a false aneurysm. These can be examined using color Doppler ultrasound. It is important to check the venous side of the fistula proximally to the subclavian vein as some stenoses which affect fistula function can occur centrally. The flow in the fistula is best assessed by measuring the flow in the brachial artery above the fistula, assuming that the bulk of blood flowing in the brachial artery will flow through the fistula. The flow can be roughly estimated by measuring the cross-sectional area of the artery and multiplying this by the time-averaged mean velocity and then by a factor of 60 to give the volume flow in milliliters per minute. Flows under 400 ml/min are inadequate for satisfactory dialysis; conversely, flows over 1200 ml/min are excessive and problems may occur with cardiac output and reserve. Dialysis is best performed with fistula flows of 500–800 ml/min.

Abdominal Vessels

In the abdomen, Doppler ultrasound can provide useful information about many of the major arteries and veins. The conditions for examination are a little more challenging than for the peripheral arteries and carotids as the vessels lie deeper, respiratory motion is present, and bowel gas interferes with the image. The examinations are best done with the patient breathing quietly, only holding his or her breath for a short time whenever necessary. Color and power Doppler ultrasound are frequently used during an abdominal examination simply to identify structures as arteries or veins and to distinguish vessels from cysts or dilated ducts.

The Liver The normal fasting diameter of the **portal vein** is less than 13 mm, but this will increase after eating. The patency of the portal vein can be confirmed and cavernous transformation identified: tumor invasion of the major portal branches in patients with hepatocellular carcinoma can also be assessed. The direction of blood flow in the portal vein and its major tributaries can be demonstrated in patients with portal hypertension and, if surgical or transjugular shunts have been created, these can be monitored using Doppler ultrasound (Fig. 25.89). In patients with intestinal ischemia, gas bubbles may be seen in the vein, or heard on Doppler ultrasound, as they pass up into the liver (Fig. 25.90). Following liver transplantation, flow in the portal vein is monitored as thrombosis or stenosis is a potential significant complication.

The **hepatic artery** normally arises from the celiac axis, but the right hepatic artery may have a separate origin from the superior mesenteric artery in some patients; this variation may be apparent on ultrasound, and is of some importance if a patient is being considered for transplantation. Flow in the hepatic artery increases in patients with portal hypertension and also in patients with liver tumors; it is also significantly increased following transplantation, and thrombosis of the artery, or one of its major branches, is a serious complication. Aneurysms of the artery can occur spontaneously but are also seen following penetrating trauma (including liver biopsy) and at the anastomosis following transplantation.

The **hepatic veins** drain into the internal vena cava. They normally show pulsatile flow, which reflects the pressure changes in the right atrium over the cardiac cycle (Fig. 25.91). If the liver becomes less compliant, these pulsatile changes are reduced or

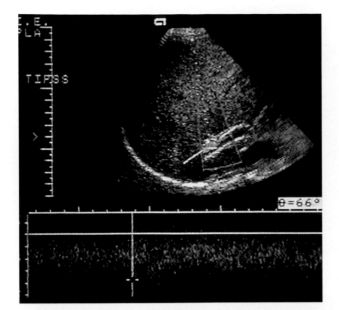

Fig. 25.89 A TIPS in a patient with portal hypertension. Spectral Doppler ultrasound shows good flow in excess of 1 m/s.

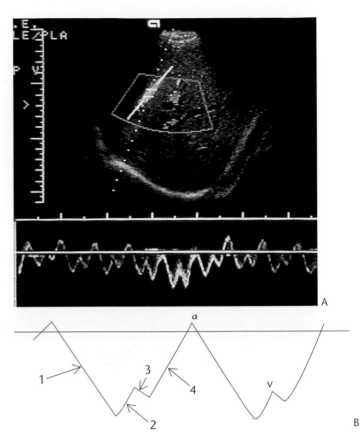

Fig. 25.91 **A**. Normal hepatic vein spectral display showing both cardiac and respiratory variations. **B**. The cardiac variations reflect the pressure changes in the right atrium during the cardiac cycle. 1, Forward flow into the atrium during diastolic relaxation; 2, reverse flow during tricuspid valve closure and ventricular systole; 3, forward flow as tricuspid valve opens; 4, reverse flow during atrial systole; a, v, the 'a' and 'v' waves, respectively, seen in the jugular venous pulse.

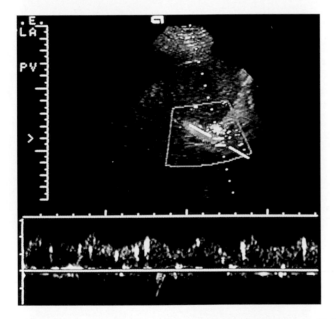

Fig. 25.90 Color and spectral Doppler images of the portal vein in a patient with ascites. The spectral display shows intermittent strong signals from gas bubbles.

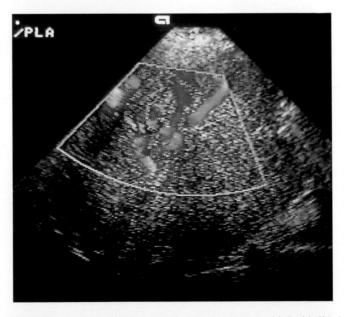

Fig. 25.92 Color Doppler image of the liver in a patient with Budd–Chiari syndrome. Instead of the normal regular pattern of hepatic veins, there is a complex network of abnormal collaterals.

lost completely. Budd–Chiari syndrome can be diagnosed using color Doppler ultrasound, which shows absence of the normal veins, together with abnormal collateral channels, some of which run out to the capsule of the liver (Fig. 25.92). In some patients the changes are only partial, affecting some of the veins, or affecting a segment of a vein. Doppler ultrasound will not diagnose microscopic veno-occlusive disease. Following transplantation, stenosis of the veins, or of the internal vena cava at the anastomosis, may result in abnormal flow or thrombosis.

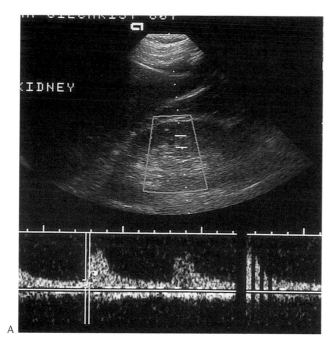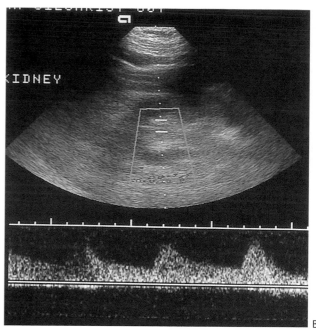

Fig. 25.93 Intraparenchymal Doppler images of a patient with renal artery stenosis show **A** a normal waveform in the right kidney but **B** a damped waveform with a prolonged acceleration time in the left kidney.

It had been hoped that patterns of flow and vascularity on Doppler ultrasound would help in the diagnosis of *benign* and *malignant tumors*. Unfortunately, although some characteristics of a malignant type of circulation can be defined, the discrimination between types of tumor is still poor and inadequate. Malignant circulation with high shifts, multidirectional flow, arteriovenous shunting, and abnormal vessels has been described in 50–80% of hepatocellular carcinomas, but many of these changes are also seen in 30–40% of metastases. Similarly, patterns of vascularity such as central disposition in a lesion, or distribution around the margin, do not allow distinction of tumor type.

The Kidneys

The renal arterial circulation has a distinctive waveform with high diastolic flow, reflecting a relatively low peripheral resistance. Various diseases produce changes in the waveform, which may be bilateral or unilateral. Unfortunately, these changes tend to be non-specific, so they are not as useful as it had first been hoped.

Renal Artery Stenoses These can be diagnosed if the stenotic segment is visualized directly; a velocity of over 1.8 m/s or a ratio of over 3.5 between the velocities in the renal artery and the aorta (the RAR) is diagnostic of a stenosis of more than 60% diameter reduction. Unfortunately, the proximal renal arteries cannot be visualized directly in a number of patients, which reduces the value of the technique as a screening test for renal artery stenosis.

The parenchymal arteries can be demonstrated in most patients, and it has been shown that significant proximal stenoses (>70%) produce changes in the waveforms in these vessels. The acceleration time is the time interval for the systolic acceleration period, an increase in this above 0.1 s is associated with a significant stenosis (Fig. 25.93). Changes to the waveform shape with loss of the early systolic complex also reflect a proximal stenosis.

Renal Vein Thrombosis This may be demonstrated directly, if the main renal veins are visible. Sometimes they are obscured, or thrombosis affects the smaller intrarenal veins. In these cases the diagnosis may be suggested by a significant reduction in diastolic flow (Fig. 25.94), or even reversed diastolic flow in the artery.

The changes in the waveform in different *diffuse parenchymal diseases* are non-specific, but an RI of over 0.7 is indicative of

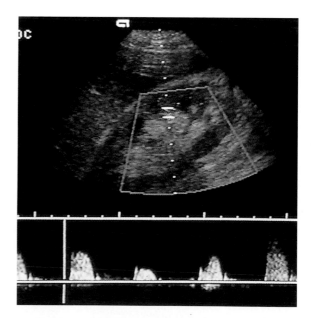

Fig. 25.94 Intra-renal Doppler image of a patient with acute renal failure shows no significant diastolic flow. This pattern may also be seen in patients with renal vein thrombosis.

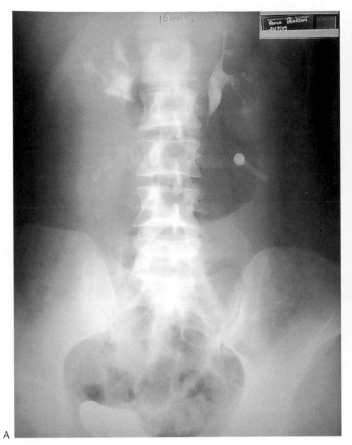

A

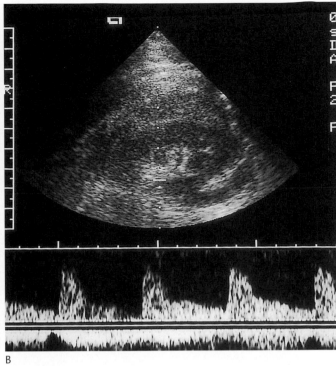

B

Fig. 25.95 **A**. A film from an intravenous urography examination in a patient who sustained right renal trauma in a road traffic accident: there is only minimal excretion of contrast from the lower fragment. **B**. Spectral Doppler ultrasound shows both arterial and venous flow in this fragment.

parenchymal change (Fig. 25.94), although it is not possible to discriminate between different types of disease and avoid the necessity for biopsy.

Ureteric Obstruction   This results in increased intrarenal pressure, which is reflected in an increase in the RI in the renal arteries. An RI of more than 0.7, or a difference between the sides of more than 0.1, is suggestive of obstruction in the appropriate clinical circumstances; these changes can be of value in the distinction between non-obstructive dilatation and obstructive dilatation in pregnant patients. Some care is needed as the changes can take several hours to develop, and underlying renal disease must also be considered; the RI in the kidneys of children under 5 years of age is normally slightly higher than in older patients.

Demonstration of arterial and venous flow in the renal fragments resulting from severe **renal trauma** allows assessment of the viability of the kidney (Fig. 25.95). Arteriovenous fistulas caused by penetrating trauma or biopsy result in increased, pulsatile venous flow; flow in the supplying artery may be increased, and color Doppler ultrasound may show the tissue vibrations which produce an audible bruit. **Renal tumors** may show typical changes of a malignant circulation, but 20% may be relatively avascular, and little or no flow is demonstrable.

Renal Transplants   Renal transplants may suffer from various vascular complications, and the relatively superficial location of the kidney makes ultrasound assessment straightforward. Stenosis of the main artery at the site of the anastomosis can be identified on color Doppler ultrasound, or because of abnormal shifts on spectral Doppler ultrasound. Distinction between acute vascular

rejection, acute tubular necrosis, and cyclosporin toxicity is not reliable, although rejection tends to produce higher resistance indices than the others. An RI of over 0.7 is a sign of abnormal circulation, and serial measurement can be used as an indicator of improving or deteriorating renal function.

The Female Pelvis

The organs of the female pelvis can be examined both transabdominally, through the full bladder, and transvaginally; the last approach allows the transducer to be positioned close to the major vessels supplying the ovaries and the uterus. The blood flow to the ovaries and uterus varies during the menstrual cycle, with increased flow and decreased pulsatility near ovulation; these changes can also be used to monitor patients undergoing *infertility* treatment and pharmacological induction of ovulation. Uterine flow is increased in cases of *trophoblastic disease*, with a low RI; return of the RI and waveform to normal correlates well with successful treatment. In *ovarian tumors* there is an increase in blood flow in the ovarian arteries but, as in the liver, the changes are not sufficiently specific to allow accurate distinction between different tumors. *Ovarian torsion* results in a significant decrease in ovarian blood flow, although some flow may still be present in a torted but salvageable ovary. Absence of flow suggests a non-salvageable gonad.

In patients with *ectopic pregnancy* the presence of active trophoblastic tissue can be demonstrated on color and spectral Doppler ultrasound as a region of increased vascularity with a low RI (<0.6). In addition, there is increased flow to the uterus

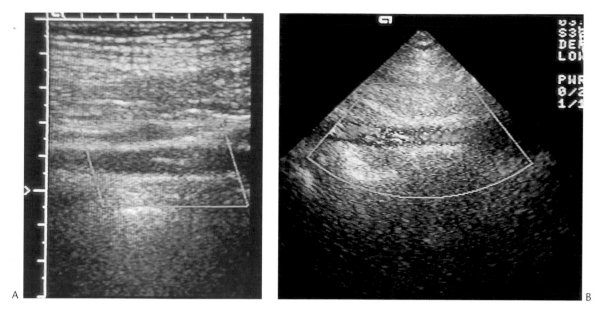

Fig. 25.96   **A**. A caval filter inserted for recurrent pulmonary emboli. **B**. Color Doppler ultrasound confirms the patency of the cava at the level of the filter. The change in color from blue to red reflects the relative change in the direction of flow in relation to the transducer as the blood flows through the sector.

and ovaries, although this is less marked than with an intrauterine pregnancy.

An increase in the uterine RI during an established pregnancy is a sign of increased resistance in the placenta, which may reflect developing *intrauterine growth retardation*; however, the changes are not sufficiently diagnostic for use as a screening technique, and need to be assessed in conjunction with other parameters. In the fetal circulation, flow to the developing brain is dominant and protected if intrauterine growth retardation develops; this is reflected in an increased RI in the abdominal aorta and branches compared with the carotids, as the cerebral circulation is maintained at the expense of the lower body.

The Male Pelvis

In patients with an acutely tender scrotum, differentiation of acute epididymo-orchitis from torsion may be aided by color Doppler ultrasound. In **epididymo-orchitis** the testis and the epididymis show increased flow, which may be generalized or focal in distribution. In cases of **testicular torsion** there is absent or markedly reduced flow to the affected side; comparison should be made with the other side if there is any doubt. After several hours, increased flow in the peritesticular tissues is seen.

The perfusion of **testicular tumors** is variable and does not allow definitive diagnosis of benign from malignant lesions. **Varicoceles** are seen as multiple serpiginous cystic areas in the epididymis, more marked on standing and coughing. If confirmation of their vascular nature is required, color Doppler ultrasound can be used in conjunction with getting the patient to cough, or to perform a Valsalva maneuver.

In prostatic disease there is increased flow on transrectal color Doppler ultrasound in areas of **prostatitis**, but this can also be seen in **prostatic carcinoma**. The presence of abnormal color Doppler findings indicates disease, but these must be considered in the light of other clinical information, and biopsy of abnormal

areas performed if malignancy is a possibility. Color Doppler ultrasound can subsequently be used to monitor the response of both conditions to appropriate treatment.

Impotence   This may be due to psychological causes or vascular disease. The vascular responses during the development and maintenance of an erection can be monitored with Doppler ultrasound after the cavernosal injection of papaverine (40–80 mg). A normal response shows an immediate, marked increase in penile arterial flow; as the erectile pressure increases, the diastolic flow decreases, becoming zero as a full erection is obtained. Peak systolic flow should then be over 0.35 m/s with a well-defined waveform of short duration. Arterial inflow disease results in a lower peak systolic velocity and a damped waveform; whereas venous leakage produces a continual high level of flow in diastole, despite a good arterial response; psychogenic or neurological impotence patients show a normal response to this test.

Aorta and Inferior Vena Cava

The most common indication for examining the **abdominal aorta** is for the diagnosis and assessment of aneurysms, and Doppler ultrasound is not usually required for this. However, if a dissection is suspected, both color Doppler and spectral Doppler ultrasound can be used to demonstrate patency or thrombosis of the channels and the branches which they supply. The *celiac axis* and its major branches can be examined as they arise from the upper aorta. The *superior mesenteric artery* also arises at this level and runs inferiorly to the left of the superior mesenteric vein; occasionally the right hepatic artery arises from the superior mesenteric artery rather than the celiac artery. The *inferior mesenteric artery* is more difficult to demonstrate, as it is smaller and more likely to be obscured by bowel gas; in suitable subjects it is best found by scanning transversely up the aorta from the bifurcation; it normally arises 3–4 cm above the bifurcation.

The waveforms in the vessels supplying the bowel vary with food, having relatively high pulsatility with low diastolic flow in fasting subjects, and higher diastolic flow following food. Stenosis of the celiac axis and superior mesenteric artery may be identified on ultrasound: peak systolic flows of over 1.8 m/s correlate with 50% stenosis, and velocities of over 2.8 m/s with stenosis of 75% or more. If both vessels are seen to be significantly narrowed, or occluded, this supports a diagnosis of **intestinal ischemia** in the appropriate clinical situation; unfortunately, the status of the inferior mesenteric artery and its contribution to bowel blood flow is difficult to assess in most patients. Other, indirect, signs of ischemia may be seen on ultrasound, including dilated, edematous, or hypoperistaltic bowel and gas in the portal vein.

The inferior vena cava and congenital variations of this can be examined with color Doppler ultrasound. The main indications are assessment for the possible extension of thrombosis or tumor from the legs or renal veins, diagnosis of compression from masses, assessment of caval filters (Fig. 25.96), and following liver transplantation.

MAGNETIC RESONANCE ANGIOGRAPHY

Jeremy P. R. Jenkins

MRI is sensitive to the detection of flow, and applications in the non-invasive assessment of vascular structures are increasing. This has been brought about by the development and implementation of multiplanar data acquisitions, sophisticated radiofrequency (RF) pulse sequences, and postprocessing of data into two- and three-dimensional display formats. The ability to acquire not only morphological but functional information non-invasively is an important advantage. Further developments are to be expected in improving spatial resolution and the postprocessing capabilities for three-dimensional display of the data. MR angiography (MRA) is now competing with conventional X-ray angiography in spatial resolution, vessel selectivity, and therapeutic (interventional) options.

An understanding of the basic processes involved in flow phenomena is required in order to interpret the MRA images obtained. Only a brief review will be given. The appearance of flowing blood is essentially a balance between those effects that produce a decrease or an increase in signal intensity. A decrease in the intensity of flowing blood can be achieved by *saturation*, *dephasing*, and *washout* effects, whereas an increase occurs with *flow-related enhancement* and *rephasing* of spins.

Protons exposed to repeated RF pulses become saturated (have a low magnetization) and produce a low signal. Unsaturated (i.e. fully magnetized) protons give a high signal when excited by an RF pulse. The *saturation* effect relates to the longer T_1 (and thus lower signal intensity) of blood compared with adjacent tissue. With appropriate T_1 weighting the intraluminal signal would be expected to be lower than that from the surrounding tissues. In conventional spin echo imaging this saturation effect is often opposed by the *flow-related enhancement* or *entry* phenomenon. This results from fresh blood (unsaturated protons) entering the imaging volume and producing a high intraluminal signal. In a multislice sequence this enhancement is more pronounced in sections nearest the entry point of the vessel into the imaging volume.

The most important process leading to a reduction in intraluminal signal is the *washout* effect. In order to generate a spin echo signal protons must receive both the 90 and 180° RF pulses. Since these pulses are usually 'slice selective' their effect is limited to the image sections. Blood flowing at above a certain velocity will have passed through the plane of section in the interval between the 90 and 180° RF pulses, and thus produce a signal void. For this to occur the average velocity within the vessel has to be equal to or greater than the slice thickness of the section divided by the time interval between the two RF pulses TE. In conventional spin echo imaging, rapidly flowing (arterial) blood is usually demonstrated as a *signal void* with slow-flowing (venous) blood as a *high signal*.

Another cause of intraluminal signal loss, particularly for inplane flow, is the spin *dephasing* effect. The moving spins in flowing blood are subjected to magnetic field gradients which lead to phase differences that are constantly changing relative to adjacent stationary spins. The greater the flow the larger the phase differences, which are also dependent on the strength and duration of the magnetic field gradients. There is thus a direct relationship between flow velocity and phase shifts which can be exploited to allow precise measurements of the former. Dephasing effects can reduce the intraluminal signal sufficiently to mask any flow-related enhancement that might be present.

Under certain circumstances, the phase differences induced by blood flowing through magnetic field gradients can be partially corrected, leading to an increase in signal from flowing blood. This *rephasing* effect is termed even-echo rephasing (gradient refocused echo imaging) and allows both the display and quantification of flow (see Ch. 20).

From the preceding discussion, it is clear that the signal intensity appearance of flowing blood is complex and dependent on several factors. These include flow velocity, repetition time (TR), echo time (TE), type of echo produced, slice thickness, and position of the section in the multislice set. Although the echo time (TE) for the MRA sequence should be as short as possible to minimize flow-related dephasing of spins, it is often desirable to increase the TE to produce an out-of-phase image (i.e. with the fat and water protons opposed, which for a 1.5 T magnet system would be 6.9 ms) in order to reduce the signal from fat.

A number of MRA methods which have exploited the above-mentioned phenomena are currently being investigated for the display and quantification of blood flow. The two techniques most widely studied are *time-of-flight* and *phase contrast*. Each has advantages and disadvantages, and can be implemented in either a two- or three-dimensional mode. Different techniques will be required for specific applications. In the *time-of-flight* (*saturation*) method the blood is modified by a selective RF pulse which then enters the region of interest. The effect is dependent on the T_1 relaxation rate of blood, which is short. This technique is thus best suited for studies of defined regions containing tortuous vessels with fast-flowing blood, such as the carotid arteries and the circle of Willis (Fig. 25.97). *Phase contrast* (*gradient refocused*) methods rely on velocity-induced phase differences to discriminate flowing blood from surrounding stationary tissue. These techniques are sensitive to the detection of slow flow in small vessels and produce a more efficient suppression of the stationary background tissue (Fig 25.98). A further advantage of the phase-sensitive methods is that a precise measure of blood flow velocity can be made (see Ch. 20). *Subtraction* techniques (analogous to DSA) can be used to provide high signal from blood with the elimination of the background signal from stationary tissue. The

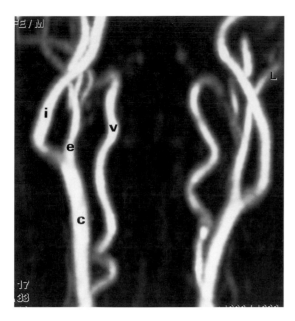

Fig. 25.97 Coronal maximum intensity projection (MIP) image of a two-dimensional time-of-flight MR angiogram showing normal bilateral neck arteries. c, common carotid artery; e, external carotid artery; i, internal carotid artery; v, vertebral artery.

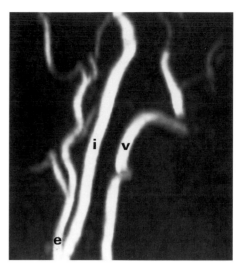

Fig. 25.99 Lateral MIP image of a two-dimensional time-of-flight MRA targeted to show the right neck arteries. (Same key as in Fig. 25.97).

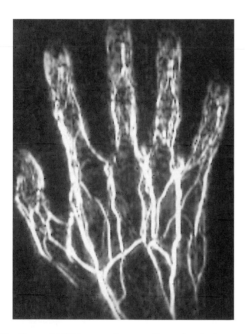

Fig. 25.98 Coronal MIP image of a two-dimensional phase contrast MR angiogram of the hand showing vessels as small as 0.2 mm in diameter. (Courtesy of IGE.)

use of *saturation RF pulses* allows tagging of particular vascular areas in order to visualize venous and arterial anatomy separately.

The source MRA data collected are computed to form projection angiograms using the maximum intensity projection (MIP) method. For each ray in the projected set only the maximum value is extracted as it is assumed that the blood in the vessel represents the highest signal in the data set. MR angiograms thus formed can be imaged as either 'black blood' or 'white blood', the former

producing an image akin to DSA (see Fig. 25.109). Postprocessing techniques also allow for improved visualization of separate vessels without overlap, for instance the targeting of the internal carotid artery branches of one side separate from the contralateral side. (Fig. 25.99)

It should be remembered, as with all techniques, that there are potential pitfalls in interpretation. Respiratory and cardiac motion can cause ghosting as well as variation in flow velocity profiles. Surgical clips can lead to signal voids which can be easily recognized on the original source MRA image, but can be mistaken on the MIP image for a stenosis, thrombus, or slow flow. It is thus imperative that the original source data set be reviewed in every case. Flow voids can occur due to turbulence (e.g. at the renal ostia on *phase contrast* MRA, or at the confluence of two tributaries such as the superior mesenteric and splenic veins). Low-signal structures can be lost using the MIP method, leading to an apparent loss of part of a vessel or overestimation of a stenosis.

A bolus intravenous injection of gadolinium-chelate, using a single or double dose (i.e. concentrations of 0.1 or 0.2 mmol/kg body weight, respectively), combined with the *time-of-flight* method is useful in producing preferential arterial enhancement. The gadolinium-chelate shortens the T_1 of blood, increasing flow-related enhancement over a large field of view, improving visualization of smaller arteries. It is thus a useful technique in patients with poor renal blood flow and renal insufficiency. The use of this technique has been described in the intracranial circulation, aorta, renal and popliteal–tibial arteries, and portal vein. The current contrast media available are extracellular space agents, but several prototypes limited to the intravascular space are under development.

Thoracic Aorta

One of the major applications of vascular MRI is in the assessment of the thoracic aorta. MRA has significant advantages over X-ray angiography and CT in the evaluation of aortic aneurysms and dissection, detecting aortic dilatations, and differentiating an aortic aneurysm from solid masses (Fig. 25.100). Advantages of MRI

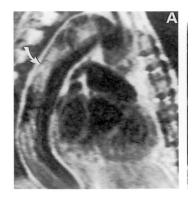
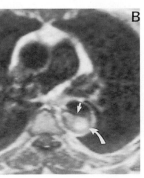

Fig. 25.100 Chronic descending aortic dissection on **A** sagittal and **B** transverse gated T$_1$-weighted spin echo (TE 26 ms). Note the signal from the slow-flowing blood in the false lumen (curved arrow), and the intimal flap (straight arrows).

include capability of topographic overview of the aorta and surrounding structures in any plane, together with visualization of the origin of arch vessels. The size of the thoracic aorta can be accurately assessed using well-defined imaging planes and true short-axis views. The following are the normal dimensions of the thoracic aorta (each with a range of ±4 mm): at the level of the sinus of Valsalva, 33 mm; mid-part of the ascending aorta, 30 mm; transverse part of the aortic arch, 27 mm; descending aorta, 24 mm. Progressive aortic dilatation, as occurs in Marfan syndrome, is easily demonstrated on follow-up MRI examinations (Fig. 25.101).

The use of phase contrast methods allows clear separation between the true and false lumens, and assessment of the re-entry site can be made in aortic dissection (Fig. 25.102). Small entry sites between true and false lumens, however, are more accurately demonstrated by transesophageal echocardiography. Knowledge

of normal anatomy (e.g. location of the left brachiocephalic vein and superior pericardial recess) and awareness of artefacts that can mimic aortic dissection are important in order to avoid any possible misinterpretation. MRI is superior to CT and transesophageal echocardiography in the assessment of the postoperative patient, and is without significant signal artefact in the majority (Fig. 25.103). Postsurgical complications include hemorrhage, hemopericardium, pseudoaneurysm formation, infection, graft occlusion, or arteriovenous fistula. In the surgically treated patient, assessment of the arch vessels and anastomoses is easily achieved by MRI, but with difficulty on transesophageal echocardiography.

The precise location, extent and severity of *aortic coarctation* can be assessed with MRI, providing information equivalent to that from X-ray angiography. The whole of the thoracic aorta can usually be demonstrated by oblique sagittal scanning along the line of the aortic arch (Fig. 25.104). In some instances the aorta is more tortuous, and multislice imaging is required for complete assessment. On MRI, the degree of stenosis of the coarctation segment, compared with the normal, correlates well with measurements made on X-ray angiography. A precise measurement of the pressure gradient and velocity across the coarctation segment can be obtained using MRA techniques (Fig. 25.105). A pressure gradient can be calculated from the measured peak flow velocity at the stenosis using the modified Bernoulli equation. Collateral vessels, including the internal mammary, intercostal, and posterior mediastinal arteries, can be visualized (Fig. 25.106). The evaluation of the descending aorta below the isthmus, which can be difficult on two-dimensional echocardiography, is also important in the preoperative assessment and can be well demonstrated on MRI.

Pulmonary Arteries

The normal dimensions of the pulmonary arteries can be well shown on transverse and coronal ECG-gated spin echo and gradient

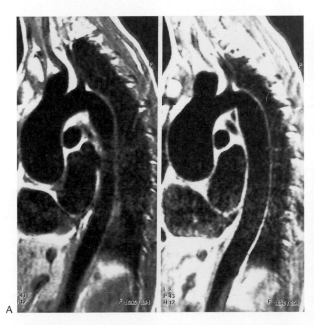
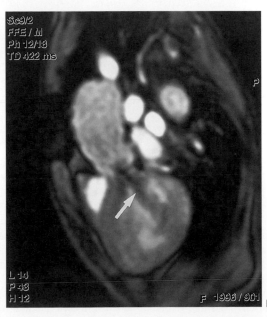

Fig. 25.101 **A**. Moderate degree of aneurysmal dilatation of the ascending aorta extending into the proximal part of the innominate artery on contiguous parasagittal T$_1$-weighted spin echo (SE 750/15) images. **B**. A sagittal–oblique phase contrast gradient echo (GE 750/7/40°) sequence in the same patient through the outflow tract shows a jet of signal void in the left ventricle (arrowed) consistent with aortic regurgitation.

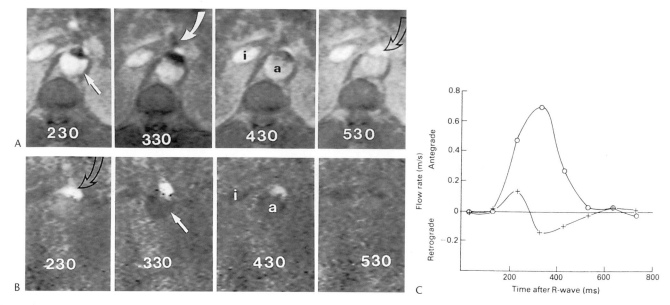

Fig. 25.102 Chronic aortic dissection on: **A** a set of four transverse cine gradient refocused (TE 28 ms) MR angiograms through the upper abdomen at the same anatomic level; **B** flow velocity maps derived from the angiograms in part A; and **C** a plot of the maximum flow rates in the true and false lumens at different times in the cardiac cycle, showing reversal of blood flow in the false lumen (○, true lumen; +, false lumen). (Same patient as in Fig. 12.14.) In part A, images have been taken at 100 ms intervals from the R-wave of the patient's ECG (indicated by the number on each image). There is a high signal within the false lumen (straight arrow) of the aorta (a) and inferior vena cava (i). Note signal loss in the true lumen (curved open arrow) and superior mesenteric artery (curved closed arrow) during systole due to high flow rates, with return of signal at 530 ms as the flow rate reduces. In part B, flow direction and velocity can be derived. Antegrade flow appears as light gray, absence of flow as mid-gray (similar to background), and retrograde flow as dark gray. The true lumen (curved arrow) shows antegrade flow during systole, whereas the false lumen (straight arrow) shows initial antegrade flow with flow reversal at 330 ms (see part C). Flow in the inferior vena cava (i) is consistently caudocranial. (Reproduced with permission from Mitchell et al. 1988.)

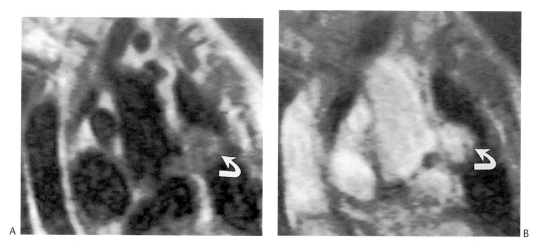

Fig. 25.103 Pseudoaneurysm of the aortic root associated with an aortic valve prosthesis on oblique-sagittal gated **A** T$_1$-weighted spin echo (TE 26 ms) and **B** gradient refocused (TE 22 ms) MR angiogram at the same anatomic level. The pseudoaneurysm (curved arrow) is clearly shown to contain flowing blood in part B.

refocused images. High signals can be seen in peripheral small branching pulmonary arteries on gated spin echo images due to slow blood flow toward end-diastole. Similar high signals can be seen in the main pulmonary arteries and aorta. These signals clear with the onset of systole. Abnormal persistence of signal in the pulmonary arteries during systole, on gated spin echo images, has been used to identify patients with pulmonary arterial hypertension.

On gradient refocused images the normal pulmonary arteries are characterized by a rapid increase in intraluminal signal intensity and diameter in systole, with a consequent decrease in diastole. In addition, branch vessels down to the subsegmental level and beyond can be delineated, extending the range of pulmonary vessels accessible to examination. By using three-dimensional MRA techniques it is possible to visualize up to the fifth and sixth branch order in the pulmonary tree. In contrast to the appearance of normal pulmonary arteries, the normal *pulmonary veins* have a distinctive signal intensity peak in both systole and diastole. These different appearances allow distinction to be made between

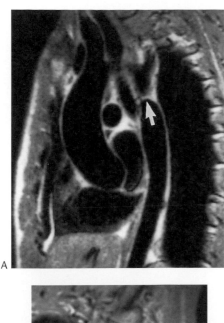

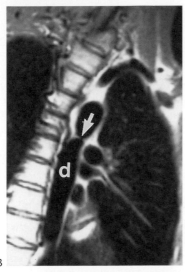

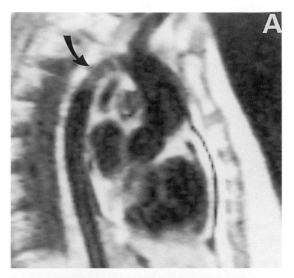

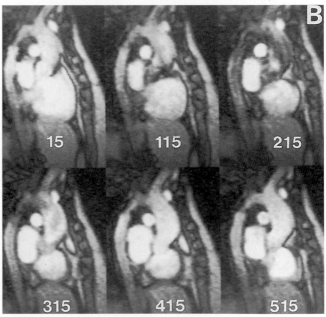

Fig. 25.104 Post-ductal coarctation of the aorta showing a narrowed diaphragm (arrowed) on **A** sagittal–oblique and **B** coronal–oblique intermediate-weighted ECG-gated spin echo (SE 1000/21) scans. Note the dilated collateral vesssels supplying the descending aorta (d) beyond the coarctation.

Fig. 25.105 Coarctation of the aorta, arrowed, previously repaired. **A**. Oblique gated T_1-weighted spin echo scan (T_E 26 ms). **B**. A set of six cine gradient refocused echo (T_E 12 ms) MR angiograms at the same anatomic level, spaced at 100 ms intervals from 15 ms from the R-wave of the ECG. At peak flow rates during systole there is some signal reduction at the repaired coarctation site (arrowed), indicating turbulence. Velocity maps (not shown) were performed at this site, giving a peak velocity (v) of 2 m/s (pressure gradient = $4v^2$, making a calculated gradient of 16 mmHg). This compared favorably with the value of 20 mmHg obtained from Doppler ultrasound.

pulmonary arteries and veins. In *pulmonary arterial hypertension* there is reduction in the normal compliance, with loss of the pulsatile systolic increase and diastolic decrease in diameter and signal intensity of the proximal pulmonary arteries.

MRI is gaining acceptance as the preferred technique for assessing pulmonary arteries in patients with pulmonary artery *atresia* or *obstruction* (Fig. 25.106). In neonates and infants, thin sections (< 5 mm) are required. Gated spin echo imaging can clearly demonstrate hypoplastic pulmonary arteries to the level of the first hilar branch. The use of MRA techniques extends the range for assessment of more peripheral branches, overcoming the limitation of two-dimensional echocardiography in depicting distal pulmonary artery branch stenoses (Fig. 25.106). Important clinical determinants in the management of patients with right ventricular outflow obstruction are the size of the pulmonary artery and the presence or absence of a pulmonary confluence.

Assessment of pulmonary artery growth following correction surgery is required to monitor and detect any developing stenoses. It should be noted that calculating vessel diameters from the intraluminal high signal obtained by MRA techniques could lead to an underestimate of true vessel size, because of magnetic susceptibility effects between the vessel wall and adjacent lung, which may lead to signal loss at the edge of the vessel. The combined use of gated spin echo imaging should overcome this problem. Difficulties in evaluating pulmonary arteries in patients

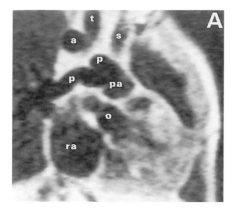
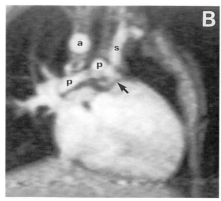
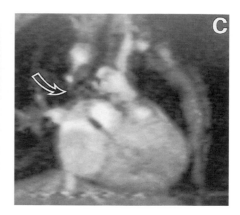

Fig. 25.106 Congenital branch pulmonary artery stenosis in an 11-year-old child with corrected Fallot's tetralogy and persistent pulmonary artery hypertension. **A**. Oblique–coronal gated T_1-weighted spin echo (TE 26 ms) image. **B,C**. Gradient-refocused echo (TE 12 ms) MR angiograms at the same anatomic level. **B**. End-diastole. **C**. In systole, showing signal loss, due to turbulence, in the right pulmonary artery (curved arrow). a, right-sided aortic arch; o, outflow tract of the left ventricle; p, right and left pulmonary arteries; pa, main pulmonary artery; ra, right atrium; s, left-sided superior vena cava; t, trachea; straight arrow in part B, position of the pulmonary valve.

with obstructive lesions have been encountered with both cine angiocardiography and two-dimensional echocardiography, and MRI should have a useful role here.

Pulmonary emboli as small as 3 mm in diameter can be detected experimentally on spin echo imaging, but may be difficult to interpret due to flow-related artefacts and poor differentiation between thrombus and areas of atelectasis or endobronchial mucous plugs. In addition, this technique does not allow acute and chronic pulmonary emboli to be distinguished. In a study of 10 patients with pulmonary embolic disease, acute and chronic emboli were distinguished using MRA techniques. On gradient refocused echo imaging, acute pulmonary embolus was recognized as a persistent low-signal intra-luminal filling defect (due to the magnetic susceptibility effect of hemosiderin) with a curvilinear capping by the high-signal intensity vascular column. Abrupt vessel cut-off without capping or the presence of webs or a narrowed and irregular vessel were interpreted as due to a chronic pulmonary embolus. No emboli distal to lobar branches, however, were demonstrated. The combination of MRA with intravenous contrast enhancement would be of benefit in these cases. MRA techniques may have a useful role in the assessment of pulmonary embolic disease, with advantages over current imaging modalities. In addition, MRI can be used to examine for the presence of deep-vein thrombosis.

Carotid Arteries

The normal carotid bifurcation can be reliably imaged on MRA (see Fig. 25.97). Both carotid bifurcations can be imaged simultaneously in less than 10 min by using a multislab three-dimensional sequence. Subsequent images can be reformatted in multiple orientations to optimize the demonstration or show both bifurcations. Patients who have undergone recent carotid endarterectomy can also be evaluated non-invasively. As indicated in the assessment of aortic coarctation, short TE values are essential to demonstrate carotid artery stenoses. In severe stenosis there may, however, be profound signal loss mimicking occlusion. Recent developments, including the use of an intravascular space contrast agent, should help to resolve this problem. In order to

demonstrate the circle of Willis, images are usually acquired in the transverse plane, where detail of the basal arterial tree and small branches can be obtained.

On MRA, aneurysms and arteriovenous malformations (including intraspinal angiomas) can be visualized together with the relative flow contribution of the individual feeding vessels, allowing improved treatment planning.

The relationship and effect of tumors on adjacent vascular structures can be more easily appreciated than with conventional spin echo imaging.

Abdominal Vessels

The normal short-axis diameter of the suprarenal abdominal aorta is approximately 25 mm, tapering down to its bifurcation, where it measures 15 mm. The indications for MRA of the abdominal aorta include patients with known iodinated contrast allergy or renal insufficiency, and those with difficult vascular access due to severe aortoiliac occlusive disease (Fig. 25.107). MRA can also be used to demonstrate arteriovenous malformations (Fig. 25.108).

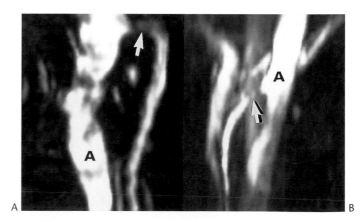

Fig. 25.107 Severe atheromatous disease of the abdominal aorta with stenosis at the origin of the superior mesenteric artery (arrowed) on sagittal MIP scans of two-dimensional **A** time-of-flight and **B** phase contrast MRAs in different patients. A, abdominal aorta.

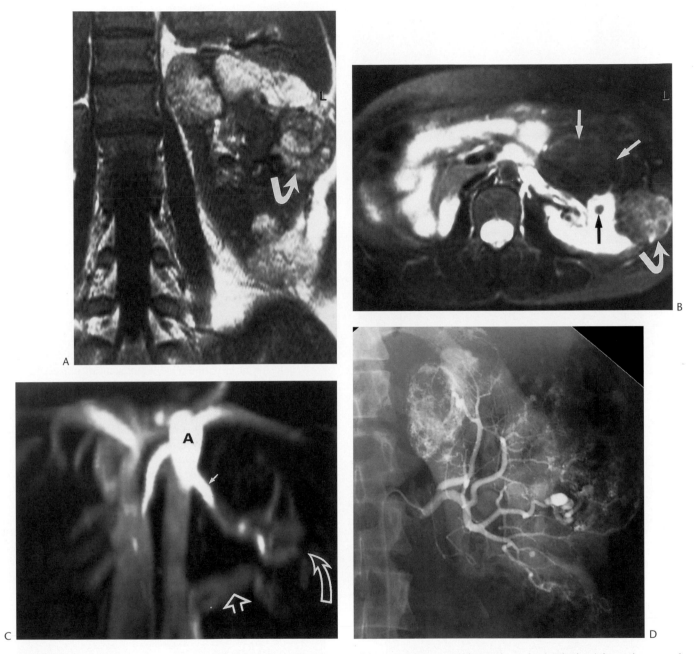

Fig. 25.108 Renal angiomyolipoma in a 35-year-old woman with recurrent left loin pain due to renal hemorrhage, having had a right nephrectomy for similar pathology. **A**. Coronal T_1-weighted spin echo (SE 603/15) image showing an enlarged left kidney with multiple lipomata and a more heterogeneous mass laterally (curved arrow). **B**. Transverse T_2-weighted turbo spin echo (TSE 1800/110) image with fat suppression demonstrates signal loss from the fatty components (straight arrows) but with a heterogeneous signal, in keeping with hemorrhage from the mass laterally (curved arrow). **C**. An off-axis coronal MIP image of a two-dimensional phase contrast MR angiogram showing a patent left renal artery (straight arrow) with an arteriovenous malformation (open curved arrow) and large draining vessel (open straight arrow). **D**. Subsequent selective renal arteriogram (arterial phase) confirming the arteriovenous malformation (curved arrow), which is amenable to embolization.

Renal Arteries Both renal arteries originate at approximately the same level, 2 cm below the origin of the superior mesenteric artery. An accessory renal artery occurs in a fifth of individuals, being commoner on the left below the level of the main renal vessel. The caliber of the renal arteries varies between 5 and 10 mm, and is dependent on the total renal blood flow indirectly reflecting renal function (Fig. 25.109).

The clinical signs of renal artery stenosis include renovascular hypertension and azotemia. Renovascular hypertension is believed to be the cause of 1–5% of all cases of hypertension. Approximately 70% of cases of renal artery stenosis are due to atherosclerosis occurring in older individuals, with the remainder due to fibromuscular dysplasia, which more often affects younger patients. Atherosclerotic renovascular lesions typically (85%) involve the

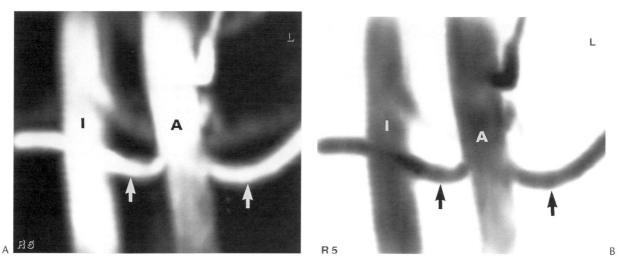

Fig. 25.109 Normal renal arteries (arrowed) on a coronal MIP image of a two-dimensional phase contrast MR angiogram with **A** white and **B** 'black' blood. A, abdominal aorta; I, inferior vena cava.

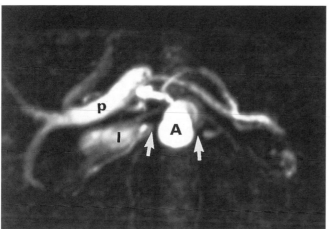

Fig. 25.110 Bilateral renal artery stenoses (arrowed) on a transverse MIP scan of a two-dimensional phase contrast MR angiogram A, abdominal aorta; I, inferior vena cava; p, portal vein.

proximal main renal arteries or the ostium (Fig. 25.110), whereas those due to fibromuscular dysplasia are usually in the more distal and segmental parts of the renal artery. Thus, MRA is indicated for the exclusion of proximal renal artery stenosis in patients with azotemic renovascular disease (Fig. 25.111), but is limited in ruling out renovascular hypertension in the younger individual.

MRA of the renal arteries poses particular problems related to cardiac, respiratory, and bowel motion artefacts, overlapping renal veins and inferior vena cava, renal vessel tortuosity, and complex flow patterns with disparate flow velocities between the aorta and renal arteries. *Phase contrast* and/or *time-of-flight* MRA can be used for detecting stenoses of the main renal artery. On *phase contrast* MRA, false ostial stenosis can be demonstrated due to loss of signal at the origin of the renal arteries from dephasing due to normal non-laminar flow at vessel origins (Fig. 25.112). Using *time-of-flight* MRA the proximal renal artery is well visualized, but visualization of the vessel more distally is hampered mainly by saturation of spins leading to fading away of the signal

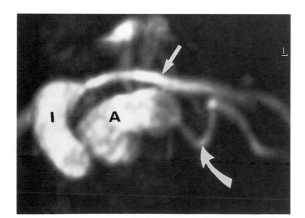

Fig. 25.111 Rotated MIP image of a two-dimensional phase contrast MR angiogram showing tortuosity and severe atheromatous disease of the abdominal aorta with occlusion of the right renal artery and normal left renal artery (curved arrow). A, abdominal aorta; I, inferior vena cava; straight arrow, left renal vein.

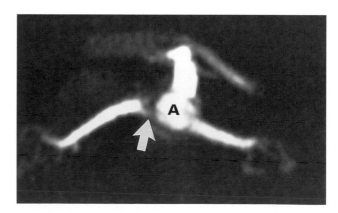

Fig. 25.112 Transverse MIP scan of a two-dimensional phase contrast MR angiogram in a normal individual showing a false renal ostial stenosis (arrowed). A, abdominal aorta; I, inferior vena cava.

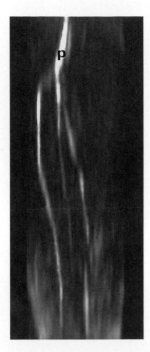

Fig. 25.113 Coronal MIP image of a two-dimensional phase contrast MR angiogram showing the normal trifurcation of arteries in the calf. p, popliteal artery.

in the vessels with slow flow. In screening for stenosis of the main renal arteries it has been shown that the combination of three-dimensional *time-of-flight* and *phase contrast* MRA sequences improved detection. Small accessory renal arteries and distal branch vessels are not visualized using current techniques, although recent advances including the use of contrast-enhanced MRA await further evaluation.

Peripheral Vessels

The absence of physiological motion in the extremities makes them ideal areas for vascular study (see Fig. 25.81). Normal and occluded popliteal trifurcation vessels can be reliably imaged using MRA techniques (Fig. 25.113). Stenotic lesions of this area, however, cannot be consistently portrayed. MRA can be used to investigate patients with claudication and in the non-invasive follow-up of patients who have undergone angioplasty, but further refinements are required if it is to compete with the more accessible and less expensive technique of Doppler ultrasound.

REFERENCES AND SUGGESTIONS FOR FURTHER READING

See end of Chapter 26.

26

PHLEBOGRAPHY

David Sutton

With contributions from P. L. Allan and Jeremy P. R. Jenkins

The types of contrast phlebography used in clinical practice include:

1. Phlebography of the lower limb
2. Pelvic phlebography and inferior vena cavography
3. Hepatic, renal, and adrenal phlebography
4. Phlebography of the upper limb and superior vena cava
5. Portal phlebography.

Intraosseous phlebography and spinal phlebography were once fairly widely practised but are now obsolete.

The investigations listed use direct contrast phlebography. Indirect phlebography can be achieved by serial filming following arteriography. The latter method is the one routinely used for the demonstration of the cerebral veins following cerebral angiography and commonly for the demonstration of the renal veins following selective renal arteriography. It is also used for portal phlebography following selective celiac or splenic arteriography—so-called *arterioportography*. Other imaging techniques have been used in the investigation of the venous system but most have only limited application.

Radioisotope Phlebography   This can be performed as a prelude to a perfusion lung scan in suspected pulmonary embolus. Half the dose of ^{99m}Tc is injected into each foot simultaneously, and the passage of the isotope up the legs and through the abdomen recorded. The resulting images may show evidence of venous obstruction or a normal deep-venous system. Delayed scans are also obtained of the calf and thigh to demonstrate local hold-up suggesting venous obstruction. Radioisotope phlebography offers an alternative technique in patients with iodine sensitivity or other contraindications to formal phlebography.

^{125}I-labeled fibrinogen has also been widely used to diagnose deep vein thrombosis. In this case, however, the isotope is injected into an arm vein and is later taken up by the developing thrombosis. Recordings are made over the calf, popliteal, and femoral veins, and will demonstrate local increase of uptake. False positives may be obtained over wounds, hematomas, and cellulitis, but the test has a high degree of accuracy with large recent thrombi, and is relatively easy to perform.

Doppler Ultrasound   This has major attractions as a non-invasive technique for diagnosing venous thrombosis. Doppler flow signals can be recognized over the femoral, popliteal, and posterior tibial veins. Deep-vein thrombosis (DVT) is suggested when signals are absent or when muscle compression of the thigh does not produce the expected increase in femoral vein blood flow. In expert hands and with the addition of color Doppler ultrasound, a high degree of accuracy is claimed, though smaller lesions in the calf are more difficult to identify by this method (see below).

Real-time or B-scan Ultrasound   This will demonstrate well such deep-seated structures as the inferior vena cava or portal vein but, generally speaking, has little place in the investigation of most of the lesions discussed in this chapter.

Computed Tomography   CT, particularly spiral CT, will demonstrate the major veins well, but usually requires contrast injections for the confirmation, of such lesions as caval thrombosis or portal thrombosis.

Magnetic Resonance Imaging   MRI also shows major veins well and does not require contrast media injections. It is further discussed below.

Digital Subtraction Angiography (DSA)   This technique is limited in the area that can be examined at one time but will reduce contrast medium dosage in areas where it can be used.

Liquid Crystal Thermography   This technique, which uses simple portable equipment, has a sensitivity of some 80% in DVT and a specificity of 57%.

D–dimer Assay   This is a simple blood test which has been shown to have a sensitivity of 95% and a specificity of 50% in DVT. A normal result can therefore exclude DVT and prevent further unnecessary investigation.

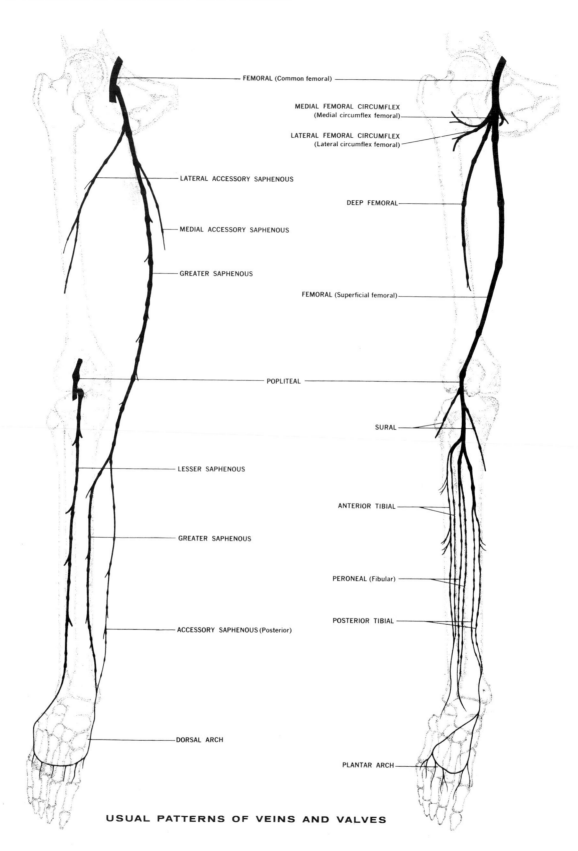

FEMORAL (Common femoral)

MEDIAL FEMORAL CIRCUMFLEX
(Medial circumflex femoral)

LATERAL FEMORAL CIRCUMFLEX
(Lateral circumflex femoral)

LATERAL ACCESSORY SAPHENOUS

DEEP FEMORAL

MEDIAL ACCESSORY SAPHENOUS

GREATER SAPHENOUS

FEMORAL (Superficial femoral)

POPLITEAL

SURAL

LESSER SAPHENOUS

ANTERIOR TIBIAL

GREATER SAPHENOUS

PERONEAL (Fibular)

POSTERIOR TIBIAL

ACCESSORY SAPHENOUS (Posterior)

DORSAL ARCH

PLANTAR ARCH

USUAL PATTERNS OF VEINS AND VALVES

Fig. 26.1 Diagram of the deep and superficial veins of the lower limb. (Copyright Eastman Kodak Co. Reprinted by courtesy of the Health Sciences Division, Eastman Kodak Co.)

THE LOWER LIMB

Indications   Phlebography of the lower limb is practised at most medical centers for the following purposes:

1. To demonstrate DVT in the calf, thigh, pelvis, or inferior vena cava

2. To show suspected venous obstruction by tumor or extrinsic pressure

3. To investigate secondary or recurrent varicose veins thought to be associated with an abnormality of the deep-venous system such as post-thrombotic destruction of valves and associated incompetent perforators, or with inadequate surgery

4. To investigate swollen legs where the differential diagnosis between lymphedema, cellulitis, and venous incompetence (or obstruction) is not clear

5. To investigate varicose ulcers in the post-thrombotic syndrome

6. To outline venous malformations.

Suspected DVT is the commonest cause for patient referral, and in most cases there is strong clinical evidence for the lesion. In some cases, however, e.g. in patients with repeated pulmonary emboli but no obvious source, the investigation may be undertaken to exclude the lower limb as a source of emboli.

Normal Anatomy   The venous drainage of the lower limb can be divided into two separate systems, the deep veins and the superficial veins. These are connected by the communicating veins (Figs 26.1 and 26.2).

The *deep* veins in the calf follow the same distribution as the main arteries but are usually double, forming the anterior tibial, posterior tibial, and peroneal veins. The calf veins, or sural veins, arise in calf muscles and emerge from them to join the peroneal, posterior tibial, or popliteal veins.

The communicating veins are usually small and paired and connect the superficial and deep veins. Normally they are extremely narrow, but they can become quite large when hypertrophied. They are valved so that blood only flows from the superficial to the deep veins. Under pathological conditions they can become incompetent, permitting reverse flow from the deep to the superficial veins (Fig. 26.3). They are most numerous and important in the calf, though there is usually one in the mid-thigh and sometimes two or three at different levels (Fig. 26.4).

The popliteal vein is a smooth large vessel lying behind the knee and passing up into the femoral vein, which follows the course of the femoral artery. The femoral vein is sometimes double, or the profunda vein, which usually lies in the upper two-thirds of the thigh, may connect in its lower part with the femoral or popliteal vein. Perforating or communicating veins in the thigh are normally small, but if incompetent may be demonstrated connecting the superficial and deep veins (Fig. 26.4).

The *superficial* leg veins drain into the saphenous veins. The short saphenous vein passes up the lateral side of the leg to the knee, where it passes deeply to join the popliteal vein. The long saphenous vein passes up the medial side of the calf and thigh and then joins the femoral vein below the groin.

The venous system can be regarded as a blood reservoir, and normally contains some two-thirds of the body blood, largely in the lower limbs. Flow to the heart depends on the pressure gradient

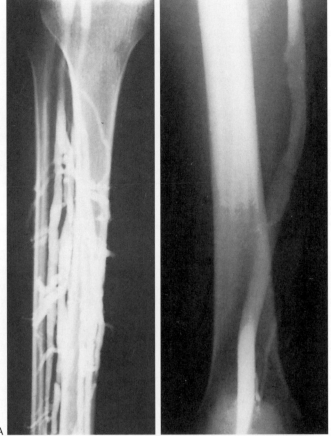

A   B

Fig. 26.2   Normal ascending phlebogram of the deep veins.

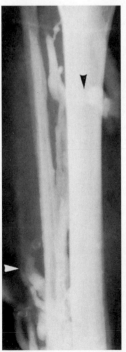   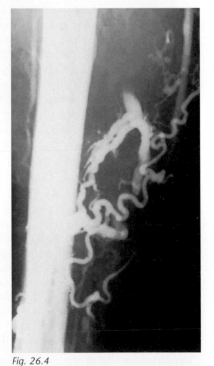

Fig. 26.3   Fig. 26.4

Fig. 26.3   Incompetent perforating veins in the calf (arrows).

Fig. 26.4   Incompetent perforating veins in the thigh.

between the veins and right atrium, and is assisted by the muscle contractions, particularly in the calf, acting as a pump. The veins themselves can also actively contract and help onward flow of blood. The valves are also of great importance in preventing retrograde flow, and their destruction or damage by thrombosis has serious hemodynamic consequences leading to venous incompetence.

Technique

1. Ascending Phlebography A large number of different techniques have been described in the literature. No standard technique has been generally accepted. The technique used by us has been modified over the years, and is as follows. A small needle is inserted percutaneously into a vein on the dorsum of the foot. Occasionally this may prove impossible, and the needle may have to be inserted by cut-down. If the foot is swollen or edematous, prior bed rest with the foot elevated is desirable to reduce the swelling. Once the needle is in position, compression is applied just above the ankle and also just above the knee by tourniquets or by inflatable cuffs. The pressure used is just sufficient to occlude the superficial veins completely without affecting the patency of the deep veins.

Contrast medium (40–50 ml) is then injected by hand pressure. In some cases more may be required to obtain adequate filling of the femoral and iliac veins, but it should rarely be necessary to use more than 80–100 ml. In the past, 65% Hypaque or an equivalent other medium has been used. However, the newer contrast media with low osmolality are now increasingly used (see Ch. 25), and these are better tolerated by the patient and less likely to produce complications.

Since the foot veins are usually punctured with small butterfly needles (21 British standard wire gauge) the injection can take 20–30 s. Flow is monitored by observation with an image intensifier, and films obtained at appropriate moments as the veins are sequentially filled. While some workers conduct the examination with the patient supine, others insist that the patient should be tilted on the table into a 30–60° feet-down position. This is mainly to prevent layering of contrast medium posteriorly, which gives rise to artefactual filling defects, and to ensure mixing of blood and contrast medium. The foot and leg should be medially rotated to separate the tibia and fibula and the deep veins of the calf. The weight should not be borne by the foot being injected, so that the calf muscles remain relaxed and their veins can be filled with contrast.

2. Descending Phlebography This is less frequently practised but is occasionally used, with the patient supine on a tilting table and the feet against the footrest. The femoral vein is punctured at the groin and, with the needle in situ, the patient is then tilted to the erect or near-erect position, and contrast medium injected. If the patient performs the Valsalva maneuver, contrast medium will reflux down an incompetent femoral vein into the popliteal vein. It has been claimed, however, that contrast will sometimes flow past competent valves, though it is usually possible to assess the degree of true incompetence and show the valves clearly, particularly when they are competent (Fig. 26.5).

Complications With the older contrast media, a few patients tolerated the procedure badly and complained of pain and discomfort in the calf with ascending phlebography. Nausea, vomiting, and minor allergic reactions were also occasionally seen, as with all contrast media. The new low-osmolality contrast media are better tolerated and give rise to little discomfort.

Care should be taken to ensure there is no contrast medium extravasation at the site of puncture, as this can be quite painful, and with a large volume of extravasation the consequences, particularly in an ischemic or edematous foot, can be serious. Skin necrosis has been recorded from this accident.

Phlebitis and postphlebography venous thrombosis can occur where large volumes of high-concentration contrast are used. This should be guarded against by flushing out residual contrast agent with saline at the end of the procedure, and by using the new low-osmolality contrast media.

Radiological Findings In the normal patient the deep veins of the calf are outlined by contrast at ascending phlebography with cuffs inflated; three paired veins accompanying the peroneal, posterior, and anterior tibial arteries can be recognized, the last being smaller than the others. There is no filling of the superficial or communicating veins (see Fig. 26.2), but with progressive injections of contrast medium there will be varying degrees of filling of the soleal muscle veins, which are typically large and valveless and drain into the peroneal and posterior tibial veins. There may also be filling of the gastrocnemius veins, which are valved and usually multiple, running a downward course from their points of entry into the upper popliteal vein.

The popliteal vein is single and commences near the knee joint, passing upwards to become the femoral vein. Views of the calf are usually obtained in both anteroposterior and lateral projections. Valves are usually obvious in the distended veins but can be accentuated by the patient performing the Valsalva maneuver.

A good-quality ascending phlebogram will also demonstrate the iliac veins and inferior vena cava, but these are best shown by releasing the tourniquet and manually compressing the calf to improve the upward flow of contrast medium at the same time as the pelvic exposure is made. This ensures a good bolus of contrast medium entering the iliac veins. If the suspected lesion affects only the pelvic veins or inferior vena cava, direct pelvic phlebography is to be preferred (see below).

Deep Vein Thrombosis

Venous thrombosis appears to be multifactorial in origin, and is associated with slowing of the blood flow and an increased liability to blood coagulation. Conditions known to predispose include malignant disease, age, obesity, trauma, and surgery, as well as prolonged immobilization, myocardial infarction, and congestive heart failure. A rare but frequently fatal condition is Hughes–Stovin syndrome, usually seen in young boys, where recurrent DVT is associated with hemoptysis from a ruptured segmental pulmonary aneurysm.

The risk of DVT is particularly high after abdominal and pelvic surgery, and even higher after operations on the hip, knee, or femur. It becomes even greater if there is associated myocardial infarction or congestive heart failure. The thrombosis may be bilateral in some 30% of patients.

Clinically, symptoms are present only if there is significant obstruction or inflammation produced by the thrombosis, and it is claimed that 50% or more of cases are silent and symptomless.

The main danger is pulmonary embolus, and the incidence in the USA of this complication is over 500 000 cases per annum. The mortality in different series ranges from 10 to 30%.

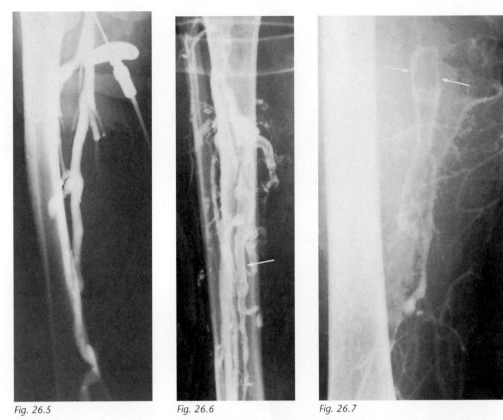

Fig. 26.5   Fig. 26.6   Fig. 26.7

Fig. 26.5 Descending phlebogram showing incompetent valves and reflux down to the popliteal vein.

Fig. 26.6 Phlebogram showing venous thrombosis in deep veins of the calf. The clot shows as a central filling defect with marginal contrast (arrow).

Fig. 26.7 Phlebogram showing venous thrombosis in the femoral vein. The clot shows as a central filling defect with marginal contrast (arrows).

The vast majority of these emboli arise from the leg veins. As already noted, half the cases show no prodromal leg symptoms before the embolus occurs.

Acute Thrombosis Acute thrombosis of the deep veins appears as filling defects within the veins, the defect often being outlined by a marginal layer of contrast. Views in more than one plane may show that the clot is adherent to the vein at some point in one or other plane. Upward extension of the clot may be seen lying more freely in the lumen, and such a floating tail is likely to embolize. Adherent clot is regarded as relatively less dangerous. Clot may be identified in calf veins only, or involving the popliteal and femoral veins, or in the iliac veins and inferior vena cava (Figs 26.6–26.9).

True clot defects should be distinguished from

1. Artefacts due to layering
2. Streaming from the entry of large non-opacified tributary veins
3. Turbulence around valves.

Films in more than one plane, the Valsalva maneuver, and multiple films all help in this respect, as do large doses of contrast medium and the semi-erect position.

Acute thrombosis is later followed by clot retraction, thrombolysis and recanalization, but the venous valves are damaged and destroyed so that the vein becomes irregular and incompetent. Some veins are severely stenosed or occluded, and in these cases

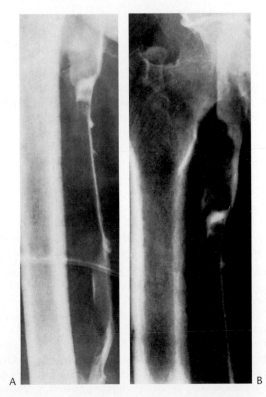

A   B

Fig. 26.8 Extensive clot in the femoral vein adherent in part.

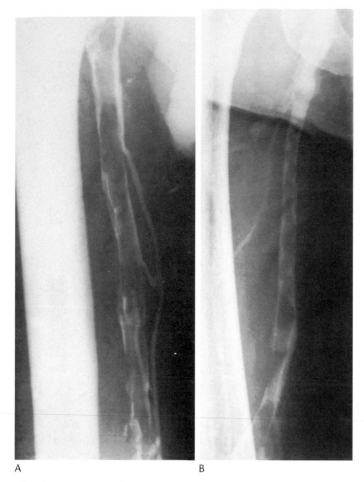

A   B

Fig. 26.9   Extensive clot in the femoral vein.

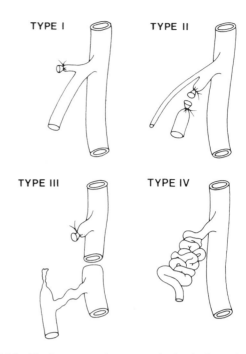

Fig. 26.10   The four types of recurrence in the thigh are shown diagrammatically. More than one type may apply in a given patient. (Reproduced from Starnes et al. 1984, with permission.)

venous return is largely by dilated collaterals. In either case a *post-thrombotic syndrome* may develop, characterized by swelling and pain in the affected leg. Eventually this may lead to induration and ulceration. This is usually on the medial aspect of the ankle, but is occasionally lateral in position. This is related to the fact that the medial aspect of the lower third of the leg just above the ankle is the site for a group of communicating veins, usually three in number. As these are at the most dependent part of the limb the increased pressure from incompetence and partial obstruction is greatest here and is accentuated by the pressure from calf muscle contractions.

Phlebography in patients with post-thrombotic states will show involved veins to be irregular and incompetent. In severe cases the major veins may be occluded in whole or in part and replaced by numerous collateral veins.

Recurrent Varicose Veins   The recurrence of varicose veins after surgery is a frequent clinical problem and may occur several years later. In these patients a useful procedure is direct injection of one or more of the superficial thigh varicose veins to demonstrate their distribution and the pattern of recurrences at the groin following the previous high ligation of the long saphenous vein. There are several mechanisms, but the most usual is a tortuous leash of recanalized vein and not a missed tributary of the long saphenous or a missed perforating vein (Fig. 26.10). The procedure may have the additional bonus of sclerosing the recanalized trunk and producing a clinical cure.

CONGENITAL ANOMALIES

Duplication   Duplication of the popliteal or femoral vein or of both is not infrequent, as is duplication of the long saphenous vein. Congenital *absence* of the posterior tibial veins is another anomaly that is not infrequent. In this case veins are usually seen passing laterally above the ankle to drain into the peroneal veins.

Congenital Absence of the Venous Valves   This is described in the major veins giving rise to venous stasis (*primary deep-venous insufficiency*) and should be considered when children or teenagers present with varicosities or chronic leg swelling. However, such a diagnosis should be made with caution as previously unrecognized DVT with recanalization cannot always be excluded. It is claimed that such recanalization can sometimes result in apparently normal-looking veins without the usual irregularities seen in the post-thrombotic syndrome.

Klippel–Trenaunay Syndrome   This is characterized by a nevus with hypertrophy of bones and soft tissues of affected limbs, usually legs, though arms may also be affected. There is venous dysplasia, and the normal venous return is replaced by persistence of a more primitive system, usually a large lateral venous channel in the leg, or a single large medial venous channel in the arm (see Fig. 26.27). These can be associated with superficial varicosities. The large drainage vein is often valveless and shows very sluggish flow. Abnormal large drainage veins also occur in the penis, resulting in erectile dysfunction and impotence.

Other Anomalies   A large *varix* or venous aneurysm can occur anywhere in the venous system. Such lesions are not uncommon at the termination of the long or short saphenous veins. Superficial or deep-venous varices or *venous angioma* are sometimes seen, such lesions having no obvious connection with an arterial lesion. Their anatomy is well shown by simple phlebography.

THE PELVIS AND ABDOMEN

As noted above, the iliac veins and inferior vena cava are quite well shown by good-quality ascending phlebograms from the foot, and their demonstration should be part of all such investigations. However, they can be more constantly and clearly demonstrated by direct femoral phlebography, which is the technique of choice where the lesion is known to be intra-abdominal. The method is also used in the occasional cases where ascending phlebography from the foot has failed to clearly exclude or confirm clot in the iliacs or inferior vena cava because of poor contrast for technical or other reasons.

The lesions shown by pelvic and inferior caval phlebography include:

1. Acute thrombosis with recent clot, or post-thrombotic sequelae with partial obstruction and collateral circulation
2. Obstruction by neoplastic or glandular masses, usually by extrinsic pressure, but also by tumor invasion as in hypernephromas
3. Extrinsic pressure from large benign tumors or other lesions, e.g. lymphocele, aneurysms, retroperitoneal fibrosis, hematoma
4. Obstruction of the left common iliac vein by pressure from the right common iliac artery (so-called 'lymphedema praecox')
5. Post-traumatic or radiotherapy venous damage
6. Pelvic varicosities
7. Congenital anomalies.

Technique The iliac veins and inferior vena cava are well shown by direct injection into the femoral veins of 30–40 ml of contrast medium on each side. Both veins are injected at the same time, unless only one iliac vein is obstructed and it is desired to show collateral and bypass drainage pathways clearly (see Fig. 26.16). A unilateral injection will also suffice if only the inferior vena cava is under examination. The injection is made through a large needle inserted into the femoral vein at the groin, or after percutaneous insertion of a catheter which is passed 5–8 cm up the vein.

To obtain good filling, contrast medium is injected rapidly as a bolus, taking 2–4 s for the 40 ml volume on each side. Serial films of the abdomen are obtained at the rate of one per second for 5 s as normal flow is rapid. Better and more prolonged filling can be obtained if the patient performs the Valsalva maneuver.

Radiographic Appearances The normal external and common iliac veins and inferior vena cava are valveless and appear as large contrast-filled tubes. There may be a slight extrinsic pressure defect at the termination of the left common iliac where it is crossed by the overlying right common iliac artery. Occasionally the artery can partially obstruct venous flow (see below). The internal iliac veins do contain valves and are not normally demonstrated. The Valsalva maneuver will fill their terminations and sometimes provides better filling, but this is unusual. Streamlining by non-opacified blood may be seen where large veins such as the renal veins enter the inferior vena cava. Figure 26.11 illustrates the normal inferior vena cava and its connections.

Congenital Anomalies Anomalies of the inferior vena cava occur in less than 1% of patients, but the incidence is higher in patients with congenital heart disease.

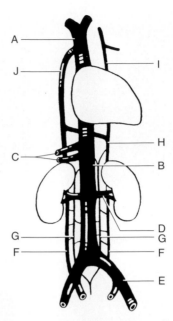

Fig. 26.11 Diagram showing venous drainage and connections of the inferior vena cava. A, superior vena cava; B, inferior vena cava; C, hepatic veins; D, renal veins; E, iliac veins; F, ascending lumbar veins; G, vertebral venous plexus; H, hemiazygos vein; I, ascending hemiazygos vein; J, azygos vein.

Left-sided inferior vena cava is the commonest of these anomalies. In these cases the left-sided vena cava terminates in the left renal vein, which then usually drains into a normally sited terminal segment of the inferior vena cava (Fig. 26.12). Less frequent is a *double inferior vena cava* with the right larger than the left, or both equal in size. The left vena cava again terminates in the left renal vein (Fig. 26.13). Occasionally a left inferior vena cava may drain into the lumbar and hemiazygos systems, the coronary sinus, or the left atrium. The suprarenal segment of a normal or abnormal infrarenal inferior vena cava occasionally drains into the azygos vein and hemiazygos vein instead of passing through the liver. This anomaly has been recognized on CT, when the dilated veins are shown behind the diaphragmatic crura adjacent to the aorta as it enters the thorax.

Both *agenesis* and *hypoplasia* of the inferior vena cava have been described. In these cases blood from the pelvis and lower limbs drains mainly into the lumbar, hemiazygos, and azygos veins, which act as collaterals.

Thrombosis Thrombosis of the iliacs or inferior vena cava in the acute phase shows similar appearances to those described above in lower-limb thrombosis, i.e. clot defect occupying most of the lumen with attachment to the vein wall (Fig. 26.14A), or, more dangerously, with a tail of clot extending into the lumen. In the latter case, surgery may be indicated to prevent emboli passing to the lung. In the past this consisted of plication of the inferior vena cava, an operation superseded by the transvenous insertion of filters (see below). Collateral bridging vessels will be seen, dependent on the site and extent of obstruction.

Complete thrombosis of the inferior vena cava is occasionally seen, and there is then a collateral circulation utilizing a wide variety of collaterals including the lumbar and azygos veins, the vertebral plexus, the anterior abdominal wall veins, and the retroperitoneal or even mesenteric veins (Figs 26.14B and 26.15). Such complete

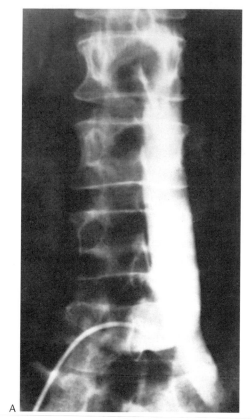

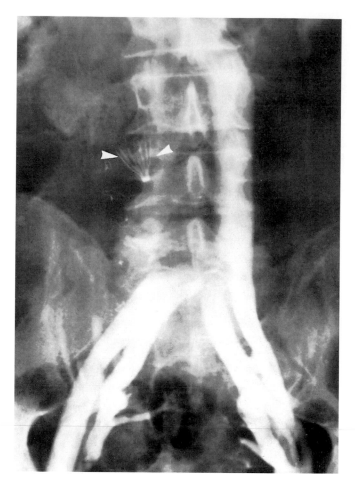

Fig. 26.13   Double inferior vena cava. A Mobin–Uddin umbrella (arrowed) has been inserted in the normal right-sided inferior vena cava. The post-operative phlebogram shows an unsuspected double inferior vena cava with the right side now occluded.

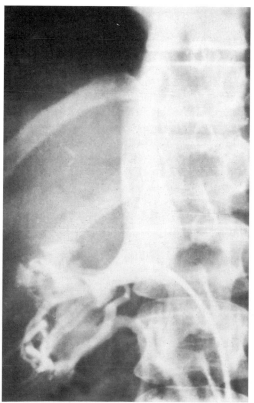

Fig. 26.12   **A**. Left-sided inferior vena cava as a chance finding in a patient undergoing renal vein catheterization. **B**. The catheter has passed over to the right renal vein through the left inferior vena cava where it joins the left renal vein; the upper part of the inferior vena cava is normally sited.

thrombosis usually extends to the level of the renal veins, which remain patent. The upper limit can be demonstrated by retrograde phlebography from above, a catheter being passed from the arm through the right auricle to the upper inferior vena cava.

Recanalization of the iliac veins and inferior vena cava may occur after complete thrombosis, when the vessels will appear smaller and more irregular with evidence of collateral vessels (Fig. 26.16).

Lipoma   Lipoma of the deep central veins is a rare intravascular tumor usually found in the inferior vena cava and occasionally in the superior vena cava. Though it can be large enough to occupy most of the lumen, it only rarely produces obstruction, and most are diagnosed as incidental findings on CT or MRI.

Glandular and Neoplastic Masses These can produce considerable distortion of the iliac veins and inferior vena cava. Large benign masses can produce marked displacement with little obstruction when only the inferior vena cava is affected (see Fig. 36.32), but the iliacs are more easily obstructed by extrinsic pressure (Fig. 26.17). In the past, inferior vena cavography was widely used to assess paraaortic glandular involvement in reticulosis in conjunction with lymphangiography, but with the development of CT and ultrasound this is no longer indicated.

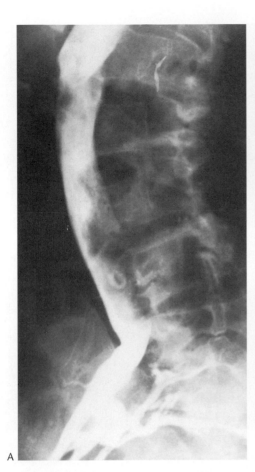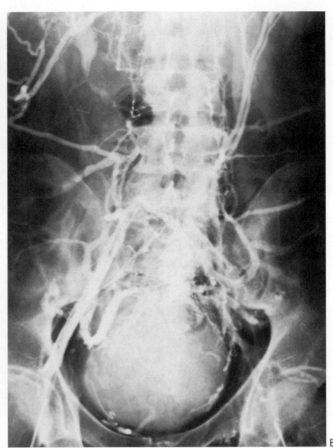

Fig. 26.14 A. Recent clot obstructing the left common iliac and partially obstructing the lower inferior vena cava. **B**. Thrombosis of the inferior vena cava and common iliacs with collateral circulation. There is some irregular recanalization of the common iliacs.

Renal vein invasion by hypernephroma is quite common, and tumor may then spread into the inferior vena cava. Such tumor spread is well shown by inferior vena cavography (Fig. 26.18) or by CT.

Spontaneous Iliac Vein Rupture   This is a very rare condition which has been reported in patients with proximal iliac obstruction (several by the common iliac artery). In one fatal case the rupture was precipitated by straining at stool. The patient presented with severe groin pain and circulatory collapse from the internal haemorrhage. Ruptured calf veins with hematoma formation are also well documented.

THERAPEUTIC INTERRUPTION OF THE INFERIOR VENA CAVA

Pulmonary embolus is a major cause of death. It is estimated that there are 630 000 cases per annum in the USA with some 200 000 deaths. In untreated cases the recurrence rate is said to be 60% with a significant further mortality rate (22%). Most cases are treated by anticoagulation, with thrombolysis by streptokinase or pulmonary embolectomy indicated in cases of massive pulmonary embolus. If anticoagulation is contraindicated, or fails to prevent recurrence, or if the patient has severe cardiac or pulmonary disease, then caval interruption should be considered, since over 90% of emboli arise from the leg veins.

Therapeutic interruption of the inferior vena cava to prevent further pulmonary emboli was first practised in 1945 by operative occlusion. Later, operative partial interruption was practised by suture partition, bead compression, and external fenestrated clipping. Because of the risks involved to seriously ill patients from general anesthesia and laparotomy, these operations were gradually replaced by a simpler technique. This involved transvenous insertion of devices from the right internal jugular vein after operative cut-down under local anesthesia. The devices used included:

1. The Mobin–Uddin umbrella filter (1967) (see Fig. 26.13)
2. The Kimray–Greenfield filter (1973)
3. The Hunter detachable balloon (1975).

A preliminary inferior vena cavogram is necessary to confirm patency, to demonstrate possible anomalies, and to show the level of the lowest renal vein. The device is passed down below the renal veins before being detached and stabilized. In some cases, filters can be introduced percutaneously from a femoral vein approach, e.g. the 'bird-nest filter' (Cook Inc.) devised by Roehm et al. This can be introduced through a sheath and an 8 French catheter. It consists of four stainless steel wires 0.18 mm wide and

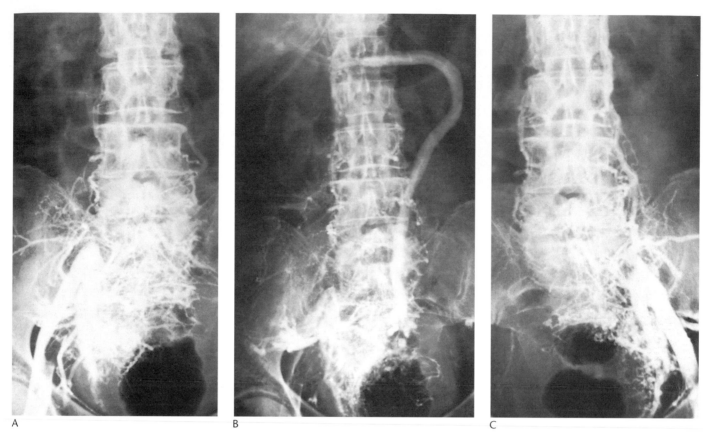

A   B   C

Fig. 26.15   A,B Thrombosis of the inferior vena cava and common iliacs. Collateral drainage from the right leg via internal iliacs and hemorrhoidal plexus → inferior mesenteric vein → portal vein. **C.** Same patient. Collateral drainage from the left leg mainly via ascending lumbar veins and vertebral venous plexus.

2.5 cm long. The filter has two fine wire hooks at each end which can be fixed to the caval wall. The whole procedure can be rapidly performed by a radiologist, but requires preliminary phlebography to ensure that the iliacs and inferior vena cava are free of clot.

There are now a wide variety of filters which can be introduced percutaneously from a transfemoral or transjugular approach, and these are listed in Chapter 25. Complications are also discussed in Chapter 25.

MISCELLANEOUS ABDOMINAL CONDITIONS

Vulval Varices   These are seen in pregnancy in 1 or 2% of patients, and persist in a small proportion, some of whom complain of discomfort requiring surgery. In some cases, phlebography by direct injection of the varix will be required to show the anatomy and drainage. This is mainly into the internal pudendal and obturator veins and thence to the internal iliac, but there may be partial drainage to the external pudendal and femoral veins.

Lymphedema Praecox   This was the term used for swelling of the left leg, usually occurring in young females and sometimes associated with partial obstruction of the left common iliac vein by the right common iliac artery passing over it (see Fig. 26.17A).

Pelvic Varicosities in the Uterovaginal Plexus   Also occurring in the broad ligament, these are said to be fairly common, and

have been cited as a cause of the *'pelvic congestion syndrome'*. They can also be associated with vulval varices. High-dose bilateral femoral phlebography with simultaneous compression of the inferior vena cava has been recommended to demonstrate these pelvic varicosities, but is not always successful.

Gonadal Veins (ovarian and testicular veins)   The right gonadal vein crosses in front of the ureter at the level of L4 as it passes up and medially to enter the inferior vena cava below the right renal vein. When hypertrophied, the ovarian vein can cause obstruction to the ureter, giving rise to the so-called *ovarian vein syndrome*. This remains a controversial subject, and the existence of this entity is not generally accepted.

The left gonadal vein usually drains into the left renal vein. Both gonadal veins can be demonstrated by passing a catheter into their upper ends from a transfemoral vein approach and injecting contrast medium. *Varicoceles,* which occur mainly on the left side, have been treated by percutaneous embolization of their drainage veins. Considerable success has been claimed for this procedure in the treatment of varicocele associated with male infertility. Another rare indication for the procedure is the localization of an *ectopic testis* which the non-invasive techniques of ultrasonography, CT and MRI have failed to locate.

Hepatic Vein Obstruction (Budd–Chiari syndrome)   Following the passage of a catheter into the upper part of the inferior vena cava, the hepatic veins can often be demonstrated by a forced

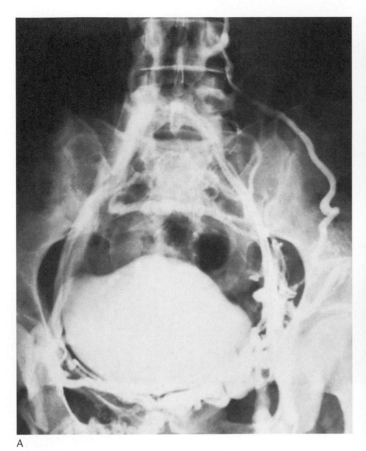
A

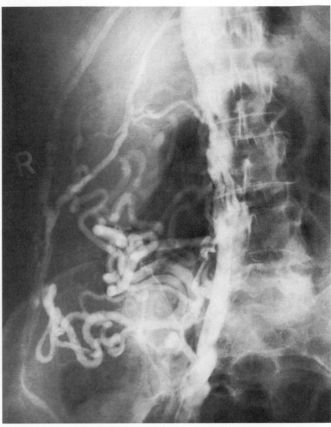
B

Fig. 26.16   **A**. Thrombosis of left iliac veins with partial recanalization and drainage of the left leg mainly by collaterals to the right iliacs via pubic veins. **B**. Thrombosis of the inferior vena cava with recanalization and collateral circulation.

injection of contrast medium, particularly if the patient performs the Valsalva maneuver during injection. Failure to fill the hepatic veins provides some evidence of thrombosis as occurs in Budd–Chiari syndrome. On inferior vena cavography, the upper inferior vena cava may be seen to be compressed or obstructed (Fig. 26.19) when a tumor is responsible.

Direct *hepatic phlebography* is performed by passing a catheter from the arm through the right auricle and into a hepatic vein. Alternatively a transfemoral vein approach is possible. In Budd–Chiari syndrome due to small-vessel disease the normal wedged hepatic vein pattern is replaced by fine collateral vessels ('spider's web network'), or actual occlusions may be shown (see Ch. 34—Figs 34.38 and 34.39).

Budd–Chiari syndrome is due to complete or partial obstruction of the venous drainage of the liver. This may be thrombotic or non thrombotic (Table 26.1), and may involve the small intrahepatic vessels, the main hepatic veins, or the intrahepatic and suprahepatic inferior vena cava, or combinations of all three. The clinical features include pain, hepatomegaly, ascites, and the development of portal hypertension and collateral circulation. Acute cases carry a high morbidity, and 86% die within 6 months unless successfully treated by surgery or interventional radiology (see Ch. 34). In Europe and North America the commonest type is idiopathic, while membranous occlusion of the vena cava (MOVC), though rare in the West, is common in Japan, Asia and South Africa. The diagnosis can be confirmed by ultrasound and/or

Table 26.1   Causes of Budd–Chiari syndrome

Thrombotic
  Idiopathic (primary veno-occlusive disease)
  Secondary to blood disorders
    Polycythemia rubra vera
    Other myeloproliferative conditions
    Paroxysmal nocturnal hemoglobinuria
    Contraceptive pill
  Post partum
  Liver abscess or other infections
  Antitumor and immuosuppressive drugs
  Graft-versus-host disease following bone marrow transplant
  Trauma

Non-thrombotic
  Tumor compression or invasion
  Congenital webs or membranous folds of the inferior vena cava
  or hepatic veins (MOVC)

phlebography. Color-coded duplex Doppler ultrasound is most helpful in assessing hepatic venous patency (see Ch. 34). The intra- and extrahepatic portal vein can be assessed at the same time for patency and direction of flow.

Surgical treatment in the past has been mainly by portosystemic shunting or by orthoptic liver transplantation. More recently, interventional radiology has provided less hazardous alternatives.

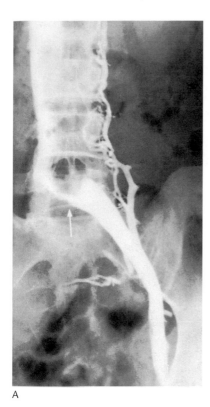
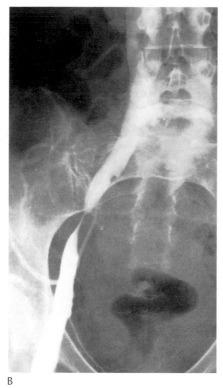
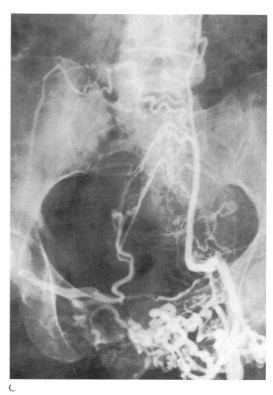

A   B   C

Fig. 26.17 **A**. Obstruction of the left common iliac vein by pressure from the right common iliac artery (arrow). Note collateral circulation via the ascending lumbar vein. **B**. Iliac vein obstruction by a glandular mass. **C**. Obstruction of the left iliac veins in a patient with carcinoma of the cervix treated by radiotherapy.

These include transfemoral thrombolysis via infusion of the hepatic artery in patients with acute venous thrombosis and normal hepatic function. In other cases, venous recanalization is attempted first by a transfemoral or transjugular approach, or, if this is not possible, by a transhepatic approach. Balloon dilatation and vein stenting can also be used if recanalization is successful, as can the TIPPS procedure. Balloon dilatation is also used with MOVC cases

Renal Phlebography The renal veins can be selectively catheterized using the Seldinger percutaneous technique. A forced injection of 10 ml of contrast medium will show the venous drainage of most of the kidney and will thus confirm or exclude a renal vein thrombosis.

The renal veins can also be shown by serial films taken after selective renal arteriography. The normal renal veins usually show well by this method. If they do not and a collateral venous drainage is also shown, this is good presumptive evidence of main renal vein occlusion.

It is important to realize that there may be more than one renal vein on either side, and attempts should always be made to identify and catheterize accessory veins. On the left side, 7% of individuals have a lower accessory vein which is smaller than the normal upper vein and is retroaortic in position. The two veins form a circumaortic ring with the lower one usually entering the inferior vena cava at L3–4 (Fig. 26.20).

Renal Vein Thrombosis This has also been investigated by inferior vena cavography. In the normal inferior vena cavagram, 'streamlining' effects are usually visible when the large renal

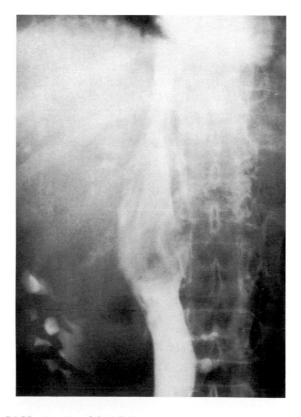

Fig. 26.18 Invasion of the inferior vena cava by hypernephroma spreading up the right renal vein.

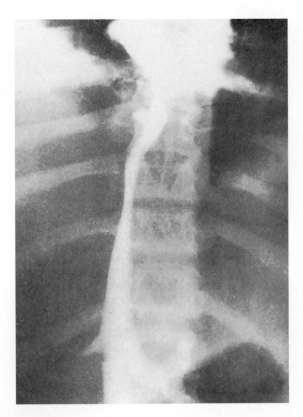

Fig. 26.19   Obstruction of hepatic veins with compression and distortion of the upper inferior vena cava by liver neoplasm resulting in Budd–Chiari syndrome. The patient was performing the Valsalva maneuver. Note reflux filling of the renal veins, but not hepatic veins.

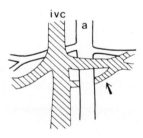

Fig. 26.20   Circumaortic ring formed by renal veins. a, aorta; IVC, inferior vena cava.

veins enter the inferior vena cava. Absence of this normal stream-lining effect is thought to be very suggestive of renal vein thrombosis, particularly when unilateral. Direct renal phlebography will prove the diagnosis conclusively.

Renal vein thrombosis is common in dehydrated infants with diarrhea. It also occurs in adults in association with inferior vena caval thrombosis, or thrombotic disease elsewhere. Occasionally, it is seen with pyelonephritis or other renal disease. The affected kidney is usually enlarged from venous engorgement, and the nephrotic syndrome may result. The vein itself is narrowed and irregular, and the small peripheral veins may be occluded.

As noted above, hypernephroma frequently involves the renal vein, and tumor may extend into the inferior vena cava (see Fig. 26.18). The renal vein may also be occluded or compressed by extrinsic tumor masses, by aneurysm, or by retroperitoneal fibrosis.

Renal Vein Renin   In cases of renal artery stenosis or suspected renal ischemia it is helpful to assay the renin in the renal venous blood from the suspected kidney. This is obtained by percutaneous catheterization of the renal veins using the Seldinger technique. Samples are obtained from an arm vein at the same time so that comparisons can be made with peripheral venous blood. A renal vein renin ratio greater than 1.5:1 is usually significant.

Adrenal Vein Phlebography   The adrenal veins can be selectively catheterized using special catheters. Small tumors have been demonstrated by this means when other methods have failed. In our experience the method has proved of most value in the diagnosis of small Conn's tumors in primary hyperaldosteronism. The method is discussed in greater detail in Chapter 36, but has now been superseded by CT. The technique is sometimes used for deliberate infarction of adrenal tumors.

UPPER LIMB AND SUPERIOR VENA CAVA

The usual indications for investigation of the venous drainage of the arm and superior vena cava are:

1. Edema of the upper limb thought to be associated with venous thrombosis or obstruction, in order to demonstrate the site of obstruction, in either the axillary, subclavian, or innominate veins
2. Superior vena caval obstruction
3. Demonstration of the full anatomy of venous angiomas or varices
4. Demonstration of congenital venous anomalies as in Klippel–Trenaunay syndrome.

Technique   A vein at the elbow is catheterized and a catheter advanced several centimeters up the arm. This can be done per-cutaneously in most cases, though occasionally a cut-down exposure may be necessary. It is best to use the median basilic vein, since this will make it possible to opacify the axillary vein. Use of the median cephalic vein will of course bypass the basilic and axillary veins, since the cephalic vein does not join the subclavian vein until it has pierced the clavipectoral fascia (Fig. 26.21).

Some 30 ml of contrast medium is injected within 2 s, using a pressure injector if necessary. A rapid rate of injection is essential, since otherwise the contrast will fail to show the superior vena cava well. It is rapidly diluted in the thorax by the large blood flow from the head and neck and contralateral upper limb.

Serial films are taken at speeds of one or two films per second.

Another technique which can be used where percutaneous puncture of an elbow vein proves difficult is similar to that used for ascending phlebography of the lower limb. A vein on the dorsum of the hand is percutaneously punctured with a fine needle of the type routinely used by anesthetists (SWG 21 or 23).

A tourniquet is applied just above the elbow, and some 30 ml of contrast medium injected. The tourniquet is then released, and the forearm massaged to ensure that a good bolus of contrast medium is delivered to the large veins in 2 s.

Radiographic Appearances   The normal findings are illustrated in Figure 26.22.

Left-sided superior vena cava is an important congenital anomaly in which the superior vena cava lies on the left and drains into the

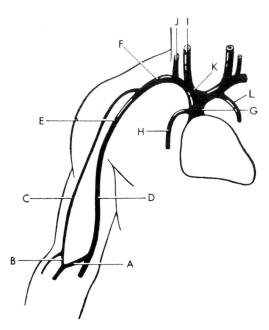

Fig. 26.21 Diagram showing venous drainage of the arm. A, median basilar vein; B, median cephalic vein; C, cephalic vein; D, basilic vein; E, axillary vein; F, subclavian vein; G, superior vena cava; H, azygos vein; I, internal jugular vein; J, external jugular vein; K, innominate vein; L, hemiazygos vein.

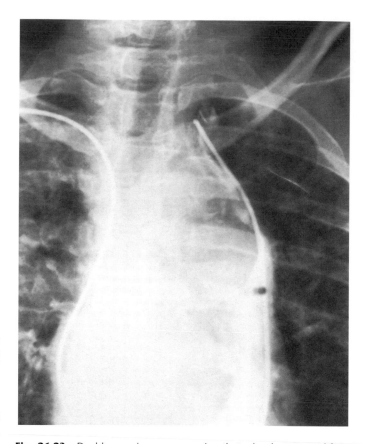

Fig. 26.23 Double superior vena cava. A catheter has been passed from the right arm for pulmonary angiography. Instead of entering the ventricle it has passed through the dilated coronary sinus and into the left superior vena cava draining into it, as evident on contrast injection. Note the widened mediastinum.

coronary sinus. It may occur alone or in association with congenital heart disease. Occasionally there is a *double superior vena cava*, the right draining normally to the right auricle, and the left into the coronary sinus (Fig. 26.23).

Where a localized thrombosis is present in a major drainage vein, such as the axillary or subclavian vein, the blockage is usually well shown, together with the collateral circulation which develops to bypass the lesion (Fig. 26.24).

Superior Vena Caval Obstruction This is characterized by venous engorgement of the head, neck, and arms. The involvement of the superior vena cava by malignant glands can be recognized well before clinical evidence of superior vena caval obstruction is seen. In these cases, extrinsic pressure defects on the vein will be seen. In the past, superior vena cavography has

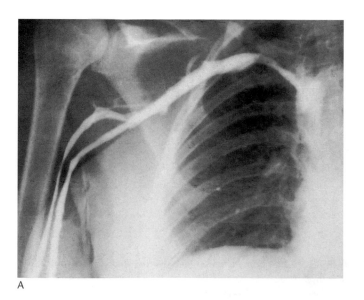

A

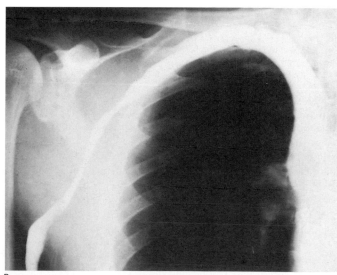

B

Fig. 26.22 **A.** Arm phlebogram showing normal appearances. **B.** Normal arm phlebogram (different case).

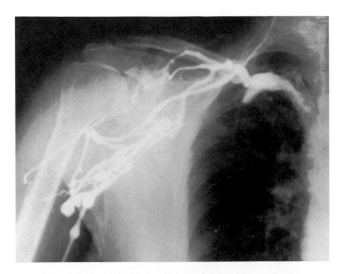

Fig. 26.24 Arm phlebogram showing obstruction in the axillary and subclavian veins.

been used to assess the suitability of cases of bronchial carcinoma for surgery, and to exclude clinically silent mediastinal glandular involvement. However, CT now provides a less invasive method of assessing mediastinal glandular involvement. Digital subtraction angiography will also enable the superior vena cava to be checked using only a small amount of low-concentration contrast medium. Radioisotope scanning can also confirm caval obstruction.

The majority of patients (over 95%) with superior vena caval obstruction are suffering from *malignant neoplasm* (Fig. 26.25). Of these, about 80% have carcinoma of the lung and about 20% are suffering from lymphomas.

The small group of patients with *benign* superior vena caval obstruction are usually suffering from *fibrosing mediastinitis* (Fig. 26.26). These patients present with a relatively slow onset, permitting the development of multiple collaterals. The etiology is either unknown (idiopathic) or it is granulomatous. In the UK the latter cases are usually *tuberculous*, but in North America *histoplasmosis* is also a cause of the syndrome. Very rarely, thrombosis of the superior vena cava is seen as a complication of ventriculoatrial shunts. Compression of the superior vena cava may also be occasionally seen with aneurysm and other non-malignant mediastinal masses.

Klippel–Trenaunay syndrome has been noted above. The appearances in the affected upper limb of a patient with this condition are illustrated in Figure 26.27. Multiple phleboliths were present in addition to the venous dysplasia.

PORTAL PHLEBOGRAPHY

Imaging of the portal system, which is illustrated diagrammatically in Figure 26.28A, is mainly requested in the investigation of portal hypertension and its complications. The causes of portal hypertension are listed in Table 26.2, and are usually classified into prehepatic, intrahepatic, and posthepatic obstruction to the portal circulation.

Imaging methods should be non-invasive where feasible (ultrasound, MRI) or minimally invasive (spiral CT), and the invasive techniques should only be used as a prelude to surgery or adjunct to interventional radiology (see Ch. 34) Figures 26.28B and 26.40 show patent portal veins imaged by spiral CT and MRI, respectively. Invasive techniques widely used in the past or currently available include:

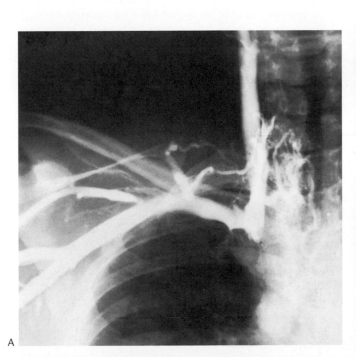

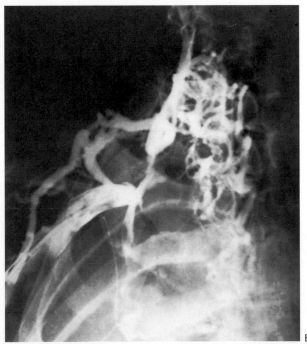

Fig. 26.25 **A**. Right arm phlebogram confirms malignant occlusion of the innominate and superior vena cava with reflux up the right internal jugular, and vertebral collaterals. **B**. Occlusion of the superior vena cava and innominate, and termination of the right subclavian vein. Collaterals are seen to the vertebral vein and vertebral plexus.

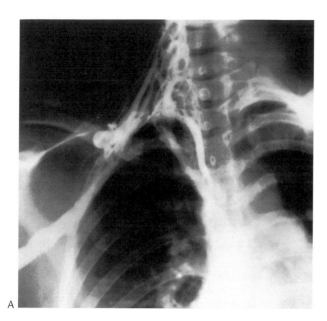

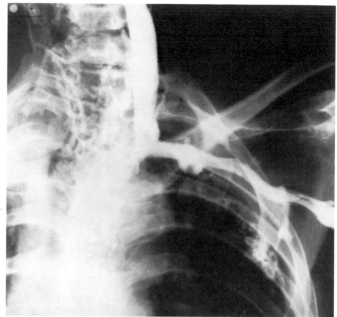

A   B

Fig. 26.26   **A**. Right arm phlebogram in fibrosing mediastinitis with involvement of the superior vena cava and the right innominate vein. **B**. Left arm phlebogram in a patient with fibrosing mediastinitis (tuberculous). Note the kinked trachea. The superior vena cava and left innominate are occluded. Collateral circulation via the left internal jugular and vertebral plexus.

1. Percutaneous splenic puncture
2. Operative mesenteric phlebography
3. Arterioportography
4. Transhepatic portal phlebography.

1. Percutaneous Splenic Puncture

This technique has been widely used in the past in the investigation of portal hypertension or suspected portal hypertension. It was also used in some cases of splenic enlargement where thrombosis in the splenic vein or portal system was thought to be a factor.

Table 26.2   Causes of portal hypertension

Prehepatic
    Portal vein thrombosis
    Portal vein compression by tumor or glandular mass
    Splenomegaly

Intrahepatic
    Cirrhosis
    Veno-occlusive disease
    Portal tract obstruction
        Parasites
        Lymphoma
        Myeloproliferative disorders
        Sarcoid
        Hepatitis
        Felty syndrome

Post-hepatic
    Budd–Chiari syndrome
    Constrictive pericarditis
    Cardiac failure

Technique   The usual landmark for percutaneous puncture of the spleen is in the 10th or 11th interspace in the mid-axillary line. The needle is passed inward and upward, and where the spleen is enlarged, puncture is fairly easy. Usually the needle point can be felt puncturing the splenic capsule, and once it is in the splenic pulp a backflow of blood into the connecting tubing takes place. If portal pressure is very high the reflux of blood may be at considerable pressure. It is possible to measure the intrasplenic pressure by attaching the connecting tubing to a manometer, and many workers practiced this routinely.

For the contrast injection, 20–50 ml of water-soluble iodide contrast medium is used.

Complications   Rupture of the spleen requiring splenectomy has been reported following the procedure. Therefore, unless laparotomy is to be proceeded with immediately after the splenic phlebogram, the patient should be carefully observed for a few days after the investigation for any sign of splenic rupture.

Occasionally the needle tip has been badly positioned and a major injection of contrast medium has been made into the subcapsular region of the spleen. Less commonly, injections have been made into the peritoneum, and even into the colon. Apart from localized pain, these accidents appear to have had no serious consequences.

Postoperative Splenic Phlebograms   These were occasionally performed to demonstrate the patency of a surgical anastomosis (Fig. 26.29).

Extrahepatic portal obstruction can result from tumors that are primary or secondary at the liver hilum. It can also result from portal vein thrombosis, and this can occur in cases of cirrhosis, as can splenic vein thrombosis. A thrombosed or partially thrombosed portal vein can result in the development of collateral veins (Fig. 26.30), a condition once thought to be congenital and termed

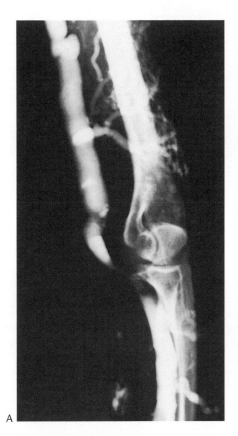

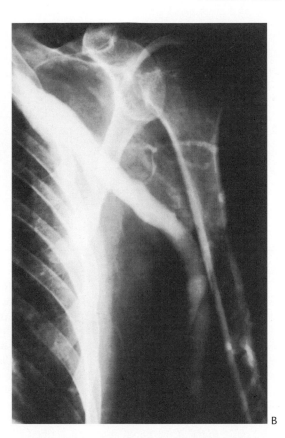

Fig. 26.27 Klippel–Trenaunay syndrome involving the left arm. Drainage is via a single medial vein which appears valveless with very sluggish flow.

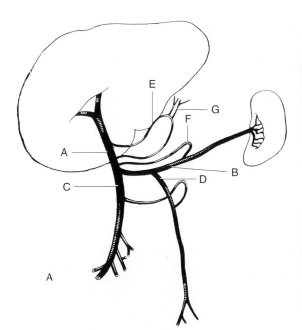

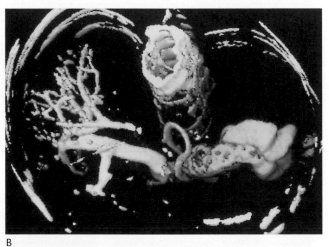

Fig. 26.28 **A**. Portal circulation. A, portal vein; B, splenic vein; C, superior mesenteric vein; D, inferior mesenteric vein; E, left gastric vein; F, gastroepiploic vein; G, esophageal vein. **B**. Spiral CT reconstruction showing a patent portal vein. (Courtesy of Dr A. Al-Kutoubi.)

'*cavernoma*' of the portal vein. It is thus clear that non-visualization of the portal vein at splenic phlebography can be due to several causes and does not exclude a diagnosis of cirrhosis.

It is also important to realize that the portal vein may occasionally fail to outline, even when patent, if there is a major

collateral circulation into which the splenic blood is being diverted. In these cases most of the portal blood is derived from the mesenteric circulation. Thus, where the portal vein failed to show at a splenic phlebogram, or where the splenic vein itself appeared obstructed, it was necessary to perform arterial portography or

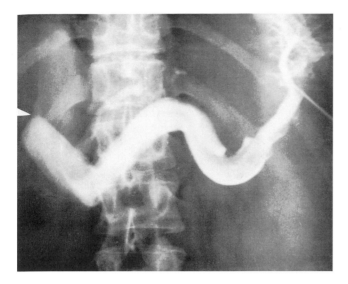

Fig. 26.29   Postoperative splenic phlebogram showing shunt of contrast from the portal vein into the inferior vena cava (arrow).

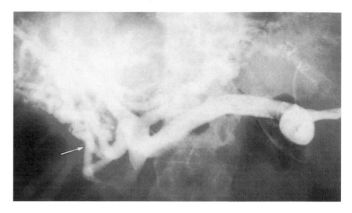

Fig. 26.30   Splenic phlebogram showing gastric varices. The portal vein is thrombosed and replaced by collaterals (arrow).

even an operative mesenteric phlebogram to decide whether or not the portal vein was patent (Fig. 26.31). This can now be done non invasively by ultrasound.

Umbilical sepsis in infants is another cause of portal vein thrombosis. Recanalization may follow, with a collateral circulation resulting in so-called cavernoma of the portal vein as described above.

Splenic phlebography has also been used in the past for demonstrating the morphology of the liver, in particular its vascular pattern in suspected neoplasms (both primary and secondary) and in cases of cirrhosis.

Radiological Appearances   In cases of portal hypertension due to cirrhosis of the liver or to posthepatic portal obstruction the splenic and portal veins are normally well demonstrated, the latter being large in caliber. The collateral circulation is usually well shown also, and where gastric or esophageal varices are present these can be clearly outlined (Fig. 26.32). In most cases, portal venography gives a better and more accurate demonstration of esophageal varices than does the simpler examination of barium swallow. Sometimes, however, cases occur with excellent demonstration of esophageal varices by barium swallow where these failed to show well at portal venography.

Distortion of the intrahepatic vascular pattern may be seen in cases of cirrhosis, but this can be difficult to interpret.

The widespread use of splenic venography in the past demonstrated the existence of numerous other collateral venous channels beside the well-recognized ones.

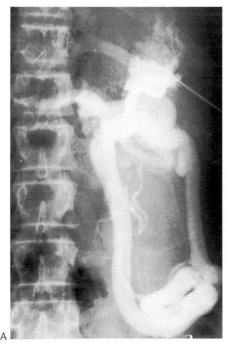

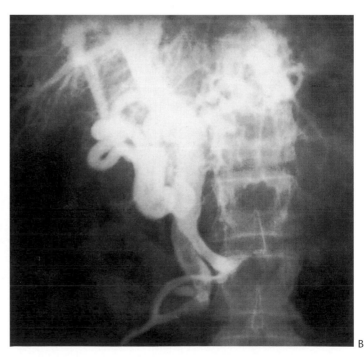

Fig. 26.31   **A**. Splenic phlebogram showing collateral circulation through a huge inferior mesenteric vein. The splenic vein was occluded distally. **B**. Operative superior mesenteric phlebogram showing a patent portal vein in the same case.

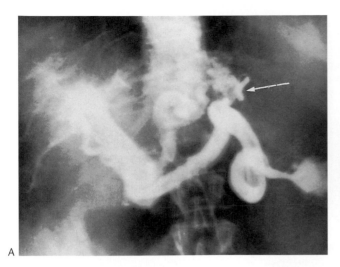
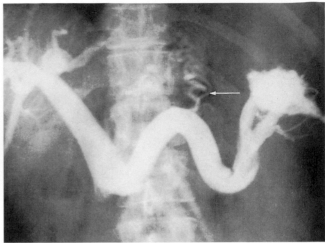

Fig. 26.32A,B   Splenic phlebograms showing gastric and esophageal varices. The portal vein is patent.

2. Operative Mesenteric Phlebography

In this method the portal system is demonstrated by injecting a mesenteric vein at laparotomy. As noted above, the technique was required in the past to prove patency of the portal vein where the findings by other techniques were inconclusive (Fig. 26.31). Today, Doppler ultrasound provides a simple non-invasive method of showing patency and direction of flow in the portal vein (see below).

Some early workers used the operative technique as a routine, but most preferred the percutaneous technique as the primary procedure.

3. Arterioportography

Advocates of this method prefer it because it obviates the dangers of direct splenic puncture and because the information obtained comprises both arterial and venous phases and can show the whole portal system. It can also contribute to the planning of shunt surgery. The normal technique is to catheterize the celiac axis and then inject from a superselective position of the catheter tip in the splenic artery. A 30–60 ml volume of contrast medium is injected at a rate of 10 ml/s, and serial films obtained in the arterial and venous phase. If the patient's condition permits, the common hepatic artery can also be injected to show the state of the liver and pancreas, with late films to demonstrate any possible hepaticofugal flow in the portal veins. If required, the left gastric artery can be injected to show varices and the superior mesenteric artery can also be injected to demonstrate the superior mesenteric vein. It may be essential to show this if mesocaval shunting is being considered.

There is no doubt that thorough arterioportography provides more information than simple splenic phlebography, but it can be a more prolonged and technically difficult procedure than simple direct splenic phlebography. It also requires good-quality subtraction films to show the portal circulation well (Fig. 26.33). Even with these, definition is never as clear as with the direct splenic method.

Digital subtraction angiography considerably improves the definition of arterioportography. It also permits adequate visualization with much smaller doses of contrast medium.

4. Transhepatic Portal Phlebography

The main collateral venous supply of gastroesophageal varices may be visualized by percutaneous transhepatic catheterization of the portal vein (Fig. 26.34). Apart from being demonstrated by injection through the percutaneous catheter, the varices can be selectively catheterized and obliterated by embolization. The major indication was severe cirrhosis in patients in whom surgery was contraindicated. After successful obliteration of varices, surgery may be performed electively or deferred.

The method of transhepatic portal phlebography has also been used for the purpose of obtaining venous samples for assay from the pancreatic drainage veins into the splenic and superior mesenteric veins. These assays are helpful in the localization of pancreatic hormone-producing tumors. The method is discussed in greater detail in Chapter 35.

DOPPLER ULTRASOUND AND THE PERIPHERAL VEINS

P. L. Allan

The indications for venous ultrasound include the diagnosis or exclusion of DVT, the assessment of chronic venous insufficiency, mapping of veins to be used in graft procedures, and locating veins for central line insertion.

Deep Vein Thrombosis

Three aspects of the ultrasound examination are used in the diagnosis of DVT: compressibility of the vein; flow on Doppler ultrasound; and visible thrombus in the lumen. A normal vein is compressible so that the lumen is obliterated with only light or moderate pressure from the transducer (Fig. 26.35), whereas thrombus will hold the vein walls apart; care must be taken as fresh thrombus is partially compressible and may be overlooked. Normally flow in the lower limb veins is spontaneous, showing respiratory variation, and a quick squeeze of the calf muscles, or getting the patient to plantar flex his or her foot, should result in a

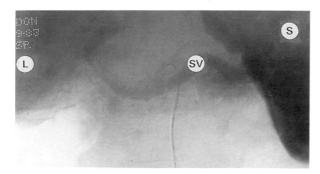

Fig. 26.33 Arterioportography—subtraction film. Venous phase of selective splenic angiogram. The portal vein is compressed by a mass of malignant glands. The spleen is grossly enlarged. SV, splenic vein; L, liver; S, spleen. (Courtesy of Dr Janet Murfitt.)

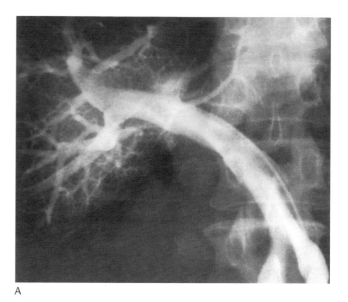

A

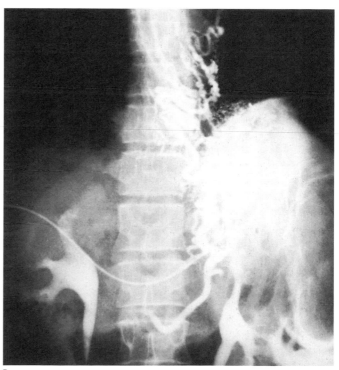

B

Fig. 26.34 **A**. Transhepatic portal phlebogram showing the main portal vein and mesenteric tributaries. (Courtesy of Dr Janet Murfitt). **B**. Gastric and esophageal varices demonstrated by transhepatic portal vein catheterization.

rapid, brief augmentation of the flow. In the presence of thrombus there will be no flow in the thrombosed segment; if there is segmental thrombus elsewhere in the main veins of the limb, then augmentation will be damped, and proximal thrombus will remove the respiratory variations normally seen in patent veins. The normal vein lumen should be anechoic and color Doppler ultrasound, or power Doppler ultrasound, should show complete fill-in across the lumen of the vein. Fresh thrombus is relatively anechoic and tends to expand the vein lumen slightly. As it matures it contracts and becomes increasingly echogenic (Fig. 26.36). Following DVT the veins usually recanalize, but they may remain occluded with collaterals forming around the occluded segment. The vein lumen may clear completely but residual wall thickening and irregularity may persist.

An advantage of ultrasound is that it may show causes for the patient's symptoms other than DVT, such as ruptured popliteal cysts, muscle hematoma, or superficial thrombophlebitis; it can also show pelvic masses which may have predisposed the patient to develop a DVT. Problems can occur if visualization of the veins is poor, as may well be the case in obese or edematous legs. Approximately 15% of the population have a dual segment of superficial femoral vein, which may cause problems if one component is thrombosed while the other is patent and the situation is not recognized (Fig. 26.37). Non-occlusive thrombus may also be missed if the failure of the color signal to fill the lumen is not appreciated. In the later stages of pregnancy the enlarging uterus may compress the iliac veins in the supine position and therefore affect the flow in the leg veins; this problem can be overcome if the patient is examined in the decubitus, or vertical position, when the uterus will be shifted off the iliac vein. If there is doubt about a segment of vein a venogram can be arranged, or a repeat scan performed 2–3 days later in order to see if any thrombus has extended from an occult point of origin into the larger, proximal veins.

Providing care and attention is taken with the examination, ultrasound has been shown to be highly accurate in the diagnosis of symptomatic DVT, with a sensitivity and specificity of over 95 and 100%, respectively, for proximal thrombus in the common femoral, superficial femoral, and popliteal veins. Flow can usually be demonstrated in the major calf veins, if these are patent. However, it is more difficult to exclude reliably small segmental calf vein thrombi, or thrombi in the muscle venous sinuses. Ultra-

sound has a sensitivity of only 60% for asymptomatic thrombus. This is not usually a problem as ultrasound can provide a clear positive or negative result in 80–85% of cases. If there is a problem area, then subsequent venography can concentrate on the particular segment concerned. In many hospitals, ultrasound has become the primary examination for the confirmation or exclusion of DVT, with venography being reserved for those cases where ultrasound does not give sufficient information for management decisions.

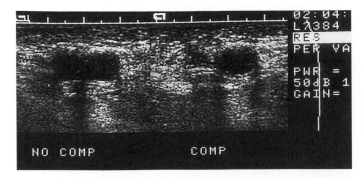

Fig. 26.35 Normal compression of the left common femoral vein. The vein is seen in the left image on the left side of the artery. On compression the vein lumen disappears and only the vein walls are visible.

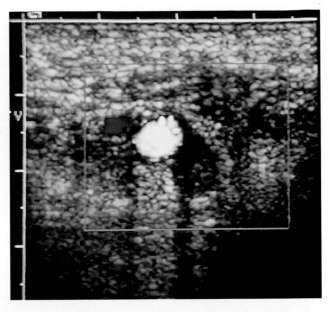

Fig. 26.37 Transverse view of the superficial femoral vessels. The artery is seen in the middle with a patent vein on the left but a thrombosed vein on the right.

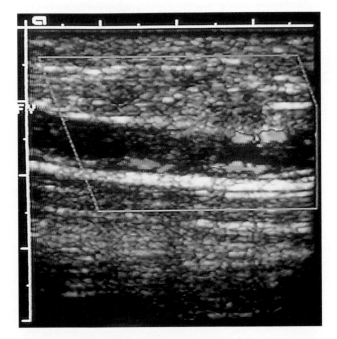

Fig. 26.36 Moderately echogenic thrombus in a superficial femoral vein. A small amount of blood flow is seen posteriorly.

Varicose Veins and Chronic Venous Insufficiency

Varicose veins are a common problem, and color Doppler ultrasound is not usually required in the diagnosis, unless there is a possibility of previous DVT damaging the deep veins, in which case removal of the superficial veins may have a major effect on the venous drainage of the limb. Most cases of primary varicose veins will be sorted out using hand-held continuous-wave Doppler ultrasound in the vascular clinic, but some patients may have atypical anatomy with unusual locations for the saphenopopliteal and saphenofemoral junctions; color and power Doppler techniques can rapidly clarify these situations.

Recurrent Varicose Veins These may show one of three patterns of recurrence: the saphenofemoral junction appears intact, suggesting that the original operation was inadequate; it may be abnormal in shape (Fig. 26.38) or show collaterals linking the saphenous vein below the point of surgical interruption to the common femoral vein; or there may be collaterals draining into other veins in the pelvis, perineum, or around the hip and buttock. Color Doppler ultrasound will allow these channels to be identified and the patterns of reflux established so that appropriate surgery can be planned.

Chronic Venous Insufficiency This can develop after DVT, or without any history of previous thrombosis. In this condition the venous valves are damaged; this leads to venous reflux, stasis, and increased hydrostatic pressure in the tissues of the lower limb. This results in leg swelling, skin changes, and ulceration. Patients are examined standing in order to demonstrate the reflux. Manual compression of the calf forces blood up the veins and, if the valves in any particular segment are incompetent, the blood subsequently falls back; this effect is seen on color Doppler ultrasound as a change of the color image from one color to the opposite color (Fig. 26.38), or on spectral Doppler ultrasound as flow above and below the baseline. A little reflux of short duration (< 0.5 s) is not significant, but more persistent reflux should be noted and the pattern of incompetent segments explored; in addition to the superficial and deep-vein systems, incompetent perforator veins linking these may be seen. Other methods of inducing reflux include pneumatic pressure cuffs and getting the patient to perform a Valsalva maneuver.

Saphenous Vein Mapping The long saphenous vein is frequently used as a conduit for bypass operations, usually for coronary artery or lower-limb arterial bypass. If there is any doubt about the suitability of one or both veins they can be examined using color Doppler ultrasound so that the length and caliber of suitable segments can be assessed. The course of the vein is marked out with an indelible marker pen, and sites of major branches and perforators indicated; this is particularly important if an in situ femoral bypass graft is being considered as arteriovenous shunts will result if any connections are left intact. The vein should be at

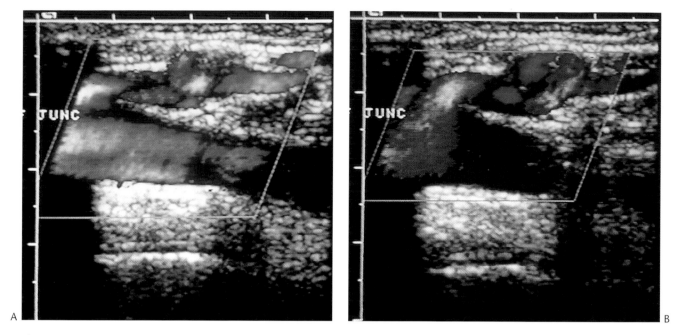

Fig. 26.38 **A**. The left sapheno femoral junction in a patient with recurrent varicose veins and reflux. The long saphenous vein is irregular, compatible with recanalization after surgery, **B** and the color flow shows reversal of colors after augmentation.

least 4 mm in minimum diameter for most of its length, but must be at least 2 mm at the ankle if a long femorodistal graft is being planned. The measurements are best done with the patient standing in order to obtain maximum distension; in addition, care should be taken not to compress the vein with the transducer.

MRI OF VEINS

Jeremy P. R. Jenkins

An understanding of the flow phenomena and MRI methodology (given in detail in Ch. 25) are applicable to the MRI study of veins. The detection and assessment of venous obstruction or thrombus is an accepted MRI technique. Thrombi in abdominal and pelvic veins can be identified on T_1- and T_2-weighted spin echo sequences (Fig. 26.39). Phlebograms, using magnetic resonance angiography (MRA) techniques, can be used to assess the deep-venous system, but are more time-consuming and often add little information compared with standard spin echo and gradient echo techniques.

A number of MRI studies in the assessment of **DVT** of the *pelvis* and *lower extremities* have shown a high sensitivity and specificity (greater than 95%) in the detection of thrombus, equivalent to that of X-ray phlebography. An advantage of MRI over X-ray phlebography is in the demonstration of thrombus within deep pelvic veins, a location where phlebography and ultrasound are ineffective. There are, however, problems with MRI in differentiating turbulent flow from thrombus. Also lack of visualization of a vein is not sufficient to diagnose an acute thrombosis, as an adjacent mass can produce venous compression without intraluminal thrombus. Phlebography remains the standard technique in the demonstration of calf DVT. MRI can, however,

identify other lesions which mimic the symptoms of a DVT such as calf hematoma, ruptured popliteal cyst, or compartment syndrome.

The presence of acute thrombus on gradient echo sequences results in a filling defect with low to almost absent signal intensity. The vessel is distended with thrombus, and there may be some high signal from flowing blood surrounding a portion of the thrombus. On spin echo imaging, an acute thrombus shows signal intensity where normally there should be a signal void (Fig. 26.39). The distinction between acute and chronic thrombus can be difficult, although a homogeneous signal is indicative of an acute clot; heterogeneity in appearance with a lower peripheral and higher central signal is in keeping with thrombus of greater age. Non-visualization of the vein, small lumen, or an irregular wall thickening in conjunction with prominent collateral vessels suggests a chronic DVT.

Improved visualization of the *calf veins* on MRI can be achieved in the majority of individuals by utilizing mechanical flow-enhancing measures. Magnetic resonance venography of the calf can be performed with the placement of a tourniquet around the thigh which, when subsequently released and combined with termination of a Valsalva maneuver by the patient, results in a transient increase in venous blood flow in the leg. Due to its expense and limited availability, MRI is unlikely to become the primary means of assessing DVT in the near future. In those individuals who are allergic to iodinated contrast medium or with limited venous access, Doppler ultrasound is recommended if the region of clinical suspicion is in the thigh. If it is suspected that a pelvic or calf vein thrombosis or other lesion is the cause of the patient's symptoms, then MRI is an alternative technique.

In the assessment of abdominal vessels there are technical difficulties due to respiratory motion with resultant reduced signal-to-noise ratio. For venous imaging, two-dimensional *time-*

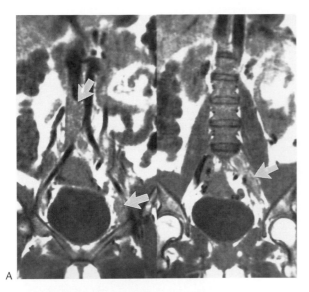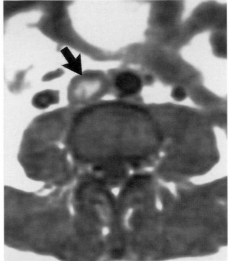

Fig. 26.39 Acute thrombosis (arrowed) within the inferior vena cava and left iliac veins on **A** coronal and **B** transverse T$_1$-weighted spin echo images (SE 560/25).

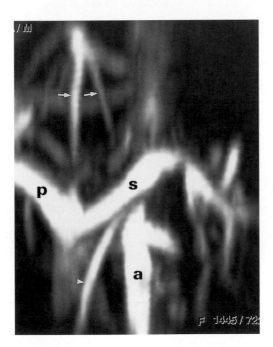

Fig. 26.40 Coronal plane maximum intensity projection (MIP) of a 2D phase-contrast MR angiogram showing normal hepatic veins (short arrows). p, portal vein; s, splenic vein; a, aorta; arrowhead, superior mesenteric artery.

of-flight angiography has advantages over *phase contrast* angiography in terms of speed and flexibility. Sequential two-dimensional *time-of-flight* imaging can be used to acquire several overlapping slices in the same breath-hold. Improved signal-to-noise and spatial resolution can also be achieved by the use of a torso array coil.

MRA is an accurate and reproducible technique for imaging the *portal vein*. The main indications for imaging are to confirm patency, show thrombus, or detect tumor invasion of the portal vein, and, in portal hypertension, to show patency of the porto-systemic shunts, varices, and collateral vessels. The presence and age of thrombus can be assessed by routine spin echo imaging as indicated above. Thrombus and tumor can be differentiated by the use of gadolinium-chelate injection. MRA, with its wide field of view, has a particular advantage over Doppler ultrasound in depicting varices and portosystemic vessels in patients with portal hypertension, which is important information in the surgical planning prior to liver transplantation. Not only can MRI provide information relating to the vascular anatomy, patency, and anomalies but it can show the hepatic parenchyma and surrounding tissues using conventional sequences.

The *major hepatic veins* are well visualized on MRA (Fig. 26.40). In liver cirrhosis the inferior vena cava and hepatic veins can appear compressed and distorted, producing a similar picture on MRA as occurs in Budd–Chiari syndrome. Comma-shaped collateral vessels which produce a 'spider-web' appearance of the collateral vessels around the obstructed vein, as depicted on X-ray contrast venography, can be demonstrated on MRA, and is suggestive of Budd–Chiari syndrome rather than cirrhosis.

MRI has been shown to be useful in assessing the patency of the thoracic inlet and mediastinal venous system. *Superior vena caval obstruction* or patients with unilateral upper extremity swelling and pain can be assessed with spin echo and gradient echo techniques with advantages over contrast-enhanced CT. Results relating to the assessment of the subclavian vein have been more variable, but the advent of newer machines with improved off-axis imaging and higher spatial resolution should improve its diagnostic value here.

REFERENCES AND SUGGESTIONS FOR FURTHER READING (Chapters 25 and 26)

References of historical interest

Berberich, J., Hirsch, S. (1923) Die roentgenographische Darstellung der Arterien und Venen am lebenden Menschen. *Klinische Wochenschrift*, pp. 2226–2228.

Brooks, B. (1924) Intra-arterial injection of sodium iodide. *Journal of the American Medical Association*, **82**, 1016–1019.

Doby, T. (1976) *Development of Angiography*. Littleton, MA: Publishing Sciences Group.

Dos Santos, R., Lamas, A. C., Caldas, J. P. (1931) *Arteriographie des Membres et de la Aorte Abdominale*. Paris: Masson.

Farinas, P. L. (1941) A new technique for the arteriographic examination of the abdominal aorta and its branches. *American Journal of Roentgenology*, **46**, 641–645.

Forssman, W. (1929) Die Sondierung der rechten Herzens. *Klinische Wochenschrift*, **8**, 2087–2089.

Gruntzig, A. (1978) Transluminal dilatation of coronary artery stenosis. *Lancet*, **i**, 263.

Gruntzig, A. et al (1978) Treatment of renovascular hypertension with percutaneous transluminal dilatation of a renal artery stenosis. *Lancet*, **i**, 801.

Haschek, E., Lindenthal, T. O. (1896) Ein Beitrag zur praktischen Verwerthung der Photographie nach Röntgen. *Wiener Klinische Wochenschrift*, **9**, 63–64.

Moniz, E. (1931) *Diagnostic des Tumeurs Cérébrals et Epreuve de l'Encephalographie Artérielle*. Paris: Masson.

Orrin, H. C. (1920) *X-ray-Atlas of the Systemic Arteries of the Human Body*. London: Baillière Tindall & Cox.

Seldinger, S. (1953) Catheter replacement of the needle in percutaneous arteriography. *Acta Radiologica*, **39**, 368–376.

Serbinenko, F. A. (1974) Balloon catheterization and occlusion of major cerebral vessels. *Journal of Neurosurgery*, **41**, 125–145.

Sicard, J. A., Forestier, J. (1923) Injections intravasculaires d'huile iodée Sous contrôle radiologique. *Comptes Rendus de la Société de Biologie*, **88**, 1200.

Sicard, J. A., Forestier, J. (1932) *The Use of Lipiodol in Diagnosis and Treatment*. London: Oxford University Press.

Sutton, D. (1962) *Arteriography*. Edinburgh: Livingstone.

References

Abrams, H. L. (ed.) (1997) *Angiography*, 4th edn. Boston: Little Brown.

Ansell, G., Wilkins, R. A. (Eds). 1996 *Complications in Diagnostic Radiology*, 3rd edn. Oxford: Blackwell.

Bell, A. M., Cumberland, D. C. (1989) Percutaneous atherectomy. *Clinical Radiology*, **40**, 122–126.

Bluth, E. I., Stavros, A. T., Marich, K. W. et al (1988) Carotid Duplex Sonography: a multicenter recommendation for standardized imaging and Doppler criteria. *Radiographics*, **8**, 487.

Carr, D. H. (Ed.) (1988) *Contrast Media*. Edinburgh: Churchill Livingstone.

Chuang, V. P., Wallace, S. (1981) Hepatic artery embolization in the treatment of hepatic neoplasms. *Radiology*, **140**, 51–58.

Debrun, G., Legre, J., Kasbarian, M. et al (1979) Endovascular occlusion of vertebral fistulae by detachable balloons with conservation of vertebral blood flow. *Radiology*, **130**, 141–147.

Ekelund, L., Gerlock, J., Ogoncharenko, V. (1978) The epinephrine effect in reneal angiography revisited. *Clinical Radiology*, **29**, 387–392.

Gregson, R. H. S., Sutton, D., Brennan, J. et al (1983) Spontaneous aortocaval fistula. *Clinical Radiology*, **34**, 683–687.

Henderson, M. J., Manhire, A. R. (1990) Cholesterol embolisation following angiography. *Clinical Radiology*, **42**, 281–282.

Herlinger, H. (1978) Arterioportography. *Clinical Radiology*, **29**, 255–275.

Hill, S., Billings, P. J., Walker, R. T. et al (1990) True spontaneous rupture of the common iliac vein. *Journal of the Royal Society of Medicine*, **83**, 117.

Hobbs, J. T. (ed.) (1977) *The Treatment of Venous Disorders*. Philadelphia: Lippincott.

Hughes, J. P., Stovin P. G. I. (1959) Segmental pulmonary aneurysms with peripheral deep vein thrombosis. *British Journal of Diseases of the Chest*, **531**, 19–27.

Lang, E. K. (1981) Transcatheter embolization of pelvic vessels for control of intractable haemorrhage. *Clinical Radiology*, **35**, 85–93.

Lea Thomas, M. (1982) *Phlebography of the Lower Limb*. Edinburgh: Churchill Livingstone.

Lee, P. H., Kellet, M. J., Bailey, J., Prior, J. P. (1996) Klippel Trenaunay syndrome as a cause of erectile dysfunction. *Clinical Radiology*, **51**, 596–597.

Lunderquist, A., Vang, J. (1974) Transhepatic catheterization and obliteration of the coronary vein in patients with portal hypertension and oesophageal varices. *New England Journal of Medicine*, **291**, 646–649.

Mandell, V. S. et al (1985) Persistent sciatic artery. *American Journal of Roentgenology*, **144**, 245–249.

Miller, D. C., Stinson, E. G., Oyer, P. E. et al (1979) Operative treatment of aortic dissections: experience with 125 patients. *Journal of Thoracic and Cardiovascular Surgery*, **78**, 365.

O'Halpin, D., Legge, D., MacErlain, D. P. (1984) Therapeutic arterial embolisation: report of five years experience. *Clinical Radiology*, **35**, 85–93.

Royal, S. A., Callen, P. W. (1979) CT evaluation of anomalies of the IVC and left renal vein. *American Journal of Roentgenology*, **132**, 759–763.

Starnes, H. F., Vallance, R., Hamilton, D. N. H. (1984) Recurrent varicose veins: a radiological approach to investigation. *Clinical Radiology*, **35**, 95–99.

Thomas, E. A., Cobby, M. J. D., Rhys Davies, E. et al (1989) Liquid crystal thermography and C-reactive protein in detection of deep venous thrombosis. *British Medical Journal*, **299**, 951–952.

Thorogood, S. V., Maskell, G. F. (1996) Case report: intravascular lipoma of the superior vena cava. *British Journal of Radiology*, **69**, 963–964.

Viamonte, M., Jr, Pereiras, R., Russell, E., Le Page, J., Hudson, D. (1977) Transhepatic obliteration of gastro-oesophageal varices. *American Journal of Roentgenology*, **129**, 237–241.

Wallace, S., Chuang, V. P., Swanson, D. et al (1981) Embolization of renal carcinomas: experience with 100 patients. *Radiology*, **138**, 563–570.

Wells, I. P., Hammonds, J. C., Franklin, K. (1983) Embolization of hypernephromas: a simple technique using ethanol. *Clinical Radiology*, **34**, 689–692.

Whitehouse, G. H. (1990) Venous thrombosis and thrombo-embolisms. *Clinical Radiology*, **41**, 77–80.

Wilbur, A. C., Woelfel, G. F., Meyer, J. P., Flanigan, D. P., Spigos, D. G. (1985) Adventitial cystic disease of the popliteal artery. *Radiology*, **155**, 63–64.

Ultrasound

Strandness, D. E., Jr (1993) *Duplex Scanning in Vascular Disorders*, 2nd edn. New York: Raven Press.

Taylor, K. J. W., Burns, P. N., Wells, P. N. T. (eds) (1995) *Clinical Applications of Doppler Ultrasound*, 2nd edn. New York: Raven Press.

Wolff, K. J., Fobbe, F. (eds) (1995) *Color Duplex Sonography: Principles and Clinical Applications*. Stuttgart: Georg Thieme.

MRI: arteries

Carr, J. J., Hatabu, H., Gefter, W. B. (1996) Thorax. In Edelman, R. E., Hesselink, J. R., Zlatkin, M. B. (eds) *Clinical Magnetic Resonance Imaging*, 2nd edn, ch. 52, pp. 1615–1682. Philadelphia: Saunders.

Chien, D., Anderson, C. M., Lee, R. E. (1996) MR angiography: basic principles. In Edelman, R. E., Hesselink, J. R., Zlatkin, M. B. (eds). *Clinical Magnetic Resonance Imaging*, 2nd edn, ch. 9, pp. 271–301. Philadelphia: Saunders.

Deutsch, H. J., Sechtem, U., Meyer, H., Theissen, P., Schicha, H., Erdmann, E. (1994) Chronic aortic dissection: comparison of MR imaging and transoesophageal echocardiography. *Radiology*, **192**, 645–650.

Finn, J. P. (ed.) (1993) Magnetic resonance angiography of the body. *Magnetic Resonance Imaging Clinics of North America*, **1**, 203–376.

Fischer, U., Vosshenrich, R., Kopka, L., Keating, D., Oestmann, J. W., Grabbe, E. (1994) Dissection of the thoracic aorta: pre- and postoperative findings on turbo-FLASH MR images obtained in the plane of the aortic arch. *American Journal of Roentgenology*, **163**, 1069–1072.

Gedroyc, W. M. (1994) Magnetic resonance angiography of renal arteries. *Urologic Clinics of North America*, **21**, 201–214.

Hartnell, G. G., Finn, J. P., Zenni, M. et al (1994) MR imaging of the thoracic aorta: comparison of spin-echo, angiographic and breath-hold techiques. *Radiology*, **191**, 697–704.

Loubeyre, P., Trolliet, P., Cahen, R., Grozel, F., Labeeuw, M., Minh, V. (1996) MR angiography of renal artery stenosis: value of the combination of three-dimensional time-of-flight and three-dimensional phase-contrast MR angiography sequences. *American Journal of Roentgenology*, **167**, 489–494.

Masaryk, T. J., Lewin, J. S., Lamb, G. (1992) Magnetic resonance angiography. In Stark, D. D., Bradley, W. G. (eds) *Magnetic Resonance Imaging*, 2nd edn, ch. 12, pp. 299–334. St Louis: Mosby.

Mitchell, L., Jenkins, J. P. R., Brownlee, W. C., Isherwood, I. (1988) Case report: Aortic dissection: morphology and differential flow patterns demonstrated by magnetic resonance imaging. *Clinical Radiology*, **39**, 458–465.

Prince, M. R. (1994) Gadolinium-enhanced MR aortography. *Radiology*, **191**, 155–164.

Ros, P. R., Bidgood, W. D. (1993) Magnetic resonance angiography. *Abdominal Magnetic Resonance Imaging*, Ch. 7 pp 134–162. St Louis: Mosby.

Sheppard, S. (1995) Basic concepts in magnetic resonance angiography (1995) *Radiologic Clinics of North America*, **33**, 91–113.

MRI: veins

Hartnell, G. G. (1993) Magnetic resonance imaging of systemic thoracic and abdominal veins. *Magnetic Resonance Imaging Clinics of North America*, **1**, 281–294.

Holtz, D. J. et al. (1996) MR venography of the calf: value of flow-enhanced time-of-flight echoplanar imaging. *American Journal of Roentgenology*, **166**, 663–668.

Spritzer, C. E. (1993) Venography of the extremities and pelvis. *Magnetic Resonance Imaging Clinics of North America*, **1**, 239–251.

Whitehouse, G. H. (1990) Editorial—venous thrombosis and thromboembolism. *Clinical Radiology*, **41**, 77–80.

27

THE LYMPHATIC SYSTEM

Graham Cherryman

In this Chapter the structure, function, and methods of imaging the lymphatic system are discussed. Benign and malignant conditions affecting the lymphatic system are reviewed, with the emphasis on the lymphomas.

STRUCTURE AND FUNCTION

The presence of a functioning lymphatic system is essential to health. The lymphatic system consists of a network of lymphatic capillaries that commence in the body tissues, freely anastomose and eventually drain back into the venous system via larger lymphatic trunks. There are lymphatics within most body tissues, although lymphatic capillaries are not found in avascular tissues such as articular cartilage. They are also not present in brain, spinal cord, bone marrow, and splenic pulp. Within these tissues there are microscopic clefts that have a similar function to lymphatics but, in contrast to lymphatic capillaries, lack an endothelial lining.

The characteristic endothelial wall seen in lymphatic capillaries is permeable to larger molecules than can pass through the endothelial lining of vascular capillaries. This allows the lymphatic system to absorb proteins and particulate matter including cell debris and micro-organisms as well as excess extracellular tissue fluid. The lymphatics draining the gut are also known as lacteals. Following a meal the lymph (chyle) within these gut lymphatics appears milky white due to the presence of fat chylomicrons being transported away from the gut wall.

In the body the larger lymphatic trunks accompany the arteries and veins. Almost all lymph in the body eventually passes into the thorax and re-enters the vascular space through either the thoracic duct or the right lymphatic duct. In the retroperitoneum the para-aortic lymphatic trunks empty into the cisterna chyli at the level of the second lumbar vertebra. The cisterna chyli may be recognized on CT sections (Fig. 27.1). Typically the cisterna chyli is a saccular structure about 5 cm long, passing up through the diaphragm to become the thoracic duct, which is smaller in diameter than the cisterna chyli and not normally identified on CT

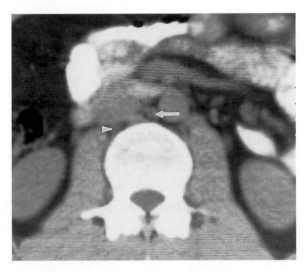

Fig. 27.1 CT section through the upper abdomen of a young male patient shows the cisterna chyli as a small (0.5 cm) low-attenuation structure lying between the aorta and inferior vena cava (arrow). The cisterna chyli may be seen on CT examination in almost all patients providing there is sufficient retroperitoneal fat. A smaller lymphatic duct may be seen behind the inferior vena cava (arrowhead).

examination. The thoracic duct may opacify after lymphography (Fig. 27.2).

The thoracic duct receives all the lymph flow from below the diaphragm as well as that from the left side of the thorax and neck. Typically the thoracic duct terminates by anastomosing with the left subclavian vein. On the right a smaller right lymphatic trunk drains lymph from the right side of the thorax and neck into the right subclavian vein. There are a number of variations in the anatomy of the larger lymphatic ducts.

The typical appearance of peripheral lymphatics at lymphography shows the arrangement of valves allowing movement of lymph in one direction only (Fig. 27.3). Lymph is propelled through the lymphatic system by the combination of filtration pressure

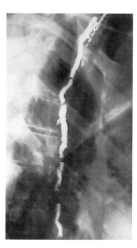

Fig. 27.2   Early phase lymphogram film with contrast medium outlining the thoracic duct.

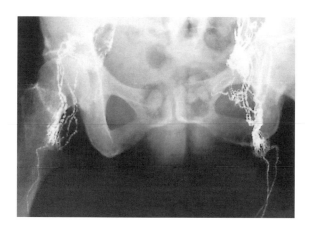

Fig. 27.3   An early phase lymphogram film showing the arrangement of valves in the lymphatic vessels.

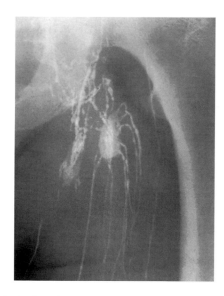

Fig. 27.4   Early phase lymphogram film with opacification of both lymph nodes and lymph vessels. There are several afferent lymphatics feeding into each lymph node. The single efferent lymphatic always leaves the lymph node through the hilum.

in the interstitial spaces, movement of the limbs and muscles, and the contraction of the smooth muscle fibers found within the wall of the larger lymphatic trunks.

Lymph from almost all parts of the body traverses one or more lymph nodes before reaching the venous circulation. Lymph nodes are encapsulated aggregates of lymphatic tissue, normally small and bean-shaped and situated in the path of the lymphatic vessels (Fig. 27.4). The outer surface of the lymph node is covered by a fibrous capsule. Fibrous tissue extends into the lymph node in the form of trabeculae arising from the undersurface of this capsule, so that the lymphoid tissue within the lymph node is supported by a fine meshwork of fibrocellular elements. A slight depression on one side of the lymph node is termed the hilum, and it is through the hilum that blood vessels enter and leave the lymph node. The single efferent lymphatic also leaves from the hilum.

Internally the lymph node contains a central medulla and a peripheral cortex; the line of demarcation between the two is often indistinct. The cortex is deficient at the hilum so that the efferent lymphatic derives its lymph from the medulla. Afferent lymphatics are usually multiple and pass through the capsule into the cortex. Lymph enters a lymph node through one of these afferent vessels

and passes onward into a subcapsular lymphatic plexus. From here the lymph passes into the sinuses of the cortex, then through the sinuses of the medulla, before leaving the lymph node through the efferent vessel. The flow of lymph in the sinuses is slightly retarded, and this encourages the deposition of particulate matter. This enables phagocytes to filter off particulate antigenic and other noxious matter from the lymph prior to drainage of lymph in the venous circulation.

The lymph node has a number of other functions, including a role in both the cellular and the humoral immune responses. Lymphocytes and other antibody-producing cells may be generated in the lymph node, usually within the cortex, where densely packed cells form follicles, often with their own germinal center. The number and size of the follicles vary and at times of great antigenic stimulation may increase to such an extent that the lymph node itself enlarges. In these circumstances the enlarged lymph node is termed reactive.

IMAGING NORMAL AND ABNORMAL LYMPH NODES

Clinical examination is the first step in the evaluation of the lymphatic system. Enlargement of neck, axillary, and groin lymph nodes may be palpable, and large abdominal nodal masses may also be palpated. Smaller volume enlargement of abdominal and pelvic lymph nodes, together with any enlargement of lymph nodes within the thorax, is impalpable. The determination of tumor extent and bulk within the body is only possible after the appropriate imaging tests have been performed.

The presence of adenopathy may be seen on plain-film examination (Fig. 27.5) and inferred from displacement of normal structures. The chest radiograph remains the most important radiological window into the thorax. Enlargement of mediastinal and hilar lymph nodes has a characteristic appearance. In many instances the information available from a chest radiograph is sufficient to plan further management of the patient. Radiographs

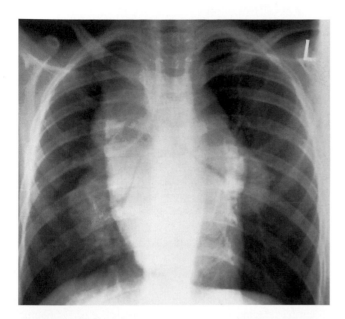

Fig. 27.5 Frontal chest radiograph. A large mediastinal nodal mass in a patient presenting with Hodgkin's disease is seen compressing the major airways.

of the abdomen are less helpful, as only large masses can be confidently recognized and the nodal nature of these masses is difficult to establish. The addition of a contrast medium (especially an IVP) to opacify the ureters is a limited but recognized method of demonstrating mass effect and the displacement of normal abdominal structures by a large abdominal mass (Fig. 27.6).

Lymphography

For many years bipedal lymphography was the standard test for the non-surgical demonstration of lymphadenopathy affecting the abdominal and pelvic lymph nodes. Although lymphography is a sensitive test that may on occasion demonstrate micrometastases in normal-sized lymph nodes, it is only moderately specific, and false-positive findings are not infrequent, especially in the elderly, in whom fibrofatty deposits within the lymph nodes may be incorrectly considered metastatic foci. This limits the value of the lymphogram technique, particularly in the staging of pelvic malignancies.

Successful lymphography depends on several sequential steps: firstly, the visualization of the lymphatics; secondly, the exposure and cannulation of the lymphatic; thirdly, the injection of a contrast material; and, finally, the taking of X-rays, both immediately after the procedure, to demonstrate the lymphatics, and again after at least 24 h delay to demonstrate the lymph nodes. Contrast medium will then remain in the lymph nodes for 6–12 months, and during this time follow-up films can be used to demonstrate changes within the opacified lymph nodes.

Lymphography may be requested when the CT examination is negative, in order to identify small deposits in normal-sized lymph nodes. However the two tests are not complementary. The value of CT is reduced if performed after lymphography. The presence of the dense oily contrast medium within the lymph nodes may cause them to enlarge in reaction, making interpretation of the CT difficult as well as creating artefacts (due to the high density of the oily contrast medium) that may degrade the CT image. There

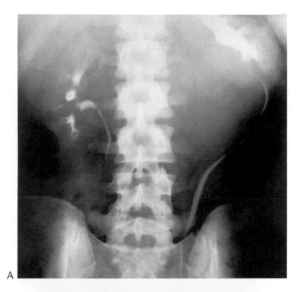

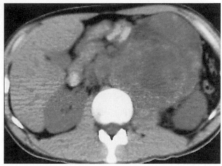

Fig. 27.6   A. The opacified ureters are seen on intravenous urography to be displaced around a large central abdominal mass. **B**. The presence of this mass is confirmed on the CT section. The final diagnosis was testicular teratoma.

is no doubt that in almost all circumstances CT has obviated the need for lymphography.

There are also practical contraindications to lymphography. These include allergies to contrast agents, vital dyes, and local anesthesia; cardiovascular or pulmonary disease, especially heart failure, angina, pulmonary fibrosis, or emphysema; and previous pulmonary irradiation. The last is a significant risk factor as the arteriovenous shunts opened up at pulmonary irradiation predispose to systemic oil embolism. Lymphography is often considered an outpatient procedure, but observation for 24 h in hospital is prudent (MacDonald 1987).

Technique   The visualization of the lymphatics prior to exposure and cannulation of the lymphatic is generally accepted as helpful. This is accomplished by the injection of 0.5 ml of patent blue violet into the first two web spaces of both feet. (At this time the patient should be warned that blue staining of the skin may persist in this area for several weeks and in addition the urine might appear blue-tinged.) The indicator dye is a large molecular compound that is absorbed into peripheral lymphatics rather than the vascular capillaries. The lymphatic may then be identified as a blue streak under the skin. The optimum time for the cut-down is within a few minutes of the injection of the indicator dye, when the blue streaks of the lymphatics first become visible. After this time the blue dye infiltrates into the skin, making it much harder to identify the opacified lymphatics.

It is easiest to expose and cannulate a single lymphatic on the dorsum of the foot. Lignocaine (1%) is injected into the skin on either side of the exposed lymphatic, making subsequent dissection easier. A longitudinal incision is made over the lymphatic, and the vessel exposed under direct vision. Fat and connective tissue is gently stripped off the lymphatic over a distance of a centimeter. The cannulation of the exposed and cleaned lymphatic is a delicate procedure, and the simplest approach is the best. A suture (4.0 silk) is loosely tied around the lymphatic proximal to the insertion point. The lymphatic is then stretched between the smooth blades of a pair of forceps, distended, and cannulated, using a purpose-made lymphogram set with a 27 gauge needle. At this time it may be helpful if an assistant can gently inject contrast medium. This, at the appropriate time, will distend the lymphatic, allowing the needle tip to be advanced a further 2–3 mm. The suture is then tightened around the needle, and the tubing of the giving set gently fastened to the patient's skin. Second punctures (if required) should be made either in a second vessel or, if that is not possible, then proximal to the initial puncture site.

To opacify the pelvic and abdominal lymph nodes, 6–7 ml of lipiodol is injected into both feet of a typical 70 kg patient. This is usually accomplished by the use of a mechanical injector which can inject the contrast medium at a rate between 0.05 and 0.1 ml/min. Too rapid an injection rate will rupture the lymphatic. Immediately after the injection commences, the lower leg is observed fluoroscopically to ensure that the needle is in a lymphatic and no lymphaticovenous communication is present.

After the injection of approximately 4 ml of contrast medium into each foot an anteroposterior (AP) radiograph of the pelvis is obtained. This acts as a check for lymphatic obstruction, crossover, or venous communication in the pelvis. After the injection of 7 ml of oily contrast medium into each foot, a supine AP radiograph of the abdomen is taken and the injection halted. The feet are then sutured and the standard radiographs obtained: AP abdomen, AP pelvis right posterior oblique (RPO), and left posterior oblique (LPO) of the abdomen and pelvis, lateral abdomen, and a chest X-ray to check for possible oil embolism. These radiographs are all repeated after 24 h, and the two series, showing initially the vessels and later the lymph nodes, are compared. Without this precaution normal lymph node hila might be mistaken for pathological filling defects. Lymphographic contrast medium still present in the lymph vessels on the delayed films may indicate lymphatic obstruction, especially if a collateral lymphatic circulation may be identified.

CT; Ultrasound; MRI

Today the formal staging of malignant disease in patients is undertaken with CT, perhaps supplemented by MRI and ultrasound examinations. The cross-sectional imaging capability of these techniques allows the direct demonstration of normal and abnormal lymph nodes. Lymph node enlargement is the imaging hallmark of metastatic involvement, and a series of size criteria for normal and abnormal lymph nodes have evolved in the different areas of the body (see below). Enlargement of the lymph nodes above these criteria is suggestive but not diagnostic of malignant involvement. The images should always be interpreted in the light of the clinical findings and the known behavior of the particular tumor.

For example, a slightly enlarged right paracaval lymph node is unlikely to be involved in a patient with a left-sided testicular teratoma, but a similarly sized para-aortic lymph node on the left may be the site of metastatic disease following spread of disease from a right testicular tumor. This is because cross-flow in the lymphatic drainage of the retroperitoneum is far more likely to occur from right to left across the midline than from left to right (Dixon et al 1986).

Radionuclide Techniques

Injected radiopharmaceuticals may collect in lymph vessels and nodes (McKusick 1985). Circulating radionuclides may be taken up by metastatic lymph nodes. This is best recognized with gallium-67. This is a tumor avid isotope taken up by tumors arising from the lymphatic system, liver or lung. Different cell types will take up the isotope differentially. The technique has been applied to patients with lymphoma. The sensitivity of the test to the presence of active lymphoma tissue is related to the volume of the tumor, the location injected, the dose, and the instrumentation. Gallium-67 imaging is sensitive to the presence of lymphoma in patients but has proved less effective than CT in determining the extent of disease site by site within individual patients. Approximately 5% of positive results with gallium-67 imaging are incorrect, usually as a result of concomitant or unsuspected infection. At present the clinical role of gallium-67 scanning in patients with lymphoma is best limited to the follow-up of patients with initial positive scans.

The lymphatics and lymph nodes may be imaged using radiopharmaceuticals. This technique is not widely used due to the high proportion of unhelpful tests. Most attention has focused on the locoregional spread of breast cancer using ^{99m}Tc human serum albumen and ^{99m}Tc antimony sulfide microcolloids. Very occasionally a lymphoscintogram is requested in patients with apparent lower limb lymphedema in whom lymphatic cannulation is technically not possible.

IMAGING NORMAL AND ABNORMAL LYMPHATICS

These may be directly opacified at lymphography. The injection of water-soluble radiological contrast media is an acceptable and safe alternative to the injection of oily contrast media but will not opacify the lymph nodes (O'Donnell & Clouse 1985). The technique of lymphography in the edematous leg is difficult, and prior elevation of the limb for 48–72 h may help reduce the amount of limb edema.

On the basis of the lymphographic appearances the **lymphedemas** may be divided into the *aplasias* with no demonstrable lymphatics, the *hypoplasias* with a reduced number of lymphatics, and the *hyperplasias* with an increase in the number of lymphatics present. Allen et al (1946) divided the lymphedemas into primary and secondary. The primary type may be further subdivided into *congenital, praecox* (before the age of 35 years), and *tarda* (after the age of 35 years).

Primary lymphedema This is a vascular dysplasia often associated with arterial and venous malformations in the same limb and other congenital defects. Most patients have aplasia or severe hypoplasia of the lymphatics. The edema may be precipitated by minor trauma or surgery. Peak incidence is seen in

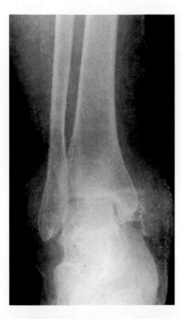

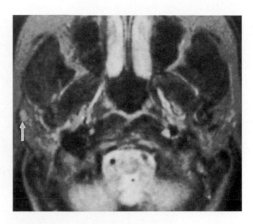

Fig. 27.8 Axial MRI examination through the neck shows a small intraparotid lymph node on the right (arrow), an incidental finding. On T_2-weighted MRI scans, lymph nodes appear white.

Fig. 27.7 Early phase lymphogram film. The limb is swollen, and when lymphography was attempted, lymphatics filled poorly. This is an example of secondary lymphedema due to filariasis.

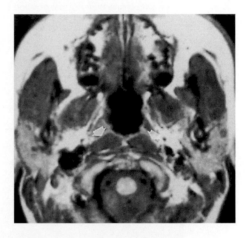

Fig. 27.9 Axial T_1-weighted MRI examination through the neck. Bilateral retropharyngeal nodes may be identified (arrows). On T_1-weighted sequences, lymph nodes appear darker than the surrounding fat. Note the flow void phenomenon—the great vessels of the neck appear black.

girls at puberty and typically involves the left leg. The term *Milroy's disease* is loosely applied to primary lymphedema, but should be limited to those few cases which are both congenital and familial.

The advent of CT has also reduced the need for lymphographic evaluation of the lymphatics as the size and number of lymph nodes parallel the size and number of lymphatics. CT assessment of the size and number of the lymph nodes can objectively classify patients into aplasia, hypoplasia, and hyperplasia of the lymphatic system.

Secondary Lymphedema This is more common than primary lymphedema, and indicates the presence of obstruction to the normal forward passage of lymph. This may be due to previous surgery or irradiation but may also result from recurrent tumor. Uncommon causes of secondary lymphedema include infection, especially with *filariasis* (Fig. 27.7). In patients with secondary lymphedema, CT is again the most useful investigation, especially when looking for new or recurrent tumor.

TOPOGRAPHY OF THE LYMPHATIC SYSTEM

The radiologist should have an understanding of the major lymphatic pathways of the body, especially those of the head and neck, thorax, abdomen, and pelvis.

Lymphatic Drainage of the Head and Neck

There are approximately 300 lymph nodes in the average adult neck, loosely arranged into several groups (Som 1987). The lymphatics and lymph nodes of the neck make up a collar of lymphoid tissue around the skull base consisting, from posterior to anterior, of the *occipital* lymph nodes, the *mastoid* lymph nodes, the *parotid* lymph nodes (and these may be extra- or intra-glandular (Fig. 27.8)), and the *submandibular, facial, submental,*

and *sublingual* lymph nodes. These lymphatic chains drain inferiorly through either the *anterior* or *lateral cervical chains* into the superior mediastinum. In addition there are also the deep and impalpable *retropharyngeal* lymph nodes (Fig. 27.9) found in the neck lateral to the longus colli and longus capitis muscles which drain lymph from the nasopharynx, oropharynx, sinuses, and middle ear to the *internal jugular chain*. Pathology in the retropharyngeal region is often associated with abnormalities of the 9th–12th cranial nerves.

The *lateral cervical lymph nodes* serve as the common drainage route for all the major head and neck structures. There are superficial and deep groups. The *superficial* group forms a chain that runs alongside the external jugular chain. Of greater importance are the lymph nodes of the deep group, in three chains forming a triangle. At the apex of the triangle lies the *jugulo-digastric* lymph node, seen in the suprahyoid compartment at the anatomic level where the posterior belly of the digastric muscle crosses the anterior jugular vein. Below this the *internal jugular chain* of lymph nodes runs forward into the anterior triangle of the neck, following the course of the internal jugular vein just behind the anterior border of the sternocleidomastoid muscle.

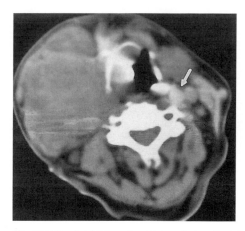
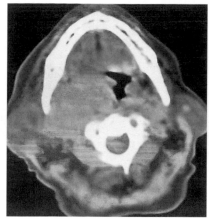

Fig. 27.10 Axial CT sections taken during the injection of intravenous contrast medium. A large malignant nodal mass is seen on the right and extending deep to compress the airway. On the left the dynamic injection of intravenous contrast medium has opacified the vessels of the carotid sheath seen in their normal position (arrow).

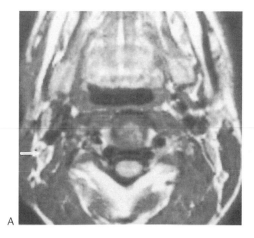
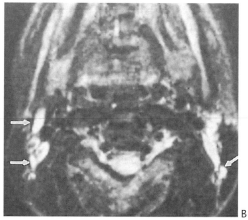

Fig. 27.11 Axial MRI examination of a boy presenting with Hodgkin's disease. **A.** The T_1-weighted image shows the posterior triangle nodes as small areas of low signal within the relatively bright signal of the fat (arrows). **B.** On the T_2 image the fat is of moderate signal intensity and the nodes show increased intensity due to their longer T_2 relaxation time (arrows).

These lymph nodes lie outside the carotid sheath, but on CT and MRI are seen to be close to the structures within the carotid sheath (Fig. 27.10). The *spinal accessory chain* runs posteriorly into the posterior triangle of the neck deep to the sternocleido-mastoid muscle. The lymph nodes of this group typically lie within fat, and in consequence are well seen on CT and MRI scans (Fig. 27.11). The extremes of the internal jugular and spinal accessory chains are joined by the *transverse cervical chain* of supraclavicular lymph nodes. The most inferior lymph nodes of the internal jugular chain are also known as the *lymph nodes of Virchow* or *Trosier*; enlargement of these lymph nodes may well be secondary to metastatic involvement from a thoracic or sub-diaphragmatic primary tumor or lymphoma or from the spread of breast malignancy (Fig. 27.12). Finally, an *anterior chain* of cervical lymph nodes accompanies the anterior cervical vein and drains the anterior neck structures, especially the infraglottic larynx and the thyroid.

There is free communication between all the lymph node groups and chains in the neck. Eventually the lymph on the left

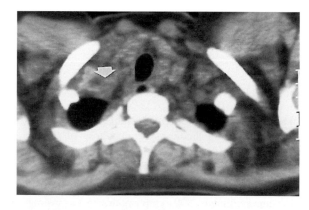

Fig. 27.12 CT scan showing a supraclavicular lymph node (arrow) on the right in this patient with Hodgkin's disease.

side of the neck flows into the thoracic duct while that on the right typically enters the venous circulation via the right lym-phatic duct. Metastatic involvement of cervical lymph nodes also

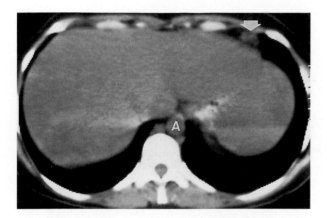

Fig. 27.13   CT scan showing enlargement and almost certain involvement of a diaphragmatic lymph node adjacent to the aorta (A). The enlargement of a diaphragmatic or paracardiac lymph node is of great importance in patients with Hodgkin's disease considered for mantle irradiation. Normal-sized lymph nodes in this area are not seen on CT examination.

results in spread of tumor along apparently illogical pathways, and this may account for 'skip lesions' often found when assessing the neck for metastatic involvement.

Lymphatic Drainage of the Thorax

The lymph nodes of the mediastinum consist of a *posterior mediastinal group* of lymph nodes found below the level of the pulmonary veins and in close relationship to the aorta and esophagus and extending inferiorly to the diaphragm. Above the posterior mediastinal lymph nodes are the *paratracheobronchial* lymph nodes. These consist of a subcarinal lymph node group, the lymph nodes of the pulmonary root, the lymph nodes between the trachea and the bronchi, and the paratracheal lymph nodes. Above these lymph nodes are the lymph nodes of the *aortopulmonary window* and the *anterior mediastinum* (Glazer et al 1985, Kiyono et al 1988). These latter lymph nodes are found in front of the great vessels. In addition, enlargement of the *internal mammary* and *diaphragmatic* lymph nodes (Fig. 27.13) should be recognized on CT examination.

The lymphatic drainage of the lungs does not strictly follow the lobar boundaries. The right upper lung drains to the right paratracheal lymph nodes, the right middle lung drains to both the right paratracheal and right subcarinal lymph nodes, while the lymphatic drainage from the right lower lung goes to the right paratracheal, subcarinal and posterior mediastinal lymph nodes. The upper portion of the left lung drains to the paratracheal lymph nodes while both the mid and lower portions of the left lung drain to the paratracheal and subcarinal lymph nodes.

Lymphatic Drainage of the Abdomen and Pelvis

This is best considered (Fig. 27.14) in relation to the appearances seen on the typical lymphogram (Harrison & Clouse 1985). Contrast medium injected into the lymphatic vessels on the dorsum of each foot will opacify the usually large and non-homogeneous lymph nodes of the groin. These are difficult to evaluate radiologically as they are frequently enlarged as a result of previous infection/reaction and often contain numerous fibrofatty filling defects. Occasionally on CT sections, pathological enlargement of

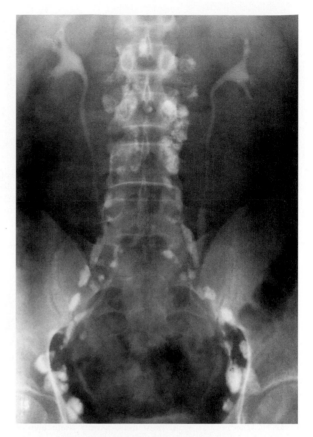

Fig. 27.14   Frontal view of a lymphogram showing opacification of the pelvic and retroperitoneal lymph nodes.

the groin lymph nodes may be seen, but in such cases the diseased lymph nodes are usually palpable (Fig. 27.15). In the pelvis, lymphographic contrast agent will opacify the *external iliac* and *common iliac* lymph nodes. The *internal iliac* and *obturator* lymph nodes are usually only seen on lymphography if there is derangement of the normal flow pattern, for example secondary to surgery, but these nodes, if enlarged, may be seen on cross-sectional imaging studies.

In the retroperitoneum the lymph nodes as high as L2 typically opacify at lymphangiography. There are lymph nodes between the

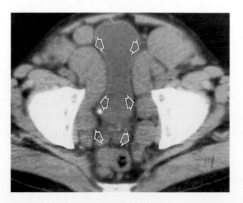

Fig. 27.15   CT section through the pelvis showing bilateral pelvic and groin lymph node enlargement in a patient with non-Hodgkin lymphoma.

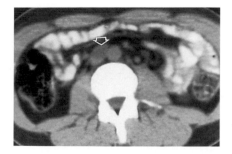

Fig. 27.16 Contrast-enhanced CT study showing enlargement and involvement of an interaorticocaval lymph node (arrow) in a patient with a right-sided testicular malignancy. Right-sided testicular tumors frequently spread to the interaorticocaval lymph nodes. This is extremely uncommon when the testicular primary is on the left.

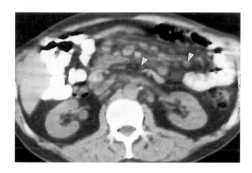

Fig. 27.17 CT section showing mesenteric lymph node involvement (arrowheads) in a patient with non-Hodgkin lymphoma. This is common in non-Hodgkin lymphoma, but seen in fewer than 5% of patients with Hodgkin's disease.

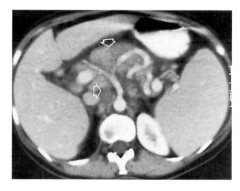

Fig. 27.18 Contrast-enhanced CT scan showing considerable enlargement of upper abdominal, peripancreatic, and portal lymph nodes (arrows). The superior mesenteric artery and the hepatic artery are outlined.

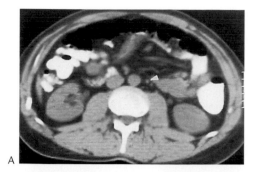

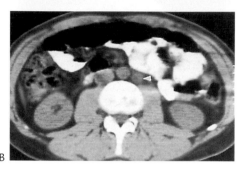

Fig. 27.19 **A**. Staging CT on this patient with a testicular primary shows no significant adenopathy. Note the 0.25 cm node in the left retroperitoneum (arrowhead). **B**. Seven months later this lymph node has enlarged (arrowhead), indicating the presence of an occult primary in the lymph node at the time of original staging.

aorta and inferior vena cava (Fig. 27.16). Mesententric lymph nodes (Fig. 27.17) and the lymph nodes around the stomach and pancreas as well as those closest to the porta hepatis and renal and splenic hila may be seen on cross-sectional imaging, but these fail to opacify at lymphography (Fig. 27.18).

LYMPH NODE ENLARGEMENT

Malignant involvement of a lymph node results in the enlargement of the affected lymph node. This may be considered to involve four stages. Firstly, the deposition of a malignant cell within the lymph node and subsequent cell division, resulting in the presence of a micrometastasis within the affected lymph node. At this stage the lymph node remains of normal size and shape and will appear normal on CT and MRI examination (Fig. 27.19). Surgical staging, with either lymph node sampling or formal lymphadenectomy, will demonstrate malignant involvement of lymph nodes before either the CT/MRI scan or the lymphogram become abnormal. Surgery and careful histology is the present 'gold standard' for evaluating lymph node involvement in patients with malignant disease. This is seen, for example, in the axillary staging of patients with breast cancer.

There is a period in which lymphography might demonstrate the presence of a micrometastasis while the lymph node itself remains of normal size. This accounts for the slightly greater sensitivity of lymphography over CT and/or MRI in evaluating the retroperitoneal lymph nodes, and is most useful in evaluating slower-growing tumors where this stage is likely to persist longer. The CT demonstration of a micrometastasis within a lymph node is more difficult but may be possible in the neck. A CT density measurement is required to differentiate a small metastasis within a lymph node from a focal deposit of fat. In the neck the incidence of fibrofatty foci within normal-sized lymph nodes is less than in the abdominal, pelvic, and axillary lymph nodes, making this a valid technique.

Eventually an involved lymph node will enlarge and become recognizable clinically and/or with cross-sectional imaging. Some tumors result in discrete lymph node metastases (Fig. 27.20) while other tumors rapidly pass onto the next phase, in which the outline of the tumor becomes blurred due to the presence of tumor

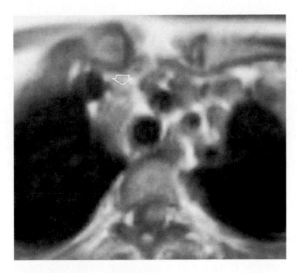

Fig. 27.20 Axial T₁-weighted MRI scan through the thorax of a patient with Hodgkin's disease showing discrete enlargement of mediastinal lymph nodes. The low-intensity lymph nodes are seen in the high-intensity fat (arrow). Note the vessels give low signal intensity, enabling them to be identified. This is an example of the flow void phenomenon.

extending into the perinodal tissues. The final or fourth stage of malignant spread of tumor to a lymph node results in a large amorphous tumor mass with infiltration of the tissue planes. At this time it is impossible to identify any residual nodal outline.

BENIGN CONDITIONS AFFECTING THE LYMPH NODES

These are important radiologically as they may result in lymph node enlargement which may be confused with malignant involvement. Benign focal lesions within the lymph nodes can also be mistaken for deposits.

Acute inflammation will enlarge lymph nodes. On lymphograms the texture of the lymph node will become more foamy, an appearance usually associated with lymphoma (Fig. 27.21). Central defects within the lymph node may also be seen. Typically it is the granulomatous or abscess-forming inflammations that produce filling defects in the lymph nodes similar to those seen in secondary deposits (Fig. 27.22). Lymph nodes may be seen to enlarge in a number of granulomatous diseases, including sarcoid and tuberculosis.

Reactive hyperplasia usually associated with a proliferation of histiocytes is another frequent cause of lymph node enlargement. This may be related to recent surgery (Fig. 27.23).

Fibrofatty deposits are seen within the lymph nodes of older patients, and these are most commonly seen in the pelvis. They may be considered a normal finding in the inguinal region, but in the remainder of the pelvis they are a source of confusion, as they may be incorrectly interpreted as secondary deposits in patients with a primary pelvic neoplasm.

MALIGNANT CONDITIONS AFFECTING THE LYMPH NODES

Lymphomas These are primary neoplasms of the immune

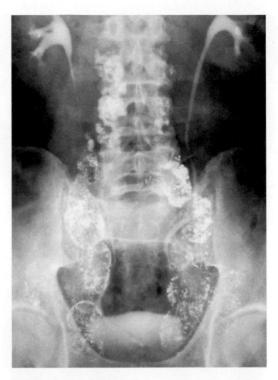

Fig. 27.21 The lymph nodes are generally enlarged and appear foamy in this patient with lymphoma.

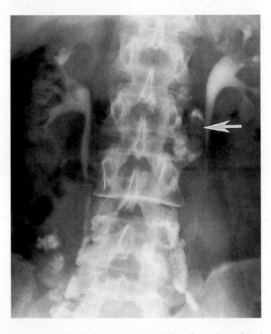

Fig. 27.22 A single focal deposit is seen within the enlarged and opacified lymph node medial to the left ureter (arrow) in this patient with an endometrial cancer.

system and arise within lymphoid tissue (Neumann et al 1985). The lymphomas are uncommon, accounting for approximately 4% of the newly diagnosed malignant tumors in the UK. Hodgkin's disease accounts for approximately 25% of newly diagnosed lymphomas, i.e. 1% of all malignancies. In children, lymphoma is the third most frequent malignancy, following

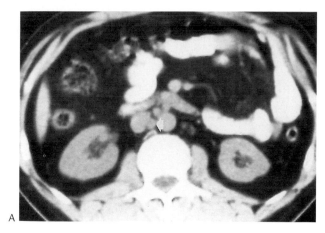

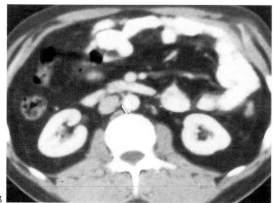

Fig. 27.23 **A**. Staging CT scans in a patient with a recently resected right-sided testicular tumor showed prominent lymph nodes between the aorta and inferior vena cava (arrow). **B**. One month later these have resolved without treatment. Reactive enlargement of lymph nodes is a possible source of error if patients are scanned too close to the date of their surgery. It is better to wait 3–4 weeks.

behind leukemia and central nervous system neoplasia. As a group the lymphomas vary enormously in outlook, but all will reduce life expectancy if untreated.

The histological subtype of the lymphoma and the anatomic extent of disease at the time of diagnosis have prognostic significance. A practicable histologic classification is the key to the appropriate investigation and management of patients with lymphoma (Callihan et al 1980). The first and most important distinction is between Hodgkin's disease and the non-Hodgkin lymphomas (NHLs).

Hodgkin's Disease

The etiology of Hodgkin's disease is obscure. The disease may present at any age, but characteristically has a peak incidence in young adulthood, with a second peak incidence in old age. The disease is slightly more common in males. The histologic diagnosis may be difficult, and the radiologist should not hesitate to question the diagnosis if the radiological findings are atypical. Fine-needle aspiration cytology is rarely helpful, and every effort should be made to obtain an adequate specimen for histologic review. This usually requires the surgical excision of enlarged lymph nodes.

The cell of origin for Hodgkin's disease is unknown, but the disease is believed to begin within a lymph node. After a time the disease begins to spread by contiguity through the lymphatic system. Hematogenous dissemination is a late phenomenon and almost invariably follows splenic involvement. The orderly spread of disease through the lymphatic system has important therapeutic considerations. Localized disease may be irradiated and cure anticipated. The radiation portals may be chosen to include both the obvious disease sites and the adjacent lymph node groups, which may in turn be the site of occult involvement. This is known as extended field irradiation, and differs from the more standard involved field techniques commonly employed in other tumors. The use of the extended field technique in Hodgkin's disease is an example of how knowledge generated by clinical, radiological, and surgical mapping of disease can be used to modify treatment successfully.

Lymph nodes involved with Hodgkin's disease will enlarge, and eventually disease will spread extranodally into the adjacent tissues. The four stages of nodal involvement described above may be recognized. True tumor invasion of surrounding organs and structures is a late phenomenon in patients with Hodgkin's disease. CT scanning will initially demonstrate contiguity between the enlarged lymph nodes and adjacent structures, but early tumor invasion of contiguous structures is difficult to recognize radiologically.

The histopathological classification of Hodgkin's disease now widely accepted was developed by Lukes et al (1966) and subsequently accepted at the Rye Conference. In essence there are four subgroups of Hodgkin's disease. Three of these are related—at least in part—to the strength of the host reaction, *lymphocyte-predominant* (LP) indicating a strong host response, *lymphocyte-depleted* (LD) indicating a very weak response, and *mixed-cellularity* (MC) indicating an intermediate group with an intermediate and moderate immune response (Castellino 1986).

Patients with the LP form almost invariably present with a localized disease, often with palpable supraclavicular lymph nodes. This variety is most frequently seen in young asymptomatic males. On histologic review of the excised lymph nodes, the characteristic Reed–Sternberg cells are scanty. This form of Hodgkin's disease has an excellent prognosis, and may be treated with local rather than systemic therapy.

The typical patient with the LD form of Hodgkin's disease is older, usually polysymptomatic, and on investigation will be found to have advanced disseminated disease. Histologic review of excised lymph nodes will show numerous Reed–Sternberg cells. The prognosis is poor.

MC Hodgkin's disease is the most frequently seen of these three histopathological subtypes. It may be seen in every age group, but is especially frequent in young adults. Patients with MC disease are often symptomatic. Three specific signs and symptoms in patients with Hodgkin's disease, known as the *B symptoms* (unexplained weight loss of more than 10% body weight in the preceding 6 months, unexplained fever above 38.4°C, and/or night sweats), are an indication that the disease may involve abdominal lymph nodes and/or the spleen. The prognosis of MC Hodgkin's disease lies between that of LP and LD disease. LP or MC variants may progress to LD or even to a NHL.

The fourth histologic subtype of Hodgkin's disease is *nodular sclerosing* (NS). This is the only subgroup more common in female patients. Typically patients present in adolescence or early adulthood, and almost invariably the mediastinal and supra-clavicular lymph node groups are involved. Histologically, lymph nodes involved with NS Hodgkin's disease will show a thick fibrous rim. Recent attention has focused on the contents within this connective tissue reaction, and it is now felt that there are subgroups within NS Hodgkin's disease. These depend on the host response, and at present are probably best regarded as a good prognosis (with a strong host response) and a poor prognosis (weak host response) subgroup. Most patients with NS Hodgkin's disease will have a good prognosis, and unlike the LP and MC subtypes, NS Hodgkin's disease rarely progresses to a stage with a less favorable histology.

The presence of fibrous stroma around the lymph nodes is important radiologically. Patients with NS Hodgkin's disease typically have large lymph nodes at presentation. These slowly reduce in size on successful therapy, and it is not uncommon for residual soft-tissue masses to persist. Interpretation of radiological findings at this time may be difficult. The temptation to over-diagnose poor response to treatment and/or residual active disease should be resisted.

The second prognostic factor in Hodgkin's disease is the anatomic extent of disease at the time of presentation. The Ann Arbor staging system (Table 27.1) has been accepted for many years (Carbone et al 1971). In this system, lymph nodes are considered part of clearly defined lymph node groups, e.g. left neck and left axilla. Involvement of one or more lymph nodes within a group is considered to represent involvement of that group.

Non-Hodgkin lymphomas

NHLs are a much more heterogeneous group of malignant tumors than the Hodgkin's lymphomas (Bragg et al 1986). They are most frequently seen in the elderly. There have been many attempts to classify the pathological appearances of the tumor, but the terminology unfortunately remains confusing. The National Cancer Institute Working Party (NCI 1981) considered all the contemporary classifications and proposed a working formulation dividing the NHLs into low-, intermediate-, and high-grade groups. Radiologists (along with most clinicians) may find this artificial and still prefer to divide their patients into two groups, the low-grade nodular or *follicular lymphomas* and the high-grade *diffuse lymphomas*.

The origin and subtypes of the NHLs may be considered as follows. In fetal life T- and B-lymphocyte precursors are formed: **T-cells** migrate to the thymus and eventually mature into helper T-cells or suppressor/cytotoxic T-cells, and leave the thymus to circulate around the body. The T-cell antigens on these cells may be recognized by monoclonal antibody techniques. After circulating around the body, T-cells accumulate in the lymph nodes and in the spleen.

B-cells are formed in the liver and migrate to bone marrow. Subsequently they may also be found in lymph nodes, but the T-cells and the B-cells are found in different parts of the lymph node. The T-cells remain paracortical while the B-cells are found within the lymphoid follicles. Depending on their nuclear morphology, two subgroups of B-cell types within the follicle may be recognized: B-cells with large round nuclei are known as centroblasts (non-cleaved), while those with irregular nuclei are known as centrocytes or cleaved cells. B-cells may be found within the circulation, where they are known as plasma cells.

Monocytes from the circulation may lodge in the body tissues, where they are known as histiocytes. Histiocytes are thought to be a third possible cell of origin for the NHLs, but *histiocytic lymphomas* account for fewer than 5% of the NHLs.

The majority of NHLs arise from the follicular cells within the lymph node follicle, and may consist of cells that appear cleaved, non-cleaved, or a mixture of the two. Although most NHLs are of B-cell origin and have a tendency to form follicles, they do not all form typical follicles. In practice, many show tumor infiltration throughout the affected lymph node. From this simple observation two important subgroups may be recognized—those that tend to remain in the follicles and are *follicular* (or *nodular*) and those which show the diffusion of tumor cells into the remainder of the lymph node and are called *diffuse*. On occasion, both diffuse and follicular features may be seen within the same excised lymph node, or within two lymph nodes excised from the same patient at the same time. Finally, follicular lymphomas may evolve into diffuse large-cell forms as part of their natural history.

Low-grade lymphomas are usually follicular while the intermediate- and high-grade tumors are usually diffuse. T-cell lymphomas (10% of the total) are found in the skin and thymus from peripheral T-cells.

NHLs frequently present as painless enlargement of lymph nodes, but the disease may also develop at a number of extranodal sites, leading to a wide variety of presenting features.

Nodal Presentations of the NHLs   The most common site is the neck, and, unlike Hodgkin's disease, the lymphoid tissue of Waldeyer's ring is usually involved. The patient will frequently have nodal enlargement at a number of palpable and radiologically obvious sites. These are often non-contiguous, and if the lymph nodes are followed up without treatment they may be found to spontaneously fluctuate in size. A patient with an NHL is much more likely to present with enlarged lymph nodes in unusual sites, for example those of the elbow or knee, than a patient with Hodgkin's disease. The secondary effects of lymph node enlargement such as limb swelling or superior vena cava obstruction are not uncommon. Backache is suggestive of retroperitoneal lymph node involvement, and constitutional symptoms, especially weight loss, fever, and anorexia, are typical.

Although designed for use in Hodgkin's disease the Ann Arbor approach to staging is frequently used for the NHLs. The majority of patients, especially those with follicular lymphomas, will have widespread disease (stage III or IV) at presentation.

Only about one-third of patients will have clinically localized disease at presentation. Of these, fewer than one-half will still

Table 27.1   Staging of Hodgkin's disease (modified from Carbone et al 1971)

Stage I	Disease confined to a single lumph node group
Stage II	Disease involving two or more lymph node groups on the same side of the diaphragm
Stage III	Disease involving lymph node groups on both sides of the diaphragm
Stage IV	Hematogenous dissemination of disease

have limited disease by the time they have been fully staged radiologically. This small subgroup (about one-sixth of the total) is important if local radiotherapy is to be considered as a curative option. With true stage I diffuse lymphoma there is a 90% chance of long-term disease-free survival. With stage II disease the proportion of patients free of relapse at 5 years falls to 40%. For this reason, chemotherapy is usually given in stage II disease unless the patient is elderly or there is some contraindication to its use. In early stage follicular lymphomas local radiotherapy will achieve symptomatic control, and over 70% of patients may well be alive after 10 years. But patients with a follicular lymphoma will relapse and cannot ever be regarded as cured. Unlike Hodgkin's disease, where there is an orderly spread of disease by contiguity through the lymph nodes, the spread of NHL does not follow a contiguous pattern, and there is no clinical advantage in planning extended rather than involved field irradiation. Palliative local radiotherapy is important, especially in the elderly, and good short-term local control is to be expected. In such patients extensive investigation is not warranted.

Most patients with NHL will have extensive disease and qualify for chemotherapy. In such instances the finer nuances of radiological staging are no longer required for treatment planning. However, some idea of tumour extent and bulk is important in assessing response to chemotherapy and for comparison of results. In most patients with diffuse NHL, combination chemotherapy is required. There are a number of different drug regimes in use, and all will produce a complete response in approximately 75% of patients; of these, three-quarters will still be alive after 5 years. The prognosis is worse in men, in patients with large abdominal nodal masses, and in those with hepatic or marrow involvement. The proportion of complete responders is greatest in those with stage II disease, and falls to 60% in those with stage III disease, and to 35% in those patients with stage IV disease. The prognosis for incomplete responders is poor, and almost all these patients will be dead in 2 years. In this group, recent attention has focused on ultrahigh-dose therapy with autologous bone marrow grafting.

Advanced *follicular (low-grade) lymphomas* are often treated expectantly, as there is little evidence that any treatment alters the outcome. Patients are usually treated symptomatically either with local irradiation and/or chemotherapy. The younger patient may occasionally be given combination chemotherapy, more in the hope than anticipation of cure. Long-term chemotherapy has been advocated in patients with low-grade lymphomas. Unfortunately, this approach may lead to bone marrow depression and drug resistance. This may be important if the disease progresses to the diffuse form, and intensive chemotherapy then offers the only hope of disease control.

The majority of *T-cell lymphomas* are seen in younger patients, often with large mediastinal masses. The tumors are aggressive, with short histories, constitutional symptoms, bone marrow involvement, and, frequently, central nervous system spread with leptomeningitis, nerve palsy, root compression, and increased intracranial pressure. The prognosis is poor, and systemic treatment is required.

Extranodal Presentations of the NHLs   Extranodal sites of disease are commonly found on detailed staging of patients with a primary nodal presentation (Glazer et al 1983). Nodal disease which has previously been treated may relapse extranodally. The NHLs may also present at an extranodal site without clinically obvious nodal disease. These patients may be difficult to diagnose and to treat.

GASTROINTESTINAL LYMPHOMA

The *small bowel* and *stomach* are the most frequent sites of involvement. In the small bowel the disease is believed to originate within the lymphoid tissue of the mucosal lining. For this reason it is most frequently seen where there is the most lymphoid tissue present. The incidence increases from the duodenum through the jejunum to the ileum. The disease may be single- or multifocal, and grows eventually to ulcerate through the mucosal bowel wall and serosa. Ultimately the regional lymph nodes are involved. The disease may progress to bowel obstruction and perforation. Most patients have *diffuse high-grade NHL of B-cell origin*. Patients with longstanding celiac disease may develop *T-cell lymphomas*, and these respond poorly to treatment. The incidence of gastrointestinal lymphoma has increased sharply over the last few years, especially those cases associated with immunosuppression (Turowski and Basson 1995).

The clinical presentation of the bowel lymphomas is varied. Many patients present acutely with abdominal pain and have urgent surgery. The diagnosis may be made after an often incomplete resection and exploration of the abdomen. Complete resection of the tumor with no evidence of spread beyond the bowel is associated with a significantly better prognosis.

NHL of the gut may present subacutely, and the diagnosis is then suggested at barium examination or CT scanning. Blackledge et al (1979) suggested a simple staging system for gastrointestinal lymphoma (Table 27.2) that is useful prognostically. Treatment of gut NHL depends on histology, stage and the presence or absence of residual disease. The present therapeutic trend is toward the use of combination chemotherapy unless the tumor is both low-grade and of limited extent. Small-bowel lymphoma is the most common pediatric bowel tumor, almost invariably involves the terminal ileum, and is of intermediate or high grade.

Stomach lymphomas often mimic adenocarcinomas clinically, with nausea and weight loss being the usual presentation symptoms (Fig. 27.24). The diagnosis may be suggested by the CT appearances (Doyle & Dixon 1994). Treatment is surgical, followed by combination chemotherapy.

MRI is increasingly used for the assessment of gastrointestinal disease. Preliminary reports are encouraging, but suggest the technique is unlikely to be tissue-specific (Chou et al 1994).

Table 27.2   CT staging of primary gut lymphomas (modified from Blackledge et al 1979

Stage	1	Confined to gut
	1A	Single tumor
	1B	Multiple tumors
Stage	2	Local extension
	2A	Adjacent nodes
	2B	Adjacent structures
	2C	With perforation and peritonitis
Stage	3	Extraregional nodal spread
Stage	4	Distant dissemination, e.g. liver or spleen

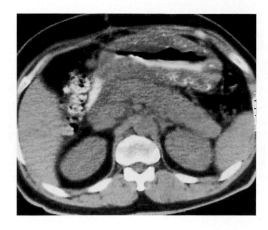

Fig. 27.24 CT scan through the abdomen of a patient with gastric NHL shows thickening of the gastric wall and prominence of the rugal folds. Note how the oral contrast medium is seen to collect in pools between the giant rugal folds.

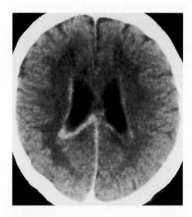

Fig. 27.25 Contrast-enhanced CT brain scan showing periventricular enhancement due to subependymal spread of NHL. This is a common appearance in central nervous system lymphoma.

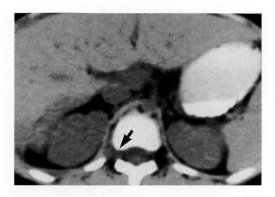

Fig. 27.26 CT scan showing normal fat and soft-tissue densities in the left paravertebral area. On the right the fat in the paravertebral area is obliterated by lymphoma tissue (arrow), which is closely applied to the nerve root exit foramen. The paravertebral tissues should be systematically reviewed when CT scanning any patient with malignant disease, so that lesions may be detected and treated prior to the onset of cord compression.

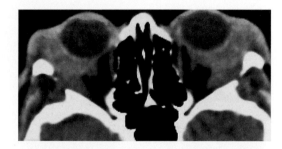

Fig. 27.27 CT scan through the orbits of a patient presenting with orbital NHL. Diffuse thickening of the tissues is seen bilaterally.

CENTRAL NERVOUS SYSTEM LYMPHOMA

Primary NHL represents about 1% of primary brain tumors (Fig. 27.25). The incidence is highest in immunocompromised patients, especially those with AIDS or renal transplants or on long-term immunosuppression for some other reason. Patients rarely develop systemic lymphoma, either at the time of diagnosis or later. Detailed systemic staging is superfluous. Treatment is primarily irradiation, and the prognosis is poor. Primary Hodgkin's disease of the brain is rare.

Secondary central nervous system lymphoma is not uncommon. It is most frequently seen in high-grade tumors, especially in children and those with T-cell disease. Approximately 50% of these patients with central nervous system involvement will develop cord compression, while the other 50% will show evidence of lymphomatous meningitis with nerve and root lesions, raised intracranial pressure, and mental confusion. Central nervous system involvement is also a feature of testicular, orbital head/neck primary sites. At all times when CT or MRI scanning any patient with a known lymphoma, the *paravertebral tissues* should be closely examined; involvement here may portend cord compression (Fig. 27.26). *Orbital lymphomas* (Fig. 27.27) almost always disseminate systemically. This is especially true if the disease is bilateral and/or involves neck lymph nodes. CT of the head and neck is the single most useful staging investigation.

HEAD AND NECK LYMPHOMAS

Primary nodal lymphomas arising in the head and neck do not require CT staging of the neck. An experienced clinician should be able to palpate enlarged lymph nodes within the neck. Abdominal CT staging is useful, as the disease often relapses outside the head and neck, typically in the gastrointestinal tract. Extranodal NHL of the head and neck is usually associated with disease dissemination in the body and a poor prognosis (Fig. 27.28).

THORACIC LYMPHOMA

Involvement of the lungs is an uncommon feature of both NHL (Fig. 27.29) and Hodgkin's disease. In high-grade NHL, pulmonary involvement may be extensive and explosive, the radiological appearances often mimicking those seen in infection. Low-grade NHL may also involve the lungs. Typically, many of these low-grade tumors are indolent, often in the past being described as pseudolymphomas. Some of these arise in the bronchus-associated lymphoid tissue.

In patients with more typical variants of NHL, CT scanning of the thorax is not rewarding, either for the assessment of the lung

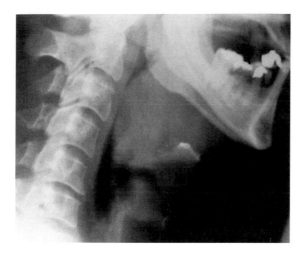

Fig. 27.28 Lateral soft-tissue radiograph of the neck showing abnormal soft tissue from a primary NHL of the neck arising in the epiglottis and presenting with dysphagia.

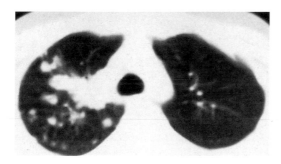

Fig. 27.29 CT scan showing pulmonary involvement in a patient with NHL. A mass of tumor tissue is seen around the right hilum. In addition, a number of ill-defined intrapulmonary nodules are seen on the right.

fields or for detecting mediastinal involvement in the presence of a normal chest radiograph. NHL involves the mediastinum less frequently than Hodgkin's disease, and mediastinal involvement in NHL typically reflects widespread disease dissemination.

Bone Bone marrow involvement is commonly found in the NHLs. On occasion a patient will present with an apparent primary bone NHL. These are most common in younger patients, and involve the appendicular skeleton, especially in the metaphyseal region. Radiologically, the most common appearance is a permeative destructive lesion. Pathologically, the lesions are typically high grade. Full radiological staging of the abdomen and chest should be undertaken, and a high percentage of patients will prove to have disseminated disease. Recent work has suggested that while MRI and CT are comparable in their ability to detect lymph-adenopathy, MRI is significantly better than CT in demonstrating occult marrow infiltration (Hoane et al 1994), and this may eventually make MRI the preferred imaging modality for the staging of lymphoma.

Testis Testicular lymphomas occur in middle-aged and elderly men. Twenty-five percent will be bilateral. Testicular NHL is aggressive, high-grade, and tends to spread not only to the regional lymph nodes in the abdomen but also to lung, the central nervous system, and in the neck to Waldeyer's ring.

CT SCANNING OF THE THORAX

CT is the current 'gold standard' for evaluating the extent of thoracic involvement in patients with Hodgkin's disease and, when required, for those with NHL. The pattern of lymphomatous involvement is different for Hodgkin's disease and NHL. In addition, the therapeutic implications of any positive findings in these two conditions also differ.

The chest should be scanned in the supine position and in held inspiration. Ideally, a modern scanner with a fast scan time of 3–4 s should be used. Contiguous sections are usual, and should be obtained at 1 cm intervals. Intravenous contrast enhancement should be dynamic, whenever possible, using at least 100 ml of contrast medium. Intravenous contrast is helpful in assessing the mediastinum, and is crucial to the complete CT evaluation of the lung hila. The presence of intravenous contrast medium is not detrimental to the imaging of the lung fields, and when it is to be used, precontrast studies are not warranted. Normal mediastinal structures, in particular blood vessels, should be routinely identified. Normal-sized lymph nodes may on occasion be seen within the mediastinal fat, but this would appear to be a less common observation in the UK than in the USA. CT sections through the mediastinum of a patient with lymphoma should clearly demonstrate the extent of adenopathy. CT identifies abnormal lymph nodes by an abnormal increase in the cross-sectional diameter of the lymph nodes. Typically, mediastinal lymph nodes more than 1 cm in diameter are interpreted as being involved. Hilar nodal enlargement usually follows mediastinal involvement, at least in Hodgkin's disease. Micrometastases occurring in normal-sized mediastinal lymph nodes cannot be diagnosed on CT, and, equally, nodal enlargement for non-malignant reasons may not be discriminated from malignant enlargement.

Hodgkin's Disease

The anterior mediastinum is the focus from which Hodgkin's disease of the chest appears to spread (MacDonald et al 1987). It is extremely uncommon to have disease at other sites within the thorax in the absence of anterior mediastinal involvement. Recognition of adenopathy at this site is the first step to successful CT scan interpretation.

Conventional radiographs will only recognize an abnormality in this region when the contour of the mediastinum and its pleural reflections is altered. In general, enlarged lymph nodes on the right side of the mediastinum are easier to identify on plain chest radiography than those on the left side, where the overlying shadow of the aortic arch makes small-volume adenopathy more difficult to recognize.

The typical CT appearance of a nodal mass in a patient with Hodgkin's disease is usually that of a homogeneous soft-tissue mass with sharply defined and often lobulated borders. Occasionally the center of the nodal mass contains an area of decreased attenuation due to necrosis. If intravenous contrast medium has been given, the lymph node may enhance.

Castellino et al (1986) reviewed the contribution that CT scanning of the thorax made in their Hodgkin's disease practice. From their study it is clear that CT will demonstrate abnormal lymph nodes more readily than conventional X-ray techniques within the thorax.

Primary Hodgkin's disease is managed by chemotherapy or

radiotherapy or a combination of both. The most profound impact on management might be expected in those patients being considered for radiotherapy. CT demonstration of the extent of disease at a particular site may influence the size of the proposed fields, and CT demonstration of disease at previously unsuspected sites, particularly in the posterior mediastinum and diaphragmatic area, may lead to a change in management from radiotherapy to chemotherapy. Thus, mediastinal CT in Hodgkin's disease is of most value when a high proportion of patients are being considered for radiotherapy. When the patient is to have chemotherapy from the start, then the more precise demonstration of disease extent within the thorax is of no immediate consequence. The value of CT scanning of the mediastinum in these patients is limited to baseline studies for the monitoring of response and assessment of residual changes. In any institution the proportion of patients considered for radiotherapy will vary, and it is this that accounts for differing opinions on the impact of mediastinal CT on the management of patients with Hodgkin's disease. Studies from different institutions confirm that the value of mediastinal CT in patients with Hodgkin's disease is maximal in those who are being considered for radiation therapy.

A decrease in size of previously enlarged lymph nodes also serves as an indicator of response to chemotherapy. In many instances this can be adequately assessed on serial chest radiographs but—especially when the chest radiograph has returned to normal—the CT scan may show residual adenopathy. Interpretation of this residual adenopathy may be difficult. Serial MRI and/or Gallium-67 studies beginning before treatment commences may help distinguish active from inactive disease following chemotherapy. This is of potential value in tailoring the chemotherapy regime (and toxicity) to the individual (Abrahamsen et al 1994).

CT scanning of the lungs may show evidence of Hodgkin's disease. The most characteristic finding is the presence of one or more nodules within the parenchyma. They are most frequently seen near the lung bases and/or the pulmonary hila, suggesting a hematogenous spread. The demonstration of these would classify the case as stage IV according to the Ann Arbor convention. As with other small pulmonary nodules, CT has a small advantage over conventional chest radiographs in the demonstration of smaller pulmonary lesions. In lymphoma these small focal changes are often poorly defined.

Lymphoma may involve the lung fields in a variety of other ways. These include patchy pulmonary shadowing, pulmonary consolidation, and lobar collapse. Pulmonary involvement is uncommon in the patient with newly diagnosed Hodgkin's disease, being seen at most in 10% of patients. Parenchymal lesions in newly presented patients who have no mediastinal or hilar adenopathy are best considered not to represent Hodgkin's disease. Pulmonary disease is a feature of recurrent Hodgkin's disease, where it may be confused not only with infection but also with the effects of treatment. These include pulmonary consolidation and fibrosis following radiotherapy, drug reactions, and opportunistic infections during or following systemic chemotherapy.

A frequent concern to the clinician is the possibility of early tumor infiltration from enlarged hilar lymph nodes into the surrounding lung tissue. This is well recognized and indicated in the Ann Arbor staging system, as, for example, stage IIE disease. Although this is a frequent indication for requesting thoracic CT, in practice it is exceptional to detect this infiltration on CT unless the chest radiograph is abnormal.

CT may be helpful in assessing the patency and diameter of airways, especially in children. Over half the children presenting with Hodgkin's disease show significant airway obstruction on CT examination, and occasionally this may require emergency treatment.

CT is ideally suited to demonstrating pleural and pleurally based lesions. These include *solid plaques* of tumor tissue and *pleural effusions*. It is important to remember that most pleural effusions seen in patients with Hodgkin's disease are benign, and are thought to be a consequence of lymphatic obstruction secondary to mediastinal and hilar lymph node involvement and enlargement.

Non-Hodgkin Lymphomas

The contribution that thoracic CT scanning might make in the management of patients with NHL is less certain, for several reasons. NHL is more likely than Hodgkin's disease to be widespread and require systemic therapy, the mediastinum is a less frequent site of disease, and in many instances the presence of mediastinal involvement will be recognized on a routine chest radiograph. Lung involvement is uncommon, and is seen in fewer than 5% of patients at diagnosis. The presence of a pleural effusion in NHL usually reflects the presence of pleural tumor. This is a reflection of the lower incidence of mediastinal adenopathy seen in NHL than in Hodgkin's disease.

A survey concluded that the addition of CT scanning to the diagnostic work-up of patients presenting with a new NHL may occasionally show additional sites of disease but does not result in a change in management.

CT SCANNING OF THE ABDOMEN

CT is now the standard method of imaging the abdomen in patients with lymphoma. In one study of 168 patients presenting with a NHL (Pond et al 1989), 29% had abdominal disease detectable only on CT scanning. Typically, CT sections are taken through the abdomen and upper pelvis at 1.5 cm intervals following opacification of the bowel with oral contrast media. Abnormal lymph nodes may be recognized by an increase in size. Retroperitoneal nodes greater than 1.5 cm in diameter are considered abnormal. Particular attention should be paid to the retrocrural region (Fig. 27.30) (where nodes greater than 0.6 cm in diameter are regarded as pathological), the retroperitoneum, the pelvic lymph nodes, and (especially in patients with NHL) the

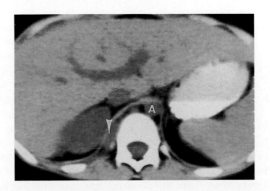

Fig. 27.30 CT scan on a patient with NHL shows enlargement of the retrocrural lymph nodes (arrowhead). A, aorta.

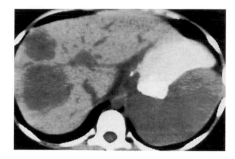

Fig. 27.31 Focal areas of low attenuation are seen in the liver of this boy with recurrent Hodgkin's disease. The spleen is enlarged and inhomogeneous.

mesenteric lymph nodes. Involvement of the spleen or liver is often difficult to detect. On occasion, focal deposits may be seen in the spleen or liver (Fig. 27.31); more typically, lymphomatous involvement results in an increase in the size of the affected organ. This may be obvious but in many cases early involvement is especially difficult to diagnose. In addition, in patients with Hodgkin's disease the spleen may enlarge in the absence of direct involvement, leading to possible radiological overstaging.

CT SCANNING OF THE HEAD AND NECK

Enlarged lymph nodes in the neck are usually palpable. CT may demonstrate non-palpable lymph node enlargement and/or central necrosis within the lymph node, the latter being a certain sign of a pathological condition. In addition, CT imaging may show that a single palpable mass consists of a conglomerate mass of several enlarged lymph nodes, an observation that may alter staging and prognosis of primary head and neck cancers. In general, the demonstration of nodal disease in the neck of patients with a primary tumor of the head and neck is of grave prognostic significance. Ipsilateral adenopathy reduces survival by 50%, and contralateral adenopathy by a further 50%. CT may also demonstrate extranodal spread of malignancy. This is associated with a further significant reduction in prognosis.

CT examination of the neck is usually performed during the dynamic infusion of intravenous contrast medium, which allows all the vascular structures to be highlighted, and in addition may demonstrate ring enhancement in patients with metastatic squamous carcinomas. At present CT remains the method of choice in staging cervical adenopathy, as it may enable small metastatic foci within normal-sized lymph nodes to be recognized—something which cannot yet be achieved with MRI. With MRI, intravenous contrast medium is not required to identify the vessels, and this may be of value in patients who are sensitive to iodine. The MRI characteristics of enlarged lymph nodes are non-specific and do not allow the cause of the enlargement, or whether the underlying pathology is benign or malignant, to be deduced.

The main criteria for abnormality when imaging the neck with CT and/or MRI is an increase in the size. Normally the lymph nodes high in the neck are larger than those lower in the neck, presumably due to benign enlargement secondary to previous recurrent throat infections. It is generally accepted that lymph nodes larger than 1 cm in diameter are abnormal, unless the lymph node is in the jugulodiagastric region, where 1.5 cm is a more reasonable upper limit of normal cross-sectional diameter.

Using these criteria, approximately 80% of the lymph nodes considered abnormal at CT and/or MRI examination will, under the appropriate clinical conditions, contain tumor.

THE GROWTH AND SPREAD OF SOLID TUMORS

There are many conventions for the staging of different tumors, and all methods reflect the bulk and distribution of tumor tissue within the body. This is of some prognostic and therapeutic significance, although in many tumors the histologic diagnosis and grading is of paramount importance. The TNM system (UICC 1987) is the most widely accepted staging system, although it is inappropriate for patients with lymphoma.

If it is assumed that a primary neoplasm starts as a single malignant cell which has the capacity to replicate itself, then it will take approximately 30 cell divisions for a tumor mass to reach a diameter of 1 cm and become radiologically visible. The doubling time of a tumor varies greatly, and may be a few days for a rapidly growing malignancy, or several months for a slow-growing tumor type. From this it may be seen that all tumors will take months or years to become radiologically detectable. For most of their life all tumors are subclinical. Once past the 30-cell division barrier it will require only a few further cell divisions for the tumor burden to become overwhelming and the untreated patient to succumb. Malignant neoplasms may metastasize at the subclinical level. In such patients, by the time the primary tumor has become apparent the patient is already incurable by local methods (surgery and radiotherapy), as these will not treat the distant tumor spread. Metastases result from lymphatic and/or vascular invasion followed by the dissemination of tumor cells within blood or lymph vessels throughout the body. As a result of the nature of vessel wall permeability discussed above, it is probable that malignant cells may be scavenged directly from the interstitial tissues into the lymphatics, passing on through the draining lymphatics into regional lymph nodes prior to any direct vascular invasion by the tumor. The detection of metastatic lymph nodes is an important component of tumor staging, as the presence of tumor within lymph nodes may herald the vascular dissemination of tumor cells.

The Primary Tumor (T-staging)

The size and location of any primary tumor should be assessed clinically and radiologically. Whenever possible, objective measurements should be taken. These measurements are invaluable in assessing response. There are recognized criteria for primary tumor or T-staging of most common tumors (UICC 1987). Knowledge of the site and extent of the primary tumor mass are valuable in predicting the likely routes of lymphatic and vascular spread.

Lymph Node Involvement (N-staging)

Similarly, criteria have evolved to determine the extent of lymph node involvement at the time of diagnosis. The regional lymph nodes for the common malignancies have been defined and stages of involvement recognized (UICC 1987).

Consider a young man presenting with a testicular teratoma. The primary tumor is removed at orchidectomy, and the specimen assessed for evidence of complete resection of the primary tumor and for lymphatic and/or vascular invasion. Teratoma typically spreads initially to to the para-aortic lymph nodes, and these then represent the first-echelon lymph nodes for testicular malignancies. Enlargement of the para-aortic lymph nodes increases the overall staging to stage II. The subscripts A, B, and C reflect the disease bulk in terms of the cross-sectional diameter of the retroperitoneal nodal mass as seen on CT: A represents a cross-sectional diameter less than 2 cm (Fig. 27.32); B a cross-sectional diameter of between 2 and 5 cm; and C a cross-sectional diameter of more than 5 cm (Fig. 27.33). The disease may then progress cephalad through the lymphatic system to involve the lymph nodes of the mediastinum (stage III disease), although more frequently involvement of the mediastinal lymph nodes in patients with testicular teratoma is associated with evidence of vascular dissemination of tumor to the lungs. The presence of pulmonary or other extranodal metastases would automatically make the disease stage IV. A further attempt is made to quantify the tumor bulk in the lung fields in terms of both the size and the number of pulmonary metastases.

Distant Metastases (M-staging)

The M-stage of malignancy recognizes the spread of tumor to distant organs. This is a result of hematogenous dissemination, and the most common sites for such involvement are the lungs, liver, and brain. These may be diagnosed several ways, but the overall information available from CT examination, often allowing a TNM (tumor, nodes, and metastases) stage to be assigned to a patient at the one examination, makes this technique supreme.

IMAGING THE LYMPHATIC SYSTEM IN PATIENTS WITH MALIGNANT DISEASE

Diagnosis CT scanning will demonstrate malignant disease within a body structure or viscus as a change in shape and/or a change in attenuation of the affected area. It is possible to propose, from the clinical details and the pattern of disease dissemination seen on CT scanning, the likely primary sites in a patient presenting with lymphadenopathy, but this speculation should never replace formal histologic investigation. On occasion the radiologist may help by providing material for pathological examination from percutaneous biopsy.

Staging As we have seen above, radiological investigation CT is essential in the TNM staging of malignant tumors and may provide information in those tumors (e.g. lymphomas) that are staged by other conventions.

Treatment Planning A patient with a fully treated primary tumor and no evidence of metastatic disease may require no further treatment unless there is evidence of disease relapse. In most circumstances, patients are watched clinically and with simple investigations such as serial chest radiographs, but there are certain tumors in which a more aggressive surveillance policy is rewarding. These are usually those tumors for which curative or salvage chemotherapy is available, and this includes testicular teratoma. Stage I teratoma patients may be placed on a surveillance protocol which includes regular clinical examination, serum marker estimation, chest radiograph, and 3-monthly CT examination of the chest, abdomen, and pelvis for 2 years (90% of relapses will occur in the first year).

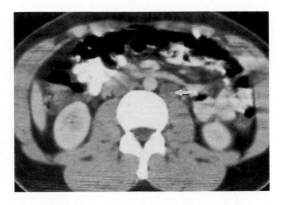

Fig. 27.32 Small-volume (<2 cm) retroperitoneal metastatic disease in a patient with a left-sided teratoma. Left-sided testicular primary teratomas almost always spread initially to a retroperitoneal lymph node under the left renal vein (arrow).

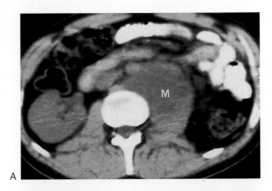

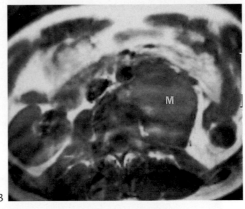

Fig. 27.33 Large retroperitoneal metastasis (M) arising from an ipsilateral testicular teratoma seen both on **A** CT and **B** MRI.

Radiotherapy Planning In patients whom it has been decided to try to cure by radiotherapy, accurate staging is essential before embarking on a course of treatment. For example, the presence of abdominal adenopathy would preclude the possibility of a cure if the pelvis is to be irradiated for a pelvic primary tumor.

The demonstration of the position, size, and extent of a localized primary tumor on CT examination may be used to plan radiotherapy fields. This is usually accomplished with special software packages, and allows dose to the tumor to be maximized while vital structures, e.g. the spinal cord or kidneys, may be partly protected.

The superior soft-tissue contrast of MRI compared to CT, especially when evaluating soft-tissue spread of tumor (e.g. in muscle), suggests that MRI depiction of radiotherapy treatment fields will have an application in the future.

The operability of tumors or residual masses may also be assessed at CT or MRI examination, and in particular the proximity of vessels and other vital structures to the tumor mass may be determined (Fig. 27.34).

Response to Treatment The treatment of any cancer is limited by the ability of the normal body tissues to withstand the treatment. There is a morbidity and a mortality associated with any treatment. Imaging is an important part of treatment evaluation. A rapid and complete response to treatment may allow a reduction in the number of treatments required, which reduces both the possible side-effects and complications (Oliver et al 1983). Alternatively, a poor or absent response to first-time treatment could lead to either a change of treatment or to a change of approach from a curative to a palliative one. The objective recording of a response to a particular treatment is also important in the evaluation of treatments and comparative treatment studies. It must be appreciated that like must be compared with like, and CT-staged patients in one arm of the study must be imaged according to the same convention in the other arm of the study. There are at present no satisfactory guidelines on when to measure a response. A reduction in tumor size at any time counts as a partial response (PR), while the objective disappearance of tumor should be regarded as a complete response (CR). On occasion a tumor may enlarge on treatment and yet still respond (Fig. 27.35).

The addition of a more sophisticated imaging modality to the initial staging protocol of a particular tumor type may also appear to alter the outcome. Previously occult metastases will be demonstrated, altering the staging typically from stage I (no metastases) to stage IV (distant metastases). This will have the effect of improving survival rates in stage I disease in the survey as some patients with metastases are now excluded from this group. The survival rate of the group of patients with stage IV disease will also apparently improve as some of them now will have very small volume metastatic disease. However, the overall survival for the

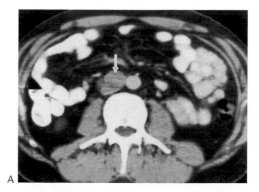

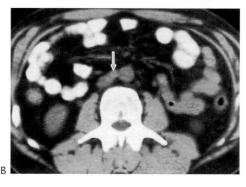

Fig. 27.34 **A**. CT scan through the abdomen of this patient with a right-sided teratoma. **B**. CT scan showing a reduction in lymph node size (arrow) following treatment.

group will not change. This is a further reason why imaging criteria for staging and restaging will need to be standardized.

Residual Masses The radiologist may be asked to comment on the possible malignant potential of any residual mass following treatment of a malignancy (Lewis et al 1982). At present it is not possible to deduce residual malignant potential from the appearances. Future possible ways of tackling this problem include functional studies using radionuclides, especially when these may be targeted to the appropriate cell type, and MRI. On MRI scans

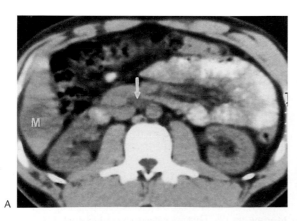

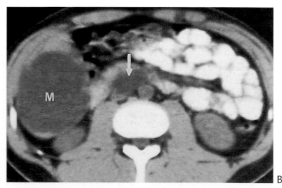

Fig. 27.35 **A**. CT scan through the abdomen of this patient with metastatic teratoma. **B**. CT scan showing an increase in tumor size, along with a decrease in attenuation following treatment, for a testicular teratoma. This almost always indicates differentiation of the tumor into a benign variant. The residuum is excised to protect the patient in the future. Note both the residual interaorticocaval lymph node (arrow) and the liver metastasis (M), both of which enlarge on treatment.

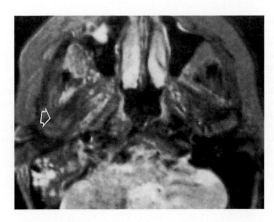

Fig. 27.36 Long-term reassessment of a patient who had previously had a parotid malignancy resected, now with clinical suspicion of recurrence, shows considerable distortion of the architecture, but the low signal intensity on T_2-weighted MRI sequences suggested the scar tissue (arrow) to be benign. This was confirmed at subsequent re-exploration.

it would appear that residual tumor masses that have a low signal on T_2-weighted images—especially when the pretreatment images show a high signal intensity on similar T_2-weighted sequences—are likely to be dormant (Fig. 27.36). Unfortunately the converse—that high signal on T_2-weighted sequences equals activity—is not true.

MAGNETIC RESONANCE IMAGING

MRI in oncology is at present of value in assessing the spinal cord, especially in patients with clinical features suggesting cord compression (see Ch. 54). In these circumstances MRI provides a more complete picture of the compressive lesion than may be obtained with myelography. MRI may also prove of value in the assessment of bone marrow involvement and complement the information available from bone marrow aspirate and trephine.

In the assessment of nodal disease, MRI is a more costly and less practical alternative to CT. MRI does not seem reliable in the recognition of splenic and/or hepatic involvement in lymphoma. A possible role for MRI is the assessment of residual masses looking for the low-T_2 signal intensity associated with fibrosis. This is occasionally useful, but, especially in the first year after treatment, high-T_2 signal intensity may persist in the residual tissue due to inflammatory rather than residual neoplastic change.

MRI is frequently used in oncology to detect and stage intra-cranial metastatic disease, and to 'problem solve' in cancer patients with pain or other focal symptoms not explained with other imaging modalities.

MRI may be used to provide biochemical rather than visual information. This may also be used to assess the response of a tumor to chemotherapy. At present this is of experimental value only.

REFERENCES AND SUGGESTIONS FOR FURTHER READING

Abrahamsen, A. F., Lien, H. H., Aas, W. et al (1994) Magnetic resonance imaging and (67) gallium scan in mediastinal lymphoma: a prospective pilot study. *Annals of Oncology*, **5**, 433–436.

Allen, E. V., Barker, N. W., Hines, E. A. (1946) *Peripheral Vascular Diseases*. Philadelphia: Saunders.

Amendola, M. A. (1986) CT staging of lymphoma. In Glazer, G. M. (ed.) *Staging of Neoplasms*, pp. 147–189. New York: Churchill Livingstone.

Blake, P. R., Carr, D. H., Goolden, A. W. G. (1986) Intracranial Hodgkin's disease. *British Journal of Radiology*, **59**, 414–416.

Blackledge, G., Bush, H., Dodge, O. G., Crowther, D. F. (1979) A study of gastrointestinal lymphoma. *Clinical Oncology*, **5**, 209–219.

Bragg, D. G., Colby T. V., Ward J. H. (1986) New concepts in the non-Hodgkin lymphomas: radiological implications. *Radiology*, **159**, 289–304.

Callihan, T. R., Berard, C. W. (1980) The classification and pathology of the lymphomas and leukemias. *Seminars in Roentgenology*, **15**, 203–218.

Carbone, P. P., Kaplan, H. S., Musshoff, K., Smithers, E. W., Tubiana, M. (1971) Report of the Committee on Hodgkin's Disease Staging. *Cancer Research*, **31**, 1860–1861.

Castellino, R. A. (1986) Hodgkin's disease: practical concepts for the diagnostic radiologist. *Radiology*, **159**, 305–310.

Castellino, R. A., Blank, N., Hoppe, R. T., Cho, C. (1986) Hodgkin disease: contributions of chest CT in the initial staging evaluation. *Radiology*, **160**, 603–605.

Chou, C. K., Chen, L. T., Sheu, R. S., Yang, C. W., Jaw, T. S., Lui, G. C. (1994) MRI manifestations of gastrointestinal lymphoma. *Abdominal Imaging*, **19**, 495–500.

Dixon, A. K., Ellis, M., Sikora, K. (1986) Computed tomography of testicular tumours: distribution of abdominal lymphadenopathy. *Clinical Radiology*, **37**, 519–523.

Dooms, G. C., Hricak, H., Moseley, M. E., Bottles, K. Fisher, M., Higgens, C. B. (1985) Characterisation of lymphadenopathy by magnetic resonance times: preliminary results. *Radiology*, **155**, 691–697.

Doyle, T. C. A., Dixon, A. K. (1994) Pointers to the diagnosis of gastric lymphoma on computed tomography. *Australasian Radiology*, **38**, 176–178.

Glazer, H. S., Lee, J. K. T., Balfe, D. M., Mauro, M. A., Griffith, R, Sagel, S. S. (1983) Non-Hodgkin lymphoma: computed tomographic demonstration of unusual extranodal involvement. *Radiology*, **149**, 211–217.

Glazer, G. M., Gross, B. H., Quint, L. E., Francis, I. R., Bookstein, F. L., Oninger, M. B. (1985) Normal mediastinal lymph nodes: number and size according to American Thoracic Society Mapping. *American Journal of Roentgenology*, **144**, 261–265.

Harrison, D. A., Clouse, M. E. (1985) Normal anatomy. In Clouse, M. E., Wallace, S. (eds) *Lymphatic Imaging*, 2nd edn, pp. 15–94. Baltimore: Williams and Wilkins.

Heron, C. W., Husband, J. E., Williams, M. P., Cherryman, G. R. (1988) The value of thoracic computed tomography in the detection of recurrent Hodgkin's disease. *British Journal of Radiology*, **61**, 567–572.

Hoane, B. R., Shields, A. F., Porter, B. A., Borrow, J. W. (1994) Comparison of initial lymphoma staging using computed tomography (CT) and magnetic resonance (MR) imaging. *American Journal of Hematology*, **47**, 100–105.

Jack, C. R., O'Neill, B. P., Banks, P.M., Reese, D. F. (1988) Central nervous system lymphoma: histological types and CT appearance. *Radiology*, **167**, 211–215.

Kaplan, H. S. (1980) *Hodgkin's disease*, 2nd edn. Cambridge, MA: Harvard University Press.

Khoury, M. B., Godwin, J. C., Halvorsen, R. A., Hanun, Y., Putman, C. E. (1984) The role of thoracic CT in non-Hodgkin's lymphoma. *Radiology*, **158**, 659–662.

Kiyono, K., Sone, S., Sakai, F. et al (1988) The number and size of normal mediastinal lymph nodes: a postmortem study. *American Journal of Roentgenology*, **150**, 771–778.

Lewis, E., Bamardino, M. E., Salvador, P. G., Cabanillas, F. F., Barnes, P. A., Thomas, J. L. (1982) Post therapy CT detected mass in lymphoma: is it viable tissue? *Journal of Computer Assisted Tomography*, **6**, 792–795.

Lukes, R. J., Butler, J. J., Hicks, E. B. (1966) Natural history of Hodgkin's disease as related to its pathological picture. *Cancer*, **19**, 317–344.

MacDonald, J. S. (1982) Lymphography in lymph node disease. In Kinmonth, J. B. (ed.) *The Lymphatics: Surgery, Lymphography and Diseases of the Chyle and Lymph Systems*, pp. 327–370. London: Edward Arnold.

MacDonald, J. S. (1987) Lymphography. In Ansell, G., Wilkins, R. A. (eds) *Complications in Diagnostic Imaging*, pp. 300–309. Oxford: Blackwell.

MacDonald, J. S., McCready, V. R., Cosgrove, D. O., Chenyman, G. R., Selby, P. (1987) Radiological and other imaging methods. In Selby, P., McElwain, T. J. (eds) *Hodgkin's Disease*, pp. 126–160. Oxford: Blackwell.

McKusick, K. A. (1985) Radionuclide lymphography. In Clouse M. E., Wallace, S. (eds) *Lymphatic Imaging*, 2nd edn, pp. 95–111. Baltimore: Williams and Wilkins.

Meyer, J. E., Linggood, R-M., Lindfors, Y. K., McLoud, T. C., Stomper, P. C. (1984) Impact of thoracic computed tomography on radiation therapy planning in Hodgkin disease. *Journal of Computer Assisted Tomography*, **8**, 892–904.

NCI (National Cancer Institute Sponsored Study of Classification of Non-Hodgkin's Lymphomas) (1981) Summary and description of a working formulation for clinical usage. *Cancer*, **49**, 2112–2135.

Neumann, C. H., Parker, B. R., Castellino, R. A. (1985) Hodgkin's disease and the non-Hodgkin lymphomas. In Bragg, D. G., Rubin, P., Youker, J. E. (eds) *Oncologic Imaging*, pp. 477–501. New York: Pergamon Press.

O'Donnell, T. F., Jr, Clouse, M. E. (1985) Abnormal peripheral lymphatics. In Clouse, M. E., Wallace, S. (eds) *Lymphatic Imaging*, 2nd edn, pp. 142–179. Baltimore: Williams and Wilkins.

Oliver, T. W., Bernardino, M. E., Sones, P. J., Jr (1983) Monitoring the response of lymphoma patients to therapy: correlation of abdominal CT findings with clinical course and histiological cell type. *Radiology*, **149**, 219–224.

Pond, G. D., Castellino, R. A., Homing, S., Hoppe, R. T. (1989) Non-Hodgkin lymphoma: Influence of lymphography, CT, and bone marrow biopsy on staging and management. *Radiology*, **170**, 159–164.

Shiels, R. A., Stone, J., Ash, D. V. et al (1984) Priorities for computed tomography and lymphography in the staging and initial management of Hodgkin's disease. *Clinical Radiology*, **35**, 447–449.

Som, P. M. (1987) Lymph nodes of the neck. *Radiology*, **165**, 593–600.

Turowski, G. A., Basson, M. D. (1995) Primary malignant lymphoma of the intestine. *American Journal of Surgery*, **169**, 4333–4341.

UICC (International Union Against Cancer) (1987) *TNM Classification of Malignant Tumours*, 4th edn. Berlin: Springer-Verlag.

Williams, M. P., Cherryman, G. R., Husband, J. E. (1989) Magnetic resonance imaging of spinal cord compression. *Clinical Radiology*, **40**, 286–290.

INDEX